SLEEP DISORDERS MEDICINE

Basic Science, Technical Considerations, and Clinical Aspects

SLEEP DISORDERS MEDICINE

Basic Science, Technical Considerations, and Clinical Aspects

THIRD EDITION

Sudhansu Chokroverty, MD, FRCP, FACP

Professor and Co-Chair of Neurology
Clinical Neurophysiology and Sleep Medicine
New Jersey Neuroscience Institute at JFK Medical Center
Edison, New Jersey

Professor of Neuroscience
Seton Hall University School of Graduate Medical Education
South Orange, New Jersey

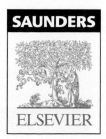

SAUNDERS

ELSEVIER

SAUNDERS
ELSEVIER

1600 John F. Kennedy Blvd.
Ste 1800
Philadelphia, PA 19103-2899

SLEEP DISORDERS MEDICINE: BASIC SCIENCE, TECHNICAL
CONSIDERATIONS, AND CLINICAL ASPECTS   ISBN: 978-0-7506-7584-0

Copyright © 2009, 1999 by Saunders, an imprint of Elsevier Inc.

Notice

Knowledge and best practice in this field are constantly changing. As new research and experience
broaden our knowledge, changes in practice, treatment and drug therapy may become necessary or
appropriate. Readers are advised to check the most current information provided (i) on procedures
featured or (ii) by the manufacturer of each product to be administered, to verify the recommended
dose or formula, the method and duration of administration, and contraindications. It is the
responsibility of the practitioner, relying on their own experience and knowledge of the patient, to
make diagnoses, to determine dosages and the best treatment for each individual patient, and to take
all appropriate safety precautions. To the fullest extent of the law, neither the Publisher nor the Editor
assumes any liability for any injury and/or damage to persons or property arising out of or related to
any use of the material contained in this book.

The Publisher

Library of Congress Cataloging-in-Publication Data

Sleep disorders medicine: basic science, technical considerations,
and clinical aspects / [edited by]   Sudhansu Chokroverty. –3rd ed.
      p. ; cm.
   Includes bibliographical references and index.
   ISBN 978-0-7506-7584-0
1. Sleep disorders.   I. Chokroverty, Sudhansu.
   [DNLM: 1. Sleep Disorders.   2. Sleep–physiology.   WM 188 S6323 2009]
   RC547.S534 2009
   616.8′498–dc22   2008037586

Acquisitions Editor: Adrianne Brigido
Developmental Editor: Arlene Chappelle
Project Manager: Bryan Hayward
Design Direction: Steve Stave

Working together to grow
libraries in developing countries

www.elsevier.com | www.bookaid.org | www.sabre.org

ELSEVIER   BOOK AID International   Sabre Foundation

Printed in the United States of America

Last digit is the print number: 9 8 7 6 5 4 3 2 1

I dedicate this book to my wife, Manisha Chokroverty, MD; my daughters, Linda Chokroverty, MD, and Keka Chokroverty-Filipowiz, BA; and my dear departed parents, Debendranath Chokroverty (1898-2001) and Ashalata Chokroverty (1910-2000).

Contributors

Vivien C. Abad, MD, MBA
Director, Sleep Disorders Center
Camino Medical Group
Cupertino, California

Richard P. Allen, PhD
Assistant Professor, Johns Hopkins University School of
*   Arts and Sciences*
Research Associate, Department of Neurology
Johns Hopkins University School of Medicine
Baltimore, Maryland

Charles W. Atwood Jr., MD
University of Pittsburgh School of Medicine
Director, Sleep Disorders Program
Veterans Affairs Pittsburgh Healthcare System
Director, Sleep Medicine Fellowship
University of Pittsburgh Medical Center
Pittsburgh, Pennsylvania

Ruth M. Benca, MD, PhD
Director, Sleep Program
Professor, Department of Psychiatry
University of Wisconsin-Madison
Madison, Wisconsin

Daniel J. Buysse, MD
Professor of Psychiatry and Clinical and Translational Science
University of Pittsburgh School of Medicine
Western Psychiatric Institute and Clinic/UPMC
Pittsburgh, Pennsylvania

Rosalind Cartwright, PhD
Professor, Department of Behavioral Sciences
Rush University Medical Center
Chicago, Illinois

Sudhansu Chokroverty, MD, FRCP, FACP
Professor and Co-Chair of Neurology
Clinical Neurophysiology and Sleep Medicine
New Jersey Neuroscience Institute at JFK Medical Center
Edison, New Jersey
Professor of Neuroscience
Seton Hall University School of Graduate Medical Education
South Orange, New Jersey

Thanh Dang-Vu, MD, PhD
Postdoctoral Researcher, Cyclotron Research Centre
University of Liege
Liege, Belgium

Yves Dauvilliers, MD, PhD
Professor of Neurology/Physiology
University of Montpellier
Montpellier, France

William C. Dement, MD, PhD
Professor of Psychiatry and Sleep Medicine
Department of Psychiatry and Behavioral Sciences
Director, Sleep Disorders Clinic and Research Center
Stanford University School of Medicine
Palo Alto, California

Martin Desseilles, MD
Research Fellow, Cyclotron Research Centre
University of Liege
Liege, Belgium

Karl Doghramji, MD
Professor of Psychiatry and Human Behavior
Professor of Neurology and Program Director
Fellowship in Sleep Medicine
Thomas Jefferson University
Medical Director, Jefferson Sleep Disorders Center
Thomas Jefferson University Hospital
Philadelphia, Pennsylvania

Helen S. Driver, PhD, RPSGT, D.ABSM
Adjunct Assistant Professor
Departments of Medicine and Psychology
Queen's University
Sleep Disorders Laboratory Coordinator
Kingston General Hospital
Kingston, Ontario, Canada

Milton G. Ettinger, MD*
Professor of Neurology
University of Minnesota Medical School
Chief of Neurology
Hennepin County Medical Center
Minneapolis, Minnesota

Richard Ferber, MD
Associate Professor of Neurology
Harvard Medical School
Director, Center for Pediatric Sleep Disorders
Children's Hospital Boston
Boston, Massachusetts

Peter L. Franzen, PhD
Assistant Professor of Psychiatry
University of Pittsburgh School of Medicine
* and Western Psychiatric Institute and Clinic/UPMC*
Pittsburgh, Pennsylvania

Christian Guilleminault, MD, DM, BiolD
Professor
Stanford University Medical School
Stanford University
Stanford, California

Wayne A. Hening, MD, PhD*
Johns Hopkins Bayview Medical Center
Baltimore, Maryland

Max Hirshkowitz, PhD
Tenured Associate Professor
Department of Medicine and Menninger Department of Psychiatry
* and Sleep Medicine Fellowship Training Director*
Baylor College of Medicine
Director Sleep Disorders and Research Center
Michael E. DeBakey Veterans Affairs Medical Center
Houston, Texas

Timothy F. Hoban, MD
Associate Professor of Pediatrics and Neurology
University of Michigan
Director, Pediatric Sleep Medicine
University of Michigan
Ann Arbor, Michigan

Sharon A. Keenan, PhD, D.ABSM, REEGT, RPSGT
Director, The School of Sleep Medicine Inc.
Palo Alto, California

John B. Kostis, MD
John G. Detwiler Professor of Cardiology
Professor of Medicine and Pharmacology and Chairman
Department of Medicine, UMDNJ-Robert Wood Johnson Medical
* School*
New Brunswick, New Jersey

Mark W. Mahowald, MD
Professor, Department of Neurology
University of Minnesota Medical School
Director, Minnesota Regional Sleep Disorders Center
Hennepin County Medical Center
Minneapolis, Minnesota

Susan Malcolm-Smith, MA
Lecturer, Department of Psychology
University of Cape Town
Cape Town, South Africa

Pierre Maquet, MD, PhD
Research Director, Cyclotron Research Centre
University of Liege
Liege, Belgium

Stéphanie Maret, PhD
Center for Integrative Genomics
University of Lausanne
Lausanne, Switzerland

Robert W. McCarley, MD
Director, Neuroscience Laboratory, and Professor and Head
Department of Psychiatry, Harvard Medical School
Veterans Affairs Boston Healthcare
Brockton, Massachusetts

Reena Mehra, MD, MS
Assistant Professor of Medicine
Case School of Medicine
Assistant Professor of Medicine and Medical Director
Adult Sleep Center Services
University Hospitals Case Medical Center
Cleveland, Ohio

Pasquale Montagna, MD
Professor of Neurology
Department of Neurological Sciences
University of Bologna Medical School
Bologna, Italy

Jacques Montplaisir, MD, PhD, CRCP
Professor, Department of Psychiatry
Université de Montréal
Director, Center for the Study of Sleep and Biological Rhythms
Hôpital du Sacré-Coeur de Montréal
Montréal, Québec, Canada

*Deceased

Robert Y. Moore, MD, PhD, FAAN
Professor, Department of Neurology
University of Pittsburgh
Pittsburgh, Pennsylvania

Charles M. Morin, PhD
Professor of Psychology and Director
Sleep Research Center
École de Psychologie
Université Laval
Québec, Canada

Tore Nielsen, PhD
Professor, Department of Psychiatry
Université de Montréal
Researcher, Center for the Study of Sleep and Biological Rhythms
Hôpital du Sacré-Coeur de Montréal
Montréal, Québec, Canada

Christopher P. O'Donnell, PhD
Associate Professor
University of Pittsburgh
Pittsburgh, Pennsylvania

Maurice Moyses Ohayon, MD, PhD, DSc
Stanford Sleep Epidemiology Research Center
Stanford University School of Medicine
Palo Alto, California

Markku Partinen, MD, PhD
Research Director
Helsinki Sleep Clinic
Vitalmed Research Centre
Adjunct Professor, Department of Clinical Neurosciences
University of Helsinki
Helsinki, Finland

Philippe Peigneux, PhD
Professor, School of Psychology
Free University of Brussels
Brussels, Belgium

Dominique Petit, PhD
Research Assistant
Department of Psychiatry
Université de Montréal
Research Assistant, Center for the Study of Sleep and Biological Rhythms
Hôpital du Sacré-Coeur de Montréal
Montréal, Québec, Canada

Timothy A. Roehrs, PhD
Professor, Department of Psychiatry and Behavioral Neuroscience
Wayne State University School of Medicine
Director of Research, Sleep Disorders and Research Center
Henry Ford Health System
Detroit, Michigan

Mary Wilcox Rose, Psy.D.
Assistant Professor
Sleep Disorders and Research Center
Baylor College of Medicine
Psychologist, Michael E. DeBakey Veterans Affairs Medical Center
Houston, Texas

Thomas Roth, PhD
Professor, Department of Psychiatry and Behavioral Neuroscience
Wayne State University School of Medicine
Sleep Disorders and Research Center
Henry Ford Hospital
Detroit, Michigan

Mark H. Sanders, MD
Retired Professor of Medicine
University of Pittsburgh School of Medicine
University of Pittsburgh Medical Center
Pittsburgh, Pennsylvania

Carlos H. Schenck, MD
Professor, Department of Psychiatry
University of Minnesota Medical School
Staff Psychiatrist, Hennepin County Medical Center
Minneapolis, Minnesota

Sophie Schwartz, PhD
Professor
University of Geneva School of Medicine
Geneva, Switzerland

Amir Sharafkhaneh, MD, PhD
Assistant Professor, Department of Medicine
Sleep Medicine Fellowship Program Director
Baylor College of Medicine
Medical Director, Sleep Disorders and Research Center
Michael E. DeBakey Veterans Affairs Medical Center
Houston, Texas

Daniel M. Shindler, MD
Professor of Medicine and Anesthesiology
UMDNJ-Robert Wood Johnson Medical School
New Brunswick, New Jersey

Eileen P. Sloan, PhD, MD, FRCP(C)
Assistant Professor, Department of Psychiatry
University of Toronto
Staff Psychiatrist, Perinatal Mental Health Program
Mount Sinai Hospital
Toronto, Ontario, Canada

Mark Solms, PhD
Professor of Neuropsychology
Department of Psychology
University of Cape Town
Cape Town, South Africa

Mircea Steriade, MD, DSc*
Professor of Neuroscience
Department of Anatomy and Physiology
Laval University Faculty of Medicine
Quebec, Canada

Robert Stickgold, PhD
Associate Professor of Psychiatry
Harvard Medical School
Associate Professor of Psychiatry and Director of the Center
for Sleep and Cognition
Beth Israel Deaconess Medical Center
Boston, Massachusetts

Ronald A. Stiller, MD, PhD
Clinical Associate Professor of Medicine
University of Pittsburgh Medical Center
Medical Director, Surgical Intensive Care Unit
UPMC-Shadyside Hospital
Pittsburgh, Pennsylvania

Kingman P. Strohl, MD
Professor of Medicine and Professor of Anatomy
Case School of Medicine
Director, Center of Sleep Disorders Research
University Hospitals Case Medical Center
Cleveland, Ohio

Patrick J. Strollo Jr., MD
Associate Professor of Medicine and Clinical
and Translational Science
University of Pittsburgh
Medical Director, UPMC Sleep Center
University of Pittsburgh
Pittsburgh, Pennsylvania

Mehdi Tafti, PhD
Associate Professor in Genomics
Center for Integrative Genomics
University of Lausanne
Lausanne, Switzerland

Michael J. Thorpy, MD
Professor of Neurology
Albert Einstein College of Medicine
Director, Sleep-Wake Disorders Center
Montefiore Medical Center
Bronx, New York

Thaddeus S. Walczak, MD
Clinical Professor of Neurology
Department of Neurology
University of Minnesota
Staff Epileptologist, MINCEP Epilepsy Care
Attending Physician, Abbott Northwestern Hospital
Minneapolis, Minnesota

Matthew P. Walker, PhD
Assistant Professor, Department of Psychology
Director, Sleep and Neuroimaging Laboratory
University of California, Berkeley
Berkeley, California

Arthur S. Walters, MD
Professor of Neurology
Vanderbilt University School of Medicine
Nashville, Tennessee

Antonio Zadra, PhD
Professor, Department of Psychology
Université de Montréal
Researcher, Center for the Study of Sleep and Biological Rhythms
Hôpital du Sacré-Coeur de Montréal
Montréal, Québec, Canada

Michael Zupancic, MD
Pacific Sleep Medicine
San Diego, California

---

*Deceased

Preface

The history of sleep medicine and sleep research can be summarized as a history of remarkable progress and, at the same time, a history of remarkable ignorance. Since the publication of the second edition in 1999 enormous progress has been made in all aspects of sleep science and sleep medicine. I am pleased to see these rapid advances in sleep medicine and growing awareness about the importance of sleep and its dysfunction amongst the public and the profession. A sleep disorder is a serious health hazard and a "sleep attack" or a lack of sleep should be taken as seriously as a heart attack or "brain attack" (stroke); undiagnosed and untreated, a sleep disorder will have catastrophic consequences as severe as heart attack and stroke. Many dedicated and committed sleep scientists and clinicians, regional, national and international sleep organizations and foundations are responsible for pushing the topic forward. I can name a few such organizations (not an exhaustive list), e.g., American Academy of Sleep Medicine (AASM), National Sleep Foundation (NSF), European Sleep Research Society (ESRS), Asian Sleep Research Society (ASRS), Federation of Latin American Sleep Society (FLASS), World Association of Sleep Medicine (WASM), World Federation of Sleep Research and Medicine Societies (WFSRMS), Restless Legs Syndrome (RLS) Foundation and International Restless Legs Syndrome Study Group (IRLSSG). Thanks to these dedicated individuals and organizations sleep medicine is no longer in its infancy stage but is now a mature, but rapidly evolving branch within the broad field of medicine, standing on its own laurels.

Rapid advances in basic science, technical aspects, laboratory tests, clinical and therapeutic fields of sleep medicine have captivated sleep scientists and clinicians. In the sphere of basic science, a discovery in 1998 of two hypothalamic neuropeptides, hypocretin 1 (orexin A) and hypocretin 2 (orexin B), independently by two groups of neuroscientists, followed by the observations of narcoleptic phenotype in hypocretin receptor 2 mutated dogs and pre-prohypocretin knock-out mice in 1999, electrified the scientific community of sleep medicine. This was rapidly followed by advances in other basic science aspects of sleep, e.g., new understanding about neurobiology of sleep-wakefulness, sleep and memory consolidation, genes and circadian clock and neuroimaging of sleep-wakefulness showing a spectacular picture of the living brain non-invasively. Some examples of advances in clinical science include new insight into neurobiology of narcolepsy-cataplexy syndrome, obstructive sleep apnea and metabolic syndrome associated with serious cardiovascular risks and heart failure, advances in pathophysiology and clinical criteria of restless legs syndrome and rapid eye movement sleep behavior disorder, genetics of sleep disorders including RLS genes, new understanding of nocturnal frontal lobe epilepsy (nocturnal paroxysmal dystonia), fatal familial insomnia and the role of the thalamus in sleep-wake mechanisms, descriptions of new disorders (e.g., propriospinal myoclonus at sleep onset, expiratory groaning or catathrenia, rhythmic foot tremor and alternating leg muscle activation [ALMA]), and the revised international classification of sleep disorders (ICSD-2). In laboratory techniques the following can be cited as recent advances: new AASM scoring guidelines, improved in-laboratory and ambulatory polysomnographic (PSG) techniques, role of peripheral arterial tonometry, pulse transit time, actigraphy in sleep medicine, identification of autonomic activation by heart rate spectral analysis and realization of the importance of cyclic alternating pattern (CAP) in the EEG as an indication of sleep stability and arousal. Rapid advances have also been made in the therapeutic field which include new medications for narcolepsy-cataplexy, insomnia, restless legs syndrome, refinements of CPAP-BIPAP, introduction of auto-CPAP, assisted servo ventilation (ASV) in Cheyne-Stokes and other complex breathing disorders and intermittent positive pressure ventilation (IPPV) in neuromuscular disorders, and phototherapy for circadian rhythm disorders. The third edition tried to incorporate most of these advances, but in a field as vast as sleep medicine—rapidly evolving and encompassing every system and organ of the body—something will always be missing and outdated.

The third edition contains seven new chapters. Chapter 3 addresses an important topic of sleep deprivation and sleepiness reflecting the controversy of sleep duration and diseases and the causes and consequences of excessive daytime sleepiness. In Chapter 9 Walker and Stickgold discuss the question of sleep and memory consolidation, focusing not only on their own original contributions but also other important research in this field. In Chapter 15 the group lead by Maquet discusses how modern neuroimaging techniques can explore the living brain in a non-invasive manner, opening a new field in our understanding of sleep and sleep disorders. Partinen summarizes the importance of understanding the role of nutrition for sleep health in Chapter 23. In Chapter 31 Solms, based on his longstanding interest and research in neurological aspects of dreaming, brings into focus dream disorders in neurological diseases, a very timely topic which remains ill understood and unexplained. Hoban, in Chapter 38, masterfully and succinctly tells us how our sleep pattern and requirement change from birth to adolescence. Finally, a very important and often neglected topic of sleep medicine in women is discussed by Driver in Chapter 39. In this edition I have invited new contributors for these seven chapters which appeared in the second edition. Hirshkowitz, Rose, and Sharafkhaneh (Chapter 6) replaced Zoltoski and co-authors for neurochemistry and biochemical pharmacology of sleep. Robert Y. Moore, one of the pioneers in circadian neurobiology, wrote Chapter 8, replacing Kilduff and Kushida. Mehra and Strohl replaced Parisi for writing the chapter (14) dealing with an essential topic of evaluation and monitoring respiratory function. Hirshkowitz and Sharafkhaneh replaced Mitler and co-workers for updating the sleep scoring technique chapter (18). Tafti and co-workers (Chapter 22) replaced Mignot, bringing together all the recent advances in human and animal genetics of sleep and sleep disorders. Morin and Benca replaced Spielman and Anderson for the insomnia chapter (26), shedding light on recent understanding about the role of non-pharmacologic and pharmacologic treatments of insomnia based on their vast experience

and original contributions to the field. Montplaisir and co-workers replaced Broughton for the chapter (35) on behavioral parasomnias, incorporating many of their original contributions in the topic. I have invited Professor Montagna to join me in revising Chapters 29 and 30. The remaining chapters have been revised and updated with new materials, references, illustrations and tables.

The purpose of the third edition remains the same as those of the previous editions, namely to provide a comprehensive text covering basic science, technical and laboratory aspects and clinical and therapeutic advances in sleep medicine so that both the beginners and seasoned practitioners of sleep medicine will find the text useful. Hence the book should be useful to internists (especially those specializing in pulmonary, cardiovascular, gastrointestinal, renal and endocrine medicine), neurologists, family physicians, psychiatrists, psychologists, otolaryngologists, pediatricians, dentists, neurosurgeons and neuroscientists, as well as those technologists, nurses and other paraprofessionals with an interest in understanding the value of a good night's sleep.

I conclude the preface for this edition with a sad note. Two of our great scientists and giants in the field (Wayne Hening and Mircea Steriade) passed away after writing their chapters but before publication. We will miss their robust scientific contributions and writings, but they remain forever in our memory and in their last and lasting contributions to this text. I am particularly devastated by the unexpected and premature death of Wayne Hening, who had been not only a longstanding colleague but also a most dear friend of my wife and me for over two decades. Our vivid memory of Wayne traveling with us, visiting cultural centers in the North and South of India, participating in vigorous discussions of many interesting and intellectually stimulating topics will never fade away.

SUDHANSU CHOKROVERTY

Acknowledgments

I must first thank all the contributors for their superb scholarly writings, which I am certain will make this edition a valuable contribution to the rapidly growing field of sleep medicine. Martin A. Samuels who wrote the foreword for this edition is a remarkable neurologist, a superb educator and a clinician with seemingly unlimited depth and breadth of knowledge not only in neurology and neuroscience but also in all aspects of internal medicine. I am most grateful to Marty for his thoughtful commentary in the foreword. I should like to acknowledge Doctor Sidney Diamond for the computer generated diagram in Chapter 12 showing components of the polygraphic circuit. I also wish to thank all the authors, editors, and publishers who granted us permission to reproduce illustrations that were published in other books and journals, and the American Academy of Sleep Medicine (formerly the American Sleep Disorders Association) for giving permission to reproduce the graph in Chapter 1, showing the rapid growth of accredited sleep centers and laboratories. This edition would not have seen the light of day without the dedication and professionalism of the publishing staff at Elsevier's Philadelphia office. Susan Pioli, as acquisitions editor first initiated the production of the third edition, and since she left Elsevier Adrianne Brigido took over from her and splendidly moved forward various steps of production. I must also acknowledge with appreciation the valuable support of Arlene Chappelle, senior developmental editor, and the staff at the Elsevier production office for their professionalism, dedication and care in the making of the book.

It is my pleasure to acknowledge Betty Coram for typing all my chapters patiently and promptly, and Annabella Drennan for making corrections, typing and editing, and for computer-generated schematic diagrams in some of my chapters without any complaints amidst her other duties as editorial assistant to *Sleep Medicine* journal. Jenny Rodriguez helped with typing some references and tables.

My wife, Manisha Chokroverty, MD, encouraged me from the very beginning to produce a comprehensive textbook in sleep medicine and continually supported my effort in each and every edition with unfailing support, love, patience and fondness throughout the long period of the book's production. I must confess that it would not have been possible for me to complete this edition without her constant support, and for that I must remain grateful to her forever.

Foreword

Oscillations and rhythms are among the most basic and ubiquitous phenomena in biology. Among them, sleep is the most salient, known to every human being but only recently yielding some of its secrets to the scrutiny of the modern tools of neurobiology. There is no clinician who is not faced daily with patients whose problems are not, at least in part, related to a disorder of the curious ultradian rhythm of sleep and wakefulness. Insomnia and excessive drowsiness are the most obvious, but equally important are phenomena, such as the early morning peak incidence of ischemic stroke, the violent acting out of dreams, hypnic headaches, seizures during sleep, nocturnal dystonias, and the relationship between iron deficiency and the Ekbom syndrome of the restless legs.

As is true of many advances in medicine, the appearance of a new insight leads one to realize how widespread a disorder is, overlooked for years because one simply did not have the insights or tools necessary to recognize it in patients. The relatively recent discovery that the REM behavior disorder is a synucleinopathy, possibly marking one of the earliest recognizable aspects of Parkinsonism, is a good example. How often did physicians of the last generation hear about violent acting out of dreams from their patients' bed partners? It seemed to be very rare, but now the history is sought and is often discovered in a very large number of people, many of whom are probably destined to develop the familiar motor syndrome of Parkinsonism. In this manner, disorders of sleep often provide critical insights into the clinical disability and often the pathogenesis of many diseases.

Sudhansu Chokroverty is a master of sleep medicine and is one of the earliest neurologists who dedicated his career to the study of this area. Given the fact that consciousness is inherently a neurological phenomenon, the contributions of Dr. Chokroverty have been critical to the understanding of sleep. His impact on the development of the field of sleep medicine and in educating generations of physicians, dentists and other health care providers about sleep disorders has been monumental. The first edition of *Sleep Disorders Medicine*, which appeared in the mid 1990s, has become the clinical gold standard for approaching sleep disorders in practice. Its combination of basic science, technical details and clinical wisdom is unique among references in the field.

The third edition of this classic work maintains its core strengths, while at the same time is dramatically updated and modernized, reflecting the enormous contributions in the field provided by neuroimaging, genetics and technical advances. One can use the book in two ways: as a reference work to look up a particular phenomenon or as a textbook, which can be read by students, residents or practicing clinicians in virtually any setting. The clinical chapters have the flavor or authenticity that can only be achieved by the fact that they are written by experienced and seasoned clinicians who understand the challenges of diagnosing and managing sleep disorders in the real world.

Dr. Chokroverty picked his authors carefully from a world cast of characters in the field. He wrote several of the chapters himself and fastidiously edited the others so that the text holds together as a single work that adheres to his vision of a book that is authoritative, while simultaneously a valuable manual for the practice of sleep medicine. The third edition of what is now the classic work in the field will undoubtedly find its way to the book shelves of everyone who sees patients.

I once asked Dr. Chokroverty what he thought the function of sleep might be. He responded that without it, we would probably become quite drowsy. His tongue in cheek answer reflects the fact that we do not yet know the full answer to this age old question. The current theories are clearly explicated in the third edition. Whether the function of sleep is to consolidate memories, to metabolize soporific compounds that are the products of brain metabolism or some other as yet unknown purpose, we can be sure that we will see the answer in authoritative form in the next edition of Chokroverty's *Sleep Disorders Medicine*.

Martin A. Samuels, MD, FAAN, MACP
Chairman, Department of Neurology,
Brigham and Women's Hospital, Professor of Neurology,
Harvard Medical School, Boston, Massachusetts

Contents

PART III
Clinical Aspects

PART I

Basic Aspects of Sleep

CHAPTER 1

Introduction

William C. Dement

Sleep disorders medicine is based primarily on the understanding that human beings have two fully functioning brains—the brain in wakefulness and the brain in sleep. Cerebral activity has contrasting consequences in the state of wakefulness versus the state of sleep. In addition, the brain's two major functional states influence each other. Problems during wakefulness affect sleep, and disordered sleep or disordered sleep mechanisms impair the functions of wakefulness. Perhaps the most common complaint addressed in sleep disorders medicine is impaired daytime alertness (i.e., excessive fatigue and sleepiness).

Critical to sleep disorders medicine is the fact that some function (e.g., breathing) may be normal during the state of wakefulness but pathologic during sleep. Moreover, a host of nonsleep disorders are, or may be, modified by sleep. It should no longer be necessary to argue that an understanding of a patient's health includes equal consideration of the state of the patient asleep as well as awake. The knowledge that patient care is a 24-hour commitment is fundamental to one aspect of sleep medicine: circadian regulation of sleep and wakefulness. It is worth suggesting that, of all industries operating on a 24-hour schedule, it is the medical profession that should lead the way in developing practical protocols for resetting the biological clock to promote full alertness and optimal performance whenever health professionals must work at night.

WHAT IS SLEEP DISORDERS MEDICINE?

"Sleep disorders medicine is a clinical specialty which deals with the diagnosis and treatment of patients who complain about disturbed nocturnal sleep, excessive daytime sleepiness, or some other sleep-related problem."[1] The spectrum of disorders and problems in this area is extremely broad, ranging from minor, such as a day or two of mild jet lag, to catastrophic, such as sudden infant death syndrome, fatal familial insomnia, or an automobile accident caused by a patient with sleep apnea who falls asleep at the wheel. The dysfunctions may be primary, involving the basic neural mechanisms of sleep and arousal, or secondary, in association with other physical, psychiatric, or neurologic illnesses. Where the associations with disturbed sleep are very strong, such as in endogenous depression and immune disorders, abnormalities in sleep mechanisms may play a causal role. These issues continue to be investigated.

In sleep disorders medicine, it is critical to examine the sleeping patient and to evaluate the impact of sleep on waking functions. Physicians in the field have an enormous responsibility to address the societal implications of sleep disorders and sleep problems, particularly those attributed to impaired alertness. This responsibility is heightened by the fact that the transfer of sleep medicine's knowledge base to the mainstream education system is far from complete, and truly effective public and professional awareness remains to be fully established. All physicians should be sensitive to the level of alertness in their patients and the potential consequences of falling asleep in the workplace, at the wheel, or elsewhere.

A BRIEF HISTORY

Well into the 19th century, the phenomenon of sleep escaped systematic observation, despite the fact that sleep occupies one-third of a human lifetime. All other things being equal, we may assume that there were a variety of reasons not to study sleep, one of which was the unpleasant necessity of staying awake at night.[2]

Although there was a modicum of sleep disorders research in the 1960s, including a fee-for-service narcolepsy clinic at Stanford University and research on illnesses related to inadequate sleep, such as asthma and hypothyroidism, at the University of California, Los Angeles,[3,4] sleep disorders medicine can be identified as having begun in earnest at Stanford University in 1970. The sleep specialists at Stanford routinely used respiration and cardiac sensors together with electroencephalography, electro-oculography, and electromyography in all-night, polygraphic recordings. Continuous all-night recording using this array of data-gathering techniques was finally named polysomnography by Holland and colleagues,[5] and patients at Stanford paid for the tests as part of a clinical fee-for-service arrangement.

The Stanford model included responsibility for medical management and care of patients beyond mere interpretation of the test results and an assessment of daytime sleepiness. After several false starts, the latter effort culminated in the development of the Multiple Sleep Latency Test,[6,7] and the framework for the development of the discipline of sleep medicine was complete.

The comprehensive evaluation of sleep in patients who complained about their daytime alertness rapidly led to a series of discoveries, including the high prevalence of obstructive sleep apnea in patients complaining of sleepiness, the role of periodic limb movement in insomnia, and the sleep state misperception syndrome first called *pseudoinsomnia*. As with the beginning of any medical practice, the case-series approach, wherein patients are evaluated and carefully tabulated, was very important.[8]

THE RECENT PAST

Nasal continuous positive airway pressure and uvulopalatopharyngoplasty replaced tracheostomy as treatment for obstructive sleep apnea in 1981.[9,10] At that time, the field of sleep medicine entered a period of significant growth that has not abated. The number of accredited sleep disorders centers and laboratories has increased almost exponentially since 1977 (Fig. 1–1). In 1990, a congressionally mandated national commission began its study of sleep deprivation and sleep disorders in American society with the goal of resolving some of the problems impeding access to treatment for millions of patients. The last decade of the 20th century, however, will be recognized

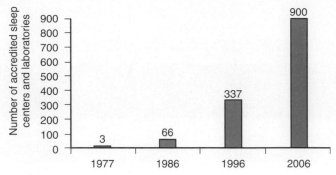

FIGURE 1–1 American Sleep Disorders Association (ASDA)–accredited sleep centers and laboratories shown graphically. *(Reprinted with permission from ASDA.)*

as a time when federal growth began to slow to a stop. Consequently, the growth of sleep medicine as a specialty practice has also slowed, although it is far from stopping. Nevertheless, the increasing competition for limited federal funds means that there is a great need for sleep disorders medicine to enter the mainstream of the health care system and for the knowledge obtained in this field to be disseminated throughout our education system.

With the incorporation of the American Academy of Sleep Medicine, the creation of the National Center on Sleep Disorders Research, the continuing strength of patient and professional sleep societies, and recognized textbooks, a healthy foundation of sleep medicine is certainly in place. The population prevalence of obstructive sleep apnea has been established—this one illness afflicts 30 million people.[11] Gallup Polls suggest that one-half of all Americans have a sleep disorder. Given the grossly inadequate public and professional awareness of sleep disorders and problems, one must conclude that most of the millions of individuals afflicted with sleep disorders, some of which can lead to death, do not recognize their disorder and therefore do not obtain the benefits available to them.

There is a continuing need for effective presentation of the organized body of knowledge of sleep disorders medicine, and this book responds to that need. Every individual involved in this field must work toward the goal of improving education on sleep disorders, work that is not only critical for medical school students, but important for all other educational levels as well.

REFERENCES

A full list of references are available at www.expertconsult.com

CHAPTER 2

An Overview of Normal Sleep

Sudhansu Chokroverty

HISTORICAL PERSPECTIVE

The history of sleep medicine and sleep research is a history of remarkable progress and remarkable ignorance. In the 1940s and 1950s, sleep had been in the forefront of neuroscience, and then again in the late 1990s there had been a resurgence of our understanding of the neurobiology of sleep. Sleeping and waking brain circuits can now be studied by sophisticated neuroimaging techniques that have shown remarkable progress by mapping different areas of the brain during sleep states and stages. Electrophysiologic research has shown that even a single neuron sleeps, as evidenced by the electrophysiologic correlates of sleep-wakefulness at the cellular (single-cell) level. Despite recent progress, we are still groping for answers to two fundamental questions: What is sleep? Why do we sleep? Sleep is not simply an absence of wakefulness and perception, nor is it just a suspension of sensorial processes; rather, it is a result of a combination of a passive withdrawal of afferent stimuli to the brain and functional activation of certain neurons in selective brain areas.

Since the dawn of civilization, the mysteries of sleep have intrigued poets, artists, philosophers, and mythologists.[1] The fascination with sleep is reflected in literature, folklore, religion, and medicine. *Upanishad*[2] (circa 1000 bc), the ancient Indian text of Hindu religion, sought to divide human existence into four states: the waking, the dreaming, the deep dreamless sleep, and the superconscious ("the very self"). This is reminiscent of modern classification of three states of existence (see later). One finds the description of pathologic sleepiness (possibly a case of Kleine-Levin syndrome) in the mythologic character

Kumbhakarna in the great Indian epic *Ramayana*[3,4] (circa 1000 bc). Kumbhakarna would sleep for months at a time, then get up to eat and drink voraciously before falling asleep again.

Throughout literature, a close relationship between sleep and death has been perceived, but the rapid reversibility of sleep episodes differentiates sleep from coma and death. There are myriad references to sleep, death, and dream in poetic and religious writings, including the following quotations: "The deepest sleep resembles death" (*The Bible*, I Samuel 26:12); "sleep and death are similar... sleep is one-sixtieth [i.e., one piece] of death" (*The Talmud*, Berachoth 576); "There she [Aphrodite] met sleep, the brother of death" (Homer's *Iliad*, circa 700 bc); "To sleep perchance to dream.... For in that sleep of death what dreams may come?" (Shakespeare's *Hamlet*); "How wonderful is death; Death and his brother sleep" (Shelly's "Queen Mab").

The three major behavioral states in humans—wakefulness, non–rapid eye movement (NREM) sleep, and rapid eye movement (REM) sleep—are three basic biological processes that have independent functions and controls. The reader should consult Borbely's monograph *Secrets of Sleep*[1] for an interesting historical introduction to sleep.

What is the origin of sleep? The words *sleep* and *somnolence* are derived from the Latin word *somnus;* the German words *sleps, slaf,* or *schlaf;* and the Greek word *hypnos.* Hippocrates, the father of medicine, postulated a humoral mechanism for sleep and asserted that sleep was caused by the retreat of blood and warmth into the inner regions of the body, whereas the Greek philosopher Aristotle thought sleep was related to food, which generates heat

5

and causes sleepiness. Paracelsus, a 16th-century physician, wrote that "natural" sleep lasted 6 hours, eliminating tiredness and refreshing the sleeper. He also suggested that people not sleep too much or too little, but awake when the sun rises and go to bed at sunset. This advice from Paracelsus is strikingly similar to modern thinking about sleep. Views about sleep in the 17th and 18th centuries were expressed by Alexander Stuart, the British physician and physiologist, and by the Swiss physician Albrecht von Haller. According to Stuart, sleep was due to a deficit of the "animal spirits"; von Haller wrote that the flow of the "spirits" to the nerves was cut off by the thickened blood in the heart, resulting in sleep. Nineteenth-century scientists used principles of physiology and chemistry to explain sleep. Both Humboldt and Pfluger thought that sleep resulted from a reduction or lack of oxygen in the brain.[1]

Ideas about sleep were not based on solid scientific experiments until the 20th century. Ishimori[5] in 1909, and Legendre and Pieron[6] in 1913, observed sleep-promoting substances in the cerebrospinal fluid of animals during prolonged wakefulness. The discovery of the electroencephalographic (EEG) waves in dogs by the English physician Caton[7] in 1875 and of the alpha waves from the surface of the human brain by the German physician Hans Berger[8] in 1929 provided the framework for contemporary sleep research. It is interesting to note that Kohlschutter, a 19th-century German physiologist, thought sleep was deepest in the first few hours and became lighter as time went on.[1] Modern sleep laboratory studies have generally confirmed these observations.

The golden age of sleep research began in 1937 with the discovery by American physiologist Loomis and colleagues[9] of different stages of sleep reflected in EEG changes. Aserinsky and Kleitman's[10] discovery of REM sleep in the 1950s at the University of Chicago electrified the scientific community and propelled sleep research to the forefront. Observations of muscle atonia in cats by Jouvet and Michel in 1959[11] and in human laryngeal muscles by Berger in 1961[12] completed the discovery of all major components of REM sleep. Following this, Rechtschaffen and Kales produced the standard sleep scoring technique monograph in 1968 (the R&K scoring technique).[13] This remained the "gold standard" until the American Academy of Sleep Medicine (AASM) published the AASM manual for the scoring of sleep and associated events,[14] which modified the R&K technique and extended the scoring rules. The other significant milestone in the history of sleep medicine was the discovery of the site of obstruction in the upper airway in obstructive sleep apnea syndrome (OSAS) independently by Gastaut and Tassinari[15] in France as well as Jung and Kuhlo[16] in Germany followed by the introduction by Sullivan and associates in 1981[17] of continuous positive airway pressure titration to eliminate such obstruction as the standard treatment modality for moderate to severe OSAS. Finally, identification of two neuropeptides, hypocretin 1 and 2 (orexin A and B), in the lateral hypothalamus and perifornical regions[18,19] was followed by an animal model of a human narcolepsy phenotype in dogs by mutation of hypocretin 2 receptors by Lin et al.,[20] the creation of similar phenotype in pre-prohypocretin knock-out mice[21] and transgenic mice,[22] and documentation of decreased hypocretin 1 in the cerebrospinal fluid in humans[23] and decreased hypocretin neurons in the hypothalamus at autopsy[24,25] in human narcolepsy patients; these developments opened a new and exciting era of sleep research.

DEFINITION OF SLEEP

The definition of sleep and a description of its functions have always baffled scientists. Moruzzi,[26] while describing the historical development of the deafferentation hypothesis of sleep, quoted the concept Lucretius articulated 2000 years ago—that sleep is the *absence of wakefulness.* A variation of the same concept was expressed by Hartley[27] in 1749, and again in 1830 by Macnish,[28] who defined sleep as *suspension of sensorial power,* in which the voluntary functions are in abeyance but the involuntary powers, such as circulation or respiration, remain intact. It is easy to comprehend what sleep is if one asks oneself that question as one is trying to get to sleep. Modern sleep researchers define sleep on the basis of both behavior of the person while asleep (Table 2–1) and the related physiologic changes that occur to the waking brain's electrical rhythm in sleep.[29–32] The behavioral criteria include lack of mobility or slight mobility, closed eyes, a characteristic species-specific sleeping posture, reduced response to external stimulation, quiescence, increased

TABLE 2–1 Behavioral Criteria of Wakefulness and Sleep			
Criteria	Wakefulness	Non–Rapid Eye Movement Sleep	Rapid Eye Movement Sleep
Posture	Erect, sitting, or recumbent	Recumbent	Recumbent
Mobility	Normal	Slightly reduced or immobile; postural shifts	Moderately reduced or immobile; myoclonic jerks
Response to stimulation	Normal	Mildly to moderately reduced	Moderately reduced to no response
Level of alertness	Alert	Unconscious but reversible	Unconscious but reversible
Eyelids	Open	Closed	Closed
Eye movements	Waking eye movements	Slow rolling eye movements	Rapid eye movements

reaction time, elevated arousal threshold, impaired cognitive function, and a reversible unconscious state. The physiologic criteria (see *Sleep Architecture and Sleep Profile* later) are based on the findings from EEG, electro-oculography (EOG), and electromyography (EMG) as well as other physiologic changes in ventilation and circulation.

While trying to define the process of falling asleep, we must differentiate sleepiness from fatigue or tiredness. Fatigue can be defined as a state of sustained lack of energy coupled with a lack of motivation and drive but does not require the behavioral criteria of sleepiness, such as heaviness and drooping of the eyelids, sagging or nodding of the head, yawning, and an ability to nap given the opportunity to fall asleep. Conversely, fatigue is often a secondary consequence of sleepiness.

THE MOMENT OF SLEEP ONSET AND OFFSET

There is no exact moment of sleep onset; there are gradual changes in many behavioral and physiologic characteristics, including EEG rhythms, cognition, and mental processing (including reaction time). Sleepiness begins at sleep onset even before reaching stage 1 NREM sleep (as defined later) with heaviness and drooping of the eyelids; clouding of the sensorium; and inability to see, hear, smell, or perceive things in a rational or logical manner. At this point, an individual trying to get to sleep is now entering into another world in which the person has no control and the brain cannot respond logically and adequately. This is the stage coined by McDonald Critchley as the "pre-dormitum."[33] Slow eye movements (SEMs) begin at sleep onset and continue through stage 1 NREM sleep. At sleep onset, there is a progressive decline in the thinking process, and sometimes there may be hypnagogic imagery.

Similar to sleep onset, the moment of awakening or sleep offset is also a gradual process from the fully established sleep stages. This period is sometimes described as manifesting sleep inertia or "sleep drunkenness." There is a gradual return to a state of alertness or wakefulness.

SLEEP ARCHITECTURE AND SLEEP PROFILE

Based on three physiologic measurements (EEG, EOG, and EMG), sleep is divided into two states[34] with independent functions and controls: NREM and REM sleep. Table 2–2 lists the physiologic criteria of wakefulness

TABLE 2–3 Summary of Non–Rapid Eye Movement (NREM) and Rapid Eye Movement (REM) Sleep States

Sleep State	% Sleep Time
NREM sleep	75–80
N1	3–8
N2	45–55
N3	15–20
REM sleep	20–25
Tonic stage	—
Phasic stage	—

and sleep, and Table 2–3 summarizes NREM and REM sleep states. In an ideal situation (which may not be seen in all normal individuals), NREM and REM alternate in a cyclic manner, each cycle lasting on average from 90 to 110 minutes. During a normal sleep period in adults, 4–6 such cycles are noted. The first two cycles are dominated by slow-wave sleep (SWS) (R&K stages 3 and 4 NREM and AASM stage N3 sleep); subsequent cycles contain less SWS, and sometimes SWS does not occur at all. In contrast, the REM sleep cycle increases from the first to the last cycle, and the longest REM sleep episode toward the end of the night may last for an hour. Thus, in human adult sleep, the first third is dominated by the SWS and the last third is dominated by REM sleep. It is important to be aware of these facts because certain abnormal motor activities are characteristically associated with SWS and REM sleep.

Non–Rapid Eye Movement Sleep

NREM sleep accounts for 75–80% of sleep time in an adult human. According to the R&K scoring manual,[13] NREM sleep is further divided into four stages (stages 1–4), and according to the current AASM scoring manual,[14] it is subdivided into three stages (N1, N2, and N3), primarily on the basis of EEG criteria. Stage 1 NREM (N1) sleep occupies 3–8% of sleep time; stage 2 (N2) comprises 45–55% of sleep time; and stages 3 and 4 NREM (N3) or SWS make up 15–20% of total sleep time.

The dominant rhythm during adult human wakefulness consist of the alpha rhythm (8–13 Hz), noted predominantly in the posterior region, intermixed with small amount of beta rhythm (>13 Hz), seen mainly in the anterior head regions (Fig. 2–1). This state, called

TABLE 2–2 Physiologic Criteria of Wakefulness and Sleep

Criteria	Wakefulness	Non–Rapid Eye Movement Sleep	Rapid Eye Movement Sleep
Electroencephalography	Alpha waves; desynchronized	Synchronized	Theta or sawtooth waves; desynchronized
Electromyography (muscle tone)	Normal	Mildly reduced	Moderately to severely reduced or absent
Electro-oculography	Waking eye movements	Slow rolling eye movements	Rapid eye movements

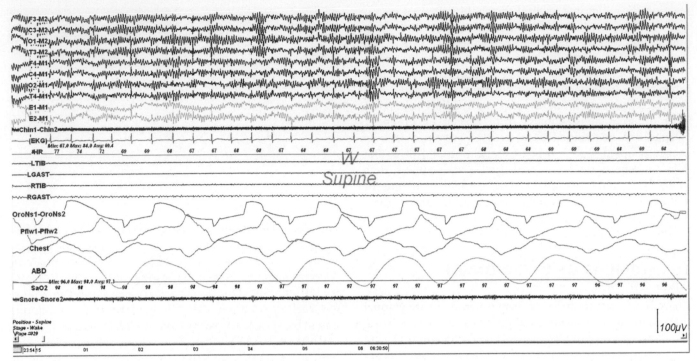

FIGURE 2–1 Polysomnographic recording showing wakefulness in an adult. Top 8 channels of electroencephalograms (EEG) show posterior dominant 10-Hz alpha rhythm intermixed with a small amount of low-amplitude beta rhythms (international nomenclature). M2, right mastoid; M1: left mastoid. Waking eye movements are seen in the electro-oculogram of the left (E1) and right (E2) eyes, referred to the left mastoid. Chin1 (*left*) and Chin2 (*right*) submental electromyography (EMG) shows tonic muscle activity. EKG, electrocardiogram; HR, heart rate per minute. On LTIB (left tibialis), LGAST (left gastrocnemius), RTIB (right tibialis), and RGAST (right gastrocnemius), EMG shows very little tonic activity. OroNs1-OroNs2, oronasal airflow; Pflw1-Pflw2, nasal pressure transducer recording airflow; Chest and ABD, respiratory effort (chest and abdomen); SaO2, oxygen saturation by finger oximetry; Snore, snoring.

stage W, may be accompanied by conjugate waking eye movements (WEMs), which may comprise vertical, horizontal, or oblique, slow or fast eye movements. In stage 1 NREM sleep (stage N1), alpha rhythm diminishes to less than 50% in an epoch (i.e., a 30-second segment of the polysomnographic [PSG] tracing with the monitor screen speed of 10 mm/sec) intermixed with slower theta rhythms (4–7 Hz) and beta waves (Fig. 2–2). Electromyographic activity decreases slightly and SEMs appear. Toward the end of this stage, vertex sharp waves are noted. Stage 2 NREM (stage N2) begins after approximately 10–12 minutes of stage 1. Sleep spindles (11–16 Hz, mostly 12–14 Hz) and K complexes intermixed with vertex sharp waves herald the onset of stage N2 sleep (Fig. 2–3). EEG at this stage also shows theta waves and delta waves (<4 Hz) that occupy less than 20% of the epoch. After about 30–60 minutes of stage 2 NREM sleep (stage N2), stage 3 sleep begins, and delta waves comprise 20–50% of the epoch (Fig. 2–4). The next stage is NREM 4 sleep (during which delta waves occupy more than 50% of the epoch) (Fig. 2–5). As stated above, R&K stages 3 and 4 NREM are grouped together as SWS and are replaced by stage N3 in the new AASM scoring manual. Body movements often are recorded as artifacts in PSG recordings toward the end of SWS as sleep is lightening. Stages 3 and 4 NREM sleep (stage N3) are briefly interrupted by stage 2 NREM (stage N2), which is followed by the first REM sleep approximately 60–90 minutes after sleep onset.

Rapid Eye Movement Sleep

REM sleep accounts for 20–25% of total sleep time. Based on EEG, EMG, and EOG characteristics, REM can be subdivided into two stages, tonic and phasic. This subdivision is not recognized in the current AASM scoring manual.[14] A desynchronized EEG, hypotonia or atonia of major muscle groups, and depression of monosynaptic and polysynaptic reflexes are characteristics of tonic REM sleep. This tonic stage persists throughout REM sleep, whereas the phasic stage is discontinuous and superimposed on the tonic stage. Phasic REM sleep is characterized by bursts of REMs in all directions. Phasic swings in blood pressure and heart rate, irregular respiration, spontaneous middle ear muscle activity, myoclonic twitching of the facial and limb muscle, and tongue movements all occur. A few periods of apnea or hypopnea also may occur during REM sleep. Electroencephalographic tracing during REM sleep consists of a low-amplitude, fast pattern in the beta frequency range mixed with a small amount of theta rhythms, some of which may have a "sawtooth" appearance (Fig. 2–6). Sawtooth waves

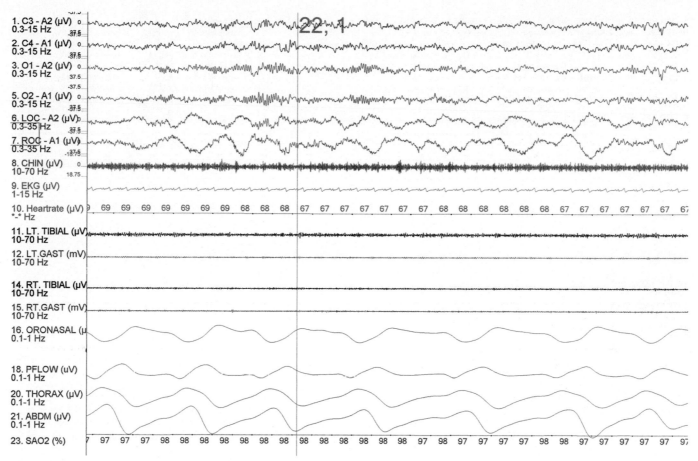

FIGURE 2–2 Polysomnographic recording shows stage 1 non–rapid eye movement (NREM) sleep (N1) in an adult. Electroencephalograms (top 4 EEG channels) show a decrease of alpha activity to less than 50% and low-amplitude beta and theta activities. Electro-oculograms (LOC: left; ROC: right) show slow rolling eye movements. A1, left ear; A2, right ear; Thorax, repiratory effort (chest). Rest of the montage is same as in Figure 2–1.

are trains of sharply contoured, often serrated, 2– to 6-Hz waves seen maximally over the central regions and are thought to be the gateway to REM sleep, often preceding a burst of REMs. During REM sleep there may be some intermittent intrusions of alpha rhythms in the EEG lasting for a few seconds. The first REM sleep lasts only a few minutes. Sleep then progresses to stage 2 NREM (stage N2), followed by stages 3 and 4 NREM (stage N3), before the second REM sleep begins.

Summary

During normal sleep in adults, there is an orderly progression from wakefulness to sleep onset to NREM sleep and then to REM sleep. Relaxed wakefulness is characterized by a behavioral state of quietness and a physiologic state of alpha and beta frequency in the EEG, WEMs, and increased muscle tone. NREM sleep is characterized by progressively decreased responsiveness to external stimulation accompanied by SEMs, followed by EEG slow-wave activity associated with sleep spindles and K complexes, and decreased muscle tone. REMs, further reduction of responsiveness to stimulation, absent muscle tone, and low-voltage, fast EEG activity mixed with distinctive sawtooth waves characterize REM sleep.

The R&K scoring system addresses normal adult sleep and macrostructure of sleep. In patients with sleep disorders such as sleep apnea, parasomnias, or sleep-related seizures, it may be difficult to score sleep according to R&K criteria. Furthermore, the R&K staging system does not address the microstructure of sleep. The details of the R&K and the current AASM sleep scoring criteria are outlined in Chapter 18. The macrostructure of sleep is summarized in Table 2–4. There are several endogenous and exogenous factors that will modify sleep macrostructure (Table 2–5).

Sleep Microstructure

Sleep microstructure includes momentary dynamic phenomena such as arousals, which have been operationally defined by a Task Force of the American Sleep Disorders Association (now called the American Academy of Sleep Medicine)[35] and remain essentially unchanged in the current AASM scoring manual,[14] and the cyclic alternating pattern (CAP), which has been defined and described in

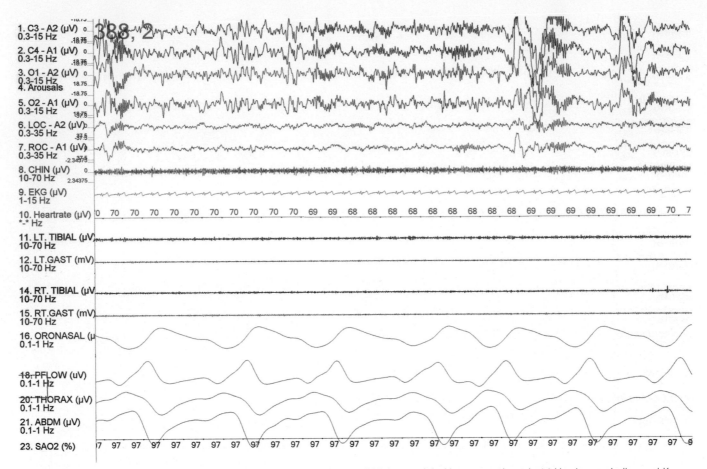

FIGURE 2–3 Polysomnographic recording shows stage 2 NREM sleep (N2) in an adult. Note approximately 14-Hz sleep spindles and K complexes intermixed with delta waves (0.5–2 Hz) and up to 75 μV in amplitude occupying less than 20% of the epoch. See Figure 2–2 for description of rest of the montage.

various publications by Terzano and co-investigators.[36–38] Other components of microstructure include K complexes and sleep spindles (Table 2–6).

Arousals are transient phenomena resulting in fragmented sleep without behavioral awakening. An arousal is scored during sleep stages N1, N2, and N3 (or REM sleep) if there is an abrupt shift in EEG frequency lasting from 3 to 14 seconds (Fig. 2–7) and including alpha, beta, or theta activities but not spindles or delta waves. Before an arousal can be scored, the subject must be asleep for 10 consecutive seconds. In REM sleep, arousals are scored only when accompanied by concurrent increase in segmental EMG amplitude. K complexes, delta waves, artifacts, and only increased segmental EMG activities are not counted as arousals unless these are accompanied by EEG frequency shifts. Arousals can be expressed as number per hour of sleep (an arousal index), and an arousal index up to 10 can be considered normal.

The CAP (Fig. 2–8) indicates sleep instability, whereas frequent arousals signify sleep fragmentation.[38] Sleep microstructure is best understood by the CAP, wherein an EEG pattern that repeats in a cyclical manner is noted mainly during NREM sleep. This is a promising technique in evaluating both normal and abnormal sleep, as well as in understanding the neurophysiologic and neurochemical basis of sleep. A CAP cycle[39] consists of an unstable phase (phase A) and relatively stable phase (phase B) each lasting between 2 and 60 seconds. Phase A of CAP is marked by an increase of EEG potentials with contributions from both synchronous high-amplitude slow and desynchronized fast rhythms in the EEG recording standing out from a relatively low-amplitude slow background. The A phase is associated with an increase in heart rate, respiration, blood pressure, and muscle tone. CAP rate (total CAP time during NREM sleep) and arousals both increase in older individuals and in a variety of sleep disorders, including both diurnal and nocturnal movement disorders. Non-CAP (a sleep period without CAP) is thought to indicate a state of sustained stability.

Summary

Sleep macrostructure is based on cyclic patterns of NREM and REM states, whereas sleep microstructure mainly consists of arousals, periods of CAP, and periods without CAP. An understanding of sleep macrostructure

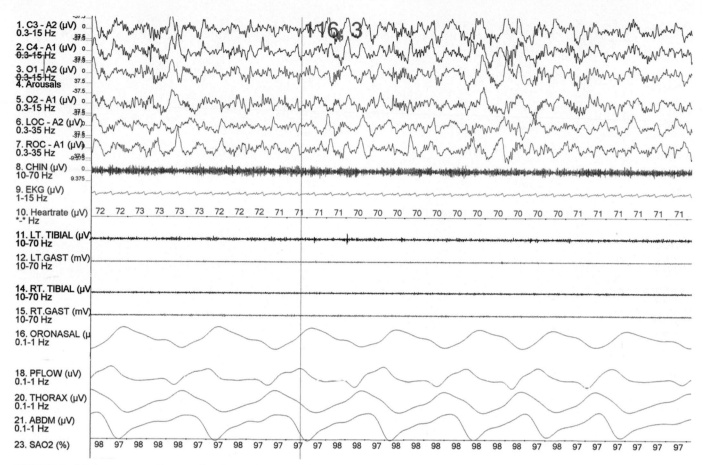

FIGURE 2–4 Polysomnographic recording from an adult showing stage 3 (N3) NREM sleep. Delta waves in the EEG (top 4 channels) as defined in Figure 2–2 occupy more than 20% of the epoch in N3 and 20–50% of the epoch in the traditional stage 3 as defined in Rechtschaffen-Kales (R&K) scoring criteria. See Figure 2–2 for description of rest of the montage.

and microstructure is important because emergence of abnormal motor activity during sleep may be related to disturbed macrostructure and microstructure of sleep.

THE ONTOGENY OF SLEEP

Evolution of the EEG and sleep states (see also Chapter 38) from the fetus, preterm and term infant, young child, and adolescent to the adult proceeds in an orderly manner depending upon the maturation of the central nervous system (CNS).[40–43] Neurologic, environmental, and genetic factors as well as comorbid medical or neurologic conditions will have significant effects on such ontogenetic changes. Sleep requirements change dramatically from infancy to old age. Newborns have a polyphasic sleep pattern, with 16 hours of sleep per day. This sleep requirement decreases to approximately 11 hr/day by 3–5 years of age. At 9–10 years of age, most children sleep for 10 hours at night. Preadolescents are highly alert during the day, with the Multiple Sleep Latency Test showing a mean sleep latency of 17–18 minutes. In preschool children, sleep assumes a biphasic pattern. Adults exhibit a monophasic sleep pattern, with an average duration from 7.5 to 8 hours per night. This returns to a biphasic pattern in old age.

Upon falling asleep, a newborn baby goes immediately into REM sleep, or active sleep, which is accompanied by restless movements of the arms, legs, and facial muscles. In premature babies, it is often difficult to differentiate REM sleep from wakefulness. Sleep spindles appear from 6 to 8 weeks and are well formed by 3 months (they may be asynchronous during the first year and by age 2 are synchronous). K complexes are seen at 6 months but begin to appear at over 4 months. Hypnagogic hypersynchrony characterized by transient bursts of high-amplitude waves in the slower frequencies appear at 5–6 months and are prominent at 1 year. By 3 months of age the NREM-REM cyclic pattern of adult sleep is established. However, the NREM-REM cycle duration is shorter in infants, lasting for approximately 45–50 minutes and increasing to 60–70 minutes by 5–10 years and to the normal adult cyclic pattern of 90–100 minutes by the age of 10 years. A weak circadian rhythm is probably present at birth, but by 6–8 weeks it is established. Gradually, the nighttime sleep increases and daytime sleep and the number of naps decrease. By 8 months, the majority of infants take two naps (late morning and early afternoon).

The first 3 months are a critical period of CNS reorganization, and striking changes occur in many physiologic

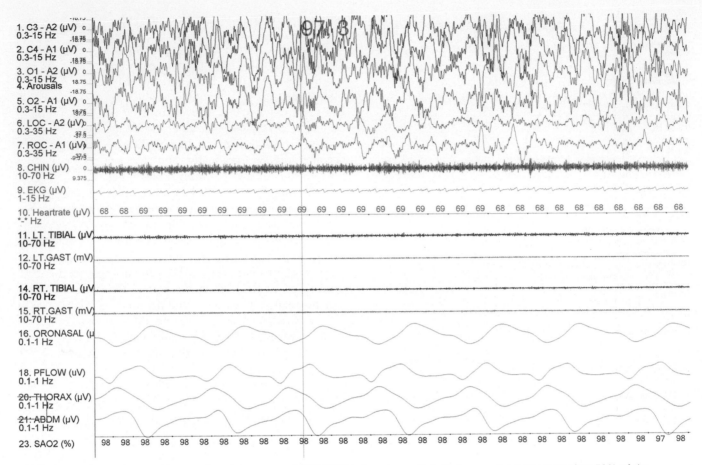

FIGURE 2–5 Polysomnographic recording shows stage 4 (N3) NREM sleep in an adult. Delta waves occupy more than 50% of the epoch in the traditional R&K scoring technique. See Figure 2–2 for description of the montage.

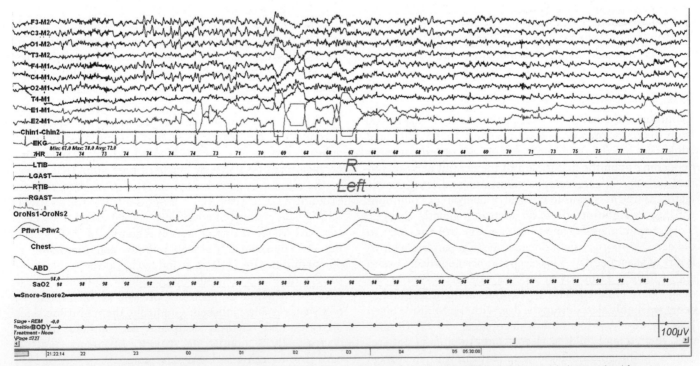

FIGURE 2–6 Polysomnographic recording shows rapid eye movement (REM) sleep in an adult. EEG (top 8 channels) shows mixed-frequency theta, low-amplitude beta, and a small amount of alpha activity. Note the characteristic sawtooth waves (seen prominently in channels 1, 2, 5, and 6 from the top) of REM sleep preceding bursts of REMs in the electro-oculograms (E1-M1; E2–M2). Chin EMG shows marked hypotonia, whereas TIB and GAST EMG channels show very low-amplitude phasic myoclonic bursts. See Figure 2–1 for description of the montage.

TABLE 2–4 Sleep Macrostructure

- Sleep states and stages
- Sleep cycles
- Sleep latency
- Sleep efficiency (the ratio of total sleep time to total time in bed expressed as a percentage)
- Wake after sleep onset

TABLE 2–5 Factors Modifying Sleep Macrostructure

- Exogenous
  - Noise
  - Exercise
  - Ambient temperature
  - Drugs and alcohol
- Endogenous
  - Age
  - Prior sleep-wakefulness
  - Circadian phase
  - Sleep pathologies

TABLE 2–6 Sleep Microstructure

- Arousals
- Cyclic alternating pattern
- Sleep spindles
- K complexes

responses. Sleep onset in the newborn occurs through REM sleep. During the first 3 months, sleep-onset REM begins to change. In the newborn, active sleep (REM) occurs 50% of the total sleep time. This decreases during the first 6 months of age. By 9 to 12 months, REM sleep occupies 30–35% of sleep, and by 5–6 years, REM sleep decreases to adult levels of 20–25%. The napping frequency continues to decline, and by age 4–6 years most children stop daytime naps. Nighttime sleep patterns become regular gradually and by age 6, nighttime sleep is consolidated with few awakenings.

Two other important changes occur in the sleep pattern in old age: repeated awakenings throughout the night, including early morning awakenings that prematurely terminate the night sleep, and a marked reduction of the amplitude of delta waves resulting in a decreased percentage of delta sleep (SWS) in this age group. The percentage of REM sleep in normal elderly individuals remains relatively constant, and the total duration of sleep time within 24 hours is also no different from that of young adults; however, elderly individuals often nap during the daytime, compensating for lost sleep during the night. Figure 2–9 shows schematically the evolution of sleep stage distribution in newborns, infants, children, adults and elderly adults. Night sleep histograms of children, young adults, and of elderly adults are shown in Figure 2–10.

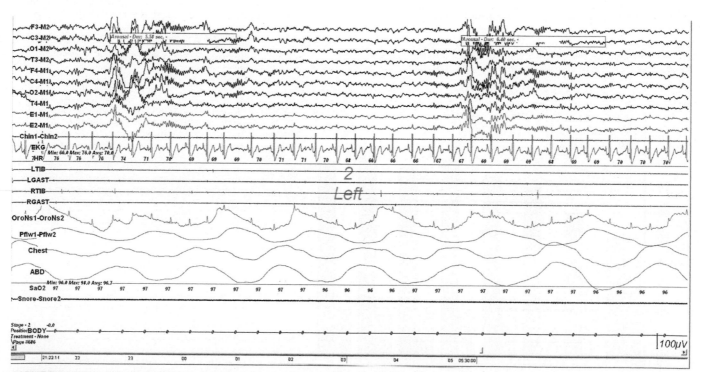

FIGURE 2–7 Polysomnographic recording shows two brief periods of arousals out of stage N2 sleep in the left- and right-hand segments of the recording, lasting for 5.58 and 6.40 seconds and separated by more than 10 seconds of sleep. Note delta waves followed by approximately 10-Hz alpha activities during brief arousals. For description of the montage, see Figure 2–1.

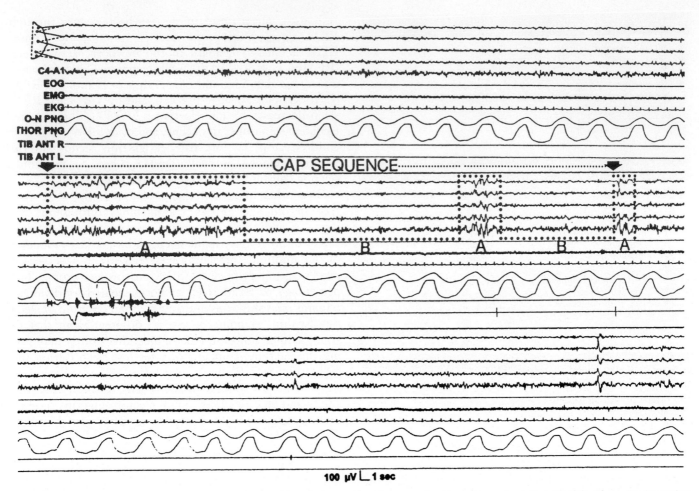

FIGURE 2–8 Polysomnographic recording showing consecutive stretches of non–cyclic alternating pattern (non-CAP) **(top),** cyclic alternating pattern (CAP) **(middle),** and non-CAP **(bottom).** The CAP sequence, confined between the two *black arrows,* shows three phase As and two phase Bs, which illustrate the minimal requirements for the definition of a CAP sequence (at least three phase As in succession). Electroencephalographic derivation (top 5 channels in top panel): FP2-F4, F4-C4, C4-P4, P4-02, and C4-A1. Similar electroencephalographic derivation is used for the middle and lower panels.*(From Terzano MG, Parrino L, Smeriari A, et al: Atlas, rules, and recording techniques for the scoring of cyclic alternating pattern [CAP] in human sleep. Sleep Med 2002;3:187.)*

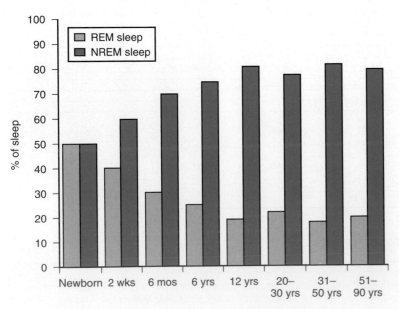

FIGURE 2–9 Graphic representation of percentages of REM and NREM sleep at different ages. Note the dramatic changes in REM sleep in the early years. *(Adapted from Roffwarg HP, Muzzio JN, Dement WC. Ontogenic development of the human sleep-dream cycle. Science 1966;152:604.)*

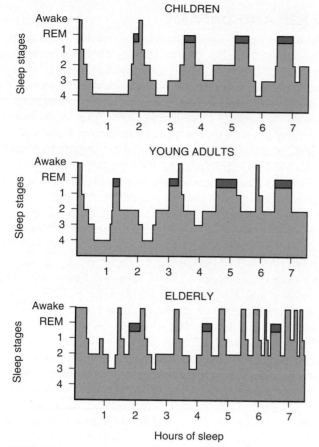

FIGURE 2–10 Night sleep histogram from a child, a young adult, and an elderly person. Note significant reduction of stage 4 NREM sleep as one grows older. *(From Kales A, Kales JD. Sleep disorders: recent findings in the diagnosis and treatment of disturbed sleep. N Engl J Med 1974;290:489.)*

There are significant evolutionary changes in the respiratory and cardiovascular functions.[42,44] Respiratory controllers are immature and not fully developed at birth. Respiratory mechanics and upper airway anatomy are different in newborns than in adults, contributing to breathing problems during sleep particularly in newborn infants. Brief periods of respiratory pauses or apneas lasting for 3 seconds or longer, periodic breathing, and irregular breathing may be noted in newborns, especially during active (REM) sleep. According to the National Institutes of Health Consensus Development Conference on infantile apnea,[45] the term *periodic breathing* refers to respiratory pauses of at least 3 seconds with less than 20 seconds of normal breathing in between the pauses. Cheyne-Stokes breathing is periodic waxing and waning of respiration accompanied by central apneas and may be noted in preterm infants. Periodic breathing and occasional central apneas of up to 15 seconds' duration in newborns may be noted without any clinical relevance unless accompanied by bradycardia or cyanosis. These

breathing events gradually disappear during the first few weeks of life. The respiratory rate also gradually slows during the first few years of life. Another important finding in the newborn, particularly during active sleep, is paradoxical inward motion of the rib cage. This occurs because of high compliance of the rib cage in newborns, a circular rather than elliptical thorax, and decreased tone of the intercostal and accessory muscles of respiration. This paradoxical breathing causes hypoxia and reduced diaphragmatic efficiency. Similar breathing in adults occurs during diaphragmatic weakness. At term the posterior cricoarytenoid muscles, which assist in maintaining upper airway patency, are not adequately coordinated with diaphragmatic activity, causing a few periods of obstructive apneas especially during active sleep. Ventilatory responses to hypoxia are also different in newborns than in adults. In quiet sleep, hypoxia stimulates breathing as in adults, but in active sleep, after the initial period of stimulation, there is ventilatory depression. Laryngeal stimulation in adults causes arousal, but in infants this may cause an apnea. Breathing becomes regular and respiratory control is adequately developed by the end of the first year.

Changes in cardiovascular function indicate changes in the autonomic nervous system during infancy and early childhood. There is greater parasympathetic control for children than infants, as assessed by heart rate low-frequency (LF) and high-frequency (HF) analysis: 0.15–0.5 Hz [HF] indicates parasympathetic and 0.04–0.15 Hz [LF] indicates sympathetic activity (see also Chapter 7). The better parasympathetic control for children than infants indicates autonomic nervous system maturity. Respiratory heart rate modulation is variable in newborns, as assessed by LF and HF heart rate spectral analysis. In active sleep, most of the power is in LF. In older infants and children, there is significant respiratory heart rate modulation, termed *normal sinus arrhythmia*. Respiratory rate during quiet sleep decreases and the respiratory variability decreases with age.

SLEEP HABITS

Sleep specialists sometimes divide people into two groups, "evening types" (owls) and "morning types" (larks). The morning types wake up early feeling rested and refreshed, and work efficiently in the morning. These people get tired and go to bed early in the evening. In contrast, evening types have difficulty getting up early and feel tired in the morning; they feel fresh and energetic toward the end of the day. These people perform best in the evening. They go to sleep late at night and wake up late in the morning. The body temperature rhythm takes on different curves in these two types of people. The body temperature reaches the evening peak an hour earlier in morning types than in evening types. What determines a morning or evening type is not known, but heredity may play a role. Katzenberg et al.,[46] using the 19-item Horne-Ostberg questionnaire to determine "morningness"/"eveningness" in human circadian rhythms, discovered a clock gene polymorphism associated with human diurnal preference. One of two human clock gene alleles (3111C) is associated with eveningness. These findings have been contradicted by later studies.[47]

Sleep requirement or sleep need is defined as the optimum amount of sleep required to remain alert and fully awake and to function adequately throughout the day. Sleep debt is defined as the difference between the ideal sleep requirement and the actual duration of sleep obtained. It has been traditionally stated that women need more sleep than men, but this has been questioned in a field study.[48] There is also a general perception based on questionnaire, actigraphy, and PSG studies that sleep duration decreases with increasing age.[49,50] This relationship, however, remains controversial. Older adults take naps, and these naps may compensate for nighttime sleep duration curtailment. Sleep is regulated by homeostasis (increasing sleep drive during continued wakefulness) and circadian factors (the sleep drive varying with time of the day). The influence of these factors is reduced in older adults but is still present. Older adults are also phase advanced (e.g., their internal clock is set earlier, yielding early bedtime and early morning awakenings).

Sleep requirement for an average adult is approximately 7.5–8 hours regardless of environmental or cultural differences.[51] Most probably whether a person is a long or a short sleeper and sleep need are determined by heredity rather than by different personality traits or other psychological factors. Social (e.g., occupational) or biological (e.g., illness) factors may also play a role. Sleep need is genetically determined, but its physiologic mechanism is unknown. Slow-wave activity (SWA) in a sleep EEG depends on sleep need and homeostatic drive. Adenosine, a purine nucleoside, seems to have a direct role in homeostasis. Prolonged wakefulness causes increased accumulation of adenosine, which decreases during sleep. SWA increases after sleep loss. Long sleepers spend more time asleep but have less SWS[52] and more stage 2 NREM sleep than do short sleepers.[53]

There is controversy whether a person can extend sleep beyond the average requirement. Early studies by Taub and Berger[54,55] showed that sleep extension beyond the average hours may cause exhaustion and irritability with detriment of sleep efficiency. The authors refer to this as the "Rip Van Winkle" effect.[55] Sleep extension studies in the past reported conflicting results regarding Multiple Sleep Latency Test scores, vigilance, and mood ratings.[56] When subjects are challenged to maximum sleep extension, there is substantial improvement in daytime alertness, reaction time, and mood.[56] Most individuals carry a large sleep debt and, as extra sleep reduces carryover sleep debt, it is then no longer possible to obtain extra sleep.[57]

SLEEP AND DREAMS

Sigmund Freud[58] called dreams the "Royal Road to the Unconscious" in his seminal book, *The Interpretation of Dreams*, published in 1900. The Freudian theory postulated that repressed feelings are psychologically suppressed or hidden in the unconscious mind and often manifested in dreams. Sometimes those feelings are expressed as mental disorders or other psychologically determined physical ailments, according to this psychoanalytic theory. In Freud's view, most of the repressed feelings are determined by repressed sexual desires and appear in dreams or symbols representing sexual organs. In recent times, Freudian theory has fallen in disrepute. Modern sleep scientists try to interpret dreams in anatomic and physiologic terms. Nevertheless, we still cannot precisely define what is "dream" and why we dream. The field of dream research took a new direction since the existence of REM sleep was first observed by Aserinsky and Kleitman[10] in 1953. It is postulated that approximately 80% of dreams occur during REM sleep and 20% occur during NREM sleep.[59] It is easier to recall REM dreams than NREM dreams. It is also easier to recall REM dreams if awakened immediately after the onset of dreams rather than trying to remember them the next morning upon getting out of bed. REM dreams are often vivid, highly emotionally charged, unrealistic, complex, and bizarre. In contrast, dream recall that sometimes may partially occur upon awakening from the NREM dream state is more realistic. People are generally oriented when awakening from REM sleep but are somewhat disoriented and confused when awakened from NREM sleep.

Dreams take place in natural color, rather than black and white. In our dreams, we employ all five senses. In general, we use mostly the visual sensations, followed by auditory sensation. Tactile, smell, and taste sensation are represented least. Dreams can be pleasant or unpleasant, frightening or sad. They generally reflect one's day-to-day activities. Fear, anxiety, and apprehension are incorporated into our dreams. In addition, stressful events of the past or present may occupy our dreams. The dream scenes or events are rarely rational, instead often occurring in an irrational manner with rapid change of scene, place, or people or a bizarre mixture of these elements. Sometimes, lucid dreams may arise in which the dreamer seems to realize vividly that he or she is actually dreaming.[60]

The neurobiologic significance of dreams remains unknown. Sleep scientists try to explain dreams in the terms of anatomic and physiologic interpretation of REM sleep. During this state, the synapses, nerve cells, and nerve fibers connecting various groups of nerve cells in the brain become activated. This activation begins in the brain stem and the cerebral hemisphere then synthesizes these signals and creates color or black-and-white images giving rise to dreams. Similarly, signals sometimes become converted into auditory, tactile, or other sensations to cause dream imagery. Why the nerve circuits are stimulated to cause dreaming is not clearly understood. Some suggestions to explain significance of dreams include activation of the neural networks in the brain,[61] and restructuring and reinterpretation of data stored in memory.[62] This resembles Jouvet's[63] hypothesis of a relationship between REM sleep and recently acquired information. According to molecular biologist and Nobel laureate Francis Crick and his colleague Graham Mitcheson,[64] the function of dreaming is to unlearn, that is, to remove unnecessary and useless information from the brain. Some have also suggested that memory consolidation takes place during the dream stage of sleep (see Chapter 9). In addition, stories abound regarding artists, writers, and scientists who develop innovative ideas about their art, literature, and scientific projects during dreams. Dream-enacting behavior associated with abnormal movement during sleep (REM sleep behavior disorder) and frightening dreams called nightmares or dream anxiety attacks constitute two important REM parasomnias.

PHYLOGENY OF SLEEP

Studies have been conducted to find out whether, like humans, other mammals have sleep stages.[1,65–68] The EEG recordings of mammals show similarities to those of humans. Both REM and NREM sleep stages can be differentiated by EEG, EMG, and EOG in animals. Dolphins and whales are the only groups of mammals showing no REM sleep on recordings.[1,69–72] Although initially thought to have no REM sleep,[73] some recent evidence suggests that Australian spiny anteaters (the monotremes, or egg-laying mammals; *echidna*) do have REM sleep.[74,75] Siegel and colleagues[75] suggest that the echidna combines REM and NREM aspects of sleep in a single sleep state. These authors further suggest that REM and NREM sleep evolved from a single, phylogenetically older sleep state.

Like humans, mammals can be short or long sleepers. There are considerable similarities between sleep length and length of sleep cycles in small and large animals. Small animals with a high metabolic rate have a shorter life span and sleep longer than larger animals with lower metabolic rates.[76] Smaller animals also have a shorter REM-NREM cycle than larger animals. The larger the animal, the less it sleeps; for example, elephants sleep 4–5 hours and giraffes sleep even less than that.

A striking finding in dolphins is that, during sleep, half the brain shows the characteristic EEG features of sleep while the other half shows the EEG features of waking.[77] Each sleep episode lasts approximately 30–60 minutes; then the roles of the two halves of the brain reverse. Similar unihemispheric sleep episodes with eye closure contralateral to the sleeping hemisphere are known to occur in the pilot whale and porpoise.[71,78,79]

Both vertebrates and invertebrates display sleep and wakefulness.[72] Most animals show the basic rest-activity rhythms during a 24-hour period. There is behavioral

and EEG evidence of sleep in birds, but the avian REM-NREM cycles are very short.[72,80] Although birds are thought to have evolved from reptiles, the question of the existence of REM sleep in reptiles remains somewhat controversial.[72] The absence of REM sleep in reptiles and the presence of NREM and REM sleep in both birds and mammals would be in favor of REM sleep being a more recent development in the phylogenetic history of land-dwelling organisms.[72] Sleep has also been noted in invertebrates, such as insects, scorpions, and worms, based on behavioral criteria.[72,81]

In conclusion, the purpose of studying the phylogeny of sleep is to understand the neurophysiologic and neuroanatomic correlates of sleep as one ascends the ladder of phylogeny from inframammalian to mammalian species. Tobler[78] concluded that sleep is homeostatically regulated, in a strikingly similar manner, in a broad range of mammalian species. These similarities in sleep and its regulation among mammals suggest common underlying mechanisms that have been preserved in the evolutionary process.

CIRCADIAN SLEEP-WAKE RHYTHM

The existence of circadian rhythms has been recognized since the 18th century, when the French astronomer de Mairan[82] noted a diurnal rhythm in heliotrope plants. The plants closed their leaves at sunset and opened them at sunrise, even when they were kept in darkness, shielded from direct sunlight. The discovery of a 24-hour rhythm in the movements of plant leaves suggested to de Mairan an "internal clock" in the plant. Experiments by chronobiologists Pittendrigh[83] and Aschoff[84] clearly proved the existence of 24-hour rhythms in animals.

The term *circadian rhythm*, coined by chronobiologist Halberg,[85] is derived from the Latin *circa*, which means *about*, and *dian*, which means *day*. Experimental isolation from all environmental time cues (in German, *Zeitgebers*), has clearly demonstrated the existence of a circadian rhythm in humans independent of environmental stimuli.[86,87] Earlier investigators suggested that the circadian cycle is closer to 25 hours than 24 hours of a day-night cycle[1,88,89]; however, recent research points to a cycle near 24 hours (approximately 24.2 hours).[90] Ordinarily, environmental cues of light and darkness synchronize or entrain the rhythms to the day-night cycle; however, the existence of environment-independent, autonomous rhythm suggests that the human body also has an internal biological clock.[1,86–89]

The experiments in rats in 1972 by Stephan and Zucker[91] and Moore and Eichler[92] clearly identified the site of the biological clock, located in the suprachiasmatic nucleus (SCN) in the hypothalamus, above the optic chiasm. Experimental stimulation, ablation, and lesion of these neurons altered circadian rhythms. The existence of the SCN in humans was confirmed by Lydic and colleagues.[93] There has been clear demonstration of the neuroanatomic connection between the retina and the SCN—the retinohypothalamic pathway[94]—that sends the environmental cues of light to the SCN. The SCN serves as a pacemaker, and the neurons in the SCN are responsible for generating the circadian rhythms.[87,95–98] The master circadian clock in the SCN receives afferent information from the retinohypothalamic tract, which sends signals to multiple synaptic pathways in other parts of the hypothalamus, plus the superior cervical ganglion and pineal gland, where melatonin is released. The SCN contains melatonin receptors, so there is a feedback loop from the pineal gland to the SCN. Several neurotransmitters have been located within terminals of the SCN afferents and interneurons, including serotonin, neuropeptide Y, vasopressin, vasoactive intestinal peptide, and γ-aminobutyric acid.[87,97,99]

Time isolation experiments have clearly shown the presence of daily rhythms in many physiologic processes, such as the sleep-wake cycle, body temperature, and neuroendocrine secretion. Body temperature rhythm is sinusoidal, and cortisol and growth hormone secretion rhythms are pulsatile. It is well known that plasma levels of prolactin, growth hormone, and testosterone are all increased during sleep at night (see Chapter 7). Melatonin, the hormone synthesized by the pineal gland (see Chapter 7), is secreted maximally during night and may be an important modulator of human circadian rhythm entrainment by the light-dark cycle. Sleep decreases body temperature, whereas activity and wakefulness increase it. It should be noted that internal desynchronization occurs during free-running experiments, and the rhythm of body temperature dissociates from the sleep rhythm as a result of that desynchronization.[1,87–89] This raises the question of whether there is more than one circadian (or internal) clock or circadian oscillator.[1] The existence of two oscillators was postulated by Kronauer and colleagues.[100] They suggested that a 25-hour rhythm exists for temperature, cortisol, and REM sleep, and that the second oscillator is somewhat labile and consists of the sleep-wake rhythm. Some authors, however, have suggested that one oscillator could explain both phenomena.[101] Recent development in circadian rhythm research has clearly shown the existence of multiple circadian oscillators functioning independently from the SCN.[102–104]

The molecular basis of the mammalian circadian clock has been the focus of much recent circadian rhythm research[105–108] (see Chapter 8). The paired SCN are controlled by a total of at least 7 genes (e.g., *Clock, Bmal, Per, Cyc, Frq, Cry, Tim*) and their protein products and regulatory enzymes (e.g., casein kinase 1 epsilon and casein kinase 1 delta). By employing a "forward genetics" approach, remarkable progress has been made in a few years in identifying key components of the circadian clock in both the fruit flies (*Drosophila*), bread molds (*Neurospora*), and mammals.[106–108] It has been established that the circadian clock gene of the sleep-wake cycle is independent of the circadian rhythm functions. There is clear

anatomic and physiologic evidence to suggest a close interaction between the SCN and the regions regulating sleep-wake states[109,110] (see also Chapter 8). There are projections from the SCN to wake-promoting hypocretin (orexin) neurons (indirectly via the dorsomedial hypothalamus) and locus ceruleus as well as to sleep-promoting neurons in ventrolateral preoptic neurons. Physiologic evidence of increased firing rates in single-neuron recordings from the appropriate regions during wakefulness or REM sleep, and decreased neuronal firing rates during NREM sleep, complement anatomic evidence of such interaction between the SCN and sleep-wake regulating systems.[110,111] Based on the studies in mice (e.g., knockout mice lacking core clock genes and mice with mutant clock genes), it has also been suggested that circadian clock genes may affect sleep regulation and sleep homeostasis independent of circadian rhythm generation.[112]

Molecular mechanisms applying gene sequencing techniques have been found to play a critical role in uncovering the importance of clock genes, at least in two human circadian rhythm sleep disorders. Mutation of the *hPer2* gene (a human homolog of the *period* gene in *Drosophila*) causing advancing of the clock (alteration of the circadian timing of sleep propensity), and polymorphism in some familial cases of advanced sleep phase state[113–115] and polymorphism in *hPer3* genes in some subjects with delayed sleep phase state,[116,117] suggest genetic control of the circadian timing of the sleep-wake rhythm. Kolker et al.[118] have shown reduced 24-hour expression of *Bmal1* and clock genes in the SCN of old golden hamsters, pointing to a possible role for the molecular mechanism in understanding age-related changes in the circadian clock. In a subsequent report, the same authors[119] found that age-related changes in circadian rhythmicity occur equally in wild-type and heterozygous clock mutant mice, indicating that the clock mutation does not make mice more susceptible to the effects of age on the circadian pacemakers. Kondratov et al.[120] reported that mice deficient in the circadian transcription factor BMAL1 have reduced life span and display a phenotype of premature aging. These findings have been corroborated by later observations that clock mutant mice respond to low-dose irradiation by accelerating their aging program, and develop phenotypes that are reminiscent of those in BMAL1-deficient mice.[121] It is important to be aware of circadian rhythms, because several other sleep disturbances are related to alteration in them, such as those associated with shift work and jet lag.

CHRONOBIOLOGY, CHRONOPHARMACOLOGY, AND CHRONOTHERAPY

Sleep specialists are becoming aware of the importance of chronobiology, chronopharmacology, and chronotherapy.[122–128] *Chronobiology* refers to the study of the body's biological responses to time-related events. All biological functions of the cells, organs, and the entire body have circadian (~24 hours), ultradian (<24 hours), or infradian (>24 hours) rhythms. It is important, therefore, to understand how the body responds to treatment at different times throughout the circadian cycle, and that circadian timing may alter the pathophysiologic responses in various disease states (e.g., exacerbation of bronchial asthma at night and a high incidence of stroke late at night and myocardial infarction early in the morning; see Chapter 33).

Biological responses to medications may also depend on the circadian timing of administration of the drugs. Potential differences of responses of antibiotics to bacteria, or of cancer cells to chemotherapy or radiotherapy, depending on the time of administration, illustrate the importance of *chronopharmacology*, which refers to pharmacokinetic or pharacodynamic interactions in relation to the timing of the day.

Circadian rhythms can be manipulated to treat certain disorders, a technique called *chronotherapy*. Examples of this are phase advance or phase delay of sleep rhythms and application of bright light at certain periods of the evening and morning.

CYTOKINES, IMMUNE SYSTEM, AND SLEEP FACTORS

Cytokines are proteins produced by leukocytes and other cells functioning as intercellular mediators that may play an important role in immune and sleep regulation.[129–137] Several cytokines such as interleukin (IL), interferon-α, and tumor necrosis factor-α (TNF-α) have been shown to promote sleep. There are other sleep-promoting substances called sleep factors that increase in concentration during prolonged wakefulness or during infection and enhance sleep. These other factors include delta sleep–inducing peptides, muramyl peptides, cholecystokinin, arginine vasotocin, vasoactive intestinal peptide, growth hormone–releasing hormone, somatostatin, prostaglandin D_2, nitric oxide, and adenosine. The role of these various sleep factors in maintaining homeostasis has not been clearly established.[129] It has been shown that adenosine in the basal forebrain can fulfill the major criteria for the neural sleep factor that mediates these somnogenic effects of prolonged wakefulness by acting through A1 and A2a receptors.[138,139]

The cytokines play a role in the cellular and immune changes noted during sleep deprivation.[129,130,140–144] The precise nature of the immune response after sleep deprivation has, however, remained controversial, and the results of studies on the subject have been inconsistent. These inconsistencies may reflect different stress reactions of subjects and different circadian factors (e.g., timing of drawing of blood for estimation of plasma levels).[129,140,145]

Infection (bacterial, viral, and fungal) enhances NREM sleep but suppresses REM sleep. It has been postulated that sleep acts as a host defense against infection and facilitates the healing process.[129,140,144,146–149] It is also believed

that sleep deprivation may increase vulnerability to infection.[150] The results of experiments with animals suggest that sleep deprivation alters immune function.[140,141,146]

There is evidence that cytokines play an important role in the pathogenesis of excessive daytime sleepiness in a variety of sleep disorders and in sleep deprivation.[151] Sleep deprivation causing excessive sleepiness has been associated with increased production of the proinflammatory cytokines IL-6 and TNF-α.[152–154] Viral or bacterial infections causing excessive somnolence and increased NREM sleep are associated with increased production of TNF-α and IL-1β.[155–157] In other inflammatory disorders such as human immunodeficiency virus infection and rheumatoid arthritis, increased sleepiness and disturbed sleep are associated with an increased amount of circulating TNF-α.[158–161] Several authors suggested that excessive sleepiness in OSAS, narcolepsy, insomnia, or idiopathic hypersomnia may be mediated by cytokines such as IL-6 and TNF-α.[162–168] In a review, Kapsimalis et al.[151] concluded that cytokines are mediators of sleepiness and are implicated in the pathogenesis of symptoms of OSAS, narcolepsy, sleep deprivation, and insomnia, and indirectly play an important role in the pathogenesis of the cardiovascular complications of OSAS.

THEORIES OF THE FUNCTION OF SLEEP

The function of sleep remains the greatest biological mystery of all time. Several theories of the function of sleep have been proposed (Table 2–7), but none of them is satisfactory to explain the exact biological functions of sleep. Sleep deprivation experiments in animals have clearly shown that sleep is necessary for survival, but from a practical point of view complete sleep deprivation for a prolonged period cannot be conducted in humans. Sleep deprivation studies in humans have shown an impairment of performance that demonstrates the need for sleep (see Chapter 3). The performance impairment of prolonged sleep deprivation results from a decreased motivation and frequent "microsleep." Overall, human sleep deprivation experiments have proven that sleep deprivation causes sleepiness and impairment of performance, vigilance, attention, concentration, and memory. Sleep deprivation may also cause some metabolic, hormonal, and immunologic affects. Sleep deprivation causes immune suppression, and even partial sleep deprivation reduces cellular immune responses. Studies by Van Cauter's group[169,170] include a clearly documented elevation of

TABLE 2–7 Theories of Sleep Function
• Restorative theory
• Energy conservation theory
• Adaptive theory
• Instinctive theory
• Memory consolidation and reinforcement theory
• Synaptic and neuronal network integrity theory
• Thermoregulatory function theory

cortisol level following even partial sleep loss, suggesting an alteration in hypothalmic-pituitary-adrenal axis function. This has been confirmed in chronic sleep deprivation, which causes impairment of glucose tolerance. Glucose intolerance may contribute to memory impairment as a result of decreased hippocampal function. Chronic sleep deprivation may also cause a detriment of thyrotropin concentration, increased evening cortisol level, and sympathetic hyperactivity, which may serve as risk factors for obesity, hypertension, and diabetes mellitus. It should be noted, however, that in all of these sleep deprivation experiments stress has been a confounding factor, raising a question about whether all these undesirable consequences relate to sleep loss only or a combination of stress and sleeplessness.

Restorative Theory

Proponents of the restorative theory ascribe body tissue restoration to NREM sleep and brain tissue restoration to REM sleep.[171–174] The findings of increased secretion of anabolic hormones[175–177] (e.g., growth hormone, prolactin, testosterone, luteinizing hormone) and decreased levels of catabolic hormones[178] (e.g., cortisol) during sleep, along with the subjective feeling of being refreshed after sleep, may support such a contention. Increased SWS after sleep deprivation[2] further supports the role of NREM sleep as restorative. The critical role of REM sleep for the development of the CNS of young organisms is cited as evidence of restoration of brain functions by REM sleep.[179] Several studies of brain basal metabolism suggest an enhanced synthesis of macromolecules such as nucleic acids and proteins in the brain during sleep,[180] but the data remain scarce and controversial. Protein synthesis in the brain is increased during SWS.[181] Confirmation of such cerebral anabolic processes would provide an outstanding argument in favor of the restorative theory of sleep. Work in animals suggests formation of new neurons during sleep in adult animals, and this neurogenesis in the dentate gyrus may be blocked after total sleep deprivation.[182]

Energy Conservation Theory

Zepelin and Rechtschaffen[183] found that animals with a high metabolic rate sleep longer than those with a slower metabolism, suggesting that energy is conserved during sleep. There is an inverse relationship between body mass and metabolic rate. Small animals (e.g., rats, opossums) with high metabolic rates sleep for 18 hr/day, whereas large animals (e.g., elephants, giraffes) with low metabolic rates sleep only for 3–4 hours. It has been suggested that high metabolic rates cause increased oxidative stress and injury to self. It has been hypothesized[184] that higher metabolic rates in the brain require longer sleep time to counteract the cell damage by free radicals and facilitate synthesis of molecules protecting brain cells from this oxidative stress. During NREM sleep, brain energy metabolism and cerebral blood flow decrease, whereas during REM sleep, the level of metabolism is similar to that of wakefulness and the cerebral blood flow increases. Although these findings might suggest that NREM sleep helps conserve energy, the fact that only 120 calories are conserved in 8 hours of sleep makes the energy conservation theory less than satisfactory. Considering that humans spend one third of their lives sleeping,[185] one would expect far more calories to be conserved during an 8-hour period if energy conservation were the function of sleep.

Adaptive Theory

In both animals and humans, sleep is an adaptive behavior that allows the creature to survive under a variety of environmental conditions.[186,187]

Instinctive Theory

The instinctive theory views sleep as an instinct,[171,188] which relates to the theory of adaptation and energy conservation.

Memory Consolidation and Reinforcement Theory

The sleep memory consolidation hypothesis is a hotly debated issue, with both proponents and opponents, and the proponents outnumber the opponents. In fact, McGaugh and colleagues[189] suggested that sleep- and waking-related fluctuations of hormones and neurotransmitters may modulate memory processes. Crick and Mitchison[64] earlier suggested that REM sleep removes undesirable data from the memory. In a later report, these authors hypothesized that the facts that REM deprivation produces a large rebound and that REM sleep occurs in almost all mammals make it probable that REM sleep has some important biological function.[190]

The theory that memory reinforcement and consolidation take place during REM sleep has been strengthened by scientific data provided by Karni and colleagues.[191] These authors conducted selective REM and SWS deprivation in six young adults. They found that perceptual learning during REM deprivation was significantly less compared with perceptual learning during SWS deprivation. In addition, SWS deprivation had a significant detrimental effect on a task that was already learned. These data suggest that REM deprivation affected the consolidation of the recent perceptual experience, thus supporting the theory of long-term consolidation during REM sleep. Studies by Stickgold and Walker[192,193] strongly supported the theory of sleep memory consolidation (see Chapter 9). There is further suggestion by Hu and colleagues[194] that the facilitation of memory for emotionally salient information may preferentially develop during sleep. Stickgold's group concluded that unique neurobiologic processes within sleep actively promote declarative memories.[195] Several studies in the past decade have provided evidence to support the role of sleep in sleep-dependent memory processing, which includes memory encoding, memory consolidation and reconsolidation, and brain plasticity (see review by Kalia[196]). Hornung et al.,[197] using a paired-associative word list to test declarative memory and mirror tracking tasks to test procedural learning in 107 healthy older adults ages 60–82 years, concluded that REM sleep plays a role in procedural memory consolidation. Walker's group concluded after sleep deprivation experiments that sleep before learning is critical for human memory consolidation.[198] Born et al.[199] concluded that hippocampus-dependent memories (declarative memories) benefit primarily from SWS. They further suggested that the different patterns of neurotransmitters and neurohormone secretion between sleep stages may be responsible for this function. Backhaus and Junghanns[200] randomly assigned 34 young healthy subjects to a nap or wake condition of about 45 minutes in the early afternoon after learning procedural and declarative memory tasks. They noted that naps significantly improved procedural but not declarative memory and therefore a short nap is favorable for consolidation of procedural memory. Goder et al.[201] tested the role of different aspects of sleep for memory performance in 42 consecutive patients with nonrestorative sleep. They used the Rey-Osterrieth Complex Figure Design test and the paired-associative word list for declarative memory function and mirror tracking tasks for procedural learning assessment. The results supported the contention that visual declarative memory performance is significantly associated with total sleep time, sleep efficiency, duration of NREM sleep, and the number of NREM-REM sleep cycles but not with specific measures of REM sleep or SWS.

In contrast to all of these studies, Vertes and Siegel[202–205] took the opposing position, contending that REM sleep is not involved in memory consolidation—or at least not in humans—citing several lines of evidence. They cited the work of Smith and Rose[206,207] that REM sleep is not involved with memory consolidation. Schabus et al.[208] agreed that declarative material learning is not affected by sleep. In their study, subjects showed no difference in the percentage of word pairs correctly recalled before and after 8 hours of sleep. The strongest evidence cited by Vertes and Siegel[202] includes examples of individuals with brain stem lesions with elimination of REM sleep[209] or those on antidepressant medications suppressing REM sleep, who exhibit no apparent cognitive deficits. Vertes and Siegel[202] concluded that REM sleep is not involved in declarative memory and is not critical for cognitive processing in sleep.

Whether NREM sleep is important for declarative memories also remains somewhat contentious.

Synaptic and Neuronal Network Integrity Theory

There is a new theory emerging that suggests the primary function of sleep is the maintenance of synaptic and neuronal network integrity.[129,185,210–212] According to this theory, sleep is important for the maintenance of synapses that have been insufficiently stimulated during wakefulness. Intermittent stimulation of the neural network is necessary to preserve CNS function. This theory further suggests that NREM and REM sleep serve the same function of synaptic reorganization.[210] This emerging concept of the "dynamic stabilization" (i.e., repetitive activations of brain synapses and neural circuitry) theory of sleep suggests that REM sleep maintains motor circuits, whereas NREM sleep maintains nonmotor activities.[210–212] Gene expression studies[213] using the DNA microarray technique identified sleep- and wakefulness-related genes (brain transcripts) subserving different functions (e.g., energy metabolism, synaptic excitation, long-term potentiation and response to cellular stress during wakefulness; and protein synthesis, memory consolidation, and synaptic downscaling during sleep).

Thermoregulatory Function Theory

The thermoregulatory function theory is based on the observation that thermoregulatory homeostasis is maintained during sleep, whereas severe thermoregulatory abnormalities follow total sleep deprivation.[214] The preoptic anterior hypothalamic neurons participate in thermoregulation and NREM sleep. These two processes are closely linked by preoptic anterior hypothalamic neurons but are clearly separate. Thermoregulation is maintained during NREM sleep but suspended during REM sleep. Thermoregulatory responses such as shivering, piloerection, panting, and sweating are impaired during REM sleep. There is a loss of thermosensitivity in the preoptic anterior hypothalamic neurons during REM sleep.

REFERENCES

A full list of references are available at www.expertconsult.com

CHAPTER 3

Sleep Deprivation and Sleepiness

Sudhansu Chokroverty

CIRCADIAN RHYTHM AND HOMEOSTASIS

Sleep and wakefulness are controlled by both homeostatic and circadian factors.[1] The duration of prior wakefulness determines the propensity to sleepiness (homeostatic factor),[2] whereas circadian factors[3] determine the timing, duration and characteristics of sleep. There are two types of sleepiness: physiologic and subjective.[4] Physiologic sleepiness is the body's propensity to sleepiness. There are two highly vulnerable periods of sleepiness: 2:00–6:00 AM (particularly 3:00–5:00 AM) and 2:00–6:00 PM (especially 3:00–5:00 PM). The propensity to physiologic sleepiness (e.g., midafternoon and early morning hours) depends on circadian and homeostatic factors.[5] The highest number of sleep-related accidents has been observed during these periods. Subjective sleepiness is the individual's perception of sleepiness; it depends on several external factors, such as a stimulating environment and ingestion of coffee and other caffeinated beverages. Homeostasis refers to a prior period of wakefulness and sleep debt. After a prolonged period of wakefulness, there is an increasing tendency to sleep. The recovery from sleep debt is aided by an additional amount of sleep, but this recovery is not linear. Thus an exact number of hours of sleep are not needed to repay a sleep debt; rather, the body needs an adequate amount of slow-wave sleep (SWS) for restoration. The circadian factor determines the body's propensity to maximal sleepiness (e.g., between 3:00 and 5:00 AM). The second period of maximal sleepiness (3:00–5:00 PM) is not as strong as the first. Sleep/wakefulness and the circadian pacemaker have a reciprocal relationship; the biological clock can affect sleep and wakefulness, and sleep and wakefulness can affect the clock. The neurologic basis of this interaction is, however, unknown. In this chapter, I briefly review experimental sleep deprivation, the population at risk of sleep deprivation, and the causes and consequences of excessive sleepiness.

SLEEP DEPRIVATION AND SLEEPINESS

Many Americans (e.g., doctors, nurses, firefighters, interstate truck drivers, police officers, overnight train drivers and engineers) work irregular sleep-wake schedules and alternating shifts, making them chronically sleep deprived.[6,7] A survey study[6] found that, compared with the population at the turn of the century (1910–1911), American adolescents ages 8–17 years in 1963 were sleeping 1.5 hours less per 24-hour period. This does not mean we need less sleep today but that people are sleep deprived. It should be noted, however, that there may be a sampling error in these surveys (e.g., approximately 2000 people were surveyed in 1910–1911, vs. 311 in the later survey). A study by Bliwise and associates[8] in healthy adults ages 50–65 years showed a reduction of about 1 hour of sleep per 24 hours between 1959 and 1980 surveys. Factors that have been suggested to be responsible for this reduction of total sleep include environmental and cultural changes, such as increased environmental light, increased industrialization, growing numbers of people doing shift work, and the advent of television and radio. A review of the epidemiologic study by Partinen[9] estimated a prevalence of excessive sleepiness in Westerners at 5–36% of the total population. In contrast, Harrison and Horne[10] argued that most people are not chronically sleep deprived but simply choose not to sleep as much as they could.

What are the consequences of sleep deprivation? This question has been explored in studies of total, partial, and selective sleep deprivation (e.g., SWS or rapid eye movement [REM] sleep deprivation). These studies have conclusively proved that sleep deprivation causes sleepiness; decrement of performance, vigilance, attention, and concentration; and increased reaction time. The performance decrement resulting from sleep deprivation may be related to periods of microsleep. *Microsleep* is defined as transient physiologic sleep (i.e., 3- to 14-second electroencephalographic patterns change from those of wakefulness to those of stage I non–rapid eye movement [NREM] sleep) with or without rolling eye movements and behavioral sleep (e.g., drooping or heaviness of the eyelids, slight sagging and nodding of the head).

The most common cause of excessive daytime sleepiness (EDS) today is sleep deprivation. In the survey by Partinen,[9] up to one-third of young adults have EDS secondary to chronic partial sleep deprivation, and approximately 7% of middle-aged individuals have EDS secondary to sleep disorders and 2% secondary to shift work. Sleep deprivation poses danger to the individuals experiencing it as well as to others, making people prone to accidents in the work place, particularly in industrial and transportation work. The incidence of automobile crashes increases with driver fatigue and sleepiness. Fatigue resulting from sleep deprivation may have been responsible for many major national and international catastrophes.[11]

SLEEP DEPRIVATION EXPERIMENTS

Although neither humans nor animals can do without sleep, the amount of sleep necessary to individual people or species varies widely. We know that a lack of sleep leads to sleepiness, but we do not know the exact functions of sleep. Sleep deprivation experiments in animals have clearly shown that sleep is necessary for survival. The experiments of Rechtschaffen and colleagues[12] with rats using the carousel device have provided evidence for the necessity of sleep. All rats deprived of sleep for 10–30 days died after having lost weight, despite increases in their food intake. The rats also lost temperature control. Rats deprived only of REM sleep lived longer. Complete sleep deprivation experiments for prolonged periods (weeks to months) cannot be conducted in humans for obvious ethical reasons.

Total Sleep Deprivation

One of the early sleep deprivation experiments in humans was conducted in 1896 by Patrick and Gilbert,[13] who studied the effects of a 90-hour period of sleep deprivation on three healthy young men. One reported sensory illusions, which disappeared completely when, at the end of the experiment, he was allowed to sleep

for 10 hours. All subjects had difficulty staying awake, but felt totally fresh and rested after they were allowed to sleep.

A spectacular experiment in the last century was conducted in 1965. A 17-year-old California college student named Randy Gardner tried to set a new world record for staying awake. Dement[14] observed him during the later part of the experiment. Gardner stayed awake for 264 hours and 12 minutes, then slept for 14 hours and 40 minutes. He was recovered fully when he awoke. The conclusion drawn from the experiment is that it is possible to deprive people of sleep for a prolonged period without causing serious mental impairment. An important observation is the loss of performance with long sleep deprivation, which is due to loss of motivation and the frequent occurrence of microsleep.

In another experiment, Johnson and MacLeod[15] showed that it is possible to intentionally reduce total sleeping time by 1–2 hours without suffering any adverse effects. The experiments by Carskadon and Dement[16,17] showed that sleep deprivation increases the tendency to sleep during the day. This has been conclusively proved using the Multiple Sleep Latency Test with subjects.[17,18]

During the recovery sleep period after sleep deprivation, the percentage of SWS (stages 3 and 4 NREM sleep using Rechtschaffen-Kales scoring criteria) increases considerably. Similarly, after a long period of sleep deprivation, the REM sleep percentage increases during recovery sleep. (This increase has not been demonstrated after a short period of sleep deprivation, that is, up to 4 days.) These experiments suggest that different mechanisms regulate NREM and REM sleep.[19]

Partial Sleep Deprivation

Measurements of mood and performance after partial sleep deprivation (e.g., restricting sleep to 4.5–5.5 hours for 2–3 months) showed only minimal deficits in performance, which may have been related to decreased motivation. Thus, both total and partial sleep deprivation produce deleterious effects in humans.[20–22]

Selective REM Sleep Deprivation

Dement[23] performed REM sleep deprivation experiments (by awakening the subject for 5 minutes at the moment the polysomnographic recording demonstrated onset of REM sleep). Polysomnography results showed increased REM pressure (i.e., earlier and more frequent onset of REM sleep during successive nights) and REM rebound (i.e., quantitative increase of REM percentage during recovery nights). These findings were subsequently replicated by Borbely[19] and others,[24,25] but Dement's third observation—a psychotic reaction following REM deprivation—could not be replicated in subsequent investigations.[24]

Stage 4 Sleep Deprivation

Agnew and colleagues[26] reported that, after stage 4 NREM sleep deprivation for 2 consecutive nights, there was an increase in stage 4 sleep during the recovery night. Two important points were raised by this group's later experiments: (1) REM rebound was more significant than stage 4 rebound during recovery nights, and (2) it was more difficult to deprive a person of stage 4 sleep than of REM sleep.[25]

Summary

The effects of total sleep deprivation, as well as of REM sleep deprivation, are similar in animals and humans, suggesting that the sleep stages and the fundamental regulatory mechanisms for controlling sleep are the same in all mammals. These experiments have proven conclusively that sleep deprivation causes sleepiness and impairment of performance, vigilance, attention, and concentration. Many other later human studies involving sleep restriction and sleep deprivation confirmed these observations and concluded that sleep deprivation and restriction cause serious consequences involving many body systems as well as affecting short- and long-term memories.

CONSEQUENCES OF EDS RESULTING FROM SLEEP DEPRIVATION OR SLEEP RESTRICTION

EDS adversely affects performance and productivity at work and school, higher cerebral functions, and quality of life and social interactions, and increases morbidity and mortality.[27–29]

Performance and Productivity at Work or School

Impaired performance and reduced productivity at work for shift workers, reduced performance in class for school and college students, and impaired job performance in patients with narcolepsy, sleep apnea, circadian rhythm disorders, and chronic insomnia are well-known adverse effects of sleep deprivation and sleepiness. Sleepiness and associated morbidity are worse in night-shift workers, older workers, and female shift workers.

Higher Cerebral Functions

Sleepiness interferes with higher cerebral functions, causing impairment of short-term memory, concentration, attention, cognition, and intellectual performance. Psychometric tests[4] have documented increased reaction time in patients with excessive sleepiness. These individuals make increasing numbers of errors, and they need increasing time to reach the target in reaction time tests.[4] Sleepiness can also impair perceptual skills and new learning. Insufficient sleep and excessive sleepiness may cause irritability, anxiety, and depression. There is a U-shaped relationship between sleep duration and depression similar to that between sleep duration and mortality. Both short (<6 hours) and long (>8 hours) sleep duration are associated with depression. Learning disabilities and cognitive impairment with impaired vigilance also have been described.[27]

Quality of Life and Social Interaction

People complaining of EDS are often under severe psychological stress. They are often lonely, and perceived as dull, lazy, and downright stupid. Excessive sleepiness may cause severe marital and social problems. Narcoleptics with EDS often have serious difficulty with interpersonal relationships as well as impaired health-related quality of life, and are misunderstood because of the symptoms.[30] Shift workers constitute approximately 20–25% of the workforce in America (i.e., approximately 20 million). The majority of them have difficulty with sleeping, and sleepiness as a result of insufficient sleep and circadian dysrhythmia. Many of them have an impaired quality of life, marital discord, and gastrointestinal problems.

Increased Morbidity and Mortality

Short-Term Consequences

Persistent daytime sleepiness causes individuals to have an increased likelihood of accidents. A study by the U.S. National Transportation Safety Board (NTSB) found that the most probable cause of fatal truck accidents was sleepiness-related fatigue.[31] In another study by the NTSB,[32] 58% of the heavy-truck accidents were fatigue related and 18% of the drivers admitted having fallen asleep at the wheel. The NTSB also reported sleepiness- and fatigue-related motor coach[33,34] and railroad[35] accidents. New York State police estimated that 30% of all fatal crashes along the New York throughway occurred because the driver fell asleep at the wheel. Approximately 1 million crashes annually (one-sixth of all crashes) are thought to be produced by driver inattention or lapses.[35a,35b] Sleep deprivation and fatigue make such lapses more likely to occur. Truck drivers are especially susceptible to fatigue-related crashes.[31,32,36–39] Many truckers drive during the night while they are the sleepiest. Truckers may also have a high prevalence of sleep apnea.[40] The U.S. Department of Transportation estimated that 200,000 automobile accidents each year may be related to sleepiness. Nearly one-third of all trucking accidents that are fatal to the driver are related to sleepiness and fatigue.[40a] A general population study done by Hays et al.[41] involving 3962 elderly individuals reported an increased mortality risk of 1.73 in those with EDS, defined by napping most of the time. The presence of sleep disorders (see *Primary Sleep Disorders Associated with EDS* later in this chapter) increases the risk of crashes. Individuals with untreated insomnia, sleep apnea, or narcolepsy and shift workers—all of whom may suffer from excessive sleepiness—have more automobile crashes than other drivers.[42]

A telephone survey[43] of a random sample of New York State licensed drivers by the State University of New York found that 54.6% of the drivers had driven while drowsy within the past year, 1.9% had crashed while drowsy, and 2.8% had crashed when they fell asleep. Young male drivers are especially susceptible to crashes caused by falling asleep, as documented in a study in North Carolina[44] in 1990, 1991, and 1992 (e.g., in 55% of the 4333 crashes, the drivers were predominantly male and 25 years of age or younger). Surveys in Europe also noted an association between crashes and long-distance automobile and truck driving.[38,45–48] A 1991 Gallup organization[49] national survey found that individuals with chronic insomnia reported 2.5 times as many fatigue-related automobile accidents as did those without insomnia. The same 1991 Gallup survey found serious morbidity associated with untreated sleep complaints, as well as impaired ability to concentrate and accomplish daily tasks, and impaired memory and interpersonal discourse. In an October 1999 Gallup Poll,[50] 52% of all adults surveyed said that, in the past year, they had driven a car or other vehicle while feeling drowsy, 31% of adults admitted dozing off while at the wheel of a car or other vehicle, and 4% reported having had an automobile accident because of tiredness during driving. A number of national and international catastrophes[11] involving industrial operations, nuclear power plants, and all modes of transportation have been related to sleepiness and fatigue, including the Exxon Valdez oil spill in Alaska; the nuclear disaster at Chernobyl in the former Soviet Union; the near-nuclear disaster at 3-Mile Island in Pennsylvania; the gas leak disaster in Bhopal, India, resulting in 25,000 deaths; and the Challenger space shuttle disaster in 1987.

Long-Term Consequences

In addition to these short-term consequences, sleep deprivation or restriction causes a variety of long-term adverse consequences affecting several body systems and thus increasing the morbidity and mortality.[51]

Sleep Deprivation and Obesity

The prevalence of obesity in adults in the United States was 15% in 1970 and increased to 31% in 2001.[52] In children, the figures for obesity were 5% in 1970 and went up to 15% in 2001. In the Zurich study,[53] 496 Swiss adults followed for 13 years showed a body mass index (BMI) of 21.8 at age 27 that increased to 23.3 at the age of 40, with concurrent decrease in sleep duration from 7.7 to 7.3 hours in women and 7.1 to 6.9 hours in men. This longitudinal study confirms the cross-sectional studies in adults[54] and children.[55] In the Wisconsin sleep cohort study[56] (a population-based longitudinal study) using 1024 volunteers, short sleep was associated with reduced leptin and elevated ghrelin contributing to increased appetite, causing increased BMI. Obesity following chronic sleep restriction was also confirmed by Guilleminault et al.[57] in preliminary observations. Short sleep duration (<7 hours) is associated with obesity defined as a BMI of 30 or more.[58]

Sleep Duration and Hypothalamo-pituitary Hormones

Elevated evening cortisol levels, reduced glucose tolerance, and altered growth hormone secretion after experimental acute sleep restriction by Spiegel et al.[59,60] suggest that participation of the hypothalamic-pituitary axis may contribute toward obesity after sleep deprivation by leading to increased hunger and appetite. There is epidemiologic evidence of reduced sleep duration associated with reduced leptin (a hormone in adipocytes stimulating the satiety center in the hypothalamus), increased ghrelin (an appetite stimulant gastric peptide), and increased BMI.[58,61–63] Spiegel et al.,[59] in studies using sleep restriction (4 hours per night for 6 nights) and sleep extension (12 hours per night for 6 nights) experiments in healthy young adults, found increased evening cortisol, increased sympathetic activation, decreased thyrotropin activity, and reduced glucose tolerance in the sleep-restricted group. Rogers et al.[64] found similar elevation of evening cortisol levels following chronic sleep restriction. In recurrent partial sleep restriction studies in young adults, the following endocrine and metabolic alterations have been documented[65]: (1) decreased glucose tolerance and insulin sensitivity, and (2) decreased levels of the anorexigenic hormone leptin and increased levels of the orexigenic peptide ghrelin. A combination of these findings caused increased hunger and appetite leading to weight gain. Because of these changes, short sleep duration is a risk factor for diabetes and obesity.

Several epidemiologic studies have shown an association between sleep duration and type 2 diabetes mellitus.[66] Ayas et al.[67] found an association between long sleep duration (≥9 hours) and diabetes mellitus. Yaggi et al.[68] reported an association between diabetes and both short (≤5 hours) and long (>8 hours) sleep duration. Gottlieb et al.[69] found a similar relationship between short (<6 hours) and long (>9 hours) sleep duration. Two recent review papers[70,71] also support this conclusion.

Sleep Duration and Mortality

Epidemiologic studies by Kripke et al.,[72] Ayas et al.,[73] Patel et al.,[74] Tamakoshi et al.,[75] and Hublin et al.[76] showed increased mortality in short sleepers (also in relatively long sleepers). There is a U-shaped association between sleep duration (both long and short) and mortality. Several studies examined sleep duration and mortality. The earliest study was by Hammond in 1964.[77] Another significant early study by Kripke et al. in 1979 found that the chances of death from coronary artery disease, cancer, or stroke are greater for adults who sleep less than 4 hours or more than 9 hours when compared to those who sleep an average of 7½–8 hours.[72] The latest studies by Kripke et al. in 2002[78] confirmed the earlier observations and documented an increased mortality in those sleeping less than 7 hours and those sleeping more than 7½ hours. Other factors, such as sleeping medication, may have confounded these issues. There is, however, insufficient evidence to make a definite conclusion about sleep duration and mortality. The underlying etiologic factors remain to be determined.

Sleep Duration and Abnormal Physiologic Changes

Several studies documented abnormal physiologic changes after sleep restriction as follows: reduced glucose tolerance,[59] increased blood pressure,[79] sympathetic activation,[80] reduced leptin levels,[81] and increased inflammatory markers (e.g., an increased C-reactive protein, an inflammatory myocardial risk after sleep loss).[82]

Sleep Restriction and Immune Responses

Limited studies in the literature suggest the following responses following sleep restriction: (1) decreased antibody production following influenza vaccination in the first 10 days[83]; (2) decreased febrile response to endotoxin (*Escherichia coli*) challenge[84]; and (3) increased inflammatory cytokines[85–87] (e.g., interleukin-6 and tumor necrosis factor-α), which may lead to insulin resistance, cardiovascular disease, and osteoporosis.

Sleep Restriction and Cardiovascular Disease

Studies by Mallon et al.[88] in 2002 addressed the question of sleep duration and cardiovascular disease. They did not find increased risk of cardiovascular disease–related mortality associated with sleep duration, but found an association between difficulty falling asleep and coronary arterial disease mortality. However, several other studies found a relationship between increased risk of cardiovascular disease and sleep duration.[73,89–92] Ayas et al.,[73] in a 2003 study, found increased risk of both fatal and nonfatal myocardial infarction associated with both low and high sleep duration. Schwartz et al.[90] stated that sleep complaints are independent risk factors for myocardial infarction. Liu and Tanaka[91] noted a risk of nonfatal myocardial infarction associated with insufficient sleep in Japanese men. Kripke et al.[78] and Newman et al.,[92] in their studies, concluded that daytime sleepiness and reduced sleep duration predict mortality and cardiovascular disease in older adults. What is the mechanism of increased cardiovascular risk after chronic sleep deprivation? This is not exactly known but may be related to increased C-reactive protein, an inflammatory marker found after sleep loss. It should be noted that, in many of the sleep restriction experiments in humans, an added stress may have acted as a confounding factor and, therefore, some of the conclusions about sleep restriction regarding mortality, cardiovascular disease, diabetes mellitus, and endocrine changes may have been somewhat flawed.

Summary

Sleep restriction and sleep deprivation are associated with short-term (e.g., increased traffic accidents, EDS, daytime cognitive dysfunction as revealed by reduced vigilance test and working memory) and long-term (e.g., obesity, cardiovascular morbidity and mortality, memory impairment) adverse effects. Thus, chronic sleep deprivation caused either by lifestyle changes or primary sleep disorders (e.g., obstructive sleep apnea syndrome [OSAS], chronic insomnia) is a novel risk factor for obesity and insulin-resistant type 2 diabetes mellitus.

CAUSES OF EXCESSIVE DAYTIME SLEEPINESS

Excessive sleepiness may result from both physiologic and pathologic causes (Table 3–1), the latter of which include neurologic and general medical disorders as well as primary sleep disorders and medications and alcohol.[93]

Physiologic Causes of Sleepiness

Sleep deprivation and sleepiness because of lifestyle and habits of going to sleep and waking up at irregular hours can be considered to result from disruption of the normal circadian and homeostatic physiology. Groups who are excessively sleepy because of lifestyle and inadequate sleep include young adults and elderly individuals, workers at irregular shifts, health care professionals (e.g., doctors, particularly the house staff, and nurses), firefighters, police officers, train drivers, pilots and flight attendants, commercial truck drivers, and those individuals with competitive drives to move ahead in life, sacrificing hours of sleep and accumulating sleep debt. Among young adults, high school and college students are particularly at risk for sleep deprivation and sleepiness. The reasons for excessive sleepiness in adolescents and young adults include both biological and psychosocial factors. Some of the causes for later bedtimes in these groups include social interactions with peers, homework in the evening, sports, employment or other extracurricular activities, early wake-up times to start school, and academic obligations requiring additional school or college work at night. Biological factors may play a role but are not well studied. For example, teenagers may need extra hours of sleep. Also, the circadian timing system may change with sleep phase delay in teenagers.

Pathologic Causes of Sleepiness

Neurologic Causes of EDS

Tumors and vascular lesions affecting the ascending reticular-activating arousal system (ARAS) and its projections to the posterior hypothalamus and thalamus lead to daytime sleepiness. Such lesions often cause coma rather than just sleepiness. Brain tumors (e.g., astrocytomas, suprasellar cysts, metastases, lymphomas, and hamartomas affecting the posterior hypothalamus; pineal tumors; astrocytomas

---

TABLE 3–1 Causes of Excessive Daytime Sleepiness

Physiological Causes

Sleep deprivation and sleepiness related to lifestyle and irregular
   sleep-wake schedule

Pathologic Causes

Primary Sleep Disorders
Obstructive sleep apnea syndrome
Central sleep apnea syndrome
Narcolepsy
Idiopathic hypersomnolence
Circadian rhythm sleep disorders
   Jet lag
   Delayed sleep phase syndrome
   Irregular sleep-wake pattern
   Shift work sleep disorder
   Non–24-hour sleep-wake disorders
Periodic limb movements disorder
Restless legs syndrome
Insufficient sleep syndrome (Behaviorally induced)
Inadequate sleep hygiene

Other Hypersomnias
Recurrent or periodic hypersomnia
   Kleine-Levin syndrome
   Idiopathic recurrent stupor
   Catamenial hypersomnia
   Seasonal affective depression
   Occasionally due to insomnia
Medication-related hypersomnia
   Benzodiazepines
   Nonbenzodiazepine hypnotics (e.g., phenobarbital, zolpidem)
   Sedative antidepressants (e.g., tricyclics, trazodone)
   Antipsychotics
   Nonbenzodiazepine anxiolytics (e.g., buspirone)
   Antihistamines
   Narcotic analgesics, including tramadol (Ultram)
Toxin and alcohol-induced hypersomnolence

General Medical Disorders
Hepatic failure
Renal failure
Respiratory failure
Electrolyte disturbances
Cardiac failure
Severe anemia
Endocrine causes
   Hypothyroidism
   Acromegaly
   Diabetes mellitus
   Hypoglycemia
   Hyperglycemia

Psychiatric or Psychological Causes
Depression
Psychogenic unresponsiveness or sleepiness

Neurologic Causes
Brain tumors or vascular lesions affecting the thalamus,
   hypothalamus, or brain stem
Post-traumatic hypersomnolence
Multiple sclerosis
Encephalitis lethargica and other encephalitides and
   encephalopathies, including Wernicke's encephalopathy
Cerebral trypanosomiasis (African sleeping sickness)
Neurodegenerative disorders
   Alzheimer's disease
   Parkinson's disease
   Multiple system atrophy
Myotonic dystrophy and other neuromuscular disorders causing
   sleepiness secondary to sleep apnea

---

of the upper brain stem) may produce excessive sleepiness. Prolonged hypersomnia may be associated with tumors in the region of the third ventricle. Symptomatic narcolepsy resulting from craniopharyngioma and other tumors of the hypothalamic and pituitary regions has been described.[94] Cataplexy associated with sleepiness, sleep paralysis, and hypnagogic hallucinations has been described in patients with rostral brain stem gliomas with or without infiltration of the walls of the third ventricle. Narcolepsy-cataplexy syndrome also has been described in a human leukocyte antigen DR2–negative patient with a pontine lesion documented by magnetic resonance imaging.

Other neurologic causes of EDS include bilateral paramedian thalamic infarcts,[95] post-traumatic hypersomnolence, and multiple sclerosis. Narcolepsy-cataplexy syndrome has been described in occasional patients with multiple sclerosis and arteriovenous malformations in the diencephalons.[94,96]

EDS has been described in association with encephalitis lethargica and other encephalitides as well as encephalopathies, including Wernicke's encephalopathy. It was noted that the lesions of encephalitis lethargica described by von Economo[97] in the beginning of the last century, which severely affected the posterior hypothalamic region, were associated with the clinical manifestation of extreme somnolence. These lesions apparently interrupted the posterior hypothalamic histaminergic system as well as the ARAS projecting to the posterior hypothalamus. Encephalitis lethargica is now extinct. Cerebral sarcoidosis involving the hypothalamus may cause symptomatic narcolepsy.[98] Whipple's disease[99] of the nervous system involving the hypothalamus may occasionally cause hypersomnolence. Cerebral trypanosomiasis,[100] or African sleeping sickness, is transmitted to humans by tsetse flies: *Trypanosoma gambiense* causes Gambian or West African sleeping sickness, and *Trypanosoma rhodesiense* causes Rhodesian or East African sleeping sickness.

Certain neurodegenerative diseases such as Alzheimer's disease, Parkinson's disease, and multiple system atrophy also may cause EDS.[101,102] The causes of EDS in Alzheimer's disease include degeneration of the suprachiasmatic nucleus resulting in circadian dysrhythmia, associated sleep apnea/hypopnea, and periodic limb movements in sleep. In Parkinson's disease, excessive sleepiness may be due to the associated periodic limb movements in sleep, sleep apnea, and depression. EDS in multiple system atrophy associated with cerebellar parkinsonism or parkinsonian-cerebellar syndrome and progressive autonomic deficit (Shy-Drager syndrome) may be caused by the frequent association with sleep-related respiratory dysrhythmias and possible degeneration of the ARAS.[103]

Sleep disorders are being increasingly recognized as a feature of Parkinson's disease and other parkinsonian disorders. Although some studies have attributed the excessive daytime drowsiness and irresistible sleep episodes ("sleep attacks") to antiparkinsonian medications,[104] sleep disturbances are also an integral part of Parkinson's disease.[105] In one study of 303 patients with Parkinson's disease, 22.6% reported falling asleep while driving.[104] Several studies also reported a relatively high prevalence (20.8–21.9%) of symptoms of restless legs syndrome in patients with Parkinson's disease.[106,107] There is also increasing awareness about the relationship between parkinsonian disorders and REM sleep behavior disorder, which may be the presenting feature of Parkinson's disease, multiple system atrophy, and other parkinsonian disorders.[108–117]

These and other studies provide evidence supporting the notion that dopamine activity is normally influenced by circadian factors.[118] For example, tyrosine hydroxylase levels fall several hours before waking and their increase correlates with motor activity. The relationship between hypocretin and sleep disorders associated with Parkinson's disease is currently being explored.[119]

Myotonic dystrophy and other neuromuscular disorders may cause EDS due to associated sleep apnea/hypopnea syndrome and hypoventilation.[120–122] In addition, in myotonic dystrophy, there may be involvement of the ARAS as part of the multisystem membrane defects noted in this disease.

EDS Associated with General Medical Disorders

Several systemic diseases such as hepatic, renal, or respiratory failure and electrolyte disturbances may cause metabolic encephalopathies that result in EDS. Patients with severe EDS drift into a coma. The other medical causes for EDS include congestive heart failure and severe anemia. Hypothyroidism and acromegaly also may cause EDS due to the associated sleep apnea syndrome. Hypoglycemic episodes in diabetes mellitus and severe hyperglycemia are additional causes of EDS.

Primary Sleep Disorders Associated with EDS

A number of primary sleep disorders cause excessive sleepiness (see Table 3–1). The most common cause of EDS in the general population is behaviorally induced insufficient sleep syndrome associated with sleep deprivation. The next most common cause is OSAS; narcolepsy and idiopathic hypersomnolence are other common causes of EDS. Most patients with EDS referred to the sleep laboratory have OSAS. Other causes of EDS include circadian rhythm sleep disorders, restless legs syndrome–periodic limb movements in sleep, some cases of chronic insomnia, and inadequate sleep hygiene.

Substance-Induced Hypersomnia Associated with EDS

Many sedatives and hypnotics cause EDS. In addition to the benzodiazepine and nonbenzodiazepine hypnotics and sedative antidepressants (e.g., tricyclic antidepressants and trazodone) as well as nonbenzodiazepine neuroleptics (e.g., buspirone), antihistamines, antipsychotics, and narcotic analgesics (including tramadol [Ultram]) cause EDS (see Chapter 33).

Toxin and alcohol-related hypersomnolence can occur as well.[123] Many industrial toxins such as heavy metals and organic toxins (e.g., mercury, lead, arsenic, copper) may cause EDS. These may sometimes also cause insomnia. Individuals working in industrial settings using toxic chemicals routinely are at risk. These toxins may also cause systemic disturbances such as alteration of renal, liver, and hematologic function. There may be an impairment of nerve conduction. Chronic use of alcohol at bedtime may produce alcohol-dependent sleep disorder. Usually this causes insomnia, but sometimes the patients may have excessive sleepiness in the daytime. Many of these patients suffer from chronic alcoholism. Acute ingestion of alcohol causes transient sleepiness.

☉ REFERENCES

A full list of references are available at www.expertconsult.com

CHAPTER 4

Neurobiology of Rapid Eye Movement and Non–Rapid Eye Movement Sleep

Robert W. McCarley

INTRODUCTION

This chapter presents an overview of the current knowledge of the neurophysiology and cellular pharmacology of sleep mechanisms. It is written from the perspective of the remarkable development of knowledge about sleep mechanisms in recent years, resulting from the capability of current cellular neurophysiologic, pharmacologic, and molecular techniques to provide focused, detailed, and replicable studies that have enriched and informed the knowledge of sleep phenomenology and pathology derived from electroencephalographic (EEG) analysis. This chapter has a cellular and neurophysiologic/neuropharmacologic focus, with an emphasis on rapid eye movement (REM) sleep mechanisms and non–REM (NREM) sleep phenomena attributable to adenosine. A detailed historical introduction to the topics of this chapter is available in the textbook by Steriade and McCarley.[1] For the reader interested in an update on the terminology and techniques of cellular physiology, one of the standard neurobiology texts could be consulted (e.g., Kandel et al.[2]). Overviews of REM sleep physiology are also available,[1,3] as well as an overview of adenosine and NREM sleep.[4] The present chapter draws on these accounts for its review, beginning with brief and elementary overviews of sleep architecture and phylogeny/ontogeny so as to provide a basis for the later mechanistic discussions. The first part of this chapter treats REM sleep and the relevant anatomy and physiology, and then describes the role of hypocretin/orexin in REM sleep control. The second part discusses NREM sleep with a focus on adenosinergic mechanisms.

Of the two phases of sleep, REM sleep is most often associated with vivid dreaming and a high level of brain activity. The other phase of sleep, called *non*–REM sleep or slow-wave sleep (SWS), is usually associated with reduced neuronal activity; thought content during this state in humans is, unlike dreams, usually nonvisual and consisting of ruminative thoughts. As one goes to sleep, the low-voltage fast EEG of waking gradually gives way to a slowing of frequency and, as sleep moves toward the deepest stages, there is an abundance of delta waves (EEG waves with a frequency of 0.5 to <4 Hz and of high amplitude). The first REM period usually occurs about 70 minutes after the onset of sleep. REM sleep in humans is defined by the presence of low-voltage fast EEG activity, suppression of muscle tone (usually measured in the chin muscles), and the presence, of course, of rapid eye movements. The first REM sleep episode in humans is short. After the first REM sleep episode, the sleep cycle repeats itself with the appearance of NREM sleep and then, about 90 minutes after the start of the first REM period, another REM sleep episode occurs. This rhythmic cycling persists throughout the night. The REM sleep cycle length is 90 minutes in humans, and the duration of each REM sleep episode after the first is approximately 30 minutes. While EEG staging of REM sleep in humans usually shows a fairly abrupt transition from NREM to

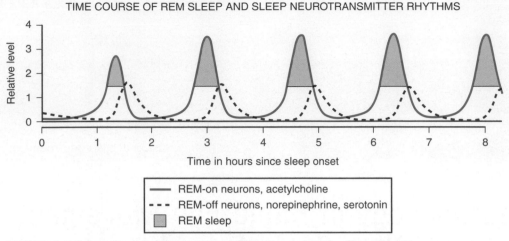

TIME COURSE OF REM SLEEP AND SLEEP NEUROTRANSMITTER RHYTHMS

— REM-on neurons, acetylcholine
- - - REM-off neurons, norepinephrine, serotonin
▨ REM sleep

FIGURE 4–1 Schematic of a night's course of REM sleep in humans. This shows the occurrence and intensity of REM sleep as dependent upon the activity of populations of "REM-on" (= REM-promoting neurons), indicated by the *solid line*. As the REM-promoting neuronal activity reaches a certain threshold, the full set of REM signs occurs (*black areas under curve* indicate REM sleep). Note, however that, unlike the step-like electroencephalographic diagnosis of stage, the underlying neuronal activity is a continuous function. The neurotransmitter acetylcholine is thought to be important in REM sleep production, acting to excite populations of brain stem reticular formation neurons to produce the set of REM signs. Other neuronal populations utilizing the monoamine neurotransmitters serotonin and norepinephrine are likely REM-suppressive; the time course of their activity is sketched by the *dotted line*. The terms *REM-on* and *REM-off* quite generally apply to other neuronal populations important in REM sleep, including those utilizing the neurotransmitter γ-aminobutyric acid (GABA). (These curves mimic actual time courses of neuronal activity, as recorded in animals, and were generated by a mathematical model of REM sleep in humans, the limit cycle reciprocal interaction model of McCarley and Massaquoi.[130,131])

REM sleep, recording of neuronal activity in animals presents quite a different picture. Neuronal activity begins to change long before the EEG signs of REM sleep are present. To introduce this concept, Figure 4–1 shows a schematic of the time course of neuronal activity relative to EEG definitions of REM sleep. Later portions of this chapter elaborate on the activity depicted in this figure. Over the course of the night, delta-wave activity tends to diminish and NREM sleep has waves of higher frequencies and lower amplitude.

REM SLEEP

REM sleep is present in all mammals, and recent data suggest this includes the egg-laying mammals (monotremes), such as the echidna (spiny anteater) and the duckbill platypus. Birds have very brief bouts of REM sleep. REM sleep cycles vary in duration according to the size of the animal, with elephants having the longest cycle and smaller animals having shorter cycles. For example, the cat has a sleep cycle of approximately 22 minutes, while the rat cycle is about 12 minutes. In utero, mammals spend a large percentage of time in REM sleep, ranging from 50% to 80% of a 24-hour day. At birth, animals born with immature nervous systems have a much higher percentage of REM sleep than do the adults of the same species. For example, sleep in the human newborn occupies two-thirds of the day, with REM sleep occupying one-half of the total sleep time,

or about one-third of the entire 24-hour period. The percentage of REM sleep declines rapidly in early childhood so that by approximately age 10 the adult percentage of REM sleep—20% of total sleep time—is reached. The predominance of REM sleep in the young suggests an important function in promoting nervous system growth and development.

Delta sleep is minimally present in the newborn but increases over the first years of life, reaching a maximum at about age 10 and declining thereafter. Feinberg and coworkers[5] have noted that the first 3 decades of this delta-wave activity time course can be fit by a gamma probability distribution and that approximately the same time course obtains for synaptic density and positron emission tomography measurements of metabolic rate in human frontal cortex. They speculated that the reduction in these three variables may reflect a pruning of redundant cortical synapses that is a key factor in cognitive maturation, allowing greater specialization and sustained problem solving.

REM Sleep Physiology and Relevant Brain Anatomy

Transection Studies

Lesion studies performed by Jouvet and coworkers in France demonstrated that the brain stem contains the neural machinery of the REM sleep rhythm (reviewed in Steriade and McCarley[1]). As illustrated in Figure 4–2,

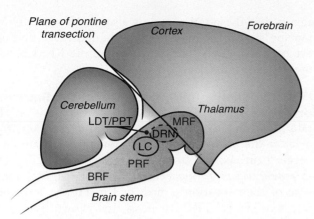

FIGURE 4–2 Schematic of a sagittal section of a mammalian brain (cat) showing the location of nuclei especially important for REM sleep. (BRF, PRF, and MRF, bulbar, pontine, and mesencephalic reticular formation; LC, locus ceruleus, where most norepinephrine-containing neurons are located; LDT/PPT, laterodorsal and pedunculopontine tegmental nuclei, the principal site of cholinergic (acetylcholine-containing) neurons important for REM sleep and EEG desynchronization; RN, dorsal raphe nucleus, the site of many serotonin-containing neurons.) The *oblique line* is the plane of transection that Jouvet[261] found preserves REM sleep signs caudal to the transection but abolishes them rostral to the transection.

a transaction made just above the junction of the pons and midbrain produced a state in which periodic occurrence of REM sleep was found in recordings made in the isolated brain stem; in contrast, recordings in the isolated forebrain showed no signs of REM sleep. Thus, while forebrain mechanisms (including those related to circadian rhythms) modulate REM sleep, the fundamental rhythmic generating machinery is in the brain stem, and it is here that anatomic and physiologic studies have focused. The anatomic sketch provided by Figure 4–2 also shows many of the cell groups important in REM sleep; the attention of the reader is called to the cholinergic neurons, which act as promoters of REM phenomena, and to the monoaminergic neurons, which act to suppress most components of REM sleep. Later sections comment on γ-aminobutyric acidergic (GABAergic) neurons, which are more widely dispersed rather than being in specific nuclei. Note that Figure 4–2 shows that the Jouvet transection spared these essential brain stem zones.

Effector Neurons for Different Components of REM Sleep: Principal Location in Brain Stem Reticular Formation

By effector neurons are meant those neurons directly in the neural pathways leading to the production of different REM components, such as the rapid eye movements. A series of physiologic investigations over the past 4 decades have shown that the "behavioral state" of REM sleep in nonhuman mammals is dissociable into different components under control of different mechanisms and different anatomic loci. The reader familiar with pathology

associated with human REM sleep will find this concept easy to understand, since much pathology consists of inappropriate expression or suppression of individual components of REM sleep. As in humans, the cardinal signs of REM sleep in nonhuman mammals are muscle atonia (especially in antigravity muscles), EEG activation (low-voltage fast pattern, sometimes termed an "activated" or "desynchronized" pattern), and rapid eye movements.

Ponto-geniculo-occipital (PGO) waves are another important component of REM sleep found in recordings from deep brain structures in many animals. PGO waves are spiky EEG waves that arise in the pons and are transmitted to the thalamic lateral geniculate nucleus (a visual system nucleus) and to the visual occipital cortex, hence the name *PGO* waves. There is suggestive evidence that PGO waves are present in humans, but the depth recordings necessary to establish their existence have not been done. PGO waves are EEG signs of neural activation; they index an important mode of brain stem activation of the forebrain during REM sleep. It is worth noting that they are also present in nonvisual thalamic nuclei, although their timing is linked to eye movements, with the first wave of the usual burst of 3–5 waves occurring just before an eye movement.

Most of the physiologic events of REM sleep have effector neurons located in the brain stem reticular formation, with important neurons especially concentrated in the *pontine reticular formation* (PRF). Thus PRF neuronal recordings are of special interest for information on mechanisms of production of these events. Intracellular recordings by Ito et al.[6] of PRF neurons show that these effector neurons have relatively hyperpolarized membrane potentials and generate almost no action potentials during NREM sleep. PRF neurons begin to depolarize even before the occurrence of the first EEG sign of the approach of REM sleep, the PGO waves that occur 30–60 seconds before the onset of the rest of the EEG signs of REM sleep. As PRF neuronal depolarization proceeds and the threshold for action potential production is reached, these neurons begin to discharge (generate action potentials). Their discharge rate increases as REM sleep is approached, and the high level of discharge is maintained throughout REM sleep, due to the maintenance of this membrane depolarization.

Throughout the entire REM sleep episode, almost the entire population of PRF neurons remains depolarized. The resultant increased action potential activity leads to the production of those REM sleep components that have their physiologic bases in activity of PRF neurons. PRF neurons are important for the rapid eye movements (the generator for lateral saccades is in the PRF) and PGO waves (a different group of neurons), and a group of dorsolateral PRF neurons just ventral to the locus ceruleus (LC) controls the muscle atonia of REM sleep (these neurons become active just before the onset of muscle atonia; see *PRF to LC* later for detailed discussion). Neurons in the midbrain reticular formation (see location in Fig. 4–2) are especially important for EEG activation, for the low-voltage fast EEG pattern. These neurons were originally described as making up the "ascending reticular activating system," the set of neurons responsible for EEG activation. Subsequent work has enlarged this original concept to include cholinergic neurons, with contributions in waking to EEG activation also coming from monoaminergic systems, neurons utilizing serotonin and norepinephrine as neurotransmitters.

REM-On Neurons and REM Promotion

Initiation and Coordination of REM Sleep via Cholinergic Mechanisms

Current data suggest cholinergic influences act by increasing the excitability of brain stem reticular neurons important as effectors in REM sleep either directly or indirectly by disinhibition due to inhibiting GABAergic neurons, which are themselves inhibitory to reticular formation neurons. The essential data supporting cholinergic mechanisms are summarized below.

Production of a REM-like State by Direct Injection of Acetylcholine Agonists into the Pontine Reticular Formation. It has been known since the mid-1960s that cholinergic agonist injection into the PRF produces a state that very closely mimics natural REM sleep (for review and detailed literature citations, see Steriade and McCarley[1]). The latency to onset and duration are dose dependent; within the PRF, most workers have found the shortest latencies to come from injections in dorsorostral pontine reticular sites. Muscarinic cholinergic receptors appear to be of major importance, with nicotinic receptors playing a lesser role. Of note, most of the in vivo cholinergic data have come from felines. A similar REM induction effect can be induced in rats and mice, although it often is less robust in these species, perhaps as a result of difficulty in localization of applications in the smaller brains and interaction with circadian control (reviewed in Steriade and McCarley[1]), as well as a perhaps different localization of GABAergic neurons inhibited by carbachol (see later). However, as described in the later section on direct excitation of PRF neurons by cholinergic agents, the in vitro evidence for carbachol excitatory effects on reticular formation neurons in the rat is undisputed. The precise site where in vivo carbachol is most effective in inducing REM or muscle atonia in the rat is disputed but appears to be within the PRF nucleus, in the pontis oralis slightly rostral to the region just ventral to the LC (the subceruleus [SubC]), or in an area neighboring the superior cerebellar peduncle (ventral tegmental nucleus of Gudden).[7–11] Recent experiments using the acetylcholinesterase inhibitor neostigmine in the mouse

suggest that the pontis oralis is also an effective REM-inducing site in the mouse,[12,13] although these findings have been disputed.[14] Of note also are the REM-reducing effects of muscarinic knockouts.[15]

LDT/PPT Cholinergic Projections to Reticular Formation Neurons. Cholinergic projections in the brain stem and to brain stem sites arise in from two nuclei at the pons-midbrain junction that contain cholinergic neurons, the *laterodorsal tegmentum* (LDT) and the *pedunculopontine tegmentum* (PPT). A sagittal schematic of their location is provided in Figure 4–2; they project to critical PRF zones, as first shown by Mitani et al.[16] and repeatedly confirmed. A similar series of studies has documented the extensive rostral projections of cholinergic neurons to the thalamus and basal forebrain, where their actions are important for EEG activation, a topic to be discussed later.

Direct Excitation of PRF Neurons by Cholinergic Agonists. In vitro pontine brain stem slice preparations offer the ability to apply agonists/antagonists in physiologic concentrations, which are usually in the low micromolar range; effective in vivo injections use concentrations that are a thousand-fold greater, in the millimolar range, and thus raise the possibility of mediation of effects by nonphysiologic mechanisms. Applications of micromolar amounts of cholinergic agonists in vitro in the rat produce excitation of a majority (about two-thirds) of medial PRF neurons. Another advantage of the in vitro preparation is the ability to use a sodium-dependent action potential blocker, tetrodotoxin; these experiments show that the excitatory effects of cholinergic agonists on PRF neurons in the rat in vitro are direct.[17] Furthermore, the depolarizing, excitatory effects of cholinergic agonist mimic the changes seen in PRF neurons during natural REM sleep.[6]

LDT/PPT Lesions and Stimulation Effects. Extensive destruction of the cell bodies of LDT/PPT neurons by local injections of excitatory amino acids leads to a marked reduction of REM sleep.[18] Low-level (10 µA) electrical stimulation of the LDT increases REM sleep.[19] In contrast, Lu et al.[20] reported that ibotenic acid lesions of the LDT did not alter REM sleep while separate ibotenic acid lesions of the cholinergic PPT produced an increase in REM sleep, an effect they attributed to including part of the medial parabrachial nucleus.

Discharge Activity of LDT/PPT Neurons Across the REM Cycle. A subset of these neurons has been shown to discharge selectively during REM sleep, and with the onset of increased discharges occurring before the onset of REM sleep,[21–23] as schematized in Figure 4–1. This LDT/PPT discharge pattern and the presence of excitatory projections to the PRF suggest that LDT/PPT cholinergic neurons may be important in producing the depolarization of reticular effector neurons, leading to production of the events characterizing REM sleep. The group of LDT/PPT and reticular formation neurons that become active in REM sleep are often referred to as *REM-on neurons*. Subgroups of PRF neurons may show discharges during waking motoric activity, either somatic or oculomotor, but a sustained depolarization throughout almost all of the population occurs only during REM sleep. Studies of expression of the immediate early gene c-*fos* have shown activation of choline acetyltransferase (ChAT)–positive neurons in REM rebound in the rat following deprivation,[24,25] although studies by Verret et al.[26] did not. It must be emphasized that c-*fos* expression, while useful, does not offer a 1:1 isomorphism with action potential occurrence (see Fields et al.[27]). Of particular note, single-unit in vivo studies in the rat strongly support cholinergic activation during REM sleep (reviewed in Steriade and McCarley[1]).

Cholinergic Neurons in Production of the Low-Voltage Fast or "Desynchronized" EEG Pattern of both REM Sleep and Waking. Rostral projections of a subgroup of LDT/PPT neurons, those with discharges during both wakefulness and REM sleep, are important for the EEG activation of both REM sleep and waking (see extensive discussion in Steriade and McCarley[1]).

Other Neurotransmitters and PRF Neurons

Peptides Co-localized with Acetylcholine. Many peptides are co-localized with the neurotransmitter acetylcholine (ACh) in LDT/PPT neurons; this co-localization likely also means they have synaptic co-release with ACh. The peptide substance P is found in about 40% of LDT/PPT neurons and, overall, more than 15 different co-localized peptides have been described. The role of these peptides in modulating ACh activity relevant to wakefulness and sleep remains to be elucidated, but it should be emphasized that the co-localized vasoactive intestinal peptide has been reported by a several different investigators to enhance REM sleep when it is injected intraventricularly. A later section of this chapter discusses GABAergic influences, as well as the role of GABAergic reticular formation neurons.

REM Muscle Atonia

This is an important REM feature from a clinical point of view because disorders of this system are present in many patients who present to sleep disorders clinicians. Work by Chase and collaborators and by Siegel and collaborators (reviewed in Steriade and McCarley[1]) suggests three important zones for atonia (listed according to their projections): PRF → bulbar reticular formation → motoneurons. We here discuss only the PRF portion of the atonia circuitry.

PRF to LC. Jouvet and colleagues in Lyon, France, reported that bilateral lesions of the pontine reticular region just ventral to the LC (termed by this group the *peri-LC alpha*) and its descending pathway to the bulbar reticular formation abolished the nuchal muscle atonia of REM sleep.[28,29] It is to be emphasized that this zone is a reticular zone, not one containing noradrenergic neurons like the LC proper, and that the name refers only to proximity to the LC. The Lyon group also reported that not only was the nuchal muscle atonia of REM suppressed, but that cats so lesioned exhibited "oneiric behavior," including locomotion, attack behavior, and behavior with head raised and with horizontal and vertical movements "as if watching something." Morrison and collaborators confirmed the basic finding of REM without atonia with bilateral pontine tegmental lesions but report that lesions extending beyond the LC alpha region and its efferent pathway to the bulbar reticular formation were necessary for more than a minimal release of muscle tone and to produce the elaborate "oneiric behaviors."[30] The exact location and numbers of inhibitory pathways is still a matter of some controversy, with all investigators agreeing on the important, if not exclusive, role of the peri-LC alpha, or, as it is often termed, the SubC.

REM-Suppressive Systems: REM-Off Neurons

The neurons described in the previous section that increase discharge rate with the advent of REM have been termed *REM-on neurons*. In contrast, groups of other neurons radically decrease and may nearly arrest discharge activity with the approach and onset of REM; these are often termed *REM-off neurons*. The typical discharge activity profile is for discharge rates to be highest in waking, then decreasing in synchronized sleep and with near cessation of discharge in REM sleep. REM-off neurons are distinctive both because they are in the minority in the brain and also because they are recorded in zones with neurons that use biogenic amines as neurotransmitters. The loci include a midline zone of the brain stem raphe nuclei, and a more lateral bandlike zone in the rostral pons/midbrain junction that includes the nucleus locus ceruleus, a reticular zone, and the peribrachial zone.

Raphe Nuclei

Neurons with a REM-off discharge profile were first described by McGinty and Harper[31] in the dorsal raphe nucleus, a finding confirmed by other workers.[32–35] Neurons with the same REM-off discharge pattern have been found in the other raphe nuclei, including the nucleus linearis centralis,[32,36] centralis superior,[37] raphe magnus,[38,39] and raphe pallidus.[40] Identification of these extracellularly recorded neurons with serotonin-containing neurons was made on the basis of recording site location in the vicinity of histochemically identified serotonin neurons and the similarity of the extracellularly recorded slow, regular discharge pattern to that of histochemically identified serotonergic neurons in vitro. Nonserotonergic neurons in the raphe system have been found to have different discharge pattern characteristics. While this extracellular identification methodology does not approach the "gold standard" of intracellular recording and labeling, the circumstantial evidence that the raphe REM-off neurons are serotonergic appears strong.

Locus Ceruleus

The second major locus of REM-off neurons is the LC, as described in the cat,[41,42] rat,[43,44] and monkey.[45] The argument that these extracellularly recorded discharges are from norepinephrine (NE)–containing neurons parallels that for the putative serotonergic REM-off neurons. Extracellularly recorded neurons that are putatively noradrenergic have the same slow, regular discharge pattern as NE-containing neurons identified in vitro and have the proper anatomic localization of recording sites, including recording sites in the compact LC in the rat, where the NE-containing neurons are rather discretely localized. Thus, while the evidence that these REM-off neurons are NE containing is indirect and circumstantial, it nonetheless appears quite strong.

Finally, the remaining groups of aminergic REM-off neurons are principally localized to the anterior pontine tegmentum–midbrain junction, either in the peribrachial zone or in a more medial extension of it—recording sites that correspond to the presence of aminergic neurons scattered through this zone. The "stray" REM-off neurons in other reticular locations also correspond to dispersed adrenergic neuronal groups, although adrenergic identification in this case is much less secure. At this point, it is noted that putatively dopaminergic (DA) neurons in the substantia nigra and midbrain *do not* alter their discharge rate or pattern over the sleep-wake cycle,[46] and thus are unlikely to play important roles in sleep-wake cycle control. However, Lu et al.[47] have found DA neurons in the rat ventral periaqueductal gray that express c-Fos during wakefulness, fulfilling c-Fos criteria for wake-active neurons. This population was localized near the dorsal raphe nucleus (DRN) and was interspersed with DRN serotonergic neurons at the ventral periaqueductal gray level of the DA neurons. Although the DRN serotonergic neurons are wake-active in unit recordings, they did not express c-FOS in the Lu et al. study with exposure to the same degree of wakefulness as the DA neurons. These DA neurons projected to cholinergic neurons in the basal forebrain and the LDT, as well as to the monoaminergic cells in the LC and DRN and to lateral hypothalamic orexin neurons, and thus have projections to zones important in sleep-wake control, as well as to the thalamus and cortex. Unit recordings will be important in confirming the wake-active nature of these DA neurons, although their admixture with serotonergic neurons will make identification difficult.

Do REM-Off Neurons Play a Permissive, Disinhibitory Role in REM Sleep Genesis by Interacting with Cholinergic REM-On Neurons?

The intriguing reciprocity of the discharge time course of REM-off and REM-on neurons led to the initial hypothesis of interaction of these two groups, as originally proposed for the REM-off adrenergic neurons.[41,42,48,49] The phenomenologic, behavioral, and cellular data have been sufficiently strong so that diverse groups of investigators have proposed that the REM-off neurons, as a complete or partial set, act in a permissive, disinhibitory way on some or all of the components of REM sleep. These postulates are summarized here, with presentation of the some of the data on which they are based. Many of these theories arose in the mid-1970s, as increased technical capability led to extracellular recordings of REM-off neurons.

Dorsal Raphe Serotonergic Neurons. The possibility that the dorsal raphe serotonergic neurons act to suppress one of the major phenomena of REM sleep, PGO waves, was explicitly proposed by Simon et al.,[50] on the basis of lesion data, and in in vivo pharmacologic experiments using reserpine,[51] which depleted brain stem serotonin and simultaneously produced nearly continuous PGO-like waves. The study of McGinty and Harper[31] was the first of many to document the inverse relationship between the discharge activity of extracellularly recorded dorsal raphe neurons and REM sleep. With respect to REM sleep onset, the decrease in discharge activity of presumptively serotonergic raphe neurons is remarkably consistent. Using a cycle-averaging technique, Lydic et al.[52] found the time course of presumptively serotonergic dorsal raphe neuronal activity over the sleep-wake cycle was very clear: waking > NREM > REM sleep. There was also a clear inverse relationship between PGO waves and dorsal raphe discharge, and a premonitory increase in dorsal raphe activity prior to the end of the REM sleep episode, a phenomenon also observed and commented upon by Trulson and Jacobs.[35]

Evidence that dorsal raphe serotonergic activity inhibits REM sleep also came from in vivo pharmacologic experiments by Ruch-Monachon et al.[53] and dorsal raphe cooling experiments by Cespuglio et al.[54] Hobson et al.[42] and McCarley and Hobson[49] originally proposed that monoaminergic neurons might inhibit REM-on cholinergic REM-promoting neurons, now known to be in the LDT/PPT. This postulate of monoaminergic inhibition of cholinergic neurons was originally regarded as extremely controversial. However, interest was quickened by the following series of findings:

1. Documentation of serotonergic projections from the dorsal raphe to the mesopontine cholinergic neurons in the LDT and PPT that are implicated in the production of REM sleep[55–57]
2. In vitro demonstration of serotonergic inhibition of mesopontine cholinergic neurons[58,59]
3. The report that microinjection of a serotonergic 5-hydroxytryptamine$_{1A}$ (5-HT$_{1A}$) agonist into the PPT inhibits REM sleep[60]
4. The finding that the level of serotonin release in the cat DRN[61] paralleled the behavioral state ordering at distant DRN projection sites (waking > SWS > REM sleep) in both rats[62,63] and cats,[64] suggesting that this would also be true at axonal release sites in the LDT/PPT

Since axon collaterals of DRN serotonergic neurons inhibit this same DRN population via somatodendritic 5-HT$_{1A}$ receptors,[65] it followed that the introduction of a selective 5-HT$_{1A}$ receptor agonist in the DRN via microdialysis perfusion should produce strong inhibition of serotonergic neural activity, which would be indicated by a reduction of 5-HT release in the DRN. Moreover, if the hypothesis of serotonergic inhibition of REM-promoting neurons were correct, the inhibition of DRN serotonergic activity should disinhibit REM-promoting neurons, producing an increase in REM sleep concomitant with the changes in DRN extracellular serotonin. Portas et al.[66] tested the effects of microdialysis perfusion of 8-hydroxy-2-(di-*n*-propylamino)tetralin (8-OH-DPAT), a selective 5-HT$_{1A}$ receptor agonist, in freely moving cats. In perfusions during waking, DRN perfusion of 8-OH-DPAT decreased 5-HT levels by 50% compared with artificial cerebrospinal fluid (Fig. 4–3), presumptively through 5-HT$_{1A}$ autoreceptor-mediated inhibition of serotonergic neural activity. Concomitantly, the 8-OH-DPAT perfusion produced a statistically significant short-latency, approximately threefold increase in REM sleep, from a mean of 10.6% at baseline to 30.6%, while waking was not significantly affected (see Fig. 4–3). In contrast, and suggesting DRN specificity, 8-OH-DPAT delivery through a probe in the aqueduct did not increase REM sleep but rather tended to increase waking and decrease SWS.

These data in the cat were confirmed in the rat by Bjorvatn et al.,[67] who found that perfusion of 8-OH-DPAT DRN led to a fourfold increase in REM sleep, while the other vigilance states were not significantly altered. In the cat, Sakai and Crochet[68] failed to replicate the findings of Portas et al.[66] in the cat and Bjorvatn et al.[67] in the rat, perhaps due to technical differences (see McCarley[3]). In contrast to the just-described positive findings related to DRN and REM control, Lu et al.[20] found that 5,7-dihydroxytryptamine lesions of the rat

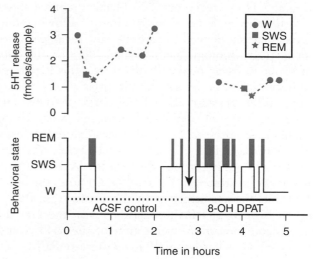

MICRODIALYSIS DELIVERY OF 8-OH DPAT
TO DORSAL RAPHE
EFFECTS ON 5HT RELEASE AND REM SLEEP

FIGURE 4–3 Time course of serotonin (5-hydroxytryptamine [5-HT]) levels and behavioral state. Time course of 5-HT levels **(top)** and behavioral state **(bottom)** during control dorsal raphe nucleus (DRN) artificial cerebrospinal fluid (ACSF) perfusion (*interrupted horizontal line*) and during DRN 8-hydroxy-2-(di-*n*-propylamino)tetralin (8-OH-DPAT) perfusion (*solid horizontal line*) in a typical experiment. Note that, prior to perfusion, waking DRN 5-HT levels (*circles*) are higher than those in slow wave sleep (SWS; *squares*) and REM sleep (*stars*). Each 5-HT value is expressed as femtomoles per 7.5-μl sample, and was obtained during an uninterrupted 5-minute sequence of the behavioral state. Upon the onset of 10-μM 8-OH-DPAT perfusion (*arrow*), the 5-HT level dropped quickly to levels as low as those normally present in SWS or REM sleep. Behaviorally, 8-OH-DPAT administration markedly increased REM sleep (*black bars* in the hypnogram). *(Adapted from Portas CM, Thakkar M, Rainnie D, McCarley RW. Microdialysis perfusion of 8-hydroxy-2-[di-n-propylamino] tetralin [8-OH-DPAT] in the dorsal raphe nucleus decreases serotonin release and increases rapid eye movement sleep in the freely moving cat. J Neurosci 1996;16:2820.)*

serotonergic DRN did not affect REM or other behavioral states.

In Vivo and In Vitro Evidence of Serotonergic Inhibition of LDT/PPT Neurons.

The data of Portas et al.,[66] however, did not directly demonstrate serotonergic inhibition of neurons in the cholinergic LDT/PPT. Moreover, the presence of some neurons with REM-on and other neurons with Wake/REM-on activity in the LDT/PPT was a puzzle in terms of the global changes in monoaminergic inhibition. McCarley et al.[69] postulated that, while monoamines might inhibit REM-on cholinergic neurons, Wake/REM-on neurons might not be inhibited, thus explaining their continued activity in waking—since serotonergic activity is highest during wakefulness, the observed high discharge rate of Wake/REM-on neurons during wakefulness would not be consistent with a high level of serotonergic inhibition from a high level of DRN activity. In vitro data were also consistent with a subset, not the entire population, of LDT/PPT cholinergic neurons inhibited by serotonin acting at 5-HT$_{1A}$ receptors.[58,59] Thakkar and collaborators[70] developed a novel methodology allowing both extracellular single cell recording and local perfusion of neuropharmacologic agents via an adjacent microdialysis probe in freely behaving cats to test this hypothesis of differential serotonergic inhibition as an explanation of the different state-related discharge activity. Discharge activity of REM-on neurons was almost completely suppressed by local microdialysis perfusion of the selective 5-HT$_{1A}$ agonist 8-OH-DPAT, while this agonist had minimal or no effect on the Wake/REM-on neurons, as illustrated in Figure 4–4. Of note, the ordering of 5-HT concentrations in the cholinergic PPT is wake > NREM > REM, consistent with the unit discharge data; moreover, application of the 5HT$_{1A}$ agonist 8-OH DPAT to the PPT suppressed REM sleep and increased wakefulness (Strecker et al.[71] and unpublished data).

The finding that only a subpopulation of the recorded LDT/PPT cells were inhibited by 8-OH-DPAT is consistent with rat pontine slice data, where, in combined intracellular recording and labeling to confirm the recorded cell's cholinergic identity, some but not all of the cholinergic neurons in the LDT/PPT were inhibited by serotonin.[59] The different percentages of LDT/PPT neurons that are inhibited by serotonin or serotonin agonists in vitro (64%) compared with the in vivo findings (36.4%)[70] may be due to anatomic differences

between species (rat vs. cat) and/or different concentrations of agents at the receptors.

Locus Ceruleus and REM Sleep Phenomena: Lesion and Cooling Studies

Lesion studies furnish an unclear picture of the role of the LC in REM sleep. *Bilateral* electrolytic lesions of the LC in the cat by Jones et al.[72] led these workers to conclude the LC was not necessary for REM sleep. However, following unilateral LC electrolytic lesions, Caballero and De Andres[73] found a 50% increase in the percentage of REM sleep ($p < 0.001$) in cats, while lesions in neighboring tegmentum and sham-operated controls showed no change. Caballero and DeAndres attributed the differences between their study and that of Jones et al.[72] to nonspecific effects, including urinary retention, of the larger lesions that may have led to a REM sleep reduction. Cespuglio et al.[74] performed unilateral and bilateral cooling of the LC in felines, using the same methodology as for the dorsal raphe cooling. In repeated cooling trials REM sleep was repetitively induced, and the percentage of REM sleep increased by 120% over control periods. However, Lu et al.[20] found that 6-hydroxydopamine lesions of the rat noradrenergic LC did not affect REM sleep or vigilance states.

Site(s) of REM-Off and REM-On Interaction

The model for REM sleep control proposed here discusses REM-off suppression of REM-on neurons. It must be emphasized that there are several, non–mutually exclusive possible sites of interaction. These include direct

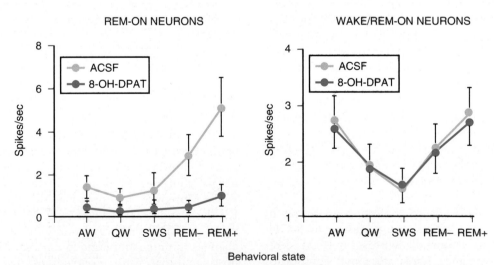

FIGURE 4–4 State-related activity of units in the cholinergic LDT and PPT and the effects of a serotonin 1A receptor agonist applied by microdialysis. **(Left)** REM-on units ($N = 9$): grand mean (±SEM) of discharge rate in each behavioral state before (*open circle*, artificial cerebrospinal fluid [ACSF]) and after (*closed circle*) 10-μM 8-OH-DPAT was added to the perfusate. Note suppression of activity (highly statistically significant). Abbreviations are defined in text. **(Right)** Wake/REM-on units ($N = 25$): grand mean (±SEM) of discharge rate of before (*light blue circle*, ACSF) and after (*dark blue circle*) 10-μM 8-OH-DPAT was added to the perfusate. Note minimal effect of 8-OH-DPAT, not statistically significant. *(Adapted from Thakkar MM, Strecker RE, McCarley RW. Behavioral state control through differential serotonergic inhibition in the mesopontine cholinergic nuclei: a simultaneous unit recording and microdialysis study. J Neurosci 1998;18:5490.)*

ACh-NE interactions in the LDT and PPT. For example, there is now evidence that ChAT-labeled fibers are present in the LC, and it has long been known that the NE-containing LC neurons also stain intensely for the presence of acetylcholinesterase (see review of NE-ACh anatomic interrelationship in McCarley[3]). NE varicosities are present throughout the reticular formation, the LDT, and the peribrachial area that is the site of ChAT-positive neurons. Thus adrenergic-cholinergic interactions may take place directly between these two species of neurons and/or may take place at reticular neurons.

GABAergic Influences and REM Sleep

In addition to the monoamines and ACh as modulators and controllers of the sleep cycle, there is accumulating, quite strong evidence that GABAergic influences may play an important role. Defining the role of GABA with certainty is difficult, however. Since GABA is a ubiquitous inhibitory neurotransmitter, purely pharmacologic experiments using agents that increase or decrease GABA do not answer a key question, namely whether the results so obtained were representative of the increases or decreases in GABA that occur naturally in the course of the sleep cycle, or were simply and trivially the result of a pharmacologic manipulation of GABA systems not naturally playing a role in sleep cycle control. Microdialysis is potentially a very useful way of sampling naturally occurring changes in GABA levels over the sleep cycle, but is often limited in sensitivity and hence in time resolution of when the changes occur in the sleep cycle.

This section surveys GABA data from the DRN, LC, and PRF that are relevant to sleep-wakefulness control. From the standpoint of sleep cycle control, one of the most puzzling as aspects has been defining what causes the "REM-off" neurons in the LC and DRN to slow and cease discharge as REM sleep is approached and entered. The reciprocal interaction model (see later) hypothesized that a recurrent inhibition of the LC/DRN might account for this. While recurrent inhibition is present, there is no clear evidence that it might be a strong causal agent in REM-off neurons turning off. Thus, the prospect that a GABAergic mechanism might be involved is of great intrinsic interest.

Dorsal Raphe Nucleus

Microdialysis in DRN. Nitz and Siegel[75] reported a significant increase in GABA levels in REM sleep compared with wakefulness, while SWS did not significantly differ from wakefulness. Moreover, there was a 67% increase in REM sleep observed with microinjections of the GABA agonist muscimol into the DRN, while reverse microdialysis of the GABA antagonist picrotoxin completely abolished REM sleep. For comparative purposes, it is noted that the approximately threefold increase in REM sleep observed with microdialysis application of the $5HT_{1A}$ agonist 8-OH-DPAT to the DRN by Portas et al.[66] described

earlier was greater, suggesting that factors other than GABA might influence serotonergic neurons. Although the data did not directly support GABAergic inhibition as a mechanism of the slowing of serotonergic unit discharge in the passage from wakefulness to SWS, Nitz and Siegel noted the possibility that a small increase in the release of GABA, possibly beyond the resolution of the microdialysis technique, might be sufficient to reduce DRN unit discharge in SWS, a suggestion indirectly supported by data from Levine and Jacobs.[76]

Microiontophoresis of DRN Neurons. Gervasoni et al.[77] reported that, in the unanesthetized but head-restrained rat, the iontophoretic application of bicuculline on rodent DRN serotonergic neurons, identified by their discharge characteristics, induced a tonic discharge during SWS and REM and an increase of discharge rate during quiet waking. They postulated that an increase of a GABAergic inhibitory tone present during wakefulness was responsible for the decrease in activity of the DRN serotonergic cells during SWS and REM sleep. In addition, by combining retrograde tracing with cholera toxin B subunit and glutamic acid decarboxylase immunohistochemistry, they provided evidence that the GABAergic innervation of the DRN arose from multiple distant sources and not only from interneurons, as classically accepted. Among these afferents, they suggested that GABAergic neurons located in the lateral preoptic area and the pontine ventral periaqueductal gray, including the DRN itself, could be responsible for the reduction of activity of the DRN serotonergic neurons during SWS and REM sleep, respectively. However, Sakai and Crochet,[68] in felines, were unable to block the cessation in vivo of the extracellular discharge of presumed serotonergic DRN neurons during REM sleep by either bicuculline or picrotoxin application via a nearby microdialysis probe. While it is entirely possible that GABA pharmacologic actions could differ radically in the cat and rat, the most parsimonious interpretation is that the two series of experiments had technical differences.

Locus Ceruleus

Microdialysis in LC. The single published study on sleep-wake analysis of GABA release in the LC region[78] found that GABA release increased during REM sleep, GABA release during SWS showed a trend-level significance ($p < 0.06$) when compared with wakefulness, and concentrations of glutamate and glycine did not change across sleep and wake states. These data, because of the SWS differences, appear to offer more direct support for LC than for DRN neurons for the hypothesis of GABA-induced inhibition causing the reduction in LC/DRN discharge in SWS and virtual cessation of firing in REM sleep.

Microiontophoresis of LC Neurons. Gervasoni et al.[79] applied their methodology of microiontophoresis and single-unit extracellular recordings in the LC of unanesthetized, head-restrained rats. Bicuculline, a GABA$_A$ receptor antagonist, was able to restore tonic firing in the LC noradrenergic neurons during both REM sleep (in contrast to its effects in the DRN) and SWS. Application of bicuculline during wakefulness increased discharge rate. These data, combined with those of Nitz and Siegel,[78] are thus consistent with GABAergic inhibition in the LC during REM and SWS.

GABA and the PRF: Disinhibition and REM Sleep

Pharmacologic Studies in Cats on the Behavioral State Effects of GABA Agents. Xi et al.[80,81] have provided pharmacologic evidence of GABA suppression of REM using agents injected into the feline nucleus pontis oralis, in a region about 2 mm lateral to the midline and more than 1 mm ventral to the LC, a region where carbachol induced a short latency (<4 min) onset of REM sleep. Here GABA receptor agonists (both A and B) induced wakefulness while antagonists (both A and B) increased REM in felines, suggesting that pontine GABAergic processes acting on both GABA$_A$ and GABA$_B$ receptors might play a critical role in generating and maintaining wakefulness and in controlling the occurrence of the state of REM sleep.

Pharmacologic Studies in Rats on the Behavioral State Effects of GABA Agents. In the head-restrained rat, Boissard et al.[82] used microiontophoresis of the GABA$_A$ receptor antagonists bicuculline and gabazine in the PRF just ventral to the LC and LDT, termed the dorsal and alpha subceruleus nuclei by Paxinos and Watson[83] and the sublaterodorsal nucleus (SLD) by Swanson[84] (see also *PRF to LC* earlier). These agents produced a REM-like state with prominent muscle atonia, but the EEG power spectrum was more similar to waking, with little theta activity, and no rapid eye movements or penile erections. In contrast to the cat, carbachol applied to the SLD in these head-restrained rats produced wakefulness and not REM sleep. These data suggested a role of GABA disinhibition in producing some REM-like phenomena, especially muscle atonia.

Sanford et al.[85] assessed REM after bilateral microinjections of muscimol (suppressed REM) and bicuculline (enhanced REM) into the reticularis pontis oralis in rats during the light (inactive) period, but they did not observe the pronounced short-latency, long-duration increase in REM seen in cats.[81] Repeating these experiments in the dark (active) phase would help determine whether the strongly circadian rat differs from the cat as a function of circadian phase.

Microdialysis Measurements of GABA in the Feline PRF. Thakkar et al.[86,87] (and unpublished data) have studied GABA release in the PRF of freely moving cats, after validating GABA measurements by pharmacologically increasing/decreasing GABA release. In four PRF sites, multiple episodes of REM sleep had consistently lower levels of GABA than wakefulness. Although wakefulness was not statistically different from SWS, there was a trend toward lower GABA levels in SWS. These data provide preliminary but direct evidence compatible with GABA disinhibition in the PRF during REM sleep.

A Model of REM Sleep Generation Incorporating GABAergic Neurons

This section briefly summarizes a structural model of REM sleep cyclicity, based on the data discussed previously; Steriade and McCarley[1] have a much more complete exposition. The history of the development of structural models encompasses the history of discovery of neurons and neurotransmitters important in REM sleep, and is one of ever-growing complexity. The first formal structural and mathematical model was presented in 1975 by McCarley and Hobson.[49] This model, termed the *reciprocal interaction model*, was based on the interaction of populations of REM-on and REM-off neurons and mathematically described by the Lotka-Volterra equations, derived from population models of prey-predator interaction. We suggest that the basic notion of interaction of REM-on and REM-off neuronal populations is a very useful one for modeling and conceptualization, even though the description of the populations of neurons characterized as REM-on and REM-off has been altered and made much more detailed. Figure 4–5 describes the "core" features of the structural and mathematical model, namely the interaction of REM-on and REM-off neurons, and provides a description of the dynamics.

Figure 4–6 identifies the neurotransmitter components of the REM-on and REM-off interaction described in Figure 4–5. Steriade and McCarley[1] provide a detailed account of the evidence supporting the model. In this model, cholinergic neurons promote REM through action on reticular effector neurons, which also provide a positive feedback onto the cholinergic neurons: LDT/PPT → PRF → LDT/PPT. (Mathematically, this is the basis of the postulate of self-excitation [positive feedback] and exponential growth of REM-on neurons—connection "a" in Fig. 4–5).

Reticular Formation and GABAergic Influences

Not only may LDT/PPT cholinergic input excite PRF neurons, but there is the intriguing possibility that inhibitory LDT/PPT projections from REM-on neurons impinge onto GABAergic PRF interneurons with projections onto PRF neurons. This would have the effect of disinhibiting glutamatergic PRF neurons as REM sleep was approached and entered. Gerber et al.[87] found that about one-fourth of PRF neurons in vitro were inhibited by muscarinic cholinergic agents. Whether these neurons that were inhibited were GABAergic or not, however, is still not known. Preliminary data in the cat support

CORE RECIPROCAL INTERACTION SCHEMATIC

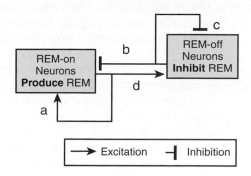

Core reciprocal interaction equations (Lotka-Volterra equations)
$X'(t) = aX - bXY$
$Y'(t) = -cY + dXY$
where
X = Time course of activity of REM-on neurons
Y = Time course of activity of REM-off neurons

FIGURE 4–5 Summary of the "core" features of the reciprocal interaction model. The REM-on neuronal population has a positive feedback so that activity grows (see connection labeled "a"). This activity gradually excites the REM-off population (connection "d"). The REM-off population then inhibits the REM-on population (connection "b"), terminating the REM episode. The REM-off population is also self-inhibiting (connection "c"), and as REM-off activity wanes, the REM-on population is released from inhibition and is free to augment its activity. This begins a new cycle of events. This interaction is formally described by the Lotka-Volterra equations, where X = REM-on activity and Y = REM-off activity:

cholinergic inhibition of GABAergic neurons, since microdialysis application of carbachol to the PRF not only induced REM but decreased GABA concentrations in samples from the same microdialysis probe.[86,87]

Moreover, as outlined earlier, there is considerable evidence that reduction of GABA inhibition in the PRF might play a role in production of REM sleep. First, there are preliminary microdialysis data in both the cat[86] and the rat[88] that GABA levels in the PRF are decreased during REM sleep compared to wakefulness; also, the Thakkar et al.[89] data indicate that levels in NREM sleep are intermediate between wakefulness and REM sleep. Second, pharmacologic experiments support this concept since GABA antagonists applied to the rostral PRF produced REM sleep in both the cat[80,81] and the rat.[85] This postulated pathway of LDT/PPT muscarinic inhibition of GABA PRF neurons during REM sleep is illustrated in Figure 4–6. The dotted lines for this and other GABAergic pathways indicate the more tentative nature of identification of both the projections and their source. This figure graphically emphasizes that inhibition of PRF GABAergic neurons that inhibit PRF neurons would "disinhibit" the PRF neurons and so constitute an additional source of positive feedback. Of note, the GABA levels in wakefulness and in REM sleep in the PRF described earlier[89] are almost the exact inverse of Nitz and Siegel's measurements of GABA in LC,[78] suggesting a possible common source in the REM neurons on neuronal activity of disinhibition in PRF and inhibition in LC REM-on neurons (PRF Wake/REM ratio = 1.7 and LC REM/Wake ratio = 1.7; also see GABA discussion earlier).

REM-Off Neurons and Their Excitation by REM-On Neurons (see Fig. 4–5, connection "d")

There is anatomic evidence for cholinergic projections to both the LC and DRN.[90] In vitro data indicate excitatory effects of ACh on LC neurons, but data do not support

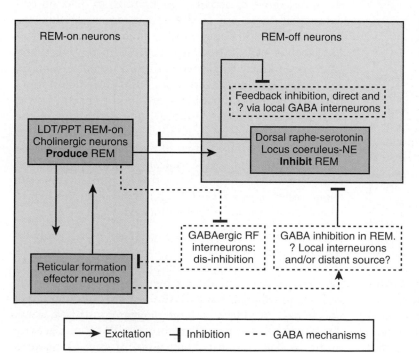

FIGURE 4–6 A structural model of REM sleep control with anatomic detail about the REM-on and REM-off populations of Figure 4–5. See text for description.

such direct effects on DRN neurons.[91] The REM-on neuronal excitation of DRN neurons may be mediated through the reticular formation; there is in vitro evidence for excitatory amino acid excitatory effects on both LC and DRN neurons.

Inhibition of REM-On Neurons by REM-Off Neurons (see Fig. 4–5, connection "b")

After the proposal of the reciprocal interaction model, this aspect was most controversial, since the indirect evidence from in vivo data, although generally supportive, was subject to alternative explanations. However, later in vitro data indicated that a subpopulation of cholinergic neurons in the LDT were inhibited by serotonin.[59] Inhibition is especially consistent for the population of LDT neurons that fire in bursts; such burst firing has been shown by in vivo extracellular recordings to be tightly correlated with lateral geniculate nucleus PGO waves, which other data indicate are cholinergically mediated. The action potential burst itself is caused by a particular calcium current, the *low-threshold spike (LTS)*, which causes calcium influx and depolarization to a level that produces a burst of sodium-dependent action potentials. Some non-burst cholinergic neurons are also hyperpolarized by serotonin. Other data indicate that effects of NE on LDT/PPT cholinergic neurons are also inhibitory.[92] Moreover, noncholinergic, presumptively GABAergic interneurons, are excited by NE[93]; GABAergic interneurons acting to inhibit cholinergic neurons would furnish yet another possible mechanism of inhibition of cholinergic mesopontine neurons by NE, thus further strengthening the model's postulates.

Inhibitory Feedback of REM-Off Neurons (see Fig. 4–5, connection "c")

There is strong in vitro physiologic evidence for NE inhibition of LC neurons and of serotonergic inhibition of DR neurons, and anatomic studies indicate the presence of recurrent inhibitory collaterals. However, there is no clear evidence that these recurrent collaterals are responsible for REM-off neurons turning off as REM sleep is approached and entered. Indeed, from the standpoint of sleep cycle control, one of the most puzzling aspects has been defining what causes the "REM-off" neurons in the LC and DRN to slow and cease discharge as REM sleep is approached and entered. Thus, the prospect that a GABAergic mechanism might be involved is of great intrinsic interest. As reviewed previously, supporting a GABAergic mechanism in the DRN is the in vivo microdialysis finding of Nitz and Siegel[75] in naturally sleeping cats that there is a significant increase in DRN GABA levels in REM sleep. Moreover, as discussed previously, the balance of pharmacologic studies support a GABA-induced suppression of DRN activity. We think it important to emphasize that the issue of GABAergic and serotonergic inhibition as important in suppression of DRN discharge is not an either/or but likely one of joint influences, since, as noted earlier, the approximately threefold increase in REM sleep observed with microdialysis application of the $5HT_{1A}$ agonist 8-OH-DPAT to DRN by Portas et al.[66] was greater than that observed with the GABA agonist muscimol by Nitz and Siegel,[78] suggesting that factors other than GABA might influence serotonergic neurons. Determination of whether the GABA time course of release parallels the decrease in activity of DRN serotonergic neurons during SWS as REM is approached awaits better technology for measurement of GABA with short duration collection periods. GABAergic influences in the LC during REM sleep have been described earlier in the microdialysis experiments of Nitz and Siegel[78] and the microiontophoresis studies of Gervasoni et al.[79]

Source of GABAergic Inputs to LC and DRN

Overall, the DRN and LC findings of increased GABA during REM are consistent with, but do not prove, the hypothesis that increased GABAergic inhibition leads to REM-off cells turning off. The increased GABAergic tone could simply be a *consequence* of other state-related changes without causing these changes. A major missing piece of evidence on GABAergic inhibition of LC/DRN and REM-off neurons is the recording of GABAergic neurons whose activity has the proper inverse time course to that of LC and DRN neurons (see review in Steriade and McCarley[1]). Figure 4–6, of the brain stem anatomy of REM sleep cycle control, suggests that GABAergic neurons in the PRF might provide the input to the DRN/LC. Certainly neurons in the PRF have the requisite time course of activity, but there is, to date, no evidence that these are GABAergic neurons. Within the LC and DRN, Maloney et al.[24] found the extent of c-Fos labeling of GAD-positive neurons in the DRN and LC to be inversely correlated with REM sleep percentage, and to decrease in recovery from REM sleep deprivation. This is of course compatible with a local source of GABA increase during REM. However, unit recordings in the DRN and LC have not found evidence for neurons with an inverse time course to that of the presumptively monoaminergic LC and DRN neurons, suggesting no local source of GABA input. Thus this section surveys data about other sites of GABAergic input with respect to where these neurons might be located.

Periaqueductal Gray. The Gervasoni et al.[77] study on the DRN pointed to the periaqueductal gray as a possible source of the GABAergic input proposed to inhibit DRN neurons. In accord with this hypothesis, both ventrolateral periaqueductal gray (vlPAG) lesions[94] and muscimol injections[95] produced a large increase in REM sleep. Thakkar and colleagues[96] recorded vlPAG unit activity in freely behaving cats, but none of the 33 neurons showed a tonic discharge increase before and during REM; rather, they were phasic in pattern and increased discharge rate too late in the cycle to be a cause of the DRN SWS suppression. These data thus suggest that, although vlPAG neurons may regulate phasic components of REM sleep, they do not have the requisite tonic pre-REM and REM activity to be a source of GABAergic tone to monoaminergic neurons responsible for their REM-off discharge pattern. The negative findings would suggest that, at a minimum, neurons with the requisite activity are not abundant in the vlPAG.

Ventrolateral Preoptic Area. This forebrain site was retrogradely labeled by Gervasoni et al.[77] as projecting to the DRN. Forebrain influences on REM sleep are discussed in Chapter 5, but the Jouvet transection experiments suggest these are not essential for the basic REM cyclicity found in the cat pontine.

GABAergic Neurons in SubC, Pontine Nucleus Oralis, and Lateral Pontine Tegmentum. Recent in vitro preliminary data from mice with a green fluorescent protein knock-in under control of the GAD67 promoter point to these locations as possible sites (see Brown et al.[97]). These mice have GABAergic neurons that are identifiable during the recording session in the in vitro slice by their fluorescence. In all of these locations, a subset of GABAergic neurons was found that was excited by the ACh receptor agonist carbachol, and thus the cholinergic activity prior to and during REM sleep would excite these GABAergic neurons, and thus inhibit target neurons in the LC and DRN. Lu et al.[20] have reported GABAergic neurons in the lateral pontine tegmentum (LPT) that express c-Fos during REM and are REM-off by c-Fos criteria, although their action potential activity has not been recorded.

An Alternative "Flip-Flop" REM-On and REM-Off Model with GABAergic Neurons

Lu et al.[20] have proposed a GABAergic model of REM sleep that has REM-off and REM-on neurons constituting a "flip-flop" model. This model is based on c-Fos expression data, lesions, and anatomic connectivity mapping, but with no cellular electrophysiologic data. The authors noted that their characterization of REM-on and REM-off neuronal activity with c-Fos must be confirmed by electrophysiologic recordings, which also are needed to determine if the time course of activity matches that of the flip-flop model. They found that REM-off (by c-Fos criteria) GABAergic neurons are present in an arc of brain stem extending from the vlPAG and continuing laterally and ventrally in a reticular area they termed the LPT. They suggested that these GABAergic REM-off neurons inhibit REM-on (c-Fos criteria) GABAergic neurons in what they term, following Luppi, the SLD (equivalent to the SubC area or peri-LC alpha in cats) and a dorsal extension of this region, termed the

preceruleus. In turn, the SLD GABAergic REM-on neurons may inhibit GABAergic REM-off neurons in the vlPAG-LPT, suggesting a flip-flop switch arrangement in which each side inhibits the other, and activity in one side is always accompanied by inactivity in the other (Fig. 4–7).

Lu et al.[20] also reported evidence that other neurons in this circuit are important in muscle atonia and hippocampal theta activity. In particular, they found that glutamatergic ventral SLD neurons have direct projections to spinal cord interneurons—apparently not requiring a relay in the medial medulla—that might inhibit spinal motoneurons. Lesions of the ventral SLD caused episodes of REM sleep without atonia, while animals with lesions of the ventromedial medulla with orexin B–saporin had normal REM atonia. In terms of EEG phenomena of REM sleep, a group of glutamatergic preceruleus neurons was found to project to the medial septum, and lesions of this region abolished REM hippocampal theta.

This paper provides a wealth of new data, but Lu et al. did not address how REM sleep periodicity might come about in this flip-flop model. Indeed, from a formal mathematical point of view, two mutually inhibitory populations will not cycle, and some external input would be required for them to get out of a state in which one inhibitory population predominates. The ecological analogy would be two populations of predators, with one

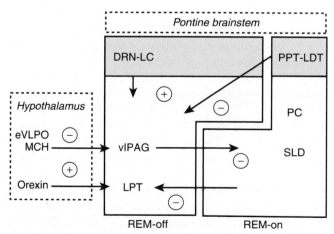

FIGURE 4–7 A GABAergic "flip-flop" model of REM sleep. In this model of Lu et al.,[20] GABAergic REM-off neurons in the vlPAG and LPT have a mutually inhibitory interaction with REM-on GABAergic neurons of the ventral SLD, but also inhibit REM generator circuitry in the remainder of the SLD and the PC in the pontine brain stem. In this model, cholinergic LDT/PPT neurons, dorsal raphe nucleus (DRN) serotonergic neurons, and locus ceruleus (LC) noradrenergic neurons are not part of the mutually inhibitory flip-flop switch, although they modulate it and are modulated by it. Also modulating this circuit are inhibitory inputs to the REM-off population from the extended ventrolateral preoptic area (eVLPO) and melanin-concentrating hormone (MCH) neurons in the hypothalamus, as well as excitatory orexinergic inputs. (GABAergic, γ-aminobutyric acidergic; LPT, lateral pontine tegmentum; PC, preceruleus; PPT, pedunculopontine tegmentum; SLD, sublaterodorsal nucleus; vlPAG, ventrolateral periaqueductal gray.)

eventually devouring the other, rather than the cycling observed in the prey-predator equations of the Lotka-Volterra equations. Moreover, the time course of pre-REM neuronal activity in the brain stem is not an immediate transition from SWS to REM, but rather a gradual change (see McCarley and Hobson[49] and Steriade and McCarley[1]).

Orexin and the Control of Sleep and Wakefulness

Background and Identification of Orexin/Hypocretin

An exciting development in sleep research in the late 1990s was discovery of the important role of neurons principally located in the perifornical and lateral hypothalamus containing the neuropeptide orexin (alternatively known as hypocretin) in behavioral state regulation and narcolepsy/cataplexy. Narcolepsy is a chronic sleep disorder that is characterized by excessive daytime sleepiness, fragmented sleep, and other symptoms that are indicative of abnormal REM sleep expression; these latter symptoms include cataplexy, hypnagogic hallucinations, sleep-onset REM periods, and sleep paralysis.[98,99] An abnormality in the gene for the orexin type II receptor has been found to be the basis of canine inherited narcolepsy,[100] whereas orexin gene knock-out mice (−/−) have increased REM sleep, sleep-onset REM periods, and also cataplexy-like episodes entered directly from states of active movement.[101] Cataplexy in canines and rodents consists of attacks of sudden bilateral atonia in antigravity muscles, with consequent collapse; these episodes last from a few seconds to a few minutes and are often provoked by emotion or excitement, such as food presentation to dogs.[101,102] Confirmation in humans of orexin's importance has been provided by Nishino et al.,[103] who reported that narcoleptic humans often have undetectable levels of orexin in the cerebrospinal fluid, and by Thannickal et al.,[104] who found an absence or greatly reduced number of orexin-containing neurons in postmortem studies of individuals suffering from narcolepsy. As well as the control of wakefulness and sleep, orexins may have a neuromodulatory role in several neuroendocrine/homoeostatic functions such as food intake, body temperature regulation, and blood pressure regulation.[101,105–107]

In late 1997, orexin/hypocretin was identified by two independent groups. De Lecea et al.[105] identified two related peptides, which they termed hypocretin-1 and -2, using a direct tag polymerase chain reaction (PCR) subtraction technique to isolate messenger RNA (mRNA) from hypothalamic tissue. Shortly thereafter, and using a different approach, Sakurai et al.[108] identified these same two peptides, which they termed orexin A (= hypocretin-1) and orexin B (= hypocretin-2). Sakurai et al.[108] used a systematic biochemical search to find endogenous peptide ligands that would bind to G protein–coupled cell surface receptors that had no previously known ligand (orphan receptors).[105] These first two reports indicated that neurons containing the orexins are found exclusively in the dorsal and lateral hypothalamic areas,[105,108] and that the orexins may function as neurotransmitters since they were localized in synaptic vesicles and had neuroexcitatory effects on hypothalamic neurons.[105] Orexin A and B are neuropeptides of 33 and 28 amino acids, respectively; they are derived from a single precursor protein.

Orexin Neuronal Projections and Orexin Receptors

Immunohistochemical studies revealed a distribution of orexin projections that is remarkable for the targeting of a number of distinct brain regions known to be involved in the regulation of sleep and wakefulness, including both brain stem and forebrain systems.[106,109–112] As illustrated in Figure 4–8, orexin projections to the forebrain include the cholinergic basal forebrain (in the rat this includes the horizontal limb of the diagonal band of Broca, the magnocellular preoptic nucleus, and the substantia innominata) and the histaminergic tuberomammillary nucleus. Brain stem targets include the pontine and medullary brain stem reticular formation, the cholinergic mesopontine tegmental nuclei (including the LDT), the LC, and the DRN.

Two orexin receptors have been identified.[108] Orexin A is a high-affinity ligand for the orexin receptor type I (orexin I), whose affinity for orexin B is 1–2 orders of magnitude lower. The orexin receptor type II (orexin II) exhibits equally high affinity for both peptides. Currently there are no ligands sufficiently specific for orexin I and II receptors to define their distribution. In situ hybridization studies of orexin receptor mRNAs[101,113] have shown a diffuse pattern, consistent with the widespread nature of orexin projections, although there was a marked differential distribution of the orexin type I and II mRNAs. Of the brain stem regions involved in state control, only the DRN and the LC appear to show a predominance of mRNA for type I receptors. While orexin A- and B-positive fibers with varicosities were detected in almost all brain stem regions, the highest densities were found in the DRN, the LDT, and the LC.[114] In vitro ^{35}S-GTPγS autoradiography for activated G proteins in the rat revealed dose-dependent increases following localized orexin A administration in brain stem LC, pontis oralis and caudalis, and DRN, and an increased ACh release in the pontis oralis following administration in this region.[115]

Actions of Orexin at the Cellular Level

Orexin A has been shown to excite the noradrenergic neurons of the LC, providing a mechanism by which orexin can promote wakefulness[116–118] and suppress REM sleep in a dose-dependent manner. In vitro work in a transgenic mouse with strong green fluorescent protein expression in the LC that was co-localized with immunoreactive

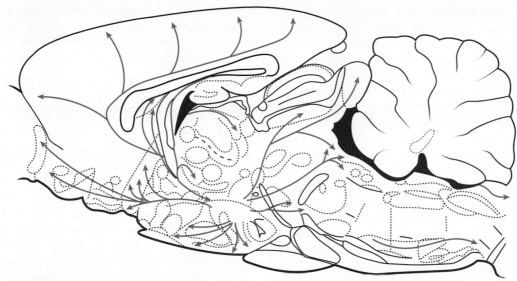

FIGURE 4–8 Location of orexin-containing neurons. Schematic sagittal section drawing of location of orexin-containing neurons (*cluster of dots* in hypothalamus) and their widely distributed projection pathways in the rat brain. *(Modified from Figure 14 of Peyron C, Tighe D, van den Pol A, et al. Neurons containing hypocretin [orexin] project to multiple neuronal systems. J Neurosci 1998;18:9996.)*

tyrosine hydroxylase showed that orexin A and B increased spike frequency, with orexin A being an order of magnitude more potent; the postsynaptic excitation was thought to be mediated by an inward cation current since effects of orexin were blocked by substitution of choline-Cl for NaCl.[119] Another report suggests excitation occurs through suppression of G protein–coupled inward rectifier potassium channel activity.[120]

In vitro work in the rat has shown that orexin rather uniformly excited GABAergic neurons of the ventral tegmental area while effects on dopaminergic neurons were more complex, with approximately one-third being excited, one-third showing development of oscillatory burst firing, and one-third showing no response.[121] Most neurons depolarized in response to both orexin A and B (100 nM), a postsynaptic effect (persisting with tetrodotoxin application). Single-cell PCR experiments showed that both orexin receptors were expressed in both dopaminergic and nondopaminergic neurons. Somewhat surprisingly, dopaminergic neurons in the substantia nigra pars compacta were unaffected by orexins, while, in contrast, bath application of orexin A (100 nM) or orexin B (5–300 nM) greatly increased the firing rate of GABAergic neurons in the pars reticulata.[122]

In the DRN, orexin A and B acting postsynaptically increased the firing rate of serotonin neurons; the excitatory effects of orexin were occluded by previous application of phenylephrine, suggesting that orexin and noradrenergic systems act via common effector mechanisms.[123] Orexin I–mediated effects appeared to be somewhat stronger than orexin II–mediated effects based on both signal strength in single-cell PCR in tryptophan hydroxylase–positive neurons and a slightly greater number of serotonin neurons responsive to orexin A than B.

Interestingly, agonists of three arousal-related systems impinging on the dorsal raphe (orexin/hypocretin, histamine, and the noradrenaline systems) caused an inward current and increase in current noise in whole-cell patch-clamp recordings from these neurons in brain slices. In most cases orexin appeared to activate a mixed cation channel with relative permeabilities for sodium and potassium of 0.43 and 1, respectively.

In an in vitro study of the tuberomammillary nucleus, both orexin A and orexin B depolarized the histaminergic neurons and increased their firing rate via an action on postsynaptic receptors.[124] The depolarization was associated with a small decrease in input resistance and was likely caused by activation of both the electrogenic Na^+/Ca^{2+} exchanger and a Ca^{2+} current. A single-cell reverse transcriptase–PCR (RT-PCR) study in this nucleus revealed that most tuberomammillary neurons express both orexin A and B, with stronger expression of the orexin II receptor. Immunocytochemistry showed that the histamine and orexin neurons were often located very close to each other, and appeared to be reciprocal. Other data suggest presynaptic effects of orexin.[125]

As noted earlier, pharmacologic, lesion, and single-unit recording techniques in several animal species have identified a region of the PRF (the SubC) just ventral to the LC as critically involved in the generation of REM sleep. However, the intrinsic membrane properties and responses of SubC neurons to neurotransmitters important in REM sleep control, such as ACh and orexins, have not previously been examined in any animal species and thus were targeted in this study.

Brown et al.[126] obtained whole-cell patch-clamp recordings from visually identified SubC neurons in rat brain slices in vitro. Two groups of large neurons were tentatively identified as cholinergic (rostral SubC) and noradrenergic (caudal SubC) neurons. SubC reticular neurons (noncholinergic, non-noradrenergic) showed a medium-sized depolarizing sag during hyperpolarizing current pulses and often had a rebound depolarization (LTS). During depolarizing current pulses, they exhibited little adaptation and fired maximally at 30–90 Hz. Those SubC reticular neurons excited by carbachol (n = 27) fired spontaneously at 6 Hz, often exhibited a moderately sized LTS, and varied widely in size. Carbachol-inhibited SubC reticular neurons were medium sized (15–25 μm) and constituted two groups. The larger group was silent at rest and possessed a prominent LTS and 1–4 associated action potentials. The second, smaller group had a delayed return to baseline at the offset of hyperpolarizing pulses. Orexins excited both carbachol-excited and carbachol-inhibited SubC reticular neurons.

SubC reticular neurons had intrinsic membrane properties and responses to carbachol similar to those described for other reticular neurons, but a larger number of carbachol-inhibited neurons were found (>50%), the majority of which demonstrated a prominent LTS and may correspond to "PGO-on" neurons. Some or all carbachol-excited neurons are presumably REM-on neurons. Elucidation of the exact mechanisms by which orexin modulates REM sleep awaits further study, given the generally excitatory effects of orexin observed thus far.

Orexin and the Control of REM-Related Phenomena and Wakefulness

The knock-out and canine narcolepsy data suggested that an absence of orexin or a defective orexin II receptor will produce cataplexy. Where might this cataplexy effect be mediated? In the absence of an effective antagonist to orexin receptors, the author's laboratory decided to use antisense oligodeoxynucleotides against the mRNA for orexin type II receptors,[127] thereby producing a "reversible knockout" or "knockdown" of the type II orexin receptor. Spatial specificity was obtained by microdialysis perfusion of orexin type II receptor antisense in the rat PRF just ventral to the LC (but presumably not affecting the LC, which has predominantly type I receptors). This treatment, as predicted, increased REM sleep two- to threefold during both the light period (quiescent phase) and the dark period (active phase). Furthermore, this manipulation produced increases in behavioral cataplexy suggesting that the REM sleep and narcolepsy-related role of orexin is mediated via the action of orexin in the brain stem nuclei that control the expression of REM sleep signs.

Chemelli et al.[101] as well as others have noted a heavy concentration of orexin-containing fibers around the somata of cholinergic neurons of the basal forebrain. This suggested that orexin might not only act on REM-related phenomena but also on wakefulness control. Indeed,

microdialysis perfusion of orexin into the cholinergic basal forebrain of the rat was found to produce a dose-dependent enhancement of wakefulness, with the highest dose producing more than a fivefold increase in wakefulness.[128]

Orexin and Modeling Circadian Control of REM Sleep

As described previously, mathematically a limit cycle model best describes the dynamics of the REM cycle, which retains its basic cyclicity no matter how it is set into motion (for discussion, see Massaquoi and McCarley[129] and McCarley and Massaquoi[130–132]). While the initial simple model[49] did not address circadian modulation, this was addressed in later modeling, and Figure 4–1 has sketched the modeling of the normal course of a night of REM activity in entrained humans. This smaller amplitude and shorter initial first cycle, as well as the absence of REM activity during the day, was modeled by having the REM oscillator shut off and modulated by excitatory input to the REM-off neurons. When this excitatory input to the REM-off neurons was not present, this allowed the REM oscillator to become active.[129–132] One of the exciting possibilities is that orexin could be the factor (or one of the factors) exciting the REM-off neurons, consistent with its effects on LC and DRN neurons. Experiments in which either the orexin ligand is knocked down or orexin neurons are destroyed are useful in determining if these manipulations destroy the circadian modulation of REM sleep, as would be predicted by this hypothesis. The breakthrough of REM-like phenomena during the day in narcolepsy, a disorder characterized by a loss of orexinergic neurons, is consistent with this hypothesis.

To provide direct evidence of orexin's effect on diurnal control of REM sleep, Chen et al.[133] microinjected short interfering RNAs (siRNA) targeting prepro-orexin mRNA into the rat perifornical hypothalamus (Fig. 4–9). Prepro-orexin siRNA–treated rats had a significant (59%) reduction in prepro-orexin mRNA compared to scrambled siRNA–treated rats 2 days postinjection, whereas prodynorphin mRNA was unaffected. The number of orexin A–positive neurons on the siRNA-treated side decreased significantly (23%) as compared to the contralateral control (scrambled siRNA–treated) side. Neither the co-localized dynorphin nor the neighboring melanin-concentrating hormone neurons were affected. The number of orexin A–positive neurons on the siRNA-treated side did not differ from the number on the control side 4 or 6 days postinjection.

Behaviorally, there was a persistent (~60%) increase in the amount of time spent in REM sleep during the dark (active) period for 4 nights postinjection in rats treated with prepro-orexin siRNA bilaterally. This increase occurred mainly because of an increased number of

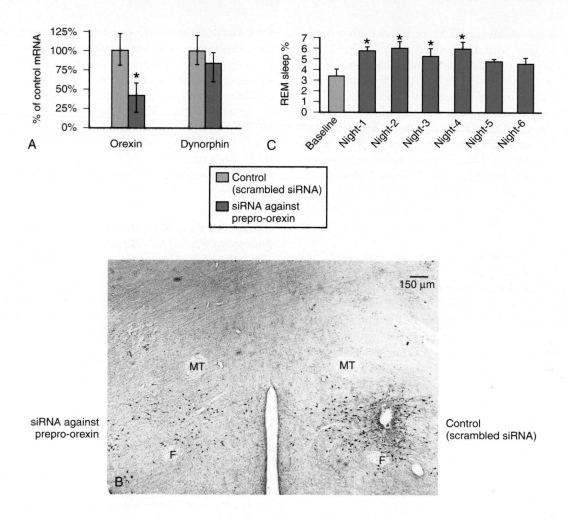

FIGURE 4–9 Short interfering RNA (siRNA) knockdown of prepro-orexin and REM sleep effects. **(Top)** Bilateral injection of siRNA against prepro-orexin into the PFH induced a significant decrease of prepro-orexin messenger RNA (mRNA) but not prodynorphin mRNA ($N = 9$) when compared to scrambled siRNA–treated (bilateral) rats ($N = 9$). Prepro-orexin and prodynorphin mRNA levels in scrambled siRNA–injected rats were normalized to 100%. Their respective levels in prepro-siRNA–injected rats were expressed as percentages of the control. Ranges of gene expression were calculated using $2^{(-\Delta\Delta Ct)\pm SEM}$. *$p < 0.05$. **(Bottom)** REM sleep percentages (*filled bars*) during the dark period after prepro-orexin siRNA injection (bilateral, $n = 6$, *top panel*) or scrambled siRNA injection ($n = 6$, *bottom panel*). There was a significant increase in full-criteria REM sleep in prepro-orexin siRNA–treated animals over the first 4 nights following injection, while scrambled siRNA–treated rats only had a transient change in REM sleep during the first postinjection night. *REM sleep values significantly different from the baseline ($p < 0.05$).

REM episodes and decrease in REM-to-REM interval. Cataplexy-like episodes were also observed in some of those animals. Wakefulness and NREM sleep were unaffected. The siRNA-induced increase in REM sleep during the dark cycle reverted back to control values on the fifth day postinjection. In contrast, the scrambled siRNA–treated animals only had a transient increase of REM sleep for the first postinjection night. These results indicate that the orexin system plays a role in the diurnal gating of REM sleep, and in the consolidation of REM sleep into the inactive phase, as well as indicting that siRNA can be usefully employed in behavioral studies to complement other loss-of-function approaches.

The siRNA knock-down data are highly compatible with other results from genetic modifications. Beuckman et al.[134] studied transgenic rats in which orexin-containing neurons were destroyed postnatally by orexinergic-specific expression of a truncated Machado-Joseph disease gene product (ataxin-3) with an expanded polyglutamine stretch under control of the human prepro-orexin promoter. Of note, in these animals, REM sleep (including sleep-onset REM) was approximately twofold increased over the wild type in the normally REM-poor dark period, arguing strongly that diurnal control of the distribution of REM sleep is under the control of orexin, and, combined with other data, indicating that orexin activity suppresses the occurrence of REM sleep during the diurnal active phase. Constitutive orexin knockouts in mice[135] showed the same level of REM-like events increase in the dark as did the Beuckmann et al.[134] animals, if all REM component events were lumped together (Tom Scammell, personal communication, August 2005). This diurnal control role is consistent with orexin levels in the squirrel monkey[136] and rat[137] and with loss of diurnal REM control in human narcoleptics,[138] as well as with anatomic data showing a suprachiasmatic nucleus–to–perifornical hypothalamus (PFH) projection.[139]

Moreover, Yoshida and colleagues[140] used microdialysis and ^{125}I radioimmmunoassay to measure changes in extracellular orexin A levels in the lateral hypothalamus and medial thalamus of freely moving rats with simultaneous sleep recordings. Orexin levels exhibited a robust diurnal fluctuation; levels slowly increased during the dark period (active phase), and decreased during the light period (rest phase). Levels were not correlated with the amount of wake or sleep in each period. Although an acute 4-hour light shift did not alter orexin levels, 6-hour sleep deprivation significantly increased orexin release during the forced-wake period. Orexin activity is, thus, likely to build up during wakefulness and decline with the occurrence of sleep. These findings, together with the fact that a difficulty in maintaining wakefulness during the daytime is one of the primary symptoms of orexin-deficient narcolepsy, suggest that orexin activity may be critical in opposing sleep propensity during periods of prolonged wakefulness.

NREM SLEEP

This section focuses on NREM sleep. It first discusses homeostatic factors, with a focus on adenosine and the basal forebrain, and then discusses hypothalamic sleep mechanisms. Steriade and McCarley[1] should be consulted for a more complete review.

Adenosine and NREM Sleep

EEG Activation

Although this is often termed *EEG desynchronization*, EEG activation is preferable, because this is the EEG pattern accompanying cortical activity and because higher frequency rhythmic activity (gamma-wave activity, about 40 Hz and higher) may be present, although the amplitude of the higher frequency is low. The early concept of the "ascending reticular activating system" has given way to the concept of multiple systems important in maintaining wakefulness and an activated EEG (see review in Steriade and McCarley[1]). Systems utilizing the neurotransmitters ACh, NE, serotonin, and histamine are also important, in addition to the brain stem reticular systems and the basal forebrain (the region emphasized in this section). The cholinergic system is likely important in activation and, as discussed earlier, we now know that a subset of the cholinergic LDT/PPT neurons has high discharge rates in waking and REM sleep and low discharge rates in SWS; this group is anatomically interspersed with the physiologically distinct REM-selective cholinergic neurons (Fig. 4–10A).[141] There is also extensive anatomic evidence that these cholinergic neurons project to thalamic nuclei important in EEG activation. In addition to brain stem cholinergic systems, cholinergic input to the cortex from the basal forebrain cholinergic nucleus basalis of Meynert is also important for EEG activation, as are GABAergic and glutamatergic cortical projections from the basal forebrain. Many neurons in this zone are active in both wakefulness and REM sleep, and both lesion and pharmacologic data suggest their importance in REM sleep (see review by Szymusiak[142]). This basal forebrain cholinergic zone is discussed next in the context of adenosine.

Adenosine as a Mediator of the Sleepiness Following Prolonged Wakefulness (Homeostatic Control of Sleep)

A growing body of evidence supports the role of purine nucleoside adenosine as a mediator of the sleepiness following prolonged wakefulness, a role in which its inhibitory actions on the basal forebrain wakefulness-promoting neurons may be especially important. Commonsense evidence for an adenosine role in sleepiness comes from the nearly universal use of coffee and tea to increase alertness, since these beverages contain the adenosine receptor antagonists caffeine and theophylline (reviewed in Fredholm et al.[143]). McCarley and coworkers[1,4] have advanced the hypothesis that, during prolonged wakefulness, adenosine accumulates selectively in the basal forebrain and promotes the transition from wakefulness to SWS by inhibiting cholinergic and noncholinergic wakefulness-promoting basal forebrain neurons via the adenosine A1 receptor.

Adenosine, a ubiquitous nucleoside, serves as a building block of nucleic acids and energy storage molecules, as a substrate for multiple enzymes, and, most importantly for this review, as an extracellular modulator of cellular activity.[144] Since its first description in 1929 by Drury and Szent-Gyorgyi,[145] adenosine has been widely investigated in different tissues. The endogenous release of adenosine exerts powerful effects in a wide range of organ systems.[146] For example, adenosine has a predominantly hyperpolarizing effect on the membrane potential of excitable cells, producing inhibition in smooth muscle cells both in the myocardium and coronary arteries, as well as in neurons in brain. From an evolutionary point of view, adenosine's postulated promotion of sleep following activity could be considered as an extension of its systemic role in protecting against overactivity, as seen most clearly in the heart.

Adenosine in the central nervous system functions both as a neuromodulator and as a neuroprotector. The modulatory function, reviewed as early as 1981 by Phillis and Wu,[147] is exerted under physiologic conditions both as a homeostatic modulator and as a modulator at the synaptic level.[148–150] Adenosine has also been implicated in neuroprotective responses to injury or hypoxia, reducing

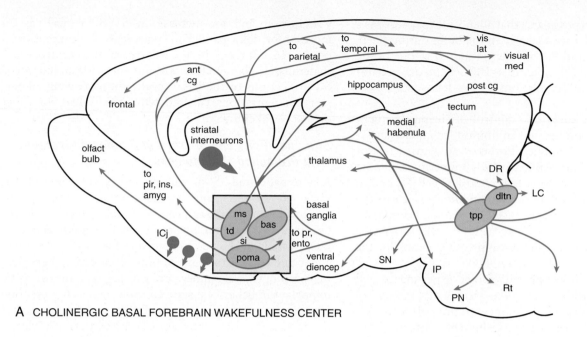

A CHOLINERGIC BASAL FOREBRAIN WAKEFULNESS CENTER

ADENOSINE METABOLISM

ADENOSINE (AD)-MEDIATED INHIBITION OF BASAL FOREBRAIN WAKE-ACTIVE NEURONS

FIGURE 4–10 Cholinergic basal forebrain and adenosine. **(A)** Cholinergic basal forebrain. **(B)** Schematic of main intra- and extracellular metabolic pathways of adenosine. The intracellular pathway from adenosine 5′-triphosphate (ATP) to adenosine diphosphate (ADP) to adenosine monophosphate (AMP) to adenosine is respectively regulated by the enzymes ATPase, ADPase and 5′-nucleotidase and extracellularly by the respective ecto-enzymes. Adenosine kinase converts adenosine to AMP, while adenosine deaminase converts adenosine to inosine. The third enzyme to metabolize adenosine is *S*-adenosylhomocysteine hydrolase, which converts adenosine to *S*-adenosylhomocysteine (SAH). Adenosine concentration between the intra- and extracellular spaces is equilibrated by nucleoside transporters. **(C)** Schematic of adenosine effects on cells in the basal forebrain. Extracellular adenosine (AD) acts on the A1 adenosine receptor subtype to inhibit neurons of various neurotransmitter phenotypes that promote electroencephalographic activation and wakefulness. *(Modified from McCarley RW. Human electrophysiology: cellular mechanisms and control of wakefulness and sleep. In S Yudofsky, RE Hales [eds], Handbook of Neuropsychiatry, 4th ed. New York: American Psychiatric Press, 2002:4.)*

excitatory amino acid release and/or Ca^{2+} influx, as well as reducing cellular activity and hence metabolism.[151] Adenosine also has been implicated in locomotion, analgesia, chronic drug use, and mediation of the effects of ethanol, topics reviewed in Dunwiddie and Masino.[152]

Initial evidence that adenosine, a purine nucleoside, was a sleep factor came from pharmacologic studies describing the sleep-inducing effects of systemic or intracerebral

injections of adenosine and adenosine agonist drugs[153] (reviewed by Radulovacki[154]). The hypnogenic effects of adenosine were first described in cats by Feldberg and Sherwood in 1954[155] and later in dogs by Haulica et al. in 1973.[156] Since then, the sedative, sleep-inducing effects of systemic and central administrations of adenosine have been repeatedly demonstrated.[153,157–159] These effects, and the fact that adenosine is a by-product of energy metabolism, led to postulates that adenosine may serve as a homeostatic regulator of energy in the brain during sleep, since energy restoration has been proposed as one of the functions of sleep.[160,161] Figure 4–10B schematizes adenosine metabolism and its relationship to adenosine triphosphate (ATP).

Reasoning that adenosine control of sleepiness might best be understood as an inhibition of wakefulness-promoting neuronal activity, Portas et al.[162] used microdialysis to apply adenosine to the cholinergic neuronal zones of the feline basal forebrain and LDT/PPT, known to be important in production of wakefulness (see earlier). At both sites, adenosine produced a decrease in wakefulness and in the activated EEG. (Fig. 4–10C provides a schematic of this wakefulness-suppressing action in the basal forebrain.)

However, these were pharmacologic experiments, and the remaining critical piece of evidence was a study of the changes in extracellular concentration of adenosine as sleep-wake state was varied. Using cats to take advantage of the predominance of homeostatic versus circadian control of sleep, Porkka-Heiskanen et al.[163] found extracellular adenosine levels in the basal forebrain were higher during spontaneously occurring episodes of wake compared with SWS. Moreover, adenosine concentrations progressively increased with each succeeding hour of wakefulness during atraumatic sleep deprivation (Fig. 4–11).

These investigators also perfused the adenosine transport inhibitor S-(4-nitrobenzyl)-6-thioinosine (NBTI, 1 mM) to produce a twofold increase in extracellular adenosine in basal forebrain, about the same as prolonged wakefulness. Both prolonged wakefulness and NBTI infusion in the basal forebrain produced the same pattern of sleep-wakefulness changes, with a reduction in

wakefulness and an increase in SWS, as well as an increase in delta-band and a decrease in gamma-band power. In contrast, in the ventroanterior/ventrolateral thalamus, a relay nucleus without the widespread cortical projections of the basal forebrain, increasing adenosine concentrations twofold with NBTI had no effect on sleep-wakefulness.

Site Specificity and Sources of Adenosine Increase with Prolonged Wakefulness

A systematic study[164] in multiple brain areas showed that sustained and monotonic increases in adenosine concentrations in the course of prolonged wakefulness (6 hours) occurred primarily in the cat basal forebrain, and to a lesser extent in the cerebral cortex (Fig. 4–12). Of note, adenosine concentrations did not increase elsewhere during prolonged wakefulness even in regions known to be important in behavioral state control, such as the preoptic anterior hypothalamus region, DRN, and PPT; nor did it increase in the ventrolateral/ventroanterior thalamic nuclei, although adenosine concentrations were higher in all brain sites sampled during the naturally occurring (and shorter duration) episodes of wakefulness as compared to sleep episodes in the freely moving and behaving animals. Not all brain sites were surveyed and so it is possible that some other site(s) might show the same pattern as the basal forebrain. For example, diurnal variations in adenosine concentrations have been found in the hippocampus,[165] although lack of sleep state recording in this study makes it difficult to know if these are primarily sleep-wake state or circadian related. It is also important to note that only 6 hours of prolonged wakefulness were studied, and some preliminary data (Basheer et al., unpublished data) suggest more widespread changes with long durations of wakefulness.

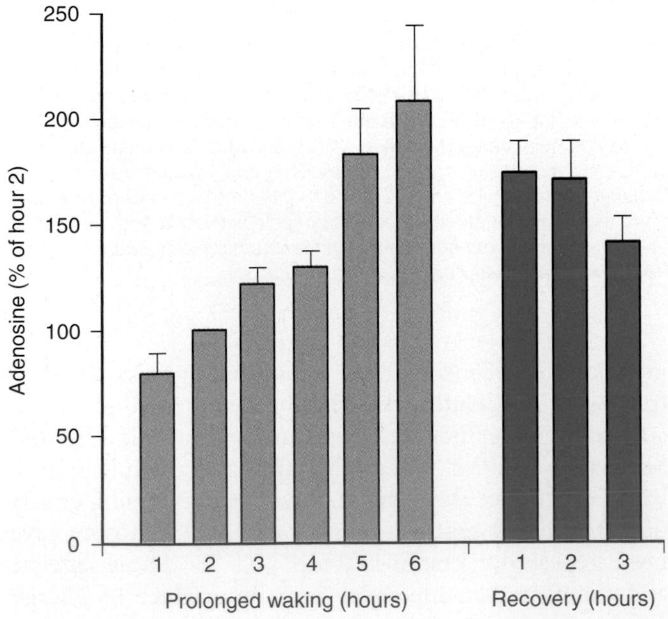

FIGURE 4–11 Adenosine concentration changes in basal forebrain during prolonged wakefulness. Mean basal forebrain extracellular adenosine values by hour during 6 hours of prolonged wakefulness and in the subsequent 3 hours of spontaneous recovery sleep. Microdialysis values in the six cats are normalized relative to the second hour of wakefulness. *(Adapted from Porkka-Heiskanen T, Strecker RE, Thakkar M, et al. Adenosine: a mediator of the sleep-inducing effects of prolonged wakefulness. Science 1997;276:1265.)*

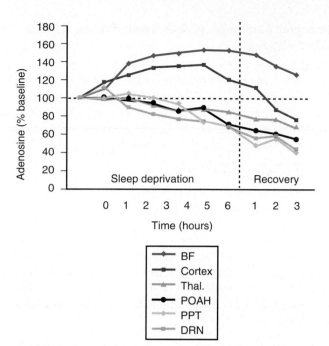

FIGURE 4–12 Adenosine concentrations in six different brain areas during sleep deprivation and recovery sleep. Note that, in the basal forebrain (BF; *top line*), adenosine levels increase progressively during the 6 hours of sleep deprivation, then decline slowly in recovery sleep. Visual cortex most closely resembles the BF, but adenosine levels decrease during the last hour and fall precipitously during recovery. Other brain areas show no sustained rise in adenosine levels with deprivation. This pattern and other data (see text) suggest the BF is likely a key site of action for adenosine as a mediator of the sleepiness following prolonged wakefulness. (DRN, dorsal raphe nucleus; POAH, preoptic anterior hypothalamus region; PPT, pedunculopontine tegmental nucleus; Thal., Thalamus.) *(Modified from Figure 6 in Porkka-Heiskanen T, Strecker RE, McCarley RW. Brain site-specificity of extracellular adenosine concentration changes during sleep deprivation and spontaneous sleep: an in vivo microdialysis study. Neuroscience 2000;99:507.)*

These data suggest the presence of brain region–specific differences in factors controlling extracellular adenosine concentration. There are several potential factors controlling the concentration of extracellular adenosine (see illustration in Fig. 4–10B).

1. *Metabolism*—First, data suggest the level of extracellular concentration of adenosine is dependent on metabolism, with increased metabolism leading to reduced high-energy phosphate stores and increased adenosine, which, via an equilibrative nucleoside transporter, might lead to increases in extracellular adenosine. For example, in the in vitro hippocampus, extracellular adenosine release, shown by ATP labeling with [3H]adenine to be secondary to ATP breakdown, was induced both by hypoxia/hypoglycemia and by electrical field stimulation.[166] Thus, when energy expenditure exceeded energy production, adenosine levels increased in the extracellular space. Of note also, pharmacologically induced local energy depletion in the basal forebrain, but

not in adjacent brain areas, induces sleep.[167] It is worth emphasizing at this point that the equilibrative transporter for adenosine is a nucleoside transporter, and in vitro data[166] suggest that the transporter inhibitor NBTI has the effect of increasing adenosine release from the cell and decreasing inosine and hypoxanthine release, in agreement with the in vivo measurements of the effects of NBTI on adenosine.[163] Support for an adenosine-metabolism link hypothesis comes from the facts that EEG arousal is known to diminish as a function of the duration of prior wakefulness and also with brain hyperthermia, both associated with increased brain metabolism. Borbely[168] and Feinberg et al.[169] reported the effect of wakefulness on reducing EEG arousal. Brain metabolism during delta-wave SWS is considerably less than in wakefulness. In humans, a 44% reduction in the cerebral metabolic rate of glucose during delta-wave sleep, compared with that during wakefulness, was determined by Maquet et al.,[170] and a 25% reduction in the cerebral metabolic rate of O_2 was determined by Madsen et al.[171] Horne[172] has reviewed metabolism and hyperthermia.

2. *ATP Release*—Another potential factor in the increase in extracellular adenosine during wakefulness is the dephosphorylation of ATP, released as a co-transmitter during synaptic activity, by ectonucleotidases.

3. *Regulatory Enzymes*—The biochemistry of enzymes responsible for adenosine production as well as its conversion to inosine or phosphorylation to adenosine monophosphate have been well characterized. In view of the observed selective increase in the levels of extracellular adenosine in cholinergic basal forebrain with prolonged waking, changes in the activity of regulatory enzymes have been examined following 3 and 6 hours of sleep deprivation in rat. None of the enzymes in the basal forebrain, including adenosine kinase, adenosine deaminase, and both ecto- and endo-5′-nucleotidases, showed any change in activity following sleep deprivation.[173,174]

4. *Nucleoside Transporters*—It is possible that adenosine concentration increases and the regional selectivity might be related to differences in activity of the nucleoside transporters in the membrane, although the lack of knowledge about these transporters and their regulation has hindered sleep-related research. The human (h) and rat (r) equilibrative (Na^+-independent) nucleoside transporters (ENTs) hENT1, rENT1, hENT2, and rENT2 belong to a family of integral membrane proteins with 11 transmembrane domains and are distinguished functionally by differences in sensitivity to inhibition by NBTI; ENT1 but not ENT2 has pharmacologic antagonists, such as NBTI.[175,176] Very little is known

about the active transporter. After 6 hours of sleep deprivation in the rat, NBTI binding to the ENT1 transporter, a possible indirect measure of ENT1 activity, was found to be decreased in the basal forebrain but not in the cortex, although ENT1 mRNA did not change.[177] Recent preliminary data from Vijay, McCarley, and Basheer (unpublished) indicate that ENT1-null mice have decreased delta-wave activity during both spontaneous sleep and sleep following deprivation, consistent with data indicating these mice have reduced adenosine tone.

5. *Nitric Oxide*—Another candidate for contributing to the increased adenosine concentration following prolonged wakefulness is the release of nitric oxide (NO) as demonstrated in hippocampal slices[178] and forebrain neuronal cultures.[179] Infusion of the NO donor diethylamine-NONOate into cholinergic basal forebrain has been shown to mimic the effects of sleep deprivation by increasing NREM sleep.[167] Recent studies by Kalinchuk and collaborators[180,181] implicate immune NO synthase in the production of NO with prolonged wakefulness and in mediating the increased extracellular adenosine.

Thus, the mechanism for sleep deprivation–induced increase in extracellular adenosine that is specific to the basal forebrain is not yet clear, but transporter differences and NO release are, in the author's opinion, excellent candidates. Of note, the observed differences in adenosine accumulation during wakefulness suggest the mechanisms responsible for these differences, such as differences in transporters or receptors, might be targets for pharmaceutical agents and a rational hypnotic.

Neurophysiologic Mechanisms of Adenosine Effects

Arrigoni et al.[182] used whole-cell patch-clamp recordings in in vitro brain slices to investigate the effect of adenosine on identified cholinergic and noncholinergic neurons of the basal forebrain. Adenosine reduced the magnocellular preoptic and substantia innominata region (MCPO/SI) cholinergic neuronal firing rate by activating an inwardly rectifying potassium current (I_{Kir}); application of the A1 receptor antagonist 8-cyclo-pentyl-theophylline blocked the effects of adenosine. Adenosine was also tested on two groups of electrophysiologically distinct, noncholinergic basal forebrain neurons. In the first group presumptively GABAergic, adenosine, via activation of postsynaptic A1 receptors, reduced spontaneous firing via inhibition of the hyperpolarization-activated cation current (I_H). Blocking the H current with ZD7288 (20 μM) abolished adenosine effects on these neurons. The second group was not affected by adenosine, and might be identified with sleep-active neurons. Of note, LDT/PPT cholinergic neurons were also found by Rainnie and coworkers[183] to be under the tonic inhibitory control of endogenous adenosine, an inhibition mediated by both I_{Kir} and I_H.

Receptor Mediation of Adenosine Effects: A1 and A2a Subtypes

To date four different adenosine receptors (A1, A2a, A2b, A3) have been cloned in a variety of species, including humans.[152,184] All of the adenosine receptors are seven–transmembrane domain, G protein–coupled receptors, and they are linked to a variety of transduction mechanisms. The A1 receptor has the highest abundance in the brain and is coupled to activation of K^+ channels (primarily postsynaptically) and inhibition of Ca^{2+} channels (primarily presynaptically), both of which would inhibit neuronal activity (see review in Brundege and Dunwiddie[185]). The A2a receptor is expressed at high levels in only a few regions of the brain, such as the striatum, nucleus accumbens, and olfactory bulb, and is primarily linked to activation of adenylyl cyclase. Evidence is available for both A1 and A2a adenosine receptor subtypes in mediating the sleep-inducing effects of adenosine.

Receptor Mediation of Adenosine Effects: The A1 Subtype. Intrapeduncular or intracerebroventricular (ICV) administration of the highly selective A1 receptor agonist N^6-cyclopentyladenosine was found to result in an increased propensity to sleep and increased delta waves during sleep, suggesting a role of the A1 adenosine receptor.[186,187] Studies in cat and in rat revealed that the somnogenic effects of adenosine in the cholinergic region of the basal forebrain appear to be mediated by the A1 adenosine receptor, since the unilateral infusion of the A1 receptor–selective antagonist cyclopentyl-1,3-dimethylxanthine increased waking and decreased sleep.[71,188] Moreover, single-unit recording of basal forebrain wake-active neurons in conjunction with in vivo microdialysis of the A1-selective agonist N^6-cyclohexyladenosine decreased, and that with the A1-selective antagonist cyclopentyl-1,3-dimethylxanthine increased, discharge activity of basal forebrain wake-active neurons[189] in a dose-dependent manner.[190]

Of particular note, blocking the expression of basal forebrain A1 receptors with microdialysis perfusion of antisense oligonucleotides, designed to hybridize with A1 receptor mRNA and thereby preventing its translation, resulted in a significant reduction in NREM sleep and increase in wakefulness in the rat (Fig. 4–13). Moreover, as illustrated in Figure 4–13, following microdialysis perfusion of A1 receptor antisense and 6 hours of sleep deprivation, the animals spent a significantly reduced (50–60%) amount of time in NREM sleep during hours 2–5 in the postdeprivation period, with an increase in delta-wave activity in each hour.[191] The absence of a sleep stage difference in postdeprivation hour 1 suggested that other regions in addition to the basal forebrain (perhaps the cortex) might mediate the immediate sleep response following deprivation. The neocortex is suggested because of the initial deprivation-induced rise in adenosine in

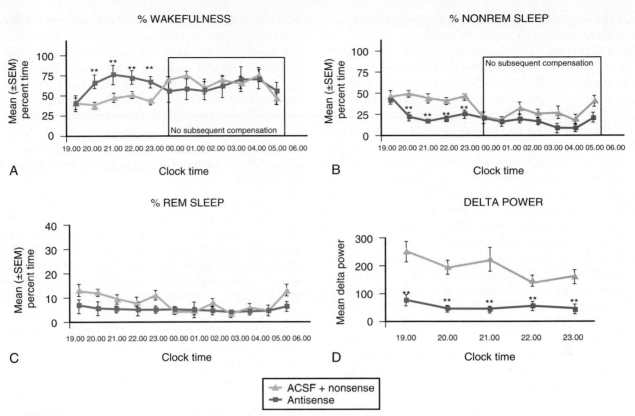

FIGURE 4–13 Effects of basal forebrain perfusion of antisense oligonucleotides against the messenger RNA (mRNA) of the adenosine A1 receptor compared with controls (artificial cerebrospinal fluid [ACSF] and Nonsense pooled) on recovery sleep following 6 hours of sleep deprivation in rats. Note increased wakefulness **(A)** and decreased NREM sleep **(B)** during the first 5 hours of the recovery sleep period in the antisense group as compared with controls. There was a significant increase in wakefulness and a decrease in NREM sleep during the second, third, fourth, and fifth hours. REM sleep **(C)** did not show significant differences. The right part of the graphs (*within box*) shows that, for the subsequent 7 hours, there was no compensation for the antisense-induced changes in wakefulness and NREM sleep. Ordinate is mean % time spent in each behavioral state (±SEM) and abscissa is time of day, with lights off occurring at 1900 hours and lights on occurring at 0700 hours. **(D)** Differences in delta-band power (1–4 Hz, mean ± SEM) for the antisense and the control groups for the first 5 hours of recovery sleep. Note the significant decrease in the delta-wave activity in antisense-treated animals during each of the 5 hours of recovery sleep as compared to the pooled controls (** = $p < 0.01$). (*Adapted from Thakkar MM, Winston S, McCarley RW. A1 receptor and adenosinergic homeostatic regulation of sleep-wakefulness: effects of antisense to the A1 receptor in the cholinergic basal forebrain. J Neurosci 2003;23:4278.*)

the neocortex, but not in other brain regions outside of the basal forebrain. Together, these observations suggested a rather strong site-specific somnogenic effect of adenosine in the basal forebrain, with a lesser effect in the neocortex. The section on adenosine A1 receptor–coupled intracellular signaling later describes the A1 selectivity of this pathway.

In contrast to the findings of the A1 receptor knockdown just described, mice with a constitutive A1 receptor knockout did not show reduced NREM sleep and delta-wave activity following deprivation.[192] Stenberg et al. noted that possible determinants of this unexpected finding were the mixed and variable genetic background of the mice and developmental compensation, perhaps with another adenosine receptor compensating.[192] Based on the presence of some overlap in the effects of the A3 and A1 receptor, this author suggests the A3 receptor might possibly compensate. An inducible knockout would help obviate developmental compensatory factors.

Receptor Mediation of Adenosine Effects: The A2a Subtype and the Prostaglandin D$_2$ System. Studies suggest the adenosine A2a receptor subtype mediates sleep-related effects not in the basal forebrain parenchyma, but in the subarachnoid space below the rostral basal forebrain. Here data suggest that there is a prostaglandin D$_2$ (PGD$_2$) receptor activation–induced release of adenosine, which exerts its somnogenic effects via the A2a adenosine receptor as documented in a series of studies by the Osaka Bioscience Institute investigators and collaborators.[193–197] Data supporting the somnogenic effects of PGD$_2$ have been reviewed by Hayaishi.[197] PGD$_2$ has been implicated as a physiologic regulator of sleep because it is the major prostanoid in the mammalian brain, and the ICV infusion of femtomolar amounts per minute of PGD$_2$ induced both NREM and REM sleep in rats, mice, and monkeys. Sleep promoted by PGD$_2$ was indistinguishable from natural sleep as judged by several electrophysiologic and behavioral criteria, in contrast to sleep induced by hypnotic drugs.

The PGD_2 link to adenosine to exert its somnogenic effects is apparently mediated by PGD_2 receptors in the leptomenenges in the subarachnoid space ventral to the basal forebrain.[195] Infusion of the A2a agonist CGS 21680 (0.02–20 pmol/min) in the subarachnoid space of rats for 6 hours during their active period (night) induced SWS sleep in a dose-dependent manner.[198–200] Infusion at the rate of 20 pmol/min was effective during the first night but became ineffective 18 hours after the beginning of infusion, resulting in a wakefulness rebound and almost complete insomnia during the first and second days of infusion, a finding attributed to A2a receptor desensitization.[201] These data provide pharmacologic evidence for the role of the A2a receptor in mediating the somnogenic effects of PGD_2.[198–200] Moreover, infusion of PGD_2 into the subarachnoid space increased the local extracellular adenosine concentration, although dose dependency was not described in this preliminary (abstract) communication.[202] Scammell et al.[196] found robust Fos expression in the basal leptomeninges, as well as the ventrolateral preoptic (VLPO) region, of rats treated with subarachnoid CGS 21680. The mediator and pathway for leptomeningeal activation of VLPO Fos expression is currently unknown. Scammell et al.[196] speculated that, "Stimulation of leptomeningeal cells by an A2a receptor agonist could induce production of a paracrine mediator that activates nearby VLPO neurons, and studying the effects of PGD2 and A2a receptor agonists on isolated or cultured leptomeningeal cells may help define this local signal." These authors suggested that presynaptic inhibition of the VLPO region might be effected by this paracrine mediator; however, the extant data on presynaptic inhibition of VLPO neurons implicate adenosine,[203] and this effect is likely A1-mediated. Scammell et al.[196] noted that data did not support an alternate hypothesis of A2a effects being mediated by the shell of the nucleus accumbens, since, in reviewing the pattern of Fos-IR neurons from previous work with PGD_2,[204] they could not identify any change in accumbens Fos expression with infusion of PGD_2.

Data indicate that the PGD_2–adenosine A2a system plays a special role in pathologic conditions affecting the leptomeninges and producing alterations in sleep. Roberts and coworkers[205] reported that the endogenous production of PGD_2 increased up to 150-fold in patients with systemic mastocytosis during deep sleep episodes. Subsequently, the PGD_2 concentration was shown to be elevated progressively and selectively up to 1000-fold in the cerebrospinal fluid of patients with African sleeping sickness.[206] It is possible that the A2a receptor system is specialized for the mediation of sleepiness that occurs with leptomeningeal inflammation, in contrast to the more homeostatically regulated A1 system.

It is useful to mention that, in the cholinergic basal forebrain, only A1 and not A2a receptor mRNA (in situ hybridization and RT-PCR studies) and protein (receptor autoradiography) have been detected.[207] These data provide strong evidence that, in the horizontal diagonal band (HDB)/SI/MCPO area of the cholinergic basal forebrain, the effects of adenosine on sleep-wake behavior are mediated through the A1 adenosine receptor, in contrast to the A2a receptor found in the leptomeninges.

Adenosine A1 Receptor–Coupled Intracellular Signal Transduction Cascade and Transcriptional Modulation

Prolonged waking or sleep restriction produces progressive, additive effects such as decreased neurobehavioral alertness, decreased verbal learning, and increased mood disturbances, often referred to as "sleep debt."[208–210] These effects are cumulative over many days and thus, unlike the shorter term effects described in previous sections, are likely to have sleep deprivation– or sleep restriction–induced alterations in transcription as a basis for these long-term effects. Figure 4–14 illustrates the adenosine signal transduction pathways that may be responsible for the relevant transcriptional alterations. Basheer, McCarley, and colleagues[4] have described an intracellular signal cascade set into motion by the prolonged presence of adenosine, acting at the A1 receptor (see Fig. 4–14). Briefly, the cascade consists of calcium mobilization from inositol triphosphate receptors on the endoplasmic reticulum, activation of the transcription factor nuclear factor-κB (NF-κB), and its translocation to the nucleus and binding to promoter regions of DNA. Genes whose transcription is control by NF-κB include the A1 receptor, and there is evidence that this signal cascade results in increased production of mRNA and functional A1 receptor. Interestingly, this signal cascade appears to be confined to cholinergic neurons in the basal forebrain.

Sleep Deprivation–Induced Increase in A1 Receptor mRNA and Functional A1 Receptors in Basal Forebrain and Elsewhere: Resetting the Sleep Homeostat Gain. In situ hybridization and RT-PCR of total RNA from the basal forebrain and cingulate cortex showed that 6 hours of sleep deprivation resulted in significant increases in A1 receptor mRNA in the basal forebrain but not in the cortex.[207] More recent work has shown that longer deprivation (12–24 hours) produces a significant increase in functional A1 receptors, as shown by increased ^{3}H-DPCPX ligand receptor autoradiography binding.[211] It seems clear that prolonged sleep deprivation and up-regulation of the A1 receptor might act to enhance the sleep-inducing effects of a given level of extracellular adenosine concentration beyond that observed before the deprivation, a "resetting of homeostat gain," and a positive feedback that would further promote sleepiness. Over very prolonged periods of deprivation (24 hours) in humans, Elmenhorst et al.,[212] using [^{18}F] CPFPX as a selective ligand in a positron emission

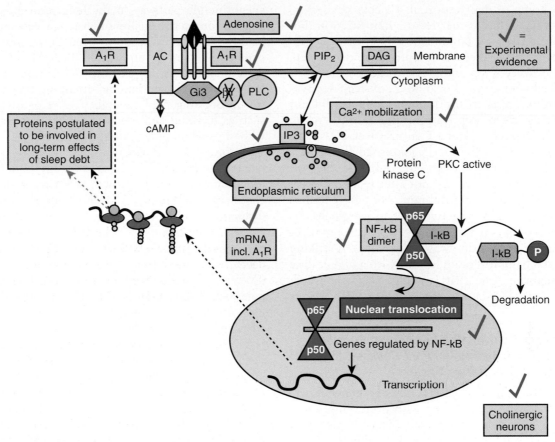

FIGURE 4–14 A1 receptor intracellular signaling pathway in cholinergic basal forebrain. In brief, adenosine binds to the A1 receptor subtype, proceeds through a second messenger pathway, producing inositol triphosphate (IP3) receptor–mediated intracellular calcium increase and leading to an activation of the transcription factor nuclear factor-κB (NF-κB). The activated NF-κB translocates to the nucleus and binds to the promoter regions of genes, one of which is the gene for A1 receptor. See text for a description of the steps in the pathway and supporting experimental evidence. The *checks* in the figure indicate steps for which supporting evidence is present.

tomography study, have shown an increase in A1 receptor binding in the frontal, orbitofrontal, occipital, and temporal cortices. This increase in A1 receptor binding (^{3}H-DPCPX ligand) in cortical areas with 24 hours of sleep deprivation is also seen in rodents (Basheer, McCarley, and Bauer, unpublished data). Not all cortical areas show increased A1 binding; the cingulate cortex, for example, does not. Thus, an important feature of the adenosine-modulated "sleep homeostat" is not only an increasing gain from A1 receptor increases in the cholinergic basal forebrain, but an extension of increases in A1 receptor binding to include many cortical regions outside of the cholinergic basal forebrain.

Basal Forebrain, Wakefulness, and Adenosine: Cholinergic Basal Forebrain Lesions

As noted earlier, the basal forebrain has cortically projecting neurons utilizing ACh, GABA, and glutamate as neurotransmitters, in addition to peptides acting as co-transmitters. One of the questions concerns the relative role of each of these neurotransmitters. The intracellular signaling pathway

with A1 receptor activation leading to increased A1 receptor production is confined to cholinergic neurons, and thus this system is of particular interest. Current findings with respect to lesion effects on the cholinergic neurons differ. The route of administration of the selective cholinergic toxin 192 IgG-saporin makes a significant difference in the results, as discussed in detail in Kalinchuk et al.[213] When saporin was administered ICV, there were very small or no effects on sleep[20,214–217] (Kalinchuk et al., unpublished). However, when saporin is administered locally into the cholinergic basal forebrain (CBF), two separate research groups found, in studies 2–4 weeks postinjection, that spontaneous sleep was decreased and recovery sleep and delta-wave activity were both profoundly reduced.[218,219] These similar results from local injections by two independent groups mitigate against technical error causing these findings.

Kaur et al.[219] found that 192 IgG-saporin injected bilaterally into the CBF transiently increased NREM sleep time predominantly during the dark (active) phase, with a decrease in recovery delta and recovery SWS time following 6 hours of deprivation at 4 weeks postlesion. Kalinchuk et al.[218] found that local administration (but not ICV administration; unpublished data) of 192 IgG-saporin decreased wakefulness and increased sleep. Moreover, recovery sleep and a rise in adenosine levels were abolished after either 3 or 6 hours of sleep deprivation. Adenosine levels in the lesioned animals did not increase during sleep deprivation, nor was there an increase in NO levels. Blanco-Centurion et al.[220] also found that ICV 192 IgG-saporin abolished the adenosine rise with sleep deprivation but, unlike in the two local administration studies, did not alter recovery sleep. Lu et al.[20] found that basal forebrain cholinergic lesions with 192 IgG-saporin or selective noncholinergic lesions with low doses of orexin-saporin did not affect spontaneous wakefulness (deprivation was not studied). A striking finding of total basal forebrain lesions with a higher dose of orexin-saporin was that waking was abolished. Kalinchuk et al.[213] discussed this issue of CBF lesions in more detail.

Sleep-Mediated Alterations in Behavior: Possible Relationship to Adenosine-Induced Changes in the Basal Forebrain Cholinergic System

In the basal forebrain, both cholinergic and noncholinergic neuronal activity is associated with promoting wakefulness.[90,141,221-224] The somnogenic effects of adenosine may be due to the inhibition of neuronal activity in both cholinergic and noncholinergic neurons of the basal forebrain. In addition, the modulatory effects of sleep deprivation on the A1 adenosine receptor mRNA and transcription factor NF-κB activation in the cholinergic basal forebrain suggest the significance of an adenosinergic pathway in the long-term effects of sleep deprivation on the quality of ensuing sleep and/or neurobehavioral alertness, cognitive functions, and mood. The cholinergic neurons in the HDB/SI/MCPO target the entorhinal cortex, neocortex, and amygdala and regulate aspects of cognition and attention, sensory information processing, and arousal.[225-230] Cognitive functions such as learning and memory show a correlated decline with degenerating cholinergic neurons, as reported in Alzheimer's disease patients.[230-233] Wiley et al.[234] developed a technique involving 192 IgG-saporin–induced lesioning of p75 nerve growth factor receptor containing cholinergic cells in rats. The cholinergic lesions using this technique resulted in severe attentional deficit in a serial reaction-time task.[235,236] The CBF is important in cortical arousal. Animals with lesioned basal forebrain show decreased arousal and increased slow waves in the cortex.[237,238] The effects of adenosine on the CBF are thus potentially important as the related sleep deprivation–induced "cognitive" effects may be mediated through adenosine.

Obviously an ability to measure cognitive effects of sleep deprivation in animals would be important. As an initial step, the effects of sleep deprivation on the 5-choice serial reaction time test (Fig. 4–15) in the rat have been examined by Cordova et al.[239] Ten hours of total sleep deprivation produced a pattern of behavioral impairments that were broadly consistent with the effects of sleep deprivation on vigilant attention performance in humans. Sleep deprivation produced a significant increase in the latency of correct responses in a dose-dependent manner, consistent with a monotonic effect of sleep debt on attention. Sleep deprivation also led to an overall

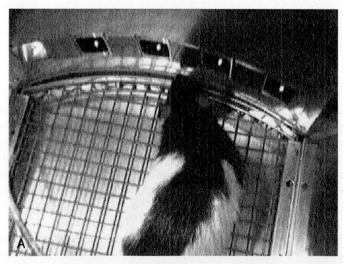

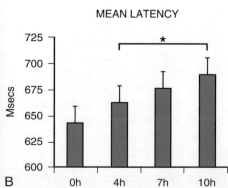

FIGURE 4–15 The 5-choice reaction time test operant chamber. **(A)** This behavioral chamber contains 5 evenly spaced ports containing a light stimulus and a sensor that registers nose entry by the interruption of an infrared beam. In each trial, a 0.5-second light stimulus is presented in 1 of 5 ports (see illuminated port on the *left*). A nose poke into the illuminated port within 3 seconds of the stimulus triggers the delivery of a sucrose pellet into a reward tray in the opposite wall of the chamber that is accessible through a flap door. **(B)** Progressively longer sleep deprivation produces a progressively increasing latency of responses, much like that seen on the human Psychomotor Vigilance Task. *(Modified from Cordova C, Said B, McCarley RW, et al. Sleep deprivation in rats produces attentional impairments on a 5-choice serial reaction time task. Sleep 2006;29:69.)*

increase in the number of omission errors, during which a rat did not respond to the stimulus within a brief period. The same measures are comparably affected in the Psychomotor Vigilance Task (PVT) following similar deprivation lengths.[240] Thus the behavioral effects of sleep deprivation closely resemble the findings in human studies using the PVT to assess vigilance and attention deficits after sleep deprivation. In the current task, care was taken to limit possible lapses of performance from sleeping by requiring the rats to behaviorally initiate each trial and by videotape evaluation of behavior.

These effects are also highly compatible with the effects of basal forebrain cholinergic lesions (saporin) in rats,[235,236] but direct microdialysis measurements of ACh in rats during sleep deprivation will be needed to prove a relationship with decreased cholinergic activity.

Adenosine and a Model of the Consequences of Obstructive Sleep Apnea

In obstructive sleep apnea, the upper airway collapses during sleep. This has two major consequences: The first is the sleep interruption, which prevents individuals from getting a normal amount of deep sleep even though there are no conscious arousals; the second is episodes of hypoxemia, whose intensity and number vary from individual to individual. One hypothesis is that the sleep interruptions might be interfering with restorative sleep and that elevations of adenosine might be responsible. To test this hypothesis, we developed a rodent model in which the animals were awakened once every 2 minutess via 30 seconds of slow movement on an automated treadmill (see description in Tartar et al.[241]). Control rats either lived in the treadmill without movement (cage controls) or had 10-minute periods of movement followed by 30 minutes of nonmovement allowing deep/continuous sleep (exercise controls). In the sleep interruption group, the mean duration of sleep episodes decreased and delta-wave activity during periods of wakefulness increased, compatible with a disturbance of deep sleep. McKenna et al.[242] (unpublished data) found that basal forebrain adenosine levels were significantly elevated in the course of sleep interruption compared to both cage and exercise controls. Adenosine rose monotonically during the sleep interruption, peaking at 220% of baseline at 30 hours of sleep interruption. The levels with sleep interruption were not statistically different from those during sleep deprivation of the same duration. These data point to adenosine as a causative factor in the sleepiness occurring with obstructive sleep apnea.

Tartar et al.[241] investigated the mechanisms by which sleep fragmentation results in memory impairment. Twenty-four-hour sleep interruption impaired acquisition of spatial learning in the hippocampus-dependent water maze test. Moreover, hippocampal long-term potentiation, a long-lasting change in synaptic efficacy thought

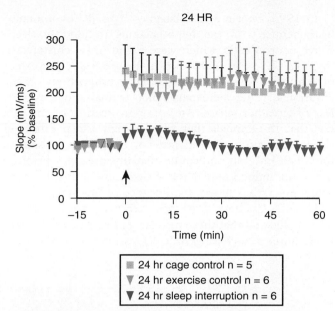

FIGURE 4–16 Effects of sleep interruption on hippocampal synaptic plasticity (long-term potentiation, LTP). Hippocampal synaptic plasticity in rats was examined after sleep interruption (SI) as compared to exercise control (EC) and cage control (CC) conditions. It was found that 24-hour SI blocks LTP ($n = 6$) compared to responses in the 24-hour EC ($n = 6$) and CC ($n = 8$) groups ($p < 0.05$). Graph shows the average responses across time for all groups. The *arrow* represents the time point of tetanic stimulation. *(Adapted from Tartar JL, Ward CP, McKenna JT, et al. Hippocampal synaptic plasticity and spatial learning are impaired in a rat model of sleep fragmentation. Eur J Neurosci 2006;23:2739.)*

to underlie declarative memory formation, was absent in rats exposed to 24 and 72 hours of sleep interruption but, in contrast, was normal in exercise control rats (Fig. 4–16). Whether increased adenosine in the hippocampus might account for these findings is now under investigation.

The VLPO Region and Active Control of Sleep

Identification of Sleep-Active Neurons in the VLPO

Based on his neuropathologic observations on patients who were victims of the encephalitis lethargica epidemic at the time of World War I, von Economo[243] predicted that the anterior region of the hypothalamus near the optic chiasm would be found to contain sleep-promoting neurons, whereas the posterior hypothalamus would contain neurons that promote wakefulness. Indeed, electrophysiologic recordings of basal forebrain/anterior hypothalamic neurons indicated that some of these neurons selectively discharge during NREM sleep, and this might represent an active sleep-promoting mechanism, although the precise anatomic localization remained unclear (for review see Szymusiak[141]).

In 1996, Sherin and colleagues[244] used Fos immunohistochemistry in the hypothalamus to identify sleep-active neuron cells, which were found to be clustered in the VLPO region. As shown in Figure 4–17, the extent of Fos immunoreactivity was directly proportional to the duration of time the experimental animals slept, regardless of circadian phase. An important feature of the data was that the animals that failed to fall asleep following sleep deprivation showed little or no Fos expression in the VLPO region, indicating that this area was involved not in the induction of NREM sleep, in contrast to adenosine, but rather in the maintenance of this state.

Double labeling with the retrograde tracer cholera toxin B showed that these neurons projected to the tuberomammillary nucleus (TMN). This nucleus is the locus of the histamine neurons that are selectively active in arousal and may comprise an important element of arousal systems. Nearly 80% of the retrogradely labeled VLPO neurons contained both the GABA-synthesizing enzyme glutamic acid decarboxylase and the peptide galanin.[245] Electron microscopy confirmed that the VLPO terminals onto TMN neurons were immunoreactive for GABA and made symmetric synapses. VLPO neurons also innervated, although less intensely, the dorsal and median raphe nuclei and the LC (see also Steininger et al.[246]).

Since Fos expression does not necessarily imply increased discharge activity, it is important that chronic microwire recordings in the lateral preoptic area found that neurons with increased discharge rates during sleep

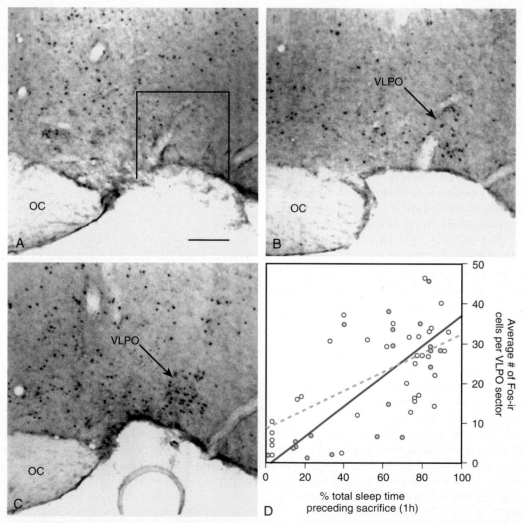

FIGURE 4–17 Ventrolateral preoptic (VLPO) region and duration of sleep. **(A–C)** Fos-immunostained coronal sections through the preoptic hypothalamus of freely behaving rats that slept 15% **(A)** and 63% **(B)** and a sleep-deprived rat that slept 83% **(C)** of the hour before they were killed. **(D)** Correlation between the number of Fos-immunoreactive cells counted in each preoptic sector containing the VLPO region (shown in **A**) and % total sleep time for the freely behaving rats (*closed circles, solid regression line, r = .74, p < 0.0001*) and sleep-deprived rats (*open circles, dashed regression line, r = .70, p < 0.0001*). (OC, optic chiasm.) *Scale = 150 µM.* (Reproduced with permission from Sherin JE, Shiromani PJ, McCarley RW, Saper CB. Activation of ventrolateral preoptic neurons during sleep. Science 1996;271:216.)

compared with wakefulness were most densely located in the same ventrolateral hypothalamic region, the VLPO, as those with Fos expression.[247] Following sleep deprivation, VLPO neuronal discharge rates during NREM sleep were increased, but discharge rates in wakefulness were not changed, thus agreeing with the Fos data indicating that VLPO neuronal activation is related to sleep occurrence and not to sleep propensity. For the group of VLPO neurons with increased discharge rate during sleep versus wakefulness, mean NREM and REM sleep discharge rates did not differ. Szymusiak and colleagues[247] noted that increased discharge from the NREM sleep–selective neurons tended to increase prior to the onset of sleep, leading to a postulate that these neurons might play a role in sleep induction. This finding is not easily reconciled with the Fos data in which animals with sleep deprivation but no sleep did not show increased Fos expression.

Lesions of VLPO and Extended VLPO Area and Effects on Sleep

To study the effects of cellular loss on sleep, Lu et al.[248] made small excitotoxic lesions in the lateral preoptic area by microinjecting ibotenic acid and comparing the numbers of remaining Fos-immunoreactive cell bodies in the VLPO cluster and the surrounding area, termed the extended VLPO area, with the changes in sleep behavior. In animals with more than 70% bilateral cell loss in the VLPO area proper, the amounts of both NREM and REM sleep were reduced by about 55%. The loss of neurons in the VLPO area proper correlated closely with the loss of NREM sleep ($r = .77$), but did not correlate significantly with loss of REM sleep. The loss of Fos-immunoreactive neurons in the extended VLPO area correlated closely with the loss of REM sleep ($r = .74$), but did not show a significant correlation with the loss of NREM sleep. Conversely, when rats were exposed to a period of darkness during the day, a condition that doubles REM sleep time, there was a concomitant increase in Fos expression in the extended VLPO area, but not the VLPO cluster.[249] Retrograde tracing from the LDT, DRN, and LC demonstrated more labeled cells in the extended VLPO area than the VLPO cluster, and 50% of these in the extended VLPO area were sleep-active. Anterograde tracing showed that projections from the extended VLPO area and VLPO cluster targeted the cell bodies and dendrites of DRN serotonergic neurons and LC noradrenergic neurons, but that the projections did not target the cholinergic neurons in the LDT. Because galanin and GABA are known to inhibit both the TMN and neurons of the LC,[250–252] these projections from the VLPO cluster and extended VLPO area are likely to be inhibitory, and, by implication, so are the DRN and cholinergic zone projections.

In summarizing their functional view of these findings, Lu and colleagues in the Saper laboratory[249] proposed that, during NREM sleep, the sleep-active neurons in the VLPO cluster inhibit the activity of the cells in the TMN, DRN, and LC by releasing galanin and GABA, thus maintaining SWS. During the transition from NREM to REM sleep, the firing of DRN and LC neurons is further decreased. Lu and colleagues proposed that this transition may be attributable at least in part to the recruitment of inhibitory neurons in the extended VLPO area that further decrease LC and DRN firing, thus disinhibiting the LDT and PPT cholinergic cells (see earlier discussion and Fig. 4–7). In addition, if extended VLPO efferents end on inhibitory interneurons in the LDT/PPT, they could further promote their firing during the transition to REM sleep. The connections of the extended VLPO neurons and their REM-active pattern would make them prime candidates to fulfill this role.

Relationship of VLPO to Other Preoptic Regions and the Suprachiasmatic Nucleus

With respect to other preoptic regions, Gong et al.[253] have reported increased Fos expression with spontaneous sleep (9:00–11:00 AM) compared with forced wakefulness in the rat median preoptic nucleus (MnPO) as well as in the VLPO region. They postulated that this area, particularly at high ambient temperatures, where Fos expression increased in the MnPO, might act in concert with the VLPO region to promote sleep. Subsequently unit recordings in MnPO by this laboratory[254] revealed that most neurons showed a heightened discharge in both NREM and REM sleep, and it was hypothesized that this region might, like the VLPO region, have GABAergic/galaninergic cells that inhibited wakefulness-promoting systems. While there is evidence for MnPO projections to monaminergic nuclei and to the VLPO region,[255] as well as preoptic projections to the CBF,[256] the neurotransmitter identity of MnPO cells is unknown.

The relationship of the VLPO region to other state control areas is currently under vigorous investigation. The suprachiasmatic nucleus projections to the VLPO region have been shown to be sparse, but the heavy input to the VLPO region from the dorsomedial hypothalamus, which receives direct and indirect suprachiasmatic nucleus inputs, could provide an alternate pathway regulating the circadian timing of sleep.[257] Other inputs to the VLPO region include histaminergic, noradrenergic, and serotonergic fibers, the lateral hypothalamic area, autonomic regions including the infralimbic cortex and parabrachial nucleus, and limbic regions including the lateral septal nucleus and ventral subiculum. Light to moderate inputs arose from orexin- and melanin-concentrating hormone neurons, but cholinergic or dopaminergic inputs were extremely sparse.

VLPO and Adenosine

In vitro studies in the rat of VLPO neurons have indicated the presence of inhibitory postsynaptic currents (IPSCs) that were fully blocked by bicuculline, suggesting they are GABA$_A$-mediated events.[188,203] Adenosine reduced the frequency of spontaneous IPSCs in 11 of 17 VLPO neurons (mean reduction 63%). Chamberlin et al.[258] confirmed and extended this effect of adenosine on IPSCs, finding it present with bath application of tetrodotoxin, and occurring in neurons expressing galanin mRNA. Thus, in addition to a possible direct action of anatomically defined inputs to the VLPO region, it is possible that adenosine might activate VLPO neurons through presynaptic inhibition of GABAergic inhibitory inputs. Microdialysis in the cat in the VLPO region provided no evidence of adenosine concentration increases with prolonged wakefulness (see Porkka-Heiskanen et al.[164]). However, the VLPO region is a small target, and it is possible the probe did not precisely or exclusively sample the small VLPO region. As discussed in the earlier section on adenosine and NREM sleep, the Hayaishi laboratory has shown that subarachnoid administration of adenosine or its agonists promotes sleep and induces expression of Fos protein in VLPO neurons.

It is possible that the VLPO GABAergic inputs arise from the lateral hypothalamus or lateral septum.[255] Although the function of the lateral septum neurons is unknown, they receive extensive inputs from the hippocampus, amygdala, midline thalamus, and brain stem monoaminergic arousal system[259] and thus may relay emotional and arousal signals that inhibit VLPO neurons during periods of stress or anxiety. Much work remains to be done to identify the sources of control of VLPO neurons.

Modeling the VLPO Region Control of Sleep

The precise mechanism controlling the "turning on" of the VLPO NREM sleep–active neurons is unknown, although adenosine is a candidate. Disinhibition of VLPO neurons by adenosine should inhibit the monoaminergic ascending arousal system, and thus induce sleep.[244–246] Chou and colleagues recently proposed that mutual inhibition between the VLPO region and ascending monoamine systems can act as a bi-stable "flip-flop" switch.[255,260] The tendency for each side of the switch to reinforce its own activity by inhibiting the other side may be a mechanism for ensuring rapid state transitions, from wakefulness to sleep and vice versa. By reducing GABAergic inhibition of the VLPO region, adenosine may act as a homeostatic sleep signal, tilting the balance toward sleep.

ACKNOWLEDGMENTS

This work was supported by awards from the Department of Veterans Affairs, Medical Research Service, and the National Institute of Mental Health (R37 MH39,683 and R01 MH40,799).

◔ REFERENCES

A full list of references are available at www.expertconsult.com

CHAPTER 5

Neurophysiologic Mechanisms of Slow-Wave (Non–Rapid Eye Movement) Sleep

Mircea Steriade

The behavioral state of sleep consists of two basic stages, as distinct as night and day. *Slow-wave* sleep (SWS), also termed *non–rapid eye movement* (NREM) sleep, and characterized by the large-scale synchronization of brain electrical activity recorded by the electroencephalogram (EEG), is antinomic to the waking state. The other stage of sleep, usually termed *rapid eye movement* (REM) sleep because of the eye movements that characterize it, is accompanied by dreaming episodes (more numerous and of different nature than those in SWS) and tempestuous activity of the brain, similar to or even exceeding the level of alertness seen during the state of wakefulness.

The dual nature of sleep is reflected by very dissimilar brain oscillations during the two sleep stages. During NREM sleep, EEG displays low-frequency (<15-Hz) thalamic and cortical rhythms that are synchronized among large neuronal populations and whose basic components are prolonged inhibitions. One of the functional roles played by these inhibitory processes is to disconnect the brain from the outside world. Both thalamic and cortical cells continue to discharge at surprisingly high rates for a presumably inactive state, however, thus suggesting that some important brain operations take place during the stage of NREM sleep. During REM sleep, the low-frequency EEG rhythms are suppressed and fast oscillations (20–40 Hz) appear. Contrary to low-frequency rhythms, the synchronization of fast rhythms is confined to more restricted territories.

This chapter deals with (1) the notion of *sleep centers* as opposed to distributed systems, in relation to the concepts of the passive or active nature of sleep; (2) the physiologic and behavioral evidence for brain deafferentation during sleep and the brain level at which the disconnection from signals arising in the outside world takes place; (3) the various types of low-frequency oscillations that appear in different SWS epochs; and (4) the cellular substrates and possible functions of these rhythms. A more detailed treatment of these topics may be found in monographs on the thalamocortical (TC) systems,[1,2] which play a major role in the generation of SWS oscillations, and the modulation of these systems by ascending brain stem reticular projections that contribute to the shift from SWS to waking and REM sleep.[3]

DISTRIBUTED SYSTEMS GENERATING THE STATE OF SLOW-WAVE SLEEP

The hypotheses postulating that sleep is a passive phenomenon due to the closure of cerebral gates (brain deafferentation) or, alternatively, an active phenomenon promoted by inhibitory mechanisms arising in some hypnogenic cerebral areas, have long been considered as opposing views. The passive and active mechanisms are probably successive steps within a chain of events, however, and they may be complementary rather than opposing.

The concept of *sleep centers* that has prevailed in the literature implies that circumscribed brain territories may generate different behavioral states of vigilance. Since the early clinical-anatomic studies of the 1920s, it has been thought that waking and sleep are generated within the posterior and anterior parts of the hypothalamus, respectively. Sleeping sickness followed lesions of the posterior hypothalamus, whereas postencephalitic insomnia was associated with prominent damage in the preoptic area of the anterior hypothalamus (reviewed in Moruzzi[4]). The clinical-anatomic observations have been followed by experimental studies suggesting the antagonistic nature of the anterior (hypnogenic) and posterior (awakening) areas of the hypothalamus[5] and proposing that an inhibitory circuit links the anterior hypothalamus to posterior arousing areas.[6] This hypothesis found support in experiments reporting long-term insomnia produced by electrolytic lesions of the preoptic area.[7] The descending circuit is now substantiated by the identification of inhibitory pathways from the anterior to the posterior hypothalamus,[8] and physiologically by the specific activation of some ventrolateral preoptic neurons during NREM sleep.[9] Recordings of neuronal activity within and around the anterior hypothalamic area, however, which includes heterogenous neuronal types using different neurotransmitters and having different projection fields, show great variability in relation to behavioral states of vigilance, with most neurons displaying an increased rate of discharge during wakefulness.[10]

That insomnia is produced by anterior hypothalamic lesions does not imply that the anterior hypothalamic area is *necessary* for sleep. After insomnia resulting from the lesion of preoptic neurons, reversible inactivation of posterior hypothalamic neurons produces recovery of sleep.[11] Thus, sleep can be restored by the removal of activating actions exerted by posterior hypothalamic histaminergic neurons, and there is no need to consider the "active inhibitory hypnogenic" properties of preoptic neurons as indispensable for NREM sleep.

Rather than being generated in discrete brain centers, waking and sleep states are produced by complex chains of interconnected systems. Most experimental data favor this contention. It follows that a lesion of one sector of interconnected neuronal groups will *not* be followed by a permanent disturbance in a given state of vigilance, but by compensatory phenomena due to the presence of remaining circuits, consisting of neurons with properties similar to those of lesioned neurons. After large chemical lesions of activating mesencephalic tegmental neurons, the state of NREM sleep increases in duration, at the expense of wakefulness, over the course of 3–4 days; however, this is followed by a period in which waking recovers and even exceeds control values, possibly due to denervation hypersensitivity in target neurons of the thalamus and nucleus basalis[12] (Fig. 5–1).

There is a redundancy of brain stem and supramesencephalic neurons that possess activating properties. Some neurotransmitters exert actions on postsynaptic targets that are very similar to those of neurotransmitters released by parallel projection pathways. For example, mesopontine cholinergic cells project to the thalamus[13,14] and exert activating effects during both waking and REM sleep.[15] However, many other brain stem reticular cells, probably using glutamate as a neurotransmitter, also project to the thalamus and similarly display increased firing rates reliably preceding brain-active states, waking, and REM sleep.[16] Acetylcholine (ACh) exerts activating effects on TC neurons partly due to the blockage of a "leak" K^+ conductance, similar to the glutamatergic action mediated by metabotropic glutamate receptors on the same neurons.[17] It is no surprise, then, that after extensive lesions of mesopontine cholinergic nuclei, TC systems continue to display signs of activation. This is due to the fact that many other brain stem systems (among them glutamatergic) remain intact. Although there is a large body of cellular studies, mainly from in vitro experiments, concerning the actions of different neurotransmitters, the synergistic or competitive effects of chemical substances released in concert on

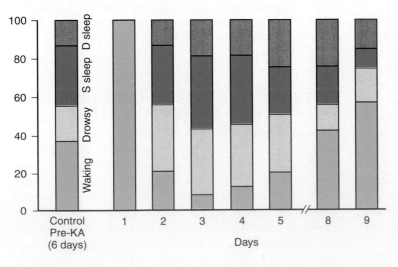

FIGURE 5–1 Evolution of wake-sleep cycle after kainate (KA) injection in the mesencephalic reticular formation in chronically implanted cat. Control was taken from average of 6 days before injection. S sleep indicates NREM sleep. D sleep indicates REM sleep. Note permanent arousal during 1 day (corresponding to the period of KA-induced excitation of midbrain reticular perikarya), diminution in waking duration for the next 4 days, and recovery, even above control value, after 8–9 days. (See histology and electrographic patterns in Steriade.[12])

natural awakening from sleep are still unknown. To give only one example, ACh inhibits thalamic reticular (RE) γ-aminobutyric acidergic (GABAergic) neurons, whereas norepinephrine and serotonin, which are simultaneously released on arousal, exert depolarizing actions on the same inhibitory neurons.[18] The study of these competitive actions remains a tantalizing task for the future.

One of the major factors accounting for sleep-inducing effects of prolonged wakefulness is adenosine (AD). Both mesopontine and basal forebrain cholinergic neurons are under the tonic inhibitory control of endogenous AD, and the extracellular concentration of AD is proportional to brain metabolic rate. AD exerts an inhibitory tone on mesopontine cholinergic neurons by an inwardly rectifying potassium conductance and by inhibition of a hyperpolarization-activated current (I_H).[19] That AD mediates the hypnogenic effects of prolonged wakefulness was demonstrated by microdialysis studies showing that an increase in extracellular AD concentration leads to a decrease in wakefulness (see details in Chapter 3). The conclusion of these experiments is that AD is a physiologic sleep factor that mediates somnogenic effects of prior wakefulness.

To summarize, the idea of *sleep centers* should be abandoned because none of the previously hypothesized centers has proved necessary and sufficient for the induction and maintenance of NREM sleep. On the basis of cellular studies indicating that some neurons display signs of increased activity preceding the electrographic signs defining various behavioral states of vigilance, the notion of *prime-mover* cells was introduced. This concept is sterile because whenever such presumptive cells are detected, the question arises: What is behind this neuronal change? The search is only transferred one synapse before, climbing a hypothetical hierarchic line.

In fact, NREM sleep is generated by a series of phenomena generated in interconnected structures, including inhibition of activating cellular aggregates, thus finally resulting in disfacilitation of target structures, as postulated by the passive theory of sleep. At this time, the best candidate for a neuronal circuit implicated in the process of falling asleep is the inhibitory GABAergic projection from the preoptic area in the anterior hypothalamus to the activating histaminergic area in the tuberoinfundibular region of the posterior hypothalamus. The rostral projections of the latter are the thalamus and cerebral cortex. Thus, the inhibition of histaminergic neurons results in disfacilitation of the thalamus and cerebral cortex. In addition to rostral targets in the diencephalon and telencephalon, the histaminergic neurons of the posterior hypothalamus also project downward to the reticular core of the upper brain stem and excite mesopontine cholinergic neurons.[20] Thus, the inhibition exerted on these posterior hypothalamic neurons by the GABAergic anterior hypothalamic cells also results in disfacilitation of mesopontine cholinergic neurons, with obvious deafferentation consequences in TC systems. All the above represent an avalanche of disfacilitory processes[15,16] (Fig. 5–2).

BRAIN DISCONNECTION FROM THE EXTERNAL WORLD DURING NREM SLEEP

The idea that sleep is essentially caused by the diminution or cessation of sensory signals assailing the brain during wakefulness is two millennia old and was substantiated more recently by transection experiments. When the brain stem is transected at the bulbospinal level, the encephalon displays fluctuations between waking and

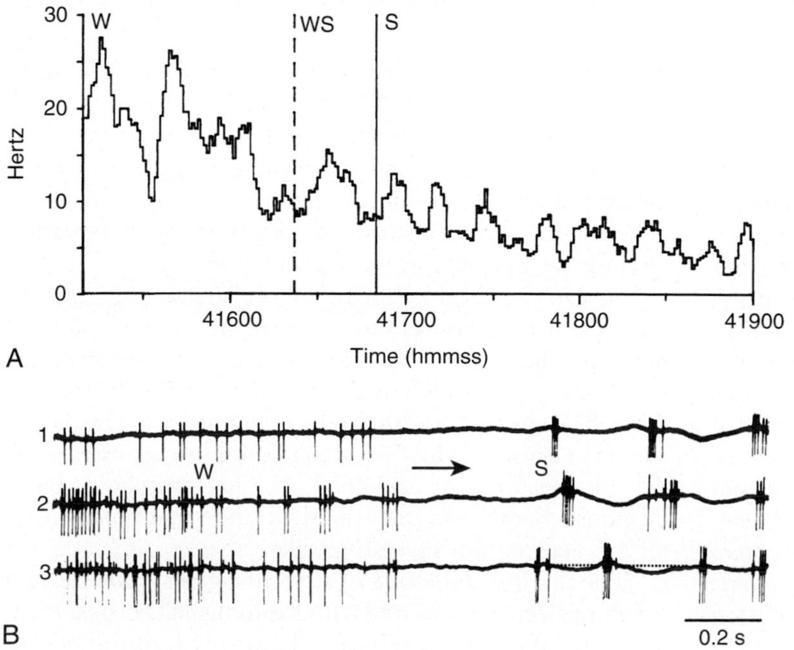

A

B

FIGURE 5–2 Neuronal activities during transition from wake (W) to sleep (S) suggests that an avalanche of disfacilitory processes underlies the process of falling asleep. **(A)** Thalamic-projecting neuron from the pedunculopontine tegmental cholinergic nucleus decreases firing rate (ordinate) from W to S (WS indicates the transitional period marked by the first EEG signs). Abscissa (~4 minutes) indicates time (hours, minutes, seconds). **(B)** Corticothalamic neuron stops firing for 0.3–0.4 seconds during transition from W to S. *(Adapted from Steriade M, Datta S, Paré D, et al. Neuronal activities in brainstem cholinergic nuclei related to tonic activation processes in thalamocortical systems. J Neurosci 1990;10:2541; and Steriade M. Cortical long-axoned cells and putative interneurons during the sleep-waking cycle. Behav Brain Sci 1978;3:465.)*

sleep, whereas a transection at the upper brain stem is followed by ocular and EEG signs resembling those of deep barbiturate narcosis.[21] The conclusion of Bremer's experiments[21] was that the cerebral tonus is maintained by a steady flow of sensory input reaching the brain stem between the medulla and midbrain, and that sleep results from the withdrawal of sensory bombardment. Subsequently, the EEG activation exerted by the ascending brain stem reticular neurons has been demonstrated.[4]

Animal experiments and clinical studies have corroborated Bremer's pioneering observations. Gross impairments of the state of vigilance, leading to hypersomnia, result from lesions of the mesopontine reticular neurons or bilateral lesions of thalamic intralaminar nuclei, which represent the rostral continuation of the brain stem reticular formation.[22] Thalamic intralaminar neurons are directly excited from the mesopontine reticular core, and they project to widespread cortical areas where they exert excitatory actions.[23] Studies of patients with prolonged lethargy led to the conclusion that the brain stem–thalamocortical circuit effectively contributes to the maintenance of alertness in higher mammals, especially in primates. The role of thalamic intralaminar nuclei in regulating arousal is also suggested by the fact that their activity increases during a task requiring alertness and attention in humans.[24] Parallel extrathalamic pathways, through which brain stem reticular neurons influence the cerebral cortex, are relayed by histaminergic projections of posterior hypothalamic (tuberoinfundibular) neurons and by cholinergic projections of the nucleus basalis.[25]

The basic mechanism of falling asleep is the transformation of a brain responsive to external signals into a closed brain. In humans, the onset of sleep is associated with functional blindness.[26] The obliteration of messages from the outside world at sleep onset is due to inhibitory processes that are reflected in peculiar EEG rhythms generated in the thalamus and cerebral cortex, as well as to the decreased excitability of both thalamic and cortical neurons.

That the transmission of afferent signals is reduced at the thalamic level from the very onset of natural sleep was first shown by recording field potentials in dorsal thalamic nuclei.[27] It was demonstrated that the thalamic responses to stimuli applied to prethalamic axon bundles are diminished from the drowsy state and that the postsynaptic waves are completely obliterated during further deepening of sleep, despite no measurable change in the presynaptic component that monitors the magnitude of prethalamic input[28] (Fig. 5–3). Indeed, simultaneous recordings from the thalamus and different relay stations in the brain stem or the retinogeniculate axons showed that, during the period of falling asleep, the diminished postsynaptic responses in dorsal thalamic nuclei are not paralleled by alterations in afferent pathways. *This demonstrates that the thalamus is the first relay station at which reduction of afferent signals takes place when falling asleep.* Intracellular recordings have shown that the diminution or suppression of the monosynaptic response of TC

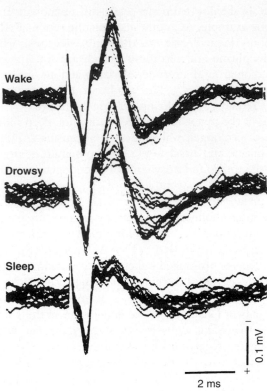

FIGURE 5–3 Blockade of synaptic transmission in thalamus at sleep onset in behaving cat with implanted electrodes. Field potentials evoked in the ventral lateral (motor) thalamic nucleus by stimulation of axons in the cerebellothalamic pathway. Evoked responses consist of a presynaptic (tract, t) component and a monosynaptically relayed (r) wave. Note progressively diminished amplitude of r wave during drowsiness, up to its complete obliteration during slow-wave sleep, despite lack of changes in afferent volley monitored by t component. *(Adapted from Steriade M. Alertness, quiet sleep, dreaming. In A Peters, EG Jones [eds], Cerebral Cortex, Vol 9: Normal and Altered States of Function. New York: Plenum, 1991;279.)*

neurons to afferent volleys occurs during the inhibitory postsynaptic potentials (IPSPs) related to sleep spindles.[29] Thalamic gating deprives the cerebral cortex of the input required to elaborate a response and is responsible for the decreased transfer of information at the cortical level. These processes constitute a necessary deafferentation prelude for deepening the state of sleep.

Instead of high-security, short-latency (1–2 msec), single-spike responses to prethalamic stimuli during waking, the same TC neuron fails to discharge or responds during SWS with occasional spike-bursts at a high frequency (200–400 Hz), occurring at longer latencies (5–12 msec). This fact, described in earlier extracellular studies,[30] was explained by low-threshold burst responses[31] that are uncovered by the hyperpolarization of TC neurons during resting sleep.[1,2]

The thalamic blockade of afferent signals from the very onset of sleep is associated with a diminished cortical reactivity to afferent stimuli. Field potential recordings in animals and humans reached similar conclusions concerning the decreased cortical responsiveness at sleep onset and during later stages of NREM sleep. With testing stimuli applied to prethalamic pathways, the earliest component of the cortical-evoked response is dramatically reduced with transition from wakefulness to drowsiness, with the consequence that the cortically elaborated postsynaptic component is also greatly diminished.[27] The decreased transfer of information through cortical circuits is not merely due to the decreased input from the thalamus, however; it also depends on intrinsic cortical events. In monkeys, the cortical field response evoked by a somatosensory stimulus consists of an abrupt surface-positive component (P1) peaking at approximately 12 msec, and a surface-negativity wave (N1) at approximately 30–50 msec after the stimulus. P1 persists in anesthetized monkeys, whereas N1 does not.[32] It seems that P1 amplitude is a simple function of stimulus intensity, whereas N1 amplitude depends on behavioral discrimination. In humans, the most sensitive components of cortical-evoked potentials during shifts in states of vigilance are fast-frequency wavelets (FFWs) superimposed on the major waves at frontal and parietal scalp electrodes. The FFWs are attenuated or totally disappear with transition from wakefulness to the early stages of NREM sleep.[33]

GROUPING OF SLEEP RHYTHMS BY THE SLOW CORTICAL OSCILLATION

Much more is known about the cellular mechanisms underlying different oscillations that characterize NREM sleep than about the functions of these oscillations or the neural and humoral processes responsible for sleep. The principal neurons involved in sleep oscillations are cortical pyramidal cells, GABAergic RE thalamic cells, and TC cells. Cortical cells project to the thalamus and excite both RE and TC cells, TC cells project to the cortex and give off collaterals to RE cells, and RE cells do not project to the cortex but project back to TC cells, thus forming an intrathalamic, recurrent inhibitory circuit (Fig. 5–4). The local-circuit GABAergic neurons, intrinsic to virtually every thalamic nucleus of felines and primates, play an important role in inhibitory processes that assist discriminatory functions but have only an ancillary role in sleep oscillations.

Three major sleep oscillations are generated in the thalamus and cerebral cortex: sleep spindles, delta oscillations, and slow cortical oscillations. Each of these can be generated in different structures, even after their complete disconnection.

- *Sleep spindles* (7–14 Hz) occur during early stages of sleep and are generated in the thalamus, even after complete decortication. Spindles are due to the pacemaking role of RE neurons that impose rhythmic IPSPs on target TC cells (see Fig. 5–4). The crucial role played by the GABAergic RE cells was demonstrated by the absence of spindles after disruption of the connection arising in the RE nucleus.[34] Moreover, spindles have been recorded in the deafferented rostral pole of the thalamic RE nucleus.[35]

- *Delta oscillations* (1–4 Hz) appear during later stages of NREM sleep and consist of two components. One of them is generated in the neocortex, demonstrated by the fact that it survives extensive thalamectomy. The other component is thalamic and can thus be recorded in vivo after decortication[36] as well as in thalamic slices.[37,38] The stereotyped thalamic delta oscillation results from the interplay between two voltage-gated currents of TC cells.[37,38] This interplay is dependent on the hyperpolarization of TC cells, which occurs during NREM sleep because of the withdrawal of brain stem–ascending, activating impulses.[3] Although the thalamic delta oscillation is generated in single TC cells, it can be expressed at the global EEG level, because TC cells can be synchronized by corticothalamic volleys, engaging RE and TC neurons.[39]

- The *slow cortical oscillation* (<1 Hz, typically 0.6–0.9 Hz) was discovered in intracellular recordings from cortical neurons in anesthetized animals.[40] It consists of prolonged depolarizations and hyperpolarizations (Fig. 5–5). The same oscillatory type was also investigated during natural NREM sleep of behaving cats[41,42] as well as during natural NREM sleep in humans.[43–46] The slow oscillation is generated within cortical networks; because it survives extensive thalamic lesions,[47] it does not appear in the thalamus after decortication,[48] and its synchronization is disrupted after disconnection of cortical synaptic linkages.[49] After preliminary data showing the presence of slow oscillation during natural sleep in humans,[40] the human slow oscillation (<1 Hz) was reported in parallel studies from four laboratories.[43–46] The different aspects of the human slow sleep oscillation are as follows: During stage II of NREM sleep, scalp recordings show a prevalent peak (0.8 Hz) within the frequency range of the slow oscillation as well as a minor mode around 15 Hz reflecting spindle waves. The depth-negative components of the slow oscillation, followed or not by spindles, represent the K complexes. The frequency of K complexes (peaks at 0.5 Hz in stage II, at 0.7 Hz in stages III and IV) is very similar, up to identity, to the frequency of the slow oscillation during natural sleep. The power spectrum reveals a major peak around <1 Hz that becomes evident from stage II and continues throughout resting sleep. The slow oscillation is particularly abundant in frontoparietal leads.

Does the slow oscillation belong to the same category of brain rhythms as sleep delta waves? Is the slow oscillation similar to the so-called cyclic alternating pattern during sleep? The reasons why the answers to these two questions are clearly negative are outlined in the remainder of this section.

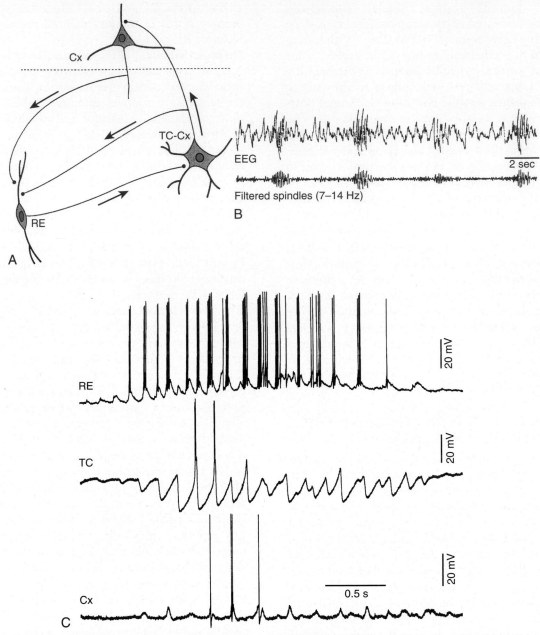

FIGURE 5–4 Generation of sleep spindles in the recurrent inhibitory circuit formed by thalamic reticular (RE) and thalamocortical (TC) neurons, and their reflection in cortical (Cx) neurons and EEG. **(A)** Network of RE, TC, and Cx neurons. **(B)** Four spindle sequences recurring rhythmically. **(C)** Intracellular recordings of RE, TC, and Cx cells during one spindle sequence. Note rhythmic spike-bursts with a depolarizing envelope in GABAergic RE cell, rhythmic inhibitory postsynaptic potentials occasionally leading to rebound spike-bursts in TC cell, and rhythmic excitatory postsynaptic potentials in target Cx cell. *(Modified from Steriade M, Deschênes M. Intrathalamic and brainstem-thalamic networks involved in resting and alert states. In M Bentivoglio, R Spreafico [eds], Cellular Thalamic Mechanisms. Amsterdam: Elsevier, 1988;37.)*

Although the delta rhythm is commonly viewed as a cortical oscillation, at least two types of rhythms are within the frequency range of 1–4 Hz, one originating in the thalamus, the other in the neocortex (as discussed earlier). We have demonstrated that cortical delta waves, associated with discharges of regular-spiking and intrinsically bursting cells, are grouped by the slow oscillation.[47] These data point to the distinctiveness of the two (slow and delta)

oscillations. The other, stereotyped (clocklike), delta oscillation is generated in the thalamus. Intracellular recordings of cortical neurons showed that clocklike delta potentials of thalamic origin occur simultaneously with, but distinctly from, the slow oscillation during a progressive increase in EEG synchronization[47] (see Fig. 5–5). Again, this indicates that the two (delta and slow) oscillations are different types of brain rhythmic activities. With the benefit of hindsight,

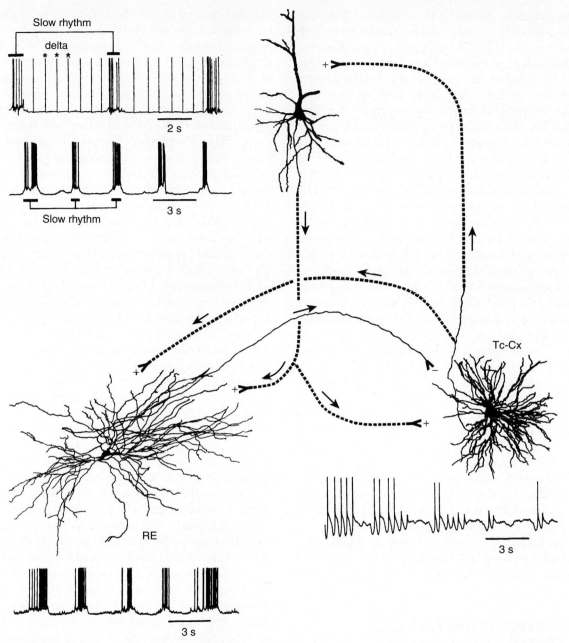

FIGURE 5–5 Slow (<1-Hz) cortical (Cx) oscillation and its effects on thalamic reticular (RE) and thalamocortical (TC) neurons. Neurons are intracellularly stained. Direction of axons is indicated by *arrows* and excitatory or inhibitory signs are indicated by + or −. Note similar slow oscillation in Cx (*second trace*) and RE neurons, combined slow rhythm and clocklike (thalamically generated) rhythm in Cx cell (*first trace*), and rhythmic disruption of clocklike delta rhythm in TC cell due to increased membrane conductance produced by slow oscillation in corticothalamic cells. *(Modified from Steriade M, Nuñez A, Amzica F. A novel slow [<1 Hz] oscillation of neocortical neurons in vivo: depolarizing and hyperpolarizing components. J Neurosci 1993;13:3266; and Steriade M, Contreras D, Curró Dossi R, Nuñez A. The slow [<1 Hz] oscillation in reticular thalamic and thalamocortical neurons: scenario of sleep rhythms generation in interacting thalamic and neocortical networks. J Neurosci 1993;13:3284.)*

one can see, in previous EEG recordings, cyclic groups of delta waves at 3–4 Hz recurring with a slow rhythm of 0.3–0.4 Hz in animals and during light sleep in humans.

As to the "cyclic alternating pattern" of EEG waves grouped in sequences recurring at intervals of 20 or more seconds,[50] it is basically different from the slow oscillation because it is associated with the enhancement of muscle tone and heart rate and was described by the term *arousal-related phasic events*. In contrast, the slow oscillation is blocked during cholinergic- and noradrenergic-mediated arousal in acute experiments[51] and during natural waking in behaving animals.[42]

The distinction of NREM sleep oscillations into three types is useful for analytic purposes. In the intact brain, however, the thalamus and cortex are interacting and their rhythms are combined in complex wave sequences in both animals and humans.[40,45,47] Thus, although spindles may be generated through the network and intrinsic properties of thalamic RE neurons, the mechanisms for the generation of spindles in the intact brain require reciprocal interactions between thalamic and cortical neurons. Indeed, spindles are evoked by corticothalamic projections[52,53] and they are grouped within periodic sequences that display a rhythm (0.2–0.5 Hz)[1,2] similar to that of the slow cortical oscillation. Although the origin of the slow rhythm of spindle sequences is still a mystery and may partially depend on intrinsic properties of thalamic neurons, each synchronous corticothalamic excitatory volley is effective in driving thalamic RE cells and in synchronizing them within the frequency range of spindles. Moreover, the spectacular synchronization and near-simultaneity of spindles in the thalamus and over the cortex is produced by corticothalamic projections, because spindles are more disorganized in decorticated animals.[54,55] Thus, although spindles appear after decortication and can even be recorded in thalamic slices,[56–58] the widespread synchronization of this thalamically generated oscillation, as seen during natural sleep in animals and humans, depends on feedback projections from the neocortex. The interaction between the cortex and the thalamus is also evident when analyzing the relation between the thalamic delta oscillation and the cortical slow oscillation. The intrinsic delta oscillation of TC neurons is periodically interrupted by excitatory impulses of cortical origin within the frequency of slow oscillation (see Fig. 5–5, lower right trace) because depolarizing input brings TC cells out of the voltage range where the stereotyped delta rhythm is generated.

The data presented in this section emphasize the necessity of investigating brains with intact circuitry when exploring the cellular mechanisms of NREM sleep rhythms.

POSSIBLE FUNCTIONS OF SLEEP OSCILLATIONS

Despite the diversity of NREM sleep rhythms, their functional outcome may be similar. As the major components of these oscillations are hyperpolarizations in thalamic and cortical neurons,[1,2] their obvious role is brain disconnection from the outside world. The reduction in neuronal responsiveness might be considered evidence for the hypothesis that the function of resting sleep is the restoration of brain energy metabolism through the replenishment of cerebral glycogen stores that are depleted during waking.[59]

The deafferentation process that occurs from the very onset of sleep and is a prerequisite to falling deeply asleep

may be just the tip of the iceberg. The high-frequency spike-bursts, repeated rhythmically during both thalamic-generated spindles and delta oscillations, may prevent the metabolic inertia that would result from complete absence of discharges in TC cells, if the hyperpolarization were to persist uninterrupted for tens of minutes or for hours during sleep. Counteraction of this metabolic inertia would favor a quick passage from SWS to either wakefulness or REM sleep.[60] Thus, the rhythmic bursts of thalamic cells may keep these cells, as well as cortical neurons, in a state of biochemical readiness for a rapid transition to an active state.[60] The flux of ions, particularly that of Ca^{2+}, across the membrane will maintain biochemical processes in the cell that are sensitive to intracellular ion concentrations.[61] Indeed, the massive fluxes of Ca^{2+} associated with the generation of rhythmic spike-bursts during NREM sleep may modulate Ca^{2+}-dependent gene expression and Ca^{2+}-dependent second messengers. Thus, the possibility exists that sleep rhythms reorchestrate the intracellular processes of neurons to perform tasks best done during quiet sleep.

Sleep oscillations may also assist the brain in complex operations, including plasticity and memory. Contrary to previous assumptions that the whole sleeping system lies dormant for the most part and that sleep is characterized by mental blankness, many cells recorded from neocortical areas of animals have been found to be firing as actively in NREM sleep as in waking, although the firing patterns change from one state to the other.[62,63] One of the mysteries of sleep is the question of why cortical cells are so active when the brain is supposed to rest. Various hypotheses propose that dreaming sleep, a behavioral state known for its association with a highly activated brain, maintains brain hardwiring[64] and consolidates the circuitry encoding memory traces.[65,66] It is now proposed that, in resting sleep—a state that is usually viewed as being associated with the obliteration of all forms of consciousness—the cyclic spike-trains or spike-bursts may reorganize and specify the circuitry and stimulate the dendrites of neocortical neurons to grow more spines, thereby leading to consolidation of memory traces acquired during wakefulness.[67] This hypothesis rests on the suggestion that the rich neuronal activity during the depolarizing components of sleep oscillations prevailingly affects certain cellular groups for which plasticity is important, as is the case for neurons from association areas.

⊘ REFERENCES

A full list of references are available at www.expertconsult.com

CHAPTER 6

Neurotransmitters, Neurochemistry, and the Clinical Pharmacology of Sleep

Max Hirshkowitz, Mary Wilcox Rose and Amir Sharafkhaneh

OVERVIEW

Many medications and other substances are used in sleep medicine. Some are specifically used to either provoke sleep or enhance wakefulness, while others may sedate or stimulate as a side effect.

The number of different pharmacologic agents available today is enormous. Attempting to remember the sleep alterations each produces as isolated pieces of information would be difficult. To facilitate a better overall understanding, as well as systematizing detailed data, we have organized this chapter according to neurotransmitter systems. In those cases in which a particular neurotransmitter system affects sleep in a reliable manner, knowing a substance's mechanism of action can help predict sleep effects. In this chapter, we endeavor to develop "rules of thumb" concerning sleep-related drug effects. Generic medication names are used throughout this chapter. However, because many medications are better known by their brand names, Table 6–1 is included for the reader as a cross-reference between generic and brand names. The table also provide classification of each pharmacologic agent discussed.

Neurotransmitter systems are the organizational backbone for this chapter (Fig. 6–1), and we begin the review by discussing those recognized as excitatory or stimulating. These are the systems that mediate arousal, alertness, activity, or responsiveness to the environment. Excitatory transmitters include dopamine (DA), norepinephrine (NE),

histamine, orexin, and glutamate. The complimentary systems—that is, systems mediating inhibition—are discussed next. These include γ-aminobutyric acid (GABA), adenosine, and glycine. Finally, we complete our discussion with a focus on brain chemistry underlying the overall regulation of sleep and wakefulness and the choreography of rapid eye movement (REM) and non–rapid eye movement (NREM) sleep. This includes the roles of acetylcholine (ACh), serotonin, and melatonin in sleep alteration.

STIMULATING TRANSMITTER SYSTEMS

Dopamine and Norepinephrine

Pharmacology

Dopamine and norepinephrine are monoaminergic neurotransmitters collectively known as catacholamines.[1] In dopaminergic neurons, synthesis begins with tyrosine from the blood that is first hydroxylated to dihydroxyphenylalanine (DOPA) and then reduced to DA. The DA is bound into vesicles and, if the vesicle fuses with the cell membrane, the DA is released to the synapse.[2] It can be catabolized intracellularly by monoamine oxidase (MAO) to 3,4-dihydroxy-phenylacetic acid or extracellularly by catechol-O-methyltransferase (COMT) into homovanillic acid (Fig. 6–2). Dopaminergic neurons project to many brain areas via several tracts. The largest amount of DA

TABLE 6–1 Medication Classifications and Names

Classification	Pharmacological Agent (Brand Name{s})
Amphetamines & congeners	Methamphetamine (Desoxyn), Adderall, dextro-amphetamine (Dexadrine), methylphenidate (Ritalin, Concerta)
DA precursor	L-DOPA (Dopar, Larodopar, Sinemet)
DA agonist	Apomorphine (Apokyn), pramipexole (Mirapex), ropinirole (Requip)
Traditional antipsychotics (D_2/D_3 antagonist)	Chlorpromazine (Largactil, Thorazine), haloperidol (Haldol), thioridazine (Mellaril)
Atypical antipsychotics	Quetiapine (Seroquel, Ketipinor), clozapine (Clozaril), risperidone (Risperdal), olanzepine (Zyprexa), ziprasidone (Geodon)
NE α_1 agonist	Phenylephrine (Ak-Dilate, Ak-Nefrin, Alcon Efrin, Alconefrin)
NE α_2 agonist	Clonidine (Catapres)
NE α_1 antagonist	Prazosin (Minipress)
NE α_2 antagonist	Yohimbine (Aphrodyne, Yocon)
NE β antagonist	Propranolol (Inderal)
NE β agonist	Isoproterenol (phenylephrine), terbutaline (Brethine, Bricanyl, Brethaire), albuterol (Ventolin, Proventil)
SNRIs	Duloxetine (Cymbalta), venlafaxine (Effexor)
TCAs	Amitriptyline (Elavil, Tryptanol, Endep, Vanatrip), doxepin (Aponal, Adapine, Sinquan, Sinequan), imipramine (Antideprin, Deprenil, Deprimin, Deprinol, Depsonil, Dynaprin, Eupramin, Imipramil, Irmin, Janimine, Melipramin, Surplix, Tofranil), clomipramine (Anafranil)
Atypical antidepressants	Bupropion (Wellbutrin, Zyban), trazodone (Desyrel, Molipaxin, Trittico, Thombran, Trialodine, Trazorel), nefazodone (Serzone), mirtazapine (Remeron, Zispin)
MAO inhibitors	Phenelzine (Nardil), isocarboxazid (Marplan), tranylcypromine (Parnate)
H_1 antagonist	Diphenhydramine (Benadryl), triprolidine (Actidil, Mydil), brompheniramine (Bromfed, Dimetapp, Bromfenex, Dimetane)
H_2 antagonist	Cimetidine (Tagamet), ranitidine (Zinetac, Zantac), astemizole (Hismanal), terfenadine (Seldane, Triludan, Teldane)
Possible histaminergic	Modafinil (Provigil)
Barbiturates	Barbital (Veronal), phenobarbital (Luminal), pentobarbital (Nembutal)
BZDs	Triazolam (Halcion), temazepam (Restoril), estazolam (ProSom), quazepam (Doral), flurazepam (Dalmane)
BZRAs	Zopiclone (Immovane), eszopiclone (Lunesta), zolpidem (Ambien), zaleplon (Sonata)
Chloral hydrate	Chloral hydrate (Aquachloral, Novo-Chlorhydrate, Somnos, Noctec, Somnote)
AChE inhibitors	Physostigmine (Antilirium, Eserine Salicylate, Isotopo Ersine), donepezil (Aricept)
ACh agonists	Arecoline, nicotine, carbachol (Carbastat, Carboptic, Isopto Carbachol, Miostat)
ACh antagonists	Scopolamine, atropine
Melatonin	Circadin
Melatonin agonist	Ramelteon (Rozerem), agomelatine (Valdoxan, Melitor)
5-HT precursor	L-tryptophan
5-HT type 2 antagonist	LSD_{25}
5-HT$_{1A}$ partial agonist	Buspirone (Ansial, Ansiced, Anxiron, Axoren, Bespar, BuSpar, Buspimen, Buspinol, Buspisal, Narol, Spitomin, Sorbon)
5-HT antagonist	Cyproheptadine (Periactin), methysergide (Sansert, Deseril)
SSRIs	Fluoxetine (Prozac), paroxetine (Paxil), sertraline (Zoloft), citalopram (Celexa), fluvoxamine (Luvox), escitalopram (Lexapro)

ACh, acetylcholine; AChE, acetylcholinesterase; BZD, benzodiazepine; BZRA, benzodiazepine receptor agonist; DA, dopamine; H_1, histamine$_1$; H_2, histamine$_2$; 5-HT, 5-hydroxytryptamine; MAO, monoamine oxidase; NE, norepinephrine; SNRI, serotonin/norepinephrine reuptake inhibitor; SSRI, selective serotonin reuptake inhibitor; TCA, tricyclic antidepressant.

projects via the nigrostriatial tract (from the substantia nigra to the striatum). The tuberoinfundibular tract runs from the hypothalamus's arcuate nucleus to the pituitary stalk. The mesolimbic tract and the mesocortical tract connect the ventral tegmentum to limbic areas and to the prefrontal area, respectively. Many structures are involved, including the hippocampus, amygdala, arcuate nucleus, periventricular hypothalamus, septum, thalamus, and frontal cortex.[3] In noradrenergic neurons, synthesis follows the same course as for DA but then, in an extra reaction, dopamine β-hydroxylase converts DA to NE. Like DA, the NE is bound into vesicles that will release if fused with the cell membrane (see Fig. 6–2). MAO will catabolize NE to normetanephrine, and COMT catabolism will result in homovanillic acid or 3-methoxy-4-hydroxymandelic acid.[4] NE synthesis occurs in several areas, including the locus ceruleus, which projects to the cerebral cortex, hypothalamus, thalamus, and hippocampus. There is a stepwise reduction in locus ceruleus activity with the levels highest during wakefulness, reduced during NREM sleep, and nearly silent during REM sleep.[5]

There are a number of pharmacologic probes that can be used to manipulate dopaminergic neurons. The precursor L-DOPA can increase the chemical needed to synthesize DA. Reuptake into the presynaptic neuron can be inhibited by traditional stimulants (e.g., amphetamines) and cocaine. Postsynaptic receptors can be agonized by apomorphine, pergolide, bromocriptine, pramipexole, and ropinirole. These are G protein–coupled receptors, and agonist action differs among drugs. Receptor antagonism can be accomplished with pimozide and any of the traditional

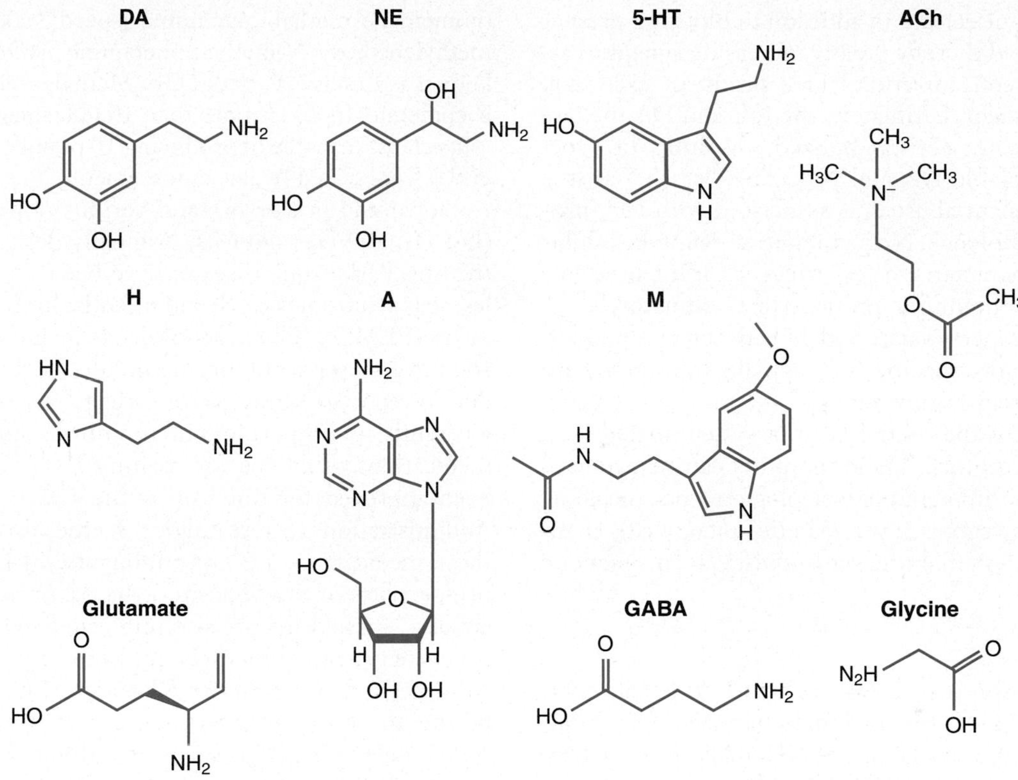

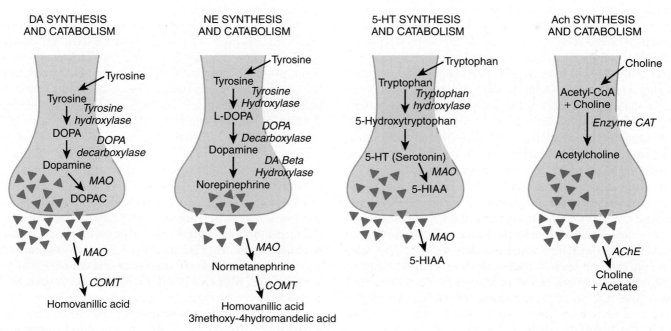

FIGURE 6–1 Neurotransmitter diagrams.

FIGURE 6–2 Monoamine and acetylcholine synthesis and catabolism.

neuroleptics (e.g., chlorpromazine, haloperidol, thioridizine). Intra- and intercellular catabolism can be diminished by MAO inhibitors (e.g., phenelzine, tranylcypromine).[6]

Norepinephrine-containing neurons can be chemically probed with a wide variety of compounds. α-Methyl-*p*-tyrosine can retard the synthesis of DA and NE by blocking the conversion of tyrosine to DOPA agents. Disulfiram also inhibits NE synthesis by blocking the final step in which DA is converted to NE. Traditional stimulants (e.g., amphetamine) cause vesicles to rupture, producing large-scale synaptic release in addition to blocking presynaptic reuptake, and thereby greatly increasing synaptic catacholaminergic concentration. This produces excitation and diminishes sleep. Ultimately, the NE and DA that are trapped synaptically get catabolized, resulting in a net depletion of available DA and NE. This "crash," as it is dubbed by stimulant abusers, is associated with very profound hypersomnolence. Norepinephrine reuptake inhibition is also characteristic of tricyclic antidepressants (TCAs; e.g., imipramine, protriptyline, amitriptyline).[7] However, this property varies widely between compounds. More recently, more specific NE reuptake inhibitors have been developed (e.g., atomoxetine).[8]

Postsynaptically, the central nervous system includes α_1, α_2, and β NE receptors. These receptors can be agonized or antagonized by different pharmacologic agents, including phenylephrine (α_1 agonist), prazosin (α_1 antagonist), clonidine (α_2 agonist), yohimbine (α_2 antagonist), and propranolol (β blocker).[9]

Sleep Effects

Patients with Parkinson's disease–related DA deficits commonly suffer from sleepiness. Some pharmacologic agents that increase synaptic availability of NE and DA tend to raise arousal level and decrease REM sleep. This is markedly true of the traditional psychostimulants. These central nervous system stimulants increase arousal level by means of autonomic sympathetic activation (and thereby decrease drowsiness). For many years, these drugs were the mainstay of therapeutics for treating disorders of excessive sleepiness. The older amphetamine formulations of benzedrine, dexedrine, and desoxyn have largely been replaced by mixtures of amphetamine salts (Adderall) and the amphetamine congener methylphenidate. Other dopaminergics with stimulant properties have also been used to treat the sleepiness associated with narcolepsy and idiopathic hypersomnia, including selegiline, pemoline, and mazindol.[10] Pemoline is seldom used today because it was "black boxed" for provoking cases of hepatic failure and jaundice; Mazindol was never very popular due to limited efficacy. Polysomnographic evaluation indicates that, by and large, compounds in this class increase time spent awake and the number of awakenings from sleep during the sleep period. They also typically prolong both latency to sleep onset and latency to REM sleep's first occurrence. In addition to decreasing total sleep time, traditional psychostimulants also suppress REM sleep and slow-wave sleep (SWS). Individuals seeking to extend the duration of their wakeful period (whether for recreational or vocational purposes) are known to abuse these medications. Trismas (lockjaw) and both sleep-related and awake teeth clenching and bruxism are associated with amphetamine and amphetamine-like stimulants. Most of the formulations also produce significant euphoria, increasing further their potential for abuse. Abused substances include both pharmaceutical and black-market products (homemade methamphetamine [speed], cocaine, and 3,4-methylenedioxy-N-methamphetamine [MDMA, commonly known as Ecstasy, X, or XTC]). Methylamphetamine abuse is epidemic. In 2003 more than 10,000 small-scale and 130 "superlabs" (capable of producing 10 pounds per production cycle) were seized by law enforcement.

Dopamine precursors and various dopamine receptor (D_2, D_3, and D_4) agonists, originally designed mainly for treating Parkinson's disease, have been used to treat restless legs syndrome (RLS) and periodic limb movement disorder (PLMD). This class of drugs includes pramipexole, ropinirole, apomorphine, pergolide (withdrawn in 2007 due to reports of heart valve damage) and bromocriptine. Currently, pramipexole and ropinirole appear to be the medications of choice for treating RLS[11] and both have been approved for this use by the U.S. Food and Drug Administration. Interestingly, at the doses prescribed, these medications are not stimulants. In fact, there have been reports of the opposite—that is, occurrence of sleep attacks. These drugs are also implicated in compulsive disorders (e.g., triggering excessive gambling, eating, and sexual urges). With respect to RLS and PLMD, medications having the opposite effect (i.e., worsening these conditions) include TCAs, selective serotonin reuptake inhibitors (SSRIs), some antiemetics (prochlorperazine, metoclopramide), lithium, some calcium channel blockers (verapamil, nifedipine, diltiazem), antihistamines, and traditional neuroleptics.[12]

Dopamine D_2 and D_3 receptor antagonists in the form of traditional neuroleptics reliably produce sedation, increase sleep efficiency, increase SWS, and usually suppress REM sleep to some degree. This holds for chlorpromazine, haloperidol, and thioridazine. The newer, non-D_2/non-D_3 neuroleptics (clozapine, olanzapine, risperidone, ziprasidone) have variable effects on SWS, with some decreasing and others (e.g., risperidone, olanzapine, ziprasidone) increasing SWS (perhaps related to their higher affinity for 5-HT$_2$ receptors). These newer atypical antipsychotics do not universally produce sedation.[13] The amount of sedation produced appears to be determined by the combination of the drug's relative potency and its affinity for the histamine$_1$ (H_1) receptor. For example, clozapine is very sedating and it has high H_1 affinity (32) and low potency (and consequently a need for large doses [50 mg]), whereas olanzapine is less sedating even with an H_1 affinity of 1149 because, with its high potency, there is need for only a low dose (4 mg). Quetiapine also falls into the low-potency (80-mg dose needed), moderate H_1 affinity (5.2) category and thus is moderately sedating. Like traditional neuroleptics, these newer drugs can increase restless legs and periodic leg movement activity during sleep.

The TCAs comprise a wide range of compounds that share a similar three-ring chemical structure. This group of agents includes imipramine, desipramine, amitriptyline, nortriptyline, clomipramine, trimipramine, doxepin, and protriptyline. Across the board, TCAs increase SWS and suppress REM sleep mildly to markedly. TCAs are generally sedating (with a few exceptions, e.g., protriptyline). The range of sedation varies greatly and is most likely a function of antihistaminergic activity (see section on histamine). Imipramine, the prototypical compound in this class, is regarded as a nonselective NE reuptake inhibitor. In vitro acute biochemical activity studies reveal that it also produces serotonin reuptake inhibition, has high α_1, and muscarinic acetylcholinergic receptor affinity, and binds somewhat to histamine receptors. In sleep medicine, imipramine is best known for its REM sleep–suppressing properties and for decades was widely used as an anticataplectic agent for treating patients with narcolepsy. Imipramine's SWS-enhancing and REM sleep–suppressing properties are illustrated in Figure 6–3. In this patient, latency to the first REM sleep episode was almost 3 hours, twice as long as normal. No REM sleep episode occurred at the usual 90- to 120-minute latency from sleep onset (the missing REM sleep episode). Additionally, REM sleep continued to be suppressed later in the night while SWS appeared to be above normal. The other popular TCA used in this manner is protriptyline. Protriptyline also has the advantage of being nonsedating; however, it can exacerbate erectile problems in men (that in turn can render therapeutic adherence problematic). The REM sleep–suppressing properties of TCAs appear to stem from a combination of aminergic (NE and serotonin) and acetylcholinergic properties. The aminergic properties theoretically provide activation of REM-off systems while the anticholinergic properties would inhibit REM-on systems. For example, clomipramine, the most REM sleep–suppressing TCA, strongly agonizes 5-HT by inhibiting reuptake of serotonin and also has moderate antimuscarinic properties. By contrast, the TCA amitriptyline, another strong REM sleep suppressor, blocks acetylcholine with its very high muscarinic binding affinity but is a weaker serotonin reuptake inhibitor.

MAO inhibitors, as a class, are the strongest suppressors of REM sleep. They, of course, alter catabolism of all biogenic amine neurotransmitters (DA, NE, and serotonin), and, like the TCAs, they can be used as antidepressants. It did not go unnoticed that, until the atypical antidepressant bupropion was developed, all known antidepressant medications suppressed REM sleep. Furthermore, even instrumentally suppressing REM sleep by awakening sleepers in the laboratory whenever they entered REM sleep improved mood in patients diagnosed with depression.[14] Thus, it was posited that REM sleep was depressionogenic in some individuals and that REM sleep suppression was necessary and sufficient to achieve an antidepressant effect. Even the atypical antidepressants venlafaxine and trazodone suppressed REM sleep (especially early in the night, with rebound toward morning). However, first bupropion and afterward nefazodone contradicted this axiom by having antidepressant properties without suppressing REM sleep. Nonetheless, while it is not necessary to suppress REM sleep, REM sleep suppression remains sufficient to produce antidepressant effects. It is also interesting to note that, unlike the TCAs, the atypical antidepressants venlafaxine, nefazodone, bupropion, and trazodone do not increase SWS.

Histamine

Histamine is an important excitatory neurotransmitter in the central nervous system. Posterior hypothalamus histaminergic neurons are thought to generate wakefulness. In particular, the tuberomammillary nucleus (TMN) is a histamine-rich structure believed to play a crucial role in maintaining alertness, and may be the brain's sole source of histamine. The TMN appears to generate physiologic "normal wakefulness" that is not associated with overactivation of motor and reward systems, and its activity follows a stepwise decreasing pattern similar to that of NE—that is, high activity during wakefulness, decreased levels during NREM sleep, and very low levels during REM sleep. This may help explain why the patients described by von Economo with posterior hypothalamic encephalitic damage were extremely sleepy but those with anterior lesions were not.

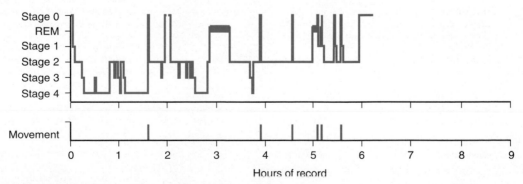

FIGURE 6–3 Imipramine and sleep macroarchitecture.

Central histaminergic effects are most well recognized for the sedation that is produced by central H_1 antagonists (that are actually inverse agonists), exemplified by the action of diphenhydramine.[15] H_1 antagonists also can decrease REM sleep or REM density. Histamine₂ (H_2) antagonists have little effect on sleep; however, cimetidine may increase SWS. Table 6–2 tabulates the main effects of antihistamines on sleep. Sedation that occurs as a side effect of other compounds often has its roots in an antihistaminergic property. Examination of in vitro acute biochemical activity reveals that the sedating TCAs amitriptyline, trimipramine, and doxepin all have high H_1 receptor affinity.[16] Other sedating medications with known antihistaminergic activity include trazodone, mirtazapine, and quetiapine. Other properties of H_1 receptor blockade are

weight gain, hypotension, and potentiating other central nervous system depressants.

Although the mechanism of action is not completely certain, the wakefulness-promoting medication modafinil is thought to act largely via a histaminergic mechanism.[17] Modafinil also activates glutamatergic circuits and appears to inhibit GABA transmission. The immediate gene product c-*fos* is activated in TMNs of cats administered modafinil.[18] Modafinil extends wakefulness and performance in normal subjects undergoing sleep deprivation, increases sleep latencies on the Multiple Sleep Latency Test in patients with narcolepsy[19] and shift work sleep disorder,[20] and increases sleep latency on the Maintenance of Wakefulness Test in patients with narcolepsy and sleep apnea (with residual sleepiness),[21–23] but does not alter nocturnal sleep when administered in the morning.[24] The American

TABLE 6–2 Medication Effects on Sleep

Classification	Pharmacologic Agent	SWS	REM	Wakefulness	Other Sleep Effects
DA agonists (traditional psychostimulants)	Amphetamines	↓↓	↓↓	↑↑↑	Severe hypersomnia and prominent REM sleep rebound on d/c after chronic use; can provoke bruxism
	Cocaine	↓↓	↓↓	↑↑↑	
DA precursor	L-DOPA	↓, ↔	↑ low dose ↓ high dose	↑	Can produce insomnia at high doses
DA agonists	Apomorphine			↑ (↓ MSLT high dose)	
	Pramipexole			↑ (↓ MSLT high dose)	
	Ropinirole			↑ (↓ MSLT high dose)	
Neuroleptics (D_2/D_3 antagonist)	Chlorpromazine Haloperidol Thioridazine	↑	↑, ↔	↓↓↓	Increase PLMs & RLS-like symptoms
NE α₁ agonist	Phenylephrine		↓ ?	↑	
NE α₂ agonist	Clonidine	↑	↓	↓↓	
NE α₁ antagonist	Prazosin		↑ ? (PTSD)	↓ (can cause daytime sedation)	Decreases nightmare distress (PTSD)
NE α₂ antagonist	Yohimbine		↔	↑	
NE α₂ antagonist (presynaptic)	Mirtazapine			↓↓	
NE β antagonist	Propranolol	↓	↓	↑	Can provoke nightmares
NE β agonist	Isoproterenol Terbutaline Albuterol	↔	↔	↔	
SNRIs	Duloxetine	↑	↓		
	Venlafaxine		↓↓	↑	
TCAs	Amitriptyline	↑	↓↓↓↓	↓↓↓↓ (↓ SL)	Tendency to increase sleep-related movements and PLM and can be associated with RLS-like symptoms
	Doxepin	↑↑	↓↓	↓↓↓↓ (↓ SL)	
	Imipramine	↑	↓↓	↓↓	
	Clomipramine	↑	↓↓↓↓	↔	
MAO inhibitors	Phenelzine		↓↓↓↓	↑	Strongest known REM suppressors; may exacerbate PLMs; prominent REM sleep rebound on discontinuation.
	Tranylcypromine		↓↓↓	↑↑↑	
H_1 antagonists	Diphenhydramine Triprolidine Brompheniramine	↑	↓ ↓ ↓	↓↓	Dream intensity rebounds when d/c
H_2 antagonists	Cimetidine	↑			Slows clearance of some BZDs; increases levels of theophylline, carbamazepine, and β blockers
	Ranitidine	No effect	No effect		
	Astemizole				Does not cross blood-brain barrier
	Terfenadine				Does not cross blood-brain barrier

Continued

TABLE 6–2 Medication Effects on Sleep—Cont'd

Classification	Pharmacologic Agent	SWS	REM	Wakefulness	Other Sleep Effects
Barbiturates	Assorted	↓	↓↓↓	↓↓↓	Severe AEs on withdrawal; high overdose liability
BZDs	Triazolam Temazepam Estazolam Quazepam Flurazepam	↓↓	↓	↓↓↓	Tolerance and rebound on d/c; low overdose liability
BZRAs	Zopiclone Eszopiclone Zolpidem Zaleplon	↔	↔	↓↓↓	Minor AE on withdraw; low overdose liability
Chloral hydrate	Chloral hydrate				
Alcohol	Alcohol		↓ acutely ↑ on withdrawal	↓	
AChE inhibitors	Physostigmine Donepezil		↑ ↑		Shorten REM latency
ACh agonists	Arecholine		↑		Can produce insomnia at high doses; shortens REM latency
	Nicotine	↑	↓	↓	Increases SL and WASO
ACh antagonists	Scopolamine		↓		Increases REM latency
	Atropine		↓ (onset)		Increases REM latency
5-HT precursor	L-tryptophan	↑	↓		Decreases SL; increases REM density
5-HT type 2 antagonist	LSD₂₅		↑		Provoked REMs in SWS; decreased REM latency; increases arousals
5-HT₁ₐ partial agonist (effects on D₂ receptors)	Buspirone		↓		No effects; reportedly an antidote for SSRI-induced bruxism
5-HT antagonist	Cyproheptadine	↑			
SSRIs	Fluoxetine	↓/=	=/↓	↑	
	Paroxetine	↓/=	↓↓	↑↑	
	Sertraline	=	↓↓	=	
	Citalopram		↓	No change	
	Fluvoxamine		↓	↑	
	Escitalopram		↓		

ACh, acetylcholine; AChE, acetylcholinesterase; AE, adverse effect; BZD, benzodiazepine; BZRA, benzodiazepine receptor agonist; DA, dopamine; d/c, discontinued; H₁, histamine₁; H₂, histamine₂; 5-HT, 5-hydroxytryptamine; MAO, monoamine oxidase; MSLT, Multiple Sleep Latency Test; NE, norepinephrine; PLM, periodic limb movement; PTSD, post-traumatic stress disorder; REM, rapid eye movement; RLS, restless legs syndrome; SL, sleep latency; SNRI, serotonin/norepinephrine reuptake inhibitor; SSRI, selective serotonin reuptake inhibitor; SWS, slow-wave sleep; TCA, tricyclic antidepressant; WASO, waking after sleep onset.

Academy of Sleep Medicine currently recommends modafinil as the first-line of treatment for sleepiness associated with narcolepsy syndrome.[25] In addition to having an indication for use in narcolepsy, the U.S. Food and Drug Administration has also approved modafinil for treating (1) residual sleepiness in patients with sleep apnea who are otherwise well treated with positive airway pressure and (2) sleepiness associated with shift work sleep disorder.[26]

Orexins (Hypocretins)

The orexins (hypocretins) are a pair of excitatory neuropeptide hormones (orexin A and orexin B or hypocretin-1 and hypocretin-2) discovered in 1998.[27,28] Produced by a small hypothalamic cell group with widespread projections throughout the brain, the orexins appear to promote wakefulness. Some researchers refer to these hormones as hypocretins because of the locus of origin. These neurons activate structures with other stimulating neurotransmitter systems, including DA, NE, ACh, and histamine.[29]

The discovery of orexins was a major breakthrough for our understanding of narcolepsy. Mutations in genes producing orexins or their receptors were found in narcoleptic mice and dogs. Humans with narcolepsy appear to have an orexin deficit produced by a degenerative process. Orexins can be deficient in cerebrospinal fluid of approximately 90% of patients with the "narcolepsy-cataplexy syndrome," as it is call in the United Kingdom.[30] Direct brain injection of orexin produces wakefulness and can reverse some of the effects of sleep deprivation.[31] A number of orexin agonists (stimulants) and antagonists (sedatives) are being developed. At this point, however, we have few data concerning the effects of orexigenic substances on human sleep.

Glutamate

The brain's most common neurotransmitter is glutamate. The N-methyl-D-aspartate (NMDA) glutamate receptor is regulated by both voltage and glutamic acid. It has binding sites for glutamate, magnesium, glycine, zinc, and phencyclidine (PCP). PCP (referred to as "angel dust" on the street) can produce hallucinations and psychosis. NMDA receptors are concentrated in the hippocampus, amygdala, basal ganglia, and cerebral cortex.

INHIBITORY TRANSMITTER SYSTEMS

GABA

GABA is one of the main inhibitory neurotransmitters in the mammalian central nervous system. It begins as glutamic acid that is catalyzed by glutamine acid decarboxylase to form γ-aminobutyric acid. GABA$_A$ agonism promotes flux in the chlorine channel. GABA, benzodiazepines (BZDs), or barbiturates can increase dilation of the ionophore and thereby promote transmission in this inhibitory pathway. Barbiturates, BZDs, benzodiazepine receptor agonists (BZRAs), alcohol, chloral hydrate, steroids, and picotoxins can all affect this system. While there are direct and partial GABA agonists, in sleep medicine the drugs traditionally used to manage the symptoms of insomnia are mainly BZDs and BZRAs. GABA neurons are widely distributed in the brain with high concentration particularly in the thalamus.

Chloral hydrate was the first pharmaceutical sleeping pill, developed circa 1860. It shortens sleep latency and initially increases sleep time. It has been described as "alcohol in pill form" because, after it passes through the gut, it forms an alcohol-like compound. Chloral hydrate is probably best known for its popularization in detective mystery stories by Dashiell Hammett and Raymond Chandler where, when mixed with alcohol, it becomes a "Mickey Finn" and is used to stupefy the gangsters' adversary. Bromides and paraldehydes followed but did not enjoy much success. At the turn of the 20th century, barbituric acid was first synthesized by Adolf von Baeyer. Derivatives were found to be extremely sedating.[32] Polysomnographic studies show that most barbiturates shorten the latency to sleep onset, increase total sleep time and sleep efficiency, and decrease wakefulness after sleep onset and the number of awakenings in patients with insomnia. They also tend to decrease REM sleep, perhaps by impairing the muscles that move the eyes and mildly decreasing SWS.[33,34] Microarchitectural sleep changes included increased fast activities (beta rhythms) in the electroencephalogram (EEG), increased sleep spindles, and decreased arousals.[35] Barbiturates, however, are extremely toxic. One popular index for toxicity is the ratio of the effective dose found for 50% of animals tested (ED$_{50}$) to the lethal dose for 50% of animals tested (LD$_{50}$). This ratio provides a safety index, with smaller numbers (larger ranges) being less dangerous. For barbiturates the ratio is only approximately 10:1 (depending on type) meaning that ingesting 10 times the effective dose confers a significant risk of death.[36] Thus, if a prescription provides the patient with more than 100 pills, it becomes a potential vehicle for committing suicide. The fact that 90% of patients with major depressive disorder have insomnia and 17% or more of patients coming to sleep disorders centers complaining of insomnia have a mood disorder sets the stage for such tragedies. There were many suicides using sleeping pills in the era of barbiturates.

In the 1960s the BZDs were developed to be sleep aids. Compared to barbiturates, BZDs were amazingly safe. In most cases it was not even possible to determine a lethal dose. Thus, it was joked at the time that the only way a BZD would kill you was if you were run over by the truck delivering them to the pharmacy. However, it soon became apparent that, when BZDs were combined with alcohol, this safety was compromised. BZDs have four major characteristics; they are (1) sedating, (2) anxiolytic, (3) myorelaxant, and (4) anticonvulsant.[37] Secondary properties include ataxia, amnesia, and potentiation of alcohol. BZDs proved very effective for treating insomnia, shortening latency to sleep onset, increasing total sleep time, and improving sleep efficiency. They did not suppress REM sleep as much as barbiturates but, on average, decreased SWS more. Sleep spindle activity is increased in a dose-response manner but without dramatic enhancement of EEG beta rhythms. Figure 6–4 shows greatly increased polysomnographic tracing sleep spindle activity in a recorded from a patient taking temazepam nightly for more than a year. Awakenings and brief arousals are reduced by most BZDs tested.[38–40] Early BZDs tended to be long acting, the champion being flurazepam with its 72- to 100-hour half-life (without counting its active

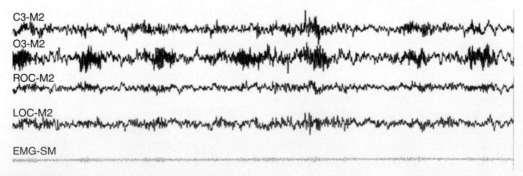

FIGURE 6–4 Temazepam and sleep microarchitecture.

metabolite). In second place, quazepam weighs in with a 27- to 43-hour half-life, followed by estazolam with a 10- to 24-hour half-life and temazepam with a 4- to 18-hour half-life.[41] Triazolam was the first short-acting BZD for promoting sleep but fell out of favor after high-profile reports of amnesia[42] (but all BZDs potentially produce amnesia).

Half-life is important for two reasons. First, in combination with the drug's minimal effective dose and the dose administered, it dictates the duration of action (or what we prefer to call the therapeutic window). If the duration of action extends beyond the individual's sleep episode, there will likely be residual sedation, commonly referred to as "hangover." Secondly, the pharmacokinetic rule-of-thumb estimates elimination time as 5 to 6 times the half-life of a compound. It should be realized that the vast majority of medications used in clinical practice are administered according to principles of the infectious disease model. The infectious disease model involves dosing a drug until it reaches therapeutic level and then maintaining it at that level until the bacterium, germ, or microorganism is eradicated. Usually, drug level is maintained for a while longer just to be certain and prevent reinfection. In some cases, as with some psychiatric medication, the drug may be kept at the therapeutic level indefinitely. By contrast, sleeping pills need to work like a switch. One wants to (1) administer the drug, (2) have it rapidly get to therapeutic level and (3) hover there for precisely 7.5 hours, and then (4) instantly disappear without a trace. Having the drug eliminated rapidly and completely helps assure there is no hangover, receptors have the maximal time to re-regulate, and there is no cascading drug level produced by adding drug into a system that already has residual drug on board. Of course, pharmacokinetics are not so well behaved. Also, we do not dose patients the way we do laboratory animals; that is, we use fixed doses rather than equivalents in milligrams per kilogram weights. Chances are that there will be undershoot and overshoot with respect to a medication's duration of action compared to the desired therapeutic window. Interestingly, if receptor systems down-regulate, adapt, or habituate, then tolerance will more likely to develop in longer acting substances, notwithstanding their potency.

In the 1980s the BZRAs, which did not have the characteristic benzene ring structure, were developed. These medications boasted generally shorter half-life, little or no alteration of sleep macroarchitecture, and greater propensity for increasing sedation than producing anxiolytic, myorelaxant, or anticonvulsant effects.[43-45] At the time it was speculated that the different characteristics associated with BZD receptor agonism were mediated by subtype receptors. The data from knock-out genetic studies in mice and rats confirmed this hunch almost 15 years later.[46] The different BZRAs boast varying degrees of greater affinity for the receptor subtype thought to mediate sedation (α_1) than other receptor subtypes (typically α_2). The receptor affinity ratio for currently marketed BZRAs with an indication for treating insomnia are 2:1 for zopiclone, 10:1 for zolpidem, and 13:1 for zaleplon.[47] Other BZRAs for treating insomnia include variants of these compounds: eszopiclone, the left-handed enantiomer of zopiclone (which turns out to be the active isomer), and zolpidem MR, a multiple-release version of zolpidem designed to extend its therapeutic window by 1–2 hours. Table 6–2 summarizes characteristics of and differences between barbiturates, BZDs, and BZRA sleep-promoting substances.

Adenosine

Nathaniel Kleitman, the dean of American sleep research, postulated that the basic rest-activity cycle was governed by the buildup of a "hypnotoxin" during wakefulness that was then eliminated during sleep.[48] This general characterization lives on today in our conceptualization of the homeostatic drive for sleep accumulating as "sleep pressure" (or "sleep debt" when unpaid and overdue). There are many possible candidates for modern-day "hypnotoxins." Perhaps the most likely candidate is adenosine. Adenosine delivered to the preoptic area and anterior hypothalamus induces NREM sleep. As an animal experiences prolonged wakefulness, basal forebrain adenosine levels rise, and they subsequently decline during recovery sleep.[49,50] Interestingly, BZDs (and GABA$_A$ receptor agonists) decrease adenosine uptake; however, caffeine (adenosine antagonist) does not alter benzodiazepine receptor action.[51]

Adenosine receptors can be antagonized by the methylxanthines caffeine (found in coffee) and theobromine (found in chocolate). Figure 6–5 shows the chemical structure for adenosine, caffeine, and theobromine. When an individual does not get enough sleep at night to rid the basal forebrain of its adenosine load, morning awakening is usually accompanied by residual sleepiness. Drinking a morning cup (or two) of coffee, or better yet coffee with chocolate in it (mocha java), provides an effective, albeit temporary, antidote. Overall, polysomnographic studies of methylxanthines show decreases in total sleep time, SWS, and REM sleep.[52] Latency to sleep onset may, or may not, be increased but, more importantly, waking after sleep onset can rise dramatically (Fig. 6–6).

According to one story, the effect of coffee beans was first noticed by a sheep herder from Caffa, Ethiopia, named Kaldi. He noticed that the sheep became hyperactive after eating the red "cherries" from a certain plant when they changed pastures. He tried a few himself and became as "hyper" as his herd.[53] The origins of chocolate remain even more obscure; however, chocolate was thought to first have been extracted from cocoa in the Amazon circa 2000 BC. Chocolate became an important part of Mayan culture in the sixth century AD. Subsequently, some 600 years later, the Aztecs attributed creation of the cocoa plant to Quetzalcoatl, who smuggled it to earth from paradise when he descended from heaven on a beam of light.[54] It was truly considered the food of the gods.

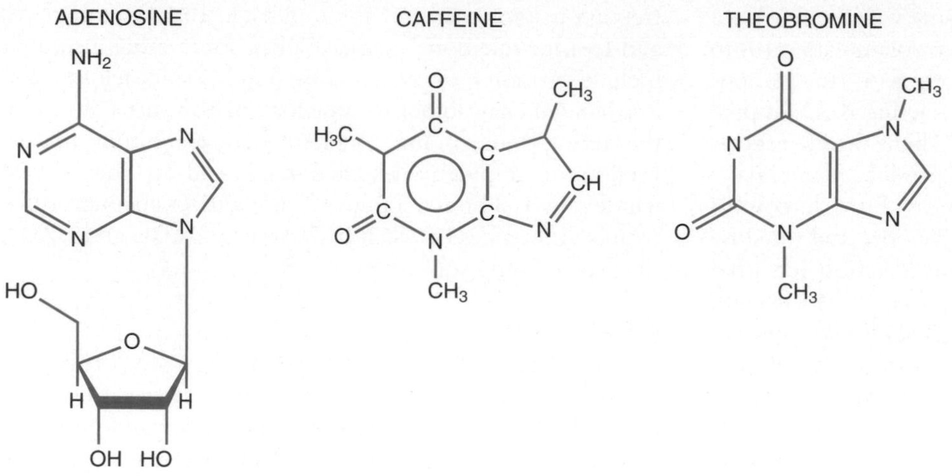

ADENOSINE   CAFFEINE   THEOBROMINE

FIGURE 6–5 Adenosine, caffeine, and theobromine.

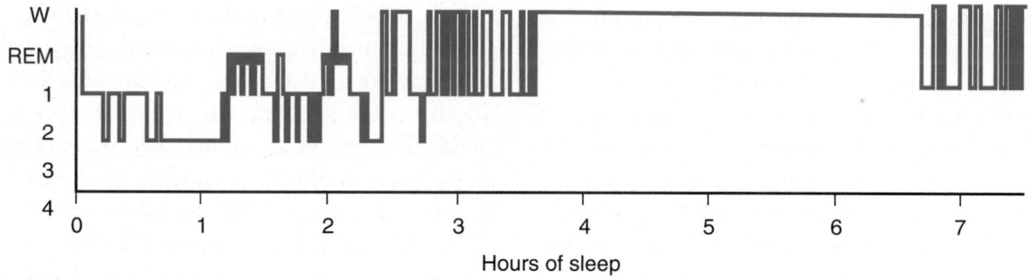

Hours of sleep

FIGURE 6–6 Caffeine and sleep macroarchitecture.

Glycine

Glycine is the simplest amino acid and can be produced by protein hydrolysis. This sweet-tasting compound was first isolated from gelatin in 1820. This central nervous system inhibitory neurotransmitter is particularly important for its role in mediating atonia occurring during REM sleep. Activation of glycine receptors produces inhibitory postsynaptic potentials that decreases spinal alpha and gamma motor neuron activity. Strychnine blocks glycine receptors. Along with glutamate, glycine's coagonist, it can activate NMDA receptors. Ingesting 3 g glycine before bedtime reportedly improves alertness and subjective feelings after awakening from sleep.[55]

REGULATING TRANSMITTER SYSTEMS

Acetylcholine

Acetylcholine begins as circulating choline in the blood. It is taken into presynaptic neurons and is combined with acetyl-coenzyme A to form ACh (reaction catalyzed by choline acetyl transferase). The ACh is then bound into vesicles that are released synaptically upon fusing with the cell wall. Synaptic ACh can be catabolized by acetylcholinesterase (AChe), rendering choline and acetate.

Acetylcholine plays a major role in regulating REM sleep.[56] There is a large concentration of ACh in the gigantocellular nucleus of the reticular formation. During the waking state, aminergic neurons are highly active and ACh is implicated in memory processes. By contrast, during SWS, cortical activity is greatly reduced. Then, during REM sleep, cortical acetylcholinergic activity returns to high levels.[57] REM sleep "on" neurons are plentiful in the laterodorsal tegmentum (LDT) and the pedunculopontine tegmentum (PPT).[58] Basal forebrain cholinergic neurons project to the hippocampus, amygdala, and cortex. Opposing these cells are the REM sleep "off" cells in the dorsal raphe (a serotonin reservoir) and the locus ceruleus (where most of the brain's NE is synthesized).

Chemical probes of ACh include the agonists arecholine, nicotine, carbachol, and pilocarpine. Antagonists include scopolamine, atropine, hyoscine, and curare. Agonism can also be achieved by using AChE inhibitors (e.g., physostigmine, donepezil). Table 6–2 shows some of the sleep changes produced by these system probes. In general, AChE inhibitors can increase REM sleep duration, hasten its appearance, or both.[59,60] ACh agonists enhance REM sleep,[61] and antagonists suppress REM sleep and its activity.[62] Administering arecholine or physostigmine intravenously can provoke REM sleep occurrence, whereas scopolamine dramatically delays REM sleep onset.

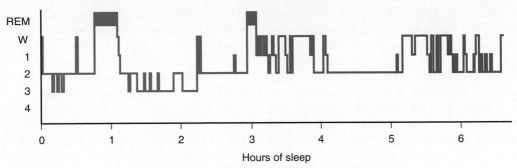

FIGURE 6–7 Fluoxetine and sleep macroarchitecture. Note the short REM sleep latency early in the night and SWS dominating the 2nd NREM-REM cycle (typical in depression). As drug becomes active later in night, REM sleep is suppressed and sleep becomes fragmented.

Serotonin

In opposition to ACh, the indoleamine serotonin serves as an inhibitor of REM sleep (Fig. 6–7). Activation of brain stem raphe nuclei suppresses REM sleep (as does locus ceruleus activation of NE areas). These biogenic amines are considered REM "off" cells responsible for reciprocal interaction with the LDT/PPT REM "on" cholinergic generators.[63] Nonetheless, serotonin raphe neurons project widely through the brain, including the hippocampus, hypothalamus, thalamus, septum, and cerebral cortex.[64] Brain stem raphe activity is highest during wakefulness, less active during NREM sleep, and nearly silent during REM sleep.

Serotonin begins with blood-borne tryptophan that is hydroxylated to 5-hydroxytryptophan, which is later reduced to 5-HT, which is serotonin. The 5-HT is bound in vesicles and can be released synaptically. Its main catabolite is MAO, which reduces it to 5-hydroxyindolacetic acid. The synthesis of 5-HT can be stimulated by L-tryptophan or inhibited with parachloralphenylalanine.[65]

Functional agonism can be achieved by inhibiting the reuptake of synaptic 5-HT into the presynaptic terminal to be re-bound in vesicles and ultimately reused. Many TCAs nonselectively inhibit serotonin reuptake along with having anticholinergic properties that produced undesirable side effects (e.g., dry mouth, ataxia, diplopia, tachycardia, constipation, memory loss, confusion). The newer SSRI antidepressants quickly became preferred because they required fewer dose adjustments and were less complicated by adverse events. By contrast, serotonin can be antagonized with methysergide and cyproheptadine (which also has antihistaminergic properties). Type 2 receptor antagonism is produced by lysergic acid diethylamide (LSD$_{25}$), and presynaptic autoreceptor partial agonism can be achieved with buspirone. Postsynaptic receptors are G protein coupled, and there is a wide array of them. Table 6–2 describes some of the changes in sleep produced by chemically probing the 5-HT system. In addition to a general REM sleep–suppressing action of 5-HT agonists,[66] these drugs sometimes unhinge the choreography of physiologic changes and activities that make up REM sleep. For example, rapid eye movements characteristically accompany wakefulness and REM sleep. However, it was noted that patients treated with SSRIs would often have rapid eye movements in sleep stages N1, N2, and N3.[67] The phenomenon was so common it developed the moniker

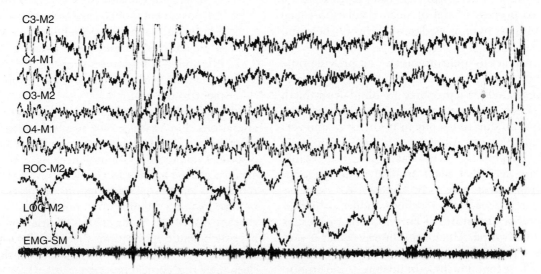

FIGURE 6–8 Fluoxetine and sleep microarchitecture.

"Prozac eyes" after the brand name of fluoxetine, the prototypical SSRI (Fig. 6–8). SSRIs also reportedly decrease the frequency of dream recall but increase the intensity of the dreams that are remembered.[68] The breakdown in coordination of gating mechanism produced by 5-HT alteration extends beyond mere eye movement activity. 5-Hydroxytryptamine agonists are noted for provoking an iatrogenic form of REM sleep behavior disorder,[69] presumably by failing to provoke or sustain striated muscle atonia when dreaming commences. Additionally, SSRIs and TCAs generally increase muscle activity and movements during sleep.[70,71]

Melatonin

Although melatonin is an endocrine secreted largely by the pineal gland, it is synthesized from 5-HT by pinealocytes. The catalyst 5-HT N-acetyltransferase transforms 5-HT first to N-acetyl-5-HT and then to hydroxyindole-O-methyltransferase, and finally is converted to melatonin, which is N-acetyl-5-methoxytryptamine.[72] Melatonin is released in response to decreasing environmental light and thus synchronizes our physiology with the light-dark cycle. In a sense, it is the "signal of darkness to the brain."[73] Therefore, if we are rats, our response to rising melatonin would be to become more alert. By contrast, if we are humans (or at least more human than rat), our response to melatonin would be to become sleepy and get ready to retire for our major sleep period. Presumably the melatonin is occupying central melatonin MT_1 and MT_2 receptors sites in the suprachiasmatic nucleus (SCN) of the hypothalamus. The SCN is a bilaterally represented structure containing several thousand cells just above the optic chiasm and to either side of the third ventricle. Thus, melatonin decreases the SCN-activating properties that hold homeostatic sleep drive (sleep debt) at bay and thereby result in sleep onset. Therefore, melatonin plays a pivotal role in the two-process model of sleep regulation (sleep drive and circadian rhythm) as described by Borbély and Achermann.[74]

Melatonin can act as a chronobiotic and provide time cues (zeitgebers).[75] The studies by Sack and colleagues clearly demonstrated this property in blind-from-birth children.[76] These patients have a chaotic circadian sleep-wake rhythm due to lesions in both visual and retinal-hypothalamic tracts. Administering melatonin daily at a set time entrains the sleep-wake cycle remarkably well. Melatonin has also been studied as a potential sleep-promoting substance.[77] It appears to decrease latency to sleep in several published studies. Whether these finding reflect hypnotic or chronobiotic properties is difficult to determine. Melatonin, however, has a very short half-life (approximately 20 minutes). This may be problematic for exogenously administered melatonin,

whereas the pineal's continual release renders the short half-life unimportant for naturally occurring endogenous melatonin. Several pharmaceutical companies make or are developing melatonin and melatonin agonists for the treatment of insomnia. Circadin is an extended-release melatonin formulation approved in Europe for treating primary insomnia in patients 55 years and older with poor-quality sleep. Ramelteon is a selective melatonin MT_1 and MT_2 agonist with a 2.6-hour half-life (and active metabolites) approved in the United States for treating insomnia.[78] In pivotal clinical trials, an 8-mg oral dose of ramelteon taken 30 minutes before bedtime shortened both objective and self-reported latency to sleep onset in adults with primary insomnia.[79] Similar results were found for individuals age 65 years and older who were diagnosed with insomnia. Agomelatine is a potent melatonin receptor agonist and $5\text{-}HT_{2C}$ antagonist with a 1- to 2-hour half-life. It appears to have antidepressant, anxiolytic, and sleep-promoting properties but has yet to be approved for use to treat insomnia in the American market.

CLINICAL PHARMACOLOGY AND SUMMARY

Overall, there appear to be several general observations we can make about drug-related changes in sleep, wakefulness, and sleep architecture. These should not be taken as hard-and-fast rules because there are exceptions. Nonetheless, these general principles may be helpful for predicting how sleep will respond to a substance, given the effects of the substance on neurotransmission. The "basic 8" rules-of-thumb are

1. Catacholamine agonists promote wakefulness and most suppress REM sleep
2. Centrally acting H_1 antihistamines are sedating
3. Orexin deficit underlies sleepiness in narcolepsy
4. $GABA_A$ agonists and BZRAs are somnogenic
5. Adenosine antagonists are somnolytic
6. Cholinergic-enhancing agents promote REM sleep while anticholinergic agents suppress REM sleep
7. NE and 5-HT agonists suppress REM sleep
8. Melatonin is the signal of darkness in the environment to the brain

Clinically, we capitalize on substance-induced sleep alterations. For example, we use wakefulness-promoting substances to bolster alertness in patients suffering from disorders of excessive somnolence. By contrast, sedating agents are used to treat insomnia. REM sleep suppression represents an approach to treating cataplexy, and chronobiotics may be helpful for individuals with circadian rhythm disorders. Additionally, a variety of medications have therapeutic applications that were determined empirically. Table 6–3 shows some of the current therapeutics in sleep medicine clinical practice.

TABLE 6–3 Clinical Pharmacology for Sleep Disorders

Sleep Disorder	Class or Disorder	Medications Used for Treatment
Insomnia	BZRA sedative-hypnotics	Zolpidem, zaleplon, eszopiclone, zopiclone
	BZD sedative-hypnotics	Flurazepam, quazepam, estazolam, temazepam, triazolam
	Hypnotics	Ramelteon
	Chronobiotics	Circadin, melatonin
	Sedating antidepressants	Trazodone, amitriptyline, doxepin
	Others—approved for other indications	Xyrem, Gabatril, mirtazapine, quatiapine
Narcolepsy	To reduce sleepiness	Modafinil, methylphenidate, amphetamines
	Anticataplectics	REM sleep–suppressing SSRIs or TCAs, GHB
Sleep-disordered breathing	Increase airway tone and/or suppress REM sleep	Protriptyline & other TCAs, medroxyprogesterone acetate, SSRIs, mirtazapine, theophylline, modafinil (as augmenting therapy)
PLMD and RLS	Assorted	Iron, pramipexole, ropinirole, propoxyphene napsylate, codeine, oxycodone, clonazepam & other BZDs
Parasomnias	Nightmares	Prazosin, quetiapine, nefazodone, mirtazapine, gabapentin
	Terrifying hypnagogia	REM sleep–suppressing Rx
	REM behavior disorder	Clonazepam, pramipexole, melatonin
	Sleep-related painful erections	Propranolol, clozapine
	Nocturnal leg cramps	Magnesium citrate (quinine no longer recommended)
	Sleep bruxism	Amitriptyline
	Enuresis	Desmopressin
	Nocturnal paroxysmal dystonia	Anticonvulsants

BZD, benzodiazepine; BZRA, benzodiazepine receptor agonist; GHB, γ-hydroxybutyrate; PLMD, periodic limb movement disorder; REM, rapid eye movement; RLS, restless legs syndrome; Rx, treatment; SSRI, selective serotonin reuptake inhibitor; TCA, tricyclic antidepressant.

ACKNOWLEDGMENT

Special thanks to Amy Hirshkowitz and Hossein Sharafkhaneh for their help with the background research.

⊙ REFERENCES

A full list of references are available at www.expertconsult.com

Physiologic Changes in Sleep

Sudhansu Chokroverty

Awareness about the importance of sleep and its effect on the human organism is growing. Adult humans spend approximately one-third of their lives sleeping, yet we do not have a clear understanding of the functions of sleep. We do know that a vast number of physiologic changes take place during sleep in humans and other mammals. Almost every system in the body undergoes change during sleep—most in the form of reduced activity, although some systems show increased activity. The physiology of wakefulness has been studied intensively, but comparatively little has been written about physiologic changes during sleep. It is important to be aware of these changes in different body systems to understand how they may affect various sleep disorders. A striking example is sleep apnea syndrome, which causes dramatic changes in respiratory control and the upper airway muscles during sleep that direct our attention to a very important pathophysiologic mechanism and a therapeutic intervention for this disorder. Similarly, physiologic changes in several other body systems are important to understanding the pathophysiology of many medical disorders, including disturbances of sleep.

Physiologic changes are known to occur in both the somatic nervous system and the autonomic nervous system (ANS) during sleep. Important changes in the endocrine system and temperature regulation are also associated with sleep. All of these factors have effects that are important for understanding clinical disorders. This chapter provides a review of the physiologic changes in the ANS, in the respiratory, cardiovascular, and neuromuscular systems, and in the gastrointestinal tract during sleep. Some attention is also given to thermal and endocrine regulation. Table 7–1 summarizes physiologic changes during wakefulness, non–rapid eye movement (NREM) sleep, and rapid eye movement (REM) sleep. For a more detailed discussion, readers are referred to excellent reviews by Orem and Barnes[1] and Lydic and Biebuyck.[2]

AUTONOMIC NERVOUS SYSTEM AND SLEEP

Central Autonomic Network

The existence of a central autonomic network in the brain stem with ascending and descending projections that are often reciprocally connected has been clearly shown by work done over the past 20 years (Figs. 7–1 and 7–2).[3–8] The nucleus tractus solitarius (NTS) may be considered a central station in the central autonomic network. The NTS, which is located in the dorsal region of the medulla ventral to the dorsal vagal nucleus, is the single most important structure of the autonomic network and is influenced by higher brain stem, diencephalon, forebrain, and neocortical regions (Fig. 7–3; see also Figs. 7–1 and 7–2). The NTS receives afferent fibers—from the cardiovascular system and the respiratory and gastrointestinal tracts—important for influencing autonomic control of cardiac rhythm and rate, circulation, respiration, and gastrointestinal motility and secretion (Fig. 7–4). Efferent projections arise from the NTS and are sent to the supramedullary structures, including hypothalamic and limbic regions, and to the ventral medulla, which exerts significant control over cardiovascular regulation.[4,9,10] The ventral medulla sends efferent

TABLE 7–1 Physiologic Changes During Wakefulness, NREM Sleep, and REM Sleep

Physiology	Wakefulness	NREM Sleep	REM Sleep
Parasympathetic activity	++	+++	++++
Sympathetic activity	++	+	Decreases or variable (++)
Heart rate	Normal sinus rhythm	Bradycardia	Bradytachyarrhythmia
Blood pressure	Normal	Decreases	Variable
Cardiac output	Normal	Decreases	Decreases further
Peripheral vascular resistance	Normal	Normal or decreases slightly	Decreases further
Respiratory rate	Normal	Decreases	Variable; apneas may occur
Alveolar ventilation	Normal	Decreases	Decreases further
Upper airway muscle tone	++	+	Decreases or absent
Upper airway resistance	++	+++	++++
Hypoxic and hypercapnic ventilatory responses	Normal	Decreases	Decreases further
Cerebral blood flow*	++	+	++++
Thermoregulation	++	+	–
Gastric acid secretion	Normal	Variable	Variable
Gastric motility	Normal	Decreases	Decreases
Swallowing	Normal	Decreases	Decreases
Salivary flow	Normal	Decreases	Decreases
Migrating motor complex (a special type of intestinal motor activity)	Normal	Slow velocity	Slow velocity
Penile or clitoral tumescence	Normal	Normal	Markedly increased

*There is in general global decrease in cerebral blood flow with regional variations during NREM sleep but this is not homogeneous. It may not decrease in some areas and may even show phasic increase in certain areas (see text and Chapter 15).

NREM, non–rapid eye movement; REM, rapid eye movement; +, mild; ++, moderate; +++, marked; ++++, very marked; –, absent.

Reproduced with permission from Chokroverty S. Sleep and its disorders. *In* Bradley WG, Daroff RB, Fenichel GM, Jankovic J (eds), Neurology in Clinical Practice. Philadelphia: Elsevier, 2008:1960.

projections to the intermediolateral neurons of the spinal cord (see Figs. 7–1 and 7–2). The final common pathways from the NTS are the vagus nerve and sympathetic fibers, which send projections to the intermediolateral neurons of the spinal cord to orchestrate the central autonomic network for integrating various autonomic functions that maintain internal homeostasis. The NTS also contains the lower brain stem hypnogenic and central respiratory neurons. Dysfunction of the ANS, therefore, may have a serious impact on human sleep and respiration.

The cardiovascular system and respiration play significant roles in the maintenance of the internal homeostasis in human beings.[9–11] Cardiovascular control in humans is maintained reflexively, involving peripheral receptors in the heart and blood vessels with afferents to the central nervous system (CNS) and efferents to the heart and blood vessels. Sympathetic preganglionic neurons regulating the cardiovascular system are located predominantly (90%) in the intermediolateral neurons of the thoracic spinal cord, with a small number (10%) in the adjacent spinal structures. Parasympathetic preganglionic neurons controlling the heart and circulation are located in the nucleus ambiguus as well as in the dorsal motor nucleus of the vagus in the medulla. Sympathetic preganglionic neurons in the intermediolateral column of the spinal cord as well as parasympathetic preganglionic neurons in the nucleus ambiguus and dorsal motor nucleus of the vagus are the central determinants of cardiovascular regulation. Both the sympathetic and parasympathetic preganglionic neurons have extensive connections to the central autonomic network, which in turn is influenced by peripheral afferents (Fig. 7–5; see also Figs. 7–1 through

7–4). There is direct projection from the hypothalamic paraventricular nucleus to sympathetic preganglionic neurons in the spinal cord (see Figs. 7–2 and 7–5).

Autonomic Changes During Sleep

During sleep in normal individuals, there are profound changes in the functions of the ANS.[3,4,6,12–16] Most of the autonomic changes that occur during sleep involve the heart, circulation, respiration, and thermal regulation. There are also pupillary changes. Pupilloconstriction occurs during NREM sleep and is maintained during REM sleep due to tonic parasympathetic drive. Phasic dilation during phasic REM sleep results from central inhibition of parasympathetic outflow to the iris.

Autonomic functions during wakefulness must be compared to those during sleep to understand ANS changes in sleep.[6,12] The basic ANS changes during sleep include increased parasympathetic tone and decreased sympathetic activity during NREM sleep. During REM sleep, there is further increase of parasympathetic tone and further decrease of sympathetic activity; intermittently, however, there is an increase of sympathetic activity during phasic REM sleep. The ANS changes during sleep can be assessed by measuring heart rate variability (HRV).[17] The indices of HRV can be documented by fast Fourier transform showing power in the following bands: high frequency (HF), low frequency (LF), very low frequency (VLF), and ultra low frequency (ULF). HF band power ranges from 0.15 to 0.4 Hz. The power in the LF band ranges between 0.04 and 0.15 Hz. The VLF band power ranges from 0.003 to 0.04 Hz and the power in the ULF band is 0.003 Hz

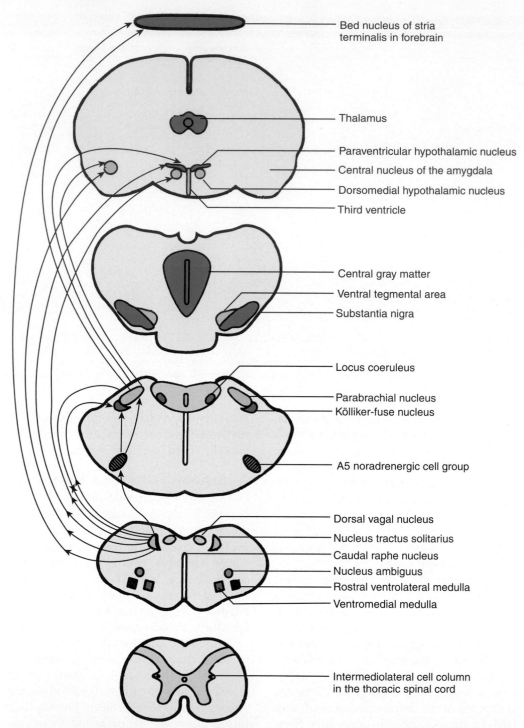

FIGURE 7–1 The ascending projections from the central autonomic network. *(Reprinted with permission from Chokroverty S. Functional anatomy of the autonomic nervous system correlated with symptomatology of neurologic disease.* In *American Academy of Neurology Course No. 246. San Diego: American Academy of Neurology, 1992:49.)*

or less. The major contributor of the HR component is the efferent vagal activity. The LF component is thought to be a marker of sympathetic modulation by some authors,[18,19] whereas others[20,21] considered this to contain both sympathetic and vagal influences. Therefore, the LF/HF ratio is thought to reflect sympathovagal balance. The significance

of VLF and ULF components remains uncertain. Both spectral components and direct nerve recordings (see below) show that the HF component predominates during NREM and the LF component predominates during REM sleep. During NREM sleep, the LF component decreases whereas the HF component increases, reflecting increased vagal

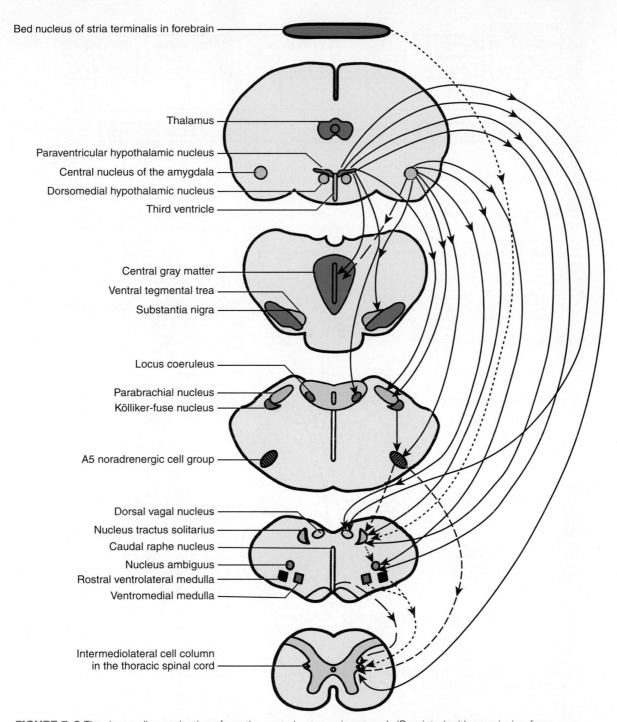

FIGURE 7–2 The descending projections from the central autonomic network. *(Reprinted with permission from Chokroverty S. Functional anatomy of the autonomic nervous system correlated with symptomatology of neurologic disease. In American Academy of Neurology Course No. 246. San Diego: American Academy of Neurology, 1992:49.)*

tone. In contrast, during REM sleep, extreme variation in LF and HF with increased LF and decreased HF components is noted. The heart rate changes precede electroencephalographic (EEG) changes during transition of sleep states. HRV is similar in presleep and intrasleep wake periods. It should be further noted that the HF component mainly reflects the respiration–vagal modulation of sinus rhythm, whereas the nonrespiratory LF component reflects

the sympathetic modulation of the heart in addition to baroreflex responsiveness to beat-to-beat variations in blood pressure (BP).[22–25] Power spectrum analysis of normal subjects at sleep onset by Shiner et al.[26] showed that the wake/sleep transition period represents a transitional process between two physiologically different states, with a decrement of LF power and unchanged HF power causing a decrement of the LF/HF ratio reflecting a shift toward

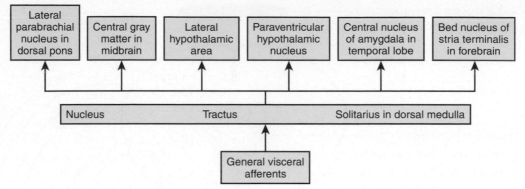

FIGURE 7–3 Schematic diagram of central autonomic network: ascending projections from nucleus tractus solitarius.*(Reproduced with permission from Chokroverty S. Functional anatomy of the autonomic nervous system: autonomic dysfunction and disorders of the CNS. In American Academy of Neurology Course No. 144. Boston: American Academy of Neurology, 1991:77.)*

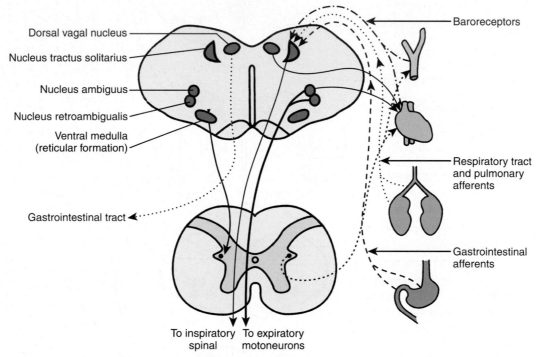

FIGURE 7–4 The visceral afferents to and efferents from the nucleus tractus solitarius.*(Reprinted with permission from Chokroverty S. Functional anatomy of the autonomic nervous system correlated with symptomatology of neurologic disease. In American Academy of Neurology Course No. 246. San Diego: American Academy of Neurology, 1992:49.)*

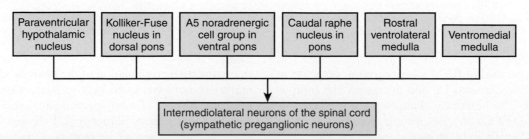

FIGURE 7–5 Schematic diagram showing descending hypothalamic and brain stem inputs to intermediolateral neurons in the spinal cord.*(Reprinted with permission from Chokroverty S. Functional anatomy of the autonomic nervous system correlated with symptomatology of neurologic disease. In American Academy of Neurology Course No. 246. San Diego: American Academy of Neurology, 1992:49.)*

parasympathetic predominance. Thus NREM sleep can be considered as a state of relative cardiorespiratory stability, whereas REM sleep is a state of profound instability with an intense autonomic and respiratory dysregulation. In a recent study, Richard et al.[27] pointed to the effect of gender on autonomic and respiratory responses during sleep. They noted that, in women, there was a greater NREM-to-REM increment in LF, a greater decrement in HF, and a greater increment in LF/HF power. NREM-to-REM excitatory cardiorespiratory responses are therefore more marked among women compared to men.

There is also a profound change of sympathetic activity in muscle and skin blood vessels. Microneurographic technique measures peripheral sympathetic nerve activity in the muscle and skin vascular beds. The technique permits direct intraneural recording of efferent sympathetic nerve activity involving the muscle and skin blood vessels by using tungsten microelectrodes.[28–32] Muscle sympathetic nerve activity is reduced by more than half from wakefulness to stage 4 NREM sleep but increases to levels above waking values during REM sleep.[31] Although sympathetic nerve activity increases in the skeletal muscle vessels (vasoconstriction) during REM sleep, the sympathetic drive decreases in the splanchnic and renal circulation (vasodilation).[31] Sympathetic nerve activity is lower during NREM sleep than during wakefulness but increases above the waking level during REM sleep, particularly during phasic REM sleep (Figs. 7–6 and 7–7). During the arousal and appearance of K complexes in NREM sleep, the bursts of sympathetic activity transiently increase (see Fig. 7–7).[31]

The implications of changes in the ANS during sleep in humans are profound. Reduced HRV may be noted in patients with myocardial infarction, cardiac transplantation, and diabetic autonomic neuropathy.[17,18,21,24,33] There is a significant relationship between the ANS and cardiovascular mortality, including sudden cardiac death. Lethal arrhythmias are related to either increased sympathetic activity or decreased vagal activity. HRV (e.g., reduced HRV) is a strong and independent predictor of mortality after acute myocardial infarction. HRV study thus has potential for assessment of ANS fluctuations in patients with cardiovascular and noncardiovascular disorders, and may help us understand physiologic phenomena, disease mechanisms, and effects of medications. Furthermore, disorders of the ANS in humans, such as multiple systems atrophy, familial dysautonomia, and secondary autonomic failure (see Chapter 29), adversely affect respiratory and cardiovascular functions during sleep. A number of human primary sleep disorders may affect autonomic functions (e.g., obstructive sleep apnea syndrome, cluster headache, sleep terrors, REM sleep–related sinus arrest and painful penile erections, and sleep-related abnormal swallowing syndrome). Thus significant sleep-related changes in the ANS affecting the circulatory, respiratory, gastrointestinal, and urogenital systems have important clinical implications in patients with central or peripheral autonomic failure (e.g., sleep-related respiratory dysrhythmias, cardiac arrhythmias, gastrointestinal dysmotility and urogenital disorders).

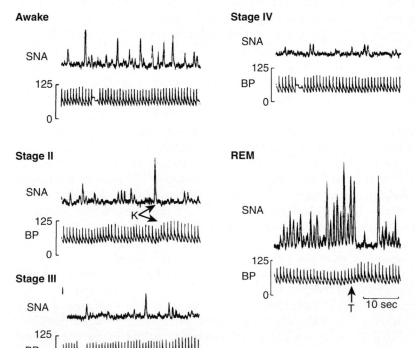

FIGURE 7–6 Symptomatic nerve activity (SNA) and mean blood pressure (BP) recordings in a normal subject while awake and during NREM stages 2, 3, and 4 and during REM sleep. Note gradual decrement of SNA during NREM stages 2–4 but profound increase of SNA during REM sleep. Arousal stimuli during stage 2 NREM sleep elicited K complexes in the EEG (not shown) accompanied by increased SNA. *(Reproduced with permission from Somers VK, Dyken ME, Mark AL, Abboud FM. Sympathetic nerve activity during sleep in normal subjects. N Engl J Med 1993;328:303.)*

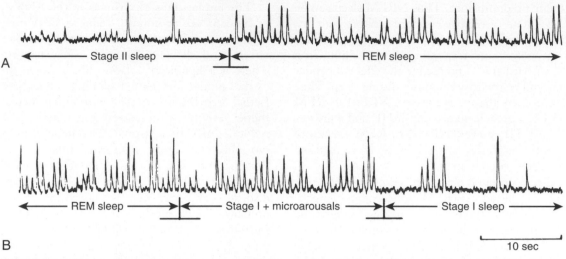

A <———— Stage II sleep ————><—— REM sleep ——————————————>

B <——— REM sleep ———><——— Stage I + microarousals ———><——— Stage I sleep ——————>

10 sec

FIGURE 7–7 Changes in sympathetic nerve activity during the transition from NREM sleep stage 2 to REM sleep **(A)** and the transition from REM sleep to NREM sleep stage 1 with microarousals, and then to regular NREM sleep stage 1 **(B).** *(Reproduced with permission from Somers VK, Dyken ME, Mark AL, Abboud FM. Sympathetic nerve activity during sleep in normal subjects. N Engl J Med 1993;328:303.)*

RESPIRATION AND SLEEP

Functional Neuroanatomy of Respiration

In order to understand the control of breathing, it is essential to have basic knowledge about alveolar ventilation and diffusion across the alveolar capillary membranes (i.e., elimination of carbon dioxide [CO_2] to and supply of oxygen [O_2] from the atmospheric air containing 21% O_2, 78% nitrogen, and 1% other inert gases). An adequate pulmonary circulation is essential to complete the processes of alveolar ventilation and diffusion. The respiratory system consists of three interrelated and integrated components: central controllers located in the medulla aided by the supramedullary structures, including forebrain influence, peripheral chemoreceptors, and pulmonary and upper airway receptors; the thoracic bellows, consisting of respiratory and other thoracic muscles and their innervation and bones; and the lungs, including the airways.

Legallois[34] discovered in 1812 that breathing depends on a circumscribed region of the medulla. After an intensive period of research in the 19th century on the respiratory centers, in the 20th century Lumsden,[35,36] and later Pitts and coworkers,[37] laid the foundation for modern concepts of the central respiratory neuronal networks. Based on sectioning at different levels of the brain stem of cats, Lumsden[35,36] proposed pneumotaxic and apneustic centers in the pons and expiratory and gasping centers in the medulla. Later, Pitts' group[37] concluded from experiments with cats that the inspiratory and expiratory centers were located in the medullary reticular formation.

There is a close interrelationship between the respiratory,[38–40] central autonomic,[5,41,42] and lower brain stem hypnogenic neurons[43–50] in the pontomedullary region. The hypothalamic and lower brain stem hypnogenic neurons are also connected.[51] Reciprocal connections exist between the hypothalamus, the central nucleus of the amygdala, parabrachial and Kölliker-Fuse nuclei, and the NTS of the medulla (see Figs. 7–1 and 7–2).[8,41,52–54] In addition, the NTS connects with the nucleus ambiguus and retroambigualis (see Fig. 7–2).[8,52–54] Thus their anatomic relationships suggest close functional interdependence among the central autonomic network and respiratory and hypnogenic neurons. In addition, peripheral respiratory receptors (arising from the pulmonary and tracheobronchial tree) and chemoreceptors (peripheral and central) interact with the central autonomic network in the region of the NTS.[38–40,55,56]

Breathing is controlled during wakefulness and sleep by two separate and independent systems[38–40,57–60]: the metabolic or automatic,[39,40] and the voluntary or behavioral.[60] Both metabolic and voluntary systems operate during wakefulness, but breathing during sleep is entirely dependent on the inherent rhythmicity of the autonomic (automatic) respiratory control system located in the medulla.[57–59] Voluntary control is mediated through the behavioral system that influences ventilation during wakefulness as well as nonrespiratory functions[61,62] such as phonation and speech. In addition, the wakefulness stimulus, which is probably derived from the ascending reticular activating system,[63,64] represents a tonic stimulus to ventilation during wakefulness. McNicholas and coworkers[65] reported that the reticular arousal system, which is probably the same as the wakefulness stimulus,[63,64,66] exerts a tonic influence on the brain stem respiratory neurons.

Upper brain stem respiratory neurons are located in the rostral pons, in the region of the parabrachial and Kölliker-Fuse nuclei (pneumotaxic center), and in the dorsolateral region of the lower pons (apneustic center).[56] These two centers influence the automatic medullary respiratory neurons, which comprise two principal groups.[38–40,55–59,67,68] The dorsal respiratory group (DRG) located in the NTS is responsible principally, but not exclusively, for inspiration, and the ventral respiratory group (VRG) located in the region of the nucleus ambiguus and retroambigualis is responsible for both inspiration and expiration (Fig. 7–8). The VRG contains the Botzinger complex in the rostral region and the pre-Botzinger region immediately below the Botzinger complex, responsible mainly for the automatic respiratory rhythmicity as these neurons have intrinsic pacemaker activity. These respiratory premotor neurons in the DRG and VRG send axons that decussate below the obex and descend in the reticulospinal tracts in the ventrolateral cervical spinal cord to form synapses with the spinal respiratory motor neurons innervating the various respiratory muscles (see Figs. 7–3 and 7–4). Respiratory rhythmogenesis depends on tonic input from the peripheral and central structures converging on the medullary neurons.[35,55,69,70] The parasympathetic vagal afferents from the peripheral respiratory tracts, the carotid and aortic body peripheral chemoreceptors, the central chemoreceptors located on the ventrolateral surface of the medulla lateral to the pyramids,

the supramedullary (forebrain, midbrain, and pontine regions) structures, and the reticular activating systems all influence the medullary respiratory neurons to regulate the rate, rhythm, and amplitude of breathing and internal homeostasis.[5,55,56,70] Figure 7–9 shows the effects of various brain stem and vagal transections on ventilatory patterns.

The voluntary control system for breathing originating in the cerebral cortex (forebrain and limbic system) controls respiration during wakefulness and has some non-respiratory functions.[55,60,70] This system descends with the corticobulbar and corticospinal tracts partly to the automatic medullary controlling system and to some degree both terminates and integrates there. However, it primarily descends with the corticospinal tract to the spinal respiratory motor neurons, in the high cervical spinal cord, where the fibers finally integrate with the reticulospinal fibers originating from the automatic medullary respiratory neurons for smooth, coordinated functioning of respiration during wakefulness.[39,40,53,59,71]

The thoracic bellows component consists of thoracic bones, connective tissue, pleural membranes, the intercostal and other respiratory muscles, and the nerves and blood vessels. Respiratory muscle weakness plays a critical role in causing sleep dysfunction and sleep-disordered breathing in neuromuscular disorders. Table 7–2 lists the respiratory muscles. The main inspiratory muscle is the diaphragm

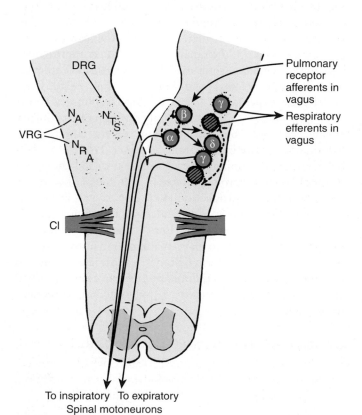

FIGURE 7–8 Schematic diagram of medullary respiratory neurons, cell types, and their interconnections. (CI, first cervical root; DRG, dorsal respiratory group; NA, nucleus ambiguus; NRA, nucleus retroambigualis; NTS, nucleus tractus solitarius; VRG, ventral respiratory group; α, β, γ, δ, designations for inspiratory cell subtypes; open circles, inspiratory cells; hatched circles, expiratory cells.) *(Reproduced with permission from Berger AJ, Mitchell RA, Severinghaus JW. Regulation of respiration. N Engl J Med 1977;297:92, 138, 194.)*

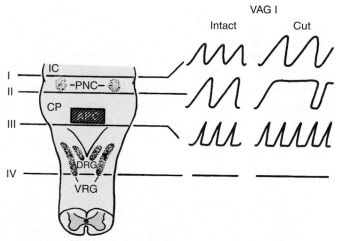

FIGURE 7–9 Effects of various brain stem and vagal (VAG) transections on the ventilatory pattern of the anesthetized animal. On the left is a schematic representation of the dorsal surface of the lower brain stem, and on the right a representation of tidal volume with inspiration upward. Transection I, just rostral to the pneumotaxic center (PNC), causes slow, deep breathing in combination with vagotomy but does not affect normal breathing. Transection II, below the PNC but above the apneustic center (APC), causes slow, deep breathing with intact vagi but apneusis (sustained inspiration) or apneustic breathing (increased inspiratory time) when the vagi are cut. Transection III, at the pontomedullary junction, generally causes regular gasping breathing that is not affected by vagotomy. Transection IV, at the medullospinal junction, causes respiratory arrest. (CP, cerebellar peduncle; DRG, dorsal respiratory group; IC, inferior colliculus; VRG, ventral respiratory group.) *(Reproduced with permission from Berger AJ, Mitchell RA, Severinghaus JW. Regulation of respiration. N Engl J Med 1977;297:92, 138, 194.)*

TABLE 7–2 The Respiratory Muscles
Inspiratory Muscles
• Diaphragm • External intercostal
Accessory Inspiratory Muscles
• Sternocleidomastoideus • Scalenus (anterior, middle, posterior) • Pectoralis major • Pectoralis minor • Serratus anterior • Serratus posterior superior • Latissimus dorsi • Alae nasi • Trapezius
Expiratory Muscles
(silent during quiet breathing but contract during moderately severe airway obstruction or during forceful and increased rate of breathing) • Internal intercostal • Rectus abdominis • External and internal oblique • Transversus abdominis

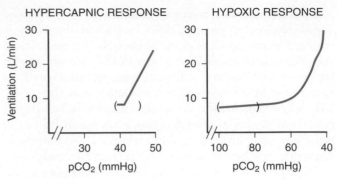

FIGURE 7–10 Schematic representation of normal hypercapnic and hypoxic ventilatory response. Normal ranges are indicated by parentheses. (Pco$_2$, partial pressure of carbon dioxide; Po$_2$, partial pressure of oxygen.) *(Reproduced with permission from White DP. Central sleep apnea. Clin Chest Med 1985;6:626.)*

(innervated by the phrenic nerve, formed by motor roots of C3, C4, and C5 anterior horn cells), assisted by the external intercostal muscles (innervated by the thoracic motor roots and nerves), which expand the core of the thoracic cavity and lungs during quiet normal breathing. Expiration is passive, resulting from elastic recoil of the lungs. During forced and effortful breathing (e.g., dyspnea and orthopnea), accessory muscles of respiration assist the breathing. Accessory inspiratory muscles include the sternocleidomastoideus, trapezius, and scalenus (anterior, middle, and posterior) as well as the pectoralis, serratus anterior, and latitissimus dorsi. Accessory expiratory muscles consist of internal intercostal and abdominal muscles (e.g., rectus abdominis, external and internal oblique, and transversus abdominis) innervated by thoracic motor roots and nerves. Normally, these three respiratory components (central controllers, chest bellows, and lungs) function smoothly in an automatic manner to permit gas exchange (transfer of O$_2$ into the blood and elimination of CO$_2$ into the atmosphere) for ventilation, diffusion, and perfusion. Minute ventilation is defined as the amount of air breathed per minute, which equals about 6 L; about 2 L stay in the anatomic dead space, consisting of the upper airway and the mouth, and 4 L participate in gas exchange in the millions of alveoli constituting alveolar ventilation. Respiratory failure may occur as a result of dysfunction anywhere within these three major components of the respiratory control systems.

Control of Ventilation During Wakefulness

The function of ventilation is to maintain arterial homeostasis (i.e., normal partial pressure of oxygen [Po$_2$] and carbon dioxide [Pco$_2$]).[72] The Pco$_2$ depends predominantly on the central chemoreceptors with some influence from the peripheral chemoreceptors, whereas Po$_2$ depends entirely on the peripheral chemoreceptors. To maintain optimal Po$_2$ and Pco$_2$ levels, the metabolic or autonomic respiratory system uses primarily the peripheral and central chemoreceptors but also to some extent the body's metabolism and the intrapulmonary receptors.[72] It is well known that hypoxia and hypercapnia stimulate breathing.[73,74] Hypoxic ventilatory response is mediated through the carotid body chemoreceptors.[75,76] Normally, this response represents a hyperbolic curve that shows a sudden increase in ventilation when Po$_2$ falls below 60 mm Hg[54–59,72] (Fig. 7–10). Conversely, the hypercapnic[72,74] ventilatory response is linear (see Fig. 7–10). It is mediated mainly through the medullary chemoreceptors[77] but also to some extent through the carotid body peripheral chemoreceptors.[75] When Pco$_2$ falls below a certain minimum level, which is called the apnea threshold, ventilation is inhibited.[72] The metabolic rate (e.g., carbon dioxide production [Vco$_2$] or oxygen consumption [Vo$_2$], particularly Vco$_2$), affects ventilation in part.[72] During sleep, metabolism slows. The intrapulmonary receptors do not seem to play a major role in normal human ventilation.[72] The Hering-Breuer reflex, important to respiration, depends on pulmonary stretch receptors. Vagal afferent stimulation by increasing lung inflation terminates inspiration.

Control of Ventilation During Sleep

In normal persons, during both REM and NREM sleep, clear alterations are noted in tidal volume, alveolar ventilation, blood gases, and respiratory rate and rhythm.[57–60,70,78–83]

Changes in Ventilation

During NREM sleep, minute ventilation falls by approximately 0.5–1.5 L/min,[72,79,80,84–87] and this is secondary to reduction in the tidal volume. REM sleep shows a similar reduction of minute ventilation, up to approximately 1.6 L/min.[72,81,85,87–89] Although there is a discrepancy in the literature regarding REM sleep–related ventilation in humans, it is generally accepted that most reduction occurs during phasic REM sleep.

The following factors, in combination, may be responsible for alveolar hypoventilation during sleep[72]: reduction of Vco_2 and Vo_2 during sleep, absence of the tonic influence of the brain stem reticular formation (i.e., absence of the wakefulness stimulus), reduced chemosensitivity (see *Chemosensitivity and Sleep* later), and increased upper airway resistance to airflow resulting from reduced activity of the pharyngeal dilator muscles during sleep.[85,90,91]

Changes in Blood Gases

As a result of the fall of alveolar ventilation, the Pco_2 rises by 2–8 mm Hg, Po_2 decreases by 3–10 mm Hg, and arterial oxygen saturation (Sao_2) decreases by less than 2% during sleep.[79,81,82,92,93] These changes occur despite reductions of Vo_2 and Vco_2 during sleep.[94]

Respiratory Rate and Rhythm

In NREM sleep the respiratory rate primarily shows a slight decrement, whereas in REM sleep the respiration becomes irregular, especially during phasic REM.[72] There is also waxing and waning of the tidal volume during sleep onset resembling Cheyne-Stokes breathing,[78,81,94–97] which is related to several factors[72]: sudden loss of wakefulness stimulus, reduced chemosensitivity at sleep onset (see *Chemosensitivity and Sleep* later), and transient arousal. During the deepening stage of NREM sleep, respiration becomes stable and rhythmic and depends entirely on the metabolic controlling system.[57–59,70,72,81]

Chemosensitivity and Sleep

Hypoxic ventilatory response in humans is decreased in NREM sleep in adult men but not in women, whereas hypoxic ventilatory response during REM sleep is significantly decreased in both men and women (Fig. 7–11).[99–102] The underlying mechanisms for this gender difference are not clear.[103] This reduction could result from two factors: (1) increased upper airway resistance to airflow during all stages of sleep[85,90,91] and (2) decreased chemosensitivity.

Hypercapnic ventilatory response also decreases by approximately 20–50% during NREM sleep[79,82,86,104,105] and further during REM sleep (Fig. 7–12).[104,105] This results from a combination of two factors: (1) a decreased number of functional medullary respiratory neurons during sleep and (2) increased upper airway resistance.[85,90,91] During sleep, the CO_2 response curve shifts to the right so that increasing amounts of Pco_2 are needed to stimulate ventilation.[93,97] These findings suggest decreased sensitivity of the central chemoreceptors subserving medullary respiratory neurons during sleep.[5] The marked blunting of the hypercapnic ventilatory response during REM sleep could be related to increasing brain blood flow during this sleep state.[103]

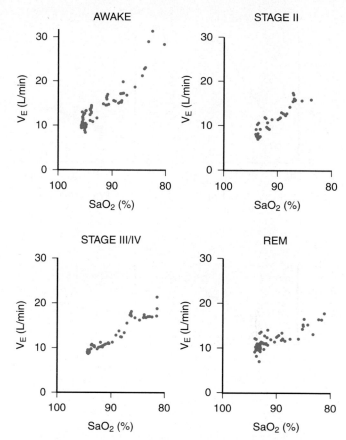

FIGURE 7–11 Hypoxic ventilatory response data show decreased responses during different stages of sleep. (Sao_2%, percentage of arterial oxygen saturation; V_E, expired ventilation [L/min].) *(Reproduced with permission from Douglas NJ, White DP, Weil JV, et al. Hypoxic ventilatory response decreases during sleep in normal men. Am Rev Respir Dis 1982;125:286.)*

Metabolism and Ventilation During Sleep

There is a definite decrease in Vco_2 and Vo_2 during sleep.[94,106,107] Metabolism slows suddenly at sleep onset and accelerates slowly in the early morning at approximately 5:00 AM.[94] During sleep, ventilation falls parallel to metabolism. The rise of Pco_2 during sleep, however, is due to alveolar hypoventilation and is not related to reduced metabolism.[72] The role of the intrapulmonary receptors during normal sleep in humans is unknown.[72]

Changes in the Upper Airway and in Intercostal Muscle and Diaphragm Tone

Upper airway resistance increases during sleep as a result of hypotonia of the upper airway dilator muscles[83,85,90,91,108,109] (see *Physiologic Changes in the Neuromuscular System* later). There is also hypotonia of the intercostal muscles and atonia during REM sleep. The phasic activities in the diaphragm are maintained, but the tonic activity is reduced during REM sleep.[59] As a result of the supine position and hypotonia of intercostal muscles, the functional residual capacity decreases.[110,111] In most normal individuals, there are

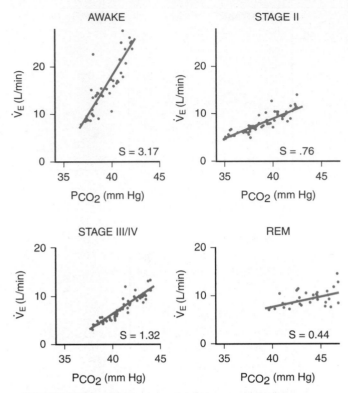

FIGURE 7–12 Hypercapnic ventilatory response data show decreased responses in sleep, the most marked one in REM sleep. (Pco2, partial pressure of carbon dioxide; V$_E$, expired ventilation [L/min].) *(Reproduced with permission from Douglas NJ, White DP, Weil JV, et al. Hypercapnic ventilatory response in sleeping adults. Am Rev Respir Dis 1982;126:758.)*

circadian changes in airway patency with mild bronchoconstriction during sleep at night.[112,113]

Arousal Responses During Sleep

Hypercapnia is a stronger arousal stimulus than hypoxemia during sleep. An increase in Pco2 of 6–15 mm Hg causes consistent arousal during sleep,[101] whereas Sao2 would have to decrease to 75% before arousing a normal person.[91,114]

Laryngeal stimulation normally causes cough reflex response, but this is decreased during both states of sleep and is more markedly decreased during REM than NREM sleep.[115] Thus, clearance of aspirated gastric contents is impaired during sleep. In infants, laryngeal stimulation causes obstructive sleep apnea (OSA), and this has been postulated as one mechanism for sudden infant death syndrome (SIDS).[116]

Summary and Conclusions

During wakefulness, both metabolic and voluntary control systems are active. In NREM sleep, the voluntary system is inactive and respiration is entirely dependent on the metabolic controller—behavioral influences and wakefulness stimuli are not controlling respiration. The nature of ventilatory control during REM sleep has not been determined definitively, but most likely the behavioral mechanism

is responsible for controlling breathing in REM sleep. Ventilation is unstable during sleep, and apneas may occur, particularly at sleep onset and during REM sleep. Respiratory homeostasis is thus relatively unprotected during sleep.

The major cause of hypoventilation and reduced ventilatory response to chemical stimuli during sleep is increased airway resistance.[85,90,91,117] The increased resistance results from reduced activity of the pharyngeal dilator muscles as well as decreased output from the sleep-related medullary respiratory neurons.[118] The reduction of the medullary respiratory neuronal activity in sleep causes a loss of the tonic and phasic motor output to the upper airway muscles, resulting in an increase in airway resistance. Other factors that contribute to sleep-related hypoventilation include the following[57–59,70,72,119]: reduction of metabolic rate by approximately 10–15%; absence of wakefulness stimuli; reduced chemosensitivity; increased blood flow to the brain during REM sleep, which may depress central chemoreceptor activity; and functional alterations in the CNS during sleep, such as cerebral cortical suppression due to reticular inhibition and physiologic cortical deafferentation (presynaptic and postsynaptic inhibition of the afferent neurons[120]) as well as postsynaptic inhibition of motor neurons during REM sleep (see *Physiologic Changes in the Neuromuscular System* later).

Sleep-related changes in breathing may have profound implications in human sleep disorders. Increased upper airway resistance, which is noted during sleep in normal individuals, may predispose to upper airway occlusion and OSA in susceptible individuals.[83] Similarly, the circadian changes of mild bronchoconstriction during sleep in normal individuals may be accentuated in patients with asthma, causing a marked decrease in peak flow rate, which may in turn cause severe bronchospasm.[83,113] As a result of the complex effects of sleep on respiration, there is an overall reduction in ventilation during sleep compared to wakefulness.[83] This may not significantly affect a normal person, but may cause life-threatening hypoxemia and abnormal breathing patterns during sleep in patients with neuromuscular disorders, chronic obstructive pulmonary disease, and bronchial asthma, especially in those with daytime hypoxemia.[83] The chemoreflex control of breathing may vary across patients with obstructive sleep apnea syndrome (OSAS). In patients with an apnea-hypopnea index of greater than 30, Mahmed et al.[121] have shown a significant overnight increase in chemoreflex sensitivity of 30%, which is another contributing factor toward destabilization of breathing during sleep in this condition.

PHYSIOLOGIC CHANGES IN THE HEART AND CIRCULATION DURING SLEEP

Physiologic changes in the heart during sleep include alterations in heart rate and cardiac output. Changes in circulation during sleep include changes in BP, peripheral vascular resistance (PVR), and blood flow to various systems and regions.[122] All these cardiovascular hemodynamic changes are controlled by the ANS. Briefly, sympathetic inhibition is associated with a decrease in BP and heart rate during NREM sleep, whereas in REM sleep, intermittent activation of the sympathetic system accounts for rapid fluctuations in BP and heart rate.[31]

Heart Rate

The heart rate decreases during NREM sleep and shows frequent upward and downward swings during REM sleep.[6,12,123–131] Bradycardia during NREM sleep results from a tonic increase in parasympathetic activity (sympathectomy has little effect).[6,123–126] Bradycardia persists during REM sleep and becomes intense owing to tonically reduced sympathetic discharge. Phasic heart rate changes (bradytachycardia) during REM sleep are due to transient changes in both the cardiac sympathetic and parasympathetic activities.[6,123–126] Thus parasympathetic activity predominates during sleep, and an additional decrease with intermittent increase of sympathetic activity is observed during REM sleep.

In several studies, the HRV during sleep stages has been documented after spectral analysis.[127–130] The documentation of the HF component of the electrocardiogram clearly indicates the prevalence of parasympathetic activity during both NREM and REM sleep. These studies also show intermittent increases of LF components in the electrocardiogram, indicating intermittent sympathetic nervous system activation during REM sleep. Studies also show that the heart rate acceleration occurs at least 10 beats before EEG arousal.[127]

Cardiac Output

Cardiac output falls progressively during sleep, with the greatest decrement occurring during the last sleep cycle, particularly during the last REM sleep cycle early in the morning.[123,132] This may help explain why normal individuals and patients with cardiopulmonary disease are most likely to die during the hours of early morning.[134] Maximal oxygen desaturation and periodic breathing are also noted at this time.

Systemic Arterial Blood Pressure

BP falls by approximately 5–14% during NREM sleep and fluctuates during REM sleep.[123,124,134] These changes are related to alterations in the ANS.[6,12] Coote[135] concluded that the fall in BP during NREM sleep was secondary to a reduction in cardiac output, whereas the BP changes during REM sleep resulted from alterations in cardiac output and PVR.

Pulmonary Arterial Pressure

Pulmonary arterial pressure rises slightly during sleep. During wakefulness, the mean value is 18/8 mm Hg; that during sleep is 23/12 mm Hg.[136]

Peripheral Vascular Resistance

During NREM sleep, PVR remains unchanged or may fall slightly, whereas in REM sleep there is a decrease in PVR due to vasodilation.[123,137,138]

Systemic Blood Flow

Cutaneous, muscular, and mesenteric vascular blood flow shows little change during NREM sleep, but during REM sleep, there is profound vasodilation resulting in increased blood flow in the mesenteric and renal vascular beds.[29–32,123,138,139] However, there is vasoconstriction causing decreased blood flow in the skeletal muscular and cutaneous vascular beds during REM sleep.[29–32,138] Mullen and coworkers[140] reported a decrease of plasma renin activity in humans during REM sleep, which indirectly suggests increased renal blood flow.

Cerebral Blood Flow

Cerebral blood flow (CBF) and cerebral metabolic rate for glucose and oxygen decrease by 5–23% during NREM sleep, whereas these values increase to 10% below up to 41% above the waking levels during REM sleep.[141–151] These data indirectly suggest[142,150] that NREM sleep is the state of resting brain with reduced neuronal activity, decreased synaptic transmission, and depressed cerebral metabolism. CBF is noted to be lower in NREM than in REM sleep, lower at the end of the night compared with that at the beginning of the night, and lower in postsleep wakefulness than presleep wakefulness.[150] Cerebral metabolic rate for oxygen and glucose also decreases in postsleep wakefulness and toward the end of the night compared with the values noted in presleep wakefulness and the beginning of the night.[150,151] This decreased metabolism, reduced CBF, and reduced anaerobic glycolysis (i.e., there is a greater decrease in glucose utilization compared with oxygen utilization) all support restorative functions of sleep.[150] In contrast, REM sleep represents an active brain state with increased neuronal activity and increased metabolism. The largest increases during REM sleep are noted in the hypothalamus and the brain stem structures, and the smallest increases are in the cerebral cortex and white matter.

In the last decade, Maquet and his group (see also Chapter 15) and others[152–169] have made significant contributions using positron emission tomography with [^{15}O]-labeled water or [^{18}F]fluorodeoxyglucose and functional magnetic resonance imaging (MRI) to understand the functional neuroanatomy in normal human sleep. These studies have shown major differences of brain activation during wakefulness, NREM sleep, and REM sleep. During NREM sleep, there is a global decrease in CBF with a regional decrement of CBF in the dorsal pons, mesencephalon, thalami, basal ganglia, basal forebrain, anterior hypothalamus, prefrontal cortex, anterior cingulate cortex, and precuneus.[159–161] These studies confirmed in humans the existence of brain stem–thalamocortical circuits responsible for the NREM sleep–generating mechanisms and correlate with the electrophysiologic findings of hyperpolarization of thalamic neurons with generation of sleep spindles, K complexes, and delta and very slow oscillations.[156,161] The pattern of deactivation in NREM sleep is not homogeneous. The least active areas in NREM sleep were noted in the dorsolateral prefrontal (DLPF) and orbito-frontoparietal and, less consistently, the temporal and insular regions.[153,156,160] The primary cortices are the least deactivated areas.[160] REM sleep is characterized by increased neuronal activity, energy requirements, and CBF with regional activations in the pontine tegmentum, thalamus, amygdala, anterior cingulate cortex, hippocampus, temporal and occipital regions, basal forebrain, cerebellum, and caudate nucleus. In contrast, there is regional deactivation in the DLPF, posterior cingulate gyrus, precuneus, and inferior parietal cortex.[152,160,162] REM sleep–related activation of the pontine tegmentum, thalamic nuclei, and basal forebrain supports the REM sleep–generating mechanisms in these regions.[166] An activation of limbic and paralimbic structures including the amygdala, hippocampal formation, and anterior cingulate cortex supports the modulatory role of these structures during REM sleep during generation of pontine-geniculate-occipital waves, a major component of phasic REM sleep and heart rate variability in REM sleep,[159] and participation of REM sleep in memory processing. REM sleep also showed regional deactivation in the DLPF, precuneus, posterior cingulate cortex, temporoparietal region, and inferior parietal lobule.[152,160,169]

There are three mechanisms controlling CBF[170]: cerebral autoregulation, cerebral metabolism, and respiratory blood gases (arterial P_{O_2} and arterial P_{CO_2}). Cerebral autoregulation is determined by the intrinsic properties of the muscles of the cerebral arterioles. Cerebral autoregulation is normally maintained between the mean arterial pressures of 150 and 60 mm Hg[170]; as the systemic BP falls, cerebral blood vessels dilate in response to changes in transmural pressure, whereas in cases of a rise in BP, the cerebral vessels constrict, thus protecting the brain from fluctuations in systemic BP. This systemic autoregulation may break down in disease states such as stroke, encephalitis, hypertensive crisis, acute head injury, and excessive antihypertensive therapy.[170] Dipping of BP up to 20% during sleep is physiologic, and these individuals are called "dippers." There are certain individuals in whom the nocturnal systolic BP during sleep does not fall below 10% of baseline waking value, and they are known as "nondippers." There are also individuals known as "reverse dippers" in whom BP does not drop but actually increases during sleep periods. Those individuals considered "extreme dippers," in whom BP falls excessively, as well as nondippers and reverse dippers, are at higher risk for stroke than dippers.[171,172] Finally, both hypercapnia and hypoxia would cause vasodilation, with hypercapnia causing stronger vasodilation in the cerebral circulation.

Summary and Clinical Implications

These hemodynamic changes in the cardiovascular system result from alterations in the ANS.[3,6,12,126,135] In general, parasympathetic activity predominates during both NREM and REM sleep and is most predominant during REM sleep. In addition, there is sympathetic inhibition during REM sleep. The sympathetic activity during REM sleep is decreased in cardiac, renal, and splanchnic vessels but increased in skeletal muscles, owing to an alteration in the brain stem sympathetic controlling mechanism. Furthermore, during phasic REM sleep, BP and heart rate are unstable owing to phasic vagal inhibition and sympathetic activation resulting from changes in brain stem neural activity. Heart rate and BP therefore fluctuate during REM sleep. Because of these hemodynamic and sympathetic alterations during REM sleep, which is prominent during the last third of total sleep in the early hours of the morning, increased platelet aggregability, plaque rupture, and coronary arterial spasm could be initiated, possibly triggering thrombotic events causing myocardial infarction, ventricular arrhythmias, or even sudden cardiac death[171,172] (see Chapter 29). As stated previously, those patients who are nondippers, extreme dippers, and reverse dippers are at higher risk for cardiovascular or cerebrovascular events causing infarctions and periventricular hyperlucencies on MRI. Meta-analysis of epidemiologic studies provides support to the circadian variation in cardiovascular and cerebrovascular events, with the highest rates of events occurring during the early morning hours.[173,174]

PHYSIOLOGIC CHANGES IN THE NEUROMUSCULAR SYSTEM

Physiologic changes have been noted during sleep in both the somatic nervous system and the ANS that in turn produce changes in the somatic and smooth muscles of the body. This section presents a discussion of the physiologic changes noted during sleep in the somatic muscles, including cranial, limb, and respiratory muscles.

Changes in Limb and Cranial Muscles

Alterations of limb and cranial muscle tone are noted during sleep. Muscle tone is maximal during wakefulness, slightly decreased in NREM sleep, and markedly decreased or absent in REM sleep. Electromyography (EMG), particularly of the submental muscle, is necessary to identify REM sleep and is thus important for scoring technique. In addition, transient myoclonic bursts are noted during REM sleep. An important EMG characteristic is documentation of periodic limb movements of sleep, which are noted in the majority of patients with restless legs syndrome; patients with a variety of sleep disorders; and normal individuals, most commonly elderly ones.

Upper Airway Muscles and Sleep

Changes occur in the function of the upper airway dilator muscles (Table 7–3) during sleep that have important clinical implications, particularly for patients with sleep apnea syndrome. The upper respiratory tract subserves both respiratory and nonrespiratory functions.[175] In experimental studies in cats, pharyngeal motor neurons in the vagus and glossopharyngeal nerves were found to be located in the medulla, overlapping the medullary respiratory neurons.[176] The experimental study by Bianchi and colleagues[177] demonstrated that, after changes induced by chemical stimuli (normocapnic hypoxia and normoxic hypercapnia), pharyngeal motor activities are more sensitive than phrenic nerve activation. The influence of sleep on respiratory muscle function has been reviewed by Gothe et al.[178] and Horner.[179,180]

Genioglossus Muscle

Genioglossal EMG activities consist of phasic inspiratory bursts and variable tonic discharges, which are decreased during NREM sleep and further decreased during REM sleep.[181–184] Selective reduction of genioglossal or hypoglossal nerve activity (i.e., disproportionately more reduction than the diaphragmatic or phrenic activities) has been noted

TABLE 7–3 Upper Airway Dilator Muscles

Palatal Muscles

- Palatoglossus
- Palatopharyngeus
- Levator veli palatini
- Tensor veli palatini
- Musculus uvulae

Tongue Muscles

- Genioglossus
- Geniohyoid
- Palatoglossus
- Hyoglossus

Hyoid Muscles

Suprahyoid

- Mylohyoid
- Hyoglossus
- Digastric
- Geniohyoid

Infrahyoid

- Sternohyoid
- Omohyoid
- Sternothyroid
- Stylohyoid

Laryngeal Muscles

- Posterior cricoarytenoid
- Lateral cricoarytenoid
- Interarytenoid
- Thyroarytenoid
- Cricothyroid
- Aryepiglottic
- Thyroepiglottic

with alcohol, diazepam, and many anesthetic agents.[181] Conversely, protriptyline and strychnine selectively increase such activity.[181]

Palatal Muscles

Levator veli palatini and palatoglossus muscles in humans show phasic inspiratory and tonic expiratory activities,[185,186] but tensor veli palatini muscle shows tonic activity during both inspiration and expiration in wakefulness and sleep.[187,188] During sleep in normal individuals, palatal muscles (palatoglossus, tensor veli palatini, and levator veli palatini) show decreased tone causing increased upper airway resistance and decreased airway space.

Masseter Muscle

Masseter contraction closes the jaw and elevates the mandible. In sleep apnea patients, masseter activation is present during eupneic episodes but decreased during apneic ones. Masseter EMG activity decreases immediately before the apnea, is absent during the early part of the episode, and increases at the end of the apneic period.[189] Based on experiments using chemical stimuli, Suratt and Hollowell[189] concluded that masseter activity can be increased by hyperoxic hypercapnia and inspiratory resistance loading. It appears that phasic EMG bursts start in the masseter at the same time as in the genioglossus and the diaphragm. Suratt and Hollowell[189] did not find phasic activity in masseter muscle in normal subjects during regular breathing, but noted such activity during inspiratory stimulation such as inspiratory resistance loading or hypercapnia. In sleep apnea patients, spontaneous phasic masseter activity was noted during regular breathing.

Intrinsic Laryngeal Muscle Activity

Intrinsic laryngeal muscles, controlled by the brain stem neuronal mechanism, play an important role in the regulation of breathing.[190–192] In addition, the larynx participates in phonation, deglutition, and airway protection.[191] The posterior cricoarytenoid (PCA) muscle is the main vocal cord abductor. Laryngeal EMG can be performed by placing hooked wire electrodes percutaneously through the cricothyroid membrane.[192]

PCA demonstrates phasic inspiratory bursts in normal subjects during wakefulness and NREM sleep.[190] In addition, there is tonic expiratory activity in wakefulness that disappears with NREM sleep. In REM sleep, PCA EMG shows fragmented inspiratory bursts and variable expiratory activity. During isocapnic hypoxia and hyperoxic hypercapnia, normal subjects show increased phasic inspiratory PCA activity but minimal increase of tonic expiratory activity.[190]

Hyoid Muscles

Suprahyoid muscles (those inserted superiorly on the hyoid bone) include the geniohyoid, mylohyoid, hypoglossus, stylohyoid, and digastric muscles.[193] Infrahyoid muscles (those that insert inferiorly) include the sterno-hyoid, omohyoid, and sternothyroid muscles.[193] The size and shape of the upper airways can be altered by movements of the hyoid bone. Motor neurons supplying these muscles are located in the pons, the medulla, and the upper cervical spinal cord. The hyoid muscles show inspiratory bursts during wakefulness and NREM sleep that are increased by hypercapnia. The relative contribution of hyoid, genioglossus, and other tongue muscles in the maintenance of pharyngeal patency needs to be clarified.[193]

It is important to understand central neuronal mechanisms and the contributions of neuromodulators and neurotransmitters involved in sleep-related suppression of pharyngeal muscle activity.[179,180] This knowledge will help in designing treatment for upper airway OSAS.

Mechanism of Mild Muscle Hypotonia in NREM Sleep

Mild muscle hypotonia in NREM sleep appears to result from a combination of disfacilitation of brain stem motor neurons controlling muscle tone (e.g., mild reduction of activity of locus ceruleus noradrenergic and midline raphe serotonergic neurons) and slight hyperpolarization of brain stem and spinal neurons.[194] In addition, there is a direct cerebral cortical mechanism to explain mild muscle hypotonia in NREM sleep, as evidenced by significant enhancement of intracortical inhibition during slow-wave sleep (SWS) after paired-pulse transcranial magnetic brain stimulation.[195] Intracellular microelectrode recording of motor neurons at the onset of NREM sleep by Chase and collaborators[194] clearly showed either no change in membrane potential or a slight hyperpolarization. It should be remembered that the resting membrane potential is determined by an unequal distribution of ions on the outside and the inside of the membrane and by differential permeabilities of the concentration of the sodium, potassium, and chloride ions.

Mechanism of Muscle Atonia or Hypotonia in REM Sleep

REM sleep is characterized by complete cessation of voluntary muscle tone in the presence of a highly active forebrain (paralyzed body with an activated brain) with inhibition of the mesencephalic locomotor region. This is nature's way of preventing abnormal movements during REM sleep in the presence of highly active cerebral cortex and forebrain regions. The dorsal pontine tegmentum appears to be an important central region responsible for limb muscle atonia in REM sleep.[44,196–198] Muscle atonia during REM sleep is initiated during activation of a polysynaptic descending pathway from the peri–locus ceruleus alpha in the region of the nucleus pontis oralis to the lateral tegmentoreticular tract, the nucleus gigantocellularis and magnocellularis in the ventral region of the medial medullary reticular formation (the inhibitory region of Magoun and Rhines),[196,197] and finally the ventral tegmentoreticular and reticulospinal tracts to the alpha motor neurons causing hyperpolarization and muscle atonia.[198–201] During REM sleep, an increased number of c-Fos (a nuclear protein synthesized during neuronal activation) labeled cells were detected by immunocytochemical techniques in the inhibitory region of Magoun and Rhines. A key element in the REM sleep–generating mechanism in the pons is the activation of γ-aminobutyric acidergic (GABAergic) neurons located in a subgroup of the pontine reticular formation as well as GABAergic neurons in the ventrolateral periaqueductal gray region in the mesencephalon.[198,201] An activation of GABAergic neurons causes excitation or disinhibition of cholinergic neurons, and inhibition of noradrenergic and serotonergic neurons, in the pons. The cholinergic neurons, in turn, excite pontine glutamatergic neurons projecting to the glycinergic premotor neurons in the medullary reticular formation, causing hyperpolarization of the motor neurons and muscle paralysis during REM sleep. This GABAergic mechanism also plays an important role in motor neuron hyperpolarization (see later). In addition, disfacilitation of motor neurons as a result of reduction of the release of midline raphe serotonin and locus ceruleus noradrenaline partially contributes to muscle atonia. Finally, a cerebral cortical mechanism may also contribute to the inhibition of spinal motor neurons in REM sleep, as evidenced by decreased intracortical facilitation in the paired-pulse transcranial magnetic brain stimulation techniques.[195]

In summary, there are four fundamental mechanisms responsible for muscle atonia in REM sleep: inhibitory postsynaptic potentials (IPSPs) causing postsynaptic inhibition of motor neurons (major mechanism); disfacilitation (i.e., a reduction of excitation of presynaptic spinal excitatory neurons); disfacilitation of brain stem motor neurons controlling muscle tone; and decreased intracortical facilitation (e.g., paired-pulse brain magnetic stimulation technique). During wakefulness and NREM sleep, there are a few spontaneously occurring low-amplitude IPSPs, but during REM sleep, in addition to an increase of these low-amplitude IPSPs, high-amplitude REM sleep–specific IPSPs are noted. These are generated by sleep-specific inhibitory interneurons located mainly in the brain stem (immunocytochemical techniques are used to prove this observation) that send long-projecting axons to the spinal cord and short axons to the brain stem motor neurons.[196–201] As a result of these IPSPs, motor neurons are hyperpolarized by 2–10 mV during REM sleep. Intracellular recordings reveal increased number and appearance of REM sleep–specific IPSPs in the lumbar motor neurons of cats.[194,202–205] Thus postsynaptic inhibition of motor neurons is responsible for the atonia of somatic muscles, as evidenced by intracellular recordings of spinal motor neurons in chronic spinal preparations of cats. These potentials are derived from inhibitory interneurons, possibly located either in the spinal cord or in the brain stem, from which long axons project to the spinal motor neurons.[196,204,206] In addition, there is also postsynaptic inhibition causing a decrease in the Ia monosynaptic excitatory postsynaptic potentials (EPSPs), resulting in motor neuron hyperpolarization. Lesions of the dorsal pontine tegmentum abolish muscle atonia of REM sleep.[203–209] Similar episodes of REM sleep without muscle atonia have also been observed in cats with localized lesions in the ventromedial medulla.[210]

Intermittently during REM sleep there are excitatory drives causing motor neuron depolarization shifts as a result of EPSPs.[194,203–206] Muscle movements caused by these excitatory drives during REM sleep are somewhat different from the movements noted during wakefulness. These movements are abrupt, jerky, and purposeless. EPSPs during REM sleep reflect increased rates of firing in the motor facilitatory pathways during REM sleep. Enhanced IPSPs during REM sleep check these facilitatory discharges, thus balancing the motor system during this activated brain state; otherwise the blind, unconscious subject will jump out of bed, as may happen in pathologic conditions such as REM sleep behavior disorders.[194,211] Facilitatory reticulospinal fibers are responsible for transient EPSP phasic discharges causing muscle twitches in REM sleep. Corticospinal or rubrospinal tracts are not responsible for these twitches because destruction of these fibers in cats[212] does not affect these twitches.

What neurotransmitters drive these IPSPs? Glycine, a major inhibitory neurotransmitter, was originally thought to be the only driving force. The elegant work by Chase and Morales[194,213] suggested that glycine is the main neurotransmitter responsible for motor neuron hyperpolarization and IPSPs. The REM sleep–specific IPSPs are reversed after strychnine (a glycine antagonist) administration by microiontophorectic application into the ventral spinal cord.[194] In contrast, picrotoxins and bicuculine (a GABA antagonist) did not abolish these IPSPs. Recent evidence, however, suggests an important contribution by GABA in addition to glycine.[214–218] It should be noted that, in the experiments by Chase and Morales, although the GABA antagonist picrotoxin did not reverse REM sleep–related IPSPs, it reduced the IPSP duration considerably. GABA suppression of muscle tone in the hypoglossal nucleus was also demonstrated by Morrison et al.[217] and Liu et al.[218] According to Nitz and Siegel,[219,220] there is a selective GABAergic inhibition of noradrenergic and serotonergic neurons during REM sleep accounting for cessation of discharge of these aminergic cells. As a result of this cessation, there is disfacilitation of motor neurons. GABA may also have a direct inhibitory effect on interneurons and motor neurons.

What is the role of hypocretin in REM motor atonia? Hypocretinergic neurons located in the lateral hypothalamus play a facilitatory role in the motor system by direct projections to the motor neurons and indirectly through projections to the monoaminergic and cholinergic neurons.[194,221–224] Hypocretinergic neurons facilitate motor activity during wakefulness but enhance motor inhibition during REM sleep. There is withdrawal of hypocretinergic activation of the locus ceruleus noradrenergic and midline raphe serotonergic neurons during REM sleep, causing disfacilitation of these aminergic neurons contributing to muscle atonia.

REM Sleep–Related Alterations in Respiratory Muscle Activity

During REM sleep, activity of upper airway muscles and the diaphragm is reduced. Three types of REM sleep–related alterations in the respiratory muscles have been described[225]:

1. *Atonia* of EMG activity throughout the REM sleep period is found. Somatic muscles characteristically show this response, which is related to glycine- as well as GABA-mediated postsynaptic inhibition of motor neurons.[194,203–206,226]
2. Rhythmic activity of the diaphragm persists in REM sleep, but certain diaphragmatic motor units cease firing. Kline and coworkers[227] described *intermittent decrement of diaphragmatic activity* during single breaths. Upper airway muscles also show similar changes.
3. *Fractionations of diaphragmatic activity* refer to pauses lasting 40–80 msec and occur in clusters correlated with pontine-geniculate-occipital waves, which are phasic events of REM sleep.[228]

What is the mechanism of muscle atonia in the upper airway muscles during REM sleep? Postsynaptic inhibition of motor neurons during REM sleep as described previously is a critical mechanism mediating suppression of hypoglossal motor neurons during REM sleep. Kodama et al.,[214] Liu et al.,[218] and Nitz and Siegel[219,220] suggested that both glycine and GABA play important roles in the regulation of upper airway and postural muscles. A combination of decreased monoamines (e.g., noradrenaline and serotonin) and increased GABA release in the motor neuron pools may be involved in the REM sleep muscle atonia. Fenik et al.[215,216] as well as several other authors[229–239] previously suggested that the suppression of upper airway motor tone, including the genioglossus muscle tone, during REM sleep is caused by withdrawal of excitation mediated by norepinephrine and serotonin. Fenik et al.[215,216] concluded that suppression of motor activity or muscle atonia of the hypoglossus and other upper airway dilator muscles is caused by all or some of the following mechanisms: the withdrawal of motor neuronal excitation mediated by norepinephrine and serotonin, and increased inhibition mediated by GABA and glycine. In summary, the selective inhibition of monoaminergic and orexinergic (hypocretinergic) systems (disfacilitation) coupled with direct active inhibition of motor neurons by GABA and glycine produces a loss of postural muscle tone.

Upper Airway Reflexes

The negative intrathoracic pressure at the onset of inspiration generates a reflex response (increased activity) to the upper airway dilator muscles. During sleep, such reflex responses are decreased, making the upper airway susceptible to suction collapse.[179,180,240] This probably results from a decrement in the excitability of the upper airway motor neurons. In this connection, the observations of McNicholas et al.[241] of increased frequency of obstructive apneas and hypopneas in normal sleeping subjects after upper airway anesthesia and increased apnea index after upper airway anesthesia in snorers[242] support the importance of the upper airway reflexes in controlling the upper airway resistance and space. However, there is no clear indication of the impairment of upper airway reflex in OSA. Patients with OSA, in contrast to snorers and normal sleepers, do not show an increase in the apnea index after upper airway anesthesia.[243,244] Alcohol, benzodiazepines, and age[179,180,245] clearly cause a decrement in upper airway reflex response.

Summary and Clinical Relevance

There is considerable reduction of the activity of the upper airway dilator muscles during NREM sleep, with further reduction in REM sleep, causing increased upper airway resistance and narrowing of the upper airway space. The site of the upper airway obstruction in OSA is usually at the level of the soft palate, but in approximately half the patients the obstruction extends caudally to the region of the tongue, with further caudal extension during REM sleep.[240,246–253] Therefore, decreased tone in the palatal, genioglossal, and other upper airway muscles causing increased upper airway resistance and decreased airway space plays an important contributing role in upper airway obstruction in OSA, particularly because many OSA patients have smaller upper airways than individuals without OSA.[240,254–256] Furthermore, sleep-related alveolar hypoventilation also predisposes such individuals to upper airway occlusion and obstructive apnea. Patients with neuromuscular disorders, chronic obstructive pulmonary disease, and bronchial asthma may be affected adversely by such hypoventilation. Asthmatic attacks may also be exacerbated at night as a result of bronchoconstriction, which is a normal physiologic change during sleep.[113]

GASTROINTESTINAL PHYSIOLOGY DURING SLEEP

A brief summary of the physiology of the gastrointestinal tract during sleep is given in this section. For a more detailed discussion, readers are referred to the writings of Orr.[257–259] Gastrointestinal changes include alterations in gastric acid secretion, gastric volume and motility, swallowing, and esophageal peristalsis and intestinal motility.

Studying the physiology of the gastrointestinal system has been difficult traditionally because of the lack of adequate technique. Techniques as well as facilities for making simultaneous polysomnographic (PSG) recordings are now available, allowing study of the alterations in gastrointestinal physiology during different stages of sleep. Before the advent of these techniques, scattered reports generally showed decreased motor and secretory functions during sleep. Subsequent methods have produced better and more consistent results, although findings are still somewhat contradictory overall. There is a dearth of adequate studies using PSG and other modern techniques to understand the physiologic alterations of gastrointestinal motility and secretions during sleep.

Gastric Acid Secretion

During wakefulness, gastric acid secretion depends on food ingestion, increased salivation, and the activity of the gastric vagus nerve. Moore and Englert[260] showed a clear circadian rhythm for gastric acid secretion in humans. These authors noted peak gastric acid secretion between 10:00 PM and 2:00 AM in patients with duodenal ulcer. Figure 7–13 (adapted from Moore and Halberg[261]) schematically shows mean 24-hour values for gastric acid secretion in patients with peptic ulcer and normal controls. Acid secretion increases considerably during the day and at night.[262,263] The importance of vagal stimulation for the control of circadian oscillation of gastric acid secretion has been demonstrated by the absence of circadian rhythm for gastric acid secretion following vagotomy.[264]

Several studies have attempted to understand gastric acid secretion during different stages of sleep, but the results have not been consistent because of methodologic flaws and cumbersome techniques.[261–269] An important

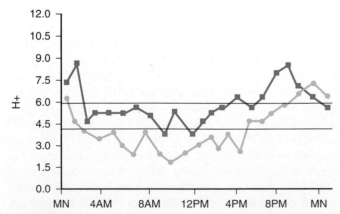

FIGURE 7–13 Mean 24-hour values for gastric acid secretion from patients with active peptic ulcer disease (dark blue rectangles) and normal controls (light blue circles) shown schematically. The ordinate shows hydrocholoric acid (H+) secretion in milliequivalents. (*Adapted from Moore JG, Halberg F. Circadian rhythm of gastric acid secretion in men with active duodenal ulcer. Dig Dis Sci 1986;31:1185.*)

study was made by Orr and colleagues,[268] who examined five duodenal ulcer patients for five consecutive nights using PSG technique and continuous aspiration of gastric contents. They found no relationship between acid secretion and different stages of sleep or REM versus NREM sleep. The most striking finding was failure of inhibition of acid secretion during the first 2 hours of sleep, a result that agrees with the previous study by Levin and associates.[262]

Gastric Motility

Findings regarding gastric motility have been contradictory. Both inhibition and enhancement of gastric motility have been noted during sleep.[269–271] Finch and coworkers[272] showed that gastroduodenal motility during sleep was related to sleep-stage shifts and body movements. Orr[257] reported that, although no definite statement regarding gastric motility can be made, there seems to be overall inhibition of gastric motor function during sleep.

Esophageal Function

There are profound alterations in esophageal function during sleep.[257–259,273–279] Gastroesophageal reflux (GER) is the most common upper gastrointestinal problem. GER occurs most commonly postprandially during wakefulness, but also occurs during sleep but is less frequent. The availability of the method to measure GER during sleep by 24-hour esophageal pH monitoring[280] has advanced our understanding of esophageal function and swallowing during sleep. Waking reflux events are rapidly cleared within 1–2 minutes, whereas sleep reflux events persist longer, causing longer acid contact. Sleep alters normal response to acid mucosal contact.[277] During wakefulness GER causes increased salivary flow and increased swallowing with the complaints of heartburn. In contrast, during sleep salivary flow and swallowing are considerably decreased, causing prolongation of acid mucosal contact. This predisposes to development of esophagitis. The refluxed acid contents are harmful not only to the esophagus but also to the tracheobronchial tree.[257–259]

There are two esophageal sphincters, the upper esophageal sphincter (UES) and the lower esophageal sphincter (LES), acting as barriers to reflux. The LES is the primary barrier to GER, and both the UES and the LES act as barriers to pharyngoesophageal reflux.[281] In a recent paper, Eastwood et al.[282] simultaneously monitored the functions of the LES and UES during PSG studies in 10 normal volunteers and found a decrement of UES pressure during SWS, particularly in the expiratory phase of breathing. In contrast to other investigators, Eastwood et al.[282] did not find an alteration of LES pressure. UES pressure is generated mainly by the cricopharyngeus and to a certain extent by inferior pharyngeal constrictor muscles.

LES pressure is generated by contractions of the esophageal smooth muscles and the diaphragm. Pandolfino et al.[283] studied 15 normal subjects using a solid-state high-resolution manometry recording from the hypopharynx to the stomach with simultaneous measurement of lower esophageal pH. These authors noted that the majority of postprandial transient LES relaxations were associated with brief periods of UES relaxations.

The relationship of GER and sleep is reciprocal: sleep affects GER and GER in turn affects sleep. Sleep-related prolonged esophageal acid clearance and acid-mucosa contact result from several sleep-related physiologic alterations, which include decreased salivary production and swallowing as well as decreased conscious perception of heartburn and arousal, and delayed gastric emptying.[257–259,279] In normal individuals who experience episodes of GER, there is generally a reduction in LES pressure.[257–259,279,281] Lipan et al.[284] postulated that reflux may advance to the laryngopharynx and into the nasopharynx and paranasal sinuses as a result of a laryngopharyngeal reflux. These authors suggested that breakdown of the following barriers to reflux may cause the laryngopharyngeal reflex: the LES and UES, esophageal motility, esophageal acid clearance, and pharyngeal and laryngeal mucosal resistance.

Intestinal Motility

Although methods are now available to accurately measure intestinal motility, the results of motility studies during sleep are contradictory.[257] A special pattern of motor activity, called *migrating motor complex* (MMC), recurs every 90 minutes in the stomach and small intestine.[285] This periodicity of the gut motor activity is similar to the cyclic REM-NREM sleep. In fact, a circadian rhythm in the propagation of the MMC has been documented with the slowest velocity occurring during sleep.[285–289] There are no clear changes in the MMC distribution between REM and NREM sleep stages. Consistent abnormalities in the MMC in different bowel diseases have not been documented.

Orr[279] summarized the studies from the literature to indicate that there is decreased colonic motility in the transverse, descending, and sigmoid colon. Rao and Welcher[290] observed increased periodic rectal motor activity during sleep; the majority of these contractions are propagated in the retrograde direction and, at the same time, the anal canal pressure is consistently above the pressure of the rectum, thus preventing the passive escape of rectal contents during sleep.

Summary and Clinical Relevance

Patients with peptic ulcer disease may have repeated arousals and awakenings as a result of episodes of nocturnal epigastric pain and failure of inhibition of gastric acid secretion that occurs after sleep onset.

Sleep-related GER, by causing marked prolongation of esophageal acid clearance time, may cause mucosal damage giving rise to esophagitis, laryngopharyngitis, pulmonary aspiration, and exacerbation of bronchial asthma.[258,259,281] GER includes esophageal syndrome and extraesophageal complications.[291] Several factors are implicated in the pathogenesis of esophageal syndrome: hiatal hernia, reduced LES pressure, prolonged esophageal acid clearance, and delayed gastric emptying. The UES prevents pharyngoesophageal reflux, and thus loss of UES pressure during sleep makes one vulnerable to reflux of esophageal contents into the pharynx and tracheobronchial tree, which is the most dreaded complication of sleep-related GER. It should be noted that OSAS also predisposes to nocturnal GER disease. Orr et al.[292] have clearly shown that sleep is a significant risk factor for acid migration to the proximal esophagus with prolongation of the acid clearance time, contributing to the extraesophageal complications of reflux such as laryngopharyngitis and pulmonary aspirations.

Patients with functional bowel disorders (e.g., irritable bowel syndrome) have increased sleep complaints, but their sleep architecture does not differ from normal controls.[279] The actual mechanism of sleep disturbance in dysfunctional bowel disorders remains to be determined. Finally, Orr[279] suggested that alterations of the periodic rectal motor contractions and anal canal pressure during sleep in sleeping individuals with diabetes may explain the loss of rectal continence in this condition.

THERMAL REGULATION IN SLEEP

Changes in Body Temperature and Circadian Rhythm

That body temperature follows a circadian rhythm independent of the sleep-wake rhythm[293] has been demonstrated in experiments involving desynchronization and resynchronization of human circadian rhythms. It has been shown that, when all environmental cues (*zeitgebers*) are removed, the endogenous rhythms are freed from the influence of exogenous rhythms and a free-running rhythm ensues. During this time, it is clear that body temperature has a rhythm independent of the sleep-wake rhythm (Fig. 7–14).[294] Nevertheless, body temperature has been linked intimately to the sleep-wake cycle.[295] Body temperature begins to fall with the onset of sleep, and the lowest temperature is noted during the third sleep cycle.[296]

Role of REM Sleep in Thermal Regulation

During REM sleep, the thermoregulating mechanism appears to be inoperative.[295,297,298] Body temperature increases during REM sleep, and cyclic changes in the temperature occur throughout this period. Thermoregulatory responses such as sweating and panting are noted in NREM sleep but are absent in REM sleep; in fact,

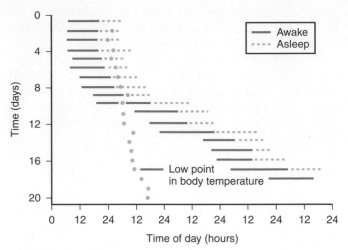

FIGURE 7–14 Synchronized (light-entrained) and desynchronized (free-running) rhythms in a person showing dissociation between body temperature and sleep-activity cycles. *(Reproduced with permission from Aschoff J. Desynchronization and resynchronization of human circadian rhythms. Aerospace Med 1969;40:847.)*

animals display a state of poikilothermia during REM sleep. Brain temperature rises during REM sleep. Szymusiak and McGinty[299] speculated that REM sleep, by elevating brain temperature or by reversing the cooling trend in SWS, prepares the body for behavioral activation. It should be noted that the loss of thermoregulation in REM sleep is not related to inhibition of motor control but is determined by central integration or thermoafferent pathways, or may be due to both mechanisms.[295]

Mechanism of Thermoregulation in Sleep

The function of sleep appears to be energy conservation, as evidenced by a reduction in body temperature and metabolism during sleep, especially NREM sleep.[296,297,300] Body temperature follows a sinusoidal rhythm with a peak around 9:00 PM and a minimum (nadir) around 5:00 AM as a result of circadian rhythmicity,[301] which is controlled by the master clock in the suprachiasmatic nucleus (SCN). The neural projections from the SCN to the ventrolateral preoptic (VLPO) nucleus of the anterior hypothalamus as well as several other brain structures participating in the regulation of sleep and wakefulness are well documented.[302] The circadian system influences core body temperature and the sleep-wake cycle through these connections. At sleep onset, there is a reduction of core body temperature. Exercise or passive body heating causes a rebound stimulating the homeostatic thermostat, permitting peripheral heat loss by vasodilation with a decline in body temperature at sleep onset. Sleep onset latency is shortened and SWS is increased by peripheral heat loss (e.g., after a hot bath).[303] This could also be achieved by simply warming the feet.[304,305] Thermoregulatory effects are also observed after sedative-hypnotic administration. The somnogenic effects of melatonin[306–308] and the benzodiazepines[309–312] are accompanied by a decrease in core body temperature. In contrast, caffeine and amphetamines decrease sleep propensity and increase body temperature.[313] The question is whether sleep onset affects body temperature or body temperature affects sleep onset. The independent circadian rhythm of body temperature appears to be unrelated to a reduction of motor activities at sleep onset.[296,312] A reduction of body temperature and peripheral heat loss promote sleep onset and amount of SWS; sleep in turn causes a further decrease in body temperature and increases heat loss, thus consolidating sleep. The body temperature and sleep regulation are therefore interrelated. The thermoregulatory changes function as physiologic triggers[293] for sleep onset.

The VLPO region of the anterior hypothalamus participates in both generation of NREM sleep and thermoregulation. Physical warming[314,315] or chemical stimulation[316] of the VLPO may initiate sleep onset. In the VLPO, warm-sensitive neurons increase firing rates at sleep onset and decrease the rates at sleep offset.[317] An immunocytochemical study by Sherin et al.[318] showed activation of VLPO neurons during sleep. These findings provide evidence for a role of temperature in sleep regulation. The conclusive evidence is provided by the observation of increased firing rates of warm-sensitive neurons in the VLPO and other brain areas participating in sleep regulation following application of heat to peripheral skin,[317,318] probably through a neural pathway between the peripheral skin and sleep-regulating regions of the brain. Van Someren[319] proposed a thermoregulatory signaling pathway to the circadian system (SCN) promoting circadian regulation of sleep and body temperature. Gilbert et al.[312] suggested a model to show how thermoregulatory changes (e.g., an increase in peripheral temperature and heat loss or a decrease in core body temperature) trigger sleep/wake–promoting areas of the brain directly or via VLPO thermosensitive neurons to initiate and consolidate sleep, taking into consideration also the circadian control of sleep and body temperature via the SCN.

MacFadyen and colleagues[320] observed increased SWS after 2–3 days of fasting in humans, suggesting that the length of hypometabolism helps conserve energy. As stated previously, the VLPO neurons participate in both NREM sleep and thermoregulation. McGinty and Szymusiak[321] also cited evidence in support of this hypothesis: VLPO warming will facilitate SWS, whereas lesions will suppress it; microinjections of putative sleep factors into the VLPO will promote SWS. Szymusiak and McGinty[299,322] also hypothesized that the neuronal mechanisms in the VLPO regions are responsible for both thermoregulation and SWS generation, and that SWS is essentially a thermoregulatory process. Although thermoregulation and sleep are clearly linked, they are also unquestionably separate.[323]

Clinical Relevance

Changes in thermoregulatory function have been noted in some insomniacs and elderly poor sleepers.[324–326] For example, in patients with sleep-onset insomnia[324] the core body temperature rhythm is delayed, suggesting that these people attempt to initiate sleep before the nocturnal dip in body temperature.[312] Similarly, in elderly poor sleepers there is advancing of the core body temperature rhythm, indicating that these individuals attempt to sleep after the decline in core body temperature[312,325] or attenuation of the circadian decline in core body temperature.[326] It has been suggested that age-related impairment of the heat loss mechanism or phase advance in body temperature rhythm may partly explain sleep initiation or maintenance difficulty in the elderly.[327] Therefore, thermal manipulation (e.g., behavior to enhance peripheral heat loss) may improve sleep.[327,328] People with cold feet (e.g., vasospastic syndrome) with impaired heat loss have also prolonged sleep onset latency.[312,329]

Jet lag and shift work may disrupt this linkage of thermoregulation and SWS generation and change the rhythms of sleep and body temperature, which may cause difficulty in initiating and maintaining sleep and disorganization of sleep architecture and daytime function.[295] Menopausal hot flashes are thought to be a disorder of thermoregulation initiating within the preoptic anterior hypothalamic area. Woodward and Freedman[330] performed 24-hour ambulatory recordings of hot flashes and all-night sleep characteristics on 12 postmenopausal women with hot flashes and 7 without hot flashes to determine the effect of hot flashes on sleep patterns. They found that hot flashes were associated with increased stage 4 sleep and that hot flashes occurring in the 2 hours before sleep onset were positively correlated with the amount of SWS. They concluded that the central thermoregulatory mechanism underlying hot flashes may affect hypnogenic pathways, inducing sleep and heat loss in the absence of a thermal load in these patients. It has been suggested that environmental temperature and hyperthermia play a role in SIDS.[331] However, multiple factors (e.g., sleep-related respiratory dysrhythmias and CNS disorders, particularly in the region of the arcuate nucleus in the medulla) are implicated in SIDS, and the primary cause of the syndrome remains unknown. Finally, the suggestion that thermoregulatory dysfunction may cause sleep disturbance in patients with depression[332] has no compelling evidence to support it.

ENDOCRINE REGULATION IN SLEEP

Neuroendocrine secretion appears to be under circadian control—that is, it shows circadian rhythm in the plasma concentrations of the hormones. The characteristic pattern of endocrine gland secretion is episodic or pulsatile secretion every 1–2 hours, which suggests ultradian rhythmicity. Hormone secretions are thus governed by both the internal biological clock located in the suprachiasmatic nuclei and the stages of sleep. For example, adrenocorticotrophic hormone (ACTH), cortisol, and melatonin rhythms are determined by the circadian clock, whereas growth hormone (GH), prolactin, thyroid-stimulating hormone (TSH), and renin rhythms are sleep related. Current evidence indicates that most likely an interaction between the circadian pacemaker and the timing of sleep/wakefulness as well as age determine the daily hormone profiles.[333–335] Changes in the secretion of some major hormones during sleep are described in the following paragraphs. Figure 7–15 shows a schematic of the patterns of neuroendocrine secretion during sleep in an adult human. It is evident from the figure that during the first part of the night the plasma GH level is high and the cortisol level is low, whereas during the later part of the night GH level is low and cortisol level is high, suggesting a reciprocal interaction of the hypothalamic-pituitary-adrenocortical axis and the hypothalamic-pituitary-somatostatin system.[336]

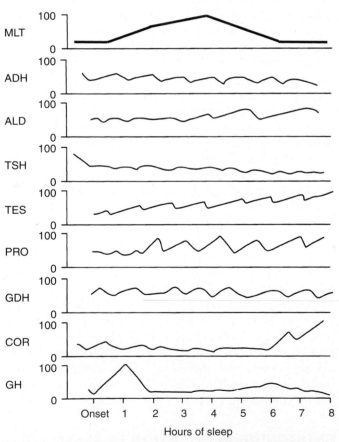

FIGURE 7–15 Schematic representation of the plasma levels of hormones in an adult during 8 hours of sleep. Zero indicates lowest secretory episode and 100 indicates peak. (MLT, melatonin; ADH, antidiuretic hormone; ALD, aldosterone; TSH, thyroid-stimulating hormone; TES, testosterone; PRO, prolactin; GDH, gonadotropic hormone; COR, cortisol; GH, growth hormone.)(*Modified from Rubin R. Sleep endocrinology studies in man. Prog Brain Res 1975;42:73.*)

Growth Hormone

Hypothalamic GH-releasing hormone (GHRH) stimulates release of GH from the anterior pituitary in a pulsatile fashion. In contrast, hypothalamic somatostatin inhibits release of GH.[336–338] Ghrelin, an appetite-stimulant gastric peptide, also stimulates GH secretion.[339] Sleep, particularly SWS, is associated with increased GH, GHRH, and ghrelin levels. GH secretion occurs shortly after sleep onset during SWS and is inhibited during awakenings and sleep fragmentation. Agents promoting SWS (e.g., γ-hydroxybutyrate) will promote GH secretion. GH has an anabolic function that is mediated by insulin-like growth factor-I produced in the liver and other organs.[336,338]

Takahashi and colleagues[340] observed that the plasma concentration of GH peaked 90 minutes after sleep onset in seven of eight normal subjects and lasted approximately 1.5–2.5 hours. The peak is related to SWS (stages 3 and 4 of NREM sleep). Several subsequent reports showed nocturnal peaks of GH in association with SWS.[336–338,341–347] Although the major peak in plasma GH occurs during the early part of nocturnal sleep, it has been shown that, in approximately one-fourth of young, healthy men, peaks in circulating GH occur before sleep onset.[346] Sleep deprivation causes suppression of GH secretion, which may be an age-dependent phenomenon that develops during early childhood. The sleep-related release of GH is absent before age 3 months and is reduced in old age.[345,347–349] It should be noted that GH secretion is regulated physiologically by opposite actions of GHRH and somatostatin.[350] It has been suggested that somatostatin may induce sleep deterioration in the elderly.[350] Van Cauter and Plat[349] suggested that age-related decrements in GH secretion play a major role in the hyposomatotropism of senescence. The timing of the release of GH shifts if sleep is phase advanced or phase delayed, suggesting a close relationship between episodic GH secretion and sleep.[351] Sadamatsu et al.[352] measured 24-hour rhythms of plasma GH, prolactin, and TSH in nine normal adult men by means of serial blood sampling at 30-minute intervals. Their findings suggested two mechanisms regulating GH secretion: one that is sleep independent and has an ultradian rhythm and another that is sleep dependent.

There is some evidence of possible circadian influences on the regulation of GH secretion from a jet lag study by Goldstein and associates[353] and a study of GH secretory rate in night workers by Weibel et al.[354] Increased GH secretion has been noted after flights both eastward and westward.[353]

The tightly linked normal relationship between GH and SWS is disrupted during sleep disturbances (see later under *Clinical Relevance*). It is interesting to note that such a tight relationship is observed only in humans and baboons, and not in rhesus monkeys and dogs,[355] a fact that may relate to the monophasic sleep patterns observed in baboons and humans.[356]

An activation of hypothalamic GHRH neurons promotes both the onset of SWS and the peak GH levels, suggesting a direct link between SWS and GH secretion.[336,338,357] Furthermore, the GHRH gene is found in the mouse in the same region regulating NREM sleep in the hypothalamus.[358] Experimentally, both intravenous[359] and intranasal[360] administration of GHRH in young men promoted sleep.[336] Many hypothalamic GHRH neurons are thought to be GABAergic.[336,361] It is notable that ventrolateral preoptic GABAergic neurons are important in initiating NREM sleep (see Chapters 4 and 5), strengthening the link between GHRH and sleep-promoting neurons in the anterior hypothalamus.

Adrenocorticotropic Hormone and Cortisol Secretion

The 24-hour ACTH-cortisol rhythm is primarily controlled by circadian rhythmicity but clearly modulated by sleep/wake state. Sleep onset is associated with a decrease in cortisol secretion but with a rapid elevation in the later part of the sleep at night and with subsequent decline throughout the day.[333,337,362–366] These effects of sleep onset and sleep offset are found to be absent during sleep deprivation. Studies have also shown that awakenings causing sleep interruption will increase the pulsatile cortisol secretion.[333] The inhibitory influence of early nocturnal sleep on ACTH-cortisol levels is most marked during SWS.[364] Some studies[367,368] have documented both a circadian and an ultradian episodic pattern of secretion for cortisol and ACTH. However, it should be noted that, in contrast to nocturnal sleep, daytime sleep fails to significantly inhibit cortisol secretion; this suggests that sleep does not suppress cortisol release at any point of its circadian rhythm, but only within a limited range of entrainment.[369,370]

In general, the circadian rhythm of cortisol secretion remains undisturbed in disease states such as Cushing's syndrome and narcolepsy.[371] With depression, the earlier occurrence of the lowest point of cortisol levels is thought to indicate a circadian phase advance.[372] The failure of dexamethasone to suppress cortisol secretion in depressed persons is not necessarily positively correlated with reduced REM latencies noted in depression.[373] Sleep deprivation itself may be responsible for such failure, as is noted in normal individuals.[374]

Sleep fragmentation is associated with pulsatile increase in cortisol secretion. Primary insomnia patients had higher mean nocturnal cortisol levels.[375,376] However, in one report[377] nocturnal cortisol levels did not differ between controls and insomnia patients. Sleep deprivation is also associated with hypercortisolism similar to that noted in normal elderly subjects, accompanied by repeated nocturnal awakenings.[378]

Prolactin Secretion

Plasma prolactin concentration has long been known to exhibit a sleep-dependent pattern, with the highest levels occurring during sleep and the lowest during waking.[371,379–381] The plasma prolactin level does not seem to have a definite circadian rhythm; it appears to be linked to sleep[379,380] but is not related to specific sleep stages.[371] The prolactin level begins to rise approximately 60–90 minutes after sleep onset and peaks in the early morning hours from approximately 5:00 to 7:00 AM.[382] Studies by Mendelson and coworkers,[371,383] Rubin et al.,[384] and Van Cauter and colleagues[385] showed no relationship between prolactin secretion and NREM-REM cycles. Subsequent studies, however, have clearly shown that prolactin secretion is also driven by a sleep-independent circadian pattern.[386,387] Waldstreicher et al.[386] studied 12 men and 10 women using a constant routine protocol, during which the subjects remained in semirecumbent wakefulness. The authors clearly documented a robust, sleep-independent, endogenous circadian rhythm of prolactin secretion in humans. The authors hypothesized that the endogenous components of the circadian rhythm of prolactin secretion, along with body temperature, urine production, and cortisol, TSH, and melatonin secretion, are driven by a central circadian pacemaker located in the SCN of the hypothalamus.[386]

Prolactin secretion is suppressed by dopamine but stimulated by thyrotropin-releasing hormone.[371] Although prolactin secretion is related to sleep, the secretory pattern of prolactin does not decline with age like that of GH.[388] In women who breastfeed and those with hyperprolactinemia, SWS is increased.

Gonadotropic Hormone (Gonadotropin)

The gonadotropin-releasing hormone (GnRH) produced by the hypothalamus stimulates the anterior pituitary gland to secrete luteinizing hormone (LH) and follicle-stimulating hormone (FSH). In men, LH is the stimulus for the secretion of testosterone by the testes, and FSH stimulates spermatogenesis. In women, the ovarian hormones estrogen and progesterone are secreted by the ovaries in response to LH and FSH, which also are responsible for ovarian changes during the menstrual cycle. It has been difficult to study the relationship between FSH and LH plasma levels because of the limitations of assay sensitivity in measurements and the inaccuracies associated with pulsatile secretion of circulating gonadotropin. A clear relationship between FSH and LH plasma levels and the sleep-wake cycle or sleep stages in children or adults has not been found.[337] In prepubertal boys and girls, FSH and LH show a pulsatile pattern of secretion. In pubertal boys and girls, however, gonadotropin levels increase during sleep.[337,389–393] By using an ultrasensitive immunofluorometric assay to measure plasma LH and deconvolution analysis to depict LH secretory characteristics, it has been possible to show an increase in sleep-associated GnRH and LH secretion during puberty and the prepubertal stage.[394] Nocturnal elevation of gonadotropins is associated with nocturnal rise of testosterone in boys at puberty.

FSH and LH show pulsatile activities throughout the night without showing any relationship to testosterone secretion. During sleep early in puberty,[389] however, there is a marked rise of plasma LH concentration, in contrast to testosterone or prolactin. Based on the observation that LH and prolactin secretion precedes testosterone secretion by 60–80 minutes, Rubin[356] suggested a relationship between these hormones. Some studies in adult men have shown a modest elevation of nocturnal LH and possibly FSH levels.[395,396] LH and FSH secretion show no distinct circadian rhythms. Plasma testosterone levels rise at sleep onset and continue to rise during sleep at night.[397] The nocturnal rise of testosterone has been found to be linked to REM sleep in some studies[398] as there was attenuation of this nocturnal rise in those who failed to have REM sleep after sleep fragmentation experiments.[399] In older men, the sleep-related rise in testosterone is reduced and the relationship to REM sleep is lost,[400] and the circadian variation of testosterone and LH is reduced.[396]

In contrast to normal men, a sleep-related inhibitory effect on LH secretion has been noted in the early parts of the follicular and luteal phases of the menstrual cycle.[401,402]

Thyroid-Stimulating Hormone

A distinct circadian rhythm has been established for the secretion of TSH in normal humans.[367,403,404] There is general agreement that sleep has an inhibitory effect on TSH secretion: TSH levels are low during the daytime, increase rapidly in the early evening, peak shortly before sleep onset, and are followed by a progressive decline during sleep.[337,371,404–406] Sleep deprivation is associated with nocturnal increase of TSH levels[333,378]; however, during SWS rebound following prior sleep deprivation, there is marked inhibition of nocturnal TSH rise, suggesting that the sleep-associated fall in TSH is related to the SWS stage.[407] The fact that TSH secretion is not suppressed significantly during daytime sleep and the fact that sleep-related inhibition of TSH secretion occurs following nighttime elevation of TSH indicate an interaction between circadian timing and sleep for the control of TSH secretion.[333] Exposure to bright light in the early evening can delay the TSH circadian rhythm, whereas exposure late at night or in the early morning can advance it.[337,406]

Melatonin

Melatonin, the hormone of darkness, is synthesized by the pineal gland and released directly into the bloodstream or cerebrospinal fluid.[408–415] The amino acid L-tryptophan, the precursor of melatonin, is converted to 5-hydroxytryptophan by the enzyme tryptophane hydroxylase, followed by decarboxylation to serotonin. The enzymes acetyltransferase and hydroxindole-O-methyltransferase then catalyze serotonin into melatonin (N-acetyl-5-methoxytryptamine). It has been clearly shown that the environment light-dark cycle and the SCN act in concert to produce the daily rhythm of melatonin production. Melatonin secretion is controlled by a complex multisynaptic pathway, which can be briefly outlined as follows: impulses from the retinal ganglion cells are transmitted via the retinohypothalamic tract to the SCN, which then sends efferent fibers to the superior cervical ganglia, which in turn transmit impulses via the postganglionic efferent fibers to the pineal gland. This complex neural pathway is activated during the night, triggering melatonin production, which is suppressed by exposure to bright light. The melatonin circadian rhythm is clearly driven by the circadian rhythm of the SCN through activation of two major melatonin receptors (MT_1 and MT_2).[416–421] Both receptors are heavily concentrated in the SCN. MT_1 receptors inhibit SCN neuronal activity and MT_2 receptors phase-shift circadian firing rhythms in the SCN. Melatonin begins to rise in the evening on attaining maximum values between 3:00 AM and 5:00 AM and then decreasing to low levels during the day.[408–410,413] The maximum nocturnal secretion of melatonin has been observed in young children, ages 1–3 years; secretion then begins to fall around puberty and decreases significantly in the elderly.[414,422,423]

Because of the important effect of melatonin on circadian rhythms and its possible hypnotic effect, there have been a few clinical applications of melatonin that appear promising.[416,417,420,424–436] Placebo-controlled, double-blind studies using a large number of subjects need to be performed, however, before accepting melatonin as a treatment for various sleep disorders. Administration of melatonin has been shown to have some beneficial effects on the symptoms of jet lag[413,424,431–433,436] and on nighttime alertness and daytime sleep of shift workers.[413,429,430,437] Administration of melatonin has been found to be beneficial in some primary circadian rhythm sleep disorders, such as delayed sleep phase syndrome[424,438,439] and non–24-hour sleep-wake syndrome.[424,426–428,440,441] In a subgroup of elderly subjects with reduced melatonin secretion at night, beneficial effects of melatonin on sleep disturbances have been noted in those with insomnia.[410,442] The hypnotic effect of melatonin has been noted in several reports.[410,443–446] Again, however, placebo-controlled, double-blind studies with large numbers of subjects are needed before considering the clinical applications of melatonin as a hypnotic agent. In conclusion, until further studies are conducted to determine the long-term effects of melatonin, its indiscriminate use (melatonin is available as a nutritional supplement without U.S. Food and Drug Administration control) should be discouraged. Furthermore, melatonin should only be administered to subjects with clearly documented melatonin deficiency.[410,411,442]

Miscellaneous Hormones

Renin-Angiotensin-Aldosterone System

The renin-angiotensin-aldosterone (RAA) system is controlled by the ANS, BP variation, and the sleep process. Renin, an enzyme secreted by the juxtaglomerular cells of the kidneys, acts upon angiotensinogen found in the α_2-globulin fraction of blood to form angiotensin I, which is then converted by a chloride-dependent converting enzyme into angiotensin II; the latter acts upon the zona glomerulosa of the adrenal cortex to stimulate aldosterone secretion. The juxtaglomerular cells act like baroreceptors responding to changes in BP variation during sleep. During NREM sleep, especially SWS, plasma renin activity (PRA) increases, associated with a fall in BP and a reduction of sympathetic activity as indicated by a significant decrement of the LF/HF power ratio in the spectral analysis of electrocardiographic R–R intervals.[447] In contrast, during REM sleep associated with fluctuating BP and intermittently increased sympathetic activity, there is a significant decrement of PRA.[140,447] Brandenberger and coworkers[448–450] demonstrated that 24-hour variations in PRA are not circadian in nature but are related to sleep processes and are dependent on the regularity and length of the sleep cycles in an ultradian manner. Thus PRA oscillations are synchronized to the NREM-REM cycles during sleep[450] (Fig. 7–16).

During sleep, aldosterone levels are increased compared with levels during wakefulness.[451] Sleep-related aldosterone levels are related to PRA oscillations, whereas during daytime waking periods aldosterone levels parallel cortisol pulses.[452] Thus the 24-hour aldosterone secretory pattern is influenced by a dual system: renin-angiotensin during sleep and ACTH during wakefulness. Sleep deprivation modifies the 24-hour aldosterone profile by preventing the rise of nocturnal sleep-related aldosterone release, causing an alteration of overnight hydromineral balance.[451]

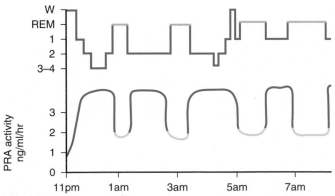

FIGURE 7–16 Plasma renin activity profiles schematically shown in a normal subject during sleep at night from 11:00 PM to 7:00 AM. Note plasma renin activity (PRA) oscillations synchronized to NREM-REM cycling, with the lowest values during REM sleep. *(Adapted from Brandenberger G, Follenius M, Goichot B, et al. Twenty-four-hour profiles of plasma renin activity in relation to the sleep-wake cycle. J Hypertens 1994;12:277.)*

Renal Excretion of Water and Electrolytes at Night. In normal persons, nocturnal urine volume and electrolytes decrease owing to decreased glomerular filtration, increased reabsorption of water, increased activation of the RAA system, and decreased sympathetic activity.[451,452] Antidiuretic hormone shows episodic secretion without any relationship to sleep, sleep stages, or circadian system, but there is a slight increase in the second half of the night.[338]

Parathyroid Hormone

In normal young men, Chapotot et al.[453] noted a significant increase in levels of plasma parathyroid hormone (PTH or parathormone) during nighttime sleep compared with waking periods but failed to find a significant association with SWS, REM sleep, or plasma ionized calcium and phosphate levels. Their findings demonstrated that the 24-hour plasma PTH profile is influenced by sleep processes with a weak circadian component. These findings of Chapotot et al.[453] of a lack of a significant association with sleep stages contradict the earlier observations by Kripke and associates[454] of PTH peaks related to cycles of SWS.

Clinical Relevance

The tightly linked normal relationship between GH and SWS is disrupted during sleep disturbances. For example, in narcolepsy,[455] depression of GH secretion is associated with sleep disturbance, and in some cases of insomnia,[456] there is a dissociation between SWS and GH secretion. Such dissociation also occurs in old age.[345,457–459] These findings suggest that there are independent mechanisms for controlling GH secretion and SWS.

In acromegaly patients, GH secretion remains high throughout sleep and has no relationship to sleep onset or SWS.[460,461] Diminished, sleep-related secretion of GH is found in both sleep apnea and narcolepsy.[462] In OSAS patients, nocturnal release of GH and prolactin is decreased in untreated apneic subjects but is increased following continuous positive airway pressure (CPAP) treatment.[333,337] Atrial natriuretic peptide (ANP) is increased in OSAS, resulting in suppression of the RAA system and increased urinary and sodium output.[463] PRA profiles show a flat oscillation in OSAS patients and are normalized after CPAP treatment. The normalization of sodium and urinary output in OSAS patients following CPAP treatment could be related to restoration of normal PRA and aldosterone oscillations as well as decreased release of ANP.[463]

The age-related decrease in GH may be related to the reduction of SWS and increased fragmentation of sleep in the elderly. Similarly, decreased prolactin levels in normal elderly subjects may cause increased awakenings and fragmented sleep. The exponential decrease of GH and linear increase of cortisol in old age correlate with age-related decrease in SWS; these changes may impair the anabolic function of sleep in the elderly.[333,337]

Glucose tolerance and thyrotropin concentrations are reduced, whereas evening cortisol concentrations and sympathetic nervous system activity are increased after sleep debt resulting from partial sleep deprivation.[378] Thus, sleep debt has a harmful effect on carbohydrate metabolism and endocrine function. These effects are similar to those noted in normal aging, thus suggesting that sleep debt may increase the severity of age-associated chronic disorders. Age-related sleep fragmentation may also cause increased nocturnal corticotrophic activity.[334,338] The pattern of GH secretion associated with clinical depression is contradictory: both impairment and normal sleep-related GH secretion have been noted.[371,456,464] GH secretion is somewhat disturbed in alcoholics.[465] Schizophrenia, alcoholism, and depression in adults are associated with impaired sleep-related GH secretion.[371] Whether the impairment is related to an associated decrease in SWS or abnormalities of biogenic amine metabolism in these disorders cannot be stated with certainty. Cushing's syndrome is associated with decreased SWS and GH secretion. Nocturnal GH secretion was found to be higher than normal, and SWS increased, in two patients with thyrotoxicosis.[466] These abnormal findings normalized in response to antithyroid medication. There is a suggestion that the shift work–related increased incidence of infertility in women may be related to a sleep-related inhibitory effect on gonadotropin release during the follicular phase of the menstrual cycle.[467]

There has been considerable progress in our understanding of how melatonin modulates sleep and circadian phase through activation of the MT_1 and MT_2 melatonin receptors, which inhibit (MT_1 receptors) neuronal activity and phase-shift (MT_2 receptors) circadian firing rhythms in the SCN.[416] This knowledge led to the development and availability of a melatonin receptor agonist (ramelteon) for the treatment of sleep-onset insomnia.[468] Additional melatonin receptor agonists are being developed for treating circadian rhythm disorders and depression.

⊘ REFERENCES

A full list of references are available at www.expertconsult. com

CHAPTER 8

Circadian Timing and Sleep-Wake Regulation

Robert Y. Moore

INTRODUCTION

In its course around the sun, the earth revolves on its axis so that, at any given moment, half the earth is in light and half in darkness. This inexorable progression of light and dark, day and night, is the most pervasive recurring stimulus in our environment and is the basis for a fundamental adaptation of living organisms, circadian rhythms ("circadian" is derived from *circa* [about] and *diem* [day]). These rhythms are expressed in nearly all forms of living organisms, from bacteria to humans, and can be observed at all levels of organization from molecular to behavioral. There are references to daily rhythms in the earliest descriptions of life and, although they were once assumed to represent a passive response to the light-dark cycle, we now know that circadian rhythms are genetically determined, endogenously generated adaptations. The fundamental properties of circadian rhythms first were observed in the 18th century, but progress in understanding their mechanisms and importance emerged slowly. Major advances in the analysis of circadian rhythms began in the mid-1950s, particularly with the work of Jurgen Aschoff[1] in humans and Colin Pittendrigh[2] in animals, and over the last 35 years we have achieved remarkable understanding of both the molecular basis and neurobiology of circadian function. In vertebrates, the major function of circadian clocks is the integration of the internal milieu with the light-dark cycle to maximize the adaptation of animals to their environment. The behavioral expression of this adaptation is daily cycles of rest and activity, sleep-wake cycles.

The intent of this review is to survey the neurobiology of circadian regulation, particularly with reference to control of the timing of sleep and wake.

CIRCADIAN RHYTHMS ARE INHERITED AND GENERATED BY MOLECULAR CLOCKS

Early studies of circadian rhythms focused on the properties of rhythms at system and behavioral levels. These expressions of circadian regulation depend, however, on events at the molecular level: gene transcription and translation. Molecular studies over the last 20 years have established that, in virtually all organisms, the fundamental clock mechanism is composed of feedback loops of gene transcription and translation that drive rhythmic, ~24-hour, expression of core clock components. The output of the molecular clock is regulation of other genes—clock-controlled genes—that establish the timing of cellular functions. Individual cells throughout the organism contain the basic clock mechanism, and molecular rhythms are exhibited both in vivo and in vitro in cells from all organs and tissues. This chapter begins with a description of the molecular basis of circadian function followed by an outline of the organization of the mammalian circadian timing system and control of the sleep-wake cycle. The references cited are to recent review articles or to papers of historical importance that, hopefully, will guide the reader to additional information.

Circadian timing in plants and animals is an inherited adaptation and, as such, is determined genetically. The discovery of clock mutants in *Drosophila* (fruit fly) by Ronald Konopka[3] and in *Neurospora* (bread mold) by Jerry Feldman[4] provided the foundation for most of our understanding of the molecular mechanisms of circadian rhythms. In *Drosophila* and *Neurospora*, the principal mutants have altered free-running periods or are arrhythmic. In *Drosophila*, the affected flies are called *per* mutants (*per* for period). *Neurospora* mutants are designated *frq* mutants (*frq* for frequency). The extensive knowledge of *Drosophila* and *Neurospora* genetics, coupled with the technology of modern molecular biology, has enabled rapid progress to be made in unraveling the molecular mechanisms of circadian function. Although molecular clock mechanisms are more complex in mammals than in *Drosophila* or *Neurospora*, the fundamental molecular mechanism, interlocked autoregulatory transcription-translation feedback loops, is similar. Seven genes—*frq* in *Neurospora*[5]; *per*, *tim* (timeless), and *cyc* (cycle) in *Drosophila*[6,7]; and *per*, *cry* (Cryptochrome), *clock*, and *bmal1* in mammals[8]—have been identified as core clock components, defined as genes whose protein products participate directly in the feedback loops. The following is a brief overview of the molecular mechanisms of clock function in mammals.

The Mammalian Molecular Clock Comprises Complex Feedback Loops

The feedback loops in mammals include positive and negative elements.[8] The positive feedback loop includes two members of the basic helix-loop-helix (bHLH)–PAS (Period-Arnt-Single-minded) transcription factor family, CLOCK and BMAL1 (Fig. 8–1). These proteins

heterodimerize and initiate transcription of E-box regulatory elements in Per 1 and Per 2 and Cry 1 and Cry 2, the beginning of the negative loop. After translation, Per and Cry are subject to post-translational modification. Casein kinase 1 epsilon (CK 1ε) and casein kinase 1 delta (CK 1δ) are important components of the post-translational modification process, and mutations in these genes produce alterations in circadian period in animals and humans. This process stabilizes and regulates Per and Cry heterodimerization and translocation back to the nucleus, where the heterodimer inhibits Per and Cry transcription through action on the CLOCK:BMAL1 complex. Per and Cry proteins are indispensable to the negative feedback loop, and Cry is the rate-limiting repressor of the molecular oscillator. Thus, the cyclic accumulation of Cry proteins must be controlled rigorously. This is accomplished by proteasomal degradation. To be recognized by the proteasome, proteins must be tagged with ubiquitin polypeptides by a ubiquitin ligase, Fbxl3. The specificity of the Fbxl3-Cry interaction was confirmed by showing that other F-box proteins did not associate with Cry proteins. This process allows rapid degradation of Cry to assure precise regulation of molecular clock processes. A further feedback loop is induced by CLOCK:BMAL1 heterodimers activating transcription of retinoic acid–related orphan nuclear receptors, Rev-erbα and Rorα. The proteins REV-ERBα and RORα compete to bind orphan receptor response elements (RORs) in the Bmal1 promoter. RORs activate transcription of Bmal1 and REV-ERBs repress transcription of Bmal1. The completion of the primary feedback loops takes approximately 24 hours.

The molecular clock is remarkably stable. Like physiologic processes under circadian regulation, it is temperature compensated; that is, timing of the clock is relatively unaffected by changes in temperature both in vivo and in vitro and is largely unaffected by rates of transcription of other genes. It is clear, however, that there is much more to be learned about regulation of the molecular clock. This includes mechanisms of entrainment, both from light and feedback from clock-regulated functions; molecular pathways by which the clock controls expression of other genes; and the role of post-translational protein modification in circadian regulation. One particularly interesting recent finding is that clock genes, *clock* and *bmal1*, are involved in histone acetylation, suggesting they participate in chromatin modification.

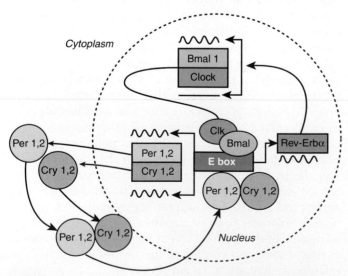

FIGURE 8–1 Molecular mechanisms of circadian function (see description in text).*(Modified from Ko CH, Takahashi JS. Molecular components of the mammalian circadian clock. Hum Mol Genet 2006;15:R271.)*

Summary

Circadian function is inherited. It is based on a highly conserved mechanism of autoregulatory feedback loops of clock gene transcription, translation, and protein production that form a molecular circadian clock regulating the expression of other genes and, hence, cellular function.

ORGANIZATION OF THE MAMMALIAN CIRCADIAN TIMING SYSTEM

Discovery of the Mammalian Circadian Timing System

The regulation of circadian rhythms is mediated by the circadian timing system (CTS), a specific set of neural structures that establishes a temporal organization of physiologic processes and behavior into precise 24-hour cycles. The fundamental properties of circadian rhythms, endogenous generation and entrainment, require that the CTS have at least three components: (1) photoreceptors and visual pathways that transduce photic entraining information, (2) pacemakers that generate a circadian signal, and (3) output pathways that couple the pacemaker to effector systems (Fig. 8–2). As described later, the circadian system in mammals is organized in a hierarchical manner. At the top of the hierarchy, an assembly of neuronal oscillators in the hypothalamic suprachiasmatic nucleus (SCN) is coupled by synaptic interaction to become a pacemaker that controls multiple effector systems via outputs to other brain areas, autonomic nervous system, and endocrine tissues and organs. The functional effect of circadian regulation is an exquisite integration of the timing of brain and peripheral system function. At the behavioral level, the principal regulatory target of the circadian system in mammals is the sleep-wake cycle. Specifically, the circadian system provides a temporal organization of behavioral state integrated with functions in other systems to maximize the effectiveness of adaptive waking behavior. Circadian timing is an important regulatory function that provides a nearly unique situation for neuroscientists in which a specialized function of the nervous system can be studied at the molecular, cellular, neural system, and behavioral levels of organization.

The systematic study of circadian rhythms began in the first half of the 20th century with observations of a wide variety of rhythms in diverse organisms. In the 1950s and 1960s, analysis of the fundamental features of circadian rhythms firmly established that they are generated by endogenous pacemakers. This work led to the discovery of neural clocks and to the elucidation and analysis of the CTS. Many individuals contributed to these advances in our understanding of circadian rhythms.[9]

In the early 1970s, a direct projection from the retina to the SCN of the hypothalamus was discovered; subsequent studies showed that this retinohypothalamic projection (RHT) is necessary for entrainment. Identification of the SCN as the site of RHT termination led directly to an initial test of the hypothesis that the SCN is the circadian pacemaker when ablation of the SCN resulted in a loss of circadian rhythms. The demonstration of the RHT and the dramatic effects of SCN ablation were the introductory events to a remarkable period of intense investigation of the mammalian circadian timing system that continues to the present.[10,11] There have also been striking advances in our understanding of the organization of the circadian timing system in invertebrates and nonmammalian vertebrates. In the sections that follow we consider the neural mechanisms of pacemaker organization and function, entrainment, and efferent output from the SCN transmitting circadian regulation.

Summary

The circadian timing system is composed of central neural elements that function to provide a precise temporal organization of physiologic and endocrine processes and behavior. Critical components include photoreceptors and visual pathways (e.g., RHT), circadian pacemakers (SCN), and output pathways that regulate the timing of functions in brain and peripheral tissues.

The SCN Is the Dominant Circadian Pacemaker

In mammals, the SCN is a paired nucleus of small neurons lying above the optic chiasm on each side of the third ventricle (Fig. 8–3). Four lines of evidence support the conclusion that the SCN is an important circadian pacemaker:

Entrainment pathway

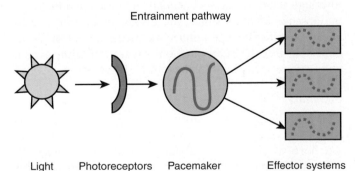

Light Photoreceptors Pacemaker Effector systems

FIGURE 8–2 Overview of the basic organization of the circadian timing system (CTS). The control feature of the CTS is the circadian pacemaker. Information from photoreceptors is conveyed by entrainment pathways to the pacemaker. The pacemaker has a rhythmic output that drives "slave" oscillators, which control functions that exhibit circadian regulation.

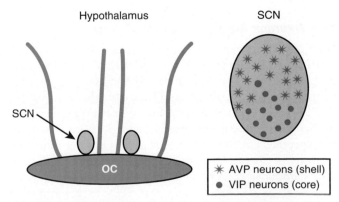

FIGURE 8–3 Diagram showing the location and organization of the human suprachiasmatic nucleus (SCN) in the anterior hypothalamus above the optic chiasm (OC) and lateral to the third ventricle. The diagram on the right shows the core–shell, with vasoactive intestinal polypeptide (VIP)–containing neurons in the SCN core and arginine vasopressin (AVP)–containing neurons in the SCN shell.

1. The SCN is the site of termination of an entraining pathway—the RHT.
2. SCN ablation abolishes many circadian rhythms, but SCN lesions typically alter only the temporal organization of a function; the function itself is unchanged.
3. Isolation of the SCN, either in vivo or in vitro, does not alter the expression of circadian rhythms in the SCN, but most circadian rhythms in other brain and peripheral areas are lost.
4. Transplantation of a fetal SCN into the third ventricle of arrhythmic hosts with SCN lesions restores the circadian rest-activity rhythm with a period that reflects donor, not host, rhythmicity.

Functional Divisions of the SCN

The SCN is made up of two distinct subdivisions, which differ in neuronal morphology, peptide phenotype, and connections. The central region of the SCN lying immediately above the optic chiasm is designated the "core," and it is surrounded by the second subdivision, the "shell." In Golgi-stained material, neurons in the shell are quite small and have sparse dendritic arbors, whereas neurons in the core are larger with more extensive dendritic arbors, often extending beyond the apparent boundary of the SCN. The majority of shell neurons contain arginine vasopressin (AVP) co-localized with the inhibitory transmitter γ-aminobutyric acid (GABA). Afferents to the SCN shell arise predominantly from the brain stem, hypothalamus, basal forebrain, and limbic cortex. Core neurons, however, typically contain vasoactive intestinal polypeptide (VIP) or gastrin-releasing peptide (GRP) co-localized with GABA. Visual afferents, the primary retinal input from the RHT, and some secondary visual projections from other visual nuclei that receive retinal afferents terminate in the core. Another important input to the core is from the serotonin neurons of the midbrain raphe nuclei. These SCN subdivisions are found in all mammals, and there is evidence that they can function as independent pacemakers.[10–16]

SCN Neurons Are Circadian Oscillators

Both physiologic and molecular studies indicate that SCN neurons are circadian oscillators that are coupled by neural connections to form a pacemaker. Individual SCN neurons maintained in cell culture each have a rhythmic firing rate that approximates 24 hours. The free-running period of SCN neurons in culture approximates 24 hours, as would be expected, but the variance in period among individual neurons is greater than that of free-running rhythms in intact animals.[17,18] The coupling of individual oscillators is critical to the function of the SCN as a pacemaker. Recent work indicates that GABA is important to the process of synchronization of SCN neurons. Evidence also suggests that gap junctions and neural cell adhesion molecules participate in the coupling of SCN neurons that underlies pacemaker function, and that these factors all interact to provide the neuronal coupling that produces an SCN pacemaker that has a reliable and uniform output that can be entrained to the solar cycle.

In Fetal Life the SCN Pacemaker Is Entrained to Maternal Rhythms

Overt circadian rhythms are typically expressed in mammals after birth. The SCN in the rat is formed in late gestation, between embryonic days 14 and 17 (E14–E17; gestation in the rat is 21 days). Circadian function in the SCN is first expressed at E19 as an intrinsic rhythm in glucose utilization, entrained to maternal rhythms. Maternal rhythmicity is not necessary, however, for the development of fetal SCN function. When the SCN of pregnant females is ablated early in gestation, before the formation of SCN neurons in the fetus, development of the fetal SCN rhythmicity progresses normally. In this situation, however, individual pups develop rhythms independent of one another and of their environment. The signal for entrainment to maternal rhythms is not known with certainty, but melatonin appears to play an important role. Limited data on development of neural mechanisms of circadian function in humans indicate that the SCN establishes circadian rhythmicity prenatally but behavioral and physiologic rhythms do not appear until after birth.

Circadian Oscillators Occur Widely in Neural and Non-neural Tissues

It was established quite early that circadian pacemakers other than the SCN are present in avian species. The evidence for non-SCN pacemakers in mammals, however, was quite limited until a circadian rhythm in melatonin production was shown in cultured hamster neural retina.[19] This study provided definitive evidence that the mammalian eye contains a circadian pacemaker, probably functioning to maintaining a circadian rhythm of visual sensitivity. With the development of understanding of the molecular basis of clock function, additional non-SCN oscillators have been described in many tissues and organs, including brain areas outside the SCN. Although these oscillators maintain circadian rhythmicity in the absence of SCN input, the timing of individual cells begins to differ and the cellular oscillators go out of phase, indicating that the SCN functions to coordinate the timing of functions throughout the body[20–23] (Fig. 8–4).

Summary

The SCN is the dominant mammalian pacemaker. It is composed of two subdivisions made up of neurons that are born as individual circadian oscillators coupled to form a pacemaker. One subdivision, the shell, contains AVP/GABA neurons and receives nonvisual input. The shell surrounds the core, which contains VIP/GABA and GRP/GABA neurons that receive visual input from the retina and from the intergeniculate leaflet (IGL) of the lateral geniculate.

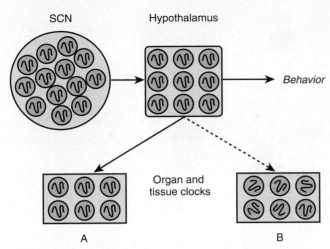

FIGURE 8–4 Diagram showing SCN control of peripheral clocks through output to brain areas controlling endocrine and autonomic function. **(A)** The peripheral clocks are under SCN control. **(B)** When that control is lost, the peripheral clocks become desynchronized.

Light Is the Principal Entraining Stimulus

Light establishes both the phase and the period of the pacemaker and, thus, is the dominant entraining stimulus, or *Zeitgeber* (time giver), of the circadian system. The pacemaker can be viewed as a somewhat inaccurate clock, which must be reset repeatedly. It free-runs with a period that is slightly off 24 hours in the absence of a light-dark cycle. The light-dark cycle sets the exact timing of the pacemaker and is best understood by looking at the phase-response curve (PRC) of the pacemaker to light (Fig. 8–5). The PRC shows that the pacemaker responds differently to light at different times of day. The process of entrainment can be envisioned in the following way. The SCN clock is an imperfect timepiece that is unable to maintain a period of exactly 24 hours and, for that reason, requires resetting on a regular basis. It is typically reset each day in the morning and the evening at the transitions between light and dark. The PRC is a description of that process.

The Circadian Retina and Retinohypothalamic Tract Are Critical to Entrainment

The SCN is a brain structure that appears exclusively to be involved in circadian function. Similarly, entrainment is mediated by specific photoreceptors, and we would expect the remaining visual structures to be unique components of the CTS. Entrainment in mammals requires the lateral eyes. As noted earlier, transection of visual pathways distal to the optic chiasm does not affect entrainment but results in blindness and loss of visual reflexes. In contrast, selective sectioning of the RHT abolishes entrainment but does not affect other visual functions. These data indicate that the RHT terminating in the SCN is the principal entrainment pathway and that it mediates only one function, circadian entrainment.[10] The circadian system is not responsive to specialized aspects of visual stimuli. It responds to changes in luminance (the total amount of light), but not to color, shape, movement, or other visual parameters. The responsiveness of the circadian system is not altered in mutant mice lacking both rod and cone photoreceptors, suggesting that other retinal photoreceptors are used for this function. Studies over the last few years have shown that circadian phototransduction occurs in a subset of retinal ganglion cells producing a photopigment (melanopsin) and projecting to the SCN[24-26] (Fig. 8–6).

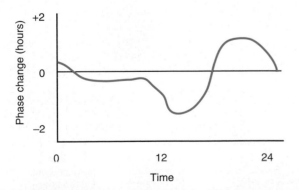

FIGURE 8–5 Diagram of a PRC to light. This shows that exposure to light in subjective day has little effect on circadian phase, but in early night it produces phase delays and late in the night it produces phase advances.

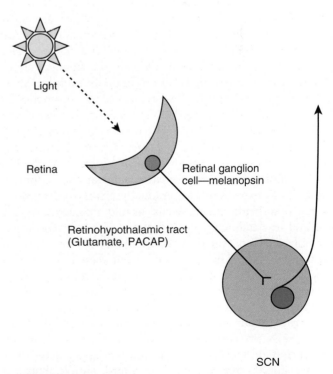

FIGURE 8–6 The organization of photic input to the SCN pacemaker. Light activates melanopsin-containing retinal ganglion cells, which project through the retinohypothalamic tract to the SCN.

Glutamate Is the RHT Transmitter

Glutamate has long been recognized as a neurotransmitter produced by most retinal ganglion cells, and glutamate is now known to mediate the entraining effects of the RHT projecting to the SCN and IGL. Stimulation of the RHT produces a PRC essentially identical to that obtained with light, as does in vitro administration of glutamate to the SCN in slices, and blocking glutamate receptors block light-induced phase shifts. Glutamate is co-localized with pituitary adenylate cyclase–activating peptide (PACAP) in the subsets of melanopsin-containing retinal ganglion cells that project to the SCN.

Summary

Entrainment is mediated by a specific photopigment, melanopsin, located in retinal ganglion cells projecting through the RHT to the SCN and the IGL independent of classic retinal efferent circuits to geniculate colliculus and accessory optic systems. The ganglion cell–SCN circuit uses Glu as a neurotransmitter with its action modulated by PACAP.

Pacemaker Output Is Local

Efferent projections of the SCN are largely to the hypothalamus, with the densest projections intrinsic to the SCN itself and to a region intercalated between the dorsal border of the SCN and the ventral border of the paraventricular nucleus, the subparaventricular zone.[27] This zone has projections that largely overlap projections of the SCN, indicating that it is coordinated by the SCN to regulate control of circadian function. The SCN also projects to other hypothalamic areas: the medial preoptic area, paraventricular nucleus, dorsomedial nucleus, and posterior hypothalamic area. Outside the hypothalamus, the SCN projects to the basal forebrain and midline thalamus. Figure 8–7 shows these relations diagrammatically.

What is the signal that SCN projections deliver to the innervated areas? SCN neurons have a circadian rhythm in the firing rate, with peak firing rates in daytime that are about twice the trough rates at night. The rhythm has a simple, nearly sinusoidal waveform; the output of the SCN is expressed as a gradually changing frequency of neuronal firing. Firing occurs at high frequency during day and low frequency during night, with the conclusion that all areas innervated by the SCN receive a stereotyped rhythmic input. Three sets of recent data indicate that this is an overly simplistic view of SCN function. First, anatomic studies show that the projections from SCN are topographically organized. There are commissural projections from one SCN to the other, and subdivisions of the SCN project largely to separate regions.[28] Second, the output of subsets of SCN neurons appears to differ among subsets over the day.[17,18] Third, simple neuronal firing with transmitter release may not be the only means by which the SCN communicates with the areas it controls. In animals in which SCN transplants restore

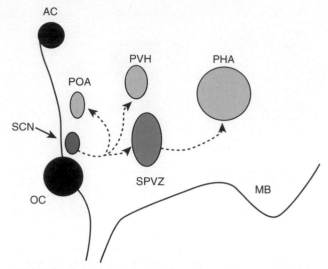

FIGURE 8–7 Output of the SCN to hypothalamic areas. This is a diagram of a sagittal view of the hypothalamus. See text for description. (AC, anterior commissure; MB, maxillary body; OC, optic chiasm; PHA, posterior hypothalamic area; POA, preoptic area; PVH, paraventricular hypothalamic nucleus.)

rhythmicity that was lost due to SCN lesions, direct connections into the host brain from the transplant, typically in the third ventricle, appear unnecessary for functional recovery.[29] This suggests that a humoral mechanism may play a role in rhythm regulation. Recent studies demonstrate that a specific peptide, prokineticin, is important in transmitting circadian information,[30] and it may be the factor mediating restoration of rhythmicity by transplants. The SCN projects densely to the subparaventricular zone and other hypothalamic areas and sparsely to nearby structures of the diencephalon and basal forebrain (Fig. 8–8). These efferent circuits control the expression of circadian rhythms in the areas innervated and throughout the body.[31]

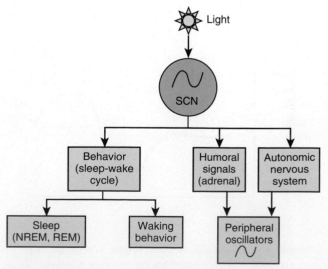

FIGURE 8–8 General organization of the circadian timing system in the control of the temporal organization of behavior.

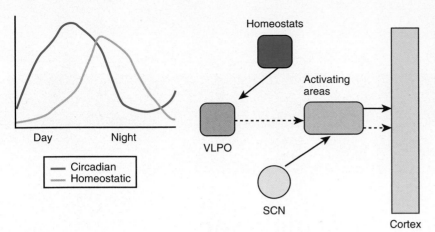

FIGURE 8–9 Diagram showing the interaction of circadian and homeostatic factors in sleep-wake regulation. **(Left)** The dark line shows the pattern of circadian output over 24 hours. The light line shows homeostatic sleep drive. **(Right)** The interaction between homeostatic and circadian regulation is shown diagrammatically. See text for description.

HUMAN CIRCADIAN TIMING SYSTEM FUNCTION AND SLEEP-WAKE REGULATION

The human CTS functions to coordinate humoral, physiologic, and behavioral mechanisms to promote maximally effective sleep and adaptive waking behavior. In the human, as in other animals, the resting state (sleep) and the active state (wake) occur in regular 24-hour epochs, a circadian rhythm. Humans are diurnal animals, so that the waking state occurs during the day and sleep, composed of non–rapid eye movement and rapid eye movement sleep, occurs at night. The underlying neural mechanisms of sleep and waking have been studied extensively over the last 3 decades and are now well understood.[32,33] The cycle of sleep and wake is controlled by two opposing factors, a homeostatic drive for sleep and circadian promotion of arousal.[34] The nature of circadian control of the sleep-wake cycle was not understood until the early 1990s, when it was shown that SCN lesions in monkeys not only alter the circadian control of sleep and wake, but also change sleep duration. Before the lesions, monkeys, like humans, slept approximately 8 hours a day and were awake for 16 hours. After the lesions, however, the monkeys slept 12 hours a day.[35] This indicates that one function of the SCN is to promote arousal. This works as follows. In the morning after awakening, there is virtually no homeostatic drive for sleep and SCN output is low, as shown by the neuronal firing rate (Fig. 8–9). As the day progresses, homeostatic drive increases and is countered by an increasing SCN output. At the end of the day, SCN output decreases and, as it becomes low, homeostatic drive results in the onset of sleep. In the morning, homeostatic drive is diminished and circadian arousal influences result in awakening.

GENERAL SUMMARY

Circadian rhythms are fundamental adaptations of living organisms to their environment. Circadian function is controlled genetically through a molecular mechanism maintained by the expression of clock genes that code for specific proteins that feed back on the nucleus to control their own production. In animals, a neural CTS establishes the temporal organization of behavior into cycles of rest and activity (sleep and wake in mammals), maximizing the adaptive success of both rest and waking behaviors. The mammalian CTS has five components: (1) specific neuronal photoreceptors that contain a novel photopigment, melanopsin; (2) entrainment pathways, an RHT arising from the photoreceptor retinal ganglion cells, and other pathways innervating the SCN, which determine the precise period and phase of the SCN circadian pacemakers; (3) the SCN, which generates circadian signals; (4) output to nearby brain areas that participate in behavioral state and autonomic and endocrine regulation; and (5) peripheral circadian clocks. Light is the dominant entraining stimulus for the CTS. The SCN controls sleep-wake cycles primarily by generating arousal to counter homeostatic drive for sleep during the wake period. The combination of autonomic, endocrine, and behavioral regulation involves coordination of circadian oscillators in tissues throughout the organism to promote restorative sleep and maximally adaptive waking behavior. Finally, disorders of circadian function are common, and research on the neurobiology of circadian timing has facilitated our understanding of the disorders and led to further insights into pathophysiology and the development of new therapies.[15,23,36]

⊙ REFERENCES

A full list of references are available at www.expertconsult.com

CHAPTER 9

Sleep and Memory Consolidation

Matthew P. Walker and Robert Stickgold

INTRODUCTION

The functions of sleep remain largely unknown, a surprising fact given the vast amount of time that this state takes from our lives. One of the most exciting, and contentious, hypotheses is that sleep contributes importantly to learning and memory processing. Over the last decade, a large number of studies, spanning most of the neurosciences, have begun to provide a substantive body of evidence supporting this role of sleep in what is becoming known as sleep-dependent memory processing.

An exciting renaissance is currently underway within the biological sciences, centered on the question of why we sleep, and focusing specifically on the consolidation of memory during sleep. But while this resurgence is relatively recent in the annals of sleep research, the topic itself has a surprisingly long history. The earliest reference to a relationship between sleep and memory is from the Roman rhetorician Quintillian, stating *"It is a curious fact, of which the reason is not obvious, that the interval of a single night will greatly increase the strength of the memory,"* and suggesting that *"the power of recollection. . .undergoes a process of ripening and maturing"* (Quintillian; first century AD). This is striking not only for the level of insight at a time when knowledge of brain function was so anemic, but also considering that it represented the first suggestion of memory requiring a time-dependent process of development, resulting in improved memory recall. Perhaps what is most surprising, however, is that these two fields of research (sleep and memory) then remained separate for almost two millennia.

In the mid-18th century, the British psychologist David Hartley proposed that the processes of dreaming might alter the strength of associative memory links within the brain.[1] Yet it was not until 1924 when Jenkins and Dallenbach performed the first systematic studies of sleep and memory to test Ebbinghaus' theory of memory decay.[2] Their findings showed that memory retention was better following a night of sleep than after an equivalent amount of time awake. However, they concluded that the memory benefit following sleep was simply a passive one due to a lack of sensory interference, in contrast to wake. They did not consider that the physiologic state of sleep itself could actively orchestrate these memory modifications. It is only in the last half-century, following the discovery of rapid eye movement (REM) and non-REM (NREM) sleep, that researchers began testing the hypothesis that sleep, or even specific stages of sleep, actively participate in the process of learning enhancement.

The following chapter explores this relationship in what has become know as sleep-dependent memory processing, and its associated brain basis, sleep-dependent plasticity. This chapter provides an overview of both sleep-dependent memory consolidation (in several memory categories), and sleep-dependent brain plasticity. It is divided into three primary sections: (1) an overview of sleep stages, memory categories, and the unique stages of memory development; (2) a review of the specific relationships between sleep and memory, both in humans and in animals; and (3) a brief survey of the wide range of evidence describing sleep-dependent brain plasticity, including human brain imaging studies as well as animal studies of cellular neurophysiology and molecular biology. We close with a consideration of unanswered questions as well as existing arguments against the role of sleep in learning and memory.

DELINEATIONS AND DEFINITIONS

Before discussing interactions between sleep and memory, we must first understand what these terms represent and encompass. The process of sleep, with its varied stages and equally diverse physiology and biology, has already been described in earlier chapters in this section, clearly demonstrating that sleep itself cannot be treated as a homogeneous state that either does or does not affect memory. Instead, sleep possesses a range of physiologic and neurochemical mechanisms that can contribute to memory consolidation. Moreover, just as sleep cannot be considered homogeneous, the spectrum of memory categories believed to exist in the human brain, and the unique stages that create and sustain memory, appear equally diverse.

Memory Categories

Although often used as a unitary term, "memory" is not a single entity. Human memory has been subject to several different classification schemes, the most popular being based on the distinction between declarative versus nondeclarative memory[3,4] (Fig. 9–1A).

Declarative memory can be considered as the consciously accessible memories of fact-based information (i.e., knowing "what"). Several subcategories of the declarative system exist, including episodic memory (memory for events of one's past) and semantic memory (memory for general knowledge, not tied to a specific event).[3] Current neural models of declarative memory formation emphasize the critical importance of structures in the medial temporal lobe, including the hippocampus,[5] a structure that is

thought to form a temporally ordered retrieval code for neocortically stored information. In contrast, nondeclarative memory can be regarded as nonconscious. The nondeclarative category includes procedural memory (i.e., knowing "how"), such as the learning of actions, habits, and skills (e.g., playing a piano, athletic sports, surgical skills, etc.), as well as implicit learning, and appears to depend on more diverse structures, depending on the task characteristics (e.g., motor, visual, etc.).

While these categories offer convenient and distinct separations, they rarely operate in isolation in real life. For example, language learning requires a combination of memory sources, ranging from nondeclarative memory for procedural motor programs to articulate speech, to memory of grammatical rules and structure, through to aspects of declarative memory for the source of word selection. This too must be kept in mind as we consider the role of sleep in learning and memory.

Memory Stages

Just as memory cannot be considered monolithic, similarly, there does not appear to be one sole event that creates or sustains it. Instead, memory appears to develop in several unique stages over time (Fig. 9–1B). For example, memories can be initially formed by engaging with an object or performing an action, leading to the formation of a representation of the object or action within the brain. Following acquisition, the "memory representation" can undergo several subsequent stages of development. The most commonly recognized next stage of memory is "consolidation." Classically the term *memory consolidation* refers to a process whereby a memory becomes increasingly resistant to interference from competing or disrupting factors in the absence of further practice, through the simple passage of time.[6] That is to say, the memory becomes more stable.

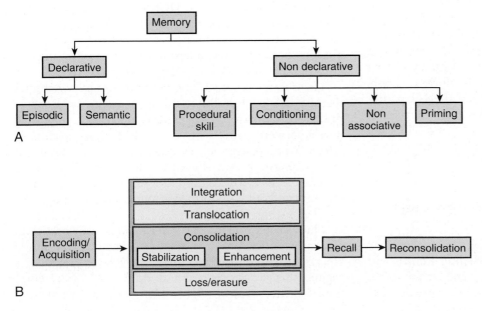

A

B

FIGURE 9–1 Memory systems and memory stages. **(A)** Memory systems. Human memory is most commonly divided into declarative forms, with further subdivisions into episodic and semantic, and nondeclarative forms, subdivided into an array of different types including procedural skill memory. **(B)** Developing stages of memory. Following initial encoding of a memory, several ensuing stages are proposed, beginning with consolidation, as well as integration of the memory representation, and translocation of the representation or erasure of the memory. Also, following later recall, the memory representation is believed to become unstable once again, requiring periods of reconsolidation.

Recent findings, however, have begun to extend this definition. For example, consolidation can be thought of as not only *stabilizing* memories, but *enhancing* them as well, two processes that may be mechanistically distinct.[7] The stabilization phase of consolidation for procedural memory appears to occur during time periods awake.[8–10] In contrast, the second enhancing stage of consolidation appears to occur primarily, if not exclusively, during sleep, either restoring previously lost memories (enhancing from a deficit)[11] or producing additional learning in the absence of further practice.[12–19] From this perspective, the enhancement phase of consolidation causes either the active retention of a memory instead of its decay, or the enhancement of a memory over and above its simple maintenance. Thus, consolidation can be expanded to include more than one phase of postacquisition memory processing, with each phase occurring in specific brain states such as wake or sleep, or even specific stages of sleep.[7]

Although this chapter focuses primarily on the effects of sleep on the postacquisition enhancement phase of consolidation, it is important to note that there are additional postacquisition stages of memory processing that perhaps should also fall under the rubric of consolidation. These include the integration of recently acquired information with past experiences and knowledge (a process of "memory association"), the anatomic reorganization of memory representations (memory translocation), reconsolidation of memory representations following conscious recall (memory reconsolidation), and even active erasure of memory representations, all of which appear to occur outside of awareness and without additional training or exposure to the original stimuli. It is interesting to note that sleep has already been implicated in all of these steps.[10,20–22]

Summary

There are a number of stages of memory processing, which use distinct brain processes to perform separate functions. When combined with the multiple classes of memories and the several stages of sleep, one is faced with a truly staggering number of possible ways that sleep might affect memory consolidation. Therefore, it is only by asking whether a specific stage of sleep affects a particular aspect of memory processing for a given type of memory that one can ask scientifically and clinically answerable question concerning sleep-dependent memory processing.

BEHAVIORAL STUDIES OF SLEEP AND MEMORY

Evidence of sleep-dependent memory processing has been found in numerous species, including human and nonhuman primates, cats, rats, mice, and zebra finch, using a variety of behavioral paradigms. For more detailed reviews, the reader is referred to the papers by Smith[23] and Peigneux et al.[24]

Human Studies of Declarative Memory

Much of the early work investigating sleep and memory in humans focused on declarative learning tasks. These studies offered mixed conclusions, some arguing for sleep-dependent memory processing and others against it. For example, De Koninck et al.[25] demonstrated significant increases in post-training REM sleep after intensive foreign language learning, with the degree of successful learning correlating with the percentage increase of REM sleep. Such findings suggest that REM sleep plays an active role in memory consolidation, and that post-training increases reflect a homeostatic response to the increased demands for REM-dependent consolidation. However, Meienberg[25] found no evidence of altered post-training sleep architecture following learning of a verbal memory task. Similar inconsistencies have been reported in the degree to which intensive declarative learning experiences can alter subsequent sleep-stage properties, as well as the learning impairments that follow selective sleep deprivation.[26–32] More recently, several studies by Born and his colleagues have shown actual improvement on a paired word association test after early night sleep, rich in slow-wave sleep (SWS),[33] and modification of sleep characteristics following intensive learning of word pairs.[34] In addition to classically defined slow delta waves (1–4 Hz), the very slow cortical oscillation (<1 Hz) also appears to be important for memory consolidation. Marshall and colleagues showed that experimentally boosting human slow oscillations in the prefrontal cortex results in improved memory performance the following day.[35] Following learning of a word-pair list, a technique called direct current stimulation (DCS) was used to induce these slow oscillation–like (in this case, 0.75 Hz) field potentials during early delta-rich sleep. The DCS not only increased the amount of delta sleep during the simulation period (and for some time after), but also enhanced the retention of these hippocampal-dependent factual memories, suggesting a causal benefit of delta sleep neurophysiology.

These findings are striking in the face of earlier studies that showed no effect. But this discrepancy may well reflect the nature of the word pairs used. While older studies used unrelated word pairs, such as dog–leaf, Born et al. used related word pairs, such as dog–bone.[33] The nature of the learning task thus shifts from forming and retaining completely novel associations (dog–leaf) to the strengthening or tagging of well-formed associations (dog–bone) for recall at testing.

Thus, sleep's role in declarative memory consolidation, rather than being absolute, might depend on more subtle aspects of the consolidation task. Indeed, several studies suggest that factors such as task difficulty[28,36] and emotional salience[37] can strongly influence the degree of sleep dependency. Furthermore, an examination of different declarative memory categories, including episodic and semantic forms, has not been fully conducted,[38] and may further clarify the apparent contradictions regarding the roles of both SWS and REM sleep in declarative memory consolidation.[23]

But such studies have only begun to test sleep-related memory processes. Indeed, all of these studies have used tasks of recall and recognition as outcome measures, thereby focusing exclusively on processes of memory enhancement and resistance to normal decay, and none has looked at such processes as memory stabilization, association, translocation, and reconsolidation, as discussed earlier. More recent studies have demonstrated that the strengths of associative memories are altered in a state-dependent manner. Several reports have shown that REM sleep provides a brain state in which access to weak associations is selectively facilitated,[21] and flexible, creative processing of acquired information is enhanced.[39] It has also been demonstrated that, following initial practice on a numeric-sequence problem-solving task, a night of sleep can trigger insight of a hidden rule and thus improve performance strategy the following morning[40]—a possible role of sleep in creativity. Moreover, a recent report demonstrated that a night of sleep not only strengthens individual item memories, but can actually build relational associations between them.[41] Indeed, the end goal of sleep-dependent memory processing may not be simply the enhancement of individual memories in isolation, but instead, the integration of these memories into a common schema and, by doing so, facilitation of the extraction of universal rules—a process that forms the basis of generalized knowledge.

Taken as a whole, these studies suggest a rich and multifaceted role for sleep in the processing of human declarative memories. While contradictory evidence is found for a role in the processing of simple, emotion-free declarative memories, such as the learning of unrelated word pairs, a substantial body of evidence indicates that both SWS and REM sleep contribute to the consolidation of complex, emotionally salient declarative memories, embedded in networks of previously existing associative memories.

Human Studies of Procedural Memory

In contrast to the declarative system, the reliance of procedural memory on sleep is a robust and consistent finding across a wide variety of functional domains, including visual, auditory, and motor systems. In this section, we review this evidence in the context of overnight learning improvements following sleep, memory deficits occurring following sleep deprivation, and learning improvements across short daytime sleep periods (naps).

Procedural Memory and Overnight Sleep

Motor Learning. Motor skills have been broadly classified into two forms: motor adaptation (e.g., learning to use a computer mouse) and motor sequence learning (e.g., learning a piano scale).[42]

Beginning with motor sequence learning and overnight sleep, we have demonstrated that a night of sleep can trigger significant performance improvements in speed and accuracy on a sequential finger-tapping task, while equivalent periods of time during wakefulness provide no significant benefit.[16] These sleep-dependent benefits appear to be specific to both the motor sequence learned and the hand used to perform the task.[17,18] Furthermore, the amount of overnight learning expressed the following morning correlated positively with the amount of stage 2 NREM sleep, particularly late in the night (Fig. 9–2). This late-night stage 2 NREM window corresponds to a time when sleep spindles, a defining electrophysiologic characteristic of stage 2 NREM, reach peak density.[43] Interestingly, spindles have been proposed to trigger intracellular mechanisms required for synaptic plasticity[44] (also see later sections), and have been shown to increase following training on a motor task.[45] As such, this late-night sleep, laden with sleep spindles, may provide a key cellular trigger initiating the required mechanisms for neural plasticity.

Using the same sequential finger-tapping task, Fisher et al. have shown that that sleep during the day triggers improvements similar to those achieved following nocturnal sleep.[17] This report, however, described a correlation with REM sleep and not stage 2 NREM, a discrepancy that remains to be resolved.

Considering, however, that the majority of skills we acquired throughout life are of a multilimb and multidigit nature, Kuriyama et al. have gone on to investigate the effects of increasing task complexity on sleep-dependent motor learning.[46] Subjects trained on a variety of task configurations involving either a short or long motor sequence, either one-handed or coordinated between two hands. Interestingly, the more complex the task became (depending on the combinations of these factors), the greater the overnight, sleep-dependent memory enhancement. This would indicate that, as task difficulty increases, the overnight sleep-dependent process responds with even greater performance improvements, further emphasizing the importance of sleep in learning many real-life motor skill routines.

From these combined findings, however, it was still unclear how the sleep-dependent process triggered significant improvements in motor performance speed and accuracy. A more detailed analysis therefore focused on performance changes within these motor sequences.[46] Prior to sleep, individual key-press transitions within the sequence were uneven (Fig. 9–3A, light circles), with some transitions seemingly easy (fast) and others problematic (slow), as if the entire sequence was being parsed into smaller subsequences during initial learning (a phenomenon termed *chunking*[47]). Surprisingly, after a night of sleep, the problematic slow transitions had been preferentially

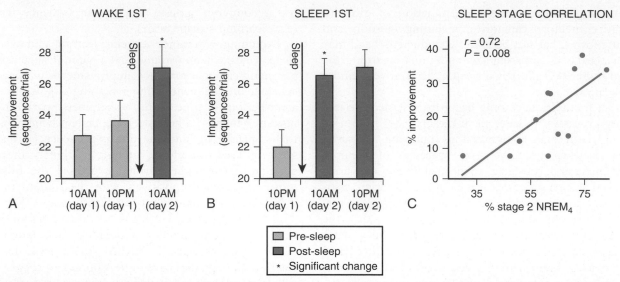

FIGURE 9–2 Sleep-dependent motor skill learning in the human brain. **(A)** Wake 1st: After morning training (10 AM, *light blue bar*), subjects showed no significant change in performance when tested after 12 hours of wake time (10 PM, *light blue bar*). However, when tested again following a night of sleep (10 AM, *dark blue bar*), performance had improved significantly. **(B)** Sleep 1st: After evening training (10 PM, *light blue bar*), subjects displayed significant performance improvements just 12 hours after training following a night of sleep (10 AM, *dark blue bar*), yet expressed no further significant change in performance following an additional 12 hours of wake time (10 PM, *dark blue bar*). **(C)** The amount of overnight improvement on the motor skill task correlated with the percentage of stage 2 NREM sleep in the last (fourth) quarter of the night (stage 2 NREM$_4$). *Significant improvement relative to training; error bars, standard error of the mean (SEM).

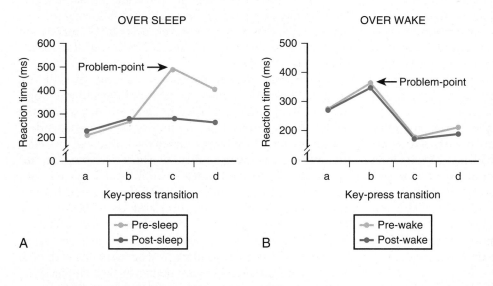

FIGURE 9–3 Single-subject examples of changes in transition speeds. Within a five-element motor sequence (e.g., "4-1-3-2-4"), there are four unique key press transitions: (1) from 4 to 1, (2) from 1 to 3, (3) from 3 to 2, and (4) from 2 to 4. **(A)** The transition profile at the end of training before sleep (*light circles*) demonstrated considerable variability, with certain transitions being particularly slow (most difficult; "problem points"), whereas other transitions appear to be relatively rapid (easy). Following a night of sleep (*dark circles*), there was a specific reduction (improvement) in the time required for the slowest problem point transition. **(B)** Similarly, at the end of training before a waking interval, transition profiles were uneven (*light circles*), with some particularly slow transitions ("problem points") and other relatively fast transitions (easy). However, in contrast to postsleep changes, no change in transition profile was observed following 8 hours of wakefulness (*dark circles*).

improved, while transitions that had already been effectively mastered prior to sleep did not change (Fig. 9–3A, dark circles). In contrast, if subjects were retested after an 8-hour waking interval across the day, no such improvement in the profile of key-press transitions, at any location within the sequence, was observed (Fig. 9–3B). These changes suggest that the sleep-dependent consolidation process may involve the unification of smaller motor memory units into one single memory element by selectively improving problem regions of the sequence. This overnight process would therefore offer a greater degree of

performance automation and effectively optimize skill speed throughout the entire motor program.

Moving from motor sequence learning to motor adaptation learning, Smith and MacNeill[48] have shown that selective sleep deprivation impairs retention of a visual-motor adaptation task. All subjects trained on the task, and were retested 1 week later. However, some subjects were either completely or selectively deprived of different sleep stages across the first night following memory acquisition. At the later retest session, not all subjects had retained the skill memory, with those subjects deprived of stage 2 NREM sleep expressing the most pronounced deficits in motor performance, again suggesting stage 2 NREM sleep to be the crucial determinant of successful motor memory enhancement.

Huber et al.[49] have similarly demonstrated that, following initial memory acquisition of a motor reaching adaptation task, delayed learning is observed exclusively across a night of sleep, and not across equivalent time periods awake. Furthermore, using high-density electroencephalography (EEG), they were able to show that daytime motor skill practice was accompanied by a discrete increase in the subsequent amount of NREM slow-wave EEG activity over the parietal cortex. It was also demonstrated that this increase in slow-wave activity was proportional to the amount of delayed learning that developed overnight, with subjects showing the greatest increase in slow-wave activity in the parietal cortex demonstrated the largest motor skill enhancements the next day.

Taken together, these reports build a convincing argument in support of overnight, sleep-dependent learning across several forms of motor skill memory. All these studies indicate that a night of sleep triggers delayed learning, without the need for further training. In addition, overnight improvements consistently display a strong relationship to NREM sleep, and, in some cases, to specific NREM sleep-stage windows at different times in the night.

Visual Perceptual Learning. Karni et al.[14] have demonstrated that learning on a visual texture discrimination task, which does not benefit from 4–12 hours of wakefulness following acquisition,[13] improves significantly following a night of sleep. Furthermore, they established that selective REM, but not NREM, sleep appears essential for these performance gains.[14] Using the same task, Stickgold et al.[13] have shown that these enhancements are specifically sleep and not time dependent, and are correlated positively with the amount of both early-night SWS and late-night REM sleep, and that the product of these two sleep parameters explains over 80% of intersubject variance, an incredibly strong correlation (Fig. 9–4A and C).

Auditory Learning. More recent studies have begun to explore sleep-dependent auditory skill learning. Using a pitch memory task, Gaab et al.[50] have shown that, regardless of whether subjects trained in the morning or evening, delayed performance improvements developed only across a night of sleep and not across similar waking time periods, whether or not the sleep episode came first. Atienza and colleagues have also described evidence of both time- and sleep-dependent auditory memory consolidation, including sleep-dependent changes in brain evoked response potentials (ERPs).[51,52] While post-training sleep deprivation did not prevent continued improvements in behavioral performance, ERP changes normally associated with the

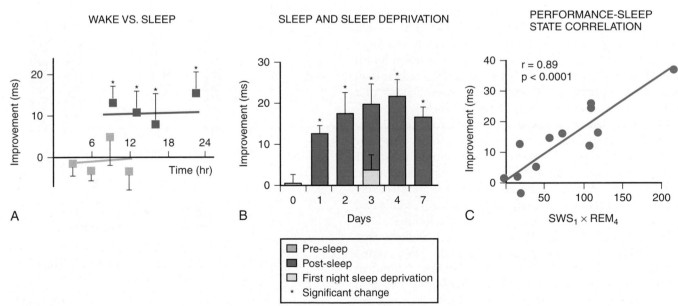

FIGURE 9–4 Sleep-dependent visual skill learning in the human brain. Subjects were trained and then retested at a later time, with the respective improvement (msec) in performance illustrated across time. Each subject was retested only once, and each point represents a separate group of subjects. **(A)** Wake *vs.* sleep. In subjects trained and then retested on the same day, after either 3, 6, 9, or 12 hours of subsequent wakefulness (*light squares*), no significant improvement was evident as a consequence of the passage of waking time across at any of the four time points. In contrast, in subjects trained and then retested 8, 12, 15, or 23 hours after a night's sleep (*dark squares*), a significant improvement occurring as a consequence of sleep. In total, $n = 57$, with $n = 7–9$ for individual points. **(B)** Sleep and sleep deprivation. Subjects ($n = 89$) trained and retested 1–7 days later (*dark bars*) continued to improve after the first night, without additional practice. Subjects ($n = 11$) sleep deprived the first night after training showed no improvement (*crosshatched bar*), even after two nights of recovery sleep. **(C)** Overnight improvement was correlated with the percentage of SWS in the first quarter of the night (SWS_1) and REM sleep in the last quarter of the night (REM_4). $*p < 0.05$; error bars, SEM.

automatic shift of attention to relevant stimuli failed to develop following a night of post-training sleep deprivation. These findings make clear the danger of presuming that a lack of change in behavioral performance is equivalent to an absence of beneficial plastic changes within the brain, and highlights the importance of using combined behavioral and physiologic analyses.

Finally, Fenn et al. have shown that periods of wakefulness following training on a synthetic speech recognition task result in a degradation of task performance, but that a subsequent night of sleep can restore performance to post-training levels. This would suggest a process of sleep-dependent consolidation capable of reestablishing previously learned complex auditory skill memory.[11]

In summary, delayed off-line learning of perceptual skills, like motor skills, also appears to develop exclusively during overnight sleep and not across equivalent time periods awake, with evidence that several different sleep-stages may be involved in triggering this form of overnight consolidation.

Sleep Deprivation and Human Procedural Memory Consolidation

Several studies have specifically investigated the effects of partial or total sleep deprivation on procedural memory consolidation. Beginning with motor skill learning, Fischer et al.,[17] using the previously described motor sequence task, have demonstrated that, if subjects are deprived of sleep the first night after training and then allowed a night of recovery sleep before being retested, normal overnight consolidation improvements are blocked. This would indicate that sleep on the first night following training is critical for consolidation and the associated delayed learning to develop. Smith and MacNeill[48] have shown that selective, rather than total, sleep deprivation also impairs the consolidation of a visual-motor adaptation task, as described earlier.

Regarding sensory perceptual learning, Karni et al. have established that selective disruption of REM, but not NREM, sleep results in a blockade of normal overnight improvements in visual skill learning.[14] Supporting these findings, and using the same task, Gais et al.[19] selectively deprived subjects of early-night sleep (normally dominated by SWS) or late-night sleep (normally dominated by REM and stage 2 NREM). Their findings indicate that consolidation is initially triggered by early SWS-related processes, while REM sleep then promotes additional enhancement late in the night. Finally, Stickgold et al. have established that obtaining less than 6 hours of sleep the night following training results in no significant overnight consolidation enhancement, and that total first night sleep deprivation, even when followed by two subsequent recovery nights of sleep, still blocks consolidation and hence normal sleep-dependent improvement (Fig. 9–4B).[12] Again these data not only highlight the importance of sleep in the evolution of delayed learning, but that adequate sleep within the first 24 hr following memory encoding is a requirement for subsequent sleep-dependent memory enhancement.

Therefore, from the perspective of procedural memory consolidation, it appears that one cannot accumulate a sleep debt and repay it at a later time. Instead, the sleep-dependent consolidation process critically depends on sleep within the first 24 hours after encoding. Furthermore, partial, selective, or total sleep deprivation all appear equally capably of blocking overnight consolidation.

Procedural Memory and Daytime Naps

While the majority of sleep-dependent memory processing studies have investigated learning across a night of sleep, several reports have begun to examine the benefits of daytime naps on perceptual and motor skill tasks. Based on evidence that motor learning continues to develop overnight, we have explored the influence of daytime naps using the sequential finger-tapping task.[53] Two groups of subjects trained on the task in the morning. One group subsequently obtained a 60- to 90-minute midday nap, while the other group remained awake. When retested later that same day, subjects who experienced a 60- to 90-minute nap displayed a significant learning enhancement of nearly 16%, while subjects who did not nap failed to show any significant improvement in performance speed across the day (Fig. 9–5). Interestingly, however, when subjects were

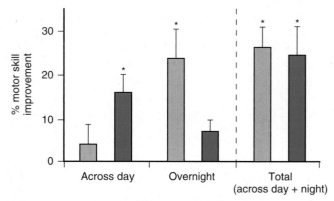

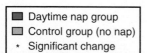

FIGURE 9–5 Daytime naps and motor skill learning. Subjects practiced the motor skill task in the morning, and either obtained a 60- to 90-minute midday nap, or remained awake across the first day. When retested later that same day, subjects who experienced a 60- to 90-minute nap (*filled bar;* "Across Day") displayed significant performance speed improvements of 16%, whereas subjects who did not nap showed no significant enhancements (*light bar;* "Across Day"). When retested a second time after a full night of sleep the next day, subjects in the nap group showed only an additional 7% increase in speed overnight (*dark bar;* "Overnight"), whereas subjects in the control group expressed a significant 24% overnight improvement following sleep (*light bar;* "Overnight"). Therefore, 24 hours later, both groups averaged the same total amount of delayed learning (*light and dark bars;* "Total"). *Significant improvement; error bars, SEM.

retested a second time following a subsequent full night of sleep, those subjects in the nap group showed only an additional 7% overnight increase in speed, while subjects in the control group, who had not napped the previous day, displayed speed enhancements of nearly 24% following the night of sleep (see Fig. 9–5).

These results demonstrate first that as little as 60–90 minutes of midday sleep is sufficient to produce large significant improvements in motor skill performance, while equivalent periods of wakefulness produce no such enhancement. Second, these data suggest there may be a limit to how much sleep-dependent motor skill improvement can occur over the course of 24 hours, such that napping changes the time course of when learning occurs, but not how much total delayed learning ultimately accrues. Thus, while both groups improved by approximately the same total amount 24 hours later (see Fig. 9–5), the temporal evolution of this enhancement was modified by a daytime nap. Such findings offer the exciting possibility that naps may protect motor skill memories against the detrimental effects of subsequent sleep deprivation.

As with motor skill learning, daytime naps also appear to benefit visual skill learning, although the characteristics of these effects are subtly different. Mednick and colleagues have shown that, if a visual skill task is repeatedly administered across the day, rather than performance improving or remaining stable, it deteriorates.[54] This may reflect a selective fatigue of brain regions recruited during task performance, a characteristic not observed in the motor system. However, if a short (30- to 60-minute) daytime nap is introduced among these repeat administrations of the visual skill task, the performance deterioration is ameliorated. If a longer nap period is introduced, ranging from 60 to 90 minutes and containing both REM sleep and NREM SWS, performance not only returns back to baseline but is enhanced.[55] Furthermore, these benefits did not prevent additional significant improvements across the following night of sleep, in contrast to findings reported previously for a motor skill task.

Together these studies build a cohesive argument, albeit from nominal studies, that daytime naps confer a robust learning benefit to both visual and motor skills, and, in the case of visual skill learning, are capable of restoring performance deterioration caused by repeated practice across the day.

Summary of Results of Human Studies

Taken as a whole, studies in humans demonstrate that sleep is a necessity for consolidation and delayed learning enhancement across a range of human procedural skills, being able to restore previously deteriorated task performance as well as trigger additional learning improvements without the need for added practice. Furthermore, different memory systems appear to require subtly different sleep stages, or even sleep-stage time windows, for consolidation and overnight improvement, and it also appears that

daytime naps may be equally capably of triggering delayed learning enhancements.

Animal Studies

Studies using animal models have provided evidence for the role of sleep in primarily hippocampus-dependent tasks. Training on both spatial and shock avoidance tasks triggers alterations in sleep-stage characteristics,[56–60] suggesting, as in humans, a homeostatic response to increased demands on sleep-dependent consolidation mechanisms. In one such study, the magnitude of change in sleep architecture demonstrated a strong relationship to initial performance during acquisition, with animals that learned quickly showing the largest change in sleep structure, while those that learned poorly showing relatively little.[61]

Datta[62] has suggested that, for at least some forms of learning, it is the ponto-geniculo-occipital (PGO) waves of REM sleep (or P waves in rats) that underlie the physiologic mechanism of consolidation. In an initial study, they reported that, following initial training on an avoidance task, both the amount of REM sleep and the density of P waves increased dramatically, and that the increased P-wave density showed a strong positive correlation with the degree of retention of presleep learning following sleep, although not with the extent of the initial learning. These findings are particularly important from the perspective of memory, since they suggest that the increase in REM sleep, and, more specifically, in the density of P waves accompanying REM sleep, is critical for the effective postsleep retention of this learning. Moreover, they emphasize the fact that simple task engagement (such as physical exertion) is not the trigger of modified sleep patterns; rather, it is the degree of learning and of successful consolidation that drives changes in physiologic sleep properties.

In a more recent report, Datta et al. have shown that the induction of PGO waves by intrapontine injection of carbachol can support postsleep retention of learning even in the face of REM deprivation, which by itself completely blocks such retention.[63] Thus, these experimentally induced PGO waves can replace the normal requirement for REM sleep, suggesting it is this cholinergically driven brain activity that is necessary for the sleep-dependent enhancement of this type of consolidation.

As with humans, sleep deprivation following task acquisition has been shown to produce learning impairments at subsequent retests.[58,64–71] Several of these early animal studies have been legitimately criticized for a failure to control for general effects of sleep deprivation on performance.[72,73] Retesting in a sleep-deprived state may mask evidence of successful consolidation due to lowered alertness and attention. Alternatively, the increased stress of prolong wakefulness, rather than the lack of sleep itself, may be the cause of unsuccessful consolidation.

More recent studies in both humans and animals have, however, demonstrated that impaired performance can still be seen several days after the end of sleep deprivation, when alertness or attention have returned to normal.[74] In addition, selective deprivation of specific sleep stages, and even specific sleep-stage time windows (some many hours to days after training), still inhibit memory consolidation,[70,75] making arguments of sleep deprivation–induced stress relatively untenable, since the stress effects would have to be uniquely produced by deprivation of specific sleep stages during specific time windows following training.

Summary

Taken as a whole, behavioral studies across phylogeny leave little doubt that sleep plays a critical role in post-training memory consolidation. Currently, the evidence is perhaps strongest for procedural learning in humans, but substantial evidence exists for conditioned learning in animals and declarative memory in humans as well. To date, all stages of sleep (except sleep-onset stage 1 NREM sleep) have been implicated in one or more aspects of memory enhancing consolidation. Still, a clear understanding of the roles of individual sleep stages remains an important future goal.

SLEEP-DEPENDENT BRAIN PLASTICITY

Memory formation depends on brain "plasticity"—lasting structural and functional changes in a neuron's response to a stimulus (such as an experience). If sleep is to be considered a critical mediator of memory consolidation, then evidence of sleep-dependent plasticity would greatly strengthen this claim. In this section, we consider a mounting wealth of data describing sleep-dependent brain plasticity at a variety of different levels in both animals and humans, complimenting evidence of sleep-dependent changes in behavior.

Neuroimaging Studies

Modification of Post-training Sleep and Brain Activation

Several studies have investigated whether initial daytime training is capable of modify functional brain activation during later sleep episodes. Based on earlier animal findings (see later in this section), neuroimaging experiments have explored whether the signature pattern of brain activity elicited while practicing a memory task actually re-emerges, or is "replayed," during sleep.

Using brain imaging, Maquet and colleagues have shown that patterns of brain activity expressed during motor skill training reappear during subsequent REM sleep, while no such change in REM sleep brain activity occur in subjects who received no daytime training[76] (Fig. 9–6). Furthermore, these researchers have gone on

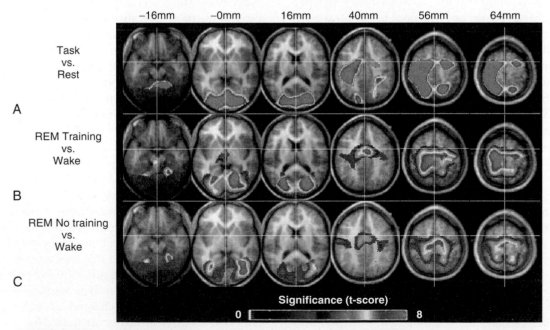

FIGURE 9–6 Task-dependent reactivation of human brain activity during REM sleep. Statistical activation maps of different experimental contrasts. Maps are displayed at six different brain levels (from 16 mm below to 64 mm above the bicommissural plane), superimposed on the average magnetic resonance imaging (MRI) scan of subjects. All maps are thresholded at $p < 0.001$ (uncorrected), except for **A,** which is thresholded at voxel-level-corrected $p < 0.05$. **(A)** Brain regions activated during daytime performance of the motor skill task (Task–Rest). **(B)** Brain regions activated during subsequent REM sleep in subjects who received daytime training (REM Sleep Training–Rest); note considerable overlap with daytime task-dependent activity patterns. **(C)** Brain regions activated during REM sleep in subjects who did not receive any daytime training (REM Sleep No Training–Rest).*(Reproduced with permission from Maquet P, Laureys S, Peigneux P, et al. Experience-dependent changes in cerebral activation during human REM sleep. Nat Neurosci 2000;3:831.) See Color Plate*

to show that the extent of learning during daytime practice exhibits a positive relationship to the amount of reactivation during REM sleep.[77] Training on a hippocampus-dependent virtual maze task during the day has similarly been associated with a subsequent increase in hippocampal reactivation in NREM SWS,[78] with the magnitude of reactivation correlating with how well subjects performed the task the following day, suggesting a function purpose/role for neuronal replay. Such findings suggest that it is not simply experiencing the task that modifies subsequent sleep physiology, but the process of learning itself, and that this reactivation can lead to next-day behavioral improvements.

The function of sleep-dependent replay may be to modify the strength of synaptic connections between neurons within specific brain networks, strengthening some synaptic connections while weakening others in the endeavor of refining memory representations.

Overnight Reorganization of Memory Representations

An alternative approach to investigating sleep-dependent plasticity is to compare patterns of brain activation before and after a night of sleep. In contrast to measuring changes in functional activity *during* sleep, this approach aims to determine if there is evidence that the neural representation of a memory has been reorganized following a night of sleep.

While the behavioral characteristics of sleep-dependent motor sequence learning are now well established, the neural basis of this overnight learning has remained unknown. Using a motor sequence task, we have recently investigated differences between patterns of brain activation before and after sleep using functional magnetic resonance imaging (fMRI).[79] Following a night of sleep, relative to an equivalent intervening time period awake, increased activation was identified in motor control structures of the right primary motor cortex (Fig. 9–7A) and left cerebellum (Fig. 9–7B)—changes that likely allow faster motor output and more precise mapping of key-press movements postsleep. There were also regions of increased activation in the right medial prefrontal lobe and hippocampus (Fig. 9–7C and D), structures that support improved sequencing of motor movements in the correct order. In contrast, decreased activity postsleep was identified bilaterally in the parietal cortices (Fig. 9–7E), possibly reflecting a reduced need for conscious spatial monitoring, together with regions of signal decrease throughout the limbic system (Fig. 9–7F–H), indicating a decreased emotional task burden. In total, these results suggest that sleep-dependent motor learning is associated with a large-scale plastic reorganization of memory throughout several brain regions, allowing skilled motor movements to be executed more quickly, more accurately, and more automatically following sleep. Furthermore, these findings hold important implications for understanding the brain basis of perfecting real-life

skills, and may also signify a potential role for sleep in clinical rehabilitation following brain damage, such as stroke.

Maquet et al.[80] have similarly demonstrated sleep-dependent plasticity using a combined visual-motor adaptation task. Subjects trained on the task and were subsequently retested 3 days later. However, half the subjects were deprived of sleep the first night following training. The remaining half, who slept all 3 nights, showed both enhanced behavioral performance at retest and a selective increase in activation in the superior temporal sulcus, a region involved in the evaluation of complex motion patterns. In contrast, subjects deprived of sleep the first night showed no such enhancement of either performance or brain activity, indicating that sleep deprivation had interfered with a latent process of neural plasticity and consolidation.

Using the sleep-dependent visual texture discrimination task described previously, Schwartz et al. have compared performance-related fMRI patterns of brain activity 24 hours after training, relative to a naive, untrained condition.[81] Significantly greater activation was observed in the 24-hours post-training condition in the primary visual cortex, suggesting that this functional area representing the visual memory had expanded. However, these findings were unable to distinguish between changes that may have occurred during training, across post-training wakefulness, or across a subsequent night of sleep.

Extending these findings, we have subsequently investigated regional brain activity patterns before and after sleep, following equivalent amounts of initial practice on this visual skill task.[82] Postsleep retesting was associated with significantly increased activity not only in the primary visual cortex, but in several downstream visual processing regions following sleep, at the occipital-temporal junction and in the medial temporal and inferior parietal lobes (regions involved in object detection and identification). In addition, there was decreased activity postsleep in the right temporal pole, a region involved in emotional visual processing. These findings strengthen the claim that a night of sleep reorganizes the representation of a visual skill memory, with greater activation throughout the visual system following sleep likely offering improved identification of both the visual stimulus form and its location in space.

Summary

Learning and memory are dependent on processes of brain plasticity, and sleep-dependent learning and memory consolidation must be mediated by such processes. Using brain imaging techniques, several studies have now identified changes in (1) the patterns of functional brain activity during post-training sleep periods (both REM and NREM), and (2) the reorganization of newly formed memories following a night of sleep. These plastic brain changes likely contribute to the refinement of the memory representations, resulting in improved next-day behavioral performance.

POST-SLEEP INCREASED ACTIVATION

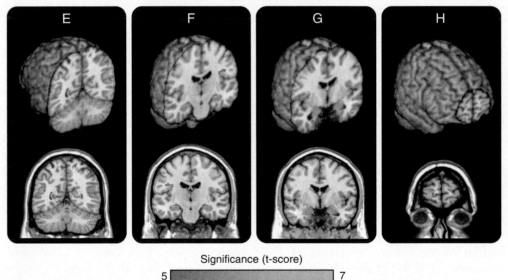

FIGURE 9–7 Sleep-dependent motor memory reorganization. Subjects were trained on a sleep-dependent motor skill task and retested 12 hours later, either following a night of sleep or following intervening wakefulness, during a functional MRI (fMRI) brain scanning session. Scans after sleep and wakefulness were compared (subtracted), resulting in regions showing increased fMRI activity postsleep (*in red/yellow;* **A–D**) or decreased signal activity (*in blue;* **E–H**) postsleep, relative to post-wakefulness. Activation patterns are displayed on three-dimensional rendered brains (*top panel* of each graphic), together with corresponding coronal sections (*bottom panel* of each graphic). Following sleep, regions of increased activation were identified in the right primary motor cortex **(B),** the left cerebellum **(A),** the right hippocampus **(C),** and the right medial prefrontal cortex **(D).** Regions of decreased activity postsleep were expressed bilaterally in the parietal lobes **(E),** together with the left insula cortex **(F),** left temporal pole **(G),** and left frontopolar area **(H),** all regions of the extended limbic system. All data are displayed at a corrected threshold of $p < 0.05$. *See Color Plate*

Electrophysiologic Studies

Throughout the sleep cycle, both REM and NREM sleep stages contain numerous unique electrophysiologic events. Many of these electrical phenomena have been implicated in the processes of plasticity by potentiating or depressing synaptic connections.[83] For example, it has been proposed that sleep spindles, seen most commonly during stage 2 NREM sleep, can provide brief trains of depolarizing inputs to targets in the neocortex that are similar to spike trains used experimentally to induce long-term synaptic potentiation.[44,84–86] Indeed, Steriade and colleagues[87] have shown that cortical neurons driven by impulse trains similar to those produced by sleep spindles can produce lasting changes in the responsiveness of these neurons. Similarly, theta waves, seen in the hippocampus during REM sleep in both humans[88] and other animals,[89] greatly facilitate the induction of long-term potentiation (LTP) in the hippocampus, believed to be a physiologic mediator of memory formation.[90,91]

Phasic events during REM sleep, specifically PGO waves, have also been associated with learning. Sanford et al.[92] have demonstrated that fear conditioning in rats can increase the amplitude of elicited P waves during REM sleep, suggesting again that they represent a homeostatically regulated component of a sleep-dependent mechanism of learning and plasticity (see Datta[62]). Interestingly, these PGO waves occur in a phase-locked manner with theta wave activity during REM sleep.[93,94] Furthermore, while experimental stimulation to several regions of the hippocampus at the peaks of theta waves facilitates LTP, the same stimulation applied at the troughs of the theta waves instead leads to long-term depression of synaptic responses.[91,95] These findings suggest that this natural REM-PGO stimulation may serve as an endogenous mediator of synaptic plasticity, based on its coincidence with theta wave oscillations, which, depending on the phase relationship of the PGO and theta waves, could lead to either strengthening or weakening of synaptic connections, both of which are necessary for efficient network plasticity.

That such selective reactivation occurs is evident not only from the human neuroimaging studies described previously, but from more precise studies of sleep-dependent network reactivation in the rat. Several groups have investigated the firing patterns of large numbers of individual neurons across the wake-sleep cycle in a variety of cortical and subcortical regions of the rat brain. The signature firing patterns of these networks, expressed during waking performance of spatial tasks and novel experiences, are replayed during subsequent SWS and REM sleep episodes, with replay during REM sleep being at speeds similar to those seen during waking, but those in SWS being an order of magnitude faster in some, but not all, studies.[89,96–99] Dave and Margoliash[100,101] have shown that waking patterns of premotor activity observed during song learning in the zebra finch are also replayed during sleep, with a temporal structural similar to that seen in wakefulness.

Together these data indicate that sleep-dependent reactivation of temporal patterns of network activity consistently occurs following learning experiences during wakefulness, across a broad spectrum of species. This replay of events is hypothesized to trigger distinct but complimentary processes within reactivated neuronal ensembles. Indeed, Ribeiro et al.[99] have suggested that SWS reinstantiates the memory representation through network reverberation, while subsequent REM sleep then potentiates the memory for subsequent postsleep recall, through gene induction–mediated synaptic plasticity.

Cellular Studies

Recently, a form of sleep-dependent plasticity at the cellular level has been elegantly demonstrated during early postnatal development of the cat visual system.[102,103] Under normal circumstances, brief periods of monocular visual deprivation during critical periods of development lead to the remodeling of synaptic connectivity, with the deprived eye's inputs to cortical neurons being first functionally weakened and then anatomically diminished.[104] Frank et al.[105] have now shown that, when 6 hours of monocular deprivation are followed by 6 hours of sleep, the size of the monocularity shift doubles. In contrast, if the cats are kept awake for these same 6 hours (in the dark, without input to either eye), a nonsignificant *reduction* in the size of the shift occurs. Thus, sleep can contribute as much to developmental changes in synaptic connectivity as does visual experience, presumably by enhancing the initial changes occurring during a prior period of monocular deprivation. In contrast, sleep deprivation results in a loss of previously formed, experience-dependent synaptic change, a pattern similar to that reported in humans, albeit at the behavioral level.[12,17]

Shaffery et al.[106] have reported complimentary findings of sleep-dependent plasticity in the rat visual cortex, suggesting that REM sleep, in conjunction with visual experience, modulates the initial time course of visual cortex maturation. In rats under 30 days of age, electrical stimulation produces increased excitability (potentiation) in specific layers of the visual cortex, while stimulation after this early developmental stage is unable to produce such potentiation. Depriving rats of REM sleep during this period can extend the window of plasticity by as much as 7 additional days, suggesting that events occurring during REM sleep normally control the duration of this period of experience-dependent plasticity.

Molecular Studies

At the molecular level, Smith et al.[107] have shown that administration of protein synthesis inhibitors to rats during REM sleep windows thought to be critical for consolidation prevents behavioral improvement following the sleep period, while rats receiving saline injections show normal sleep-dependent learning. Such protein synthesis could reflect a fundamental mechanism regulating plasticity, namely the activation of genetic cascades that produce key molecules for synaptic remodeling. Our understanding of such gene inductions during sleep is only now being unraveled. In their initial studies, Cirelli and Tononi reported that several of the known "immediate early genes" (IEGs) are specifically down-regulated during sleep.[108–110] These findings have been used subsequently to argue that sleep is incapable of supporting plasticity and hence memory consolidation.[72] Since then, however, Cirelli et al.[111] have described approximately 100 genes that are specifically up-regulated during sleep—almost the same number that are up-regulated during wakefulness. Moreover, up-regulation of these genes during sleep was seen only in brain tissue.

This extensive up-regulation of genes during sleep is particularly striking, as it was seen in the absence of any specific learning tasks being performed prior to sleep. Insofar as this up-regulation is related to learning and memory consolidation, one might expect that such gene induction would only be seen after training on tasks that undergo sleep-dependent consolidation. Indeed, Ribeiro and colleagues have found up-regulation in rats of zif-268, a plasticity-associated IEG, during REM sleep following exposure to a rich sensorimotor environment, but its down-regulation during both SWS and REM sleep in the absence of such exposure.[112] Thus, there appears to be a window for increased neuronal plasticity during REM sleep periods following enriched waking experience (Fig. 9–8).

This rich environment effect can be mimicked by brief electrical stimulation of the medial perforant pathway.[113] Unilateral stimulation results in a wave of zif-286 expression during subsequent REM sleep, with expression seen predominantly in the ipsilateral amygdala and entorhinal and auditory cerebral cortices during the first REM sleep episodes after LTP induction, but extending into somatosensory and cerebral cortices during subsequent REM

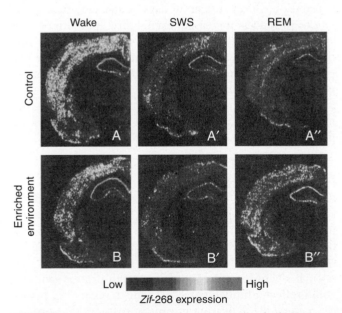

FIGURE 9–8 Experience-dependent up-regulation of zif-268 gene expression during wakefulness (WAKE) and slow-wave sleep (SWS) and REM sleep (REM) states in the rat. Autoradiograms of frontal coronal brain sections whose gene expression levels best represent the means for each group studied. In controls, zif-268 expression decreased from WAKE **(A)** to SWS **(A')** and REM **(A")**. In enriched-environment animals, zif-268 levels decreased from WAKE **(B)** to SWS **(B')**, but increased from the latter to REM **(B")**. This effect was particularly noticeable in the cerebral cortex and the hippocampus. (Reproduced with permission from Ribeiro S, Goyal V, Mello CV, Pavlides C. Brain gene expression during REM sleep depends on prior waking experience. Learn Mem 1999;6:500.) See Color Plate

periods.[113] These distinct phases of induction may correspond to the unique stages of consolidation previously reported from behavioral studies.[10]

Summary

Learning and memory are dependent on processes of brain plasticity, and sleep-dependent learning and memory consolidation must be mediated by such processes. Many examples of such sleep-dependent plasticity have now been reported, with several of them specifically induced by waking experiences. But while the existence of sleep-dependent plasticity is no longer in doubt, what remains to be demonstrated is that these specific components of brain plasticity, aside from their overall requirement for protein synthesis, actually mediate sleep-dependent learning and memory consolidation. Such evidence would require elegant interventions in the cellular and molecular processes of brain plasticity during the normal course of sleep-dependent consolidation, studies that most likely are already in progress.

UNRESOLVED QUESTIONS

Over the last several years, as evidence of sleep's role in learning and memory consolidation has grown, several researchers have raised questions concerning the nature or even existence of this relationship. Having focused our attention so far on the evidence in support of sleep's role, we turn now to objections, many of which hold clinical relevance.

Fear Conditioning and REM Sleep in Rodents

Studies described earlier have reported increases in REM sleep in rats following fear conditioning using a shuttle-box avoidance task. Such increases have been taken as indications of homeostatic increases in REM sleep driven by an increased demand on REM-dependent consolidation. In contrast, Sanford and colleagues[92,114] have reported *decreases* in REM sleep in mice following fear conditioning. At first glance, these findings appear contradictory, but differences in protocol suggest a more parsimonious explanation. While the shuttle-box avoidance task used in the studies showing increases in REM sleep involved training the animals how to successfully avoid future shocks, Sanford et al.'s studies[92,114] involved training animals to expect future unavoidable shocks. These learned helplessness protocols permit no useful learning, and the decrease, rather than increase, in REM sleep makes perfect sense within this context since, for example, the magnitude of the post-training increase in REM sleep has, in some cases, been proportional to the amount of learning.[61] It also provides an exemplary demonstration of the inability of stress per se to adequately explain REM increases.

Stress, REM Sleep, and Memory Consolidation

As noted earlier, several of the early findings of REM sleep–related alterations in memory have been criticized as possible confounds of stress induced both by fear conditioning paradigms and by sleep deprivation. This argument was originally presented in a comprehensive review by Horne and McGrath,[115] who made clear that they considered this was an alternative interpretation and not evidence against sleep-dependent consolidation. A more extreme stance has since been adopted by some authors,[72,73] who have used these arguments as strong evidence against any role for REM sleep in memory consolidation and learning. Two distinct objections have been raised: first, that the increase in REM sleep seen after training is induced by the stress of the training and not by a need for REM-dependent consolidation, and, second, that the deterioration in performance after REM deprivation is due to stress produced by sleep deprivation. However, several findings—including the previously discussed delayed "REM windows,"[116] the persistence of sleep deprivation effects for up to a week,[74] the correlation of the magnitude of the REM increase with the degree of prior learning[61] and subsequent retention,[62] and the decreased REM sleep following learned helplessness training[92,114]—all make it very unlikely that stress alone can explain these effects. Furthermore, the findings of performance enhancement seen in humans after a nap with REM sleep[55] as well as in rats after various procedures that increase REM sleep,[117] or even increase just PGO waves in the absence of REM sleep,[63] along with the suppression of enhancement by protein synthesis inhibition during REM windows,[107] cannot be explained in any way by these arguments.

Antidepressants, Sleep, and Memory

A recurring issue in the sleep and memory debate has been the REM sleep–suppressant effects of monoamine oxidase inhibitors (MAOIs) and other antidepressants and the impact, or lack thereof, on memory functioning. It has been suggested that these findings argue that such REM suppressants can be taken for years with no deleterious effects on learning.[72,73] First, while MAOIs appear to reduce REM sleep to a greater or lesser extent early in medication,[118,119] REM sleep re-emerges later in the course of medication,[120–122] suggesting a strong REM compensatory mechanism. Furthermore, there is a potent REM rebound during periods when medication is paused—the so-called drug holidays.[121,123,124] As such, the claim that patients live for years without REM sleep is unfounded.

Second, most of these studies use a simple one-off test of memory, which unfortunately does not address the question of intact or impaired sleep-dependent learning, since this obviously requires a retest following sleep. Even when a memory retest has been performed, almost all studies have retested memory within minutes of initial training. No studies to date have involved retesting following sleep, or recorded subjects' sleep to determine the extent of REM suppression. As a result, these findings provide little useful information regarding the role of post-training REM sleep in memory consolidation, let alone the role of sleep in general. A systematic study focusing on the effects of antidepressant medication on memory consolidation represents an important future goal, particularly considering the implications of such sleep-dependent memory impairment as a consequence of these drugs.

Sleep and IQ

An alternate discussion has focused on sleep and IQ. Based on the premise that REM-dependent memory consolidation exists, it has been suggested that species with greater intelligence should therefore have more REM sleep than others, and individuals with higher IQs should have more REM sleep than others.[72,73] But there are several difficulties with such an inference:

1. It is unclear whether IQ and intelligence have any correlation with the efficacy of memory consolidation.
2. If such a correlation did exist, it is unclear whether it would predict that lower IQ should correlate with less REM sleep (since less REM sleep produces less consolidation) or more REM sleep (since greater demands produce more REM sleep).
3. Given that there are also positive correlations between SWS and stage 2 NREM sleep and memory consolidation, these should also increase, which would lead to the unreasonable conclusion that the more intelligent an individual or species, the more they would sleep.
4. Since REM sleep is thought to mediate additional functions besides that of memory consolidation, it is not clear that IQ or intelligence should be the dominant determinant of baseline REM sleep amounts.

With this kaleidoscope of possible interpretations, the meaning of IQ and its relationship to sleep in discussing memory consolidation remains unclear.

Future Questions

This being said, there remain numerous important and unanswered questions regarding sleep-dependent learning and memory consolidation. Four broad categories of questions represent obvious future goals. First, it remains unclear exactly which types of memory undergo sleep-dependent consolidation. While procedural learning (both perceptual and motor), is clearly enhanced by post-training sleep, the forms of declarative memory that are similarly affected are less well resolved. Second, sleep's contribution to the processes of stabilization, enhancement, reconsolidation, integration, translocation, and active erasure require further elucidation. Third, the actual processes within sleep that effect consolidation are almost completely unknown. Candidate mechanisms—including (1) synchronous brain activity, such as that of PGO waves, sleep spindles, and theta rhythms; (2) changes in regional brain activation and inter-regional communication; and (3) shifts in global concentrations of neuromodulators, including acetylcholine, norepinephrine, and serotonin, and more classic hormones such as cortisol and even growth hormone—are all only beginning to be adequately investigated.[83,125,126] Finally, almost nothing is known about how these processes are altered in various populations, whether related to normal aging or to psychiatric and neurologic disorders. Much of the excitement over the next decade will be in beginning to address these questions more fully.

SUMMARY

Over the last 25 years, the field of sleep and memory research has grown exponentially, with the number of publications per year doubling every 9–10 years, faster than the growth for either sleep or memory alone. These reports, ranging from studies of cellular and molecular processes in animals to behavioral studies in humans, have provided a wealth of converging evidence that sleep-dependent mechanisms of neural plasticity lead to the consolidation of learning and memory across a range of animal species.

At the molecular level, significant number of genes appear to be up-regulated specifically in brain tissue during sleep, and at least one immediate early gene related to synaptic plasticity, *zif*-286, is up-regulated during REM sleep expressly in response to environmental or direct electrical stimulation of the hippocampus. In rats, patterns of neuronal activation expressed during waking exploration reappear during subsequent sleep, and, in humans, patterns of regional brain activation seen during daytime task training are repeated during subsequent REM sleep.

At the electrophysiologic level, studies in rats have shown that retention of learning of a shuttle-box avoidance task increases subsequent P-wave density, and is strongly correlated with this increase. In humans, spindle density increases following training on a declarative memory task, and, again, this increase correlates with subsequent improvement on the task.

At the behavioral level, animal studies have found robust increases in REM sleep following task training, and decrements in performance after REM deprivation, even when retesting is delayed until a week after the end of deprivation. In contrast, several animal studies have failed to find evidence of either increased REM sleep or deterioration following deprivation. Most likely this reflects a combination of methodologic problems and conditions under which consolidation is, in fact, not sleep dependent. Similarly, human studies have provided examples where increases in REM sleep are seen following training; where REM, SWS, or stage 2 NREM deprivation diminishes subsequent performance; and where overnight improvement correlates with REM, SWS, or stage 2 NREM sleep.

In the end, the question appears not to be whether sleep mediates learning and memory consolidation, but instead, how it does so. The future of the field is truly exciting, and the challenge to neuroscience will be to both uncover the mechanisms of brain plasticity that underlie sleep-dependent memory consolidation, and to expand our understanding of sleep's role in memory processes beyond simple consolidation, into the constellation of additional processes that are critical for efficient memory development. Work across the neurosciences will be necessary to answer these questions, but with the current rate of growth of research in the field, the next decade should provide important advances in our understanding of this critical function of sleep. By way of this multidisciplinary approach, and with a measured appreciation that sleep plays a fundamental role in consolidating and reforming memories, we can look forward to new advances in treating disorders of memory, and perhaps even improving the capacity of our own.

ACKNOWLEDGMENTS

This work was supported by grants from the National Institutes of Health (MH48,832, MH65,292, MH06,9935, and MH67,754) and the National Science Foundation (BCS-0121953).

⊘ REFERENCES

A full list of references are available at www.expertconsult.com

POST-SLEEP INCREASED ACTIVATION

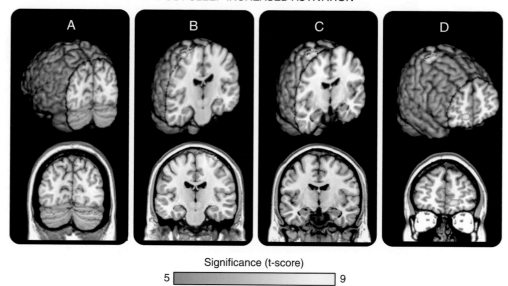

Significance (t-score)

5   9

POST-SLEEP DECREASED ACTIVATION

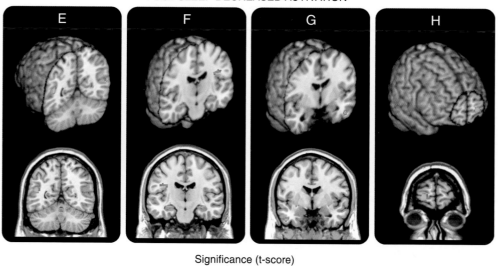

Significance (t-score)

5   7

FIGURE 9–7 Sleep-dependent motor memory reorganization. Subjects were trained on a sleep-dependent motor skill task and retested 12 hours later, either following a night of sleep or following intervening wakefulness, during a functional MRI (fMRI) brain scanning session. Scans after sleep and wakefulness were compared (subtracted), resulting in regions showing increased fMRI activity postsleep (*in red/yellow;* **A–D**) or decreased signal activity (*in blue;* **E–H**) postsleep, relative to post-wakefulness. Activation patterns are displayed on three-dimensional rendered brains (*top panel* of each graphic), together with corresponding coronal sections (*bottom panel* of each graphic). Following sleep, regions of increased activation were identified in the right primary motor cortex **(B),** the left cerebellum **(A),** the right hippocampus **(C),** and the right medial prefrontal cortex **(D).** Regions of decreased activity postsleep were expressed bilaterally in the parietal lobes **(E),** together with the left insula cortex **(F),** left temporal pole **(G),** and left frontopolar area **(H),** all regions of the extended limbic system. All data are displayed at a corrected threshold of $p < 0.05$. (See page 122)

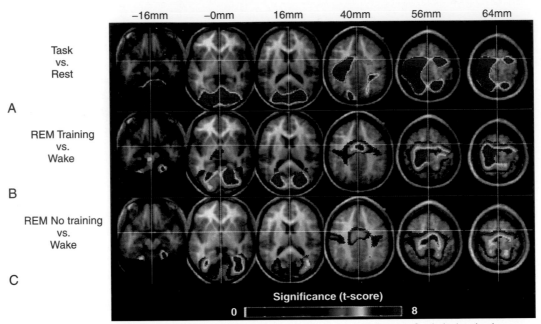

| | −16mm | −0mm | 16mm | 40mm | 56mm | 64mm |

A Task vs. Rest

B REM Training vs. Wake

C REM No training vs. Wake

Significance (t-score)

0 ⬛ 8

FIGURE 9–6 Task-dependent reactivation of human brain activity during REM sleep. Statistical activation maps of different experimental contrasts. Maps are displayed at six different brain levels (from 16 mm below to 64 mm above the bicommissural plane), superimposed on the average magnetic resonance imaging (MRI) scan of subjects. All maps are thresholded at $p < 0.001$ (uncorrected), except for **A,** which is thresholded at voxel-level-corrected $p < 0.05$. **(A)** Brain regions activated during daytime performance of the motor skill task (Task–Rest). **(B)** Brain regions activated during subsequent REM sleep in subjects who received daytime training (REM Sleep Training–Rest); note considerable overlap with daytime task-dependent activity patterns. **(C)** Brain regions activated during REM sleep in subjects who did not receive any daytime training (REM Sleep No Training–Rest).*(Reproduced with permission from Maquet P, Laureys S, Peigneux P, et al. Experience-dependent changes in cerebral activation during human REM sleep. Nat Neurosci 2000;3:831.)* (See page 120)

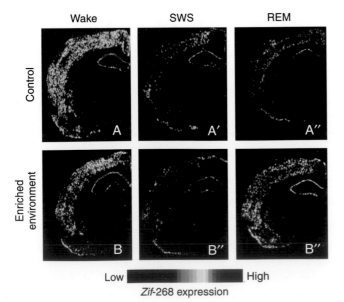

Wake   SWS   REM

Control

A   A'   A''

Enriched environment

B   B''   B''

Low ⬛ High

Zif-268 expression

FIGURE 9–8 Experience-dependent up-regulation of *zif*-268 gene expression during wakefulness (WAKE) and slow-wave sleep (SWS) and REM sleep (REM) states in the rat. Autoradiograms of frontal coronal brain sections whose gene expression levels best represent the means for each group studied. In controls, *zif*-268 expression decreased from WAKE **(A)** to SWS **(A')** and REM **(A'').** In enriched-environment animals, *zif*-268 levels decreased from WAKE **(B)** to SWS **(B'),** but increased from the latter to REM **(B'').** This effect was particularly noticeable in the cerebral cortex and the hippocampus.*(Reproduced with permission from Ribeiro S, Goyal V, Mello CV, Pavlides C. Brain gene expression during REM sleep depends on prior waking experience. Learn Mem 1999;6:500.)* (See page 124)

CHAPTER 10

Dreaming in Sleep-Disordered Patients

Rosalind Cartwright

A BRIEF HISTORICAL INTRODUCTION

Sleep disorders medicine is a direct descendent of the discovery of rapid eye movement (REM) sleep in the early 1950s. At that time, sleep was assumed to be a time of physical rest and recuperation but without psychological activity of any importance. The recall of dreams was too irregular, both within and between persons, and too difficult to decode for meaning, for dreams to be a good candidate for research effort. The REM discovery changed all that: the regular and close association of the distinctive brain state to the presence of the psychological experience of dreaming meant that the elusive unconscious mind was now open to systematic investigation. This, in turn, it was believed would lead to new insights into the "mental disorders" whose etiology was frequently modeled as an under- or overcontrol of unconscious motives (wishes) from early childhood. These were believed to surface in dreams, when the learned controls (defenses) are loosened and input from external stimuli is reduced. This new accessibility to reports of dreams, close to the time these are occurring, promised a more direct approach to their understanding through the methods of science than had been achieved through the theory-based method of psychoanalytic interpretation.

However, well-controlled studies of the dreams of psychiatric patients proved to be difficult, and laboratory-based dream research, in the first 2 decades following the discovery of REM, was most often conducted on normal samples. By the 1970s, when sleep clinics began to open, the focus of sleep research shifted from what was happening in the mind to the body, to studies of patients with sleep disorders. Dreams were rarely collected on these patients who were seen as suffering from a medical disorder requiring a medical diagnosis and treatment.

Now, however, there is a renewal of interest in the unconscious mind and in dream function. This is partly driven by the availability of more sophisticated technology such as brain imaging conducted during sleep.[1] Positron emission tomography (PET) scans, for example, have identified the areas of the brain that are more or less active in different sleep states relative to their activity in waking, as well as differences between sleep-disordered patients and controls. Functional magnetic resonance imaging,[2] too, is helping to map various functional relations. Specifically, the ventral visual pathway, which is selective for faces, has been of recent interest as this is relevant to sleepwalking, in which faces are reported not be recognized. Spectral analysis scoring[3–5] of the sleep studies also gives a more fine-grained ability to compare patient groups to healthy controls than the traditional sleep stage scoring has been able to do.

Another stimulus for the revival of interest in dreaming comes from new research on sleep-related learning and memory,[6] showing the continuity of information processing throughout all of sleep.[7,8] These studies demonstrate that the cooperation between non-REM (NREM) and REM sleep is essential to the retention of new learning in memory, and thus to improving waking performance in both animals and humans. In addition, the overnight regulation of negative emotion in normal individuals and the failure to regulate mood in the depressed suggested the content of the intervening dreams be addressed. And then there are the patients presenting at sleep centers whose

TABLE 10–1 REM/Dream Characteristics of Four Sleep Disorders

Disorder	REM	Recall	Affect
Major depression	Early	Poor	Absent
NREM parasomnia	Delayed	Poor	Acted out
Nightmares	Interrupted	Vivid	Strong
Dream enactment	Interrupted	Good	Strong and acted out

NREM, non–rapid eye movement.

complaints hint that the source of their sleep disturbance may not lie in a physical problem but in malfunctioning of REM sleep and their dreams. Those suffering from sleep-disturbing nightmares[9] following major disasters such as 9/11[10] are one such group.

This chapter reviews the characteristics of dreaming as an activity, and the nature of the dreams of patients who fall into four diagnostic categories (Table 10–1): (1) those with insomnia complaints associated with major depressive disorder; (2) those complaining of frequent nightmares, including those with post-traumatic stress disorder (PTSD); (3) adults who present with sleepwalking or fear-driven arousals from delta sleep (NREM parasomnias); and (4) those who enact their disturbing dreams with vivid recall (REM parasomnia). These four groups are chosen to look into the effect of specific abnormalities. In major depression, REM occurs too early and dreams are bland and poorly recalled. In nightmares, REM is interrupted with an abrupt awakening and vivid recall of a frightening nature. In the NREM parasomnia of sleep terrors, there is a motor arousal from delta sleep that delays REM sleep with physiologic manifestations of fear but no dream content and very limited recall. In the NREM parasomnia of sleepwalking, the basic survival drives are enacted with no recall. In the REM parasomnia of dream enactment, there is both the motor arousal from REM sleep and the enactment of a dream with good recall. The emphasis in this discussion will be on how these various abnormalities contribute to our understanding of mental activity occurring during sleep and its place in the 24-hour sleep-wake cycle. Dreams are an important piece of that cycle, and the information from individuals with various sleep disorders illuminates the workings of the mind both in sickness and in health.

What We Know of Dreams 50 Years After REM

The early laboratory work on dreams was for the most part descriptive, conducted on small samples usually drawn from young, healthy, predominantly male medical or undergraduate psychology students. Most of the core knowledge about dreams either has never been replicated or has failed to be confirmed on replication. Only Snyder's[11] analysis of the content of the dreams reported by 56 subjects over 250 nights produced a database from a fairly homogeneous sample, large enough to inspire confidence in the reliability of the findings. Although he reported that negative emotions were twice as common as positive feelings, with fear and anxiety predominating followed next by anger, his overall conclusion was that the typical dream is a "clear, coherent, and detailed account of a realistic situation involving the dreamer and other people caught up in very ordinary activities and preoccupations." This was not at all what had been anticipated on the basis of dreams reported during psychoanalytic sessions.

Snyder suggested an explanation for this discrepancy: dreams reported to a therapist are a highly selected sample and perhaps are more memorable because they are more dramatic, vivid, and emotionally rich. Furthermore, he suggested, the dreams of people who are emotionally disturbed most likely reflect this disturbance, and therefore will differ from the ordinary dreams of nonpatient samples. He also pointed out that, even within the relatively homogeneous sample in his study, there were marked individual differences in dreams, just as there are in waking cognition. Some subjects always had interesting dreams to report, and others' reports were consistently dull. In this view, Snyder anticipated the current model of dreaming as part of the continuity of information processing across all states in the 24-hour sleep-wake cycle. However, it may be argued that continuity of dream content is an experimental artifact. Waking a sleeper to full consciousness in order to retrieve a report from the first period of REM sleep (REM_1) may have an effect on the content of the following REM period. In other words, a continuous theme during sleep within a night from REM period to REM period may not have been present if the awakenings had not brought the initial dream into waking awareness.

Despite this difficulty, the laboratory-based dream collection protocol has clear advantages over those dreams spontaneously remembered at home. Not only is there the much higher yield, given that three to five reports can be collected on any one night, but their relation to the characteristics of the REM state from which they are drawn can be examined. Does the density of the eye movements or the heart rate that precedes the awakening relate to the emotionality of the content, for example? These are interesting questions. Collecting dreams in the laboratory does mean an investment in time. Most patients do not sleep well on their first night of monitored sleep. The first REM period is often skipped altogether or sustained for only a minute or two before another descent into an NREM cycle takes place. Also, the REM reports from a first night often reflect the laboratory setting and the experience of being observed.[12] These "laboratory effects" discouraged early researchers who complained that these dreams were not representative of "natural" dreams. Comparing dreams collected in the laboratory to the home dream reports of the same subjects proved the point: home dreams were more emotional and contained more sex and aggression. To obtain a representative sample of a night's dreams therefore requires at least a second laboratory night. This presents a problem of cost for clinical patients unless the second night is supported by a funded study, and has no doubt limited dream research on sleep-disordered patients.

Those who undertake to collect dreams need to follow a standardized awakening procedure. If the experimenter waits to ask for a report until a REM period is over, and stage 2 sleep has returned, the percentage of awakenings yielding recall of a dream drops markedly.[13] To ensure that differences between groups, or within groups over time, are not due to differences in the method of their retrieval, it is recommended that a protocol for making the awakening after a set number of consecutive epochs of REM be carefully followed. This, of necessity, truncates the dream story before a natural ending. Nonetheless, the ability to follow a formal design with appropriate controls makes the laboratory the preferred setting for studies investigating the function of dreaming and the nature of dream content in various disorders.

REVIVAL OF DREAM STUDY

Sleep and Dreaming in Insomnia and Depression

Originally the investigation of the dreams of psychiatric patients was hampered by the difficulty of controlling for the effects of their treatment. Most often these patients are treated with many different kinds and amounts of antidepressants, antipsychotics, and other medications that cannot be discontinued safely, and that might have effects on REM sleep and on the dreams themselves. However, some promising work was done in the past. In the depressed, it was noted that these patients had poor recall from REM awakenings, and that when dreams were reported, they were notably short, stark, and bland in affect.[14] This state of affairs did not change until shortly before remission from the depression. At that point, dream reports become longer with stronger affect. Although this return of recall of strongly emotional dreams—often nightmares—also posed an increased risk of suicide,[15] it also hinted that dreams might be predictive of a return to mental health.

In Snyder's[11] study of healthy subjects whose dreams were more likely to express negative emotion, they nonetheless tested as being in a better mood in the morning than they were the night before. Perhaps when the affect was not too extreme, experiencing negative emotion in dreams has a mood-regulating effect. The ideal sample on which to test this hypothesis is one known not to wake in a positive mood.

Kupfer[16] laid the groundwork for testing whether the dreams of the depressed were "malfunctioning" and so responsible for their low morning mood. His research established that the depressed had an abnormally reduced latency to the first REM period (65 minutes or less) in comparison to the approximate 90 minutes in normal

controls, and that the more severe the depression the shorter that latency. This was so reliable a finding he called it a "biological marker." Support for this assertion came from Giles et al.'s sleep studies of first-degree relatives of depressed patients.[17] The early REM marker was found in many, even in those who had no history of any depression episodes. Those with early onset of REM sleep frequently also had an early offset of sleep (an early morning awakening) and a complaint of insomnia. Sleep centers were finding that many of their insomnia patients had both the early REM period and the shortened total sleep time with inability to get back to sleep once waking too early.

The Ford and Kamerow[18] study of insomnia in the general population added further to the relation of insomnia and depression. Those subjects meeting insomnia criteria at both the first and second testing who were untreated, and had no depression at the first testing, were likely to meet criteria for a new diagnosis of depression at the 1-year follow-up point. This, the authors suggested, represented a challenge for preventive intervention. These results led to a debate about whether insomnia precedes or follows the onset of depression or whether the two are independent of each other.[19]

One way to untangle these possibilities is to manipulate the major sleep symptom of depression: the early REM period. The landmark study by Vogel and colleagues[20,21] did just that. The protocol employed several weeks of nightly REM deprivation for 6 consecutive nights followed by a seventh uninterrupted night. They were able to carry out this extended suppression because they established a ceiling of 30 awakenings per night. The alternating routine of 6 nights of REM suppression and one of uninterrupted sleep was repeated until there was a clinical response. This typically took three repetitions. When this was effective in restoring patients to normal functioning, it appeared to do so by resetting the timing of REM sleep within the night, from preponderance in the first half of the night to the usual balance of the majority occurring in the second half of the night. Those patients who went into remission stabilized their improved mood well enough to be discharged from the hospital with no other treatment. Was this lifting of the depressed mood due to the repeated suppression of abnormal dreams, or was the corrected sleep architecture, on the seventh recovery night, responsible for the change? Perhaps the shifting of slow-wave sleep back to its rightful place before the first REM period may be the variable worthy of further investigation. Whether the improved mood could be attributed to preventing abnormal dreams could not be investigated in Vogel et al.'s study as no dreams were collected before the deprivation manipulation or after.

What might be wrong with the REM dreams of the depressed, besides their timing, was suggested by brain imaging as reported by Nofzinger et al.[22] The PET scans of patients with major depression, in comparison to matched controls, show higher brain activation in the limbic and paralimbic areas during their REM sleep than in their waking scans, and this activity is higher than it is in the REM sleep of controls. The hyperarousal of areas associated with emotion suggests that the dream content might be more emotionally toned rather than less. However, depressed patients also show greater activation of the executive cortex during their REM sleep. Nofzinger et al. stated that this neocortical activity may have a dampening effect on the dream construction process and so account for the blandness of the affect and lack of thematic development in their dreams.

Kramer[23] filled in some of the gaps in the emerging picture connecting dream content to change in overnight mood by testing the mood of healthy volunteers before and after sleep using the Clyde Mood Scales and collecting the dreams from REM awakenings in between. He reported a significant decrease in the morning score of the "Unhappiness" scale, and that this is a robust finding consistent in several samples. The improvement in morning mood was found to be correlated with the number of characters included in the preceding dreams. Given the social withdrawal of the depressed in wakefulness, Kramer's finding suggests that a lack of dream characters may reflect this and perhaps contributes to the failure to improve their unhappy morning mood.

Taking these suggestive findings into account, Cartwright[24–27] addressed the relation of dream content to overnight mood regulation in a series of longitudinal laboratory studies of untreated depressed subjects and not depressed controls. All were volunteers undergoing an emotional event (a marital dissolution). This life event is known to be highly related to an episode of major depression.[28] The most recent of these studies[27] involved a sample of 30 subjects, 20 who met depression criteria and 10 who did not. These were studied longitudinally over a 5-month period. The design involved three daytime evaluations for depression—at screening, at month 3, and at month 5—and three sleep and dream assessments in the laboratory at months 1, 2, and 4. The depression status was assessed by the Structured Clinical Interview for DSM-IV,[29] the Hamilton Depression Rating Scale,[30] and the self-administered Beck Depression Inventory.[31] On each of the laboratory nights, the volunteers also completed a Profile of Mood States (POMS)[32] scale before and after sleep and a Current Concerns[27] rating form before each REM collection night. Two nights were involved in each of the three occasions of laboratory sleep. The first was always a baseline night of uninterrupted sleep, and the second a night of REM interruption to collect reports of whatever mental activity they could recall. The aim was to differentiate those who remained depressed from those who no longer met depression criteria at month 5, and to investigate the contribution of some sleep and dream variables to this difference. The overnight improvement in negative mood, as assessed by

the change on the Depression scale of the POMS was one such variable. A second was the quality of the intervening dream reports collected from each REM interruption on the three laboratory occasions, as well as their complexity and affect component. A third was the effect of the degree of waking concern about the former spouse on their inclusion in dream reports, and whether dreams of the spouse were related to an immediate change of morning mood and a long-term lifting of the depression.

As many of the results of these studies have been published, this chapter focuses on new data analyses comparing the dream content in depressed subjects who remit and those who do not. Of the 20 volunteers who met depression criteria on all three measures at screening, 12 were in remission (R group) at the end of the study. The difference between the R group and the eight who remained depressed (NR group) was strongly related to the dreamlike quality of their reports even at month 1, the first occasion of REM awakenings. The measure used was a five-category system developed by Foulkes[33] to differentiate NREM (thought-like) reports from REM (dreamlike) reports. Each report was scored as follows:

1. a failure to recall anything
2. the report is a "thought" rather than an image
3. there is one or more image
4. the images have a story-like connection between them
5. the report has many images and a well-developed story linking them

The percentage of REM reports judged to be 4 or 5 at month 1 for the R group was 53% and for the NR group 21%, a significant difference. The mean percentage of REM awakenings scoring 4 or 5 over the three occasions was 57% for the R subjects, 25% for the NR subjects, and 31% for the controls. Those in the R group created more dreamlike scenarios in REM periods throughout the study than did those not depressed, and twice as many as those who remained depressed when untreated. The two groups had not differed at intake in the severity of their depression on the clinician-rated Hamilton scale but the NR group was significantly more depressed on the self-rated Beck Depression Inventory.

The pattern of overnight mood change on the Depression scale of the POMS is very different for the two depressed groups.[34] Although both groups reduced the morning Depression scores from night 1 to morning 1, the R group remained at the reduced score when tested again before the second lab night. Those in the NR group relapsed to their night 1 level of depressed mood on night 2. This pattern repeated each month. The R group maintained overnight gains during the day and made further reductions each night. The NR group reverted to the high scores each night and made no overall progress in mood reduction. What was happening in the intervening dreams that might contribute to this difference was explored next.

A Current Concerns test was completed prior to each sleep-through night. There were 15 items, including "ex-spouse." The subject was asked to rate how concerned he or she has been over the past week about each item. The correlation between the rating of the ex-spouse (on a five point scale with 1 = not at all concerned to 5 = very concerned) at month 1 and the total number of times that person was named as a character in the dream reports was significant ($r = .56$, $p < 0.01$). This correlation was also significant at the end of the study. The score on concern about the ex-spouse at month 4 and number of incorporation dreams correlated at $r = .67$ ($p < 0.00$). The higher the waking concern, the more likely it was for that person to be included in the dreams. The degree of depression on the Hamilton scale at screening is positively correlated with the degree of concern about the spouse at month 1 ($r = .54$, $p < 0.00$) and this relation was less strong but was still significant at the end of the study (Hamilton scale at month 5 and the last Current Concern score on the ex-spouse item at month 4: $r = .39$, $p < 0.03$). Those more depressed subjects were more concerned about the ex-spouse, and the more concerned they were about that person, the more often that person was directly included in the dream story.

There were too few dream reports when the ex-spouse was directly named to do formal tests of differences between groups on the nature of these dreams. By inspection by independent raters, there were differences in both the affect and complexity. The ex-spouse dreams of the NR group were short and barren of any affect, while these dreams of the R group expressed negative feelings of unhappiness, rejection, and embarrassment in relation to the former spouse and were more complex in their structure. They included more changes of scene, more dream characters, and images drawn from both current experience and the past. Here is an example from a woman in the depressed group who was no longer depressed at the end of the study. She was strictly raised, was of mixed ethnicity, and had emigrated from South Africa with her husband, who shortly after left her:

> I dreamed I was fleeing from something with my son and my daughter on a dark street in a suburban area but in an Indian or Asian community with barbed wire around the fence. My son needed to use the bathroom and my daughter needed water for her dog. We knocked on the door of this house and an old woman answered. I asked her for help but a man came to the door and said "No." I asked "Why not?" and the man said "You would have to be my wife." I didn't know what to do. Then we were backtracking through a field and there were shots being fired all around. Then we were in a room where a dance was being planned. I was telling my ex-husband that I would only be staying for five minutes and he said "Fine" like he didn't care. I knew that his new girl friend would be there and they would be dancing. I felt resentful. I didn't want to see that.

In contrast is a dream of a very traditional stay-at-home woman who remained depressed:

> My husband was dating this girl that he works with and him taking her out. He was meeting her at our house. I was just sitting in my house in my living room and he was just going out the door with this girl. I was reading a newspaper. I was just looking at them.

Both women dream of losing the husband to another woman, but the first, although she pictures herself in a hostile setting, is actively seeking help, whereas the second is passive. The first recognizes her feelings of resentment, the second expresses no feelings. The first includes more characters and she herself is in several different roles, while the second is unrelated to others. The first is made up of two scenes, the second of a single one. The first links the past to the present, the second is static in present time.

The overnight mood regulation was progressive over time for those who would no longer meet depression criteria at the end of the study. For those remaining depressed, the negative mood improved following sleep, but this did not change the way the intervening waking experience was processed, leading them to become re-depressed by the POMS test that night. One clear difference that may account for this is how poorly constructed the dreams were, especially those related to the loss of the marriage partner and their lack of relevant affect. These subjects may create images representing the present ("my ex-husband has a new girlfriend") but do not link these to older memory material ("I do not have the right to expect help from older people back home"). It is this linkage that is apparent in the spouse dreams of the R group and is absent in the NR group's dreams. Learning to cope successfully with this loss is impaired in the absence of a constructive dream process, one that changes the structural organization of the related memory system, which is what guides behavior choices in waking. Processing waking experience in the same way leads to an unchanged emotional state.

Sleep and Dreaming in Nightmare Patients

Nightmares are defined as abrupt awakenings from REM sleep with a clear recall of a frightening dream.[9] In contrast to the dreams of depressed persons, the dreams in this disorder have too much affect. Rather than the REM period coming too early in the sleep cycle, nightmares most often occur toward the end of the night when REM episodes are longer and the eye movement density higher. Chronic nightmares are a relatively common parasomnia, with a prevalence of 6% reporting as many as one per week. They are more frequent in women than in men, in children than adults, and in psychiatric samples than in those with no mental health diagnosis. They are found less often in the elderly. This distribution suggests that it is those with fewer coping skills who are more prone to nightmares.

Repetitive dreams that replay some trauma along with the accompanying emotions of rage, fear, or grief are one of the defining diagnostic symptoms of PTSD. These nightmares are more likely to occur at any time of night in both NREM and REM sleep. Lavie and Kaminer[35] studied 23 survivors of the Holocaust and 10 controls, more than 40 years after their traumatic experiences during World War II. Their findings support Vogel et al.'s[21] study that perhaps it is better to have no dreams than it is to experience and remember bad dreams.

Lavie and Kaminer divided the sample of survivors into a well-adapted group and those who were not. All were studied for 4 nights in the sleep laboratory, with dreams collected on nights 1, 3, and 4. In waking, the well-adjusted survivors had fewer PTSD symptoms, greater ego strength, and less manifest anxiety, and their defensive style was characterized as "repression." Their sleep differences included lower eye-movement density counts and a lower rate of dream recall. The dreams that were retrieved were less complex with lower salience and less dream anxiety than those reported by the subjects who were poorly adjusted. The authors interpret these results as demonstrating that repression of dreams and of waking negative memories works to protect the mental health of the individual by sealing off the traumatic past, thus allowing a better waking life adjustment.

This conclusion calls into question the emotional information processing model of dream function, in which waking emotional experience evokes a dream response that integrates the new experience with previous emotional experiences that have had successful resolutions in the past. This model is challenged by long-lasting, highly stressful experiences, like the Holocaust, that have no precedent in the life of the sleeper, and for which there is no reality solution. Under these circumstances, different personalities may respond differently. Perhaps Hartmann's[36] concept outlined in his book *Boundaries in the Mind* is applicable. He describes people with thick boundaries between reality and fantasy as being able to live with their unresolved, negative experiences because they successfully compartmentalize their memories and the dreams that evoke them, while those whose boundaries are "thin" may continue to have trouble adapting because they are less successful at suppressing their nightly reminders of negative life experiences in dreams.

The difficulty in interpreting the results of Lavie and Kaminer's study, and generalizing from these, is the length of time between the initial traumatic experience and the dream collection study. It is possible that those who made a good life adjustment were those who experienced adaptive dreaming at the time, and that this was a major factor in their better level of waking adaptation many years later. This can only be assessed by longitudinal studies following a recent trauma.

Some studies have been carried out close to the time of a crisis. The response to the San Francisco earthquake,[37] for example, had a geographic control. The authors compared the nightmare frequency in a sample living in the affected area to those living remotely in Arizona. They reported that the closer subjects were to the event, the higher the nightmare rate.

A review of the findings to date from studies of Vietnam veterans with traumatic dreams by Domhoff[38] points out the differences in characteristics between those combat veterans who did and did not develop PTSD with traumatic dreams. Those who developed this syndrome are younger, less well-educated, and more likely to have experienced the death of a friend than those who did not develop the syndrome. Those who escaped this disorder resemble the description of Lavie and Kaminer's well-adjusted Holocaust survivors, and Hartmann's subjects with thick boundaries. They "put up a wall between themselves and others while in Vietnam."

Over time, traumatic dreams become less like the original experience as the memory is merged with other memories. However, if events that resemble the original trauma occur, the old nightmares may return. Kramer et al.[39] reported that a later loss of a spouse due to death or divorce will trigger a resurgence of dreams of the original war trauma. These PTSD-related traumatic dreams occur earlier in the night than do the traumatic dreams of patients who suffer from chronic nightmares. Kramer et al.[39] suggested that the emotion engendered by the traumatic event overwhelms the person's ability to assimilate the experience at the time, and this allows the original trauma to re-emerge from the memory networks in dreams when a new traumatic event occurs that matches the original loss in some way. This fits the hippocampal-neocortical dialogue model of how sleep processes new emotional learning and retains it in memory.[6–8,40]

The 9/11 disaster is another recent event that is being studied currently.[10,41] Children who were at a preschool just across from the World Trade Center are being followed. Some of these children, who witnessed frightening scenes of people jumping from the windows of the towers, have had persistent nightmares, while others have not. It is those who had previous frightening experiences, such as a dog bite or a tonsillectomy, who are more likely to have continuing nightmares.[41] They have been sensitized to attend to frightening events.

Laboratory studies of PTSD patients are difficult to carry out, given the frequency of dual diagnoses with depression and chronic alcoholism, the need to discontinue medication, the effects of its withdrawal, and the difficulty of obtaining a traumatic dream in the sleep laboratory, which is often experienced as a protective environment. There is clearly a need for further work in this area, particularly longitudinal studies that reveal the course of changes in sleep and in dreaming over time. The data currently available appear to support the emotional information processing model of dreaming with the caveat of personality trait and context differences. When strong negative affect is engendered in someone who has been sensitized by previous traumas, and who must remain in the disturbing conditions over time, that person is more likely to have heightened arousal levels throughout all sleep. This makes it possible for nightmares to occur in NREM as well as REM sleep, and for the dream content to mirror older traumatic memories. Patients who present with recurrent nightmares may have been PTSD patients years ago and are now experiencing a relapse due to some new stress with a similar psychological meaning to them.

Dreams in Sleep Terrors

Sleep terrors, one of the NREM parasomnias, have been well described by Broughton[42] as an arousal, usually from the first or second delta sleep cycle of the night, accompanied by a confusional state and the behavior and physiologic manifestations of terror. Sleep terrors are more common in children than adults. Since they happen during the transition from delta to REM sleep, they typically delay the appearance of the first period of REM sleep and may reduce the total amount of REM sleep on the nights they occur. The sleeper is usually inconsolable at the time and may engage in complex behaviors believing they must rescue someone, escape from some threat, or fight an enemy. There is little or no recall once the episode is over and rarely any morning recall even of the event itself.

Children who experience sleep terrors rarely have any associated psychopathology, but adults who continue to have these experiences are more likely to have some personality disturbance. The Minnesota Multiphasic Personality Inventory[43] profiles of some of these patients seen in our laboratory show them to have elevated scores on the Psychopathic Deviant scale, which measures impulses to act out with antisocial behaviors. This tendency is often tightly controlled by the patient during waking.

There has been only one laboratory study reporting the recall of what 12 adults with night terrors believed during an episode recorded in the laboratory.[44] Their report is a single image, which has a strong emotional basis, of being crushed or trapped, or that they are choking or being stepped on. There has been a debate over whether this perception is present before the arousal or is constructed postarousal to account for the high heart rate and feelings of terror. A common observation is that the report often contains curses and foul language in even the most polite patients—a breakthrough of defenses. A case example illustrates this:

> The patient is a well-mannered, mild young man, not at all psychologically minded. His presenting complaint was of sleep terrors with a single image of a bus about to run him over. He would jump out of bed to run out of the way of the oncoming bus. When asked during a treatment session to change the image to one with a more positive conclusion, he stated with strong affect that he would "turn around and shoot the son of a bitch." This

alerted the therapist to note that the threat was from a male, and came from the rear, perhaps a homosexual threat. His sleep terrors had re-emerged in adulthood, after a long period of quiescence, following his marriage to a robust, warm, womanly bride. The interpretation of the meaning of his bus image is highly speculative.

Further work is needed to collect examples from these patients of what they recall of their episodes in comparison to the content of their REM dreams following arousal and on non–sleep terror nights. They share sleep characteristics with sleepwalkers, narcoleptic patients, and those suffering REM sleep behavior disorder, a genetic defect[45] associated with a failure to maintain reduced motor activity during NREM sleep that allows behavioral arousals into confusional states. In sleep terrors, the arousal from delta sleep aborts the first REM period and the chance for down-regulation of the fear to take place in a dream.

Sleepwalking differs from sleep terrors in having less autonomic arousal. However, there is a good deal of overlap in these two disorders.[46] The behaviors that take place during the confused brain state of partial waking and partial sleep include eating, and even cooking; aggressive behaviors against the self, others, or objects; sexual acts of self-stimulation, or involving the bed partner or a sleeping child; exploring the environment; and attempts to rescue others from danger. All of these can be classed as primitive survival drives. The fact that these are enacted prior to REM sleep gives us a window into what emotion-driven necessity precedes a dream that, given the muscle atonia of REM sleep and imagery rather than action, might have been expressed safely. The lack of studies of the dreams of sleepwalkers following an episode in the laboratory or on a nonwalking night is a gap in the literature.

Dream Enactment

Dream enactment is another REM parasomnia. It differs from nightmares in that there is motor behavior appropriate to the dream and a failure of full consciousness during the arousal. This symptom is most often part of the REM sleep behavior disorder[47] syndrome and closely associated in the elderly with a neurodegenerative disorder, most often Parkinson's disease (PD). However, it may be found in young, otherwise healthy patients who are under stress and sleep deprivation. Although it is possible that this is a prodrome for the later development of PD or some other neurologic disorder,[48] it is also possible that it is a standalone disorder in some cases. This may be the case in a 25-year-old medical student who presented with this complaint. He described his problem as sitting up in bed and talking in an agitated manner four to six times per night on about 5 or 6 nights a week for the last 3 months. In a recent episode, he thought there was an anaconda in the bed: "I yelled to my wife: 'You grab the tail. I'll grab the head.'" In another episode he recalled that he acted out carrying the Olympic torch.

His sleep study showed the presence of periodic leg movements scattered throughout the night and clustering before arousals in REM sleep. The patient was unaware that the history of his dream enactment coincided with his marriage, just 3 months ago, and with the stress and loss of sleep during his preparation for his upcoming board examinations. The images of his dreams may be interpreted as concerns with his masculine prowess. In treating him, it was important for him to learn relaxation techniques and to allow himself to get adequate amounts of sleep regularly.

CONCLUSION

This chapter has reviewed four sleep disorders, highlighting their abnormality of REM timing in the night's sleep, or the arousal from NREM or REM sleep, in order to consider the behavior or mental content associated with these disorders in relation to the putative mood-regulating function of dreaming. REM sleep provides the conditions that allow the ongoing stream of affect-related thought to occupy awareness. Those persons in a state of hyperarousal due to strong negative affect may experience an early onset of REM sleep (as in depression), develop the conditions for dreaming in NREM sleep (as in PTSD), delay REM sleep (as in sleep terrors and sleepwalking), or interrupt REM sleep with an arousal (into a nightmare or dream enactment). All of these conditions are less efficient for morning mood regulation. Dreaming is a natural part of a continuous 24-hour system of mental activity. The disturbance of dreaming in sleep-disordered patients provides an opportunity to understand more fully the nature and function of their personal dreams and the general function of dreaming.

⊙ REFERENCES

A full list of references are available at www.expertconsult.com

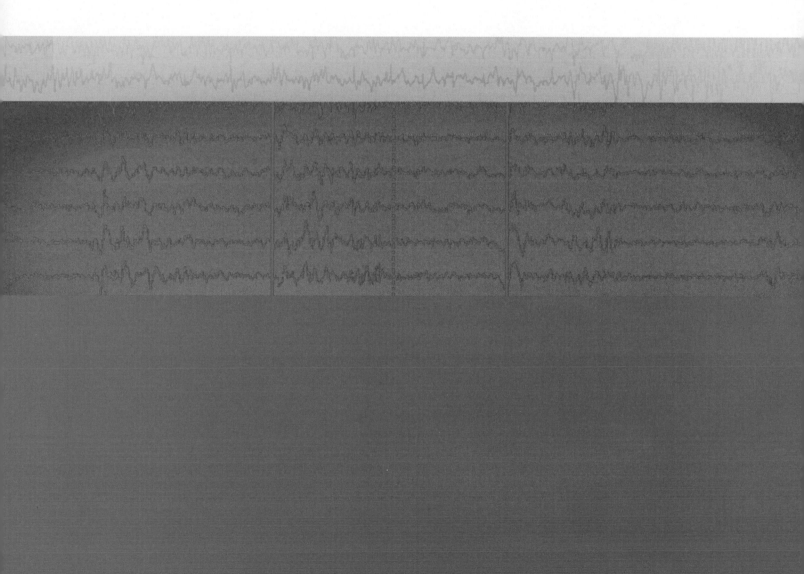

PART II

Technical Considerations

CHAPTER 11

Polysomnographic Technique: An Overview

Sharon A. Keenan

INTRODUCTION

The term *polysomnography* (PSG) was proposed by Holland, Dement, and Raynal[1] in 1974 to describe the recording, analysis, and interpretation of multiple, simultaneous physiologic parameters during sleep. PSG is an essential tool in the formulation of diagnoses for sleep disorders patients and in the enhancement of our understanding of normal sleep.[2–14] It is a complex procedure that should be performed by a trained technologist. Innovations for monitoring changes in physiology during sleep continue to hold great promise in the quest to understand healthy sleep and to diagnose sleep disorders.

Recent publications in polysomnography include the 2005 American Academy of Sleep Medicine (AASM) standards of practice and practice parameters guidelines for polysomnography.[15] As well, the *International Classification of Sleep Disorders: Diagnostic & Coding Manual*[16] describing more than 85 sleep disorders was revised in 2005. In the same year, an AASM task force was established to review and revise scoring of PSG data. The first papers from that process are published (see Chapter 18). Numerous atlases of PSG data have been published, expanding the knowledge of PSG, normal sleep, and sleep disorders.[17–23] The reader is directed to other references[24–38] for current indications and standards of practice articles that have appeared in the literature since the previous edition of this text. Summaries of key relevant points have been incorporated into this chapter. Currently, the Board of Registered Polysomnographic Technologists reports more than 7000 registered PSG technologists around the world. In January 2006, the AASM established an accreditation program for training PSG technologists.

This chapter is a review of the technical aspects of PSG, providing a step-by-step approach to traditional, classic in-laboratory PSG recording techniques. Problems likely to be encountered during a recording are examined, as are ways to alleviate them. Figures and actual tracings augment the text and help identify artifacts. An entire chapter in this text (see Chapter 18) is dedicated to the use of digital PSG systems. A brief discussion of digital recording and comparisons between analog and digital systems are made throughout this chapter. Digital systems have become the primary tool to collect, manipulate, display, and store data from sleep studies. Elsewhere in this volume, specified protocols are discussed and physiologic recording techniques are reviewed in detail. Recent advances include sleep studies transmitted over the Internet for scoring and final interpretation, wireless PSG systems, and studies validating alternative technologies in comparison to PSG.[39] Technological advances have enabled increased possibility of monitoring sleep and enhanced ability to deliver sleep health care. PSG continues to be held as the gold standard for diagnosis of sleep disorders.

Clinical Indications for PSG

According to the 2005 AASM proposed guidelines,[15] an attended PSG is considered the standard of practice for

- Diagnosis of sleep-related breathing disorders (SRBD)
- Positive airway pressure titration
- Preoperative assessment before snoring or obstructive sleep apnea (OSA) surgery
- Evaluating results of the following treatments:
  - Oral appliances for moderate to severe OSA
  - Surgical procedures for moderate to severe OSA
  - Surgical or dental procedures in SRBD for return of symptoms
- Treatment results requiring follow-up PSG:
  - Substantial weight loss or gain (10% of body weight)
  - When clinical response is insufficient or when symptoms return
- Patients with systolic or diastolic heart failure and nocturnal symptoms of SRBD
- Patients whose symptoms continue despite optimal management of congestive heart failure
- Neuromuscular disorders with sleep-related symptoms
- Narcolepsy (Multiple Sleep Latency Test [MSLT] after PSG)
- Periodic limb movement disorder in cases secondary to complaints by patient or observer (movements during sleep, frequent awakenings, excessive daytime sleepiness)

PSG is not required to diagnose

- Parasomnias
- Seizure disorders
- Restless legs syndrome
- Common, uncomplicated, noninjurious events (arousals, nightmares, enuresis, sleeptalking, bruxism)
- Circadian rhythm disorders

Diagnosis with clinical evaluation alone is the standard in these cases. Standard evaluation includes history, details of behavior, age of onset, time, frequency, regularity, and duration.

PATIENT CONTACT

A number of factors need to be kept in mind when a PSG is scheduled. Issues such as shift work, time zone change, or suspected advanced or delayed sleep phase syndrome should be taken into consideration. The study should be conducted during the patient's usual, major sleep period, to avoid confounding circadian rhythm factors.

When the PSG is scheduled, the patient is sent a questionnaire about his or her sleep-wake history and a sleep diary that solicits information about major sleep periods and naps for 2 weeks prior to the study (Appendix 11–1). Information is provided for the patient about the purpose and procedures of the sleep study. The goal is to make the patient's experience of the sleep study as uncomplicated and comfortable as possible.

In sleep laboratory settings, the technologist should ensure that patients are familiar with the surroundings and that they receive explicit information about the process. Patients should be shown to a bedroom and through the laboratory. They are made aware that someone will be monitoring their sleep throughout the entire study and told how to contact the technologist if necessary.

Before the study is undertaken, a full medical and psychiatric history should be completed and made available to the technologist performing the study. This information is necessary for correct interpretation of the data, and it allows the technologist to anticipate difficulties that may arise during the study. Technologists must also understand what questions the study seeks to answer. This enhances their ability to make protocol adjustments when necessary, and ensures that the most pertinent information is recorded.

Prestudy Questionnaire

It is not uncommon for patients, particularly those with excessive sleepiness, to have a diminished capacity to evaluate their level of alertness.[28] In addition, patients with difficulty initiating and maintaining sleep often report a subjective evaluation of their total sleep time and quality that is at odds with the objective data collected in the laboratory. For these reasons, it is recommended that subjective data be collected systematically as part of the sleep laboratory evaluation.

The Stanford Sleepiness Scale (SSS)[40,41] (Appendix 11–2) is an instrument used to assess a patient's subjective evaluation of sleepiness prior to the PSG. The SSS is presented to the patient immediately before the beginning of the study. Patients respond to a series of phrases by selecting the set of adjectives that most closely corresponds to their current state of sleepiness or alertness. The scale is used extensively in both clinical and research environments. However, it has two noteworthy limitations: it is not suitable for children who have a limited vocabulary or for adults whose primary language is not English. In these situations, a linear analog scale is recommended to provide an introspective measure of sleepiness (see Appendix 11–2). One end of the scale represents extreme sleepiness and the other end alertness. Patients mark the scale to describe their state just prior to testing.

Another instrument, the Epworth Sleepiness Scale,[42] lends information about chronic sleepiness. Patients are asked to report the likelihood of dozing in situations such as riding as a passenger in a car, watching television, and the like.

Patients are also asked about their medication history, smoking history, any unusual events during the course of the day, their last meal prior to the study, alcohol intake, and a sleep history for the last 24 hours, including naps.

Involvement of the patient in providing this information usually translates into increased cooperation for the study. A technologist's complete awareness of specific patient idiosyncrasies, in the context of the questions to be addressed by the study, ensures a good foundation for the collection of high-quality data.

Nap Studies

A proposed alternative to nocturnal PSG has been the nap study (to be distinguished from the MSLT). The rationale is that, if a patient has a sleep disorder, it will be expressed during an afternoon nap, not just during a more extensive PSG. The nap study approach has been used most frequently for the diagnosis of SRBDs and was proposed in an effort to reduce the cost of the sleep laboratory evaluation. The short study in the afternoon avoids the necessity of having a technologist present for an overnight study. There are serious limitations to the use of nap studies, however, including the possibility of false-negative results or the misinterpretation of the severity of SRBDs if the patient is sedated or sleep deprived prior to the study. When a nap study is performed, it should follow the guidelines published by the American Thoracic Society[43]:

> Although minimal systematic data exist on the value of nap recordings, nap studies of 2 to 4 hours' duration may be used to confirm the diagnosis of sleep apnea, provided that all routine polysomnographic variables are recorded, that both non-REM and REM sleep are sampled, and that the patient spends at least part of the time in the supine posture. Sleep deprivation or the use of drugs to induce a nap are contraindicated. Nap studies are inadequate to definitively exclude a diagnosis of sleep apnea.

Preparation of the Equipment

This chapter describes the polygraph, an instrument in which the main component is a series of amplifiers (see also Chapter 12). Usually there is a combination of alternating current (AC) channels and direct current (DC) channels; some amplifiers may be able to function in either AC or DC mode. Typically, at least 12 to 16 channels are available for recording, though many systems offer more channels. The data from the amplifiers were historically written to a moving chart. In modern digital systems, the analog signal is converted to a digital signal, which is stored by the computer for subsequent manipulation and analysis. A complete discussion of digital systems appears in Chapter 18, and a brief discussion appears near the end of this chapter. Currently, the data are reduced via a human visual pattern recognition process. However, some aspects of PSG data readily lend themselves to automatic analysis, and the use of sophisticated frequency analysis, such as fast Fourier transform analysis.[44]

Equipment for recording polysomnograms is produced by a number of manufacturers. Each may have a distinctive appearance and some idiosyncratic features, but there is a remarkable similarity when the basic functioning of the instrument is examined.

Equipment preparation includes an understanding of how the filters and sensitivity of the amplifiers affect the data collected. Decisions regarding sensitivity, filters, and channel selection are often predetermined by default software settings. Inasmuch as the major difference between classic analog PSG and computer-based systems lies principally in data storage and display, it is important that all technologists, regardless of the system used, have adequate knowledge of the operation of the equipment.

The amplifiers used to record physiologic data are very sensitive, so it is essential to eliminate unwanted signals from the recording. By using a combination of high- and low-frequency filters, and appropriate sensitivity settings, it is possible to maximize the likelihood of recording and displaying the signals of interest and decrease the possibility of recording extraneous signals. When using the filters, however, care must be taken to ensure that an appropriate window for recording specific frequencies is established and that the filters do not eliminate important data.

Alternating Current Amplifiers

Differential AC amplifiers are used to record physiologic parameters of high frequency, such as the electroencephalogram (EEG), the electro-oculogram (EOG), the electromyogram (EMG), and the electrocardiogram (ECG). The AC amplifier has both high- and low-frequency filters. The presence of the low-frequency filter makes it possible to attenuate slow potentials not associated with the physiology of interest; these include galvanic skin response, DC electrode imbalance, and breathing, any of which may be reflected in an EMG, EEG, or EOG channel. Combinations of specific settings of the high- and low-frequency filters make it possible to focus on specific bandwidths associated with the signal of interest. For example, respiration is a very slow signal (roughly 12–18 breaths/min) in comparison with the EMG signal, which has a much higher frequency (~20–200 Hz or cycles/sec). In the sleep lab, the bandwidth of interest for EEG data is 0.5–25 Hz.

Direct Current Amplifiers

In contrast to the AC amplifier, the DC amplifier does not have a low-frequency filter. DC amplifiers are typically used to record slower moving potentials, such as output from the oximeter or pH meter, changes in pressure in positive airway pressure treatment, or output from transducers that record endoesophageal pressure changes or body temperature. Airflow and effort of breathing can be successfully recorded with either AC or DC amplifiers.

An understanding of the appropriate use of filters in clinical PSG is essential to proper recording technique.[45] Table 11–1 provides recommendations for filter settings for various physiologic parameters.

TABLE 11–1   Recommendations for Filter Settings and Sensitivity for Various Physiologic Parameters

Channel*	Low-Frequency Filter (Hz)	Time Constant (sec)	High-Frequency Filter (Hz)	Sensitivity
EEG	0.3	0.4	35	50 (μV/cm)
EOG	0.3	0.4	35	50 (μV/cm)
EMG	5[†]	0.03	90–120	20–50 (μV/cm)
ECG	1.0	0.12	15	1 MV/cm
Index of airflow	0.15[‡]	5[‡]	15	[§]
Index of effort	0.15[‡]	5[†]	15	[§]

*EEG includes C3/A2, C4/A1, O1/A2, and O2/A1 (or any other EEG derivation). EOG includes right outer canthus and left outer canthus referred to opposite reference (or any other EOG derivation).
[†]If shorter time constant or higher low-frequency filter is available, it should be used. This includes settings for all EMG channels, including mentalis, submentalis, masseter, anterior tibialis, intercostal, and extensor digitorum.
[‡]Because breathing has such a slow frequency (as compared to the other physiologic parameters), the longest time constant available, or the lowest setting on the low-frequency filter options, would provide the best signal. It is also possible to use a DC amplifier (with no low-frequency filter, time constant = infinity) to record these signals.
[§]It is common in clinical practice to index changes in airflow and effort to breathe by displaying qualitative changes in oral/nasal pressure, temperature, and chest and abdominal movement. It is well recognized that quantitative methods (such as endoesophageal pressure changes) provide a more sensitive and accurate measure of work of breathing. Ideally, a multimethod approach is used to increase confidence in detecting events of sleep-related breathing anomalies.
ECG, electrocardiography; EEG, electroencephalography; EMG, electromyography; EOG, electro-oculography.
Modified from Keenan SA. Polysomnography: technical aspects in adolescents and adults. In C Guilleminault (ed), Clinical Neurophysiology of Sleep Disorders (Handbook of Clinical Neurophysiology Series). Amsterdam: Elsevier, 2005:33.

Calibration of the Equipment

Ideally, any recording instrument is calibrated prior to a test. The calibration ensures adequate functioning of amplifiers and appropriate settings for the specific protocol. Historically, in analog systems, a series of calibrations was performed and documented. The first calibration is an all-channel calibration (Fig. 11–1). During this calibration, all amplifiers are set to the same sensitivity, high-frequency filter, and low-frequency filter settings, and a known signal is sent through all amplifiers simultaneously. The proper functioning of all amplifiers is thus demonstrated, ensuring that all are functioning in an identical fashion.

A second calibration is performed for the specific study protocol. During this calibration, amplifiers are set with the high-frequency filter, low-frequency filter, and sensitivity settings appropriate for each channel; the settings are dictated by the requirements of the specific physiologic parameter recorded on each channel (Fig. 11–2; see also Table 11–1). The protocol calibration ensures that all amplifiers are set to ideal conditions for recording the parameter of interest. Filter and sensitivity settings should be clearly documented for each channel. Epoch lengths and clock times should be verified.

Digital systems generally do not require day-to-day adjustments; however, the calibration procedures should be performed before each study to document the selected filter and sensitivity settings and to confirm appropriate signal response for each channel.

"Paper Speed"

Historically, the speed of the chart drive for the recording instrument established the epoch length (amount of time per page) of the recording. A common paper speed for traditional polysomnography was 10 mm/sec, providing a 30-second epoch. Another widely accepted paper speed was 15 mm/sec, a 20-second epoch length. For patients with suspected sleep-related seizure activity, a paper speed of 30 or 60 mm/sec enhanced the ability to visualize EEG data. Data such as oxygen saturation, respiratory signals, or changes in penile circumference, however, were more easily visualized with slower paper speeds. The issue of selecting the appropriate paper speed became moot when digital systems became the norm. The ability to manipulate the display of data after collection is a major advantage of the digital systems.

Sleep stage scoring requires epoch-by-epoch review of the data. The AASM Task Force[46] recommends a 30-second epoch as the standard unit of time for analysis of sleep stages. Analysis of anomalies in movement or cardiac rhythms are counted and described in terms of their relation to stage of sleep.

THE STUDY

Electrode/Monitor Application Process

The quality of the tracing generated in the sleep laboratory depends on the quality of the electrode application.[47] Before any electrode or monitor is applied, the patient should be instructed about the procedure and given an opportunity to ask questions. The first step in the electrode application process involves measurement of the patient's head. The International 10–20 System[48] of electrode placement is used to localize specific electrode sites (Fig. 11–3). The following sections address the application process for EEG, EOG, EMG, and ECG electrodes.

Electroencephalography

As noted in the Rechtschaffen and Kales manual,[49] standard electrode derivations for monitoring EEG activity during sleep are C3/A2 or C4/A1 for central EEG activity, and O1/A2 or O2/A1 for occipital EEG activity.

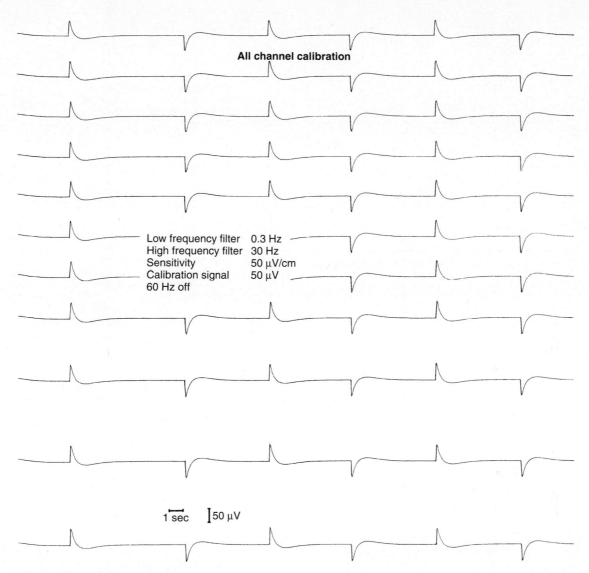

All channel calibration

Low frequency filter   0.3 Hz
High frequency filter   30 Hz
Sensitivity   50 µV/cm
Calibration signal   50 µV
60 Hz off

1 sec   50 µV

FIGURE 11–1 All-channel calibration. All amplifiers have the same sensitivity and high- and low-frequency filter settings.

The AASM Task Force terminology includes the terms "M1" and "M2" instead of "A1" and "A2" for the reference electrodes placed on the mastoid process.[46] In this case, the derivations would be C3/M2 or C4/M1, and O1/M2 or O2/M1. In some situations there may be a need for additional electrodes. For example, to rule out the possibility of epileptic seizures during sleep, or to detect the presence of other sleep-related EEG abnormalities, it may be necessary to apply the full complement of EEG electrodes according to the International 10–20 System (see Fig. 11–3). An abbreviated montage to screen for EEG abnormalities during PSG is discussed in Appendix 11–3. Also, the AASM Task Force pointed to the importance of frontal derivations (Fp1/M2, Fp2/M1) when considering decisions regarding K complexes and/ or slow-wave activity.

For recording an EEG, a gold cup electrode with a hole in the center is commonly used. Silver–silver chloride electrodes are also useful to record an EEG, though they may have limitations such as increased maintenance (evidenced by the need for repeated chloriding) and the inability to attach these electrodes to the scalp.

The International 10-20 System of electrode placement determines the placement of EEG electrodes. Reference electrodes are placed on the bony surface of the mastoid process. A description of the measurement procedure appears in Appendix 11–4.

The collodion technique[47] has long been an accepted and preferred method of application for EEG scalp and reference electrodes. This technique ensures a long-term placement and allows for correction of high impedances (>5000 ohms) after application. Other methods using

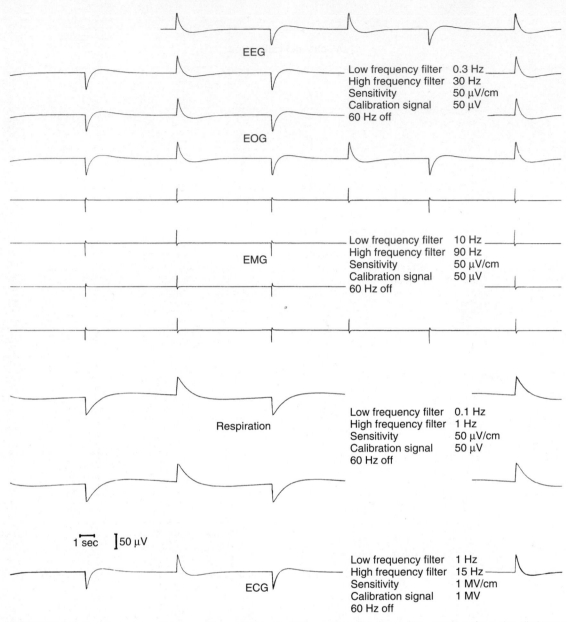

FIGURE 11–2 The montage calibration shows changes in high- and low-frequency filter settings from the all-channel calibration to accommodate the display of a variety of physiologic signals for the polysomnograph. (ECG, electrocardiogram; EEG, electroencephalogram; EMG, electromyogram; EOG, electro-oculogram.)

electrode paste and a conductive medium are acceptable and often preferred in certain conditions.

Electro-oculography

The EOG is a recording of the movement of the corneo-retinal potential difference that exists in the eye. It is the movement of this dipole with respect to the eye movement electrodes that is recorded. Gold cup electrodes or silver–silver chloride electrodes can be used to monitor the EOG. An electrode is typically applied at the outer canthus of the right eye (ROC) and is offset 1 cm above the horizontal. Another electrode is applied to the outer canthus of the left eye (LOC) and is offset by 1 cm below

the horizontal. The previously mentioned A1 and A2 (M1, M2) reference electrodes are used as follows: ROC/A1 (or M1) and LOC/A2 (or M2). Additional infra-orbital and supraorbital electrodes enhance the ability to detect eye movements that occur in the vertical plane, and can be particularly useful in the MSLT[50,51] (Fig. 11–4). It should be noted that many variations of electrode placement and recording derivations have been used in a variety of clinical and research settings. In an attempt to standardize procedure, the AASM Task Force has recently made recommendations[46] regarding eye movement recording, naming of references (M1, M2 vs. A1, A2), and the use of frontal derivations to enhance

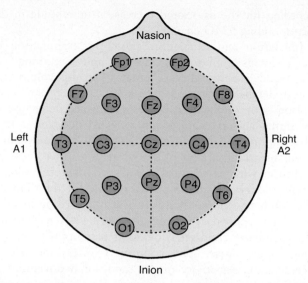

FIGURE 11–3 The complete International 10-20 System of electrode placement.

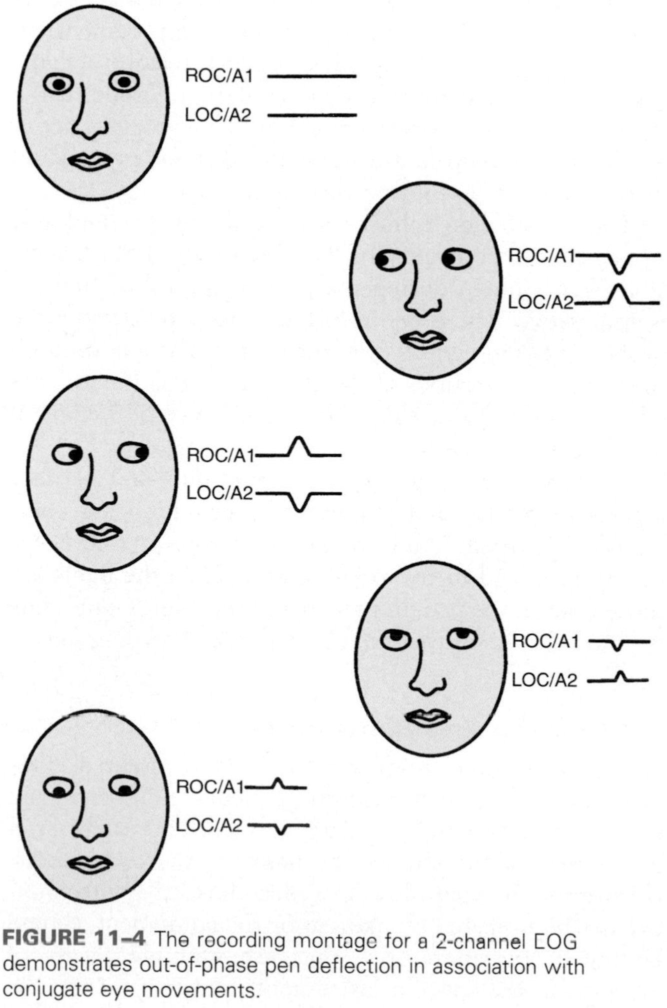

detection of EEG waveforms such as K complexes and slow-wave activity.

EOG electrodes are typically applied to the surface of the skin with an adhesive collar; this method avoids the risk of collodion contacting the patient's eyes.

Given the existing variations in methodology within the clinical and research environments, it is important to know exact electrode placement and inputs to EOG channels when interpretation of EOG activity has significant impact on diagnosis or treatment outcome.

Electromyography

A gold cup or a silver–silver chloride electrode attached with an adhesive collar is used to record EMG activity from the mentalis and submentalis muscles. Two of the electrodes are used to create a bipolar EMG recording. At least three EMG electrodes are applied to allow for an alternative electrode to be used in the event that artifact develops in one of them. The additional electrode can be placed over the masseter muscle to allow for detection of bursts of EMG activity associated with bruxism (Fig. 11–5).

Electrocardiography

There are a variety of approaches for recording the ECG during PSG. The simplest approach involves use of standard gold cup electrodes. However, disposable electrodes are also available to record ECG.

ECG electrodes are applied with an adhesive collar to the surface of the skin just beneath the right clavicle and on the left side at the level of the seventh rib ("modified lead II"). A stress loop is incorporated into the lead wire to ensure long-term placement.

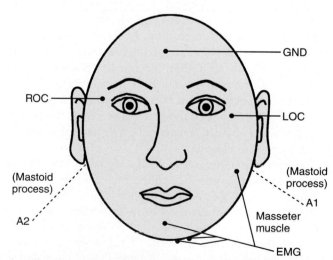

FIGURE 11–5 Schematic diagram showing placement of the electromyography (EMG) electrodes to record activity from the mental, submental, and masseter muscles. (GND, ground [earth]; LOC, left outer canthus [of the eye]; ROC, right outer canthus.)

FIGURE 11–4 The recording montage for a 2-channel EOG demonstrates out-of-phase pen deflection in association with conjugate eye movements.

Impedances

Before recording, electrodes should be visually inspected to check the security of their placement and an impedance check should be performed and documented. An impedance meter is ideally part of the recording system. Alternatively, a separate device can be used. Adjustment should be made to any EEG, EOG, or chin EMG electrode with an impedance greater than 5000 ohms. Higher impedances (20–30 kohm) are tolerated for ECG electrodes and for other EMG (anterior tibialis, extensor digitorum) derivations.

Physiologic Calibrations

Physiologic calibrations are performed after the electrode and monitor application is complete. This calibration allows for documentation of proper functioning of the electrodes and other monitoring devices, and provides baseline data for review and comparison when scoring the PSG. The specific instructions given to the patient for this calibration include

- Eyes open, look straight ahead for 30 seconds.
- Eyes closed, look straight ahead for 30 seconds.
- Hold head still, look to left and right, up and down. Repeat.
- Hold head still, blink eyes slowly, five times.
- Grit teeth, clench jaw, or smile.
- Inhale and exhale slowly, three times.
- Hold breath for 10 seconds.
- Flex right foot, flex left foot.
- Flex right hand, flex left hand.

As these instructions are given to the patient, the technologist examines the tracing and documents the patient's responses. When the patient stares straight ahead for 30 seconds with eyes open, the background EEG activity is examined. As the patient looks right and left, the tracing is examined for out-of-phase deflections of the signals associated with recording the EOG. Out-of-phase deflection occurs if the inputs to consecutive channels of the polygraph are ROC/M1 for the first EOG channel and LOC/M2 for the second. It is also important, when the patient closes his or her eyes, to observe the reactivity of the alpha rhythm seen most prominently in the occipital EEG; alpha rhythm is usually best visualized when the patient's eyes are closed.

The mentalis/submentalis EMG signal is checked by asking the patient to grit the teeth, clench the jaws, or yawn. The technologist documents proper functioning of the electrodes and amplifiers used to monitor anterior tibialis EMG activity by asking the patient to dorsiflex the right foot and the left foot in turn. If rapid eye movement (REM) sleep behavior disorder is suspected, additional electrodes should be applied to the surface of the skin above the extensor digitorum muscles of each arm. Patients are asked to extend their wrists while the technologist examines the recording for the associated increase in amplitude in the corresponding EMG channel.

Inhalation and exhalation allow for examination of the channels monitoring airflow and breathing.[52,53] The reader is referred to Chapter 14 in this volume for a more detailed discussion of this topic. A suggested convention is that inhalation causes an upward deflection of the signal and exhalation a downward deflection. It is most important that the signals on all the channels monitoring breathing are in phase with each other to avoid confusion with paradoxical breathing. The technologist should observe a flattening of the trace for the duration of a voluntary apnea. (Note: It is strongly recommended to include end-tidal or transcutaneous CO_2 monitoring when studying children,[24] or adult patients with underlying lung disease. The addition of CO_2 monitoring increases the sensitivity of the study of hypoventilation [see Fig. 11–7 later].)

If the 60- or 50-Hz notch filter (also called "line filter" or "AC filter") is in use, a brief examination (2–4 seconds) of portions of the tracing with the filter in the "out" position is essential. This allows for identification of any 60- or 50-Hz interference that may be masked by the filter. Care should be taken to eliminate any source of interference and to ensure that the 60- or 50-Hz notch filter is used only as a last resort. This is most important when recording patients suspected of having seizure activity, because the notch filter attenuates the amplitude of the spike activity seen in association with epileptogenic activity. If other monitors are used, the technologist should incorporate the necessary calibrations.

The physiologic calibrations enable the technologist to determine the quality of data before the PSG begins. If artifact is noted during the physiologic calibrations, it is imperative that every effort be made to correct the problem, as the condition is likely to get worse through the remaining portions of the recording. The functioning of alternative (spare) electrodes should also be examined during this calibration.

When a satisfactory calibration procedure and all other aspects of patient and equipment preparation are completed, the patient is told to assume a comfortable sleeping position and to try to fall asleep. Then the lights are turned out in the patient's room and the "lights-out" time is noted clearly on the tracing or in the recording log.

Monitoring and Recording

Complete documentation for the PSG is essential. This includes patient identification (patient's full name and medical record number), date of recording, and a full description of the study. The name of the technologist performing the recording, as well as those of any technologists who prepared the patient or the equipment, should be noted. In laboratories that use multiple pieces of equipment, the specific instrument used to generate the recording should be identified. This is particularly useful in the event that artifact is noted during the analysis portion (scoring) of the sleep study.

Specific parameters recorded on each channel should be clearly noted, as should a full description of sensitivity, filter, and calibration settings for each channel. Information regarding epoch length should be clearly visible. The time of the beginning and end of the recording must be recorded, as well as specific events that occur during the night. Any changes made to filter, sensitivity, or paper speed settings should be clearly noted in the study.

The technologist is also responsible for providing a clinical description of unusual events. For example, if a patient experiences an epileptic seizure during the study, the clinical manifestations of the seizure must be detailed: deviation of eyes or head to one side or the other, movement of extremities, presence of vomiting or incontinence, duration of the seizure, and postictal status. Similar information should be reported on any clinical event observed in the laboratory, such as somnambulism or clinical features of REM sleep behavior disorder. Physical complaints reported by the patient are also noteworthy.

Troubleshooting and Artifact Recognition

In general, when difficulties arise during recording, the troubleshooting inquiry begins at the patient and follows the path of the signal to the recording device. More often than not, the problem can be identified as a difficulty with an electrode or other monitoring device. It is less likely that artifact is the result of a problem with an amplifier. If the artifact is generalized (i.e., on most channels), then the integrity of the ground electrode and the instrument cable should be checked. If the artifact is localized (i.e., on a limited number of channels), then the question should be: which channels have this artifact in common and what is common to the channels involved? The artifact is probably the result of a problem located in an electrode or monitoring device that is common to both channels. If the artifact is isolated to a single channel, the source of artifact is limited to the inputs to the specific amplifier, the amplifier itself, or to display of the channel.

Figures 11–6 through 11–15 depict some frequently encountered artifacts seen during PSG.

Ending The Study

Often, clinical circumstances and laboratory protocol dictate whether the patient is awakened at a specific time or allowed to awaken spontaneously. Deviations from the patient's usual sleep period must be clearly noted. After awakening at the end of the study, the patient should be asked to perform the physiologic calibrations to ensure that the electrodes and other monitoring devices are still functioning properly. Ideally, the equipment should be calibrated at the settings used for the study. Last, the

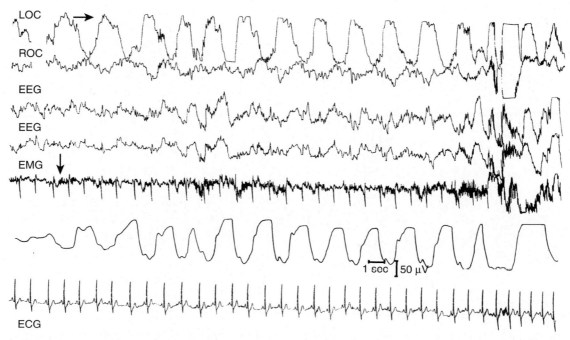

FIGURE 11–6 Artifact in left outer canthus (LOC) channel (LOC/A1) can be localized to the LOC electrode. The EEG channels in the trace are C3/A2 and O2/A1. Since the artifact does not appear in the O2/A1 channel, it is localized to the LOC electrode. The electrode placement may be insecure or the patient may be lying on the electrode and producing movement of the LOC electrode in association with breathing. Additional artifact is noted in the EMG channel. This signal is contaminated with ECG artifact, and the intermittent slower activity as well as the wandering baseline are most likely due to a loose lead. The ECG channel also shows a pattern consistent with a loose electrode wire.

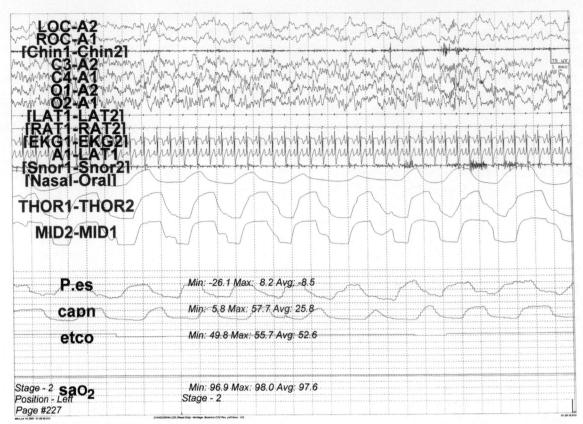

FIGURE 11-7 Sleep-disordered breathing: hypopnea. Note that end-tidal carbon dioxide (etco2) channel shows CO_2 retention while arterial oxygen saturation (SaO_2) channel shows normal values. *(Reproduced with permission from Chokroverty S, Thomas RJ, Bhatt M. The Atlas of Sleep Medicine. Philadelphia:Elsevier Butterworth-Heinemann, 2005:338.)*

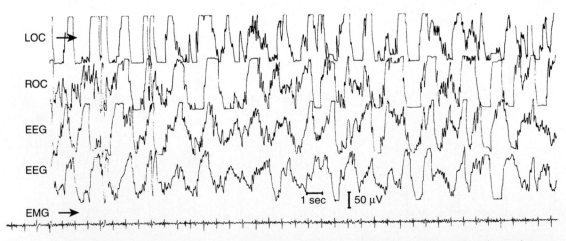

FIGURE 11-8 The blocking artifact seen with inappropriate sensitivity settings can be alleviated by decreasing sensitivity. If adjustments to sensitivity are made, they should be clearly noted, and the same adjustments should be made on all channels displaying EEG data. It is common procedure to calibrate the equipment with decreased sensitivity (i.e., 100 µV/cm) for children's studies or increased sensitivity (i.e., 30 µV/cm) for older patients. Typically, sensitivity settings are not changed frequently during the recording (as they may be in routine EEG). As a result, it is not uncommon to see this artifact when the patient enters slow wave sleep. This is not a common problem with digital systems because of the user's ability to manipulate sensitivity after data collection.

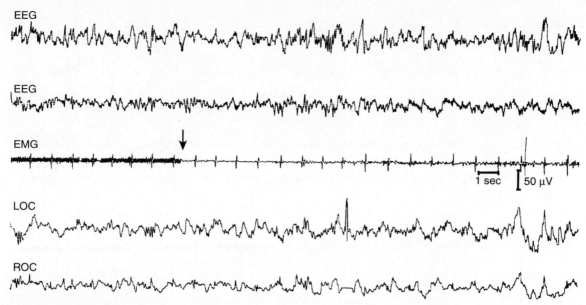

FIGURE 11–9 A 60-Hz artifact exists in the EMG channel. At the *arrow,* the 60-Hz filter is turned on. However, there is continued evidence of difficulty with electrodes on this channel, as evidenced by the ECG artifact and occasional spike-like activity. Turning on the 60-Hz filter is not the correct response to eliminate the artifact. If possible, the technologist should switch to an alternative electrode or fix the one involved.

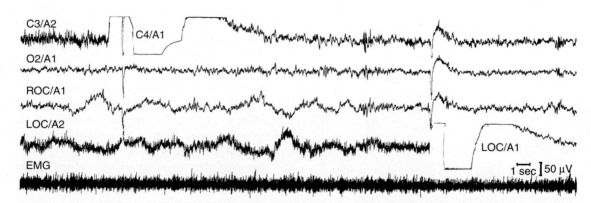

FIGURE 11–10 The high-frequency (probably EMG) artifact noted in the C3/A2 and LOC/A2 channels can be localized to the A2 electrode. This problem can be solved by switching to the alternative reference (A1) electrode. A high-amplitude discharge is noted during the switch from C3/A2 to C4/A1 and LOC/A2 to LOC/A1. This can be avoided by placing the amplifier in standby mode, if possible, while making the change.

amplifiers should be set to identical settings for high- and low-frequency filters and sensitivity and an all-channel calibration should be performed. This is essentially the reverse of the calibration procedures outlined for the beginning of the study.

A subjective evaluation is made by the patient. The patient is asked to estimate how long it took to fall asleep, the amount of time spent asleep, and if there were any disruptions during the sleep period. Patients should also report on quality of sleep and the level of alertness upon arousal.

For patient safety, a plan needs to be made for patients leaving the laboratory after a study. A patient who has a severe sleep disorder should avoid driving. An arranged ride or public transportation should be used, particularly

if the patient has withdrawn from stimulant medications for the purpose of the study.

DIGITAL SYSTEMS

The first digital EEG systems,[20,44] which became available in the late 1980s, revolutionized EEG and PSG by increasing the flexibility and sensitivity of data analysis. Significant advantages of digital systems include autocorrection of amplifier gains, self-diagnostic tests of amplifier functions, and software-controlled in-line impedance testing. The use of the computer has facilitated storage of data, manipulation of data after collection, and the presentation of different views of the data. Despite these

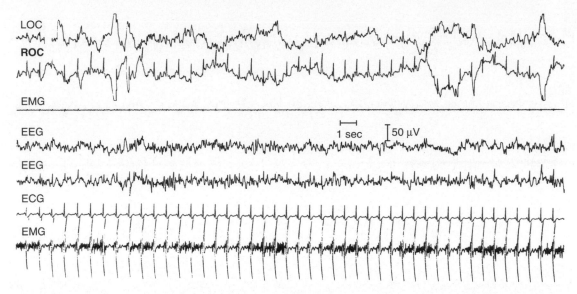

FIGURE 11–11 The ROC channel (ROC/A1) and the second EEG (O2/A1) channels are contaminated with ECG artifact. The artifact can be identified by aligning the spike-like activity noted in these channels with the R wave on the ECG channel. Because it is seen in both ROC/A1 and O2/A1, and A1 is common to both channels, it must be localized to the A1 electrode. It should be noted that the high-amplitude ECG artifact, seen in the EMG channel below the ECG channel, is unavoidable. This artifact is due to the proximity of EMG electrodes to the heart, which creates a robust signal superimposed on the intercostal EMG signal.

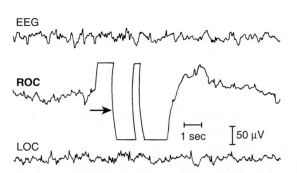

FIGURE 11–12 The high-amplitude deflection in the ROC (ROC/A1) channel is associated with an electrode artifact commonly referred to as an "electrode pop." This can be the result of a compromised electrode placement or insufficient electroconductive gel under the electrode. When this artifact is observed, the electrode involved should not be trusted to give reliable data.

changes, however, users of digital systems must still adhere to the rigorous standards that ensure high-quality data in analog recordings. Both analog and digital systems require electrodes and other sensors to be applied with the greatest of care. Ideally, calibration procedures should be performed to document and ensure the collection of high-quality data at the beginning and end of the recording. Knowledge of the specifics of the equipment and of the physiology of interest are important to ensure accurate signal processing.

Some of the main differences noted between analog and digital systems include the following:

- The size of the display of the data is a function of the size of the computer monitor.
- The ability to view data in retrospect may not be available during collection in digital systems.

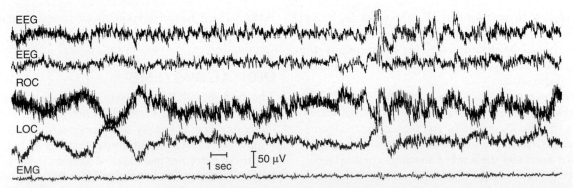

FIGURE 11–13 The generalized, high-frequency activity superimposed upon the EEG and EOG channels is most likely secondary to muscle activity. The EMG channel shows only artifact. In addition, there appears to be a slant to the left, particularly in channels 1 through 4, which is probably secondary to difficulty with the mechanical baseline of the pens.

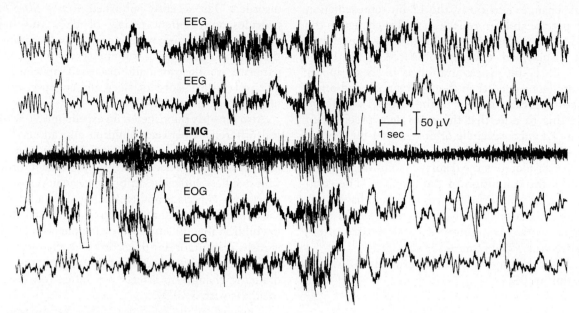

FIGURE 11–14 This burst of high-frequency artifact, superimposed on the EEG and EOG channels, is due to a brief movement by the subject. As in Figure 11–13 this is a superimposition of EMG activity on the EEG and EOG channels. It should also be noted that there is an electrode pop in the first EOG channel. The EMG channel in this tracing is of good quality and should be compared to Figure 11–13.

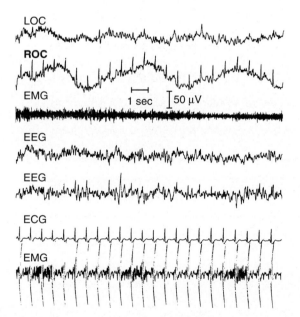

FIGURE 11–15 A high-amplitude, slow artifact is noted in the ROC (ROC/A1) channel. This is most likely associated with the patient's breathing and is secondary to a loose electrode or the patient lying on the right side and disturbing the electrode in synchrony with breathing. A relatively high-amplitude ECG artifact is also seen. The artifact can be localized to the ROC electrode. The EMG tracing noted at the bottom of this example is an intercostal EMG. The high amplitude ECG spike in this channel is impossible to eliminate; however, brief bursts of EMG activity can be noted in association with the artifact seen in the ROC/A1 channel. This suggests that the artifact noted in the ROC electrode is associated with breathing, since the bursts of intercostal EMG activity are seen in association with the effort of breathing.

- Annotation of the recording requires the use of the mouse or a keyboard, which can be more difficult than using a pen.
- Pen noise is absent, which prevents auditory perception of movement, entry into REM sleep, or other events.

In digital systems, it is rare to encounter breakdown of any mechanical component; the most frequently encountered problems have to do with disk drives or cables. To ensure trouble-free operation, it is important to avoid mechanical shock, dust, or static electricity.

An important factor for understanding the digital systems is the concept of sampling rate. Sampling rate can be understood as the frequency with which the signal is reviewed for conversion to the digital signal. Currently, 100 Hz is regarded as the minimum acceptable sampling rate for EEG, EOG, and EMG with high-frequency filters set at 35 Hz. A sampling rate of 200 Hz would be required if the high-frequency filter were set at 70 Hz.[54]

Another issue unique to digital systems is the precision of recordings. The resolution of the signal is a function of the number of binary bits used to represent the digital values. Readers will recall that a bit is a value of 1 or 0. Thus, in binary, 8 bits is equal to 2^8 (2 to the eighth power), or 256. For example, if we assume an EEG voltage change of 256 μV (from −128 μV to +128 μV) this would result in a resolution (using an 8-bit system) of 1 μV difference being represented by 1 bit. Among the digital systems that are currently available, 8-bit systems provide the lowest degree of precision. Usually, a 10- or 12-bit system is preferred to give increased resolution. For example, at 12 bits, successive digital values represent a 0.0625-µV change. Obviously, the 12-bit representation is far more precise and can reflect a smaller change in the signal. Additionally, the 8-bit resolution may appear jagged on the display screen when compared to the 12-bit waveform. The 12-bit representation is likely to appear smoother and less jagged than the 8-bit signal, and offers a signal that has greater fidelity to the original waveform. (It is interesting to note that the equivalent precision of paper tracings is approximately 6 bits, and 64-bit systems are now available at low cost!)

Also to be considered is the display resolution, which is determined by the resolution of the monitor. The computer screen for review of the recording should have a sufficiently high resolution. Ideally, the screen should be at least 20 inches with a resolution of 1280 × 1024 pixels, and flicker free (i.e., 75-Hz monitor scan rate).[44]

Figures 11–16 through 11–19 are examples of digital recordings during PSG.[17]

PERSPECTIVE ON POLYSOMNOGRAPHY

Technical advances and increases in clinical knowledge provide great potential for our ability to monitor physiologic changes in our quest to understand sleep and its

disorders. The recently published *Atlas of Sleep Medicine*[18] provides an excellent review of PSG and hypnogram analysis. Specialized techniques, including pulse transit time, peripheral arterial tonometry, and cyclic alternating patterns, are illustrated and discussed. Special attention is given to motor disorders, sleep and epilepsy, and a variety of other neurologic disorders.

Also recently published is an excellent review of the critical differences between children and adults[24] who have SRBD and restless leg syndrome. It is imperative that we identify sleep disorders as early as possible in order to prevent needless suffering. In order to achieve this goal, it is crucial for clinicians and technologists to understand that the clinical presentation of sleep disorders may be different in children than in adults. For example, as mentioned previously, it is important to record CO_2 changes in children as they may show retention of CO_2 more commonly than dramatic changes in arterial O_2 saturation (as compared to adults with SRBD).

Throughout its evolution, PSG has proven a robust tool for enhancing understanding of sleep and its disorders. It is an essential diagnostic procedure. Increased public awareness of sleep disorders as a major public health concern will drive the need for diagnosis and treatment. We must be effective and efficient in providing the

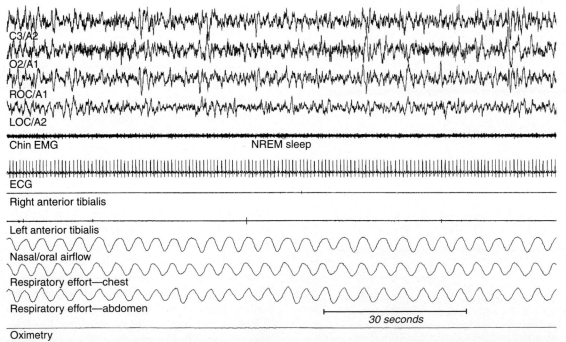

FIGURE 11–16 Digital recording sample of non–rapid eye movement (NREM) sleep using time-scale compression. Digital data can be further compressed to display several epochs on a screen simultaneously. This sample, and the recordings shown in Figures 11–17 through 11–19, have been compressed to accommodate 4 epochs of data (2 minutes) to a page. This type of display offers the scorer or interpreter a general overview of the sleep recording, as well as a practical method of counting any prominent sleep-related events such as obstructive apneas, hypopneas, or body movements. The resolution of the data is inadequate, however, for precise EEG evaluation or sleep-stage scoring. This sample shows a normal respiratory pattern during NREM sleep, without any apparent evidence of arousal, movement, or other form of sleep disturbance. *(Reprinted with permission from Butkov N. Atlas of Clinical Polysomnography. Ashland, OR: Synapse Media, 1996.)*

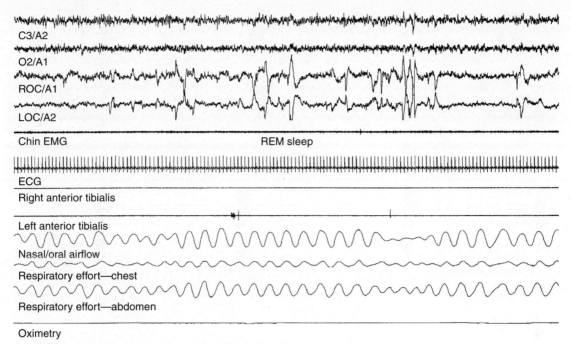

FIGURE 11–17 Digital recording sample of REM sleep. Although altered by time-scale compression, the sleep-stage pattern can readily be identified as REM. Note the mild respiratory irregularity, which is a normal variant of REM sleep physiology. *(Reprinted with permission from Butkov N. Atlas of Clinical Polysomnography. Ashland, OR: Synapse Media, 1996.)*

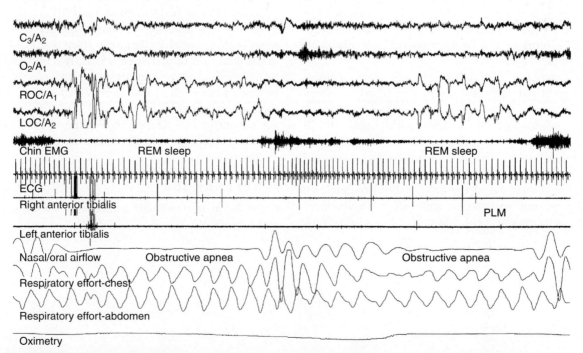

FIGURE 11–18 Digital recording sample showing a compressed display of repetitive obstructive apneas occurring during REM sleep. These represent the extreme end of the sleep-disordered breathing continuum. In this example, all the features of classic obstructive sleep apnea are present, including distinct paradoxic (out-of-phase) respiratory effort, instances of complete cessation of airflow, subsequent EEG arousals, and cyclic oxygen desaturations. *(Reprinted with permission from Butkov N. Atlas of Clinical Polysomnography. Ashland, OR: Synapse Media, 1996.)*

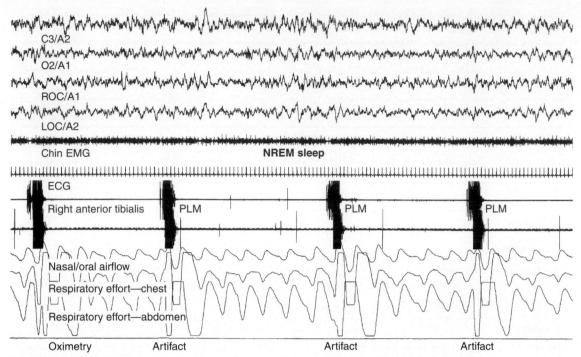

C3/A2

O2/A1

ROC/A1

LOC/A2

Chin EMG   **NREM sleep**

ECG

Right anterior tibialis   PLM   PLM   PLM

Nasal/oral airflow
Respiratory effort—chest
Respiratory effort—abdomen

Oximetry   Artifact   Artifact   Artifact

FIGURE 11–19 Digital recording sample of periodic limb movements, which often generate artifacts in the respiratory channels that appear similar to cyclic hypopneas. This sample shows a compressed version of the characteristic pattern of periodic limb movement (PLM), recorded by the right and left anterior tibialis EMG. Note that the respiratory channel artifact appears almost identical to the cyclic hypopneas seen in Figure 11–18. *(Reprinted with permission from Butkov N. Atlas of Clinical Polysomnography. Ashland, OR: Synapse Media, 1996.)*

highest quality of patient care. It is well recognized that questionnaires[55] have proven to be excellent tools in helping to triage patients in need of further evaluation. Polysomnography remains the "gold standard" for diagnosis when indicated.

PSG is complex and labor intensive. It requires specialized technical skills and knowledge of normal sleep and sleep disorders. Technologists need to be experts with equipment, competent in dealing with medically ill patients, and capable of dealing with emergencies that may be encountered. The establishment of accredited training programs and licensure are tangible signs of the growth and development of the field of PSG technology. New Jersey became the second state after Louisiana to license an independent profession of PSG technology.

This legislation, known as the PSG Practice Act, became effective as of as of December 15, 2005.

Recent publications[56-58] and changes in reimbursement policies are clear demonstration that PSG is moving in the direction of increased access. It is our responsibility to millions of patients awaiting optimal sleep health care to demand that all studies performed during sleep meet the highest standards of practice. With this commitment, we maximize our ability to facilitate improved patient health outcomes for all those suffering from sleep disorders.

✪ REFERENCES

A full list of references are available at www.expertconsult.com

Template for 24-Hour Sleep-Wake Log

This log should be completed by the patient for a period of 2 weeks prior to the study.

	Date				Date				Date		
Time	Awake	Asleep		Time	Awake	Asleep		Time	Awake	Asleep
12:00				12:00				12:00		
13:00				13:00				13:00		
14:00				14:00				14:00		
15:00				15:00				15:00		
16:00				16:00				16:00		
17:00				17:00				17:00		
18:00				18:00				18:00		
19:00				19:00				19:00		
20:00				20:00				20:00		
21:00				21:00				21:00		
22:00				22:00				22:00		
23:00				23:00				23:00		
24:00				24:00				24:00		
01:00				01:00				01:00		
02:00				02:00				02:00		
03:00				03:00				03:00		
04:00				04:00				04:00		
05:00				05:00				05:00		
06:00				06:00				06:00		
07:00				07:00				07:00		
08:00				08:00				08:00		
09:00				09:00				09:00		
10:00				10:00				10:00		
11:00				11:00				11:00		
Exercise				Exercise				Exercise		
Treatment				Treatment				Treatment		
Sleep Quality				Sleep Quality				Sleep Quality		
Medications				Medications				Medications		
Comments				Comments				Comments		

For each hour of the day:

- *indicate sleep or wake time with an (X) in the appropriate box(es)*
- *indicate naps with an (N) in the appropriate box(es)*
- *indicate periods of extreme sleepiness with an (S) in the appropriate box(es)*

Subjective Evaluation of Sleepiness

Stanford Sleepiness Scale

1. Feeling active and vital; alert; wide awake.
2. Functioning at a high level, but not at peak; able to concentrate.
3. Relaxed; awake; not at full alertness; responsive.
4. A little foggy; not at peak; let down.
5. Fogginess; beginning to lose interest in remaining awake; slowed down.
6. Sleepiness; prefer to be lying down; fighting sleep; woozy.
7. Almost in reverie; sleep onset soon; lost struggle to remain awake.

Linear Analog Scale/Introspective Measure of Sleepiness

Ask patient to make a mark on the scale that corresponds to state (level of alertness versus sleepiness) prior to testing.

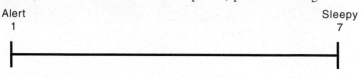

Alert   Sleepy
1   7

Adapted from Hoddes E, Dement WC, Zarcone V. The development and use of the Stanford Sleepiness Scale (SSS). Psychophysiology 1972;9:150.

Suggested Montages for Recording Sleep-Related Seizure Activity

Montage for a 12-Channel Study

1. Fp1–C3
2. C3–O1
3. Fp1–T3
4. T3–O1
5. Fp2–C4
6. C4–O2
7. Fp2–T4
8. T4–O2
9. EMG: submentalis–mentalis
10. Right outer canthus–left outer canthus
11. Nasal/oral airflow
12. ECG

Montage for a 21-Channel Study

1. Fp1–F3
2. F3–C3
3. C3–P3
4. P3–O1
5. Fp2–F4
6. F4–C4
7. C4–P4
8. P4–O2
9. Fp1–F7
10. F7–T3
11. T3–T5
12. T5–O1
13. Fp2–F8
14. F8–T4
15. T4–T6
16. T6–O2
17. EMG: mentalis–submentalis
18. Right outer canthus–A1
19. Left outer canthus–A2
20. Nasal/oral airflow
21. ECG

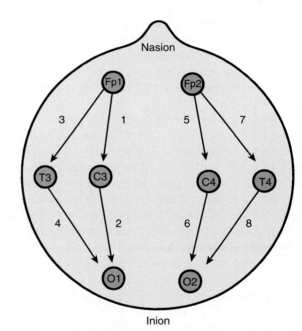

FIGURE 11–A1 Suggested montage to be used to screen for possible seizure activity during sleep. Use of wide interelectrode distance affords for a global view of EEG activity and conserves the channels. To more adequately localize epileptogenic activity, a full complement of electrodes should be used. For a more comprehensive review of montages, the reader is referred to Standard EEG Montages as proposed by American EEG Society Guidelines No. 7, Grass Instruments (1980).

Measuring the Head for C3, C4, O1, and O2

Before measuring the head, it is helpful to make an initial mark at the inion, the nasion, and the two preauricular points.

1. Measure the distance from the nasion to inion along the midline through the vertex. Make a preliminary mark at the midpoint (Cz). An electrode will not be placed on this spot, but it will be used as a landmark.

2. Center this point in the transverse plane by marking the halfway point between the left and right preauricular points. The intersection of marks from steps 1 and 2 gives the precise location of Cz.

3. Reposition the measuring tape at the midline through Cz and mark the points 10% up from the inion (Oz) and nasion (Fpz).

4. Reposition the measuring tape in the transverse plane, through Cz, and mark 10% (T3) and 30% (C3) up from the left preauricular point and 10% (T4) and 30% (C4) up from the right preauricular point.

5. Position the tape around the head through Fpz, T3, Oz, and T4. Ten percent of this circumference distance is the distance between Fp1 and Fp2 and between O1 and O2. Mark these four locations on either side of the midline.

6. The second marks for O1 and O2 are made by continuing the horizontal mark for Oz. Do this by holding the tape at T3 and T4 through Oz, and extend the horizontal mark to intersect the previous O1 and O2 marks.

7. To establish the final mark for C3, place the tape from O1 to Fp1 and make a mark at the midpoint of this line. When extended, this mark will intersect the previous C3 mark. Repeat on the right side for C4.

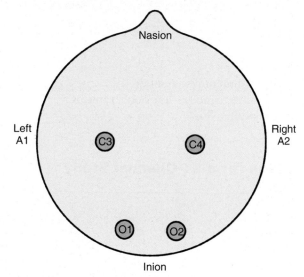

FIGURE 11–A2 The International 10-20 System of EEG electrode placement for sleep recordings.

CHAPTER 12

Electroencephalography, Electromyography, and Electro-Oculography: General Principles and Basic Technology

Thaddeus S. Walczak and Sudhansu Chokroverty

INTRODUCTION

Electroencephalography (EEG) has played a central role in the beginnings and evolution of sleep medicine. Many would agree that modern sleep medicine started with the prolonged EEG studies of sleep by Kleitman, culminating in the historic discovery (with Aserinsky) of rapid eye movement (REM) sleep in 1953.[1] This and other seminal early reports emphasized that studying sleep required measurement of electrocerebral activity as well as other physiologic functions such as eye movements and axial electromyography; thus traditional EEG was extended into polysomnography (PSG). As sleep pathology became better defined, the need to measure other physiologic function such as respiratory parameters, limb movements, gastric pH, and penile tumescence, among others, became clear. In the process, EEG received less and less attention.

Early studies of sleep typically devoted 2 channels to monitoring eye movement and 1 channel each for electromyography (EMG) and EEG. This was largely due to the limited amount of channels in the machines available at that time. Increasing numbers of channels were available in subsequent polygraphs, but these were utilized for measuring other physiologic parameters of interest as

understanding of sleep pathology grew. Unfortunately, even in modern times EEG recording often remains confined to 2 channels, though 32 channels are often available in contemporary recording systems. We believe that this tendency to neglect cerebral electrophysiology in contemporary polygraphy is unfortunate. Various central nervous system and metabolic disorders may result in a syndrome mimicking excessive daytime somnolence. Unusual nocturnal spells may be seizures. EEG findings during PSG may be the first indication of these medical disorders. Furthermore, EEG findings associated with epilepsy may be confined solely to sleep. Thus, we believe a thorough sampling of electrocerebral activity with multiple channels covering both sides of the scalp should be performed during routine PSG, especially if seizures are suspected. Similarly, multiple EMG channels may provide a more accurate understanding of muscle tone or periodic movments. In summary, the broad availability of multiple polygraphic channels increases the information these studies can provide and so requires a more complete understanding of normal and abnormal EEG, EMG, and electro-oculographic (EOG) patterns.

A complete description of the technical and interpretive issues in EEG, EMG, and EOG is not possible in a single chapter. The reader is referred to several excellent monographs[2–6] for more detail. The discussion presented in this chapter starts with basic technical and safety issues. The polygraphic circuit and differences between analog and digital recording are discussed. Measurement and interpretation of EOG and EMG is then briefly reviewed. The bulk of the chapter is devoted to normal EEG findings in wakefulness and sleep as well as frequently encountered abnormalities. The discussion is limited to findings in humans ages 2 months and older. Several useful sources are available for the reader interested in neonatal wake and sleep EEG.[2,3,5,7]

ELEMENTARY CONCEPTS OF ELECTRICITY

It is useful to begin with a review of some elementary concepts of electricity. Electricity is largely the study of the concentration and flow of charged particles. A fundamental principle of electricity states that like charges repel and unlike charges attract. Thus, if particles of like charge are allowed to move freely, they will quickly reach a relatively uniform distribution. The flow of charged particles is called *current* (I). Various features of biological systems, such as equilibrium constants of reactions or membrane permeability, often result in a concentration of particles of like charge. This concentration is a store of potential energy that is released when the charged particles are allowed to move and achieve a more uniform distribution. *Voltage* (V) measures how much energy is released when a set amount of charge is allowed to move as current flow. Voltage, also known as *potential difference*, is always measured between two points. Because the concentration of charge may differ at any two points, the potential energy contained in a given concentration of charge can only be measured by relating it to the concentration of charge elsewhere. Charges experience *resistance* (R) as they move through a conducting medium. The resistance is measured in *ohms*. Current, voltage, and resistance are related by *Ohm's law*, which states that I = V/R. The law makes intuitive sense: The higher the voltage (V) between two points, the more "pressure" there is for the charges to move, and so one would expect flow of charge (I) to be higher. Conversely, if there is more resistance (R) to the movement of charge, one would expect the flow of charge (I) to be less.

Concentrations of charges of different polarity are often separated by a poorly conducting medium. This situation can be modeled by an electrical device known as a *capacitor*. Capacitors can be thought of as two conducting plates separated by insulation. The ability of the capacitor to store charge is measured by the capacitance, which equals the amount of charge the device can store for a given voltage. When a capacitor is connected to a source of constant voltage such as a battery, positive charges will flow from the positive pole of the battery to one plate and flow from the positive pole of the battery to one plate and

negative charges will flow from the negative pole of the battery to the other plate. Charges will continue flowing until the mutual repulsion of the accumulated charges on each plate equals the potential difference of the battery. At this point, current flow will cease.

The situation is different when the source of voltage varies with a predictable frequency. Voltages generated by the brain and recorded by the EEG do not stay constant but vary continuously within certain limits. In a circuit with such a voltage source and a capacitor, it can be shown that the current flow at any time equals the capacitance multiplied by the change in voltage with respect to time.* Thus, the capacitor will influence and resist the flow of current in a circuit with a varying voltage. The resistance to current flow exerted by the capacitor is measured by the *capacitative reactance* (X_C). It is clear that the concept of resistance must be expanded to include capacitative reactance in circuits with a voltage source that varies. *Impedance* (Z) is a measure of resistance that includes reactive capacitance and is therefore appropriate in circuits with varying voltages. In these situations, Ohm's law takes the form I = V/Z. Because cerebral voltages vary with time, impedance is the proper measure of how well electrodes and gel transmit brain activity.

PHYSIOLOGIC BASIS OF ELECTROENCEPHALOGRAPHY

An EEG record is essentially a measure of the changes of electrocerebral voltages over a period of time. To interpret an EEG, it is important to understand the source of the voltages recorded at the scalp and how these voltages are organized into normal cerebral rhythms.

Electrocerebral activity measured by EEG does not appear to be caused by individual or summed action potentials. Action potentials are too short (usually <1 msec), and synchronized bursts of action potentials have too limited a distribution, to account for the rhythms seen in a normal EEG. Excitatory and inhibitory postsynaptic potentials, in contrast, last much longer (15–200 msec or more). These synaptic potentials induce more extensive voltage changes in extracellular space. Scalp-recorded EEG activity results from extracellular current flow induced by summated excitatory or inhibitory postsynaptic potentials.

Figure 12–1 illustrates, in a simplified fashion, how synaptic potentials induce voltage changes recorded at the scalp. An excitatory input on a deep dendrite causes positive ions to flow into the pyramidal neuron, resulting in a lack of positive charges, or negativity outside the neuron. Everywhere else, including at the superficial dendrite, positive ions flow out of the cell into the

---

*Capacitance (C) is defined as the amount of charge (Q) the capacitor can store for a given voltage (V), or Q/V. Presuming that C is constant, and differentiating with respect to time (t), we find that dC/dt = 0 = −[(Q/V2) (dV/dt)] + [(1/V) (dQ/dt)]. Rearranging, dQ/dt = (Q/V) (dV/dt). Current flow (I) = dQ/dt. Hence, I = C(dV/dt).

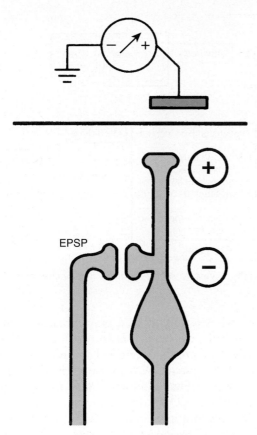

FIGURE 12–1 Scalp EEG voltage recordings resulting from an excitatory input on a deep synapse. (EPSP, excitatory postsynaptic potential.) *(Modified from Kandel ER, Schwartz JH [eds]. Principles of Neural Science, 4th ed. Amsterdam: Elsevier, 2000.)*

extracellular space to complete the current loop. This results in a relative positivity in the superficial extracellular space. Because the superficial dendrite and surrounding extracellular space are closer to the scalp electrode, a positive deflection is recorded. The separation of superficial positive and deep negative charges allows one to view the pyramidal neuron as a dipole. This permits a more complete analysis of how synaptic potentials result in scalp EEG changes.[8-10]

EEG voltage recordings are rhythmic (i.e., they are regularly recurring waveforms of similar shape and duration). It is important to understand how voltage changes induced by individual neurons are organized into the widely distributed rhythms recorded with EEG. The dominant theory of EEG rhythmicity was advanced by Andersen and Andersson[11] and is based on studies of barbiturate-induced spindle activity. These investigators recorded synchronous rhythmic spindles from the cerebral cortex and thalamus. Neither removal of the cerebral cortex nor transection of the brain stem below the thalamus eliminated thalamic spindles. Ablation of the entire thalamus, however, abolished spindle activity. These findings led to the proposal that rhythmic oscillations of

thalamic neurons induced synchronous synaptic excitatory or inhibitory potentials over broad areas of the cortex, and thus the rhythmic voltage changes recorded with scalp EEG. Diffuse thalamocortical neuronal projections were known to exist and could mediate this thalamic influence. This model was expanded to explain most EEG rhythmic activity.

More recent work has emphasized the fact that barbiturate-induced spindles differ significantly from other cerebral rhythms.[12] The role of the thalamus in synchronizing barbiturate spindle activity over broad areas of cortex may not be relevant to other EEG rhythms. Neurons in other brain structures, including the inferior olive, hippocampus, and temporal neocortex, exhibit oscillatory behavior and may play a role in generating EEG rhythms.[13] Although widespread subcortical influences probably play an important role in organizing EEG rhythms, it is premature to conclude that all EEG rhythms are induced by oscillations of thalamic neurons.

Cerebral activity recorded at the scalp has approximately one-tenth the voltage of activity simultaneously recorded at the cortical surface. This attenuation is largely due to the cerebrospinal fluid, dura, and skull overlying the cortical surface. The area and location of the cortex generating the activity also play a role.

COMPONENTS OF THE POLYGRAPHIC CIRCUIT

Voltages and current flows generated by the cortex, eyes, and heart during PSG studies are exceedingly small. The function of the polygraph is to transform these tiny voltages into an interpretable record. The major components necessary to accomplish this are illustrated in Figure 12–2. Two types of polygraphic machines are in use: analog polygraphs based on solid-state circuitry and digital polygraphs based on digital circuits, computers, and, increasingly, network technology (see Fig. 12–2). As one may suspect, analog polygraphs are becoming replaced by more contemporary digital machines. However, study of signal flow through analog systems remains important because it provides a fundamental understanding of how brain signals need to be modified so that clinical interpretation is possible. To start with, we discuss electrodes and the scalp-electrode interface. We then discuss the components of the analog polygraph. Finally we discuss how the functions of the polygraphic circuit are carried out by the digital polygraph. The discussion is based on idealized systems rather than polygraphs provided by any specific vendor.

Electrodes and the Scalp-Electrode Interface

Electrodes and conducting gel transmit biological voltages from skin or muscle to the polygraphic circuit. Various types of electrodes have been designed.[4,14] Disk electrodes are preferred for recording EEG, EOG, and

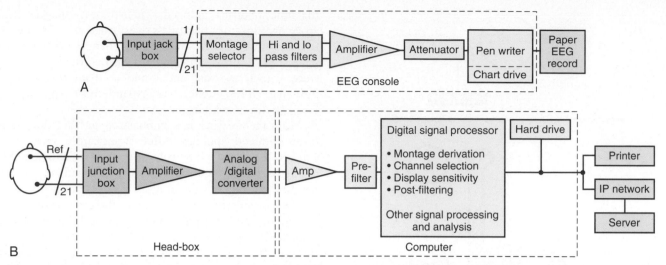

FIGURE 12–2 Computer-generated components of an analog **(A)** and a digital **(B)** polygraph. *(Courtesy of Dr. Sidney Diamond.)*

electrocardiography, and may be used to record EMG as well. These are typically made of chlorided silver or noble metals such as gold or platinum.

The critical component of the conducting gel is an electrolyte, usually sodium chloride, that easily dissociates into its ionic components. The anions and cations establish a layer of positive and negative charges between the scalp and recording electrode. This charged double layer allows transmission of scalp voltage changes to the electrode and the rest of the polygraphic circuit.

The electrode-electrolyte interface is the most critical link in the polygraphic circuit. Most artifact originates here; consequently, careful technique in electrode application largely determines the quality of the recording. The impedance in any electrode pair should not exceed 10 kohm. High impedance can decrease the amount of signal the electrode presents to the amplifier. Methods to achieve low impedance are described in Chapter 11. In addition, the impedance in the two electrode inputs into the amplifier should not differ by more than 10 kohm. Higher values will degrade the ability of a differential amplifier to eliminate environmental noise and will increase artifact (see *Artifacts* later). Impedance varies with composition and surface area of the electrode as well as with the surface area of the conducting gel beneath the electrode. Thus, these factors should be held constant in an electrode pair attached to the same amplifier. For example, a disk electrode and needle electrode have different surface areas, and conducting gel is not used with needle electrodes. Therefore, impedances of the two electrodes will be significantly different. If the two electrodes are attached to the same amplifier, environmental artifact is likely to contaminate the recording.

The Analog Polygraphic Circuit

Electrodes are attached to electrode wires, which conduct the EEG signal to the electrode box or jackbox. The

electrode wires terminate in a pin that is plugged into a receptacle in the electrode box known as a *jack*. The jacks are usually numbered or identified according to the International 10-20 System. Wires from each of the jacks run together in a shielded conductor cable to the polygraph. Here, wires from each of the jacks are connected to a specific point on a multiple contact switch known as the electrode selector. The selector contains rows of switches, arranged in pairs corresponding to the two inputs of an amplifier. Depressing the switches allows the technician to select which two electrodes will contribute signal to each amplifier.

The amplifiers used in both analog and digital polygraphic recording have several important features. *Differential* amplifiers are usually used. These amplify the *difference* in voltage between the two amplifier inputs. Figure 12–3 provides an illustration. Let us assume that T3 is connected to input 1 of an amplifier and C3 is connected to input 2 of the same amplifier. The amplifier would determine the difference between the two inputs (5 µV) and the galvanometer pen would register a deflection of 5 units. The actual amount of the deflection in millimeters would depend on the sensitivity used (see next paragraph). The fact that the differential amplifier amplifies the difference between electrode inputs rather than the absolute voltage at any electrode is a useful feature, because environmental noise, which is likely to be the same at the two electrodes, is "subtracted out" and therefore does not contaminate the recording. The *common mode rejection ratio* measures the ability of the amplifier to suppress a signal, such as noise, that is present simultaneously at both electrodes. This ratio should exceed 1000:1; most amplifiers currently in service have values that exceed 10,000:1.

A differential amplifier multiplies the small difference in cerebral voltages by a constant, referred to as *gain*. This multiplication is necessary because the recording galvanometer pen requires voltages much higher than those generated by the brain to generate an EEG record.

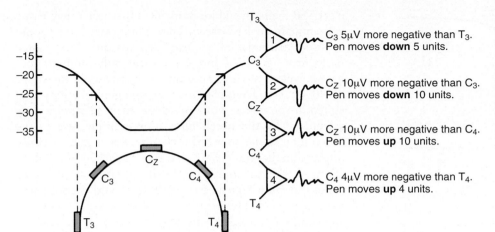

FIGURE 12–3 Scalp voltage distribution of a vertex wave. A plot of hypothetical absolute voltages at various electrode positions is shown on the left, and resulting EEG tracing with explanation is shown on the right. A transverse bipolar chain is used with amplifiers connected from left to right. The same electrode is connected to input 2 of an amplifier and input 1 of the next amplifier in the chain.

C₃ 5µV more negative than T₃. Pen moves **down** 5 units.

C_Z 10µV more negative than C₃. Pen moves **down** 10 units.

C_Z 10µV more negative than C₄. Pen moves **up** 10 units.

C₄ 4µV more negative than T₄. Pen moves **up** 4 units.

Analog-to-digital converters also require higher voltages to perform digitization. Amplifiers can faithfully amplify input voltages only within a certain range known as the *dynamic range*. Input voltages below the lower limit of the dynamic range are lost in noise; voltages above the upper limit result in a distorted EEG output. Flexible control of amplification within the dynamic range is achieved by manipulating the sensitivity switch. The sensitivity switch is connected to a series of voltage dividers that attenuate the amplified cerebral voltages sufficiently for the EEG record to be interpretable. *Sensitivity* is defined as the amount of voltage necessary to produce a set deflection of the pen. The usual units are microvolts per millimeter or millivolts per centimeter. One of the technologist's most important tasks during analog recording is to maintain sensitivity settings low enough for the input voltage to result in a pen deflection of sufficient amplitude to be detectable. However, the sensitivity cannot be so low that the amplitude of pen deflection interferes with or "blocks" pen movements in adjacent channels. Because the voltage of electrocerebral activity varies during the study, sensitivity settings may need to be adjusted to maintain an appropriate amplitude of recorded EEG activity. Because amplitude of various waveforms is an important consideration in scoring sleep stages, these adjustments must be carefully documented.

Whereas the sensitivity settings determine the *amplitude* of pen deflection, the polarity of the cerebral activity determines the *direction* of the pen deflection. The differential amplifier compares polarity at the two electrodes. The resulting pen deflection is determined according to the *polarity convention*. The pen moves up if input 1 is negative relative to input 2, or if input 2 is positive relative to input 1. The pen moves down if input 1 is positive relative to input 2, or if input 2 is negative relative to input 1. It follows that *phase reversals* of EEG waveforms can be used to roughly localize the scalp distribution of those waveforms. The scalp voltage distribution of a typical vertex wave is illustrated in Figure 12–3, where hypothetical absolute voltages at several electrode positions are shown.

The electrodes are linked in serial pairs from left to right. When C3 is connected to input 1 and Cz is connected to input 2 in amplifier 2, the amplifier determines that the difference between the two electrodes is 10 µV. Input 2 is more negative than input 1. Thus, the galvanometer pen recording from this amplifier registers a downward deflection of 10 units. In amplifier 3, Cz is connected to input 1 and C4 to input 2. The amplifier determines that the difference in voltages is also 10 µV. However, input 1 is now more negative than input 2. Consequently, the galvanometer pen recording from this amplifier registers an upward deflection of 10 units. The phase reversal in the adjacent channels marks the electrode where the vertex wave is most negative. This is the electrode shared by both amplifiers, Cz. Because most cerebral activity is negative at the scalp, phase reversals with the pen deflections pointing toward each other (see Fig. 12–3) are encountered most commonly. Positive cerebral activity would result in a phase reversal with the pen deflections pointing away from each other at the electrode that was most positive. Note that localization by phase reversal is accurate only when electrodes spaced at relatively short distances are serially linked in adjacent amplifiers. This is known as a *bipolar montage*.

After voltages at the two inputs are subtracted and amplified, the result is passed through a series of filters. The goal of filtering is to attenuate voltages occurring at undesirable frequencies (e.g., environmental noise) without disturbing frequencies found in the biological signal of interest. A frequency-response curve measures the ability of a filter to attenuate various frequencies. Frequency-response curves for two types of analog filter included in many polygraphs are presented in Figures 12–4 and 12–5. A *high-pass filter* (also known as a *low-frequency filter*) allows higher frequency activity to pass unchanged while progressively attenuating lower frequencies (see Fig. 12–4). A *low-pass filter* (also known as a *high-frequency filter*) allows lower frequencies to pass unchanged while progressively attenuating higher frequencies (see Fig. 12–5). Analog filters are defined by *cutoff frequency* and *roll-off*. The filter with a given

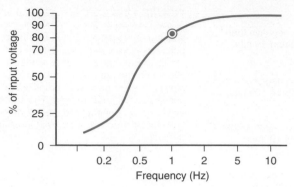

FIGURE 12–4 Frequency-response curve of a hypothetical high-pass filter with a cutoff frequency of 1 Hz and a roll-off of −6 dB per octave. *(Modified with permission from Tyner F, Kott J, Mayer W Jr. Fundamentals of EEG Technology, Vol 1. New York: Raven, 1983.)*

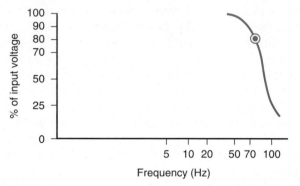

FIGURE 12–5 Frequency-response curve of a hypothetical low-pass filter with a cutoff frequency of 70 Hz and a roll-off of −6 dB per octave. *(Modified with permission from Tyner F, Kott J, Mayer W Jr. Fundamentals of EEG Technology, Vol 1. New York: Raven, 1983.)*

cutoff frequency will attenuate voltage of that frequency by 20%* (e.g., the high-pass filter in Figure 12–4 has a cutoff frequency of 1 Hz, so a 100-μV, 1-Hz wave passed through this filter will have an amplitude of 80 μV). Attenuation of frequencies above the cutoff frequency is more or less linear for the high-pass filter. Attenuation of frequencies below the cutoff frequency is progressively more severe as lower frequencies are encountered. This progressively more severe attenuation is defined by the filter's roll-off. Roll-off for most analog EEG filters is −6 dB per octave. For the high-pass filter, this means that the voltage of activity is decreased by half for every halving of the frequency.

The *60-Hz* or *notch* filter is also present in most polygraphic amplifiers.[†] This filter is designed to attenuate mains frequency very harshly while attenuating activity of surrounding frequencies less extensively.[4] Because

electrical mains are ubiquitous, 60-Hz artifact may easily contaminate an EEG recording. The notch filter should be used sparingly for at least two reasons. First, some biological signals of interest to the polysomnographer have waveforms with important components in the range of 40–80 Hz. Examples include myogenic activity and epileptiform spikes, both of which may be significantly attenuated by the notch filter. For example, use of the notch filter in the chin EMG channel may result in a false impression that tonic EMG has significantly decreased. In addition, the capability of the differential amplifier to reject common signals (see earlier) should be sufficient to suppress 60-Hz artifact in most cases. Thus, the appearance of 60 Hz usually signals a problem somewhere in the polygraphic circuit that needs to be resolved. Most often the culprit is high impedance at the electrode-scalp interface. Less frequently, defects in the amplifier or grounding of the polygraph are responsible. In these cases, addressing the cause of the 60 Hz rather than using the notch filter is the appropriate course. There are circumstances in which a nearby source of 60 Hz (e.g., a critical piece of medical equipment that cannot be disconnected) renders the EEG uninterpretable. Use of the 60-Hz filter may be justified in these circumstances but must be clearly documented.

A writer unit transforms the amplified and filtered signal into a written record. The writer unit consists of an oscillograph and chart drive. A *galvanometer pen unit* is a widely used oscillograph (Fig. 12–6). A specially designed coil of wire and a pen stylus are mounted on a rod. The coil of wire is placed between the two poles of a permanent magnet. Current flow from the amplifier enters the coil and induces a magnetic field. The induced magnetic field interacts with the field of the permanent magnet, resulting in a deflection of the pen stylus on the paper. The amount of deflection is proportional to the magnetic field, which is proportional to the current from the amplifier, which in turn is proportional to the biological signal. A spring attached to the rod returns the pen stylus back to baseline after the current responsible for the deflection has ceased. This spring, together with the friction of the pen stylus against the paper and the inertia of the galvanometer, are collectively known as *damping* and resist the pen movement. Very rapid signal changes (high-frequency signal) require very rapid galvanometer movement, increasing disproportionately the amount of energy necessary to overcome damping. Because more energy is required to write out high-frequency signals, the galvanometer pen unit, in effect, acts as a high-frequency filter. Galvanometer pen writer units usually do not faithfully reproduce signals with frequencies higher than 80–90 Hz.

The *chart drive* pulls the paper below the pens at a constant speed to provide a continuous record of pen deflections (voltage changes) over time. Paper speeds slower than 10 mm/sec save paper but cannot be recommended

---

*In electrophysiology, a widely used convention dictates that voltage at the cutoff frequency is attenuated by 20%. In electrical engineering, voltage at the cutoff frequency is attenuated by approximately 30%.

[†]Because mains frequency is 50 Hz, a 50-Hz notch filter is widely available.

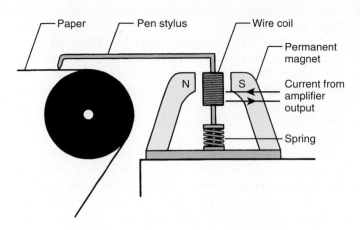

FIGURE 12-6 Hypothetical galvanometer pen writer unit (not to scale). *(Modified with permission from Tyner F, Kott J, Mayer W Jr. Fundamentals of EEG Technology, Vol 1. New York: Raven, 1983.)*

because resolution of faster waveforms necessary for scoring sleep stages is impossible. When suspicious waveforms such as epileptiform spikes are noted, increasing paper speed to 30 mm/sec can aid interpretation.

Components of the Digital Polygraphic Circuit

Modern digital communications technology has allowed miniaturization of what had been much bulkier (if somewhat hardier) solid state components. It has also resulted in some reorganization of the functions of the polygraphic circuit. Digital polygraphs perform all of the functions of the analog polygraphic circuit. However, the ability to digitize the EEG signals allows easier manipulation, transmission, display, and storage, conferring some distinct advantages.

Many contemporary systems have folded jackbox inputs, amplification, and sampling/analog-to-digital conversion into one box, approximately the size of the jackbox in analog systems (see Fig. 12–2B). In addition to inputs for the standard 10-20 scalp electrode postions, electrode inputs for digital systems always include one or more additional inputs for reference electrodes. A location between Fpz and Fz is often chosen for the reference electrode, but any location on the scalp that is relatively noise free and where firm attachment to the scalp is possible can be used. Reference electrodes are necessary because digital EEG recording is always referential. In other words, signal recorded from any given electrode is presented to input 1 of the differential amplifier assigned to that electrode, while signal recorded from the reference electrode is always presented to input 2. Referential recording allows easy re-montaging later in the polygraphic circuit. This contrasts with analog EEG machines, in which signal from each electrode is presented to the montage selector switch; in the latter situation, the technician decides on the montage at the time of recording and changing montages later is not possible. However, referential recording can cause significant confusion if the reference electrode becomes disconnected.

The signal (still an analog signal) is next presented to an amplifier assigned to that particular input. The principles of differential amplifiers and common mode rejection described previously also pertain to digital machines. Amplifiers are smaller and typically are part of the box containing the inputs.*

Amplified inputs are next presented to the *analog-to-digital converter* (ADC). The ADC is the heart of the digital EEG machine. Conceptually, the ADC has several parts: a clock, a voltmeter, and memory. Simply put, the ADC assesses (samples) the voltage (amplitude) of the continuous analog EEG, creates a numeric value corresponding to this voltage, and stores this value in memory. The ADC then repeats this process at a uniform interval (intersample interval). In this manner, a continuous (analog) EEG signal is converted into a series of numeric values representing the voltage of the signal at serial moments in time. Thus the signal is commonly referred to as "digitized" or a "digital signal."

For the digitized EEG signal to be clinically useful, it has to be a faithful representation of the "real" analog signal. Two features of the ADC determine how accurately digitized signal reflects the original analog waveform: (1) the sampling rate of the ADC ("horizontal resolution"), and (2) the number of bits in the ADC ("vertical resolution"). The number of times the EEG amplitude is sampled in a period of time is called the *sampling rate*. Intuitively, the more often the ADC samples an analog waveform, the more accurately the digitized output reflects the analog waveform. For example, a sampling rate of 256 per second means that the voltage of the analog waveform is sampled (assigned a numerical value) every 1/256 of a second (the intersample interval). This intersample interval indicates the horizontal (time)

---

*Amplifiers in contemporary systems (and in most analog systems) perform amplification in multiple stages. Usually the last (and most significant) stage incorporates analog filters. These attenuate frequencies that can potentially damage the analog-to-digital converter but that are not physiologically relevant. Analog filters at this stage are "wide open"; that is, they do not attenuate clinically relevant activity. They cannot be modified by technicians or interpreters. Filtering of clinically relevant material is performed later in the polygraphic circuit (see later).

resolution and is a typical value for contemporary polygraphs. If the digitized signal is to reflect the analog signal faithfully, the sampling rate must be at least two times the highest frequency in the analog signal. Frequencies in the analog signal exceeding half the sampling rate will appear in the digitized signal at a lower frequency than in the analog signal. This is known as *aliasing* because the faster frequencies in the analog signal appear under the "alias" of a lower frequency in the digitized signal (see Ebersole and Pedley,[2] page 47, for further discussion).

The number of discrete numeric levels that the voltage of the analog signal can potentially be assigned indicates the vertical resolution. Intuitively, the more numeric levels the ADC has available to assign a voltage reading of an analog waveform at any point in time, the more accurately the digitized signal represents the "real" analog waveform. Vertical resolution of the analog-to-digital converter is measured in "bits" or powers of 2. For example, a 10-bit converter can assign 2^{10}, or 1024, levels to the voltage of a signal at any point in time. Vertical resolution of the converter should be higher than the noise level of the amplifier so that all signals exceeding noise level can be represented. Because noise level of contemporary amplifiers is approximately 1 μV, a 10-bit converter is usually adequate for EEG signals. A 10-bit converter would allow amplitude at any point in an analog signal to be assigned a value in 1-μV steps from −511 to +512 μV ($2^{10}/2 - 1$ level assigned to 0 μV). This range encompasses the vast majority of EEG voltages recorded from the scalp. This is usually adequate for EMG and EOG signals as well. Contemporary digital polygraphic systems typically utilize ADC with vertical resolution ranging from 16 to 22 bits.

The digitized signal is now passed to a computer for storage in memory and further manipulation by a software program. Sofware programs perform many of the functions of the solid state components of the analog polygraph (see Fig. 12–2B).

Montage selection is performed by software manipulation of the digitized signal. Because the analog EEG signal is recorded referentially (see earlier), montage selection can occur by simple subtraction of the digitized outputs of amplifiers corresponding to the individual electrodes. For example, a patient undergoing a sleep study may have a full complement of electrodes attached. The amplifiers in the digital headbox amplify the signal from each of these relative to the reference electrode (Fp1-R, T3-R, O1-R, C3-R, A2-R, etc.), and this signal is digitized and recorded in computer memory. The interpreter desires to display C3-A2 and sends the appropriate command to the software. The software subtracts C3-R from A2-R and the screen displays C3-A2. This recording displays unusual activity, and there is concern that this may represent a seizure. The interpreter requests the software to display Fp1-T3, T3-O1, Fp1-C3, and C3-O1.

Digitized referential output from these amplifiers was being recorded to the computer hard drive throughout the study but was not being displayed. The interpreter can now use this information to address concerns that the unusual EEG activity was an epileptic seizure. In a similar manner, a variety of montages can be accessed by the interpreter to address other concerns provided that a broad range of information is recorded referentially throughout the study.

Filtering is another function performed by software on the digitized EEG signal. Digital filters are computer algorithms that transform a digitized EEG by filtering out designated frequencies. Digital filtering can be performed in the frequency domain by computing the Fourier transform of a segment of an EEG, replacing coefficients at the frequency one wishes to eliminate by zero, and then reconstituting the EEG by computing the inverse Fourier transform.[15] (See further discussion of Fourier analysis later.) Digital filtering can also be performed in the time domain by using a moving average method.[15] Such finite impulse response[12] filters are increasingly used in digital EEG machines and allow filtering without phase distortion, an advantage over traditional analog filters.

Software can manipulate and analyze digitized EEG signal in more sophisticated ways as well. Spectral analysis is a commonly employed technique relying on the Fourier theorem and forms the basis of sleep stage scoring software. Pitfalls and limitations of this technique are discussed later. Algorithms designed to detect seizures and epileptiform abnormalities are also commercially available.[16] The clinical utility of these is variable, and they do not replace a thorough analysis of the original record by a qualified interpreter.

Modified and organized digital signal can be directed from computer memory to a variety of destinations. Polygraphic data must be presented to the interpreter for visual inspection. Polygraphic data in digital systems is typically displayed on monitors. Monitor resolution must be sufficient so that the degree of resolution provided by the ADC is not significantly compromised. For example, if 1024 pixels (a common horizontal resolution in "off-the-shelf" computer monitors) are available to display 30 seconds of EEG, at most 1024/30 or 34 pixels can be devoted to display 1 second of EEG. This is far less than the 256 samples/sec horizontal resolution provided by ADCs typically used in contemporary polygraphic systems. While this degree of horizontal resolution may be adequate for sleep stage scoring, it is not sufficient for analysis of epileptiform activity or electrographic seizures. Changing the time base of the display so that 10-second epochs are displayed on the monitor will triple the horizontal resolution of the monitor in the previous example and bring it more into line with the resolution provided by the ADC. Similar considerations pertain to the vertical resolution of the monitor, though this is of less concern in polygraphy, in which fewer channels of polygraphic recording are typically presented at any time. In general, larger monitors with higher monitor resolution better reflect all the information present in the digitized signal.

Digitized polygraphic data can be transmitted to a printer to generate a "hard copy" polygraphic tracing of selected epochs. Printing an entire polygraph is rarely necessary with digital systems. Digitized data in computer memory must ultimately be transmitted to peripheral devices for storage. A variety of digital storage media are available, all of which are less expensive and more convenient than the paper and microfilm required for analog EEG. After security and privacy issues are addressed, digitized polygraphic data can be transmitted via network or the Internet to other computers in the clinic, the interpreter's home, or another continent.

Advantages and Limitations of Digital Recording Systems

The advantages of digital recording are leading to the obsolescence of analog polygraphic systems. Advantages include decreased size and weight, the ability to record vast amounts of data cheaply and efficiently, and the ability to re-montage digitized data post hoc as needed. Digitized polysomnograms can be analyzed, transmitted, and stored more cheaply, quickly, and efficiently than analog studies. For these reasons, digital recording will continue to replace analog polygraphic systems over time.

The reliance of digital polygraphic systems on referential recording (see earlier) leads to a vulnerability that is important to remember. If the reference electrode becomes detached, the EEG signal from the recording electrode may be overwhelmed by the environmental noise from the open reference input. When inputs from individual channels are subtracted to display a montage, the record may appear identical to a low-voltage EEG. An unsuspecting technician may think nothing is amiss when in fact no EEG signal at all is being transmitted to the digital headbox and potentially clinically important activity is being missed. Checking impedance of the reference electrode and displaying all electrodes to reference at the beginning and end of the study will address this weakness. In general, it is important to remember that the analog electrophysiologic signal is closer to the clinical phenomena that interest the practitioner of sleep medicine than the digital signal interpreted on the monitor. Understanding how the original analog signal is transformed is therefore important.

SPECTRAL ANALYSIS

Spectral analysis is probably the most widely used computerized analysis of a digitized EEG.[15,17,18] Spectral analysis is based on the Fourier theorem, which states that any waveform can be decomposed into a sum of sine waves at different frequencies with different amplitudes and different phase relationships. When summed, these waves reconstitute the original waveform. The Fourier transformation is a mathematical operation that provides the frequency, amplitude, and phase parameters of each of these component sine waves. Fourier coefficients represent the amplitude and phase relationship at each of the component sine wave frequencies. Squaring and summing the Fourier coefficients at each frequency provides the power at that frequency. A plot of power at each of the component frequencies is called the *power spectrum*. The power spectrum allows determination of relative amounts of given frequencies in the waveform over the time segment analyzed.

The fast Fourier transform algorithm[19] allows real-time spectral analysis with contemporary personal computers. Commercially available software packages offer straightforward presentation of the power contained in the traditional frequency bands during a set period of EEG. This allows detection and quantification of frequencies not detected with visual inspection. However, there are many potential pitfalls.[17,18] Theoretically, the power spectrum is a faithful representation of the original signal only if the original signal is stationary (has stable statistical properties). The EEG signal is clearly not stationary over long periods, although it appears reasonably stationary over brief epochs.[20] In practice this means that the EEG segment selected for analysis should not include obvious changes such as those due to alerting or drowsiness. In addition, the Fourier theorem assumes that an infinitely long sample is available for analysis. Because even long samples are clinically impractical, tapering or "windowing" of the end points of the sample is necessary to attenuate the spurious frequencies (leakage) arising from the segmentation of the signal. Windowing is never completely successful—some leakage is unavoidable. This may affect clinical interpretation when power is displayed in the traditional frequency bands; for example, a reasonable amount of alpha power may leak to the theta or beta bands. Nonsinusoidal rhythms such as "spiky alpha" are common in routine EEG. Fourier analysis of a nonsinusoidal rhythm of a set frequency often shows a large peak at that frequency with smaller peaks at harmonics of the frequency. These smaller, higher frequency peaks may lead the interpreter to conclude that cerebral activity at the higher frequency is actually present. The most common pitfall in interpreting power spectra is artifact. Artifact is ubiquitous, often subtle, and can take an almost infinite variety of forms. The computer cannot separate artifact from EEG and includes artifact in the computation of the power spectrum. This can lead to significant misinterpretation. Artifact is much more difficult to recognize in the power spectrum than in the unprocessed EEG. It is therefore very important to review an EEG before spectral analysis or interpretation of the power spectrum to prevent analysis of segments contaminated by artifact.

Despite these limitations, spectral analysis can play a useful role in the operating room and in routine scoring of sleep studies (see Chapter 18). A basic understanding of the principles of signal processing and thorough experience in the appearance of various cerebral activities after spectral analysis is necessary. Unprocessed "real" physiologic signal must always be reviewed. Spectral analysis has not demonstrated any consistent clinical utility in routine EEG despite almost 2 decades of active research. Because the potential for misinterpretation and abuse is high, the major neurologic and neurophysiologic professional organizations have taken strong positions against the use of spectral analysis during routine EEG.[21,22]

ELECTRICAL SAFETY

Contemporary polygraphic and EEG studies are very safe procedures. Nevertheless, the possibility of electrical injury exists whenever a patient is connected to an electrical apparatus. Thus, technicians performing studies and physicians supervising sleep laboratories must understand the basic principles of electrical safety.

Electrical injury is caused by excessive current flow through biological tissue. Such electrical injury includes burns, seizures, and irreversible damage to nervous tissue. When excessive current flows through the heart, potentially fatal arrhythmias may occur. The amount of current necessary to induce ventricular fibrillation is dependent on skin impedance, the mass of tissue the current must traverse before reaching the heart, the health of the heart, and the general health of the patient, among other factors. In a healthy adult with dry intact skin, 100–300 mA delivered at 60 Hz will induce fibrillation (macroshock).[4] Smaller amounts of current (microshock) will induce fibrillation in electrically susceptible patients. These include patients with wet skin or wounds, as well as patients with pacemaker electrodes inserted in the ventricular myocardium. Dry intact skin offers high impedance to current flow, as technicians well appreciate. Increased skin moisture or skin interruption significantly reduces this impedance, allowing current to flow toward the heart more readily. Pacemaker wires allow the current to flow directly into the vulnerable myocardium rather than through the high impedance offered by the chest wall and pleural cavities. When a 60-Hz current is applied directly to the heart, intensities as low as 100 μA can result in fibrillation, although higher values are necessary in most cases.[23–25]

Current flow requires a source of current and the formation of a complete circuit. Thus, electrical safety has two goals: (1) the polygraph must not become a source of excessive current, and (2) the polygraph and patient (or technician) must not form a complete circuit through which excessive current may flow and cause electrical injury. Proper maintenance, proper grounding, and use of isolation devices accomplish these goals.

The power unit of the polygraph is a potential source of excessive current. A fault in the power unit may result in a short circuit that would allow a *fault current* to flow to the polygraph chassis (Fig. 12–7A). If the machine ground were disabled and the patient were touching a pipe or some other conducting substance, current would flow through the electrodes and the patient to the pipe, possibly causing electrical injury. Current would also flow through a technician touching the polygraph and a conducting substance. To guard against this possibility, the chassis of the polygraph is connected to the building ground through a three-pronged outlet (Fig. 12–7B). Should a current-bearing element contact the chassis, the current would be shunted through machine ground to the building ground because this path has the least resistance. The sudden high-current flow would blow a fuse in the power unit or open a circuit breaker, stopping further current flow. A brief period is necessary for the excessive current to blow the fuse and, if the patient is touching a conducting substance during this period, current will still flow through the patient. The duration of the current flow would be briefer, however, and the danger to the patient decreased.

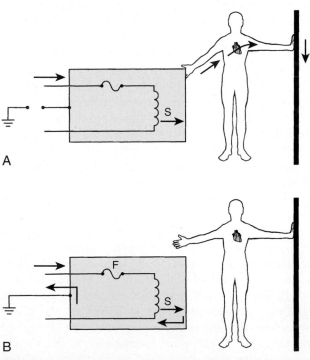

FIGURE 12–7 (A) Technician touches polygraph chassis and water pipe. Polygraph chassis is ungrounded because of interruption in ground wire. A short circuit (S) in the power supply unit allows current to flow to the chassis, through the technician's heart, and to the water pipe. *Arrows* trace path of current flow. **(B)** A short circuit in the polygraph with an intact chassis ground. A short circuit (S) in the power supply allows current to flow to the chassis. The low-resistance chassis ground allows unimpeded flow of current to the building ground. The current surge blows a fuse (F), quickly stopping further current flow. Bystanders are safe unless they touch the chassis at the moment of the short circuit.

It follows that the connection between the polygraph and building ground must not be compromised. Electrical outlets powering appliances connected to patients must have documented secure connection to building ground. Technicians should ensure good contact between the ground pin of the power cord and the outlet. Three- and two-pronged adapters do not provide secure contact with building ground and must not be used. Resistance of the ground circuit in the polygraph should be checked periodically to detect interruptions. Fuses should never be defeated (i.e., short-circuited). Repeatedly blown fuses may indicate fault currents and potential danger to the technician and patient. Finally, regular maintenance may prevent potentially dangerous fault currents.

Even in the absence of a fault, the complicated circuitry of the polygraph generates lower intensity currents known as *leakage currents. Stray capacitance* is a major source of leakage current. Any circuit with current flow that is insulated from other conducting substances can be viewed as a capacitor. The current-carrying circuit can be considered one plate of a capacitor, the insulation and surrounding space can be considered the dielectric, and the other conducting substances can be considered the other plate of the capacitor. Alternating current flowing through any insulated circuit will therefore generate currents in other conducting substances in the area. One pertinent example is the power cord of the polygraph. Alternating current flow in the insulated "hot" wire of the power cord will induce a lower amount of current flow in the neutral and ground wires. Although leakage currents are much smaller than fault currents, they can cause injury in electrically susceptible patients. Acceptable limits for leakage currents have been defined.[4,26] Adequate grounding protects both patient and technician in this circumstance. The leakage current is shunted to the low-resistance machine ground and then to the building ground. Extension cords increase stray capacitance, and thus leakage currents and should never be used during PSG. Isolation jackboxes that limit the amount of possible current flow through electrodes, and therefore prevent currents generated from the machine from reaching the patient, are widely used. These offer additional protection in electrically susceptible patients and should be employed wherever possible.

Current flow can also occur when machinery attached to the patient draws power from different outlets or when multiple grounds are attached to the patient. The voltage of the ground contact at different outlets may be quite different, resulting in current flow. Multiple grounds can result in a *ground loop*, which can act as a secondary coil of a transformer and generate current flow. A ground loop also acts as an antenna that will pick up ubiquitous environmental electromagnetic radiation and will increase artifact. These potentially dangerous situations can be avoided by plugging in all machinery attached to the patient to the same outlet cluster and using only one patient ground.

ELECTRO-OCULOGRAPHY

The electrical field generated by the eye approximates a simple dipole (Fig. 12–8A) with a posterior negativity centered at the retina and a relative positivity probably centered at the cornea. Eye movements change the orientation of this dipole. Polygraphic recording from strategically placed electrodes can detect these changes and can therefore be used to monitor eye movements. The Rechtschaffen and Kales (R&K) standard sleep scoring manual[27] (see also Chapter 18) recommends that an EOG use at least 2 channels (Fig. 12–8B). One electrode is placed 1 cm superior and lateral to the outer canthus of one eye. This electrode is input 1 to an amplifier; input 2 to this amplifier is an electrode attached to one ear or the mastoid. Another electrode is placed 1 cm inferior

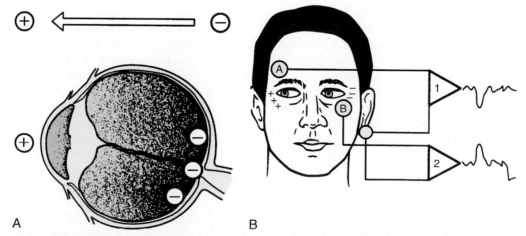

A   B

FIGURE 12–8 (A) The voltage field generated by the eye can be represented by a simple dipole, the cornea being positive and the retina negative. **(B)** Use of two polygraphic channels to detect conjugate eye movements according to the scheme suggested in the EOG sleep scoring manual.[18] Eye movements result in out-of-phase potentials in the 2 channels.

and lateral to the outer canthus of the other eye. This electrode forms input 1 to a second amplifier; input 2 to this amplifier is attached to the same ear as input 2 of the first amplifier. This placement scheme will detect conjugate horizontal and vertical eye movements. For example, when the eyes look to the right (see Fig. 12–8B), the cornea of the right eye approaches electrode A and electrode A becomes positive relative to the inactive ear. According to the polarity convention, amplifier 1 will register a downward deflection. Simultaneously, the retina of the left eye approaches electrode B. Consequently, electrode B becomes negative relative to the inactive ear and amplifier 2 registers an upward deflection. The out-of-phase deflections in the two adjacent channels indicate that a conjugate eye movement has occurred. Similarly, an upward eye movement results in an downward deflection in amplifier 1 and a upward deflection in amplifier 2. Eye blinks will produce an identical pattern because eye closure results in an upward rotation of the eyeball (Bell's phenomenon) (see also Chapter 11).

Some laboratories attach electrodes to both ears and refer the periocular electrodes to the contralateral ear (e.g., right upper canthus to left ear and left lower canthus to right ear). This minor change has several advantages. The longer interelectrode distances increase the amplitude of the deflections. The amplitude of the deflections generated by the movement of each eye is more likely to be equal because the interelectrode distances are equal. Finally, if one of the ear electrodes comes off during the study, the technician can refer both periocular electrodes to the remaining ear electrode and avoid waking the patient. Whereas these montages detect both horizontal and vertical eye movements, they cannot distinguish between them. This can be easily accomplished by recording inputs from supraorbital and infraorbital electrodes with a third amplifier.[4,14]

Several varieties of eye movements are recorded during routine PSG. Although the patient is awake, saccadic eye movements as well as eye blinks are noted. Saccadic eye movements are rapid and can point in any direction. Eye blinks produce the same EOG pattern as vertical eye movement. One of the first signs of drowsiness is the cessation of any eye movements. Somewhat later in drowsiness, slow eye movements are seen. These usually have a frequency of less than 0.5 Hz,[28] are most consistently recorded in the horizontal axis, gradually increase in amplitude as background alpha activity drops out, and usually disappear in stage 2 sleep. REMs occur during REM sleep. Movements along the horizontal axis are the most common, although oblique and vertical movements occur as well. REMs typically occur in bursts and may be preceded by characteristic sawtooth waves on the EEG. There is no widely accepted definition of REMs that would serve to distinguish these from slow eye movements. Parameters useful for computerized quantification of REMs have been reported,[29] but these are not directly applicable to visual scoring. Radtke[30] has suggested a reasonable, clinically applicable definition for REM, namely that the duration of the initial pen deflection is less than 200 msec and that the duration of the entire waveform is less than 1 second.

In a study of drowsiness in normal subjects, Santamaria and Chiappa[28] recorded eye movements with a sensitive motion transducer attached over the globe as well as with the traditional EOG. They found two types of eye movements not previously reported. What were named *small fast irregular eye movements* were found in 60% of normal subjects in early drowsiness, before the occurrence of slow eye movements. They did not appear in the routine EOG channels. What were called *small fast rhythmic eye movements* were found in 30% of normal subjects, usually associated with the traditional slow eye movements. These occasionally appeared in the routine EOG channels, although usually with a very low amplitude. If confirmed, these findings could be useful for determination of early stages of drowsiness.

ELECTROMYOGRAPHIC RECORDINGS IN SLEEP DISORDERS

EMG activities are important physiologic characteristics that need to be recorded for diagnosis and classification of a variety of sleep disorders. An EMG represents electrical activities of muscle fibers resulting from depolarization of the muscles after transmission of nerve impulses along the nerves and neuromuscular junctions.[6] An EMG could represent tonic, phasic, and rhythmic activity. Physiologically, there is a fundamental tone in the muscles, at least throughout the period of wakefulness and non-REM (NREM) sleep, but it is markedly diminished or absent in major muscle groups during REM sleep. Maintenance of muscle tone is a complex physiologic phenomenon that depends on suprasegmental, segmental, and peripheral afferent mechanisms.[31] Tone, therefore, may be influenced by a variety of extrinsic and intrinsic stimuli. After a nerve impulse, the resting muscle membrane potential is altered, and when it reaches a threshold level, depolarization of the muscle results from a change in the external and internal ionic balance and muscle calcium channel alterations.[6] The threshold depolarization causes an action potential to develop in the muscle. A compound muscle action potential represents summation of the action currents in many muscle fibers. Surface EMG recordings are of many muscle fibers, bundles, and groups; needle EMGs record approximately 15–20 muscle fibers near the needle tip.[6] Phasic EMG represents activities related to some physiologic alterations, either spontaneous or induced. Examples of phasic EMGs are EMG activities phasically related to inspiratory bursts and myoclonic muscle bursts that occur spontaneously or in response to some stimuli. If there are rhythmic activities (e.g., tremor), EMG bursts have a rhythm. In sleep disorders medicine, the tonic and phasic EMG bursts are usually the most important ones. As sometimes happens, however, rhythmic EMG bursts are noted in certain sleep disorders, such as patients with restless legs syndrome or other sleep-related movement disorders (see Chapter 28).

Method of Recording

EMG recordings from submental muscles using surface electrodes are routinely performed in PSG and multiple sleep latency tests. Electrodes placed in this area record mostly the activities of the mylohyoid and the anterior belly of the digastric muscles, which are innervated by the motor Vth cranial nerve. The electrodes also record some activities from the genioglossus and hyoglossus muscles (innervated by the XIIth cranial nerve) by volume conduction. This recording is important for identifying the presence or absence of muscle tone for sleep stage scoring.

In a patient suspected of restless legs syndrome, tibialis anterior muscles must be recorded, preferably bilaterally, because sometimes the periodic movements of legs alternate between the two legs. Ideally, the recording should also include 1 or 2 EMG channels from the upper limb muscles, as occasionally movements are noted in the upper limbs.

To understand the pathophysiology of sleep apnea, it is important to record the respiratory muscle activities (see also Chapter 14). These should include not only the intercostal muscles but also the diaphragmatic muscle, a variety of upper airway muscles, and the facial muscles. The true diaphragmatic activities are typically recorded by intraesophageal bipolar electrodes, which can also quantitate the diaphragmatic EMG activity.[32–34] This technique as well as esophageal pressure recording by inserting an esophageal balloon transnasally (which provides respiratory muscle mechanical activity) are invasive and uncomfortable. The noninvasive technique of placing surface electrodes to the right or left of the umbilicus or over the anterior costal margin may also pick up diaphragmatic activity, but the admixture of intercostal muscle activity makes this noninvasive technique unreliable for quantitative assessment of diaphragmatic EMG.[35] The intercostal EMG recorded from the seventh to the ninth intercostal space[36] with active electrodes on the anterior axillary line and the reference electrodes on the midaxillary line may record some diaphragmatic muscle activity in addition to the intercostal activity. Sharp et al.[37] compared data from chest wall surface electrodes (surface electrodes over the sixth and seventh intercostal space just above the right costal margin) with simultaneous data obtained from a swallowed bipolar electrode double-balloon catheter similar to that described by Onal and coworkers.[38] After performing power spectral analysis of diaphragmatic EMGs from surface electrodes and esophageal electrodes, Sharp et al.[37] concluded that thoracic surface recordings of the diaphragmatic EMG do not accurately reflect frequency information. Esophageal balloon manometry is important for a definite diagnosis of upper airway resistance syndrome.[39] In this condition, a narrowed upper airway results in increased work necessary to move air through a constricted airway but does not cause apneas or hypopneas.[39,40] Esophageal balloon manometry in this condition documents abnormally increased negative intrathoracic pressure during inspiration associated with repeated arousals and fragmentation of sleep that are responsible for daytime hypersomnolence. Esophageal balloon manometry has been superseded by the use of a thinner and better tolerated water-filled catheter connected to a transducer.[40,41]

An important muscle for recording respiratory activity is the alae nasi muscle.[34] This muscle picks up not only inspiratory activity but also some expiratory activity. Many upper airway muscles are accessory muscles of respiration. All the facial muscles, including the masseter muscles, show inspiratory bursts during EMG recordings.[36] To show the decrease of tone in the genioglossus and other oropharyngeal and laryngeal muscles, it is important to record EMGs from them. Intramuscular electrodes in humans are typically used to record inspiratory-related genioglossal muscle activity.[42–44] For many of these upper airway muscles, however, recordings can be made in a noninvasive manner by means of intraoral surface electrodes.[36,45] For some laryngeal muscles, an invasive technique using fine-wire electrodes is required.[42] To record the muscle activity from an individual muscle only, wire electrodes must be inserted into that particular muscle only.

For patients with suspected REM sleep behavior disorder (RBD), multiple muscle EMGs from all four limbs are essential—there is often dissociation in the activities between upper and lower limb muscles with these patients. Hence, if upper limb EMGs are not included in the recording, REM sleep without atonia may be missed in some cases.[46] Polysomnographic documentation of REM sleep without muscle atonia associated with excessive tonic and phasic EMG activities is a requirement in the second edition of the International Classification of Sleep Disorders for diagnosis of RBD.[47] This is, however, a qualitative documentation and there is no standardized, generally acceptable quantitative scoring method available.[48–51] A quantitative standardized scoring method is essential to determine the severity of RBD, monitor the effectiveness of therapy, and understand the pathophysiology of RBD.

In patients with nocturnal paroxysmal dystonia, which is now thought to be a form of nocturnal frontal lobe epilepsy, multiple muscle EMGs including all four limbs are required. In this condition, the patient displays dystonic-choreoathetoid movements; surface EMGs in addition to the video recordings are necessary to record these activities.

Clinical Significance of EMG Recording

EMG shows decreasing tone from wakefulness through stages 1–4 of NREM sleep. In REM sleep, the EMG tone is markedly diminished or absent. It is important to use the appropriate filters and very high gain at the beginning of the recording to appreciate the decreasing muscle tone during REM sleep. In certain pathologic conditions (e.g., RBD), the EMG tone may persist or phasic muscle bursts may be seen repeatedly during REM sleep. This may also happen in patients being treated for narcolepsy-cataplexy syndrome, and may represent a medication (e.g., selective serotonin reuptake inhibitors or tricyclic antidepressants being used to treat cataplexy) side effect.

EMG recordings of the tibialis anterior muscles are essential for the diagnosis of periodic limb movements in sleep (PLMS), which are seen in most of the cases of restless legs syndrome, a variety of other sleep disorders, and normal individuals, particularly older ones. Characteristics of the EMG bursts in PLMS are described in Chapter 28. In upper airway obstructive apnea, the EMG of the upper airway muscles shows marked decrease of tone during the apneic episodes, whereas the diaphragmatic and intercostal muscle activity persists.[36] During REM sleep, however, intercostal and even diaphragmatic EMGs show marked diminution of the tonic activity.[52]

In certain neurodegenerative diseases such as multiple system atrophy (Shy-Drager syndrome), laryngeal EMG

recording may be important to detect vocal cord paralysis causing upper airway obstructive apnea.[53]

Multiple muscle EMG recordings are also important in patients with restless legs syndrome because of the presence of a variety of EMG activity types in these patients, including PLMS (predominantly dystonic), myoclonic bursts during both wakefulness and sleep, and a mixture of myoclonic and dystonic EMG bursts (Fig. 12–9) (see Chapter 28). Restless legs syndrome patients often have PLMS in the agonist and antagonist muscles (see Fig. 12–9), occasionally in the arms and rarely in the submental muscles (Fig. 12–10).[54]

Multiple muscle EMGs may also be required for evaluation of propriospinal myoclonus at sleep onset, hyponic jerks, rare parasomnias such as sleep-related faciomandibular myoclonus,[55] and other sleep-related movement disorders (e.g., rhythmic movement disorder).

EMG recordings are needed to score excessive fragmentary myoclonus, hypnagogic foot tremor, and alternating leg muscle activation.[56] For research purposes, multiple muscle EMGs, including those of cranially innervated muscles, are necessary to understand the pathophysiology of post-polio syndrome,[57,58] neuroleptic-induced akathisia,[59] and tardive dyskinesias.[60,61]

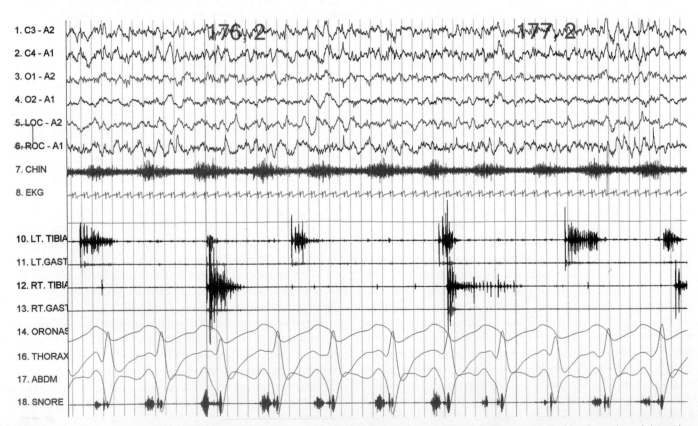

FIGURE 12–9 Polysomnographic (PSG) recording showing periodic limb movements in sleep (PLMS) characterized by dystonic and dystonic-myoclonic electromyographic (EMG) bursts in left (LT) and right (RT) tibialis (TIBIA) and gastrocnemius (GAST) muscles during stage 2 (N2) non–rapid eye movement (NREM) sleep in an adult patient with restless legs syndrome (RLS). Top 4 channels show electroencephalograms (EEG) using international nomenclature. (A1, left ear; A2, right ear; ABDM, abdominal respiratory effort; CHIN, submental EMG; EKG, electrocardiogram; LOC, left electro-oculogram; ORONAS, oronasal airflow; ROC, right electro-oculogram; THORAX, chest respiratory effort.)

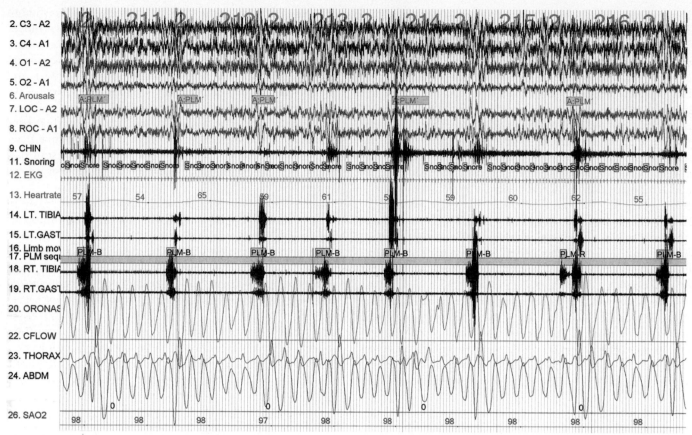

FIGURE 12–10 Overnight PSG recording from an adult patient with RLS showing PLMS in tibialis and gastrocnemius muscles bilaterally synchronous with EMG bursts in submental (CHIN) muscles. (A:PLM, arousal with PLMS; Limb mov, limb movements; PLM seq, PLMS sequence; PLM-B, PLMS in right and left limbs; PLM-R, PLMS in right limb seen independently; SaO₂, oxygen saturation (%) by finger oximetry.) For description of the montage, see Figure 12–9.

ELECTROENCEPHALOGRAPHY

An EEG is recorded in sleep studies mostly to assist scoring of sleep stages. Obviously, EEGs can provide other useful information as well. Routine diagnostic EEGs usually sample at most 1 hour of electrocerebral activity. The PSG records EEG activity for much longer periods, increasing the likelihood that abnormalities will be recorded. Consequently, the polysomnographer must be familiar with the broad range of normal EEG findings and the abnormalities encountered in the various age groups. The following is at best an incomplete review of some of the major patterns encountered in routine EEG.

Normal Waking Rhythms

Individual waves recorded on the EEG can be characterized by their frequency (i.e., how many of that wave would be required to occupy a given period of time, typically 1 second). Frequency of EEG activity has been divided into four bands, assigned the Greek letters beta, alpha, theta, and delta. Scoring of sleep is largely based on the amplitude and frequency of EEG waves. Human electrocerebral activity is better characterized, however, by the broader concept of EEG *rhythms*. EEG rhythms can be defined as sustained periods of electrocerebral activity of similar frequency with a stereotyped distribution, reactivity, symmetry, and synchrony, and are associated with specific physiologic states. These rhythms have also been assigned Greek letters that correspond, in part, to the letters assigned to frequency.

Several rhythms characterize the awake adult EEG. The most obvious is the *alpha rhythm*. Alpha rhythm frequency varies between 8 and 13 Hz. This rhythm is distributed over the parieto-occipital regions bilaterally. A normal alpha rhythm is synchronous and symmetric over the two hemispheres. Frequency of the rhythm should not vary by more than 1 Hz, and amplitude should not vary by more than 50%. The alpha rhythm is best seen during quiet alertness with eyes closed. Various maneuvers cause alpha rhythm to react or decrease in amplitude. The most effective is opening the eyes, but any sort of intense stimulation produces some degree of amplitude attenuation. Up to 10% of normal adults will show no alpha rhythm during quiet wakefulness. The low-voltage EEG in these subjects is characterized by poorly sustained beta and theta frequencies with amplitudes between 10 and 20 μV. Occasionally, hyperventilation elicits a typical alpha rhythm in such patients.

Low-voltage EEGs have not been recorded in normal subjects less than 10 years old.

Beta rhythms are present in virtually all adults, although they are usually less striking than alpha rhythms. Frequency of the beta rhythm is by definition above 13 Hz but typically ranges between 18 and 25 Hz. There are probably at least two beta rhythms, one distributed over the frontal and central regions and the other with a more diffuse distribution. Beta rhythms are present during wakefulness and drowsiness. They may appear more persistent during drowsiness, drop out during deeper sleep, and reappear during REM sleep. Amplitude over the two hemispheres should not vary by more than 50%. Amplitude of beta activity is less than 20 μV in 98% of normal drug-free subjects. A persistent beta rhythm with higher amplitude suggests use of sedative-hypnotic medications because most such medications increase amplitude of beta activity.

Mu rhythms are recorded in approximately 20% of routine daytime EEGs and are most common in young adults. This rhythm consists of brief trains of 7- to 11-Hz waves over the central regions, often with phase reversals over C3 or C4. The waves have a wicket or arciform shape (Fig. 12–11). Mu may occur synchronously or independently over the two hemispheres. This rhythm shows a characteristic reactivity. Active or passive movement of the limbs or even an intention to move a limb attenuates mu activity. Mu is seen during wakefulness and may become more prominent during stages 1 and 2 of NREM sleep. It typically disappears in slow-wave sleep and may reappear during REM sleep.[62] Direct EEG recordings from the human motor cortex have demonstrated superharmonics of mu activity that react to limb movement.[63] This has led to the conclusion that mu is a "ubiquitous rhythm of the sensorimotor cortex at rest."[64]

Lambda rhythm is present in approximately 75% of young adults and becomes somewhat less common as individuals age. Lambda consists of a diphasic or triphasic waveform with the most prominent phase being a positivity at O1 or O2. The lambda rhythm is elicited by saccadic eye movements and appears to be an evoked response. It is present only during wakefulness with eyes open.

The EEG in infants and children undergoes significant evolution with increasing age. This paragraph emphasizes a few major points; the reader is referred to other sources for details.[65–67] A sustained parieto-occipital, alpha-type

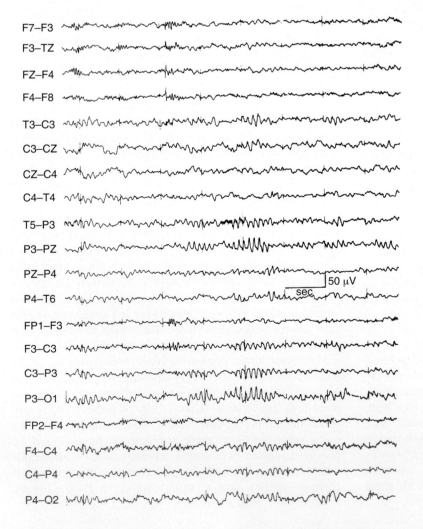

FIGURE 12–11 Mu rhythm in the left parietal region (P3). Note phase reversal of the 7- to 8-Hz comblike rhythm at P3 with spread of activity to C3.

rhythm is not seen until approximately 3 months of age. At that time, reactive 3-Hz waves are recorded during wakefulness. Frequency of the parieto-occipital rhythm increases rapidly over the next several years, reaching adult values in most children by 3 years of age. *Polyphasic slow waves* (slow waves of youth) are found in the occipital regions bilaterally after 2 years in as many as 10% of normal subjects. Prevalence is highest at approximately age 10 and gradually decreases afterward. These waveforms rarely occupy more than 25% of the record, and they do not significantly exceed the amplitude of other background rhythms. Polyphasic slow waves react to eye opening in the same manner as the alpha rhythm; these waves are in fact considered a variant of the alpha rhythm. Greater amounts of random frontocentral theta activity are seen in children than in adults, but this decreases as the child ages. Brief runs of more sustained low-amplitude (15-μV) frontal 6- to 7-Hz waves are seen in as many as 35% of adolescents. This rhythm is present during quiet wakefulness with eyes open and may be related to affective arousal.

In the elderly, frequency of the alpha rhythm slows somewhat from a population mean of approximately 10.5 Hz to approximately 9 Hz. However, an alpha rhythm with a dominant frequency of less than 8 Hz is abnormal in adults. Focal temporal theta activity is seen in as many as 35% of asymptomatic individuals older than 50 years. Such activity is more commonly noted over the left temporal regions and should probably occupy no more than 5% of the tracing. Slower frequency or more persistent temporal slowing is considered abnormal by the authors. The exact point at which temporal slowing in the elderly can be considered unequivocally abnormal, however, remains controversial.[68-70]

Sleep Electroencephalography in Adults

The R&K standard scoring manual[27] divides sleep into four stages (see the American Academy of Sleep Medicine modification in Chapters 2 and 18). EEG findings in each of these stages are discussed in this section.

Drowsiness or *stage 1 NREM sleep (N1)* is used to designate the transition between wakefulness and stage 2 sleep and beyond. Stage 1 sleep is also briefly seen after arousals from other sleep stages and often transiently precedes and follows periods of REM sleep. Because this is a transitional sleep stage, it occupies a relatively small percentage of a normal night's sleep, generally less than 5%.[71]

A number of studies have emphasized the fact that EEG activity recorded during the transition between wakefulness and stage 2 NREM (N2) sleep is variable and complex. EEG and physiologic changes that are inconsistent with wakefulness clearly occur before stage 1 as defined in the R&K sleep scoring manual. Santamaria and Chiappa[28] identified several phases of drowsiness and more than 20 distinct EEG patterns in a careful study of 55 normal adults. The patterns of drowsiness varied in different subjects and varied in the same subject at different times.

An early phase was characterized by changes in the alpha rhythm that persisted throughout this phase. Alpha may shift from its characteristic parieto-occipital distribution to the frontocentral or temporal regions. Amplitude of alpha activity may either increase or decrease, and frequency of the alpha rhythm may slow. Slower theta and delta frequencies may be superimposed in the central or temporal regions. These may have a paroxysmal or sharpish character and be confused with epileptiform potentials. Paroxysmal theta bursts may predominate in one temporal region and be misinterpreted as the temporal sharp waves often associated with complex partial seizures. Criteria for distinguishing these benign potentials from genuine focal epileptiform discharges have been outlined.[72]

As the alpha rhythm disappears, bursts of frontocentral beta and generalized delta slowing may appear. Frankly paroxysmal but nonetheless benign patterns are occasionally seen in normal adults at this time as well. *Benign epileptiform transients of sleep* (BETS) are seen in 5–24% of normal subjects.[28,73] These are spiky, often diphasic transients with a broad field of distribution, usually involving both hemispheres. They typically shift from side to side and become less frequent during deeper sleep stages. Although BETS may superficially resemble epileptiform spikes, they are not associated with seizure disorders. White and coworkers[73] have outlined useful criteria distinguishing BETS from genuine epileptiform discharges. Less frequently, paroxysms of 6-Hz spike-and-wave discharge (Fig. 12–12) may be noted in either the frontal or temporal regions. The spike component usually has a relatively low amplitude, whereas the following slow wave is more prominent. Paroxysms of such activity rarely last longer than 3 seconds,[74] have an evanescent quality, and are less common during deeper sleep. Despite their paroxysmal quality, they are not associated with seizures either.[74]

Eventually, the alpha rhythm disappears altogether. *Vertex waves* are now frequently present. These are high-voltage sharp transients, surface negative, followed by a lower voltage, surface-positive component. They have maximal voltage at the Cz electrode. Mild asymmetry between the two hemispheres and extension of the field to Fz, or less frequently Pz, is not uncommon. Vertex waves occur spontaneously or in response to stimuli that are insufficient to fully arouse the subject. *Positive occipital sharp waves of sleep* (POSTS) appear in post–transitional stage 1, although these potentials are more common in deeper sleep stages (Fig. 12–13). These are diphasic or triphasic sharp waves with a predominant positive phase at the occipital electrodes. They have a triangular appearance similar to lambda waves. POSTS are noted synchronously over the two hemispheres and may occur singly or in runs. Occasional shifting amplitude asymmetry is noted in normal controls; however, persistent significant asymmetry should raise suspicion of a posterior lesion. Because these potentials have a paroxysmal sharpish appearance, they may be confused with epileptiform discharges.

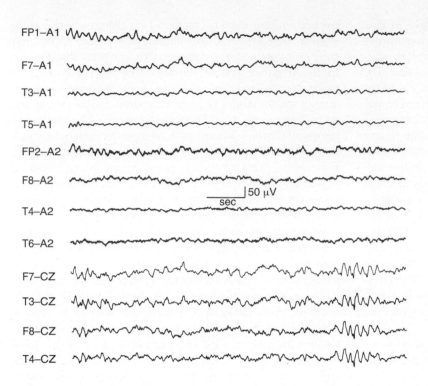

FIGURE 12–12 Spike-and-wave discharge of 6 Hz (phantom spike and wave) seen in the last 4 channels.

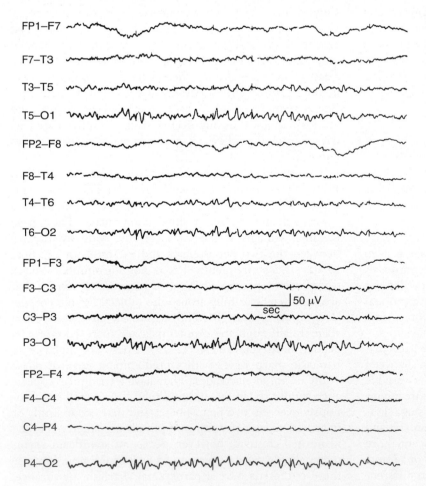

FIGURE 12–13 Positive occipital sharp transients (T5-O1, T6-O2, P3-O1, P4-O2 channels) during stage 1 NREM sleep.

To summarize, drowsiness, or stage 1 (N1), is a transitional state with many shifting and variable EEG patterns. Some of these resemble abnormal patterns, and determining whether an individual potential is normal may be difficult with the limited EEG montages typically used in PSG. It is important not to overinterpret. If there is uncertainty, routine EEG with a full complement of electrodes and multiple montages often clarifies the issue.

The R&K standard sleep scoring manual defines *stage 2 NREM sleep (N2)* by the presence of sleep spindles of at least 0.5-second duration or K complexes, as well as the absence of the features of slow-wave sleep (N3). Stage 2 sleep (see Fig. 2–3) comprises the bulk of a normal night's sleep (approximately 50% in normal adults).[71] Sleep spindles consist of a sequence of 12- to 14-Hz sinusoidal waves typically lasting a second or more. Voltage is usually maximal over the central regions. There is a high degree of symmetry and synchrony between the two hemispheres in normal subjects older than 1 year. Some investigators have proposed a classification of spindles based on topography and frequency,[64,75,76] but it is not clear that this has clinical utility at this time.

K complexes have been defined differently by sleep disorder specialists and electroencephalographers, which may confuse those trained in both disciplines. The R&K sleep scoring manual[27] defines the K complex as a well-delineated negative sharp wave followed by a positive component. The K complex must exceed 0.5 seconds in duration and may or may not be accompanied by sleep spindles. Vertex waves are not specifically defined in the manual or the sleep disorders glossary of terms.[77] Most polysomnographers accept that vertex waves have a duration of less than 0.5 seconds and distinguish vertex waves from K complexes on the basis of duration, although this may be difficult at the slow paper speeds often used. This distinction is important when scoring sleep because K complexes, even without spindles, are sufficient for scoring stage 2 sleep, whereas vertex waves alone do not allow the scoring of stage 2 sleep. Glossaries of EEG terminology,[78] in contrast, insist that K complexes always have associated sleep spindles and do not specify a duration.

The EEG in *stages 3 and 4 NREM sleep (N3)* (see Figs. 2–4 and 2–5) is marked by high-amplitude slow waves. The R&K sleep scoring manual[27] requires that more than 20% of any epoch be occupied by slow waves slower than 2 Hz and greater than 75 μV for stage 3 and that more than 50% of any epoch be occupied by slow waves with these characteristics for stage 4. Computerized analyses indicate that sleep spindles, vertex waves, and POSTS[79,80] are abundant in stages 3 and 4, although they may be less discernible to the interpreter's eye because of the abundant slow activity.

During *REM sleep* (see Fig. 2–6), the background EEG is characterized by low-voltage, mixed-frequency activity similar to early stage 1. Alpha frequencies are often present and may be more persistent than in stage 1. The alpha frequencies are usually 1–2 Hz less than the subject's waking rhythm.[81] Vertex waves, sleep spindles, and K complexes are absent. Characteristic *sawtooth waves* are frequently recorded. These are 2- to 3-Hz sharply contoured triangular waves, usually occurring serially for several seconds with highest amplitude over the Cz and Fz electrodes. A series of sawtooth waves typically precedes a burst of REM.[82,83] REM sleep occupies 20–25% of a night's sleep in a normal subject.[71] Brief periods of stage 1 sleep typically precede and follow a period of REM sleep. Detailed rules for demarcating onset and termination of REM sleep in these and other circumstances have been outlined in the R&K sleep scoring manual.[27]

Various *atypical PSG patterns* have been described. These usually occur in various sleep pathologies or when sleep has been significantly disrupted in normal individuals. *Alpha-delta sleep* (see Fig. 33–1) is characterized by persistence of alpha activity during stages 3 and 4. Excessive alpha intrusion may be seen in stage 2 as well, and the abundance of spindles appears to be decreased. This pattern appears to be associated with nonrestorative sleep and is seen in a variety of conditions.[84,85] It may signal the fibromyalgia syndrome. Moldovsky and Scarisbrick[86] have elicited this EEG pattern in normal subjects by selectively depriving them of stage 4 sleep. Deprivation of stage 4 sleep also elicited complaints of diffuse arthralgias, myalgias, and fatigability, similar to the complaints of the fibromyalgia syndrome. *REM-spindle sleep* (Fig. 12–14) is characterized by the intrusion of sleep spindles into portions of the PSG that otherwise meet all criteria for REM sleep. This pattern may be seen in 1–7% of normal subjects[87] but is more common when sleep is disrupted and after the first night of continuous positive airway pressure treatment. Broughton[88] reviewed other atypical patterns that occasionally occur during REM sleep.

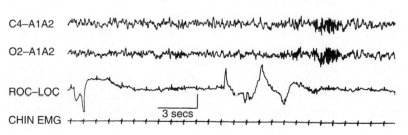

C4–A1A2

O2–A1A2

ROC–LOC

CHIN EMG

3 secs

FIGURE 12–14 REM-spindle sleep. Note intrusion of sleep spindles in the EEG channels of a portion of a polysomnography that meet all criteria for REM sleep. REM is present in the eye channel—outer canthus of the right and left eye (ROC-LOC)—and atonia in the chin electromyography (CHIN EMG). Calibration (*vertical bar*) is 50 μV for the top 3 channels and 20 μV for the bottom channel.

Normal Sleep Electroencephalography in Pediatrics

The transition from neonatal to infantile EEG sleep patterns occurs between 1 and 3 months. Even after this period, there is a great deal of change in the EEG patterns until the adult patterns are reached. The major points are emphasized in the following paragraphs; the reader is referred elsewhere for more detailed discussion (see also Chapters 2 and 38).[65–67,89]

Drowsiness in the pediatric age group differs from the adult patterns in several ways. Before 8 months of age, drowsiness is marked by a progressive slowing of EEG frequencies until delta waves predominate. After 8 months, the onset of drowsiness is marked by long runs of continuous, generalized, high-voltage, rhythmic theta or delta rhythms that have been called *hypnagogic hypersynchrony*. Three types have been described in normal subjects.[66,67,89] In the most common type, the rhythmic slow waves have highest amplitude in the frontal and central regions. The continuous rhythmic slowing may persist for several minutes. Less commonly, amplitude is highest in the parieto-occipital regions. Finally, a paroxysmal type occurs in approximately 10% of normal children. With this pattern, the alpha rhythm is gradually replaced by mixed frequencies. Diffuse bursts of 2- to 5-Hz slow waves, a few seconds in duration, then appear intermittently. Occasionally, random, poorly developed, sharpish waveforms are noted amid the slow waves. These may be random, superimposed alpha transients and should not be confused with epileptiform spike-and-wave discharge. The first two types of hypnagogic hypersynchrony are rarely recorded after age 10. The paroxysmal type persists into the mid-teens or, rarely, into adulthood.[66,67] In infancy and early childhood, 20- to 25-Hz beta activity is also a prominent feature of drowsiness. The beta rhythm may have maximum voltage anteriorly or posteriorly or have a diffuse distribution. The amplitude may reach 60 μV. This pattern appears at 6 months and is seen most frequently from 12 to 18 months. Prevalence decreases subsequently, and prominent beta activity during drowsiness is rarely seen after 7 years.[89]

Vertex waves and K complexes appear at age 6 months. These potentials are rather blunt and may reach amplitudes exceeding 200 μV in infancy and early childhood. By age 5, both vertex waves and K complexes have an increasingly spiky configuration. Mild asymmetry is quite common. They may occur repetitively in brief bursts.

Sleep spindles appear at approximately 3 months of age. Between 3 and 9 months of age, spindles occur in wicket-like trains often exceeding several seconds. These potentials are common at this age, often occupying as much as 15% of stage 2 (N2) sleep. Asynchrony between the hemispheres is the rule, with only half of the trains demonstrating interhemispheric synchrony at 6 months.[90,91] Interhemispheric synchrony increases to 70% by 12 months, and the duration and frequency of the spindle bursts gradually decrease. By 2 years of age, virtually all spindle trains are synchronous; however, spindles are much less frequent, occupying only 0.5% of stage 2 sleep.[90,91] Spindles remain infrequent until approximately 5 years of age.[91]

Stages 3 and 4 (N3) sleep are marked by high-amplitude, slow activity, as in adults. However, amplitude of the slow activity is usually higher. An occipitofrontal gradient is often present, with the very-high-amplitude, slower frequencies predominating posteriorly and lower amplitude, faster frequencies predominating anteriorly.[92] This gradient becomes less striking with age, so that by 5 years, the slow waves are distributed more diffusely.

The EEG during REM sleep in infants and children is characterized by a greater amount of slow activity than is seen in adults. The mature desynchronized EEG with scattered alpha rhythms emerges during the mid-teens.[93] The percentage of a normal night's sleep occupied by REM gradually decreases from 40% at ages 3–5 months to 30% at ages 12–24 months and then gradually assumes adult values after puberty.[94] REM onset latency gradually lengthens over the first year of life as well.

Abnormal Electroencephalographs

Many abnormal EEG patterns have been described. Only frequently encountered abnormalities are discussed in this section. *Diffuse slowing of background activity* (Fig. 12–15) is probably the most commonly recorded EEG abnormality. It can take several forms. One may see slowing of the parieto-occipital, alpha-type rhythm to a frequency below that allowable for the patient's age. Alternatively, frequency of the alpha-type rhythm may be normal but excessive, and diffuse theta and delta activity may be recorded. Finally, one may see both a slowing of the alpha-type rhythm and excessive, diffuse slower frequencies. Before concluding that an EEG has excessive slowing of background frequencies, the polysomnographer must consider the patient's age and state of alertness. More diffuse theta activity is seen in normal children than is acceptable for adults. Frequency of background rhythms must be assessed while the patient is clearly awake. As noted earlier, both slowing of alpha-type rhythms and diffuse slower frequencies are commonly found in drowsiness in normal subjects. Consequently, the polysomnographer must be certain that the background frequencies are slow during wakefulness. Unfortunately, diffuse slowing of background frequencies is a very nonspecific pattern. It is commonly interpreted as being consistent with a variety of diffuse encephalopathies, including toxic, metabolic, and degenerative encephalopathies, among others.

Focal slowing (Fig. 12–16) means that slow frequencies predominate over one region of the brain. Electrocerebral activity elsewhere is normal, or generalized slowing is

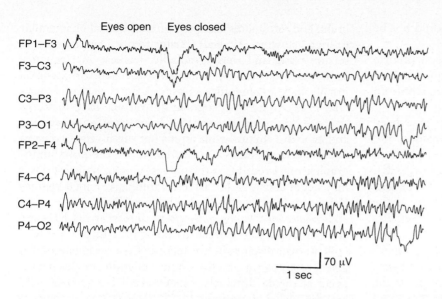

Eyes open   Eyes closed

FP1–F3
F3–C3
C3–P3
P3–O1
FP2–F4
F4–C4
C4–P4
P4–O2

70 µV

1 sec

FIGURE 12–15 Diffuse slowing in a 67-year-old patient with dementia. Activity of 6–7 Hz predominates over the parieto-occipital regions. Although it is reactive to eye closure, the frequency of this rhythm is abnormally slow. Calibration: vertical bar = 70 µV, horizontal bar = 1 sec. *(Reproduced with permission from Emerson RE, Walczak TS, Pedley TA. EEG and evoked potentials. In LP Rowland [ed], Merritt's Textbook of Neurology. Philadelphia: Lippincott Williams & Wilkins, 2000:64.)*

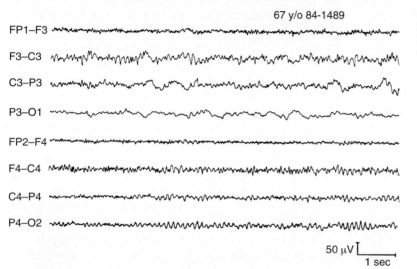

67 y/o 84-1489

FP1–F3
F3–C3
C3–P3
P3–O1
FP2–F4
F4–C4
C4–P4
P4–O2

50 µV

1 sec

FIGURE 12–16 Focal left hemispheric slowing in a 67-year-old (y/o) patient with a large left hemispheric infarction. Left hemispheric alpha rhythm is also attenuated. *(Courtesy of Dr. Timothy Pedley.)*

present but is relatively mild. In experimental models, focal slowing is produced by focal white matter lesions, even when the cerebral cortex remains intact.[95] Focal cerebral lesions often involve both white matter and cortex, however, so the usefulness of this distinction is blurred in practice. A structural lesion must always be suspected when persistent focal slowing is recorded. Not all patients with focal slowing, however, will have neuroradiologically demonstrable lesions.[96] Patients with transient ischemic attacks or focal epilepsy often have focal EEG slowing even when complete neuroimaging evaluations are normal. In epilepsy patients, this slowing may be due to ongoing local inhibitory phenomena or may be a transient postictal finding.

Focal attenuation of background rhythms means that frequencies in one region of the brain have significantly lower amplitude than elsewhere. In experimental models, focal attenuation of background is produced when the gray matter is lesioned and the underlying white matter remains intact.[95] Consequently, focal attenuation is often

interpreted as indicating focal cortical dysfunction. In practice, attenuation of background frequencies is usually seen in combination with focal slowing (see Fig. 12–16). Neuroradiologic investigations usually reveal large lesions involving both cortex and white matter.[97,98] Any fluid collection between the cortex and the recording electrode attenuates the recorded EEG activity. Thus, subdural fluid collections and subgaleal hematomas may result in a focal attenuation of background, although the cortex may not be damaged.

The detection of *epileptiform discharges* is important because these potentials have close association with epilepsy. Pedley[99] suggested that an epileptiform discharge should meet several criteria:

1. It must be paroxysmal, which means that it must clearly stand out from the background.
2. An epileptiform discharge must be spiky, which means that the transition from ascending to descending phase is abrupt and the duration of the discharge is short (by convention, 200 msec).

3. It must have a clear field—that is, it should not be confined to one electrode.
4. It should have negative polarity, because epileptiform discharges with positive polarity are uncommon.*
5. Finally, a slow wave often follows an epileptiform discharge.

Several varieties of epileptiform discharges have been described and associated with epilepsy syndromes.[99,100] A basic distinction is made between generalized and focal epileptiform discharges. Generalized epileptiform discharges indicate that the patient's seizure is likely to start simultaneously throughout the brain. An example is the generalized 3-Hz spike-and-wave discharge (see Fig. 30–2) that is characteristic of petit mal absence seizures. Focal epileptiform discharges indicate that the patient's seizure is likely to start in a restricted area of the brain, although it may subsequently spread. An example is the anterior temporal sharp wave that is characteristic of complex partial seizures of temporal lobe origin (Fig. 12–17). This is an important distinction because the treatment and prognosis in these two epilepsy syndromes are very different.[100] Approximately 90% of adults with epileptiform discharges will have a history of seizures,[101,102] and incidental epileptiform discharges are very uncommon in normal adults.[103] The association of epileptiform discharges with seizures in the pediatric age group is not as strong and varies with patient age and type of epileptiform discharge.[104]

The polysomnographer must be able to recognize *electrographic seizures* (see Fig. 30–10). These may occur in patients with epilepsy or in patients with sleep apnea during severe hypoxia. The EEG patterns associated with seizures are extremely variable. In general, an electrographic seizure has abrupt onset, has sustained and rhythmic evolution of frequencies, spreads to contiguous areas of the brain, and terminates abruptly, often followed by irregular postictal slowing. Typically, faster frequencies are seen at seizure onset and these gradually decrease in frequency as the seizure continues. Seizures associated with hypoxia usually have a generalized onset. A good deal of experience is necessary to recognize the various EEG patterns that can occur during a seizure. In practice, any sustained and evolving rhythm with an abrupt onset raises concern about electrographic seizures. However, the polysomnographer must recall that drowsiness and arousal responses may begin abruptly and have rhythmic, sustained characteristics as well, especially in children.

Periodic lateralizing epileptiform discharges (PLED) are another important pattern to recognize. In this pattern, epileptiform discharges are recorded continuously over a given region (Fig. 12–18). The epileptiform discharges occur at regular intervals, usually every 1–2 seconds, and are thus labeled periodic.[105,106] Background activity is usually significantly attenuated on the side with the discharges, and excessive slow frequencies are often seen bilaterally.[105,106] This pattern is usually associated with an acute focal cerebral insult. In a review of 586 cases reported in the literature,[107] 35% were related to an acute cerebral infarction, 26% to other sorts of mass lesions, and the remainder to infection, anoxia, or other causes. Clinically, PLED is associated with obtundation, seizures, and focal neurologic deficits. Seventy to 90% of patients with PLED have seizures during the acute stage of their illness.[105–107] Twenty-five to 40% of patients with this pattern die in the hospital or shortly after discharge. Mortality may be especially high in patients with acute stroke and PLED.[105,106,108] PLED is almost always a transient phenomenon. The discharges become less frequent and lower in amplitude over the 2 weeks after the acute insult and are gradually replaced by focal delta slowing.[109]

Polysomnography typically does not utilize a full complement of scalp electrodes because the major clinical issue is scoring of sleep stages rather than detection of electrocerebral abnormalities. Distinguishing EEG abnormalities

---

*Positive rolandic sharp waves are occasionally recorded in premature infants with intraventricular hemorrhage or periventricular leukomalacia. Otherwise, positive sharp waves are very uncommon in older patients.

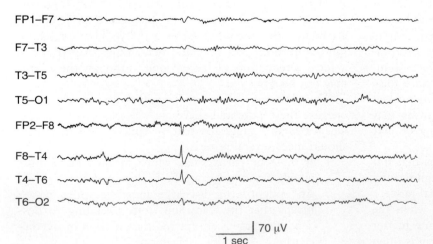

FIGURE 12–17 Right temporal interictal epileptiform discharge in a 32-year-old patient with complex partial seizures. Calibration: vertical bar = 70 μV, horizontal bar = 1 sec. (*Reproduced with permission from Emerson RE, Walczak TS, Pedley TA. EEG and evoked potentials. In LP Rowland [ed], Merritt's Textbook of Neurology. Philadelphia: Lippincott Williams & Wilkins, 2000:64.*)

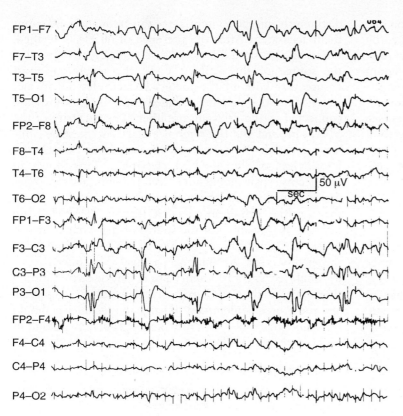

FIGURE 12-18 Periodic lateralized epileptiform discharges at a rate of 0.8/sec arising from the left parietal and posterior temporal regions (P3, T5) in a 72-year-old woman with a history of confusion and falling episodes.

such as persistent focal slowing may be difficult if only a few electrodes are devoted to EEG. Nonetheless, the polysomnographer should be thoroughly familiar with common EEG abnormalities. Suspicious activity should prompt re-montaging and further examination. If this is unrevealing and suspicions remain high, routine EEG with a full complement of electrodes should be performed.

Artifacts

The polygraph is designed to record the relatively small voltages generated by the human brain, muscles, eyes, and heart. Unfortunately, the remainder of the human body and the surrounding environment are not electrically silent. These generate abundant electrical activity that may obscure the biological signals of interest. This extraneous electrical activity is called *artifact* (see also Chapter 11).[2-5] Making the distinction between the signal of interest and artifact is a central task for the polysomnographer, and the task is most difficult when interpreting an EEG. Because high sensitivities are required to record the relatively low voltages generated by the brain, extraneous voltage sources are especially likely to contaminate the EEG recording.

Four sources of artifact exist: (1) irrelevant physiologic signals, (2) environmental signals, (3) aberrant signals due to faulty or improperly applied electrodes, and (4) aberrant signals produced by the polygraph. More than one of these sources can contribute to a particular artifact. The following discussion summarizes frequently encountered artifacts and is by no means exhaustive.

Irrelevant Physiologic Signals

Irrelevant signals may contaminate recording of biological signals of interest, especially EEGs. *Myogenic potentials* originating from scalp muscles may obscure EEG recording (see Figs. 11-9 and 11-11). Myogenic activity may be difficult to distinguish from electrocerebral activity in the beta frequency range, especially at slow paper speeds. It may obscure lower amplitude electrocerebral activity.

Head movement also causes artifacts, frequencies of which are usually in the delta range (see Fig. 11-13). These artifacts are due to changes in electrode impedance, together with spurious static and capacitative potentials. Head movement artifacts are induced by slight movement of the electrodes on the scalp and the swaying of wires. The head movements associated with respiration often elicit movement artifact on the EEG, especially when the patient is lying on the recording electrodes. Correlating the spurious delta waves on the EEG with a respiratory monitor establishes their artifactual source. This may be important because these spurious potentials should not be used to score slow-wave sleep.

Sweating may result in very slow frequencies and changes in baseline, especially when direct current amplifiers are used in the polygraph. The salt content of sweat changes the ionic composition of the conducting gel, resulting in this particular artifact. Potentials that arise from the sweat glands also play a role. Sweating may be asymmetric, and the resulting EEG asymmetry may mislead the interpreter.

Pulse artifact occurs when an electrode is placed on one of the scalp arteries. The electrode movement caused by the pulsations produces a delta wave. The regular relationship of the delta wave to the electrocardiogram (ECG) indicates the extracerebral origin of this activity.

The electrical fields generated by *ECG* and eye movements are commonly recorded from scalp electrodes (see Fig. 11–10) and may be confused with electrocerebral activity. Again, referring to the channels that are recording ECG and eye movements demonstrates whether suspicious activity recorded at the scalp is caused by these extracerebral sources.

Environmental Signals

The hospital environment contains many sources of electrical signals that may mimic electrocerebral or other physiologic activity. The *circulation of moistened air* through a respirator tube may induce bursts of alpha or theta frequencies at scalp electrodes. The electrostatic charges on drops entering an intravenous cannula—*intravenous drop artifacts*—may cause periodic spike-like artifacts. *Intravenous infusion pumps* can cause bursts of spiky transients followed by slower components. These artifacts are thought to be due to electromagnetic (rather than electrostatic) sources. *Telephones and pager systems* are among the other potential sources of environmental artifacts. The interpreter relies on the technician to correlate unusual recorded potentials with specific events in the environment, thereby establishing the artifactual nature of the potentials.

Sixty-hertz electromagnetic radiation due to alternating current in power lines is ubiquitous in the hospital environment and may contaminate the recording (in Europe, mains frequency is 50 Hz). The resulting 60-Hz artifact may be impossible to distinguish from myogenic activity at the slow paper speeds commonly used for PSG. The presence of this artifact in EMG leads may persuade the interpreter that tonic EMG activity is at a high level when it is actually low. The 60-Hz artifact is verified when 60 cycles are counted in 1 second of recording. Usually, paper speed must be increased to at least 60 mm/sec to distinguish adjacent potentials of this frequency and count them accurately. After the presence of 60 Hz is verified, the technician should proceed systematically to determine the source of the artifact. First, the technician must ensure that both of the involved electrodes are in fact attached to the patient, plugged into the jackbox, and connected to the relevant amplifier. The integrity of the patient ground and the reference electrode must be similarly ensured. Next, the technician should check the impedances of the involved electrodes. Impedances in any electrode pair should not exceed 10 kohm, and the impedances of the two electrodes should be roughly equal. Only then can the technician conclude that the electrode-scalp interface is probably not the source of the artifact. At this point, the technician should search for 60-Hz sources in the environment. A "dummy patient," consisting of two leads shorted with a 10-kohm resister, may be carried around the room until the 60-Hz artifact reaches maximal amplitude and the source is identified. Finally, the technician should remember that faults with instrument ground may result in 60-Hz activity as well.

Aberrant Signals from Faulty Electrodes

Improperly applied electrodes or electrode faults may result in other sorts of artifact.

Electrode "pops" are the most common electrode artifact. These are abrupt vertical transients (Fig. 12–19), usually of positive polarity, that are confined to one electrode. They are superimposed on but do not modify ongoing recording. Pops are due to abrupt changes in impedance and usually indicate either that the electrode is not securely attached or that electrolyte gel is insufficient. When confronted with a popping electrode, the technician should reset the electrode and apply more gel. If popping persists, the electrode needs to be changed. Occasionally the electrode impedances change more gradually, mimicking slow activity. Again, the observation that the slow activity is confined to one electrode indicates that the electrode, rather than the body, is the source of the potential.

Other electrode faults may result in artifact even if the electrode-scalp interface is intact. An interruption in the

FIGURE 12–19 Electrode pops at P3 electrode.

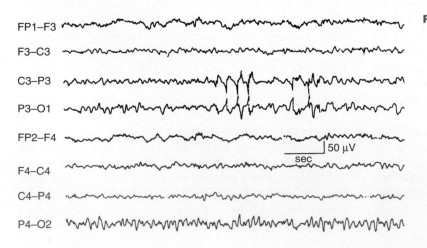

plating of the electrode may result in battery potentials, which can appear as bizarre, high-amplitude discharges confined to the faulty electrode. A similar artifact may occur when electrode gel connects the disk electrode and the wire lead, which are usually made of different metals.

Aberrant Signals from the Polygraph

Finally, the polygraph can be a source of artifact. Random fluctuation of charges in any complicated recording instrument results in some spurious output. In contemporary digital equipment, this *instrument noise* is infrequent and has low amplitude. It should not contaminate recording at standard sensitivities but may occasionally appear when sensitivities greater than 2 μV/mm are required.

Corrosion or loosening of contacts in switches or wires may cause abrupt changes in voltage or sudden loss of signal. The nonphysiologic nature of such potentials is usually readily apparent, but finding the source in the instrument may be difficult, especially if the artifact is intermittent. Again these issues are rare in digital polygraphs.

A meticulous, alert, and experienced technician is the first and best defense against artifact. The critical importance of properly applied and gelled electrodes cannot be overemphasized for PSG, because adjusting or changing electrodes usually means waking the patient. The technician should be on the lookout for bizarre potentials and seek to determine whether these are physiologic or artifactual. Observation of the patient and environment, correlations with the recorded activity, and careful documentation are critical. The technician must then decide whether the artifact significantly interferes with recording of the signal of interest. Deciding whether to change an electrode and possibly wake the patient, or allow a partially interpretable recording to continue, requires seasoned judgment. Technicians should be aware of the major issues involved in interpreting a PSG so they can make these on-the-spot decisions wisely.

CONCLUSION

The interpretation of a PSG can be considered a pattern-recognition task. The EEG is the most complicated and variable recording the polysomnographer interprets. Several issues continuously preoccupy the polysomnographer when interpreting the EEG. One question is whether the recorded signal is a true cerebral potential or whether it represents artifact. Another is whether the signal is present throughout the scalp or whether it is confined to a single region of the scalp. The use of multiple channels for EEG recording allows the polysomnographer to answer these questions with greater certainty. Unfortunately, even in today's digital environment, EEG recorded during routine PSG is often limited to a few channels. Limited montages and slow paper speeds often do not allow confident interpretation of unusual activity. This is especially unfortunate because EEG abnormalities important to the patient's care are more likely to occur during the longer PSG recordings than during routine EEG. The cost of a few additional EEG channels is more than repaid by the greater certainty in interpretation and the greater likelihood that important abnormalities will be found. Sometimes a confident decision regarding the nature of suspicious potentials cannot be made, even when several EEG channels are available. It is important not to overinterpret suspicious events. The polysomnographer should not be afraid to admit uncertainty in a situation in which data are insufficient. Referral for routine sleep EEG is usually appropriate in these circumstances. The full complement of scalp EEG channels often provides the necessary information. Similarly, information from additional EMG and EOG channels often clarify ambiguities. Equivocal changes are often interpreted more confidently when more data are available.

⊗ REFERENCES

A full list of references are available at www.expertconsult.com

CHAPTER 13

Electrocardiographic Technology of Cardiac Arrhythmias

Daniel M. Shindler and **John B. Kostis**

A wealth of information is available about cardiac rate and rhythm disturbances during sleep. Twenty-four-hour ambulatory electrocardiography (ECG) has made it possible to study cardiac rhythm in both awake and sleeping subjects. For most practical purposes, it is possible to think about cardiac rhythm during sleep in the same way as during wakefulness, although the average heart rate is slower during sleep. As a result, escape-type arrhythmias may appear or become more frequent. One should first be familiar with the normal behavior of the heart and subsequently become familiar with a simple classification of cardiac arrhythmias.

NORMAL CARDIAC RHYTHM

The normal cardiac rhythm is defined as a normal sinus rhythm—that is, the cardiac rate is between 60 and 100 bpm and the cardiac impulse originates in the sinus node. This is best confirmed by identifying a normal-looking P wave that is followed by a normal and constant PR interval and is always succeeded by a single QRS complex. It is quite normal for cardiac cycle length (R–R interval) in a given patient to be somewhat variable. This is referred to as *sinus arrhythmia* (Fig. 13–1).[1–3] The heart rate of children and infants is faster than the heart rate of adults. The rate of the sinus node is influenced by the autonomic nervous system.

CARDIAC ARRHYTHMIAS

Arrhythmias are due to disturbances of impulse formation, impulse conduction, or a combination of the two. Arrhythmias can be separated into two large groups.

Those that originate in the sinus node, atria, or atrioventricular (AV) node are referred to as *supraventricular arrhythmias*; those that originate in the ventricles are classified as *ventricular arrhythmias*. Figures 13–2 to 13–18 illustrate a variety of cardiac arrhythmias.

Supraventricular Arrhythmias

When the QRS complex is narrow, the arrhythmia is, with few exceptions, supraventricular. Unfortunately, when the QRS complex is wide, it is often impossible to determine conclusively whether an arrhythmia is supraventricular or ventricular. Inspection of the ECG is the first step in evaluating an arrhythmia. If the arrhythmia is considered potentially life threatening, a specialized electrophysiologic study may be required to further assess its significance.

Sinus Tachycardia

The most common rhythm disturbance (which may not be abnormal), sinus tachycardia, is an acceleration of the sinus heart rate above 100 bpm.[4] In most cases sinus tachycardia does not exceed 180 bpm. Sinus tachycardia is best diagnosed by identifying P waves, determining that they are of normal morphology, subsequently establishing that the PR interval is normal and constant, and determining that each QRS complex is preceded by the P wave and each P wave is followed by a normal QRS. In the course of normal daily activity, the heart rate rises in a gradual fashion and subsides in a gradual fashion.[5] Sinus tachycardia can occur during rapid eye movement

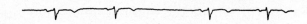

FIGURE 13–1 Normal sinus rhythm with sinus arrhythmia.

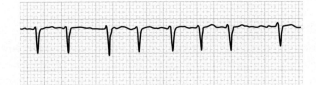

FIGURE 13–2 Atrial fibrillation.

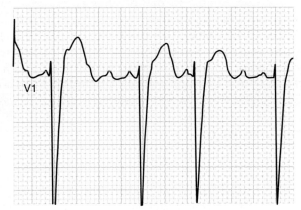

FIGURE 13–3 Atrial flutter with variable ventricular response.

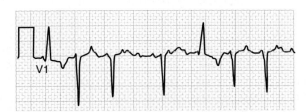

FIGURE 13–4 Atrial flutter. The first and fifth QRS complexes are aberrantly conducted.

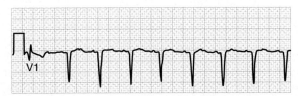

FIGURE 13–5 Atrial tachycardia with 2:1 block.

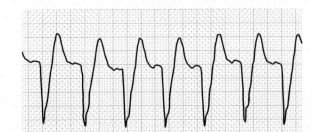

FIGURE 13–6 Undetermined wide-complex rhythm, rate 100 bpm.

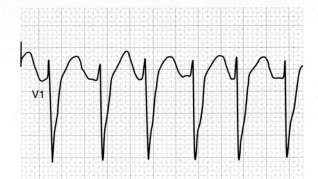

FIGURE 13–7 Undetermined wide-complex tachycardia, rate 145 bpm.

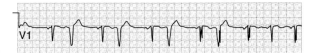

FIGURE 13–8 Ventricular tachycardia.

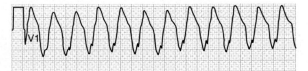

FIGURE 13–9 Normal sinus rhythm. Premature ventricular contractions in bigeminy.

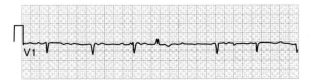

FIGURE 13–10 Atrial fibrillation. Premature ventricular contraction.

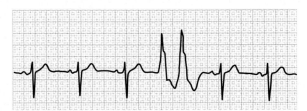

FIGURE 13–11 Normal sinus rhythm. Premature ventricular couplet.

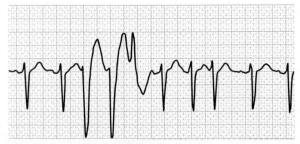

FIGURE 13–12 Normal sinus rhythm. Three-beat multifocal ventricular tachycardia salvo. The eighth QRS complex is a premature atrial contraction.

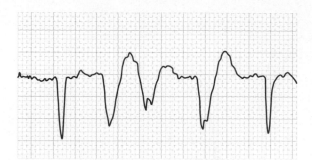

FIGURE 13–13 Three-beat ventricular salvo resembling baseline artifact. Artifacts do not have T waves.

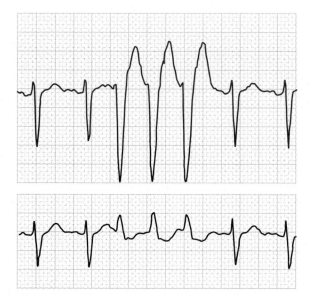

FIGURE 13–14 Three-beat ventricular salvo demonstrated in two simultaneous leads.

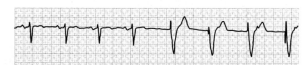

FIGURE 13–15 Sinus rhythm with a demand pacemaker taking over in the last 4 beats. Note the disappearance of P waves.

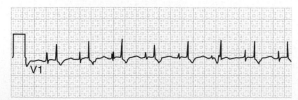

FIGURE 13–16 AV sequential pacemaker. The sixth QRS complex is a native nonpaced premature beat. The pacemaker is programmed to deliver a ventricular pacing spike anyway.

(REM) sleep. Yet, patients suffering from REM sleep behavior disorder can have violent body movements without an increase in the heart rate due to the absence of autonomic arousal.

Sinus Bradycardia

The opposite boundary of normal heart rate is sinus bradycardia. Sinus bradycardia is defined as a rate slower than 60 bpm.[6] Again, it is manifested by a normal P wave appearance; a normal and constant PR interval; and a normal relationship of the P wave to the QRS complex, with a 1:1 sequence similar to that of sinus tachycardia. One observational pitfall in the patient with sinus bradycardia is the fact that, at times, U waves become very prominent and can easily be confused with P waves. As a result, blocked premature atrial contractions can be misdiagnosed. Use of β blockers can slow the heart rate as well as cause nightmares and sleep disruption.

Sinus Arrhythmia

Sinus arrhythmia is especially easy to notice with slowing of the heart rate during sleep. The P-wave morphology usually does not change. If it does change, the changes are phasic and the P waves do not appear retrograde. There should be a 10% difference between the maximum and minimum cardiac cycle length. Atrioventricular conduction is normal. This is manifested as a PR interval greater than 120 msec. A shorter PR interval with an abnormal P wave would indicate that the beats are not of sinus origin. The variations in sinus cycle length may be phasic, with respiration becoming shorter with inspiration due to reflex inhibition of vagal tone. This form of sinus arrhythmia disappears with apnea.

Premature Atrial Contractions

Premature atrial contractions are observed frequently in normal subjects and patients with a variety of diseases. They are manifested as an interruption in the heart rhythm with a premature beat having a narrow QRS complex. Because the origin of the atrial impulse is ectopic, the appearance of the P wave is abnormal, denoting its abnormal early origin. There is quite a wide spectrum in the incidence and frequency of premature atrial contractions. Their nature is classified as follows: If the premature atrial contractions occur singly, they are classified according to their incidence per period of time. Therefore, an ambulatory ECG report commonly describes how many premature atrial contractions were observed in a given time, such as an hour, a minute, or 24 hours, according to how common they are. When premature atrial contractions are frequent, it is customary to further describe their nature (cyclic or noncyclic) and rate. For example, when premature atrial contractions occur cyclically, they may show a bigeminal pattern.

FIGURE 13–17 Aberrant conduction.

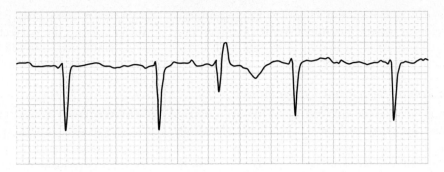

FIGURE 13–18 Torsades de pointes.

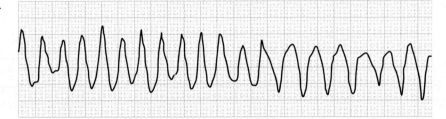

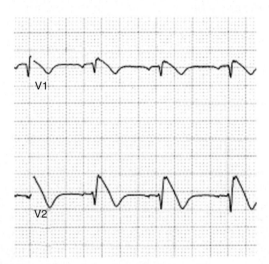

FIGURE 13–19 Brugada syndrome: leads V₁ and V₂ show an rSR′ QRS complex with ST-segment elevation in both leads.

Multifocal Atrial Tachycardia

A variant of frequent premature atrial contractions is tachycardia, which is called *multiform atrial tachycardia* or *chaotic atrial tachycardia*.[7] This is a rhythm disturbance with definite clinical significance. It is identified by an irregular heart rhythm with narrow QRS complexes and rates in excess of 100 bpm. As the name implies, it is multifocal: The atrial beats originate in multiple sites in the atria. Consequently, the appearance of the P waves varies with the point of origin. There is variability in both the P-wave morphology and the PR interval. Multifocal atrial tachycardia is an arrhythmia that may have significant consequences. It is particularly common in patients with significant lung disease. These same patients often suffer sleep disorders. When analyzing ECG recordings, multifocal atrial tachycardia should not be confused with atrial fibrillation.

Atrial Fibrillation

Atrial fibrillation is a very common rhythmic disturbance that is important to diagnose, as the initial heart rate can be quite fast and drug therapy (usually digitalis) may be required to slow it down. Patients with chronic atrial fibrillation are at increased risk for thromboembolic phenomena and are therefore often admitted to the hospital for further management when this rhythm is diagnosed.[8] The ECG hallmark of atrial fibrillation is a completely random and irregular heart rhythm with no reproducible R–R interval. Because the atria are fibrillating at a rate of 500 bpm, there are no P waves. The ECG baseline may appear irregular and erratic. This should not be confused with the variable P waves of chaotic atrial tachycardia or with U waves, as mentioned earlier. The ventricular rate in patients with atrial fibrillation tends to be fast when it first occurs. The rate may range around 150 bpm. A clue to underlying conduction system disease is a slow ventricular rate. In this case, caution needs to be exercised with therapeutic modalities, because therapy with an agent such as digitalis may produce undesirable AV conduction problems.[9,10]

Atrial Flutter

A variant of atrial fibrillation is a rhythm disturbance known as *atrial flutter*.[11] Atrial flutter differs in that atrial activity can be diagnosed as occurring 300 times per minute. At this rate, the ECG hallmark is a characteristic sawtooth pattern at a rate of 300 bpm. The usual presentation of atrial flutter is an atrial rate of 300 bpm with some degree of block between the atria and ventricles (the usual block is 2:1). Therefore, it is quite typical to recognize atrial flutter by the presence of a sawtooth baseline with a ventricular response of 150 bpm. The therapeutic goal in atrial flutter (similar to atrial fibrillation) is to slow down the ventricular response when it is fast. Again, caution is exercised when the initial ventricular response (with no medication) is an unduly slow rate with a conduction block of 4:1 or greater.

Automatic Versus Re-entrant Tachycardia

The rhythm disturbances referred to earlier are classified as automatic rhythm disturbances. If properly diagnosed, they can be classified as disorders of cardiac automaticity. The warmup phenomenon (gradual, nonabrupt increase in heart rate) is a hallmark of automatic tachycardia. Usually, an automatic tachycardia requires a search for its cause, which is then treated. For example, multifocal atrial tachycardia is typically seen in patients with lung disease, and improvement of hypoxemia often results in the return of the cardiac rhythm to normal. Sinus tachycardia frequently indicates a metabolic disturbance such as fever, thyrotoxicosis, or hypovolemia. Again, therapy of the cause is the proper approach rather than addressing the mechanism of the rhythm disturbance itself.[12,13] Conversely, a group of tachycardias referred to as *re-entrant* are treated by addressing the mechanism of re-entry. When this is corrected, the rhythm is restored to normal.

Paroxysmal Atrial Tachycardia

Paroxysmal atrial tachycardia is the classical re-entrant tachycardia treated with medications that interrupt the mechanism of re-entry.[14] As the name implies, a paroxysmal atrial tachycardia begins abruptly. There is no warmup phenomenon, and the heart rate instantly increases to between 140 and 180 bpm. It may cease spontaneously and, just as abruptly, return to sinus rhythm. It is quite common to observe these salvos of atrial tachycardia in patients, whether they are awake or asleep. When paroxysmal atrial tachycardia is persistent, it warrants treatment because of the unduly fast heart rate. Several maneuvers that increase vagal tone, such as a Valsalva maneuver or carotid sinus massage, can break the arrhythmia.[15] When these are ineffective, it becomes necessary to use medication. The calcium channel blocker verapamil is quite useful for this purpose. More recently adenosine, an agent that causes complete but very transient AV block, has emerged as the modality of choice.[16]

Sick Sinus Syndrome

Various combinations of tachycardia with bradycardia may suggest the diagnosis of sick sinus syndrome. Ambulatory ECG monitoring may be required to demonstrate the presence of sinus node dysfunction.[17–20]

Aberrant Supraventricular Conduction

A transient delay in intraventricular conduction can be seen in patients with supraventricular tachycardias. If the P waves are not clearly identifiable, the rhythm may be misdiagnosed as ventricular tachycardia (see *Ventricular Tachycardia* later). QRS complex morphology may be useful in making the correct diagnosis. The initial aberrant conduction occurs in the QRS complex, which terminates a short cardiac cycle immediately preceded by a long cardiac cycle.[21,22]

Ventricular Arrhythmias

The next group of rhythm disturbances, the ventricular arrhythmias, may be more hemodynamically significant and can be associated with clinically important heart disease. They can also be seen in normal patients.

Premature Ventricular Contractions

A very common rhythm disturbance often felt by patients is the premature ventricular contraction. It is most commonly an early beat that is easily recognized on the ECG as a wide QRS complex with abnormal repolarization.[23] The incidence on 24-hour ECG monitoring can be reported according to how often this finding is present; therefore, premature ventricular contractions are reported as occurring a certain number of times per hour. If rare, they are classified by how many times they occur in 24 hours; if very common, they may be classified in terms of occurrence per minute.[24]

Ventricular Bigeminy

A very common rhythm disturbance is a sustained rhythm, especially at night, consisting of an alternating normally conducted QRS complex with a premature ventricular contraction followed by a pause and a resumption of the sequence. This is referred to as *ventricular bigeminy*. It is benign for most practical purposes, but it has some clinical implications. For example, a clinician taking a pulse may notice only the normally conducted beats. The pulse deficit might then result in a mistaken diagnosis of bradycardia.

Ventricular Tachycardia

The finding of three or more premature ventricular contractions in a row (at a heart rate faster than 100 bpm) is referred to as *ventricular tachycardia*,[25] and it may be brief or sustained.[26] The most important distinction that needs to be made when ventricular tachycardia is suspected is the alternate diagnosis of supraventricular tachycardia with aberrant ventricular conduction. The diagnostic approach to this critical differential diagnosis is multifaceted. The diagnosis begins at the bedside. If the patient is hemodynamically decompensated, it is necessary to act rapidly.[27,28] Multiple ECG leads should be used to identify P waves that mark atrial activity. Atrial P waves that are unrelated to ventricular QRS complexes make ventricular tachycardia more likely than aberrant conduction. The appearance of the QRS complex has been useful in the recognition of a ventricular origin for tachycardia. Sustained ventricular tachycardia often degenerates into ventricular fibrillation, resulting in death.[29]

Ventricular Fibrillation

Ventricular fibrillation is a lethal terminal dysrhythmia that requires immediate electrical defibrillation.[11] There are no identifiable QRS complexes. It may begin on a T wave (this is referred to as *R on T*). It may also be seen in association with a unique ventricular tachyarrhythmia called *torsades de pointes*.

Torsades de Pointes

The morphology of torsades de pointes is unique. The points of the ventricular complexes vary in their height, appearing to turn around a central axis, the baseline of the ECG tracing. It is important to measure the QT interval. QT prolongation can be caused by electrolyte disturbances, antiarrhythmic drugs, or central nervous system or congenital disease.[30–34]

Accelerated Idioventricular Rhythm

The law of the heart states that the fastest pacemaker is the one that governs the heart. Accelerated idioventricular rhythm (AIVR) is a slow ventricular rhythm that captures the heart because the sinus rate is even slower. The rate of AIVR is less than 100 bpm. It is usually faster than the typical 40-bpm ventricular escape rate (thus the term *accelerated*). This is typically an escape rhythm that should not be suppressed with antiarrhythmic agents such as lidocaine. AIVR is often short lived and has no hemodynamic consequences. In this setting, it does not require treatment. When AIVR is sustained and hypotension is observed, an agent such as atropine may be useful in overdriving the AIVR by accelerating the sinus node. The ECG diagnosis of AIVR consists of establishing the ventricular origin of the rhythm.

Brugada Syndrome

Patients with a structurally normal heart may have syncopal episodes and/or sudden cardiac death due to Brugada syndrome. This genetically determined syndrome is rare. There may be a family history of sudden death. Ventricular fibrillation may occur during sleep and may be related to nighttime bradycardia.[35] The ECG hallmark of the Brugada syndrome is a combination of right bundle branch block and ST-segment elevation in leads V_1 to V_3 (Fig. 13–19). This diagnostic ECG pattern can be evanescent, and may not be present in patients at all times.

PACEMAKER RHYTHM

Pacemaker rhythms are identified by the pacemaker spike preceding the wide QRS complex. It is necessary to determine proper capture as well as proper sensing. Dual-chamber pacemakers are designed to restore the normal sequence of AV contraction. They are also associated with pacemaker-induced arrhythmias.[36] Some patients may have a pacemaker or defibrillator implanted to treat life-threatening ventricular arrhythmias.[37,38]

INTRACARDIAC RECORDINGS

Certain patients may be referred for electrophysiologic study to further evaluate their arrhythmia. The tracings obtained during those studies may demonstrate ECG information about the heart that is unobtainable from surface ECG studies. It is possible to record the electrical activity of the bundle of His. This may help decide which patients require a permanent pacemaker. The sinus node recovery time can be measured in patients with sick sinus syndrome. Ventricular arrhythmias can be induced to assess efficacy of antiarrhythmic therapy.[39]

SIGNAL-AVERAGED ELECTROCARDIOGRAM

It is possible to amplify the ECG complex by as much as 1000 times with the use of signal averaging. The signal-averaged ECG can demonstrate the presence of late potentials (high-frequency, low-amplitude signals). Their absence is associated with a more favorable prognosis after myocardial infarction.

MANAGEMENT OF ARRHYTHMIAS DETECTED DURING SLEEP

The sophisticated monitoring equipment available today permits detection of cardiac arrhythmias and conduction disturbances as they occur during sleep. Sustained ventricular arrhythmias require immediate attention. The patient needs to be awakened, and blood pressure and mental status must be determined. If the ventricular arrhythmia causes hypotension or the patient is unarousable, emergency measures may be required, but this is extremely rare. Nonsustained ventricular arrhythmias are a more common finding. Typically, by the time the patient is aroused, blood pressure is normal. The patient needs to be monitored, however, for recurrence of the arrhythmia. Conduction disturbances can also be detected. Sinus arrest is manifested by the disappearance of P waves and an area other than the sinus node taking over the cardiac rhythm. This can be a junctional, ectopic atrial, or ventricular rhythm. It is important to ascertain by ECG whether arrhythmias are, as mentioned, sustained or nonsustained. It is also worthwhile to determine whether a newly detected rhythm disturbance is a consequence of a conduction abnormality followed by an escape mechanism, rather than a premature mechanism for arrhythmia initiation such as a premature ventricular contraction. The hemodynamics, as measured by blood pressure, are the most important indicators of the significance of an arrhythmia as it is occurring. It is also important to take into account the underlying cardiac status of the particular patient in whom the arrhythmia is observed.

✪ REFERENCES

A full list of references are available at www.expertconsult.com

CHAPTER 14

Evaluation and Monitoring of Respiratory Function

Reena Mehra and **Kingman P. Strohl**

INTRODUCTION

As a high proportion of patients referred to the sleep clinic are evaluated for the possibility of sleep-disordered breathing (SDB), it is very important to perform a comprehensive assessment of the patient's baseline pulmonary status by obtaining a thorough medical history and performing a complete physical examination geared toward pulmonary-based issues. Medical history should focus particularly on symptoms including dyspnea with exertion or at rest, cough, sputum production, stridor, and wheezing; smoking history/illicit drug use; occupational exposures; and family history of pulmonary disorders/sleep apnea. Physical examination should include an assessment of the airway (Mallampati classification, tonsillar hypertrophy, retrognathia, micrognathia, thyromegaly), lung auscultation (including with forced expiration) and percussion, evaluation of clubbing/cyanosis, upright to supine nasality of voice, and the like. If clinical suspicion of impaired pulmonary function is suspected based on initial evaluation, then testing to assess the type and severity of limitation is warranted.

The American Academy of Sleep Medicine (AASM) *International Classification of Sleep Disorders: Diagnostic & Coding Manual* outlines criteria and definitions for sleep-related hypoventilation and hypoxemic syndromes, including sleep-related nonobstructive alveolar hypoventilation, sleep-related hypoventilation/hypoxemia due to pulmonary parenchymal or vascular pathology, sleep-related hypoxemia due to lower airways obstruction, and sleep-related hypoxemia/hypoventilation due to neuromuscular and chest wall disorders.[1] The diagnostic criteria for these disorders incorporate the degree of hypoxia as ascertained from oxygen saturation monitoring during polysomnography (PSG), and hypercapnia determined by carbon dioxide level based on arterial blood gas measurements obtained during sleep, thereby highlighting the need to understand respiratory monitoring methods and techniques. This chapter focuses upon specific aspects of diagnostic testing performed in the evaluation of pulmonary disease that may be of concern in the context of SDB assessment, and also reviews facets of respiratory monitoring performed during polysomnographic appraisal of sleep disorders.

EVALUATION OF BASELINE PULMONARY FUNCTION AND PHYSIOLOGY

Although the testing discussed in this section is not warranted in the routine evaluation of sleep disorders, if a provocative history of baseline pulmonary abnormality is elicited in the context of a sleep disorder evaluation, then further pulmonary disorder diagnostic workup is indicated.

Radiographic Testing

Static and dynamic imaging studies both have roles in investigating the structure and function of the upper airway during wakefulness and sleep. These studies have demonstrated the role of not only the tongue and soft palate, but also of the lateral pharyngeal walls, in exerting alterations in upper airway shape and caliber. Upper airway imaging has also been used to elucidate changes in upper airway anatomy occurring in the context of weight loss, oral appliances, and upper airway surgery. In patients undergoing upper airway surgery, and potentially in those being fitted for oral appliances, upper airway imaging or cephalometrics should be considered.[2]

Radiographic assessment of the lung fields may be helpful in the context of a concerning cardiopulmonary or smoking history to identify concomitant disorders that may play a role in exacerbating pathophysiologic consequences of SDB. Radiographic review of enlarged pulmonary arteries, reticulonodular densities, emphysematous changes, lung mass, mediastinal lymphadenopathy, and interstitial/alveolar processes can be done.

Spirometry/Pulmonary Function Testing

Spirometry

Pulmonary function testing allows for the ascertainment of lung physiology and mechanics. Spirometry with flow-volume loops assesses the mechanical properties of the respiratory system by measuring expiratory volumes and flow rates. This test requires the patient to make a maximal inspiratory and expiratory effort. The patient, in a sitting position, breathes into a mouthpiece, and nose clips are placed to prevent air leak. At least three tests of acceptable effort are performed to ensure reproducibility of results.

Spirometry is typically reported both in absolute values and as a predicted percentage of normal. Normal values vary depending on sex, race, age, and height. The following are some of the measured values by spirometry:

- *Forced vital capacity (FVC):* After a deep inhalation, the volume of air that can be forcibly and maximally exhaled out of the lungs until no more can be expired (usually expressed in liters).
- *Forced expiratory volume in 1 second (FEV$_1$):* The volume of air that can be forcibly exhaled from the lungs in the first second of a forced expiratory maneuver (measured in liters).
- *FEV$_1$/FVC:* The ratio of FEV$_1$ to FVC, indicating what percentage of the total FVC was expelled from the lungs during the first second of forced exhalation.

Flow-volume loops provide a graphic illustration of a patient's spirometric efforts. Flow is plotted against volume to display a continuous loop from inspiration to expiration. The overall shape of the flow-volume loop is important in interpreting spirometric results (Fig. 14–1). In healthy subjects, maximal expiratory flow is highest at total lung capacity and progressively is reduced until residual volume is reached, while inspiratory flow is more even throughout the maximal effort of breathing in from residual volume to total lung capacity. (Total lung capacity is the volume of air in the lungs when the patient has

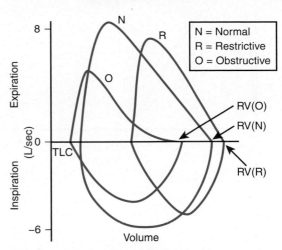

FLOW-VOLUME LOOPS

N = Normal
R = Restrictive
O = Obstructive

FIGURE 14–1 Example of flow-volume loops demonstrating normal, restrictive, and obstructive physiology.

taken a full inspiration.) In addition, the flow patterns are a rather smooth progression during either expiration or inspiration. One feature of the loop that was thought to represent sleep apnea was a flutter on inspiration (as well as on expiration) believed to represent unstable upper airway structures (sawtooth sign)[3] (Fig. 14–2). Although the precise mechanism may differ among individuals, fluttering on inspiration is not routinely seen in sleep apnea and can be present in those patients with motor disease, such as Parkinson's disease, and may also be seen in normal patients.[4] Another feature is the proportion of flow between inspiration and expiration, especially at midlung volumes, halfway between residual volume and total lung capacity. At this point, expiratory flow is less than inspiratory flow in health and in intrathoracic airway disease, such as asthma, chronic obstructive pulmonary disease (COPD), or tracheomalacia. If flows are equal *and*

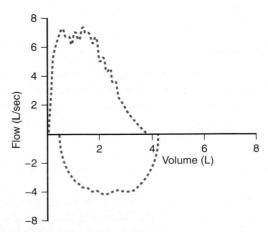

FIGURE 14–2 Sawtooth appearance of expiratory limb of flow-volume loop, which may be observed in the setting of sleep apnea or neuromuscular disease.

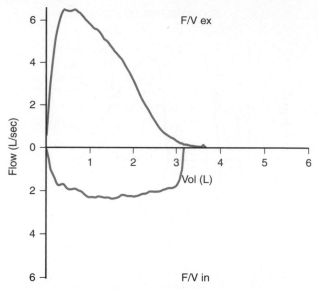

FIGURE 14–3 Flow-volume loop demonstrating flattened appearance of the inspiratory limb of the loop, suggesting variable extrathoracic obstruction.

reduced, there is the possibility of a fixed upper airway obstruction, such as tracheal damage from prior surgery or airway tumor/foreign body. If inspiratory flow exceeds expiratory flow at midlung volume, this physiology is one of a variable extrathoracic obstruction, seen in people with tracheal injury, vocal cord paralysis, and other conditions in which the act of breathing in restricts the size and flow of inspiration while breathing out opens the segment that has dynamic collapse during inspiration (Fig. 14–3).

Reversibility of airway obstruction can be assessed with the use of bronchodilators. After spirometry is completed, the patient is given an inhaled bronchodilator and the test is repeated. The purpose of this is to assess whether a patient's pulmonary process is bronchodilator responsive by looking for improvement in the expired volumes and flow rates. In general, a >12% increase in the FEV_1 (an absolute improvement in FEV_1 of at least 200 ml) or in the FVC after inhaling a β-agonist is considered a significant response.

Lung Volumes

In contrast to spirometry, a dynamic test of airflow function, measurement of lung volumes is designed to collect values relating to the size of the lung as a gas-exchanging unit. These volumes are indirectly calculated from measures of a slow inspiration (or expiration) and a direct measure of thoracic gas volume at functional residual capacity (FRC), with a subsequent derivation of a number of values.

FRC is usually measured by a gas dilution technique or body plethysmography. Gas dilution techniques are based on a simple principle, are widely used, and provide a good measurement of all air in the lungs that communicates with the airways. A limitation of this technique is that it does not measure air in "noncommunicating" bullae and, therefore, may underestimate total lung capacity, especially in patients with severe emphysema.

Body plethysmography is a second method of measuring lung volume that takes advantage of the principle of Boyle's law, which states that the volume of gas at a constant temperature varies inversely with the pressure applied to it. The primary advantage of body plethysmography is that it can measure the total volume of air in the chest, including gas trapped in bullae. Another advantage is that this test can be performed quickly. Drawbacks include the complexity of the equipment as well as the need for the patient to sit in a small enclosed space. From the FRC, the patient pants against a closed shutter to produce changes in the box pressure proportionate to the volume of air in the chest. The volume measured by this technique is referred to as thoracic gas volume and represents the lung volume at which the shutter was closed, typically FRC.

After measurement of FRC, the patient would exhale fully and then take a large breath to total lung capacity. The difference between FRC and residual volume is called the expiratory reserve volume (ERV), and the difference between the slow vital capacity from residual volume and FRC is called the inspiratory capacity. The ERV is reduced in obesity, in which the chest wall mass makes for a smaller FRC.

The interpretation of lung volumes is coordinated with that of spirometry to allow one to distinguish between obstructive lung physiology, restrictive lung physiology, and a mixed picture (see Fig. 14–1). An obstructive pattern may be seen most commonly if there is narrowing of the airways due to bronchial smooth muscle contraction (i.e., asthma), or to inflammation and swelling of bronchial mucosa and the hypertrophy and hyperplasia of bronchial glands (i.e., bronchitis). In some patients obstructive sleep apnea may coexist with COPD, which has been coined the "overlap syndrome." Patients with the overlap syndrome have been shown to have a higher frequency of breathing and lower tidal volume than patients with sleep apnea. Increased mean inspiratory flow and increased mouth occlusion pressure have been noted in overlap syndrome compared to controls, indicating higher neuromuscular output.[5,6] Although epidemiologic data do not support an association between mild obstructive airway disease and SDB,[7] those patients with overlap syndrome have more pronounced oxygen desaturation, hypercapnia, and higher mean pulmonary artery pressures compared to individuals with SDB without accompanying obstructive lung disease.[8] "Restriction" in lung disorders always means a decrease in lung volumes. This term can be applied with confidence to patients whose total lung capacity has been measured and found to be significantly reduced. There are a variety of restrictive disorders, such as intrinsic lung disease (sarcoidosis, interstitial lung disease), extrinsic restrictive lung disorders (morbid obesity, kyphosis/scoliosis), and neuromuscular restrictive disorders (myasthenia gravis, muscular dystrophy, post-polio syndrome, amyotrophic lateral sclerosis). There is currently no correlation between these patterns that is specific or sensitive for any certain sleep disorder.

Diffusing Capacity

Diffusing capacity measures the features at work involving movement of oxygen from the alveolar surface through to the hemoglobin molecule. The clinical test that determines diffusing capacity of the lung most commonly uses carbon monoxide (CO) as the tracer gas for measurement because of its high affinity for binding to the hemoglobin molecule. This property allows a better measurement of pure diffusion, such that the movement of the CO is in essence only dependent on the properties of the diffusion barrier and the amount of hemoglobin. The properties of oxygen and its relatively lower affinity for hemoglobin compared with CO also make it more perfusion dependent; thus cardiac output may influence actual measurement of oxygen diffusion measurements.

Diffusing capacity of the lung for CO (DL_{CO}) is the measure of CO transfer. DL_{CO} is a measure of the interaction of alveolar surface area, alveolar-capillary perfusion, the physical properties of the alveolar-capillary interface, capillary volume, hemoglobin concentration, and the reaction rate of CO and hemoglobin. The most widely used and standardized technique is referred to as the single-breath breath-holding technique. This technique relies on a patient inhaling a known volume of test gas (usually helium); the patient inhales the test gas, holds his or her breath for 10 seconds, and then exhales to "wash out" mechanical and anatomic dead space. DL_{CO} is calculated from the total volume of the lung, the breath-holding time, and the initial and final alveolar concentrations of CO. Alveolar volume is estimated by the test gas dilution and the initial alveolar concentration of CO. The driving pressure is assumed to be the initial alveolar pressure of CO.

Because the level of hemoglobin present in the blood and diffusing capacity are directly related, a correction for anemic patients is used to further delineate whether DL_{CO} is decreased due to anemia or due to parenchymal or interface limitation. Diseases such as interstitial pulmonary fibrosis or any interstitial lung disease may make the DL_{CO} abnormal long before spirometry or volume abnormalities are present. Low DL_{CO} is not only an abnormality of restrictive interstitial lung disease but may also occur in the presence of emphysema. On the other end of the spectrum, alveolar hemorrhage or congested capillary beds may actually increase the DL_{CO}. As for spirometry, predicted formulas have been established for DL_{CO} and DL_{CO} corrected for alveolar volume. It is important to note, however, that differences in race have been observed in normal subjects, and a race correction of 7% is allowed for African American patients.[9] The

diffusing capacity, if reduced, may be a reason for oxygen levels to be low even when there are relatively normal values on spirometry or lung volumes. Such a circumstance is found with pulmonary vascular disease.[10] To the extent that a reduced diffusing capacity affects oxygen levels, it can be one reason for excess hypoxemia during sleep, even in the absence of apneas or hypopneas.

Arterial Blood Gases

A sample of blood is drawn anaerobically from a peripheral artery (radial, brachial, femoral, or dorsalis pedis) via a single percutaneous needle puncture, or from an indwelling arterial cannula or catheter for multiple samples. A resting arterial blood gas measurement may be considered in the setting of hypoxia out of proportion to the degree of SDB, thereby suggesting underlying possible cardiopulmonary disease, or to obtain a sense of resting hypercapnia if underlying obesity-hypoventilation syndrome, obstructive lung disease, or neuromuscular disease is known or suspected.

The arterial blood gas sample allows for the measurement of partial pressures of arterial carbon dioxide ($PaCO_2$) and arterial oxygen (PaO_2), hydrogen ion activity (pH), total hemoglobin, oxyhemoglobin saturation, carboxyhemoglobin, and methemoglobin. Table 14–1 presents the approach to acid-base determination. Arterial blood gases permit another assessment of gas exchange and of ventilation. One can derive a value of the alveolar-arterial (A-a) gradient to determine a problem in gas exchange at the alveolar level:

$$P_{(A-a)}O_2 = [FiO_2(P_B - P_{H_2O}) - PaCO_2/RQ] - PaO_2$$

where

- $P_{(A-a)}O_2$ = alveolar-arterial oxygen gradient
- FiO_2 = fraction of inspired oxygen
- P_B = barometric pressure of oxygen
- P_{H_2O} = partial pressure of water
- RQ = respiratory quotient: the amount of CO_2 relative to the amount of O_2 consumed (in normal situations this is approximately 0.8)

An increased A-a gradient would cause a reduction in arterial blood oxygen levels and be the result of a ventilation-perfusion mismatch (most common, and most commonly the result of obstructive diseases such as COPD or asthma) or an anatomic shunt (as in liver disease). A second pattern seen is a normal A-a gradient with the hypoxemia explained by hypoventilation of lung units, retention of carbon dioxide, and elevated arterial $PaCO_2$. As anything that produces hypoxemia during wakefulness is likely to produce lower oxygen saturation levels during sleep when the FRC is lower and there is reduced ventilation; the presence of hypoxemia or hypoventilation in an arterial blood gas measurement is predictive of greater hypoxemia during a sleep study. Hypercapnia determined by arterial blood gas measurement may be helpful in clarifying situations in which obesity-hypoventilation

TABLE 14–1 Determination of Acid-Base Status

Step I: Determine Primary Acid-Base Status Disorder

A. Determine Acidosis versus Alkalosis
pH <7.35: Acidosis

pH >7.45: Alkalosis

B. Determine Metabolic versus Respiratory

Primary Metabolic Disorder
- pH changes in same direction as bicarbonate, $Paco_2$
- Metabolic Acidosis
  - Serum pH decreased
  - Serum bicarbonate and $Paco_2$ decreased
- Metabolic Alkalosis
  - Serum pH increased
  - Serum bicarbonate and $Paco_2$ increased

Primary Respiratory Disorder
- pH changes in opposite direction of bicarbonate, $Paco_2$
- Respiratory Acidosis
  - Serum pH decreased
  - Serum bicarbonate and $Paco_2$ increased
- Respiratory Alkalosis
  - Serum pH increased
  - Serum bicarbonate and $Paco_2$ decreased

Step II: Determine Compensation

Metabolic Acidosis:
$Paco_2$ decreases 1.2 mm Hg per 1 mEq/L bicarbonate fall
Metabolic Alkalosis:
$Paco_2$ increases 6 mm Hg per 10 mEq/L bicarbonate rise

Acute Respiratory Acidosis:
Bicarbonate increases 1 mEq/L per 10 mm Hg $Paco_2$ rise
Chronic Respiratory Acidosis:
Bicarbonate increases 4 mEq/L per 10 mm Hg $Paco_2$ rise
Acute Respiratory Alkalosis:
Bicarbonate decreases 2 mEq/L per 10 mm Hg $Paco_2$ fall
Chronic Respiratory Alkalosis:
Bicarbonate decreases 4 mEq/L per 10 mm Hg $Paco_2$ fall

syndrome, overlap syndrome, or concomitant neuromuscular disease in the context of SDB is suspected.

MONITORING OF RESPIRATORY FUNCTION DURING SLEEP

Most airflow sensors detect apneas reliably, but the detection and quantification of decreased flow needed to diagnose hypopneas depend on the type of sensor used. Hypopneas make up the majority of obstructive respiratory events,[11] and therefore measurement needs to be reliable.

Pneumotachometer

Pneumotachometry is considered the reference standard for obstructive apnea and hypopnea detection. This method of airflow monitoring provides a direct quantitative measurement of airflow or tidal volume; however, it requires connection to a sealed mask placed over the nose or mouth, which may be obtrusive and disrupt sleep. Therefore, although this provides a beneficial and accurate research tool, in the clinical setting this technique is somewhat cumbersome, with the exception of application or titration of positive pressure therapy. The pneumotachometer measures the flow rate of gases during breathing. The breath is passed through a short tube in which there is a fine metal mesh, which presents a small resistance to the flow. Flow is derived from the pressure difference over the small, fixed resistance offered by the metal mesh. The pressure drop across the resistance relates linearly to flow at relatively low flows, when the flow pattern is laminar. Higher flows give rise to a turbulent flow pattern, when the pressure drop across the resistance changes more than proportionally with flow.

Accurate measurements are best performed when the flow pattern is laminar and flow linearly related to pressure drop.

Intranasal Pressure Transducer

Intranasal pressure transducers provide an indirect measurement of airflow by detecting pressure changes, with an excellent response to airflow profile, and are capable of detecting airflow limitation. Changing pressures require a transducer that can respond to rapid changes. Nasal pressure transducers provide a significantly more sensitive measure of airflow than temperature-based transducers, and many believe that pressure transducers may provide a measure of upper airway resistance as inspiration and expiration provide transducer signal fluctuations similar to airflow.[12] In one study, the nasal cannula/pressure transducer was found to be a noninvasive, reproducible detector of all events in SDB—in particular, it detected the same events as esophageal manometry (respiratory effort–related arousals [RERAs]) with an intraclass correlation coefficient of 96.[13,14] The newer transducers provide additional information for scoring hypopneas (Fig. 14–4). If used for evaluation of sleep-related breathing disorders, the new level of sensitivity may lead to scoring of many more events than are typically scored with other methods of airflow detection (Figs. 14–5 and 14–6). These events may be as significant as conventionally scored apneas, but at present virtually all of the clinical literature is based on temperature-based airflow transduction.

Nasal pressure monitoring is not recommended for patients who are predominantly mouth breathers or have nasal obstruction, in which case airflow may be underestimated.[15] Nasal pressure sensors connected to the nose

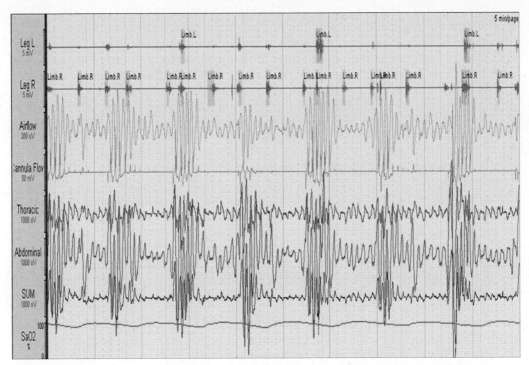

FIGURE 14–4 Respiratory monitoring polysomnography data shown at 5 min/page demonstrating recurrent episodes of obstructive respiratory hypopneic events, with persistence of effort on thoracic and abdominal respiratory inductance plethysmography signals. Also note the temporal and nontemporal relationship of periodic limb movements with respiratory events. Note increased reduction in flow detected by nasal cannula (transducer) compared to airflow monitored by nasal thermistor.

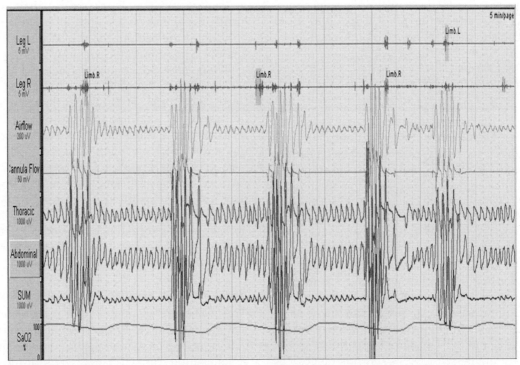

FIGURE 14–5 Respiratory monitoring polysomnography data shown at 5 min/page demonstrating recurrent episodes of obstructive apneic events, with persistence of effort noted on thoracic and abdominal respiratory impedance plethysmography monitoring. Note increased reduction in flow detected by nasal cannula (transducer) compared to airflow monitored by nasal thermistor.

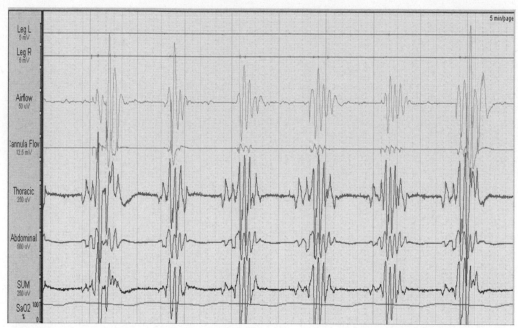

FIGURE 14–6 Respiratory monitoring polysomnography data shown at 5 min/page demonstrating recurrent episodes of central/mixed apneic events, as shown by initial absence of effort on abdominal and thoracic respiratory impedance plethysmography signals.

via nasal prongs are more accurate than thermoelements in detecting hypopneas.[15] However, nasal pressure is falsely increased in the presence of nasal obstruction, and there is a nonlinear relation between nasal pressure and nasal flow. Square root linearization of nasal pressure greatly increases the accuracy for quantifying hypopneas and detecting flow limitation.[16,17] Mouth breathing can affect the measurement, but pure mouth breathing is uncommon.[18,19]

Nasal Thermocouple/Thermistor

A nasal and/or oral thermocouple is an inexpensive way to assess airflow via indirect semi-quantitative assessment detecting increased temperature of expired air, with only directional changes providing reliable results. Thermocouples are commonly used for temperature measurement as they are highly accurate and operate over a broad range of temperatures. They consist of two different metal wires that are welded together at one end (A). These wires generate a thermoelectric voltage between their open ends that changes according to the temperature difference between the two ends, that is, between the junction (A) and the reference (R). Thermistors consist of an electronic component (semiconductor material) that exhibits a large change in resistance in proportion to a small change in temperature. In comparison to thermocouples, thermistors have a limited (smaller) temperature range; however, they are highly sensitive within this range. The resistance of these devices often changes in a nonlinear fashion with temperature, and additional instruments are required to linearize the reading.

In laboratory models that have compared thermistors and thermocouples to a pneumotachograph, the thermal sensors have been shown to be nonlinearly related to airflow, generally providing an overestimation of ventilation.[18] Therefore, they cannot be used to determine hypopneas reliably. Furthermore, their accuracy varies greatly depending on the position of the sensors, the sleep position of the patient, the presence of nasal obstruction, and the type of thermoelement used.[20]

Thermistors are commonly included as a part of PSG, and are likely to have the longest history of use in clinical sleep laboratories of all the airflow sensors. Given the limitations of thermal sensors in accurately detecting quantitative measures of airflow, with measures correlating poorly with pneumotachography,[18,21] these sensors have been determined not to provide quantitative measures of airflow for detection of hypopneas. However, they may be a fairly reliable method to detect complete airflow cessation (i.e., apneas). The AASM Respiratory Task Force has recently recognized the oronasal thermal sensor as the sensor to detect absence of airflow for apnea identification.[22]

Respiratory Inductance Plethysmography

The literature supports that respiratory inductance plethysmography (RIP) is acceptable for the semi-quantitative measurement of ventilation assessed by thoracic and abdominal pressure changes.[20] With this technique, transducers are placed at the level of the nipples and at the umbilicus to monitor cross-sectional changes reflected by changes in inductance or resistance to change in flow of the transducers.[23] The sum of the signals may provide an estimate of tidal volume and respiratory pattern during sleep. RIP is based upon the two-compartment model of thoracoabdominal movement during respiration.[24] Accurate initial calibration, and constancy during body movements and changes during respiration, are imperative to obtaining valid measurements.[25] Measurement inaccuracies may occur due to slippage (displacement of transducer bands) and position changes.[23] RIP detects changes in the volume of the chest and abdomen during inspiration and expiration, and, when properly calibrated, the sum of the two signals can provide an estimate of tidal volume.[26] However, calibration may be difficult to maintain throughout the night.[27] RIP allows an acceptable semi-quantitative measurement of ventilation and therefore hypopneas. The AASM Task Force recommends the use of RIP or measurement of nasal pressure using nasal cannulas to detect airflow and ventilation.[28]

Snore Monitoring Microphone

A microphone is used to detect snoring during PSG, providing an output signal with easily identifiable waveforms. This tracing, in conjunction with sleep technician comments, may assist in the diagnosis of primary snoring when evidence for SDB is lacking. In addition, snore monitoring is of use during positive pressure titration to determine the optimal pressure setting.[13]

Respiratory Muscle Monitoring: Surface Diaphragmatic Electromyography

This modality provides an indirect measurement of respiratory effort via electrodes placed on the chest wall; however, it is not an ideal measurement for detecting RERAs or central respiratory events.[28] Reliable recordings are difficult to obtain, it is prone to electrocardiography artifact, and nonrespiratory muscle electromyography is difficult to eliminate. There are no data on accuracy, reliability, or correlation with long-term outcomes with respect to this technique.[28]

Esophageal Balloon Manometry

The measurement of esophageal pressure with continuous overnight monitoring is the reference standard for measuring respiratory effort during PSG. Respiratory efforts are associated with changes in pleural pressure that can be accurately measured using esophageal manometry. This method is useful when distinguishing central versus obstructive apneas, and is useful for detecting RERAs in the setting of upper airway resistance syndrome, during which there is increasingly more negative esophageal pressures immediately preceding an arousal, subsequent to which the esophageal pressure fairly rapidly returns to normal levels.[29,30]

Piezo Sensors, Strain Gauges, Magnetometers, Impedance Pneumography

Other methods that have been used to assess airflow include piezo sensors, strain gauges, and magnetometers. Piezo sensors may measure qualitative changes in airflow; however, they are not reliable in distinguishing central from obstructive respiratory events. In one study, 37% of the apneas scored as central based on strain gauge measurements were reclassified as obstructive or mixed based on esophageal balloon measurements, indicating a high misclassification rate.[31] Mercury strain gauges generate qualitative data rather than quantitative data and have the following limitations: difficulty with calibration, slippage, and development of bubbles within the mercury in the tubing that may compromise signal quality. Magnetometers can measure the anterior-posterior diameter of the rib cage (fifth intercostal space) and the abdominal wall surface (2 cm above umbilicus); however, they also have the limitation of providing qualitative rather than quantitative data.

Impedance pneumography involves placement of two or three electrodes on the rib cage. However, it is limited by providing only qualitative data as there is no direct relationship to the volume of air, there are no standards for precision/reliability, signal degradation occurs with changes in body position, and signals are susceptible to cardiogenic/motion artifact.

Pulse Oximetry Monitoring

The fundamental physical property that allows the measurement of arterial oxygen saturation is that blood changes color with saturation. Hemoglobin, in its reduced form or oxygenated state, absorbs light at wavelengths below approximately 630 nm, which includes the entire part of the visible spectrum aside from the red region. The opposite situation occurs in the near-infrared region (810–1000 nm), where hemoglobin absorbs more light when it is desaturated. Pulse oximeters usually are designed with two emitters (usually light-emitting diodes): one designed to emit light in the red region (~660 nm), and the other in the near-infrared region (~925 or 940 nm). In order to measure absorption of arterial blood only, without interference from venous blood, skin, bone, and the like, and to minimize scatter effect, a differential absorption is calculated by dividing the small change in intensity by the total intensity of the output light. Chromophores other than oxyhemoglobin and reduced hemoglobin, such as carboxyhemoglobin and methemoglobin, may cause falsely elevated readings for the arterial oxygen saturation. Of note, oximeters may be calibrated using functional or fractional oxygen saturation, with the former reading slightly higher (1–3%). Oximeters may be prone to artifact, such as during states of poor perfusion, excessive patient motion (particularly at the probe site), and electrical noise, and also may be affected by changes in heart rate and circulation time.[32]

Overall, pulse oximetry is easy to use, inexpensive, readily available, and noninvasive, and it permits continuous monitoring of oxygen saturation. Pulse oximetry sensitivity is improved with shorter sampling intervals, and minimal filtering in order to achieve the most rapid response. The utility of pulse oximetry in clinical decision making in the realm of sleep/pulmonary medicine has been assessed by a recent study, and determined to be an area in need of further standardization and refinement of physician interpretation.[33]

Carbon Dioxide Monitoring

Expired End-Tidal CO_2 Monitoring

This modality works by a drawing a stream of air from the nose or the mouth to a chamber in which a light is shone through the air. The degree of absorption at a certain frequency of infrared light is proportional to the concentration of CO_2. The light may be split, with half passing through a reference cell. The light may also be "chopped" so that it is not continuously heating the gas in the reference cell.

Continuous measurement of CO_2 reflects the excretion pattern of CO_2 from the lung. Values for CO_2 are at or near zero on inspiration and show an abrupt rise until the end of expiration, when there is a plateau in the CO_2 level. The end-expiratory value is correlated with $PaCO_2$ provided that there is complete gas emptying to functional residual capacity, and little effect of ventilation-perfusion mismatch. End-tidal CO_2 monitoring may help in identifying hypoventilation in obesity-hypoventilation syndrome, as well as COPD, congestive heart failure, and neurologic diseases that produce neuromuscular weakness. In addition, end-tidal CO_2 values can be helpful in assessing disorders of chronic hyperventilation, distinguishing pathophysiologic from psychogenic causes by the persistence or resolution of hypocapnia during sleep.

A limitation of end-tidal CO_2 monitoring includes the inability to measure levels in the setting of continuous positive airway pressure or bilevel pressure therapy in order to assess response to treatment. The value of capnography (breath-by-breath CO_2 measurements) is twofold, but limited in scope compared to direct measures of airflow. First, capnography may detect absence of expiratory airflow and signal an apnea. There are no established criteria, but an apnea event is considered to occur when end-expiratory CO_2 fails to fall after expiration, with subsequent decline in CO_2 over the next 10 seconds to values at or near zero. The end of the apnea is heralded by the occurrence of a rapid rise in CO_2 with expiration; the length of an event is from the peak of the last CO_2 rise to the peak of the next CO_2 rise, if greater than 10 seconds. A cardiac oscillation in the capnography signal indicates a patent airway during a central apnea (but the frequency of this is only recorded at an anecdotal level of evidence). There can be expiratory puffs after an obstructed inspiratory effort, but again the frequency of this is only recorded at an anecdotal level of evidence. Second, capnography can be used to identify obstructive hypopneas. In this instance there are persistent efforts characterized by asynchronous chest wall movements of the rib cage and abdomen with a rising end-tidal CO_2 over time. Again the frequency of this kind of pattern is only recorded at an anecdotal level of evidence.

Scoring of events from the CO_2 monitor should be directed at apneas, and to the extent possible correlated with rib cage/abdominal movements and CO_2 fluctuation in synchrony with electrocardiography (central event) or with respiratory efforts (expiratory puffs signaling an obstructive event). Obstructive hypopneas would be detected by a series of breaths with asynchronous rib cage/abdominal motion associated with an increasing end-expiratory CO_2 level. In general, studies appear to indicate that end-tidal CO_2 values tend to underestimate arterial CO_2, with the largest discrepancies occurring in hypercapnic subjects or in subjects with respiratory disease.[34–36]

Transcutaneous CO_2

Two methods may be employed in transcutaneous CO_2 monitoring; the first uses a silver electrode that measures CO_2 that has diffused from the skin through a gas-permeable membrane into solution (response time <1 minute), and the other uses an infrared capnometer that anlyzes CO_2 in the gas phase (response time more than 2 minutes). Studies have assessed end-tidal and transcutaneous monitoring of CO_2, and concluded that neither of these measurements was an accurate reflection of CO_2 levels, and therefore they should not be used during routine PSG.[37] The transcutaneous values tended to have a smaller bias compared to arterial values than do the measurements of end-tidal partial pressure of CO_2 (PCO_2), with a tendency for overestimating PCO_2 values.[34,38]

AASM Definition And Scoring Of Respiratory Events

Obstructive Apneas

The most recent AASM scoring rules define an obstructive apnea as a drop in peak thermal sensor excursion by $\geq 90\%$ of baseline lasting at least 10 seconds, with at least 90% of the event's duration meeting the amplitude reduction criteria for apnea, and with continued or increased inspiratory effort noted throughout the entire period of absent airflow. The event duration is measured from the nadir preceding the first breath that approximates the breathing amplitude. When baseline breathing amplitude cannot be easily determined, an event may be terminated when either there is a clear and sustained increase in breathing amplitude or if there is an accompanying desaturation, or if an event-associated resaturation of at least

2% is observed. Obstructive apnea identification does not require a minimum desaturation criterion.[22]

Central Apneas

Central apnea is defined as a drop in peak thermal sensor excursion by ≥90% of baseline lasting at least 10 seconds, with at least 90% of the event's duration meeting the amplitude reduction criteria for apnea, and with absent inspiratory effort noted throughout the entire period of absent airflow. The event duration is measured from the nadir preceding the first breath that approximates the breathing amplitude. When baseline breathing amplitude cannot be easily determined, an event may be terminated when either there is a clear and sustained increase in breathing amplitude or there is an accompanying desaturation, or if an event-associated resaturation of at least 2% is observed. Central apnea identification does not require a minimum desaturation criterion.[22]

Mixed Apneas

Mixed apnea is defined as a drop in peak thermal sensor excursion by ≥90% of baseline lasting at least 10 seconds, with at least 90% of the event's duration meeting the amplitude reduction criteria for apnea, and with absent inspiratory effort noted during the initial portion of the respiratory event, followed by resumption of inspiratory effort during the latter part of the event. The event duration is measured from the nadir preceding the first breath that approximates the breathing amplitude. When baseline breathing amplitude cannot be easily determined, an event may be terminated when either there is a clear and sustained increase in breathing amplitude or there is an accompanying desaturation, or if an event-associated resaturation of at least 2% is observed. Mixed apnea identification does not require a minimum desaturation criterion.[22]

Hypopneas

The AASM recommended definition of hypopnea as a drop of ≥30% of the nasal pressure signal compared to baseline lasting at least 10 seconds, accompanied by a >4% oxygen desaturation from pre-event baseline, and with at least 90% of the event's duration meeting the amplitude criteria for hypopnea. An alternative definition is also provided, characterized by a drop of ≥50% of the nasal pressure signal compared to baseline lasting at least 10 seconds, accompanied by a ≥3% oxygen desaturation from pre-event baseline (or associated with an arousal), and with at least 90% of the event's duration meeting the amplitude criteria for hypopnea.[22]

Respiratory Effort–Related Arousal

A RERA is scored when there is a sequence of breaths lasting for at least 10 seconds, characterized by increasing respiratory effort or flattening of the nasal pressure waveform leading to an arousal from sleep, when the sequence of breaths does not meet criteria for an apnea or hypopnea.[22]

Cheyne-Stokes Respirations

Cheyne-Stokes respirations are scored when respiratory monitoring indicates at least three consecutive cycles of cyclical crescendo-decrescendo change in breathing amplitude and at least one of the following: (1) five or more central apneas or hypopneas per hour of sleep, or (2) the cyclical crescendo-decrescendo change in breathing amplitude has a duration of at least 10 consecutive minutes.[22]

Sleep-Related Hypoventilation

Sleep-related hypoventilation is defined as a ≥10 mm Hg increase in $Paco_2$ during sleep in comparison to an awake supine value.[22]

❂ REFERENCES

A full list of references are available at www.expertconsult.com

CHAPTER 15

Neuroimaging in Sleep and Sleep Disorders

**Martin Desseilles, Thanh Dang-Vu, Sophie Schwartz,
Philippe Peigneux** and **Pierre Maquet**

Functional neuroimaging is a powerful tool to explore regional brain activity in humans. It includes a variety of metabolic and hemodynamic techniques such as positron emission tomography (PET), single-photon emission computed tomography (SPECT), functional magnetic resonance imaging (fMRI), and near-infrared spectroscopy. Neurophysiologic techniques such as electroencephalography (EEG) and magnetoencephalography (MEG) are not reviewed here.

Neuroimaging in patients suffering from sleep disorders may serve several purposes. First, it can help characterize the cerebral consequences of sleep disruption due to intrinsic sleep disorders, or to extrinsic environmental or medical causes. For instance, neuroimaging studies have shown that chronic sleep fragmentation in sleep-disordered patients (e.g., patients with obstructive sleep apnea syndrome)[1] or acute sleep deprivation in normal subjects[2–4] eventually leads to impaired cognitive functioning associated with significant changes in the underlying pattern of regional brain activity.

Second, neuroimaging may serve to better characterize the pathogenic mechanisms of sleep disorders, or at least their cerebral correlates. This endeavor is hindered by the fact that, from the practical and methodologic points of view, scanning patients during their sleep is not easy. However, alternative approaches are available, as the functional and structural consequences of these sleep disorders can also be assessed during wakefulness. For instance, voxel-based morphometry analysis can be used to detect structural brain changes typical of specific sleep disorders. Likewise, cardiovascular regulation can be assessed by probing important reflexes, as during the Valsalva maneuver.

Third, neuroimaging might help to establish the nosography of sleep disorders. For instance, neuroimaging could help classify different subtypes of insomnia in terms of their underlying characteristic patterns of regional brain activity, an approach that may prove complementary to clinical observation.

Finally, functional neuroimaging can also be used to assess the effects of hypnotic drugs on regional brain function. This may enhance our understanding of their effects, assuming that hypnotic medications inducing typical patterns of brain activation rely on cellular mechanisms similar to those prevailing in normal sleep.

This chapter reviews attempts made in these various directions. To set the stage for the study of sleep disorders, we first describe recent contributions of neuroimaging techniques to the functional neuroanatomy of normal sleep in humans.

NEUROIMAGING IN NORMAL HUMAN SLEEP

Sleep profoundly impacts the activity of numerous physiologic systems (see, e.g., Kryger et al.[5]). PET, SPECT, or fMRI studies reviewed in this section have demonstrated that global and regional patterns of brain activity during sleep are remarkably different from those during wakefulness. These studies have also shown the persistence of brain responses to external stimuli during sleep, and plastic changes in brain activity related to previous waking experience.

Functional Neuroimaging of Normal Human Sleep

Noninvasive functional neuroimaging with PET brought an original description of the functional neuroanatomy of human sleep. These studies described a reproducible regional distribution of brain activity during sleep stages (rapid eye movement [REM] and non-REM [NREM] sleep) that largely differs from wakefulness, as expected from animal data. More recent data, using event-related fMRI, have also assessed the brain activity related to spontaneous neural events within sleep stages, such as sleep spindles.

NREM Sleep

In mammals, the neuronal activity observed during NREM sleep is sculpted by a cortical slow oscillation that alternates short bursts of firing ("up" states) and long periods of hyperpolarization ("down" states).[6] Slow oscillations organize the synchronization of other NREM sleep rhythms (spindles and delta waves),[7] and should also have a major impact on regional cerebral blood flow (rCBF), which when averaged over time decreases in the areas where they prevail. Taking into account that PET measurements average cerebral activity over 45–90 seconds, decreases in cerebral blood flow (CBF) and cerebral glucose metabolism during NREM sleep are thought to underlie a change in firing pattern, reflected by the slow oscillation and characterized by synchronized bursting activity followed by long hyperpolarization periods.[8] Accordingly, as compared to wakefulness, the average cerebral metabolism and global blood flow levels begin to decrease in light (stage 1 and stage 2) NREM sleep,[9–11] and reach their nadir in deep (stage 3 and 4) NREM sleep, also named slow-wave sleep (SWS).[12,13]

In animals, the cascade of events that generates NREM sleep oscillations among thalamo-neocortical networks is induced by a decreased firing in the activating structures of the brain stem tegmentum.[6] In agreement with animal data, humans PET studies show that brain stem blood flow is decreased during light NREM sleep[14] as well as during SWS.[14–17] During light NREM sleep, the pontine tegmentum appears specifically deactivated, whereas the mesencephalon seems to retain an activity that is not significantly different from wakefulness.[14] In SWS, both pontine and mesencephalic tegmenta are deactivated.[16]

The thalamus occupies a central position in the generation of NREM sleep rhythms, due to the intrinsic oscillating properties of its neurons and to the intrathalamic and thalamo-corticothalamic connectivity. As expected, in humans, regional activity decreases have been found in the thalamus during both light and deep NREM sleep in PET[14–16] and block-design fMRI[18] studies; rCBF decreases in the thalamus have also been evidenced in proportion to the power density of the EEG signal in the spindle and delta frequency range[19] (but see Dang-Vu et al.[20] for a critical discussion of these findings).

The role of the cortex in the generation of NREM sleep oscillations is equally important but not yet fully understood,[21] especially at the neuronal level. Electroencephalographic power density maps have revealed a relatively typical predominance of the delta frequency band in the frontal regions, whereas sigma power predominated over the vertex.[22] Human PET data similarly showed that the pattern of cortical deactivation was not homogeneously distributed throughout the cortex. As compared to wakefulness, the least active areas in SWS were observed in various associative cortices of the frontal (in particular in the dorsolateral and orbital prefrontal cortex) and parietal, and to a lesser extent in the temporal and insular, lobes.[14–16,23] In contrast, the primary cortices were the least deactivated cortical areas.[15] Finally, a meta-analysis of our own data[20] showed a linear (inverse) relationship between EEG spectral power within the delta frequency band and rCBF in ventromedial prefrontal regions during NREM sleep in non–sleep-deprived normal subjects. This result suggests an important role of medial prefrontal cortices in the modulation of delta waves.

The reasons for this heterogeneous cortical distribution remain unclear. One hypothesis is that, since polymodal association cortices are the most active cerebral areas during wakefulness, and because sleep intensity is homeostatically related to prior waking activity at the regional level,[24] these cortices might be more profoundly influenced by SWS rhythms than primary cortices.[8]

The predominance of rCBF decreases in prefrontal regions may be functionally important since these cortical regions are involved in mood regulation and in various cognitive functions (e.g., planning or probability matching)[25] that help adaptation of individual behaviors. Studies of the deleterious effects of sleep deprivation on human cognition also pointed to a high sensitivity of these association cortices to sleep deprivation (see later).

The previous functional brain imaging studies have compared periods or "blocks" of brain activity averaged over several tens of seconds or minutes between NREM sleep and wakefulness. Because hyperpolarization phases may predominate over these periods, the resulting picture emerging from these studies is decreasing brain activity during NREM sleep in the areas where slow oscillations are most prevalent. While NREM sleep is consistently characterized by a global and regional net decrease of brain activity over several seconds or minutes, the concept of NREM sleep as a stage of brain quiescence is not accurate, as we know from animal studies that NREM sleep is also characterized by transient bursts of neuronal discharge ("up" states) organized by NREM sleep oscillations. We conducted an event-related fMRI study during NREM sleep in normal non–sleep-deprived human volunteers and showed that the occurrence of the phasic sleep spindles was associated with increases of brain activity in a specific set of cortical and subcortical structures, including the thalamus, paralimbic areas, and superior temporal gyri.[26] Moreover, beyond this general activation pattern, we also demonstrated that slow and fast spindles could be differentiated in terms of their macroscopic hemodynamic responses: slow spindles were specifically associated with activation of the superior temporal gyrus, and fast spindles preferentially recruited hippocampal and sensorimotor cortical areas. Besides bringing further evidence that spindles can be divided in two biologically distinct subtypes, this study demonstrates that NREM sleep cannot be reduced to a state of sustained brain deactivation but is characterized by phasic increases in brain activity triggered by NREM sleep oscillations, such as spindles, in agreement with animal data.

REM Sleep

REM sleep is characterized by desynchronized neuronal activity[27,28] and, correspondingly, by high cerebral energy requirements[12] and blood flow.[13,29] In this active but sleeping brain, some areas are particularly active, even more than during wakefulness, while others have lower than average regional activity.

PET studies have shown significant rCBF increases during REM sleep in the pontine tegmentum, thalamic nuclei, limbic and paralimbic areas, amygdaloid complexes,[30,31] hippocampal formation,[15,31] anterior cingulate cortex,[15,30,31] and orbitofrontal and insular cortices[31] (Fig. 15–1). Posterior cortices in temporo-occipital areas were also found to be activated,[15] although less consistently. In contrast, the inferior and middle dorsolateral prefrontal gyri, the inferior parietal cortex, and the posterior cingulate cortex and precuneus were the least active brain regions.[15,30]

Functional connectivity between remote brain areas is also modified during human REM sleep. The functional relationship between striate and extrastriate cortices, usually excitatory, is reversed during REM sleep.[15,32] Likewise, the functional relationship between the amygdala

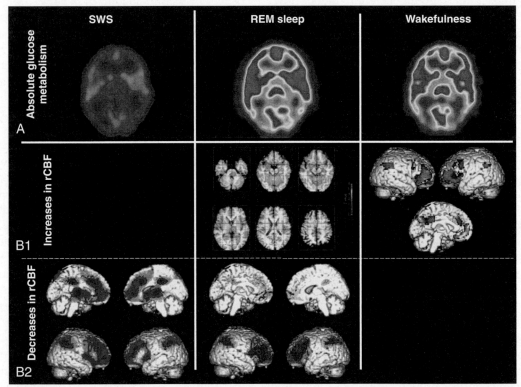

FIGURE 15–1 Cerebral glucose metabolism (CGM) and regional cerebral blood flow (CBF) during deep NREM sleep (*first column*), REM sleep (*second column*), and wakefulness (*third column*). **(Row A)** CGM quantified in the same individual at 1-week interval, using FDG and PET. The three images are displayed at the same brain level using the same color scale. The average CGM during deep NREM sleep (versus wakefulness) is significantly decreased. During REM sleep, the CGM is as high as during wakefulness. **(Row B1)** Distribution of the *highest* regional brain activity, as assessed by CBF measurement using PET, during wakefulness and REM sleep. The most active regions during *wakefulness* are located in the polymodal associative cortices in the prefrontal and parietal lobes (both on the medial wall and convexity). During *REM sleep,* the most active areas are located in the pontine tegmentum, thalami, amygdaloid complexes, and anterior cingulate cortex. Other data (not shown) have shown a large activity in the occipital cortices, insula, and hippocampus.[15] **(Row B2)** Distribution of the *lowest* regional brain activity, as assessed by CBF measurement using PET, during NREM and REM sleep. In both sleep stages, the least active regions are located in the polymodal associative cortices in the prefrontal and parietal lobes (convexity). During *NREM sleep,* the brain stem and thalami are also particularly deactivated. *See Color Plate*

and the temporal and occipital cortices is different during REM sleep than during wakefulness or NREM sleep.[33] This pattern suggests that functional interactions between neuronal populations are different during REM sleep than during wakefulness.

Regional brain activity in subcortical mesopontine and thalamic regions during human REM sleep[14,30,31] is in keeping with our current understanding of sleep generation in animals. REM sleep is generated by neuronal populations of the mesopontine reticular formation that monosynaptically activate the thalamic nuclei, which in turn activate the cortex.[27]

In contrast, the neurobiologic basis of the regional pattern of cortical activity during REM sleep remains unclear. Modifications of forebrain activity and responsiveness during REM sleep might rely on neuromodulatory changes. In cats, neurons in the raphe nuclei (serotonergic neurons) and locus ceruleus (noradrenergic cells) remain silent during REM sleep; simultaneously, mesopontine tegmentum cholinergic cells maintain a high firing rate.[27,34] To the best of our knowledge, there is still no report characterizing these neuromodulatory changes and their effect on regional brain function during human REM sleep.

Pontine waves, or ponto-geniculo-occipital (PGO) waves, are also primary features of REM sleep. In rats, the generator of the pontine waves projects to a set of brain areas shown to be active in human REM sleep: the occipital cortex, the entorhinal cortex, the hippocampus, and the amygdala as well as brain stem structures participating in the generation of REM sleep.[35] In cats, although most easily recorded in the pons,[36] the lateral geniculate bodies,[37] and the occipital cortex,[38] PGO waves are observed in many parts of the brain, including limbic areas (amygdala, hippocampus, cingulate gyrus).[39] Several observations suggest that PGO waves also occur during human sleep. In epileptic patients, direct intracerebral recordings in the striate cortex showed monophasic or diphasic potentials during REM sleep, isolated or in bursts.[40] In normal subjects, surface EEG revealed transient occipital and/or parietal potentials time-locked to the REMs.[41] Source dipoles of MEG signal were localized in the brain stem, thalamus, hippocampus, and occipital cortex during REM sleep.[42,43] Using PET, we showed that the rCBF in the lateral geniculate bodies and the occipital cortex is tightly coupled to spontaneous eye movements during REM sleep, but not during wakefulness.[44] This finding has been confirmed by an fMRI study.[45] Although fully conclusive components are still awaited, these various elements support the hypothesis that PGO-like activities participate in shaping the distribution of regional brain activity during human REM sleep.

Brain Reactivity to External Stimulation During Sleep

Electrophysiologic studies have demonstrated that sleep is not a state of complete unresponsiveness to external stimuli (see, e.g., Perrin et al.[46]). Early studies have shown that external stimuli can induce an autonomic or electrophysiologic response during human sleep, in particular after a relevant or meaningful stimulus presentation.[47] The analysis of event-related potential components could distinguish between different levels of external input processing during sleep. Middle-latency evoked potentials were found to be reduced during deep sleep, whereas brain stem auditory evoked potentials are not modulated by the vigilance state but rather by the circadian variations of body temperature.[48] As for long-latency components (P300), they are modulated by the sleep stage. During NREM sleep (and especially in stage 2 sleep), sensory stimulation triggers K complexes that are differentially affected by some stimulus features, with the later components of K complexes being more connected to the physical attributes of the stimulus and the early ones to its intrinsic significance.[19] In REM sleep, the evoked potential signs of stimulus discrimination differ from those observed during waking.[50] Indeed, words devoid of meaning were detected as anomalous and evoked N400 during waking, and yielded responses similar to those of congruous words in REM sleep.[50] Even if the information processing is quite comparable during stage 2 NREM and REM sleep (persistence of a differential response to the subject's own name, relative to any other proper name in both conditions), the electrophysiologic counterparts of these sleep phases show that their underpinning neural mechanisms are different.[48,50]

Available PET and fMRI data globally suggest that the processing of external stimuli can proceed beyond the primary cortices during NREM sleep. However, the mechanisms by which salient stimuli can recruit associative cerebral areas during sleep remain unclear. A pioneering fMRI study found that, during NREM sleep as during wakefulness, several areas continue to be activated by external auditory stimulation: the thalamic nuclei, the auditory cortices, and the caudate nucleus.[51] Moreover, the left amygdala and the left prefrontal cortex were found to be more activated by subjects' own names than by pure tones, suggesting the persistence during sleep of specific responses for meaningful or emotionally laden stimuli.

Other groups observed that auditory stimulation induced a decreased response in the auditory cortex and was related to negative signal in the visual cortex and precuneus.[52] Intriguingly, visual stimulation during SWS in adults elicited a decrease in activity in the occipital cortex.[53] This decrease was more rostral and dorsal compared to the relative rCBF increase along the calcarine sulcus found during visual stimulation in the awake state. The origin of this negative blood oxygenation level is still unclear despite recent replication.[54]

Sleep and Brain Plasticity

Evidence accumulates suggesting that sleep participates in the consolidation of recent memory traces.[55] Accordingly, PET studies have shown that waking experience influences regional brain activity during subsequent REM and NREM sleep. Several brain areas, activated during procedural motor sequence learning (using a serial reaction time task) during wakefulness, have been found to be significantly more activated during subsequent REM sleep in subjects previously trained on the task than in nontrained subjects.[56] Furthermore, this effect is not observed in subjects trained to a task with similar practice requirements but devoid of any sequential content.[57] These findings speak against use-dependent changes in regional brain activations. Additionally, functional coupling between learning-related areas was found to be enhanced during post-training REM sleep.[58] Another PET study demonstrated that hippocampal and parahippocampal areas, which are activated during a spatial memory task, can be reactivated during post-training NREM sleep and that the amount of hippocampal activity during SWS positively correlated with overnight improvement in the memory for spatial locations.[59] Collectively, these findings suggest that reactivations of regional activity and modifications of functional connectivity during post-training sleep reflect the off-line processing of recent memory, which eventually leads to improved performance the next day. Moreover, these results are in line with behavioral data suggesting that NREM sleep and REM sleep differentially modulate the consolidation of declarative and nondeclarative memories, respectively.[60,61] However, they do not rule out an alternative hypothesis that natural succession of NREM sleep and REM sleep is also mandatory for memory consolidation. Additionally, these results are consistent with a recent intracranial EEG study in epileptic patients showing that, during sleep, functional connectivity between rhinal and hippocampal structures was larger for patients with good dream recall than for those with poor recall after they were awaked during REM sleep.[62]

Finally, recent fMRI studies demonstrated that sleep deprivation hinders the plastic changes that normally would occur during post-training sleep.[63] In this study, the effects of normal sleep or sleep deprivation on learning-dependent changes in regional brain activity were assessed after the subjects were trained on a pursuit task, in which they had to hold a joystick position as close as possible to a moving target, whose trajectory was predictable on the horizontal axis but not on the vertical axis. The time on target was used as the behavioral performance parameter. In the first group, subjects were totally sleep-deprived during the first post-training night, while in the second group, they were allowed to sleep. Both groups were then retested after 2 more nights of normal sleep in order to recover a similar state of arousal across the two groups and between the training and retest sessions. The fMRI scanning session was recorded during the retest, while subjects were exposed to the previously learned trajectory and also to a new one in which the predictable axis was vertical. Behavioral results showed that the time on target was larger for the learned trajectory

than for the new one in both groups during the retest, and that this performance gain was greater in the sleeping group than in the sleep deprivation group. The fMRI data showed a significant effect of learning, irrespective of the group, in two regions: the left supplementary eye field and the right dentate nucleus. A region of the right superior temporal sulcus, close to regions coding for motion processing (biologic motion, smooth pursuit, etc.), was found to be more active for the learned than for the new trajectory, and more so in the sleeping group than in the sleep deprivation group. The functional connectivity also showed that the dentate nucleus was more closely linked to the superior temporal sulcus, and the supplementary eye field to the frontal eye field, for the learned than for the new trajectory, and more so in the sleeping group. Moreover, interactions between the temporal cortex and cerebellum, as well as between the frontal eye field and the supplementary eye field, are both known to be implicated in the standard pursuit eye movement pathways.[64] These results therefore suggest that the performance on the pursuit task relies on the subject's ability to learn the motion characteristics of trajectory in order to program optimal motor pursuit execution. Sleep deprivation during the first post-training night would disturb the slow processes that lead to the acquisition of this procedural skill and alter related changes in functional connectivity that were reinforced in subjects allowed to sleep.[63]

Recently, Orban et al.[65] used fMRI in order to map regional cerebral activity during place-finding navigation in a virtual town, immediately after learning and 3 days later, in subjects either allowed regular sleep (RS) or totally sleep-deprived (SD) on the first post-training night. Results showed that, at immediate and delayed retrieval, place-finding navigation elicited increased brain activity in an extended hippocampo-neocortical network in both RS and SD subjects. Moreover, behavioral performance was equivalent between groups. However, striatal navigation-related activity increased more at delayed retrieval in RS than in SD subjects. Furthermore, correlations between striatal response and behavioral performance, as well as functional connectivity between the striatum and the hippocampus, were modulated by post-training sleep. Overall, these data suggest that brain activity is restructured during sleep in such a way that navigation in the virtual environment, initially related to a hippocampus-dependent spatial strategy, becomes progressively contingent in part on a response-based strategy mediated by the striatum. Interestingly, both neural strategies eventually relate to equivalent performance levels, indicating that covert reorganization of brain patterns underlying navigation after sleep is not necessarily accompanied by overt changes in behavior.[65] Further studies have also evidenced a reorganization of brain activity when post-training sleep is allowed both for neutral[66] and emotional[67] verbal material. In addition, exposure to an odor during SWS that had been presented as context during prior learning improved the retention of hippocampus-dependent declarative memories and elicited a significant hippocampal activation during SWS.[68]

In addition, EEG and MEG studies have provided robust evidence for the "sleep and memory consolidation" hypothesis by focusing on more specific sleep features and mechanisms that are regarded as important for different types of memory, including sleep spindles,[69–72] slow waves,[73] or the actual number of rapid eye movements.[74] For instance, sleep homeostasis has a local synaptic component, which can be triggered by a learning task involving specific brain regions. The local increase in slow-wave activity after learning correlated with improved performance of the task after sleep.[73] Moreover, the induction of slow oscillation–like potential fields by transcranial application of slowly oscillating potentials (0.75 Hz) during early nocturnal NREM sleep (i.e., a period of emerging SWS) enhanced the retention of hippocampus-dependent declarative memories in healthy humans. This kind of stimulation induced an immediate increase in SWS, endogenous cortical slow oscillations, and slow spindle activity in the frontal cortex.[75] Last but not least, it has been suggested that sleep may promote "creativity" or "insight".[76,77]

Alertness, Performance, and Sleep Deprivation

Sleep deprivation or fragmentation is increasingly common in industrialized societies (noisy environments, shift work). Likewise, many sleep disorders tend to become more frequent (e.g., insomnia, anxiety disorders). The considerable proportion of vehicle accidents related to sleep loss is now viewed as a serious concern for public health.[78] The impact of sleep deprivation on cognition and brain functions has been assessed mainly in healthy subjects. By comparison, studies on the consequences of sleep disorders on behavior and cerebral activity remain scarce.

Basal Metabolism

An early study investigated the effect of total sleep deprivation (about 32 hours) on brain metabolism.[79] Although global brain metabolism was not affected by sleep deprivation, absolute regional glucose metabolism significantly decreased in the thalamus, basal ganglia, and cerebellum. A significant reorganization of regional activity was observed after sleep deprivation, with relative decreases in the cerebral metabolic rate of glucose (CMRglu) within the temporal lobes and relative increases in the visual cortex.[79] Additionally, sleep deprivation significantly reduced performance in an attentional continuous performance test, and this decrease was significantly correlated with reduced metabolic rate in thalamic, basal ganglia, and limbic regions.[79]

Cognitive Challenges

Sleep deprivation is known to alter alertness and performance in a series of cognitive tasks. Several neuroimaging studies have tried to determine the underlying patterns of cerebral activity during different cognitive tasks. The cerebral responses to sleep deprivation seem to depend on the type of task and also on its level of difficulty. Both decreases and increases in responses were reported. The former were interpreted as metabolic impairments related to sleep deprivation, whereas the latter were viewed as compensatory responses.

A recent study showed that, even after as little as 24 hours of continuous wakefulness, significant decreases in global CMRglu are observed with [^{18}F]2-fluoro-2-deoxy-D-glucose (^{18}FDG) PET.[3] When subjects performed a sleep deprivation–sensitive serial addition/subtraction task (which combines arithmetic processing and working memory), significant decreases in absolute regional CMRglu were found in several cortical and subcortical structures, whereas no areas of the brain showed any significant increase in regional metabolism. Alertness and cognitive performance scores declined in parallel with deactivations in the thalamus and in the prefrontal and posterior parietal cortices.[3]

The same group of researchers characterized the cerebral effects of 24, 48, and 72 hours of sleep deprivation during the same task performance in 17 healthy subjects using correlations with performance measures outside of the scanner and metabolism during resting state assessed by ^{18}FDG PET.[4] Results showed that absolute CMRglu and relative regional CMRglu (rCMRglu) decreased further at 48 and 72 hours of sleep deprivation primarily in the prefrontal and parietal cortices and in the thalamus, the same areas that showed decreases at 24 hours of sleep deprivation. The authors proposed that the decreases in CMRglu induced in the prefrontal-thalamic network by sleep deprivation underlie the progressive impairment in cognitive performance and alertness and the progression toward sleep onset. In contrast, increased activity in visual and motor areas would reflect voluntary attempts to remain awake and perform despite a continuing decline in prefrontal-thalamic network activity.[4]

In these CMRglu studies, metabolism during resting state was correlated with performance measures obtained outside of the scanner. However, a different picture emerges when subjects are scanned during task performance.

Drummond and colleagues used fMRI on normal subjects while those subjects performed different cognitive tasks after a normal night of sleep or following 35 hours of sleep deprivation. In a first report,[2] the study used a serial subtraction task. Bilateral activations in the prefrontal, parietal, and premotor cortices were found during task practice after a normal night of sleep, whereas activity in these regions declined markedly after sleep deprivation, mainly in the prefrontal cortex,[2] which is in agreement with the hypothesis of prefrontal cortex vulnerability to sleep deprivation.[80] Likewise, Mu and colleagues[81] found reduced activations in several frontal and parietal regions (left dorsolateral prefrontal cortex, right ventrolateral prefrontal cortex, supplementary motor area, Broca's area, bilateral posterior parietal cortices) but no significant increased activations during practice of the Sternberg working memory task (SWMT) after 30 hours of sleep deprivation compared to normal sleep. However, a very different pattern emerged when using other types of tasks. For example, the effects of 35 hours of continuous wakefulness on cerebral activation during verbal learning (memorizing a list of words) was also investigated using fMRI.[82] The authors found that the prefrontal cortex and parietal lobes were more activated during verbal learning after 1 night of sleep deprivation than after normal sleep. In addition, increased subjective sleepiness in sleep-deprived subjects correlated significantly with the amount of prefrontal cortex activation, while stronger parietal lobe activation was linked to less impairment in the free recall of words. It has been suggested that these results reflect dynamic, compensatory changes in cerebral activation during verbal learning after sleep deprivation.[82] Likewise, another study found stronger correlation between difficulty in a logical reasoning task and increased activity in the bilateral inferior parietal lobes, bilateral temporal cortex, and left inferior and dorsolateral prefrontal cortex following 35 hours of continuous wakefulness than after normal sleep.[83] This suggests that compensatory mechanisms may lead to activation in regions that do not show significant responses to task demands in the well-rested condition, as well as to stronger responses within regions typically underlying task performance.[83]

Neurobehavioral (fMRI) effects of 24 hours of continuous wakefulness were assessed using two verbal working memory tasks of different difficulty levels, known to induce responses in frontal-parietal networks in normal, non–sleep-deprived conditions. After sleep deprivation, activity was reduced in the medial parietal, anterior medial frontal, and posterior cingulate regions in both tasks, and disproportionately greater activation of the left dorsolateral prefrontal cortex and bilateral thalamus was observed when additional manipulation of information in working memory was required[84] (see also Choo et al.[85]).

Other cognitive domains seem to be impaired by sleep deprivation. For instance, competent decision making was impaired after sleep deprivation, which induced a modulation of activation in the nucleus accumbens and insula, brain regions associated with risky decision making and emotional processing.[86]

These data suggest that decreases in regional brain activity could contribute to cognitive impairment after sleep deprivation and that increased prefrontal and thalamic activation may represent compensatory adaptation. In a similar attempt to better consideration how sleep deprivation might interact with task difficulty, the effects of normal sleep and 36 hours of total sleep deprivation were assessed by fMRI during a verbal learning task with two levels of difficulty (easy and difficult words).[87] A set of regions showed increased response to difficult words after sleep deprivation compared with normal sleep (inferior frontal gyrus, dorsolateral prefrontal cortex and inferior parietal lobe, bilaterally). While better free recall performance on the difficult words following sleep deprivation was positively related to activation within the left inferior and superior parietal lobes and left inferior frontal gyrus, it was negatively related to activation within the right inferior frontal gyrus. Consequently, the performance relationships are thought to be both beneficial (as a compensatory function) and deleterious (as an interference with task performance), depending on the brain regions implicated.

Since prefrontal cortex functioning appears to be affected by sleep loss, processes mediated by this region should be altered after sleep deprivation (e.g., attention, emotion, motivation, feeding, olfaction). In order to asses the effects of sleep deprivation on olfaction, which is mediated by the orbitofrontal cortex, a region known to have decreased activity after sleep deprivation,[3] Killgore and McBride[88] studied 38 healthy subjects at rest and after 24 hours of sleep deprivation. Relative to rested baseline performance, sleep-deprived subjects showed a significant decline in the ability to identify specific odors on the Smell Identification Test.

Duration of Sleep Deprivation

Chronic restriction of sleep to 6 hours or less per night produces cognitive impairments similar to up to 2 nights of total sleep deprivation. Thus, it appears that moderate sleep restriction can seriously impair waking neurobehavioral functions in healthy adults, who are very often unaware of such deficits.[89] Sleep debt could be better understood as a consequence of extended wakefulness, with a neurobiologic "cost" that could accumulate over time.[89] However, rapid sleep loss has been shown to produce significantly more impairment on tests of alertness, memory, and performance compared to the slow accumulation of a comparable amount of sleep loss.[90] Some authors have proposed that this may reflect some mechanism(s) of adaptation to chronic sleep deprivation.[90] While the majority of the neuroimaging studies on sleep deprivation have used 1 night of sleep deprivation (24 hours of continuous wakefulness), neuroimaging studies that systematically assess what happens following shorter or longer sleep deprivation duration are still awaited.[4]

Personal Vulnerability to Sleep Deprivation

People may be differently affected by the same sleep-depriving environmental conditions. Results from one study suggest that brain responses to sleep deprivation for a given task are modulated by individual vulnerability to sleep deprivation.[91] In this study, subjects were divided into two groups, a sleep deprivation (SD)–resilient group and an SD-vulnerable group, according to their performance on the SWMT after sleep deprivation. In the SD-resilient group, significant activations were found in several cortical areas (left dorsolateral prefrontal cortex, left ventrolateral prefrontal cortex, left supplementary motor area, left posterior parietal cortex) during practice of the SWMT after sleep deprivation. By contrast, in the SD-vulnerable group, only the left dorsolateral prefrontal cortex was found to be activated after sleep deprivation. The patterns of brain activation after sleep deprivation may therefore differ as a function of the subjects' individual vulnerability to sleep deprivation.[91] The same group conducted another fMRI study on fatigue vulnerability in military pilots. Pilots were scanned during the SWMT under non–sleep-deprived conditions and individual fatigue vulnerability was quantified using performance on a flight simulation during 37 hours of continuous wakefulness. Correlation analyses revealed that global cortical activation was significantly related to fatigue vulnerability on flight-simulator performance. The authors therefore proposed that baseline fMRI scan activation during the SWMT may provide a good index of individual fatigue susceptibility.[92]

Recently, interindividual differences in working memory performance were evaluated in 26 healthy subjects both after normal sleep and after 24 and 35 hours of sleep deprivation using fMRI.[93] In both sleep deprivation sessions, there was reduced task-related activation in the superior parietal regions and left thalamus, as compared to normal sleep. Moreover, activation of the left parietal and left frontal regions after normal sleep was negatively correlated with individual performance decline from normal sleep to 24 hours of sleep deprivation. Thus, frontoparietal activation after normal sleep could differentiate individuals who will maintain working memory performance following sleep deprivation from those who will be vulnerable to its effects.

In another study, individuals better able to maintain inhibitory efficiency in a go/no-go task after sleep deprivation could be distinguished by lower stop-related, phasic activation of the right ventral prefrontal cortex during rested wakefulness.[94] These individuals also showed a larger rise in such activation both in that region and in the right insula after sleep deprivation relative to people whose inhibitory efficiency declined.

Interestingly, the most robust behavioral marker of vulnerability to sleep deprivation was the change in the intraindividual variability of reaction times. This was shown both to be stable over time and to be correlated with the drop in left parietal activation from rested wakefulness to sleep deprivation.[95] The modulation of this parietal activation may provide a good physiologic marker of vulnerability to sleep deprivation because of its reproducibility.

Functional Imaging and Drug Response

Functional neuroimaging can also be used to explore the effect of drugs on brain function and vigilance states and the influence of several neurotransmitter systems in the regulation of human sleep. Several examples are available in studies on assessment of muscarinic cholinergic receptors[96] and modafinil[97] in narcolepsy, use of bupropion in depression,[98] and assessment of opioid receptor agonists in restless legs syndrome.[99]

Several studies assessed the effects of benzodiazepines and sedative-hypnotics on brain function.[100–104] For instance, lorazepam administration markedly decreases regional brain glucose metabolism in the thalamus and occipital cortex during wakefulness.[100] It was suggested that benzodiazepine-induced changes in thalamic activity may account for the sedative properties of these drugs, since changes in metabolic activity in the thalamus correlated to lorazepam-induced sleepiness. During sleep induced by zolpidem (an imidazopyridine hypnotic relatively selective for the BZ1 or omega receptor), rCBF was found to decrease in the anterior cingulate cortex during REM sleep while it decreased in the prefrontal cortex and the insula during NREM sleep.[103] Finally, blood flow decreased in the basal forebrain and amygdaloid complexes during NREM sleep induced by triazolam (a short-acting benzodiazepine).[105] These results suggest that hypnotic effects of the benzodiazepines may be mediated mainly by deactivation of forebrain control systems that are usually strongly activated during active wakefulness, and also by the anxiolytic effect induced by deactivation of the amygdaloid complexes.[105]

NEUROIMAGING IN SLEEP DISORDERS

Sleep may be disrupted in a number of conditions ranging from medical diseases (e.g., endocrine disorders, chronic pain, brain lesions, sleep apnea) and psychiatric disorders (e.g., anxiety, depression, schizophrenia) to environmental situations (e.g., jet lag, shift work, noisy environment).

In this section, we consider several primary sleep disorders (narcolepsy, periodic limb movement disorder, idiopathic insomnia, recurrent hypersomnia, and obstructive sleep apnea) as well as specific parasomnia syndromes (sleepwalking, REM sleep behavior disorder) and several sleep disorders associated with psychiatric or neurologic disorders (psychoses, mood disorders, fatal familial insomnia, Landau-Kleffner syndrome and related disorders). We do not review sleep disorders due to disturbances from external, environmental sources.

Idiopathic Insomnia

Idiopathic insomnia is a lifelong inability to obtain adequate sleep that is presumably due to an abnormality in the neurologic control of sleep-wake regulation systems.[106] This disorder is thought to reflect an imbalance between the arousal system and the various sleep-inducing and sleep-maintaining systems. Neuroanatomic, neurophysiologic, or neurochemical dysfunctions or lesions within the sleep-wake systems are suspected in some of these patients.[106]

Theoretically, either hyperactivity within the arousal system or hypoactivity within the sleep system may cause idiopathic insomnia, but hyperarousal is believed to be the final common pathway of the disorder.[106] Increased arousal might be of a physiologic, cognitive, or affective nature; it is likely that these categories overlap,[5,107] since several studies have reported increased alertness on the Multiple Sleep Latency Test, increased heart rate during the sleep period, increased anxiety on rating scales, and increased tension during wakefulness.[107–109] In addition, poor sleep leads to altered mood and motivation, decreased attention and vigilance, low levels of energy and concentration, and increased daytime fatigue.[106]

Quantitative EEG recordings suggest an overall cortical hyperarousal in insomnia. However, hyperarousal in primary insomnia was also found to be associated with greater increase in beta/gamma activity at sleep onset, followed by a decline of high-frequency EEG activity leading to a period of hypoarousal.[110] This could explain why some neuroimaging studies showed a cortical hyperarousal pattern in insomnia while others reported a decrease in cortical functions. In the latter case, decreased metabolism might originate from time-window coincidence of the cortical hypoarousal period to neuroimaging acquisition, and therefore does not discard the hyperaousal hypothesis of primary insomnia.

Only a few studies tried to characterize the functional neuroanatomy of idiopathic insomnia disorder (referred to as primary insomnia in these reports). rCBF was estimated using technetium-99m–labeled hexamethylene-propyleneamine oxime (^{99m}Tc-HMPAO), a gamma-emitting radionuclide imaging agent used in the evaluation of rCBF, in five insomniacs and four normal sleepers. Patients with insomnia showed major rCBF decrease in the basal ganglia, medial frontal cortex, occipital cortex, and parietal cortex. These results suggest that idiopathic insomnia is associated with an abnormal pattern of regional brain activity during NREM sleep that particularly involves a dysfunction in the basal ganglia.[111]

More recently, ^{18}FDG PET was used to measure regional CMRglu of 7 patients with idiopathic insomnia and 20 healthy age- and gender-matched subjects during waking and NREM sleep.[112] Insomniac patients showed increased global CMRglu during sleep as compared to healthy subjects, suggesting an overall cortical hyperarousal in insomnia. Moreover, insomniac patients had a smaller decline, related to healthy subjects, in relative CMRglu from waking to sleep states in the ascending reticular activating system, hypothalamus, thalamus, insular cortex, amygdala, hippocampus, anterior cingulate, and medial prefrontal cortices (Fig. 15–2). During wakefulness, reduced relative metabolism, as compared to healthy subjects, was found in the prefrontal cortex bilaterally, in the left temporal, parietal, and occipital cortices, and in the thalamus, hypothalamus, and brain stem reticular formation. These findings confirm that regional brain activity does not normally progress from waking to sleep states in patients with insomnia. Additionally, it was proposed that daytime fatigue resulting from inefficient sleep may be reflected by decreased activity in the prefrontal cortex.[112]

Four of the insomnia patients from the Smith et al. study were rescanned after they had been treated with cognitive behavioral therapy.[113] After this psychotherapeutic

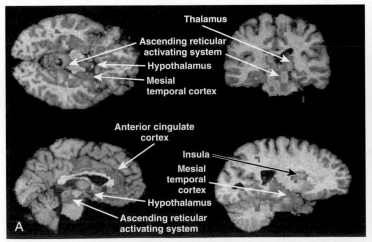
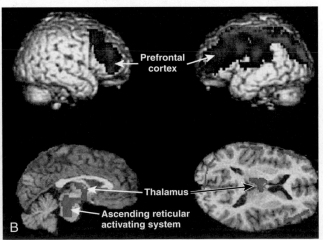

FIGURE 15–2 CMRglu assessed by ^{18}FDG PET in insomniacs (versus healthy subjects) during waking and NREM sleep. **(A)** Brain structures that did not show decreased cerebral metabolic rate of glucose (CMRglu) from waking to sleep states in patients with idiopathic insomnia. **(B)** Brain structures where relative metabolism while awake was higher in healthy subjects than in patients with insomnia. Differences in all regions shown reached statistical significance ($p < 0.05$), corrected at the cluster level. *(Reproduced with permission from Nofzinger EA, Buysse DJ, Germain A, et al: Functional neuroimaging evidence for hyperarousal in insomnia. Am J Psychiatry 2004;161:2126. Copyright 2004, American Psychiatric Association.) See Color Plate*

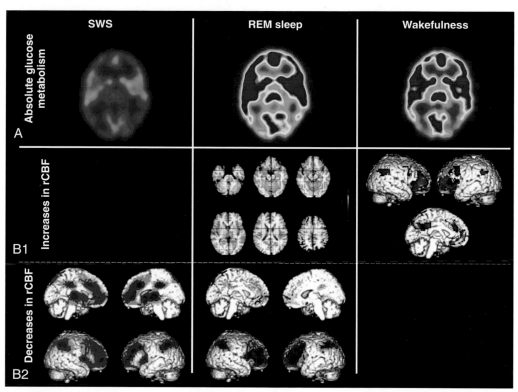

FIGURE 15–1 Cerebral glucose metabolism (CGM) and regional cerebral blood flow (CBF) during deep NREM sleep (*first column*), REM sleep (*second column*), and wakefulness (*third column*). **(Row A)** CGM quantified in the same individual at 1-week interval, using FDG and PET. The three images are displayed at the same brain level using the same color scale. The average CGM during deep NREM sleep (versus wakefulness) is significantly decreased. During REM sleep, the CGM is as high as during wakefulness. **(Row B1)** Distribution of the *highest* regional brain activity, as assessed by CBF measurement using PET, during wakefulness and REM sleep. The most active regions during *wakefulness* are located in the polymodal associative cortices in the prefrontal and parietal lobes (both on the medial wall and convexity). During *REM sleep,* the most active areas are located in the pontine tegmentum, thalami, amygdaloid complexes, and anterior cingulate cortex. Other data (not shown) have shown a large activity in the occipital cortices, insula, and hippocampus.[15] **(Row B2)** Distribution of the *lowest* regional brain activity, as assessed by CBF measurement using PET, during NREM and REM sleep. In both sleep stages, the least active regions are located in the polymodal associative cortices in the prefrontal and parietal lobes (convexity). During *NREM sleep,* the brain stem and thalami are also particularly deactivated. (See page 200)

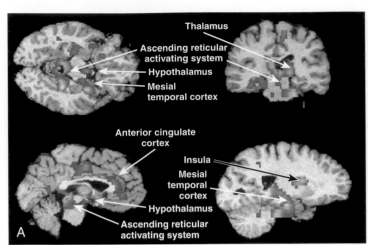

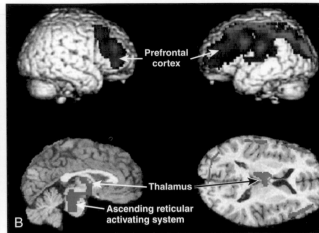

FIGURE 15–2 CMRglu assessed by [18]FDG PET in insomniacs (versus heathy subjects) during waking and NREM sleep. **(A)** Brain structures that did not show decreased cerebral metabolic rate of glucose (CMRglu) from waking to sleep states in patients with idiopathic insomnia. **(B)** Brain structures where relative metabolism while awake was higher in healthy subjects than in patients with insomnia. Differences in all regions shown reached statistical significance ($p < 0.05$), corrected at the cluster level.*(Reproduced with permission from Nofzinger EA, Buysse DJ, Germain A, et al: Functional neuroimaging evidence for hyperarousal in insomnia. Am J Psychiatry 2004;161:2126. Copyright 2004, American Psychiatric Association.)* (See page 206)

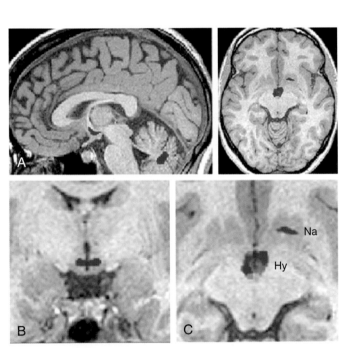

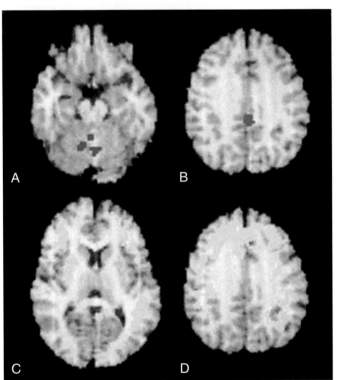

FIGURE 15–3 Statistical parametric maps demonstrating the structural difference in gray matter between narcolepsy patients and healthy control subjects. Differences are shown superimposed in red on a normalized image of a healthy control subject. The *left panel* in *A* is the left side of the brain. A significant decrease in gray matter concentration was found in the hypothalamus (Hy) (*A-C*) and in the area of the right nucleus accumbens (Na) (*A and C*) *(Reproduced with permission from Draganski B, Geisler P, Hajak G, et al: Hypothalamic gray matter changes in narcoleptic patients. Nat Med 2002;8:1186. Copyright 2002, Nature Publishing Group.)* (See page 207)

FIGURE 15–4 SPECT findings during sleepwalking after integration into the appropriate anatomic magnetic resonance image. The highest increases of regional CBF (>25%) during sleepwalking compared with quiet stage 3 to 4 NREM sleep are found in the anterior cerebellum (i.e., vermis) **(A)**, and in the posterior cingulate cortex **(B)**. However, as compared to data from normal volunteers during wakefulness, large areas of frontal and parietal association cortices remain deactivated during sleepwalking, as shown in the corresponding parametric maps. Note the inclusion of the dorsolateral prefrontal cortex **(C)**, mesial frontal cortex **(D)**, and left angular gyrus **(C)** within these areas. *(Reproduced with permission from Bassetti C, Vella S, Donati F. et al. SPECT during sleepwalking. Lancet 2000;356:484. Copyright 2000, The Lancet.)* (See page 211)

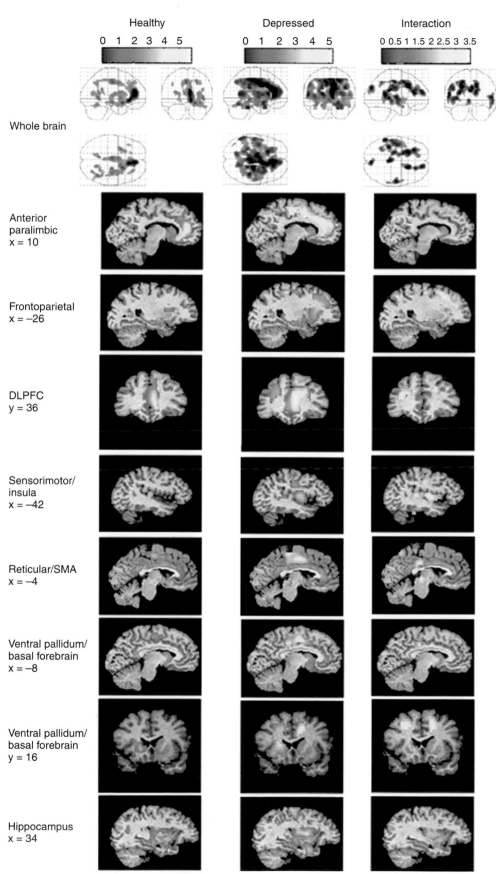

FIGURE 15–5 rCMRglu from waking to REM sleep in depression. Waking-to–REM sleep activation in healthy subjects (*column 1*) and depressed subjects (*column 2*), and interactions showing regions where the depressed subjects' waking-to–REM sleep activations are greater than those of healthy subjects (*column 3*). (DLPFC, dorsolateral prefrontal cortex; SMA, supplementary motor area; x and y, Talairach x and y coordinates.) *(Reproduced with permission from Nofzinger EA, Buysse DJ, Germain A, et al: Increased activation of anterior paralimbic and executive cortex from waking to rapid eye movement sleep in depression. Arch Gen Psychiatry 2004;61:695. Copyright © 2004, American Medical Association. All rights reserved.)* (See page 215)

treatment, sleep latency was reduced by at least 43% and there was a global 24% increase in CBF, with significant increases in the basal ganglia. Smith and collaborators proposed that such increase in brain activity might reflect the normalization of sleep homeostatic processes. These encouraging initial results will certainly inspire further investigations on the effects of psychotherapy on brain functioning in insomnia.

Narcolepsy

Narcolepsy is a disorder characterized by excessive sleepiness that is typically associated with several manifestations of so-called dissociated or isolated REM sleep features, such as muscle atonia (i.e., cataplexy), sleep paralysis, and hallucinations.[106,114] Human narcolepsy has recently been found to be associated with reduction in or loss of the hypothalamic peptide hypocretin (also called orexin) implicated in arousal systems.[115-119]

Anatomic Neuroimaging Studies of Narcolepsy

The pontine tegmentum controls transitions between sleep states and was therefore first proposed as a possible main site of anatomic or functional impairments in narcolepsy. While Plazzi and coworkers had reported pontine tegmentum abnormalities in three narcoleptic patients,[120] two other structural magnetic resonance imaging (MRI) studies[121,122] found no pontine abnormalities (except in 2 of 12 patients who had long-standing hypertension[122]). The MRI abnormalities found in Plazzi et al.'s study could reflect nonspecific age-related pontine vascular changes rather than a narcolepsy-related phenomenon.[120]

More recently, studies tried to find evidence for hypothalamic abnormalities using voxel-based morphometry (VBM). VBM is a neuroimaging analysis technique that allows the investigation of focal differences in tissue composition (gray and white matter) based on high-resolution scans. To date, VBM studies have reported equivocal results in narcoleptic patients. An early study found no structural change in brains of patients with hypocretin-deficient narcolepsy.[123] Two subsequent studies did find cortical gray matter reduction predominantly in frontal brain regions,[124] as well as in inferior temporal regions.[125] Interestingly, relative global gray matter loss was independent of disease duration or medication history, and there were no significant subcortical gray matter alterations.[125] Significant gray matter concentration decreases were found in the hypothalamus, cerebellum (vermis), superior temporal gyrus, and right nucleus accumbens in 29 narcoleptic patients relative to unaffected healthy controls (Fig. 15–3).[126] Given the major projection sites of hypocretin-1 (the hypothalamus among others) and hypocretin-2 (the nucleus accumbens among others), the decreases in gray matter could thus reflect secondary neuronal losses due to the destruction of specific hypocretin

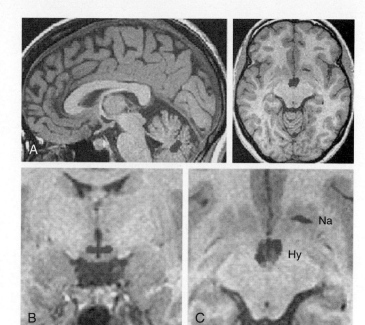

FIGURE 15–3 Statistical parametric maps demonstrating the structural difference in gray matter between narcolepsy patients and healthy control subjects. Differences are shown superimposed in red on a normalized image of a healthy control subject. The *left panel* in **A** is the left side of the brain. A significant decrease in gray matter concentration was found in the hypothalamus (Hy) (**A-C**) and in the area of the right nucleus accumbens (Na) (**A** and **C**) *(Reproduced with permission from Draganski B, Geisler P, Hajak G, et al: Hypothalamic gray matter changes in narcoleptic patients. Nat Med 2002;8:1186. Copyright 2002, Nature Publishing Group.) See Color Plate*

projections. The results of this study were recently corroborated by another VBM study.[127]

Proton magnetic resonance spectroscopy (^{1}H-MRS) was also used to assess the *N*-acetylaspartate (NAA) and creatinine plus phosphocreatinine (Cr+PCr) content in the specific brain areas of narcoleptic patients. A reduced NAA/Cr+PCr ratio indicates reduced neuronal function, which could reflect neuronal loss (i.e., fewer neurons) but could also be due to reduced activity of existing neurons. An analysis of spectral peak area ratios revealed a decrease in the NAA/Cr+PCr ratio in the hypothalamus[128] and the ventral pontine areas[129] of narcoleptic patients compared with control subjects. Several factors can explain equivocal results across both VBM and spectroscopy studies, such as inhomogeneous patient groups, history of treatment, or, for VBM, prestatistical image processing and limited sensitivity of this technique. In conclusion, VBM studies with larger samples of drug-naive patients are required to identify reliably structural abnormalities in narcolepsy.

Functional Neuroimaging Studies of Narcolepsy

Early functional observations using ^{133}Xe inhalation showed that, during wakefulness, brain stem and cerebral blood flow was lower in narcoleptic patients than in normal subjects.[130] However, after sleep onset (3 of

13 cases in REM sleep), the CBF increased in all regions, particularly in temporoparietal regions. This pattern was supposedly attributed to dreaming activity, in line with prior reports showing increased regional blood flow in temporoparietal areas during visual dreaming and hypnagogic hallucinations.[130,131]

More recently, a ^{99m}Tc-HMPAO SPECT study in six narcoleptic patients found similar HMPAO uptake in the waking state and REM sleep,[132] suggesting a similar overall cortical activity. Data analysis using regions of interest additionally indicated an activation of parietal regions during REM sleep.[132] The latter result is intriguing given the parietal deactivation usually observed by PET studies during normal REM sleep.[8] Further studies are needed to confirm these results in a larger population.

There are very few data describing the neural correlates of cataplexy in narcoleptic patients. One SPECT study was conducted on two patients during a cataplexy episode compared to REM sleep or a baseline waking period.[133] During cataplexy, perfusion increased in limbic areas (including the amygdala) and the basal ganglia, thalami, premotor cortices, sensorimotor cortices, and brain stem, whereas perfusion decreased in the prefrontal cortex and occipital lobe. Increased cingulate and amygdala activity may relate to concomitant emotional processing that is usually reported as a powerful trigger of cataplexy. However, such hyperperfusion in the pons, thalami and amygdaloid complexes was not found in a recent single case report.[134]

Based on the clinical observation that cataplexy episodes are often triggered by positive emotions (e.g., hearing or telling jokes), an event-related fMRI study was performed on narcoleptic patients and controls while they watched sequences of humorous pictures. A group comparison revealed that humorous pictures elicited reduced hypothalamic response together with enhanced amygdala response in the narcoleptic patients. These results suggest that hypothalamic hypocretin activity physiologically modulates the processing of emotional inputs within the amygdala, and that suprapontine mechanisms of cataplexy might involve a dysfunction of hypothalamic-amygdala interactions triggered by positive emotions.[135,136]

Neurotransmission in Narcolepsy

Given the role of acetylcholine as an important neurotransmitter in the generation of REM sleep (see earlier), it was hypothesized that disturbances in the cholinergic system might underlie narcolepsy. However at present, there is no existing evidence for a change in muscarinic cholinergic receptors in narcoleptic patients.[96]

Likewise, the dopamine system has been probed by PET and SPECT in narcoleptic patients because increased dopamine D_2 receptor binding was shown in the brains of deceased narcoleptic patients.[137,138] The results from these neuroimaging studies remain mostly inconsistent. One SPECT study showed elevated D_2 receptor binding in the striatal dopaminergic system, correlating with the frequency of cataplectic and sleep attacks in seven patients with narcolepsy.[139] However, other PET[140–142] or SPECT[143,144] ligand studies did not find such change in D_2 receptor binding. A potential explanation for this discrepancy might be related to the drug treatment of narcoleptic patients. Indeed, considerable increase in the uptake of ^{11}C-raclopride, a specific D_2 receptor ligand, was observed in the putamens of narcoleptic subjects older than 31 years who underwent various regimens of prolonged treatment.[145] Likewise, despite the fact that the binding of iodobenzamide (IBZM, a highly selective CNS dopamine D_2 receptor ligand), was similar in narcoleptic patients and normal controls, treatment by stimulants and/or antidepressants for 3 months significantly changed ligand uptake in four of five patients.[144] Therefore, elevated postmortem dopamine binding might be due to the long-term effect of prior treatment rather than intrinsic modifications.

Brain Response to Drug Probe in Narcolepsy

The effects of stimulant drugs on cerebral function in narcoleptic patients was assessed in two fMRI studies. The first one tested the effect of modafinil, a wakefulness-promoting drug.[97] In normal subjects, larger brain responses to a multiplexed visual and auditory stimulation paradigm were found at 10:00 AM than at 3:00 PM in visual areas, but not in auditory areas, suggesting time-of-day influences. Surprisingly, the reverse pattern of activity was observed in a group of 12 narcoleptic patients, with higher activity at 3:00 PM than 10:00 AM. Critically, modafinil administration did not modify the average level of activation either in normal subjects or in narcoleptics ($n = 8$), but postdrug activation level was inversely proportional to the predrug activation level. These findings are not easy to interpret but might suggest that modafinil can modulate brain activation in response to external stimuli.

Another fMRI study assessed the effects of amphetamines in two patients with narcoleptic syndrome.[146] The extent of the brain response to auditory and visual stimulation decreased after amphetamine administration in normal subjects. The reverse pattern was observed in the narcoleptic patients. Once again these findings remain difficult to interpret, and larger samples of patients should be studied. The apparent disparity of these results indicates that, despite recent breakthroughs in the pathophysiology of narcolepsy, more studies using state-of-the-art technology of acquisition and analysis of functional neuroimaging data are needed to better characterize the functional organization of the narcoleptic brain during wakefulness and sleep.

Recurrent Hypersomnia

Recurrent hypersomnia is a disorder characterized by recurrent episodes of hypersomnia that typically occur weeks or months apart.[106] One SPECT study in a

24-year-old male with recurrent hypersomnia showed decreased blood flow in the left thalamus during the hypersomnolent period, but failed to report any abnormal activation during recovery or remission periods.[147] This case report neuroimaging study provides only limited information about possible pathophysiologic mechanisms of this disorder. By contrast, other clinical and electrophysiologic studies clearly point toward a hypothalamic rather than a thalamic dysfunction.[148–150]

Obstructive Sleep Apnea Syndrome

Obstructive sleep apnea syndrome (OSAS) is characterized by repetitive episodes of upper airway obstruction that occur during sleep, usually associated with a reduction in blood oxygen saturation.[106] Population-based epidemiologic studies have revealed a high prevalence (1–5% of adult men) of OSAS. They also associate OSAS with significant morbidity, such as hypertension, cardiovascular disease, stroke, and motor vehicle accidents.[151] OSAS may lead to functional and structural brain alterations. Functional alterations such as sleep fragmentation are often associated with neuropsychological deficits that can be reversible after treatment of OSAS. Structural alterations may indicate irreversible consequences on brain integrity and suggest permanent cognitive impairment, although this proposal remains a matter of debate in the literature.

The pathophysiology of OSAS is complex and not yet completely understood. Several studies suggest that OSAS across all age groups is due to a combination of both anatomic airway narrowing and abnormal upper airway neuromotor tone. Notwithstanding the known anatomic factors, such as craniofacial anomalies, obesity, and adenotonsillar hypertrophy, that contribute to OSAS, clear anatomic contributing factors cannot always be identified.[106] This suggests that alterations in upper airway neuromuscular tone also play an important role in the etiology of OSAS.[152] The pathophysiology of OSAS also includes enhanced chemoreflex sensitivity and an exaggerated sympathetic response during hypoxemic episodes.[153]

OSAS has been associated with distinctive cognitive alterations in various domains. Both hypoxemia and fragmented sleep are proposed as the main factor leading to neurocognitive impairments during wakefulness.[154–161] Several studies emphasized the deterioration of executive functions in OSAS patients, including the inability to initiate new mental processes[162,163] and deficits in working memory,[162,163] analysis and synthesis,[162,164] contextual memory,[165] selective attention,[166] and continuous attention.[166] A recent meta-analysis showed that untreated patients with OSAS had a negligible impairment of intellectual and verbal functioning but a substantial impairment of vigilance and executive functioning.[167]

Structural changes in brain morphology were assessed using VBM in 21 patients with OSAS and in 21 control subjects.[168] Gray matter loss was apparent in patients with OSAS in multiple brain sites involved in motor regulation of the upper airway as well as in various cognitive functions, including the frontal and parietal cortices, temporal lobes, anterior cingulate, hippocampus, and cerebellum. Another VBM study conducted in seven OSAS patients and seven controls showed a significantly lower gray matter concentration restricted to the left hippocampus in the OSAS patients.[169] There was no difference in total gray matter volume between the two groups.

Another study compared both neuropathologic and neuropsychological effects of hypoxia in patients with either carbon monoxide poisoning or OSAS.[170] Brain imaging showed a hippocampal atrophy in both groups. Interestingly, a linear relationship between hippocampal volume and memory performance selectively in the OSAS group was found for a subset of tests (the delayed recall or the Rey-Osterrieth Complex Figure Design and Trail 6 of the Rey Auditory Verbal Learning Test among others). Moreover, hippocampal volume was related to performance on nonverbal information processing (Wechsler Adult Intelligence Scale–Revised Block Design) in both groups. Further investigation will be necessary to better delineate the specificity and contribution of hippocampal atrophy in OSAS.

Single-voxel ^{1}H-MRS has also been used to assess whether OSAS can induce axonal loss or dysfunction, or myelin metabolism impairment. An early study using this technique showed that the NAA/Cr ratio in cerebral white matter was significantly lower in patients with moderate to severe OSAS than in patients with mild OSAS and healthy subjects.[171] In a more recent study, the NAA/Cr and choline/creatine (Cho/Cr) ratios as well as absolute concentrations of NAA and choline were significantly lower in the frontal white matter of OSAS patients when compared to controls.[172] Even if these findings may explain some of the deficits in executive function associated with OSAS, it remains unclear whether hypoxia or sleep fragmentation is the primary cause of such dysfunction.

Consistent with the VBM results noted previously, decreases in absolute creatine-containing compounds in the left hippocampal area correlated with increased OSAS severity and worse neurocognitive performance.[173] In addition, a study by Halbower et al.[174] showed a decrease in NAA/Cho ratio in the left hippocampus and in the right frontal cortex using the same technique in a pediatric population with OSAS. Together, VBM and spectroscopy studies point to an atrophy and/or dysfunction of hippocampal regions in OSAS.

Long-term consequences of OSAS have been more rarely assessed after nasal continuous positive airway pressure (nCPAP) treatment. An early ^{99m}Tc-HMPAO SPECT study in 14 adult OSAS patients reported a marked frontal hyperperfusion in 5 patients.[175] In contrast, regional analysis showed reduced perfusion in the left parietal region. All these changes were reversed by effective nCPAP therapy, suggesting that the main deleterious effects of OSAS on brain activity are reversible. According to the authors, there might be an apnea-associated effect of local vascular autoregulation mechanisms acting to compensate systemic blood flow alterations or blood gas changes in OSAS. In a ^{1}H-MRS study, NAA in the parieto-occipital cortex was reduced significantly more in 14 OSAS patients than in controls but, this reduction persisted after nCPAP therapy despite clinical, neuropsychological, and neurophysiologic normalization.[176] Mandibular advancement led to decreased fMRI response in the left cingulate gyrus and the bilateral prefrontal cortices in 12 healthy subjects during induced respiratory stress.[177] Simultaneously, the subjective effects of this treatment were assessed by a visual analog scale that confirmed successful reduction of respiratory stress.

Apnea episodes in OSAS patients have considerable hemodynamic consequences, which are mediated by a complex cascade of physiologic events. Repetitive episodes of apnea trigger marked fluctuations in both blood pressure and heart rate, with consequent effects on the estimates of cardiovascular variability.[5] Several important regulatory mechanisms in cardiovascular homeostasis seem to be impaired in OSAS patients. Specific chemoreceptors seem to be implicated in the pathophysiology of OSAS.[178] For instance, the ventilatory response to carbon dioxide is elevated in OSAS patients[178] due to an elevation of the partial pressure of carbon dioxide that delimits carbon dioxide ventilatory recruitment threshold. An altered autonomic balance has been suggested as one possible pathogenic factor. This autonomic dysfunction has been thought to be implicated in the subsequent development of cardiovascular diseases in patients with OSAS.

Several fMRI studies have been conducted in OSAS patients to characterize the neural correlates of integrated afferent airway signals with autonomic outflow and airway motor response.[179-182] For instance, altered response after a Valsalva maneuver involves cerebellar, limbic, and motor area gray matter loss. Enhanced sympathetic outflow after a forehead cold pressor challenge results in both diminished and exaggerated responses in the limbic area, cerebellum, frontal cortex, and thalamus.

Altogether, these findings suggest that neuropsychological deficits in OSAS might relate to various alterations in the prefrontal cortex, hippocampus, and parietal cortex. Even if abnormal brain activations are reversible under nCPAP, several studies have suggested that not all neuropsychological impairments disappear after nCPAP.[163,183,184] Although the basic pathophysiologic mechanisms are not completely understood, a dysregulation in autonomic control seems to play an important role. However, some peripheral factors may also contribute to the deficits observed in OSAS patients, including exaggerated mass index and motivational problems.[185,186]

Periodic Limb Movements

Periodic limb movement disorder (PLMD) during sleep and restless legs syndrome (RLS) are distinct but overlapping disorders. PLMD is characterized by periodic episodes of repetitive and highly stereotyped limb movements that occur during sleep.[106] RLS is a disorder characterized by disagreeable leg sensations, usually prior to sleep onset, that cause an almost irresistible urge to move the legs.[106]

The diagnosis of PLMD does require the presence of periodic limb movements in sleep (PLMS) on polysomnography as well as an associated sleep complaint. A diagnosis of RLS, however, is essentially made on clinical grounds. Moreover, PLMS are themselves nonspecific, occurring both with RLS and with other sleep disorders (e.g., narcolepsy, sleep apnea syndrome, REM sleep behavior disorder) as well as in normal individuals.[187] Thus, the diagnosis of PLMD requires the exclusion of other potential causes for the associated sleep complaint.[188]

An inhibition of descending inhibitory pathways implicating dopaminergic, adrenergic, and opiate systems is thought to be involved in PLMS pathogenesis.[189] Patients' condition worsens when dopamine antagonists are given,[190] whereas dopaminergic drugs have been shown to relieve PLMS.[191-193] Staedt et al. have tested the hypothesis of a decrease dopaminergic activity in PLMS patients. In a series of SPECT studies, they report a decreased IBZM striatal uptake, indicating a lower D_2 receptor occupancy in PLMS patients.[194-197] Treating patients with dopamine replacement therapy increased the IBZM binding and improved the sleep quality in these patients.[196]

As RLS responds to dopaminergic medications, an etiologic link between RLS and Parkinson's disease (PD) has been hypothesized. However, a study demonstrated that RLS was present in only 15.2% of PD patients. Moreover, the prevalence of RLS in PD patients was very similar to the prevalence in the general population or a clinic population, suggesting that these two diseases may not share the same pathophysiologic mechanisms.[198]

Fourteen patients with idiopathic RLS and PLMS with a good response to dopaminergic and nondopaminergic treatment were investigated while off medication by using ^{123}I-IBZM and SPECT.[199] They were compared to 10 healthy, sex- and age-matched control subjects. The patients presented sleep disturbances, severe PLMS, and severe RLS symptoms during the period of scanning and did not show any significant differences in striatal-to-frontal ^{123}I-IBZM binding to D_2 receptors compared to controls, contrary to the previous study. These findings suggest the recovery of normal D_2 receptor function in successfully treated patients with idiopathic RLS and PLMS.[199]

One study evaluated the striatal pre- and postsynaptic dopamine status in 10 drug-naive patients suffering from both RLS and PLMS and 10 age-matched controls, by means of ^{123}I methyl-3β-(4-iodophenyl)tropane-2β-carboxylate (^{123}I-β-CIT), a ligand of dopamine transporter, and ^{123}I-IBZM SPECT, respectively.[200] There was no difference in dopamine transporter (^{123}I-β-CIT) binding between RLS-PLMS patients and controls. The study of the striatal D_2 receptor binding (^{123}I-IBZM) revealed again a significantly lower binding in patients as compared with controls. Numerous mechanisms may be responsible for the decrease of the D_2 receptor binding. Since ^{123}I-β-CIT binding is normal, a decreased number of D_2 receptors or a decreased affinity of D_2 receptors for ^{123}I-IBZM is more likely than a down-regulation of D_2 receptors due to an increased level of synaptic dopamine.[200]

Structural cerebral abnormalities have recently been reported in patients with idiopathic RLS.[201] High-resolution T1-weighted MRI of 51 patients and 51 controls analyzed using VBM revealed a bilateral gray matter increase in the pulvinar in patients with idiopathic RLS. These authors suggest that changes in thalamic structures are either involved in the pathogenesis of RLS or may reflect a consequence of chronic increase in afferent input of behaviorally relevant information. Finally, an fMRI study also attempted to localize some cerebral generators of leg discomfort and periodic limb movements in RLS.[202] During leg discomfort, the study showed a bilateral activation of the cerebellum and contralateral activation of the thalamus in patients. During a second condition combining periodic limb movements and sensory leg discomfort, patients also showed activity in the cerebellum and thalamus with additional activation in the red nuclei and brain stem close to the reticular formation. Interestingly, when subjects were asked to voluntarily imitate PLMS, there was no activation in the brain stem, but rather additional activation in the globus pallidus and motor cortex. These results suggest an involuntary mechanism of induction and a subcortical origin for RLS.

Taken together, these studies support the hypothesis that a central dopamine dysfunction is involved in the pathophysiology of RLS and PLMS, although more recent studies specifically implicate the cerebral metabolism of iron.[203] However, iron and the dopaminergic system are linked since iron is an important cofactor for tyrosine hydroxylase, the step-limiting enzyme in dopamine synthesis, and also plays a major role in the functioning of postsynaptic D_2 receptors.[5] Consistent with a link between the dopaminergic system and iron, Allen et al.[204] found decreased regional iron concentrations in the substantia nigra and putamens of five patients with RLS, both in proportion to RLS severity. In addition, Earley et al.[205] found diminished iron concentration across 10 brain regions in early-onset RLS patients but not in late-onset RLS patients when compared to controls.

Sleepwalking

Sleepwalking is an arousal parasomnia consisting of a series of complex behaviors that result in large movements during sleep.[206] It is perceived as a dissociation state whereby most of the brain sleeps except motor-related areas. One 16-year-old male subject was studied during sleepwalking using ^{99m}Tc-labeled ethyl cysteinate dimer SPECT.[207] Compared to awake normal volunteers ($n = 24$), a decrease in rCBF in the frontoparietal associative cortices and an increase in rCBF in the posterior cingulate cortex were found, suggesting that this state dissociation arose from combined activation of thalamocingulate pathways and persisting deactivation of other thalamocortical arousal systems (Fig. 15–4).

REM Sleep Behavior Disorder

This condition, initially described by Schenck et al.,[208] is characterized by brisk movements of the body associated with dream mentation during REM sleep that usually disturbs sleep continuity. During the nocturnal spells, patients behave as if they were acting out their dream.[106]

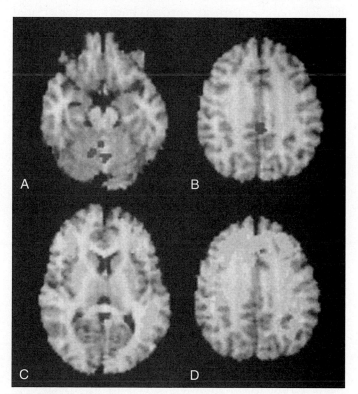

FIGURE 15–4 SPECT findings during sleepwalking after integration into the appropriate anatomic magnetic resonance image. The highest increases of regional CBF (>25%) during sleepwalking compared with quiet stage 3 to 4 NREM sleep are found in the anterior cerebellum (i.e., vermis) **(A),** and in the posterior cingulate cortex **(B)**. However, as compared to data from normal volunteers during wakefulness, large areas of frontal and parietal association cortices remain deactivated during sleepwalking, as shown in the corresponding parametric maps. Note the inclusion of the dorsolateral prefrontal cortex **(C)**, mesial frontal cortex **(D)**, and left angular gyrus **(C)** within these areas. *(Reproduced with permission from Bassetti C, Vella S, Donati F, et al. SPECT during sleepwalking. Lancet 2000;356:484. Copyright 2000, The Lancet.) See Color Plate*

This disease may be idiopathic (up to 60%) or associated with other neurologic disorders. A sizeable proportion of patients with REM sleep behavior disorder (RBD) will develop extrapyramidal disorders,[209–211] Lewy body dementia,[212] and multiple system atrophy (MSA).[213,214] More recently, a strong association between RBD and α-synucleinopathies has been observed, with the parasomnia often preceding the clinical onset of the neurodegenerative disease.[212]

Interestingly, an early experimental model of RBD in the cat has shown that lesions in the mesopontine tegmentum can lead to the disappearance of muscle atonia during REM sleep together with dream-enactment behavior.[215]

A study combining MRI and ^{123}I-IMP SPECT in 20 patients with RBD and 7 healthy controls during REM sleep reported significantly decreased blood flow in the upper portion of both sides of the frontal lobe and pons in patients with RBD, in comparison with normal elderly subjects.[216] Another SPECT study in eight RBD patients during waking rest showed decreased activity in the frontal and temporoparietal cortices but found increased activity in the pons, putamen, and right hippocampus.[217] In addition, an increased Cho/Cr ratio in the brain stem suggesting local neural abnormalities was revealed by ^{1}H-MRS in a 69-year-old man with idiopathic RBD as compared with healthy adults.[218] In contrast, one ^{1}H-MRS study, conducted in 15 patients with idiopathic RBD and 15 matched control subjects, failed to reveal any difference in metabolic peaks of NAA/Cr, Cho/Cr, and myoinositol/creatine ratios in the pontine tegmentum and the midbrain.[219] Whether idiopathic RBD involves mesopontine neuronal loss or ^{1}H-MRS–detectable metabolic disturbances therefore remains unsettled.

Using SPECT and IPT (a ligand of striatal presynaptic dopamine transporter), IPT binding in RBD patients (n = 5) during wakefulness was found to be lower than in normal controls but higher than in PD patients (n = 14).[220,221] These results suggest that the number of presynaptic dopamine transporters is decreased in both PD and RBD patients. Other studies probed the density of striatal dopaminergic terminals using PET and ^{11}C-dihydrotetrabenazine (^{11}C-DTBZ, a monoamine vesicular transporter inhibitor used as an in vivo marker for dopaminergic nerve terminals). Significant reductions in striatal ^{11}C-DTBZ binding characterized 6 elderly subjects with chronic idiopathic RBD, as compared to 19 age-matched controls, particularly in the posterior putamen.[222] Likewise ^{11}C-DTBZ binding in the striatum was decreased in 13 patients with MSA.[214] Striatal ^{11}C-DTBZ uptake was inversely correlated with the severity of symptoms in this MSA group. Moreover ^{123}I-iodobenzovesamiol (^{123}I-IBVM) binding was reduced in the thalamus in this MSA population. ^{123}I-IBVM is a radiotracer that selectively binds to the intraneuronal storage vesicles of cholinergic nerve endings, and is used as a highly specific marker for cerebral cholinergic neurons.

It remains to be shown whether theses alterations play a causal role in the pathophysiology of RBD or reflect functional consequences and adaptations to the pathologic conditions. Although there is evidence that some PD patients do show excessive nocturnal movements,[197,223] it is interesting that only a small percentage of PD patients develop full-blown RBD. This suggests that modifications of other systems of neurotransmission are probably necessary for full-blown RBD to occur.

Sleep Functional Imaging in Mental Disorders

Psychoses

Psychoses are psychiatric disorders characterized by the occurrence of delusions, hallucinations, incoherence, catatonic behavior, or inappropriate affects that cause impaired social or work functioning. Insomnia or excessive sleepiness is a common feature of psychoses.[106]

Schizophrenia is a major, devastating psychosis that affects approximately 1% of the population irrespective of culture, social status, or gender. The pathophysiology of schizophrenia is complex and remains poorly understood. There are different, nonexclusive, pathophysiologic theories of schizophrenia, including neurotransmitter dysfunction, developmental abnormalities, and genetic susceptibilities.[224] The most robust theory has focused on dysfunction of the neurotransmitters dopamine and glutamate.[224]

Schizophrenia, as a syndrome, is composed of a variety of relatively specific core symptoms.[225] These can be divided into positive and negative symptoms. The former include hallucinations, delusions, and disorganization, and the latter comprise anergia, flattening of affect, and poverty of thought content. Additional characteristics are disorganization (including bizarre thoughts and behavior) and cognitive function disturbances.

The negative symptoms of schizophrenia have been related to the decrease of cerebral activity in frontal areas.[226] It was suggested that each characteristic symptom reflects a specific pattern of abnormal cerebral activity in associative frontal, parietal, or temporal regions, and in related subcortical structures. During the performance of executive tasks, schizophrenic subjects exhibit impaired frontal activation, and during memory tasks they show impaired temporal lobe activation. However, abnormalities seem to be mainly subtended by a disturbed connectivity between cerebral areas rather than by specific regional dysfunctions.[227] Sleep problems are common in schizophrenia. Polysomnographic abnormalities seem to occur consistently in schizophrenic patients, including sleep-onset and maintenance insomnia, reduced amounts of SWS, reduced REM sleep latency, and defective REM rebound following REM deprivation.[228,229]

However, these findings are not specific to schizophrenia. Furthermore, only a subgroup of schizophrenic patients presents these abnormalities. Reduced SWS is thought to reflect a neurodevelopmental disorder,[228] and was linked to impairments in visuospatial memory in schizophrenics.[230]

It remains controversial whether reduced SWS in schizophrenia relates either directly or indirectly to an underlying brain dysmorphology. In schizophrenic patients, a close association between SWS and ventricular volume was found in one study[231] but not in another study.[232]

Finally, similarities between dreams and schizophrenia delusions and hallucinations might suggest that cerebral activity in schizophrenia is comparable to cerebral activity during REM sleep.[233] However, this hypothesis is not supported by a PET study that investigated the relationship between REM sleep and schizophrenia.[234] Glucose consumption during REM sleep in 12 controls was found to differ largely from cerebral activity in 49 awake schizophrenic patients and 30 awake controls.

Mood Disorders

Mood disorders constitute a psychiatric condition that is characterized by either one or more episodes of depression, or partial or full manic or hypomanic episodes. Typical sleep disturbances in mood disorders are insomnia and, more rarely, excessive sleepiness.[106] The association between insomnia and depression is not clearly understood.

Depression is the most common primary diagnosis in patients suffering from insomnia.[235] In addition, depressed patients frequently report increased daytime fatigue and tend to compensate with daytime napping. However, sleep disturbances appear to vary even across depression subtypes. For instance, patients with bipolar disorder report insomnia while depressed, but also hypersomnia, with extended nocturnal sleep periods, difficulty awakening, and excessive daytime sleepiness.[235] In addition, depression is associated not only with insomnia but also with other sleep disorders such as OSAS and hypersomnolence.[236] Here, we only focus on the links between depression and insomnia.

Neuroimaging studies in depressed patients during wakefulness suggest that dysfunctions within the prefrontal cortical and striatal systems that normally modulate limbic and brain stem structures play a role in the pathogenesis of depressive symptoms.[237] Abnormalities within orbital and medial prefrontal cortex areas persist following symptom remission.[237] These findings involve interconnected neural circuits in which dysfunction of neurotransmission may result in depressive symptoms.[237,238]

We first present the hyperarousal hypothesis, which links depression to insomnia. Next, we review studies conducted during NREM and REM sleep in depressed patients. Finally, we discuss results pertaining to the use of sleep deprivation as a treatment in depression.

Hyperarousal Hypothesis. In depressed patients, modifications of sleep architecture are characterized by reduced SWS, early onset of the first episode of REM sleep, and increased phasic REM sleep.[239] In addition to daytime tiredness, patients often report persistent and disturbing mental activity when getting asleep. In addition to cognitive and emotional hyperarousal, physiologic hyperarousal has been described. According to Clark and Watson, this physiologic hyperarousal reflects an anxiety component in anxiety-depression disorder.[240–242] Interestingly, hyperarousal has been described in idiopathic insomnia (see earlier). Moreover, risk of depression as a comorbid state appears to be particularly strong in insomnia patients.[243]

Intriguingly, sleep deprivation has rapid beneficial effects on about 60% of depressed patients.[244] Responders to sleep deprivation are usually patients with high behavioral activation and low levels of tiredness.[245,246] These findings suggest increased arousal in depressed patients,[240,245,247] a hypothesis that found some support in functional neuroimaging data. Beta activity was proposed as an EEG marker of arousal during sleep. In an [18]FDG PET study,[248] beta power was negatively correlated with subjective sleep quality in both normal and depressed subjects, although depressed patients exhibited increased beta activity during the night versus normal controls. Interestingly beta power was correlated with glucose metabolism levels in the ventromedial prefrontal cortex, a region among the most deactivated during consolidated SWS (see earlier).[248]

These clinical, electrophysiologic, and neuroimaging studies indicate hyperarousal in depressed patients. Nevertheless, the exact pathophysiologic mechanisms linking hyperarousal and insomnia to depression are still unclear.

NREM Sleep Neuroimaging in Depression. An early study indicated that whole-brain absolute CMRglu during NREM sleep is higher in depressed patients than in normal subjects.[249] The greatest increases were observed in the posterior cingulate, amygdala, hippocampus, and occipital and temporal cortices. Significant reductions of relative CMRglu were found in the prefrontal and anterior cingulate cortices, caudate nucleus, and medial thalamus.

In a more recent study, depressed patients showed less decrease than controls in relative rCMRglu from presleep wakefulness to NREM sleep in the left and right laterodorsal frontal gyri, right medial prefrontal cortex, right superior and middle temporal gyri, insula, right posterior cingulate cortex, lingual gyrus, striate cortex, cerebellar vermis, and left thalamus.[250] This finding suggests that transition from wakefulness to NREM sleep in depressed patients might be characterized by relatively persistent "elevated" activity in the frontoparietal regions and thalamus. Intuitively, it is as if the low frontal metabolism during wakefulness could not be further decreased during NREM sleep, as is the case for normal subjects. These findings suggest that abnormal thalamocortical network function may underlie sleep anomalies and nonrestorative sleep complaints in depressed patients.[250]

REM Sleep Neuroimaging in Depression. All the available data to date have been obtained by using the [18]FDG PET method. Due to radiation exposure limitation, a restricted number of scan can be acquired in a single patient, which limits the statistical power of the results. Therefore, great care must be taken in the interpretation of the results, which should be viewed as preliminary.

During REM sleep as compared to wakefulness, anterior paralimbic areas (anterior cingulate cortex, right insula, right parahippocampal gyrus) were found to be less active in depressed patients than in normal subjects.[251] Conversely, another study by the same group showed that, while both healthy and depressed patients activate anterior paralimbic structures from waking to REM sleep, the spatial extent of this activation was greater in depressed patients (Fig. 15–5).[252] Moreover, depressed patients showed greater activation in the bilateral dorsolateral prefrontal, left premotor, primary sensorimotor, and left parietal cortices, as well as in the midbrain reticular formation[252] and in the tectal area, inferior temporal cortex, amygdala, and subicular complex[251] from waking to REM sleep.

The severity of the depression has been found to correlate with the density of rapid eye movement (number of such movements per minute of REM sleep).[253,254] In depressed patients compared to healthy controls, average REM count (an automated analog of REM density) was positively correlated with rCMRglu bilaterally in the striate cortex, the posterior parietal cortices, and the medial and ventrolateral prefrontal cortices and negatively correlated with rCMRglu in areas corresponding bilaterally to the lateral occipital cortex, cuneus, temporal cortices, and parahippocampal gyri.[255] For the authors, these results suggested that average REM count may be a marker of hypofrontality during REM sleep in depressed patients.

Bupropion, an antidepressant drug, increased activity in the anterior cingulate, medial prefrontal cortex, and right anterior insula from waking to REM sleep in depressed patients, due to a reduction in waking relative metabolism in these structures following treatment in the absence of a significant effect on REM sleep–related metabolism.[98]

Sleep Deprivation in Depression. Sleep deprivation has profound effects on brain metabolism in both normal and depressed subjects. As stated previously, sleep deprivation relieves acute depressive symptoms in 60% of patients. In depressed patients responding favorably to sleep deprivation, baseline brain activity during wakefulness was reported to be higher in responders than in nonresponders in the anterior cingulate cortex[256,257] and/or the nearby mesial frontal cortex.[257–260] This activity was significantly decreased after sleep deprivation. A similar profile of brain activation was observed in elderly depressed patients, including normalization after total sleep deprivation associated with antidepressant treatment.[261] Moreover, the normalization of anterior cingulate metabolism persisted even after recovery sleep.[261] It was also shown that sleep deprivation responders exhibit a significant decrease in relative basal ganglia D_2 receptor occupancy after sleep deprivation, as compared to nonresponders.[262] These results suggest that the antidepressant benefits of sleep deprivation are correlated with enhanced endogenous dopamine release in responders. These results corroborate previous hypotheses about the role of dopaminergic response in the therapeutic action of sleep deprivation, and indirectly support a dopamine hypothesis of depression.[262]

In combination with data obtained during REM sleep in depressed patients, sleep deprivation data suggest a tight link between mood alteration and activity in limbic and paralimbic structures. The data suggest that anterior cingulate hyperactivity in depressed patients during wakefulness may hinder further increases during REM sleep. Hence, sleep deprivation may alleviate depression symptoms by decreasing abnormally elevated activity in the anterior cingulate cortex during wakefulness. However, available data remain limited, and further studies are needed to understand the causes and consequences of these mesial frontal metabolic disturbances.

Sleep Functional Imaging in Neurologic Disorders

Fatal Familial Insomnia

Fatal familial insomnia (FFI), a hereditary or sporadic disease caused by prion-protein gene mutation, is characterized by insomnia, autonomic hyperactivity and motor abnormalities.[263,264] This disease is invariably lethal.[263] The disrupted sleep profile is characterized by a loss of sleep spindles and SWS, and enacted dreams during REM sleep.[264] In four awake patients investigated using [18]FDG PET, a prominent hypometabolism was observed in the anterior part of the thalamus.[265] Two patients exhibited symptoms restricted to insomnia and dysautonomia. Thalamic hypometabolism was found isolated in one subject, accompanied by frontal, anterior cingulate, and temporal polar hypometabolism in the other. In the two patients who had a more complex clinical presentation, hypometabolism was more widespread and involved many cortical areas, the basal ganglia, and the cerebellum. This widespread pattern was already present at an early stage of the disease and was found to be significantly aggravated as the disease progressed in one patient examined twice several months apart. However, it is not known

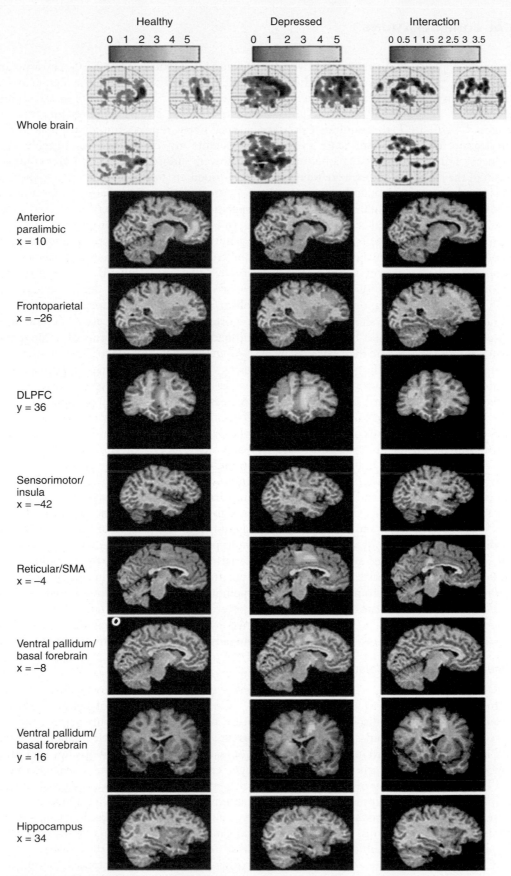

FIGURE 15–5 rCMRglu from waking to REM sleep in depression. Waking-to–REM sleep activation in healthy subjects (*column 1*) and depressed subjects (*column 2*), and interactions showing regions where the depressed subjects' waking-to–REM sleep activations are greater than those of healthy subjects (*column 3*). (DLPFC, dorsolateral prefrontal cortex; SMA, supplementary motor area; x and y, Talairach *x* and *y* coordinates.) *(Reproduced with permission from Nofzinger EA, Buysse DJ, Germain A, et al: Increased activation of anterior paralimbic and executive cortex from waking to rapid eye movement sleep in depression. Arch Gen Psychiatry 2004;61:695. Copyright © 2004, American Medical Association. All rights reserved.) See Color Plate*

whether this widespread hypometabolism is indicative of the more advanced stages of the disease or whether it indicates two forms of this disorder, one thalamic and the other disseminated.

Another study used [18]FDG PET to examine regional cerebral glucose utilization in seven patients with FFI.[266] Severely reduced glucose utilization in the thalamus and a mild hypometabolism in the cingulate cortex were found in all FFI patients. In six of these subjects, brain hypometabolism also affected the basal and lateral frontal cortex, caudate nucleus, and middle and inferior temporal cortices. Further comparison between homozygous ($n = 4$) or heterozygous ($n = 3$) patients at codon 129 showed that the hypometabolism was more widespread in the heterozygous group, which had a significantly longer symptom duration at the time of [18]FDG PET study. Comparison between neuropathologic and [18]FDG PET findings in six patients showed that areas with neuronal loss were also hypometabolic. However, cerebral hypometabolism was more widespread than expected by histopathologic changes, and significantly correlated with the presence of a protease-resistant prion protein. Neuroimaging results indicated that hypometabolism of the thalamus and cingulate cortex is a common feature of FFI, while the involvement of other brain regions depends on the duration of symptoms and some unknown factors specific to each patient.[266] Even in a case of atypical FFI, thalamic hypometabolism was confirmed as an early marker while cortical changes varied with clinical presentation and stage.[267]

More recently, serotonin function was examined in two FFI patients with ^{123}I-β-CIT SPECT and compared to age-expected control values.[268] This study showed a dramatic reduction in serotonin transporter availability in a diencephalic region for both FFI patients. Although this finding suggests an involvement of serotonin neurotransmission, it is not clear whether it is causal in the FFI pathogenesis.[268]

The Landau-Kleffner Syndrome and Related Disorders

The Landau-Kleffner syndrome (LKS) and the syndrome of continuous spike-and-wave discharges during SWS (CSWS) were originally described separately and are still considered as distinct pathophysiologic entities. LKS is characterized by acquired aphasia and paroxysmal sleep-activated EEG predominating over the temporal or parieto-occipital regions. Paroxysmal events are spike-and-wave discharges that are activated by SWS. Secondary symptoms include psychomotor or behavioral disturbances and epilepsy, with a favorable outcome for seizure control.[269] CSWS is characterized by continuous spike-and wave discharges during SWS, usually combined with global intellectual deterioration and epileptic seizures.[270] Both syndromes share many features in common, including early onset during childhood, deterioration of cognitive function (previously acquired

normally), seizure type, EEG pattern, and pharmacologic reactivity. They also have in common the regression of neuropsychological symptoms, EEG abnormalities, and seizures before the end of adolescence. Early reports found no structural brain lesions detectable by computed tomography or MRI.[269–272] However, more recent MRI volumetric analyses performed in four children with typical LKS revealed volume reduction in bilateral superior temporal areas, specifically the planum temporale and superior temporal gyrus, where receptive language is localized.[273,274]

Initial functional imaging studies using PET[269,275–278] and SPECT[277,279–285] described metabolic abnormalities in LKS that predominantly involved the temporal lobes. Focal or regional areas of decreased and increased metabolism were reported. A normal distribution of CBF was reported in one isolated case.[286] These early results were difficult to interpret in terms of pathogenesis.

Later on, cerebral glucose metabolism was investigated using [18]FDG PET in a larger population of asleep and awake patients.[287,288] Again regional increases and decreases in cerebral glucose metabolism were observed. The metabolic patterns were found to be variable from one patient to another, and grossly related to the neuropsychological deterioration. Moreover, metabolic patterns in individual patients were reported to change over time. Interestingly, another PET study showed that residual impairment in verbal short-term memory after recovery was probably linked in two of three LKS patients with significantly less activation than controls in their left and right posterior superior temporal gyrus during immediate serial recall of lists of 4 words, compared to single-word repetition. One patient having near-normal short-term memory performance showed increased activity in the posterior part of the right superior temporal gyrus. According to the authors, these results suggested that impaired verbal short-tem memory at late outcome of LKS might be related to a persistent decrease of activity in those posterior superior temporal gyri that were involved in the epileptic focus during the active phase.[289]

Voxel-based analyses of cerebral glucose metabolism were performed in a group of 18 children with CSWS using statistical parametric mapping. Each patient was compared with a control group, and the influence of age, epileptic activity, and corticosteroid treatment on metabolic abnormalities was assessed. Cerebral metabolic patterns were heterogeneous across patients with CSWS. Age and intensity of awake interictal spiking did not significantly differ in patients showing focal hypermetabolism compared with the others. Treatment with corticosteroids corrected focal hypermetabolism. Altered parietofrontal connectivity observed in patients with hypermetabolism was interpreted as a phenomenon of remote inhibition of the frontal lobes induced by the highly epileptogenic and hypermetabolic posterior cortex.[290]

Studies in LKS patients indicated four basic metabolic characteristics. First, LKS patients have a higher rate of metabolism in the cortical mantle than in the thalamic nuclei. This metabolic pattern is characteristic of an immature brain. Second, they show focal or regional metabolic abnormalities of the cortex, suggesting a focal origin of the spike-and-wave discharges. Third, they have metabolic disturbances predominantly involving associative cortices, suggesting deterioration of cognitive function only. Fourth, glucose metabolism in thalamic nuclei remains symmetric despite significant cortical asymmetries, suggesting that corticothalamic neurons either do not participate in the generation of spike-and-wave discharges or are being inhibited by pathologic mechanisms.

These studies also suggest that CSWS is produced by an alteration in the maturation of one or more associative cortices, potentially leading to disturbed neuronal wiring. An imbalance of inhibitory and excitatory drives would lead to deterioration in associated higher cerebral functions and would create conditions contributing to the production of neuronal discharges. Discharges expressed during waking would be activated during SWS because of the physiologic reinforced synchronization of neuronal firing characteristic of that type of sleep.[291]

CONCLUSIONS

Functional neuroimaging provides unprecedented possibilities to explore brain function during normal and pathologic sleep. Nevertheless, neuroimaging in sleep is still in its infancy, at present mostly restricted to research purposes. A major research effort should be developed in order to better characterize pathophysiologic mechanisms of sleep disorders, teasing apart functional causes from consequences. Functional neuroimaging could also be helpful to assess the functional and structural consequences of long-term sleep disruption. These efforts should benefit from advanced multimodal neuroimaging and improved experimental designs.

ACKNOWLEDGMENTS

M.D., T.D., and P.M. are supported by the Fonds National de la Recherche Scientifique (FNRS), Belgium (grant number 3.4516.05 to M.D.). Additional support for the work presented here comes from the research funds of the University of Liège, the Queen Elisabeth Medical Foundation, and the Interuniversity Attraction Pole program. S.S. is supported by the Swiss National Science Foundation (grants #310000–114008 and #3200B0–104100).

⊗ REFERENCES

A full list of references are available at www.expertconsult.com

CHAPTER 16

Measurement of Sleepiness and Alertness: Multiple Sleep Latency Test

Thomas Roth and **Timothy A. Roehrs**

INTRODUCTION

Daytime sleepiness as a consequence of inadequate sleep the previous night is a common experience for most adults. Because of the universality of the acute experience of daytime sleepiness, it is typically minimized as a health problem within the general population; in a 1997 Gallup Poll of Americans, only 6% of those reporting impairing sleepiness considered it medically serious.[1] Although minimized by laypeople, increasingly chronic excessive daytime sleepiness is recognized as an important and significant symptom in medicine. Furthermore, excessive daytime sleepiness can and should be distinguished from fatigue, tiredness, and lassitude, although many patients may not make such distinctions themselves unless they are carefully queried.

Representative surveys of the populations of industrialized countries have found that between 11% and 32% of respondents report that sleepiness interferes with activities almost daily.[1-5] Sleepiness is associated with a number of medical, behavioral, and pharmacologic causes, and, regardless of its cause, has serious social and medical consequences. Nearly half of the patients with excessive sleepiness seen at sleep disorders centers report automobile accidents; more than half report occupational accidents, some life threatening; many have lost jobs because of their sleepiness; and the impact of sleepiness on family life is disruptive.[6] Information on traffic and industrial accidents in the general population suggests a link between sleepiness and life-threatening events. For example, the highest rate of automobile accidents occurs in the early morning hours, which is remarkable because fewer automobiles are on the road during these hours.[7] Shift workers, a particularly sleepy subpopulation, have the poorest job performance and the highest rate of industrial accidents among all workers.[8]

Problems in assessing sleepiness became evident during early research on the daytime consequences of sleep loss before the clinical significance of sleepiness was recognized. Sleep loss compromises daytime functions. Virtually all individuals experience dysphoria and reduced performance when they do not sleep adequately. The majority of performance tasks are insensitive to the effects of sleep loss,[9] but long and monotonous tasks are reliably sensitive to changes in the quantity and quality of nocturnal sleep. Using various measures of mood, including factor analytic scales, the most consistent and systematic response to sleep loss is increased sleepiness. Among the various subjective measures of sleepiness, the Stanford Sleepiness Scale (SSS) is the best validated.[10] Yet clinicians have found that patients may rate themselves alert on the SSS even as they are falling asleep.[11] The likely reason for such discrepancies is that subjective daytime sleepiness has multiple dimensions.[12]

Normal and pathologic variations in daytime sleepiness and alertness can now be directly assessed and quantified by the Multiple Sleep Latency Test (MSLT), a test of the rapidity with which a subject falls asleep in a standardized, sleep-conducive setting, repeated at 2-hour intervals throughout the day. The MSLT uses standard sleep recording methods to document both the rate of sleep onset and the appearance of rapid eye movement (REM) episodes at sleep onset. Other procedures that have been used to quantify sleepiness and alertness (but that, because of a variety of shortcomings, are not widely used), including pupillometry, subjective rating scales, and tests of vigilance or reaction time, are all correlated to some extent with the MSLT. The MSLT has become the standard method in clinical sleep disorders medicine for documenting complaints of excessive daytime sleepiness and to document treatment success. It is also used to document sleep-onset REM periods, a diagnostic sign of narcolepsy. The American Academy of Sleep Medicine has indicated that the MSLT should be used as part of an evaluation of suspected narcolepy and may be helpful in evaluation of suspected idiopathic hypersomnia.[13] Since the development of the MSLT by Carskadon and Dement[14] in the late 1970s, enormous progress has been made in the scientific investigation and understanding of both normal and pathologic variations in sleepiness and alertness.

MULTIPLE SLEEP LATENCY TEST METHODS

Recording Montage

General and specific technical guidelines for the administration of the MSLT have been published.[15] Briefly, the guidelines require that the standard Rechtschaffen and Kales recording montage be used in performing the MSLT.[16] The montage includes the referential electroencephalogram (EEG) from a central (C3 or C4) placement, two horizontal referential electro-oculograms (EOGs) from the right and left outer canthi, and a mental or submental electromyogram. Also helpful in the determination of sleep onset is a referential occipital EEG lead, which shows alpha activity in relaxed wakefulness with eyes closed and is followed by a characteristic change to mixed-frequency EEG activity at the onset of sleep. An EOG recording with filters set to allow visualization of slow rolling eye movements (e.g., 250 msec) is another sign of sleep onset.

General Procedures

As indicated in the guidelines, to ensure a reliable and valid MSLT, a number of general procedures are necessary.[15] A 1- or 2-week sleep diary recorded before the test that includes information on usual bedtime, time of arising, napping, and drug use (i.e., caffeine, alcohol, illicit and licit drugs) is very helpful. Deviations from the subject's habitual sleep behavior should be noted, because sleep time accumulated or lost over the week before an MSLT can significantly affect the result. Some controversy has arisen regarding what defines adequate sleep

prior to the MSLT.[16,17] The critical point is that the sleep prior to the MSLT should represent a patient's habitual sleep at home. Central nervous system (CNS)–active drugs, as well as their discontinuation, can alter sleep and REM latencies, and therefore these drugs should be discontinued sufficiently well in advance of the test. The sleep of the night preceding an MSLT should be documented with a standard nocturnal sleep recording. This nocturnal sleep recording should be scheduled to coincide with the timing and amount of the subject's usual sleep, as revealed in the diary.

The reliability of the MSLT is based on multiple determinations of sleep latency, as the studies discussed in the following sections have shown. Consequently, as indicated in the guidelines, four or five tests of sleep latency at 2-hour intervals throughout the day should be conducted.[15] Testing should be initiated from 1.5 to 3 hours after the nocturnal sleep period has been terminated, typically at 9:30 or 10:00 AM. The MSLT should be conducted in a sleep-conducive environment that is quiet, dark, and controlled at a comfortable temperature. Any potentially arousing stimuli should be removed from the test area.

Specific Procedures

The following procedures are specified by the guidelines for conducting the MSLT.[15] After arising from nocturnal sleep, the subject should toilet, dress in street clothes, and eat the usual breakfast (avoiding caffeinated beverages). Between the latency tests, the subject should be kept out of the bed and monitored by technical staff to assure that no napping occurs. A small retrospective study of patients being evaluated for excessive daytime sleepiness monitored the patients telemetrically between tests, and brief inadvertent napping did occur.[18] However, the naps occurred among the sleepiest patients and did not alter the clinical results appreciably. Preparations before each latency test include smoking cessation 30 minutes before lights out, bedtime preparation (removing shoes and restrictive clothes such as belts or neckties) at 10 minutes before lights out, all electrode connections and calibrations completed at 5 minutes before lights out, and the instructions to relax and fall asleep given 5 seconds before lights out.

Ending a Test

According to the guidelines, if sleep does not occur, each test is concluded 20 minutes after lights out.[15] For the clinical version of the MSLT, in which the occurrence of REM sleep is in question, the test is concluded 15 minutes after the first 30-second epoch of sleep. In a research version of the MSLT, the test is concluded after three consecutive 30-second epochs of stage 1 sleep or one 30-second epoch of another sleep stage. When the recording is equivocal, it is safer to allow clearer signs of sleep (i.e., spindles and K complexes) to emerge rather than to terminate the test prematurely.

Scoring and Interpretation

Criteria for scoring sleep onset differ from criteria for test termination.[15] There has been some confusion in the MSLT literature in this regard. Furthermore, it should be noted that the MSLT sleep latency criteria differ from the typical definition of nocturnal sleep onset (stage 2 sleep or 10 continuous minutes of sleep) in much of the all-night sleep literature. MSLT sleep latency is the elapsed time in minutes from lights out to the first 30-second epoch scored as sleep. According to the scoring criteria of Rechtschaffen and Kales,[19] this implies that 16 seconds of sleep (i.e., >50% on a given epoch of the recording) is sufficient to score a sleep onset. REM sleep latency in a clinical test is scored as minutes from sleep onset (as defined earlier) to the first epoch of REM sleep.

Average sleep latency (in minutes) for the four or five latency tests is the parameter typically used to express the level of sleepiness. In some of the clinical literature, the MSLT result is expressed as a median sleep latency or a sleepiness index, which is merely the average latency subtracted from 100 and multiplied by 100% (and corrected if fewer than five tests are conducted). In population studies, survival analyses have been used to examine predictors of sleep onset during the MSLT.[20] The occurrence of REM sleep within 10–15 minutes of sleep onset is generally defined as a sleep-onset REM period (SOREMP), and the frequency of such SOREMPs is also tabulated.

Sources of Error

The level of sleepiness (defined as the average sleep latency) observed on the MSLT is affected by the sleep of the previous night and weeks. Any deviation from the subject's habitual sleep schedule (as revealed in the sleep diary) and sleep quality (as seen in the nocturnal sleep recording and the individual's estimate of its consistency with usual sleep) is likely to overestimate or underestimate the usual level of daytime sleepiness. Similarly, the timing of the nocturnal sleep and daytime MSLT assessment relative to the subject's circadian phase is a potential source of error that is an issue in studying shift and night workers. Out-of-phase sleep is likely to be disturbed and associated with shorter MSLT latencies. Moreover, sleep latency itself varies as a function of circadian phase.

Sedating or alerting effects of drugs or discontinuation of long-term drug use can also be a source of error in documenting sleepiness. For some patients, a urine drug screen may be necessary to confirm the absence of drugs. A noisy, bright, or stimulating test environment invalidates an MSLT result. As well, stimulating activity immediately prior to a latency test will increase sleep latency on the subsequent test.[21] Instructions given to the subject at the initiation of the test are also important. Subjects should be aware that they are to close their eyes, lie still, and allow sleep to occur. Excessive tossing and turning are to be avoided. It should be recognized that the instruction "relax and fall asleep" may be emotionally loaded for patients with insomnia. This issue is discussed in the section on Determinants of Daytime Sleepiness later.

Finally, a "last test" effect might be observed (this has not yet been systematically studied). In anticipation of going home for the day, subjects may remain awake for the 20 minutes of the last latency test. This last test effect could elevate the average sleep latency for the day. It can be avoided by scheduling other nonarousing activities after the last latency test. Patient feedback sessions with the clinician either before or after the last test can be disruptive to that test and should be avoided.

REM sleep can occur on latency tests of the MSLT as a result of a number of factors. Many drugs suppress REM sleep, and discontinuing them increases the likelihood of SOREMPs on an MSLT. For example, a study of cocaine addicts found an average of 2.8 SOREMPs on five test MSLTs conducted on the first 2 days after discontinuing the cocaine use.[22] By days 13 and 14 of discontinuation, the average number had dropped to 0.2 SOREMPs. The circadian-phase timing of the MSLT is also important with respect to the occurrence of REM sleep. REM sleep can occur on early-morning latency tests in a person who is a late-morning sleeper. Excessive disturbance of the sleep of the previous night also has the potential to result in REM sleep on early-morning latency tests. For example, it has been suggested that apnea patients with highly fragmented sleep may have more SOREMPs than the general population. SOREMPs should be re-evaluated in patients suspected of narcolepsy, but who show apneas in the nocturnal sleep recording. It is rare for sleep restriction the week previous to an MSLT to alter REM occurrence on the MSLT.

RELIABILITY AND VALIDITY

Reliability

Several studies of the reliability of the MSLT have been conducted. In healthy normals who maintained consistent sleep-wake schedules, the test-retest reliability of a four-test MSLT was 0.97 over a 4- to 14-month test-retest interval.[23] The test-retest interval (~6 months vs. >6 months) and the level of sleepiness (average latency of ~5 minutes vs. 2:15 minutes) did not affect this MSLT reliability. The *number* of latency tests did alter MSLT reliability: The coefficient dropped to 0.85 for three tests and 0.65 for two tests. Another study of patients with insomnia over an interval of 3–90 weeks found a test-retest correlation of 0.65 on a five-test MSLT.[24]

There has also been interest in the test-retest reliability of SOREMPs in patients with narcolepsy. The current criteria require two or more SOREMPs out of five possible sleep onsets. In the only study done to date, 28 of 30 patients had two or more SOREMPs when retested

(K = 0.93, $p < 0.05$). Of particular interest is the finding that the REM latency on SOREMPs during the initial evaluation was also correlated to that during retesting ($r = 0.64$, $p < 0.02$).[25]

Strength of test-retest reliability for mean sleep latency and SOREMPs on the MSLT is dependent on test-retest scoring reliability. Several studies have demonstrated strong scoring reliability in clinical populations. The intrarater scoring reliability for mean sleep latency on MSLTs from 200 patients was 0.87 and the interrater coefficient was 0.90.[26] The intrarater and interrater scoring reliabilities for one or more SOREMPs were 0.78 and 0.91, respectively.

Validity

The MSLT measures the speed of falling asleep on repeated tests conducted in a sleep-conducive setting, as described earlier. The validity of the MSLT as a measure of sleepiness rests on its response characteristics to known determinants of sleepiness, which are discussed in the following section. Additionally, in evaluating its validity, the parametric limits of average sleep latency as measured on the MSLT must be discussed.

The first issue is the two anchors of the scale. By scoring definition (i.e., sleep onset is scored in 30-second epochs), one cannot fall asleep in less than 30 seconds, often referred to as a "floor" effect. Thus, a brief (<15 seconds) attention lapse or microsleep, which emerges in continuous performance assessments of excessively sleepy individuals,[27] is not scored on the MSLT. Similarly, by the standard MSLT procedure, the test is terminated after 20 minutes of continuous wakefulness. Thus, average sleep latencies can be no longer than 20 minutes, which has been referred to as a "ceiling" effect. Consequently, alerting drug effects in nonsleepy individuals can be difficult to detect, although, as discussed later, studies have shown alerting drug effects in volunteers whose basal average sleep latency is within a standard deviation of population norms.

Second, the linearity of average sleep latency across the 0.5- to 20-minute range of the MSLT cannot be assumed, an issue that has received little investigation. A study in healthy normals compared the alerting effects of caffeine (0, 75, and 150 mg) after 8 hours' or 5 hours' time in bed (TIB) the previous night.[28] Average sleep latency was increased by 2 minutes with 75 mg and 4 minutes with 150 mg regardless of the placebo baseline, which was 6 minutes and 10 minutes, respectively, for the 5- and 8-hour TIBs. Conversely, in patients with excessive sleepiness and MSLT scores of <6 minutes, an increase due to treatment in average sleep latency from 2 to 6 minutes may be quite different than that from 6 to 10 minutes.

The validity and clinical utility of the MSLT was recently reviewed.[29] It was concluded that average sleep latency and multiple SOREMPs "do not discriminate well between patients with sleep disorders and normal populations." As the next section indicates, a number of factors cause sleepiness and multiple SOREMPs in both patients and normals. Furthermore, the excessive sleepiness of a given patient may have multiple causes. Thus, the MSLT would not be expected to have good diagnostic specificity. As to sensitivity, the review suggested that most patients with complaints of excessive sleepiness do show short average sleep latencies, although establishing the limits of normal and pathologic is complex (see *Multiple Sleep Latency Test Norms* later).

DETERMINANTS OF DAYTIME SLEEPINESS

Quantity and Continuity of Sleep

A number of different causes of sleepiness have been identified. The degree of daytime sleepiness is directly related to the amount of nocturnal sleep. Habitual bedtime is predictive of median sleep latency on the MSLT, with short bedtimes predictive of short latencies.[30] Partial or total sleep deprivation in normal subjects is followed by increased sleepiness the following day, which can reach pathologic levels.[31] Furthermore, modest sleep deprivation (as little as 1 hour per night) accumulates over time to progressively increase daytime sleepiness, again to pathologic levels.[32] In normal young adults, however, increased sleep time—extending TIB beyond the usual 7 or 8 hours per night—produces increased alertness (i.e., reduction in sleepiness).[33] Daytime sleepiness also relates to the quality and continuity of a previous night's sleep. Sleep in patients with a number of sleep disorders is punctuated by frequent, brief arousals of 3–15 seconds' duration. The arousals typically do not result in awakening, as judged either by Rechtschaffen and Kales sleep staging criteria[19] or by behavioral indicators, and the arousals recur in some conditions as often as one to four times per minute. The arousing stimulus differs in various disorders and can be identified in some cases (e.g., apneas, leg movements, pain). The critical point is that the arousals generally do not result in shorter sleep, but rather in fragmented or discontinuous sleep, and this fragmentation produces daytime sleepiness.[34]

Correlational evidence suggests a relationship between sleep fragmentation and daytime sleepiness. Fragmentation, as indexed by the number of brief EEG arousals, number of shifts from other sleep stages to stage 1 sleep or wake, and percentage of stage 1 sleep, correlates with excessive sleepiness in various patient groups.[34] Fragmentation of the sleep of healthy normals has been produced by inducing 3- to 15-second arousals with an auditory stimulus. Studies have shown that subjects aroused at various intervals during the night demonstrate performance decrements and increased sleepiness on the following day[35–38] and that fragmented sleep is nonrecuperative.[39]

CNS-Acting Drugs

CNS-depressant drugs, as might be expected, increase sleepiness. The benzodiazepine hypnotics hasten sleep onset at bedtime and shorten the latency to return to sleep after an awakening during the night, as demonstrated in a number of objective studies.[40,41] If taken at bedtime, long-acting benzodiazepines continue to shorten sleep latency on the MSLT the next day.[42] Ethanol administered at bedtime and during the day reduces sleep latency as measured by the MSLT.[43,44] One of the most commonly reported side effects associated with the use of H_1 antihistamines is daytime sleepiness, and studies with objective measurement of sleepiness have confirmed the effect.[45,46]

CNS-stimulant drugs reduce sleepiness. In healthy volunteers, 75–300 mg of caffeine, compared to placebo, increased average sleep latency on the MSLT by 2–4 minutes during a simulated night shift or during the day after 4 hours' TIB the previous night.[27,47] Even after a night of "normal" sleep, average sleep latency was increased from 10.7 to 17.8 minutes by 400 mg of caffeine four times daily.[48] In healthy volunteers, 20 mg of methylphenidate increased average sleep latency after both 8 and 0 hours TIBs, and 10 mg of methylphenidate similarly increased average sleep latency after both 8 and 4 hours TIBs.[49,50] In patients with narcolepsy, 60 mg of methylphenidate increased average sleep latency.[51] Finally, in three studies of patients with excessive sleepiness associated with narcolepsy, sleep apnea, and muscular dystrophy, modafinil increased average sleep latency.[52–54]

Sleep Disorders

Disorders of the CNS are assumed to be another determinant of daytime sleepiness. A deficiency in the hypothalamic hypocretin system is the putative cause of excessive sleepiness in patients with narcolepsy.[55] Another sleep disorder associated with excessive sleepiness and thought to be due to an unknown disorder of the CNS is idiopathic CNS hypersomnolence.[56] In both conditions, excessive sleepiness has been well documented, although the pathophysiology for idiopathic CNS hypersomnolence has not been definitively established.

Several case series have presented MSLT results in patients with complaints of excessive daytime sleepiness.[57,58] These series have clearly shown that patients experiencing difficulties with excessive sleepiness show MSLT average sleep latencies of 8 minutes or less, although questions regarding the degree to which their diagnoses were based on the MSLT result have to be raised.[28] As noted previously in the validity discussion, short average sleep latencies on the MSLT do not differentiate normals from patients (norms and deviations from the norm in healthy adults are discussed later). However, multiple SOREMPs are infrequent (i.e., rates of 5–10% in population-based studies[59,60]) in normal individuals, whereas the occurrence of two or more is considered suggestive of narcolepsy.[28]

Furthermore, the data have shown that differences in the severity of some sleep disorders are reflected in different levels of sleepiness on the MSLT. For example, patients with obstructive sleep apnea syndrome who have 40 or more apneas per hour of nocturnal sleep usually have average sleep latencies of 5 minutes or less, whereas those with fewer apneas per hour (20–40) have average latencies of 5–8 minutes and sometimes more. Finally, among sleep disorders associated with excessive daytime sleepiness, a differentiation in levels of sleepiness and frequency of SOREMPs can be seen. Patients with chronic insufficient sleep usually have a more moderate level of sleepiness (5–8 minutes) than do patients with narcolepsy or severe obstructive sleep apnea syndrome (no more than 5 minutes).[28] Among sleep disorders patients, only those with narcolepsy show two or more SOREMPs.

The relationship between nocturnal sleep and daytime sleepiness (i.e., MSLT scores) in insomnia patients is not as clearly established. Insomnia patients do not necessarily complain of daytime sleepiness as the consequence of their perceived inadequate nocturnal sleep. Often the complaint is fatigue, tiredness, and dysphoria. In fact, some data suggest that insomnia patients may be hyperalert. Although showing shortened nocturnal sleep compared to age-matched, healthy controls, this group of insomnia patients has unusually high average sleep latencies (i.e., >15 minutes).[61]

Evaluation of Therapeutic Interventions

A number of studies have shown that MSLT levels in various sleep disorders are improved after appropriate therapeutic intervention. Two current treatments of obstructive sleep apnea syndrome are continuous positive airway pressure (CPAP) and uvulopalatopharyngoplasty (UPPP). CPAP provides a pneumatic splint of the airway, eliminating the upper airway obstructions and thus the brief arousals that fragment sleep. This improved sleep is associated with normalization of the MSLT,[62] and the duration of nightly use predicts sleepiness on the MSLT.[63] UPPP, a surgical treatment aimed at removing excess upper airway tissue and thus establishing a patent airway, is less consistently successful. In those patients who benefit from the surgery, apneas are reduced, sleep is improved, and the MSLT level of sleepiness is normalized[64]; however, in patients whose apnea does not improve, the MSLT result remains at presurgery levels, even though patients perceive a subjective improvement in alertness. This once again indicates the inaccuracy of subjective assessments of sleepiness and alertness.

MODIFICATIONS OF THE MULTIPLE SLEEP LATENCY TEST

The basic MSLT procedure has been modified in various ways, with no clear improvement. The first such modification was a change in the instructions to "try to stay awake" while lying in bed in a quiet, dark room.[65] The instruction does produce longer sleep latencies, but the change did not increase sensitivity of the MSLT.[66] A subsequent variation, the Maintenance of Wakefulness Test, instructs the subject to stay awake while seated in a chair.[67] Again, longer sleep latencies result from the change, but improvement in sensitivity over the MSLT has not been documented. Finally, the Modified Assessment of Sleepiness Test (MAST) has been offered as an alternative to the MSLT.[68] It consists of three standard sleep latency tests (with a "try to sleep" instruction) alternating with two tests of the subject's ability to remain awake while seated in a chair reading a book. As indicated earlier, MSLT reliability begins to decline as the number of tests is reduced; this is also found with the MAST. Improved sensitivity has not been established for the MAST.

The intent of the MSLT modifications is to measure a subject's ability to remain awake. It is argued that, clinically, the patient's problem is remaining awake (which adds a certain face validity to the instruction to remain awake). The ability to stay awake is a function of many factors that can momentarily override the underlying physiologic state, including the motivation to remain awake, presence of competing motives, the environment, and time of day. Consequently, the ability to maintain wakefulness varies significantly between individuals and hour to hour within an individual. No single laboratory test is generalizable to the variety of circumstances under which wakefulness is to be maintained. The MSLT attempts to remove the confounding factors and measure the underlying physiologic state, thus defining the patient's maximal risk.

Correlations among the standard MSLT and these modified versions of the MSLT—and also with two widely used subjective measures of sleepiness, the Epworth Sleepiness Scale and the Sleep-Wake Activity Inventory—are relatively weak.[69,70] This has led some to argue that there are different types of or dimensions to sleepiness. A more parsimonious and valid explanation, however, is that the methodologies differ in sensitivity. Another more plausible explanation is that, rather than different kinds of sleepiness, there are different levels of ability to detect sleepiness, different environmental demands for alertness, and different abilities to counteract sleepiness. Additional constructs have utility and become meaningful when the same variable affects the constructs in different ways. This has not been demonstrated for the various versions of the MSLT.

MULTIPLE SLEEP LATENCY TEST NORMS

Enough data on the MSLT have now been collected to describe the range of values. The previously described 2005 review of the MSLT calculated a weighted mean across a total of 27 studies that presented control or healthy normal data.[28] Across studies, the mean daily sleep latency for studies presenting four-test MSLT data was 10.4 ± 4.3 minutes, and for those studies presenting five-test data it was 11.6 ± 5.2 minutes. These studies selected their participants as healthy normals. From a representative U.S. population-based sample of 1648 adults, 157 randomly chosen volunteers with a 68% response rate underwent a five-test MSLT conducted on the day after an 8.5-hour overnight polysomnogram.[71] The population mean daily sleep latency was 11.3 ± 4.5 minutes. These data, both selected and unselected, suggest that the population mean for a five-test MSLT is about 11 minutes, with an approximate 5-minute standard deviation.

Clinically, evidence of pathologic sleepiness is considered to be an average daily sleep latency of 5 minutes or less. An average latency of 6–8 minutes is considered borderline pathologic, and latencies of 9 minutes and greater are considered normal. In samples of healthy, normal individuals, some have latencies in the pathologic range (no more than 5 minutes). These normative data (in a statistical sense) do not help in differentiating normals without complaints from sleep disorders patients with excessive sleepiness. What appears to be the critical difference is that the sleepiness in the normals is not persistent. With adequate sleep over a number of nights, the average daily sleep latency increases, reaching the population norm (see the discussion of sleep disorders under *Determinants of Daytime Sleepiness* earlier).

A final issue is the degree to which average sleep latency changes as a function of age. In several reports of healthy, noncomplaining adults using a four-test MSLT, younger subjects (ages 21–35 years) had an average daily sleep latency of 10 minutes, adults ages 30–49 years had an average latency of 11–12 minutes, and subjects 50–59 years old averaged a latency of 9 minutes.[72,73] For the older subjects, nocturnal sleep efficiency was lower than that of the other age groups, and periodic leg movements during sleep were observed in 50% of the sample. In the 2005 MSLT review, just the opposite age effect on MSLT values was found: With age, average daily sleep latency increased. The difference probably relates to the fact that, in those studies, participants were selected for their normal nocturnal sleep. Finally, preadolescent children rarely fall asleep on a sleep latency test, and hence average sleep latencies are close to 20 minutes.[74,75]

REFERENCES

A full list of references are available at www.expertconsult. com

CHAPTER 17

The Maintenance of Wakefulness Test

Karl Doghramji

INTRODUCTION

Daytime sleepiness is associated with a variety of impairments, including social and occupational deficits, accidents, and catastrophes. Its detection and quantification are, therefore, important goals in clinical and occupational settings. The Maintenance of Wakefulness Test (MWT) is a polysomnographic procedure that is utilized to evaluate the extent of daytime somnolence. It assesses an individual's ability to successfully resist the urge to fall asleep (i.e., the ability to remain awake) during soporific circumstances and thus provides an objective measure of *wake tendency*. The instructions to the patient comprise a key difference between this procedure and the Multiple Sleep Latency Test (MSLT), which is also utilized for the evaluation of daytime somnolence. Whereas, during the MWT, patients are instructed to resist the urge to fall asleep, during the MSLT they are instructed to yield to this urge. It follows that the MSLT measures an individual's ability to fall asleep, or *sleep tendency*. Therefore, the MWT and the MSLT differ substantially in the functions that they assess.

HISTORICAL OVERVIEW

Daytime nap studies have been utilized extensively for the quantification of daytime somnolence.[1-5] The first such procedure to be utilized in clinical settings was the MSLT,[6] the primary application of which was the confirmation of narcolepsy and the quantification of daytime somnolence in narcolepsy and other disorders such as obstructive sleep apnea syndrome.[7] Shortly after its introduction, however, questions were raised as to whether the MSLT accurately measures the clinical function of greatest interest in some sleepy patients. The MSLT assesses how easily patients succumb to sleep (i.e., sleep tendency). However, the function of greater relevance in some situations is how successful they are in resisting this urge, inasmuch as the latter more closely reflects the challenge that they face in the soporific situations of everyday life such as driving and reading. Additionally, the MSLT did not appear to be sensitive in detecting changes in levels of sleepiness following therapeutic interventions in highly sleepy populations.

Hartse et al.[8] addressed this issue and noted that, in a multiple nap study in normal subjects, sleep latency increased by changing instructions from "try to sleep" to "try to stay awake." They then developed the Repeated Test of Sustained Wakefulness (RTSW), which involves instruction to remain awake while lying in bed. Soon thereafter, Mitler et al.[9,10] developed the MWT, which is similar in its instructions to the RTSW, yet patients are positioned in a comfortable, partially reclining chair or propped up in bed. Mitler et al. reported both the methodology and results in 10 narcoleptics and 8 control subjects. Mean sleep latency differed significantly between the two populations (9.9 vs. 17.9 minutes, respectively). Narcoleptics also exhibited an average of 3.2 sleep-onset rapid eye movement (REM) episodes over the five sessions versus none for the controls. Sleep latency increased by 300% when instructions were changed from "try to sleep" to "try to remain awake." Nevertheless, eight narcoleptics who were retested following treatment did not exhibit a significant increase in MWT sleep latency.

In the intervening years, the MWT has been utilized clinically to quantify the extent of daytime somnolence, to assess the effects of treatment in sleepy patients, and to determine patients' suitability for performing tasks at home and in the workplace. Despite diversity in methodology, the core aspects of the test have remained constant. Following a night of polysomnography, and while being monitored polysomnographically, patients are given four to five opportunities, at 2-hour intervals, to remain awake while comfortably reclining in a bed or armchair. The first trial begins at 10:00 AM. Patients are instructed to remain awake as long as possible. Depending on the application, trials are terminated either at sleep onset or following a constant period of sleep. Sleep latency is calculated for each wakefulness opportunity and an average sleep latency score is reported, which is regarded as being inversely proportional to the extent of daytime somnolence.

Methodologic uniformity is clearly desirable for those who wish to compare results of various trials and assess clinical results in the context of normative data. However, methodologic diversity has existed in various areas. These include polysomnographic montage, illuminance level, seating position, room temperature, meal timing, and patient instructions, among others. The effect of many of these factors on sleep latency in nap test protocols has been demonstrated.[11,12] The two areas of greatest variability have been the definition of sleep onset and duration of each wakefulness opportunity. The initial studies of Mitler et al.[9,10] utilized a stringent definition of sleep onset: three 30-second epochs of stage 1 or one epoch of any other sleep stage. Later studies of patients with obstructive sleep apnea syndrome[13,14] undergoing treatment utilized a more lenient definition of sleep onset (one 30-second epoch of any sleep stage). The former, stricter, definition of sleep onset would be anticipated to yield longer sleep latency scores than the latter. Similarly, wakefulness opportunity durations have varied between 20 minutes and 40 minutes. Scores for the 40-minute trial would be anticipated to be longer. To a certain extent, methodologic variations have resulted from attempts to adapt the MWT to a variety of situations depending on the degree of sleepiness and motivational characteristics of the population to be studied. As examples, with extremely somnolent subjects such as patients with narcolepsy, a shorter trial duration—say, 20 minutes—can be used with minimal ceiling effects. In individuals who are only moderately sleepy (say, MSLT sleep latencies in the 6- to 10-minute range), as opposed to extremely sleepy (say MSLT sleep latencies in the 0- to 5-minute range), MWT trial durations of 30 minutes or 40 minutes are needed to reduce problems with ceiling effects.[15–17]

NORMATIVE DATA

A few studies have provided normative data on the MWT.[18–20] The largest of these provided data on 64 healthy subjects (27 males and 37 females) whose ages ranged between 30 and 70 years.[19] Test conditions were kept uniform across sites and subjects, including polysomnographic montage, illuminance level, seating position, room temperature, meal timing, and subject instructions. Subjects were given four 40-minute MWT trials at 2-hour intervals with the first trial beginning at 10:00 AM. Bedrooms were dimly lit and illuminance was measured at 0.10 to 0.13 lux at the corneal level. Subjects sat up in bed with their backs and heads supported by a bed-rest cushion. Ambient temperature was kept at 72° F. Meal timing was set at 1 hour prior to the first MWT trial, and immediately after the termination of the noon trial. Instructions to the subjects were "Please sit still and remain awake for as long as possible. Look ahead of you, and do not look directly at the light." Subjects were not allowed to maintain wakefulness by using extraordinary measures such as slapping the face or singing.

Each wakefulness trial was terminated either at the first onset of sleep or, if sleep onset was not achieved, after a maximum in-bed duration of 40 minutes. For the purposes of trial termination, sleep onset was defined as the first occurrence of sustained sleep, defined as three consecutive 30-second epochs of stage 1 or any single 30-second epoch of another sleep stage (2, 3, 4, or REM). However, in an effort to understand the effects of variations in trial duration and definition of sleep onset, sleep latency scores were also calculated on the basis of a sleep onset defined as the first epoch of any sleep stage. Similarly, although the study was conducted with a maximum wakefulness trial duration of 40 minutes, sleep latency scores were also calculated on the basis of 20-minute trial durations. Therefore, the study not only yielded normative data, but also allowed for comparison of these data to those of prior studies utilizing various methods. In summary, results were calculated utilizing the following four protocols:

1. SUSMWT40: 40-minute MWT trials with sleep onset defined as three continuous epochs of stage 1 sleep or any single epoch of another sleep stage
2. MWT40: 40-minute MWT trials with sleep onset defined as the first epoch of any sleep stage
3. SUSMWT20: 20-minute MWT trials with sleep onset defined as three continuous epochs of stage 1 sleep or any single epoch of another sleep stage
4. MWT20: 20-minute MWT trials with sleep onset defined as the first appearance of any sleep stage

Normative data obtained from this trial are summarized in Table 17–1. As anticipated, longer maximum trial durations yielded longer sleep latency scores. However, average scores were not affected by the definition of sleep onset.

CLINICAL APPLICATIONS

A Task Force of the Standards of Practice Committee of the American Academy of Sleep Medicine (AASM) recently reviewed the database derived from studies utilizing the

TABLE 17–1 Normative and Clinically Derived MWT Data

Study	Sample	N	Sleep Onset Criteria*	Trial Duration (min)	Protocol[†]	Mean Sleep Latency (min ± SD)	p[‡]
Doghramji et al.[19]	Normals	64	A	40	SUSMWT40	35.2 ± 7.9	
			A	20	SUSMWT20	18.7 ± 2.6	
			B[§]	40	MWT40	32.6 ± 9.9	
			B[§]	20	MWT20	18.1 ± 3.6	
Poceta et al.[17]	OSA	322	A	40	SUSMWT40	25.9 ± 11.8	<0.0001
Sangal et al.[35]	Excessive daytime sleepiness	258	B	20[¶]	MWT20[¶]	15.9 ± 5.0	<0.001
	Excessive daytime sleepiness	258	B	40	MWT40	26.5 ± 12.4	<0.001
Browman et al.[34]	Narcolepsy	11	A	20	SUSMWT20	10.7 ± 5.3	<0.001
	Normal controls	11	A	20	SUSMWT20	19.0 ± 1.5	≥0.05
Browman et al.[33]	Narcolepsy	12	A	20	SUSMWT20	11.0 ± 5.6	<0.001
	OSA	12	A	20	SUSMWT20	11.0 ± 4.8	<0.001
	Normal controls	10	A	20	SUSMWT20	18.3 ± 4.0	≥0.05
Mitler et al.[10]	Narcolepsy	10	A	20	SUSMWT20	9.9 ± 6.1	<0.001
	Normal controls	8	A	20	SUSMWT20	17.9 ± 4.4	≤0.05

*A, three 30-second epochs of stage 1 or one epoch of any other sleep stage; B, one 30-second epoch of any sleep stage.
[†]See text for definitions of protocols.
[‡]Compared with corresponding measure of sleep latency in Doghramji et al.[19]
[§]Or 10 seconds of microsleep.
[¶]Data based on a 40-minute protocol were recalculated for the 20-minute protocol.
OSA, obstructive sleep apnea; SD, standard deviation.

MWT,[21] on the basis of which the AASM set forth practice parameters for the use of the MWT.[22] These practice parameters propose two indications for the MWT:

1. The MWT 40-minute protocol may be used to assess an individual's ability to remain awake when his or her inability to remain awake constitutes a public or personal safety issue.
2. The MWT may be indicated in patients with excessive sleepiness to assess response to treatment.[22]

Assessment of the "Normality" of an Individual

The problem of defining normal and abnormal performance on tests such as the MWT has no universal solution. Some have advocated the use of standard deviation criteria; threshold values for normality are often considered to be 2 standard deviations from the mean.[23] Applying this definition to normative data yields low limits for normality, which appear in Table 17–2. Depending on

TABLE 17–2 Lower Limits for Normality as Assessed by 2 Standard Deviations Lower than the Mean for Various MWT Protocols

Protocol*	Lower Limit (Mean − 2 SD in Min)	% Subjects Scoring Less than Lower Limit
SUSMWT40	19.4	8
MWT40	12.9	9
SUSMWT20	13.5	6
MWT20	10.9	8

*See text for definitions of protocols.
SD, standard deviation.
Reproduced with permission from Doghramji K, Mitler M, Sangal RB, et al. A normative study of the Maintenance of Wakefulness Test (MWT). Electroencephalogr Clin Neurophysiol 1997;103:554.

the protocol utilized, therefore, individuals scoring below these cutoff points would be considered to be "too sleepy." The use of standard deviation criteria is, however, problematic since normative MWT sleep latencies form a skewed distribution that is truncated at 40 minutes (Fig. 17–1), with most subjects able to maintain wakefulness on each trial, but with a few subjects failing to maintain wakefulness after as little as 10 minutes.

In contract, the AASM practice parameters advocate the use of a percentile cutoff score.[22] They recommend the use of the MWT40 protocol since the longer opportunity to nap provides for a less of a "ceiling effect" than the

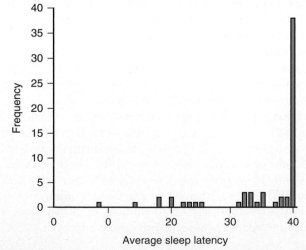

FIGURE 17–1 Normative MWT data. Average sleep latencies over four 40-minute-long MWT trials were calculated for each of 64 healthy volunteers and plotted in frequency histogram format. See text for details. *(Reproduced with permission from Doghramji K, Mitler M, Sangal RB, et al. A normative study of the Maintenance of Wakefulness Test (MWT). Electroencephalogr Clin Neurophysiol 1997;103:554.)*

20-minute protocol and since the utilization of a sleep onset criterion of any epoch of any sleep stage also provides for a more normal range of scores than the more rigorous (sustained) definition of sleep onset. Additionally, they recommend a threshold percentile of 97.5%. Accordingly, since 97.5% of the normal subjects in the normative study by Doghramji et al.[19] had a mean sleep latency of >8.0 minutes, a mean sleep latency <8.0 minutes on the 40-minute MWT is considered abnormal; values greater than this but less than 40 minutes are of uncertain significance.

Others have suggested that the number of trials in which a subject fails to maintain wakefulness should define pathology. The normative data indicate that, on average, for both the 40-minute and 20-minute trials, that number is less than 1 (0.81 ± 1.25 and 0.56 ± 1.02, respectively). Requiring that an individual stay awake on all trials on the MWT appears to provide the strongest evidence of an individual's "normality."

Closely related to the assessment of normality is the assessment of safety in occupations in which daytime alertness is critical, such as airline pilots and truck drivers. The assessment of safety in driving is also of great importance for most patients with disorders of daytime somnolence. Unfortunately, no physiologically based test, including the MWT, has been shown to be a valid predictor of operator errors on the highway or in the workplace. In addition, in spite of normal MWT values at any given point in time, levels of sleepiness during everyday life may change due to the influence of noncompliance with treatment, the effects of sedating medications, the quantity and quality of prior night's sleep, prior work hours, and circadian variations. Therefore, the use of the MWT as a stand-alone tool in determining safety and fitness for duty cannot be supported. That having been said, ignoring poor performance on the MWT also seems inappropriate. No cutoff points with respect to average sleep latency or number of failed MWT trials are suggested here. However, it is wise to consider several MWT parameters (e.g., average sleep latency, number of failed trials) as part of a comprehensive clinical evaluation, which includes the interview, examination, other laboratory tests, and so forth. It may also be useful to establish, with the participation of relevant stakeholders, guidelines for pass/fail ranges.

Detecting the Effect of Therapeutic Interventions

The MWT has also proven to be sensitive in assessing treatment efficacy of continuous positive airway pressure in obstructive sleep apnea syndrome[13] and of various pharmacologic agents in narcolepsy.[24–26] The MWT and the RTSW have been shown to be sensitive to pharmacologic interventions aimed at reducing sleepiness.[26–28] Data on the ability to sustain wakefulness during the night and the remedial effects of napping and caffeine on functioning during simulated shiftwork are also available.[27,29–32]

Providing a Profile of Sleepiness for Groups with Certain Disorders

It is useful to describe the characteristic degree of impairment in alertness for disorders of excessive somnolence. The MWT has been utilized in this capacity for narcolepsy and sleep apnea syndrome, as summarized in Table 17–1.[14,17,33–35] All studies also include a comparison with healthy controls.

MWT VERSUS MSLT

The MWT can be conceptualized as an outgrowth of the MSLT with altered instructions and body position. Some studies have shown that the MSLT and MWT produce similar data when detecting remedial interventions.[28] However, other studies have failed to show a consistent relationship between the two tests when applied to the same patient groups.[16,19,35,36] Such data suggest that the MSLT and the MWT assess fundamentally separate functions (i.e., waking ability and sleeping ability). Discordance between the MSLT and the MWT may also be partially understood, as Bonnet and Arand suggested,[11] in terms of the additive effects of instruction and posture. Another potential explanation is that the MWT, because of its instruction to remain awake, adds a nonlinear motivational factor that is not present with the MSLT. The MWT often reveals improvement in treated patients who continue to be physiologically sleepy on the MSLT. Thus, the MWT is sometimes considered to be a way of extending the sensitivity range of the MSLT.[37] Such reasoning is complicated, however, by the possibility that the MSLT may also incorporate nonlinear motivational factors.

The MSLT and the MWT may have a unique set of clinical applications. Various studies have indicated that, whereas the MSLT is not particularly sensitive in detecting treatment effects in patient groups,[34,38] the MWT is. The MWT is also sensitive in detecting the effects of manipulation of the prior night's sleep quality and quantity on daytime alertness.[27] It also stands to reason that the MWT may be more accurate in assessing the risk of falling asleep unintentionally during soporific activities where individuals are attempting to stay awake, such as driving, reading, and other activities of daily life. However, no such comparisons between the two tests have been yet performed. Clearly expanded studies are needed to explore the reasons for the discordance between the two tests and the relative utility of each.

PROTOCOL RECOMMENDATIONS

As noted earlier, various definitions of sleep onset and trial duration have been utilized for the MWT since its introduction. Regardless of definition, however, the MWT appears to be capable of separating sleepy from healthy individuals. Therefore, the determination of which of these protocols should be utilized in each individual case can be based on the specific clinical need and the nature of practical constraints. For example, if the sample being tested is likely to have subjects with a low level of sleepiness, maximizing the test's sensitivity in detecting sleep onset and maximizing the duration of each trial may minimize the potential for a ceiling effect and, in turn, allow for more meaningful comparison among subjects tested. In this case, therefore, utilizing the 40-minute trial duration and the first appearance of any epoch of sleep as the definition of sleep onset may be optimal. The same protocol may be best suited for assessing treatment response. If the population under investigation is highly sleepy, or if accuracy is critical, the more stringent definition of sleep onset (three epochs of stage 1 or one epoch of any other sleep stage) may be preferred. Practical, economic, limitations may favor the use of the 20-minute duration.

For routine clinical applications, authors of the normative trial recommended the use of the 20-minute protocol with sleep latency measured to the onset of any sleep stage.[19] They noted that the 20-minute protocols are more cost effective, and, unlike the 40-minute protocol, are not affected by age. However, the AASM practice parameters, which were developed subsequently, and which were based on the methods of the normative trial of Doghramji and colleagues[19] but modified by collective expert opinion using Rand/UCLA Appropriateness Method, favored the 40-minute protocol with sleep latency measured to the onset of any sleep stage, noting that the longer nap opportunity offers a more normal distribution of the data.[22] The following are the AASM protocol recommendations:

1. The four-trial MWT 40-minute protocol is recommended. The MWT consists of four trials performed at 2-hour intervals, with the first trial beginning about 1.5–3 hours after the patient's usual wake-up time. This usually equates to a first trial starting at 0900 or 1000 hours.
2. Performance of a polysomnogram prior to the MWT should be decided by the clinician based on clinical circumstances.
3. Based on the Rand/UCLA Appropriateness Method, no consensus was reached regarding the use of sleep logs prior to the MWT; there are instances, based on clinical judgment, when they may be indicated.
4. The room should be maximally insulated from external light. The light source should be positioned slightly behind the subject's head such that it is just out of his or her field of vision, and should deliver an illuminance of 0.10–0.13 lux at the corneal level (a 7.5-W night light can be used, placed 1 foot off the floor and 3 feet laterally removed from the subject's head). Room temperature should be set based on the patient's comfort level. The subject should be seated in bed, with the back and head supported by a bedrest (bolster pillow) such that the neck is not uncomfortably flexed or extended.

5. The use of tobacco, caffeine, and other medications by the patient before and during the MWT should be addressed and decided upon by the sleep clinician before the test is conducted. Drug screening may be indicated to ensure that sleepiness/wakefulness on the MWT is not influenced by substances other than medically prescribed drugs. Drug screening is usually performed on the morning of the MWT, but its timing and the circumstances of the testing may be modified by the clinician. A light breakfast is recommended at least 1 hour prior to the first trial, and a light lunch is recommended immediately after the termination of the second noon trial.
6. Sleep technologists who perform the MWT should be experienced in conducting the test.
7. The conventional recording montage for the MWT includes central (C3–A2, C4–A1) and occipital (O1/A2, O2/A1) electroencephalography derivations, left and right eye electro-oculograms, mental/submental electromyogram, and electrocardiogram.
8. Prior to each trial, the patient should be asked if he or she needs to use the bathroom or needs other adjustments for comfort. Standard instructions for biocalibrations (i.e., patient calibrations) prior to each trial include: (1) sit/lie quietly with your eyes open for 30 seconds; (2) close both eyes for 30 seconds; (3) without moving your head, look to the right, then left, then right, then left, then right, and then left; (4) blink eyes slowly five times; and (5) clench or grit your teeth tightly together.
9. Instructions to the patient consist of the following: "Please sit still and remain awake for as long as possible. Look directly ahead of you, and do not look directly at the light." Patients are not allowed to use extraordinary measures to stay awake such as slapping the face or singing.
10. Sleep onset is defined as the first epoch of greater than 15 seconds of cumulative sleep in a 30-second epoch.
11. Trials are ended after 40 minutes if no sleep occurs, or after unequivocal sleep, defined as three consecutive epochs of stage 1 sleep, or one epoch of any other stage of sleep.
12. The following data should be recorded: start and stop times for each trial, sleep latency, total sleep time, stages of sleep achieved for each trial, and the mean sleep latency (the arithmetic mean of the four trials).
13. Events that represent deviation from standard protocol or conditions should be documented by the sleep technologist for review by the sleep specialist.

⊘ REFERENCES

A full list of references are available at www.expertconsult.com

CHAPTER 18

Clinical Polysomnography and the Evolution of Recording and Scoring Technique

Max Hirshkowitz and Amir Sharafkhaneh

INTRODUCTION

Sleep can be defined many ways. Behaviorally, it is a reversible state of inactivity associated with decreased responsiveness. In humans, sleep usually begins in the late evening or early night. During sleep, our bodies cool and remain mostly immobile. As in coma, responsiveness to environmental stimuli declines, but unlike coma, the state can rapidly change to wakefulness, usually without lingering cognitive impairment. Coma passively results from brain stem and cortical metabolic depression; however, sleep is an active process.[1]

Although most often described as a "state," sleep represents an essential brain process. As such, the traditional approach for investigating sleep involves comparing brain activity during sleep to brain activity accompanying wakefulness. One of the earliest tools available for investigating brain activity was electroencephalography (EEG). Thus, studying the EEG correlates of normal sleep was a logical place for the scientific study of sleep to begin.

ELECTROENCEPHALOGRAPHIC AND ELECTRO-OCULOGRAPHIC WAVEFORMS IN SLEEP

Descriptions and Examples

Hans Berger, the father of EEG, made the first sleep recordings.[2] EEG activity during relaxed wakefulness (with eyes closed) was a nearly sinusoidal pattern in the frequency range of 8–13 cycles/sec. Berger named this

rhythm "alpha" and found that it would diminish when the subject opened his or her eyes or engaged in mental arithmetic. Berger also discovered that alpha activity was replaced by low-voltage mixed frequency activity at sleep onset. Even to this day, this finding remains as the foundation of sleep-wake classification, with EEG alpha cessation defining the transition from wakefulness to sleep (Fig. 18–1). The low-voltage, mixed-frequency activity associated with sleep onset is also marked by a general slowing of EEG frequency and the appearance of a 4- to 7-cycle/sec waveform called EEG *theta activity*. By contrast, the abrupt diminution of alpha activity provoked by eye opening is usually characterized by high-frequency EEG beta activity (>13 cycles/sec), rapid eye movements associated with changes in direction of gaze, and/or blinking.

The first continuous all-night EEG recordings of human sleep were not made until almost 3 decades after Berger first recorded the brain's electrical activity during sleep.[3] It became immediately apparent that sleep was not a single homogeneous process. The low-voltage, mixed-frequency activity seen at sleep onset would sometimes contain single, high-amplitude, negative-going, high-frequency wave bursts. These waveforms are known as *vertex sharp waves* and are commonly observed near sleep onset (Fig. 18–2). As sleep further progresses, there begin to appear short phasic bursts of discrete 12- to 16-cycle/sec waveforms typically lasting 0.5–1.5 seconds. The waveform envelope is "spindle" shaped, and consequently these bursts

FIGURE 18–1 Transition from wakefulness to sleep. (C3, left central; EMG-SM, electromyogram-submentalis; F3, left frontal; LOC, left outer canthus; M2, right mastoid; O1, left occipital; ROC, right outer canthus.)

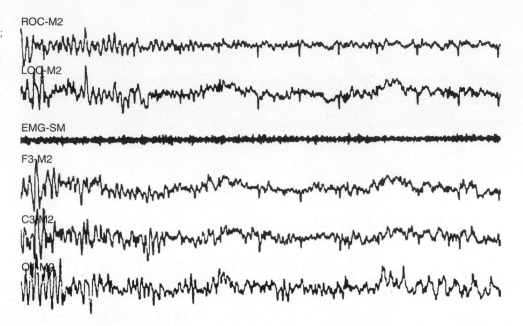

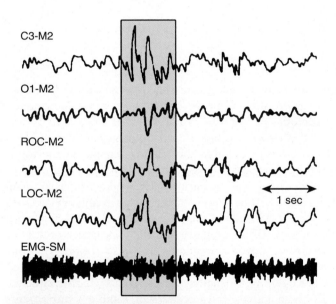

FIGURE 18–2 Vertex sharp wave. (C3, left central; EMG-SM, electromyogram-submentalis; LOC, left outer canthus; M2, right mastoid; O1, left occipital; ROC, right outer canthus.)

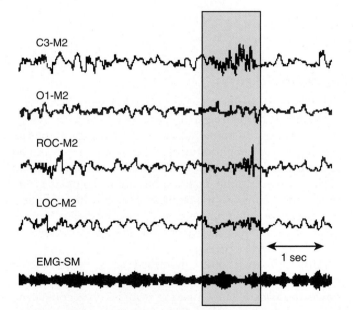

FIGURE 18–3 Sleep spindle. (C3, left central; EMG-SM, electromyogram-submentalis; LOC, left outer canthus; M2, right mastoid; O1, left occipital; ROC, right outer canthus.)

were named *sleep spindles* (Fig. 18–3). Sometimes in concert with or proximal to a sleep spindle, a high-amplitude, negative-going sharp wave appears and is immediately followed by a positive component. This waveform, referred to as a *K complex*, stands out from the background activity and has a total duration greater than 0.5 seconds (Fig. 18–4).

Over the course of the first hour of sleep, most individuals will gradually have increasing amounts of high-amplitude, low-frequency activity called EEG *delta rhythm* (with frequencies <4 cycles/sec). In the young

adult, delta rhythm and a subset called *slow waves* (with frequencies <2 cycles/sec) usually increase to the point that the low-voltage, mixed-frequency activity is completely replaced by these high-voltage synchronized waves (Fig. 18–5). Sleep spindles may persist, occurring in conjunction with the slow-wave activity, and can sometimes be seen "riding" on the slow waves. When the bout of delta and slow-wave activity subsides, a period of low-voltage, mixed-frequency activity re-emerges. During this period, theta activity is often observed. This theta rhythm's morphology differs slightly from that seen near

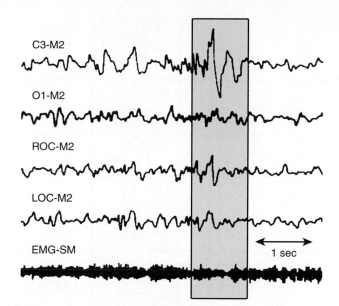

FIGURE 18–4 K complex. (C3, left central; EMG-SM, electromyogram-submentalis; LOC, left outer canthus; M2, right mastoid; O1, left occipital; ROC, right outer canthus.)

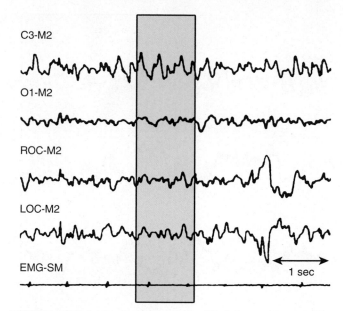

FIGURE 18–6 Sawtooth theta activity. (C3, left central; EMG-SM, electromyogram-submentalis; LOC, left outer canthus; M2, right mastoid; O1, left occipital; ROC, right outer canthus.)

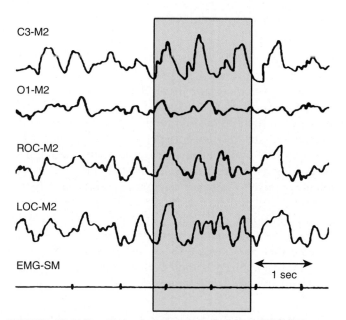

FIGURE 18–5 Slow-wave activity. (C3, left central; EMG-SM, electromyogram-submentalis; LOC, left outer canthus; M2, right mastoid; O1, left occipital; ROC, right outer canthus.)

sleep onset in that the waves have a notched appearance, resembling the teeth on a saw. These *sawtooth theta waves* (Fig. 18–6) usually do not occur interspersed with sleep spindles and K complexes but rather appear in conjunction with rapid eye movements.

Eye movements can easily be recorded by placing an electrode on the face near the eye. The cornea has a positive charge and, as the eye moves toward an electrode, a large voltage change occurs. By making recordings with electrodes placed near the outer canthus of each eye,

horizontal eye movements can be recorded. As one eye is moving toward its proximal electrode and the other eye is moving away from the other electrode, voltage deflections are in opposite directions (out of phase) on the recording. Consequently, these eye movements can be easily differentiated from EEG and in particular delta EEG activity (which is in phase).

Eye movements occur during both wakefulness and sleep. The saccade is a very rapid eye movement in which the brain moves the eye from one target to another (with ocular suppression occurring during the actual transit). The *rapid eye movements* (REMs) that accompany the low-voltage, mixed-frequency background EEG that are thought to correspond to direction of gaze during dreaming[4,5] are slightly slower than eyes-open saccades. It has been demonstrated that volitional saccades in a dark field are of equivalent speed; therefore, the velocity loss appears to be visual field dependent rather than state dependent. Additionally, there are slow, rolling, almost pendular eye movements that can occur in the drowsy awake state, at sleep onset, and/or for up to several minutes after sleep has become well established. These *slow eye movements* in some instances may be correlated with hypnagogic or hypnapompic imagery. Rapid and slow eye movements during sleep are illustrated in Figure 18–7.

Summarizing Waveforms

Waveforms, like most physiologic parameters, can be characterized along the standard dimensions: frequency, magnitude, and duration. For example, sleep spindle density (the mean number of spindles per minute) is a common frequency index. Magnitude could be quantified in terms of the average peak amplitude or area under the

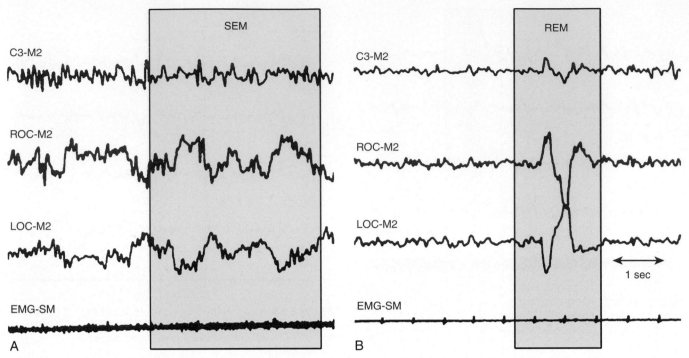

FIGURE 18–7 Sleep-related eye movements. **(A)** A typical slow eye movement (SEM) of the type usually seen at sleep onset. **(B)** A rapid eye movement (REM) characteristic of REM sleep. (C3, left central; EMG-SM, electromyogram-submentalis; LOC, left outer canthus; M2, right mastoid; O1, left occipital; ROC, right outer canthus.)

curve normalized for overall duration. Mean spindle length would exemplify a duration measure. Obviously, because the number of waveforms occurring during a single night may be very large, hand measuring, tabulating, and statistically summarizing the frequency, magnitude, and duration of each could amount to a Herculean task. Therefore, automation was embraced early in sleep research laboratories. Using computers to perform complex EEG analysis (e.g., Fourier transforms, period-amplitude analysis, and complex demodulation) to characterize sleep EEGs and plot spectral arrays long predates their use as digital polysomnographs.[6]

Waveform analysis has been used to study sleep physiology,[7] psychiatric illness,[8] clinical pharmacology,[9] sleep disorders,[10] and aging.[11] Other computerized techniques examining connectivity between waveform events (e.g., Markovian chain analysis) attempt to understand the behavior of the underlying physiology. To date, there has not been any large-scale organized attempt to standardize sleep signal processing recording method, detection technique, quantitative analysis, or summarization. Each researcher tailors his or her technique to meet the particular investigative needs.

Waveform Changes Across the Night

Certainly the most profound intranight waveform change is the progressive decrease in delta (and slow-wave) activity observed in most individuals.[12] Commonly quantified as delta power (a measure combining magnitude and

duration), some researchers posit delta activity as a measure of sleep homeostatic drive. The prototypical record shows rapid evolution of delta and slow waves dominating the EEG in the first 60–90 minutes of sleep. After a brief interval marked by low-voltage, mixed-frequency EEG activity, delta power again rises, but neither as high or for as long as in the first cycle. Another interval of low-voltage, mixed-frequency activity intervenes before another round of delta activity commences. Through each cycle, delta power diminishes. By contrast, REM activity generally increases as the night progresses. This gradual increase may also involve theta, and especially sawtooth theta, activity. Sleep spindles, theta activity, and other waveforms remain fairly stable across the night of sleep.

Changes as a Function of Age

Of all the age-related phenomena revealed by polysomnography, the decline in delta and slow-wave activity is perhaps the most striking.[13] Not only does the duration of slow-wave activity decline, but the amplitude of the waveforms declines as well. The extent of the decline is what makes it dramatic. Sophisticated analytic tools are not required to visualize the changes; they are apparent to the naked eye (Fig. 18–8). Not surprisingly, most of the other waveforms also show age-related decline. Studies of K complexes, sleep spindles, and theta activity reveal age-related alterations in density and amplitude. Similarly, REM density may be lower in some samples of elderly individuals.

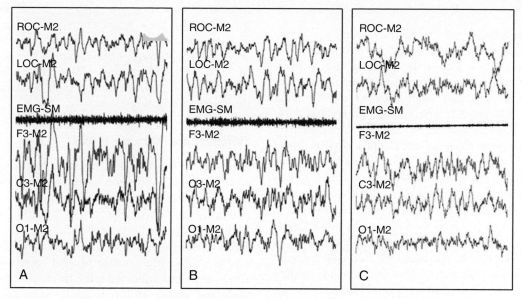

FIGURE 18–8 Slow Wave Activity in a Child (**A**), Young Adult (**B**), and Very Healthy Older Adult (**C**). This figure illustrates that in addition to decreased duration of sleep stages 3 and 4 (slow wave sleep), amplitude of slow activity also declines with age. (C3, left central; EMG-SM, electromyogram-submentalis; F3, left frontal; LOC, left outer canthus; M2, right mastoid; O1, left occipital; ROC, right outer canthus.)

SLEEP STAGING

Recording and Scoring Techniques

It is hard to imagine how overwhelming the enormity of the data must have seemed to early researchers when they first began collecting continuous all-night polysomnographic recordings from human subjects. Information needed to be summarized into a manageable form. From the very start, schemes were developed to reduce data within a time domain; thus, *sleep staging* was invented.

Staging's basic principle involves nominally classifying a recording segment of set duration according to the activity observed during that time interval. In this case, the nominal classifications are categories called "stages" and the set duration is called an "epoch." Also, until the mid-1980s, sleep studies were mainly recorded on paper. The duration of an epoch varied in different laboratories, undoubtedly influenced mainly by paper chart speed and paper size. Early fan-fold paper was 30 cm wide and came in boxes of 1000 sheets. If the chart speed was 10 mm/sec (as was common in many sleep laboratories), then one page of recording was 30 seconds in duration and one box of paper would hold 8 hours and 20 minutes worth of tracings. Designating one page as one epoch was very convenient, and it quickly became a de facto standard.

Categorizing each epoch as one or another sleep stage is based on similarities and differences in the activity present. An assortment of rules can be developed to guide categorization (re: staging). But how many categories are needed? How well do the generalizations work? Does sleep staging really characterize the bioelectrical activity associated with normal sleep? To explore these questions, consider the following exercise the senior author (M.H.) regularly conducts on the first day of class before the medical students, residents, and fellows have been taught anything about sleep medicine. Each student is given 100 randomly selected, 30-second pages selected from five different normal polysomnographic 4-channel (C3-A2 EEG, ROC-A2, A2-LOC, and submentalis EMG) recordings. Students are instructed to sort the pages into piles, based on similarities of the squiggly lines decorating each page. Recording channels, recording speed, and even page orientation remains unspecified. No other directions are given. Groups of two and three individuals are formed and the exercise is performed three times, each time with different partners. The first two trials are considered practice and the results of the third are tabulated. On the third trial of blindly categorizing paper tracings, novices create 5–10 categories and REM sleep is recognized with near universality. Pages with low-voltage, mixed-frequency activity that also have sleep spindles are grouped with great regularity. Furthermore, one to three categories containing slow waves are derived. Overall, the majority of pages are sorted into categories that roughly correspond to one or another stage definition. Thus, even with all the arbitrariness of the staging rules' specific details, every time we experimentally invent sleep staging we produce similar results. Therefore, the reader should not be surprised by the remarkable comparability of the different sleep staging systems described below.

Loomis (1936)

Recording Montage. As the first researchers to make continuous all-night sleep recordings, Loomis and colleagues[14] were also the first to face the daunting task of quantifying miles of paper tracings for summary analysis. They developed a data reduction scheme called sleep staging (*stages A, B, C, D, and E*). Staging was largely based on the presence of particular EEG activity. EEG activity included beta activity, sleep spindles, alpha rhythm, theta rhythm, delta rhythm, and slow waves recorded from three electrodes pairs.[14] One electrode was place above and to the left of the left eye and referenced to the mastoid behind the ear. This derivation was used to detect eye movements and frontal lobe activity. A second electrode, placed midline at the top of the head (roughly corresponding to Cz) was referenced to the left mastoid and was used to score sleep spindles and K complexes. The final active recording site was midline on the occiput (mastoid referred) and was used to maximally visualize alpha activity.

Sleep Staging. *Stage A (Alpha)* is described as containing alpha "trains" of varying durations possibly accompanied by slow, rolling eye movements. *Stage B (Low Voltage)* has neither alpha activity nor spindle activity; however, rolling eye movements may occur. *Stage C (Spindles)* is defined by the presence of sleep spindle activity with mostly low-voltage background. *Stage D (Spindles plus random)* is scored when sleep spindles occur together with large "random" waves (corresponding to delta and slow wave activity). Finally, *Stage E (Random)* is when delta and slow waves dominate the recording, or, as the authors put it "large random potentials persist and come from all parts of the cortex." Interestingly, when sleep is graphically represented over the course of a night with stages arrayed from A through E on the y axis and time on the x axis, the histograms look remarkably similar to what is used today. Also noted on the histograms were subject reports of dreaming that occurred when subjects awoke from stage B.

Dement-Kleitman (1957)

Dement and Kleitman[15] developed criteria for classifying epochs of sleep according to EEG criteria. To a large degree, this technique was the foundation for most scoring systems used throughout the world, up to and including the present time. Noteworthy was the fact that it was the first scoring system that incorporated REM sleep, the new sleep stage recently discovered in their laboratory by Eugene Aserinsky. Essentially, each recording epoch was classified as awake or sleep stage 1, 2, 3, or 4. *Stage 1* was classified when a nonawake EEG with a low-voltage, mixed-frequency background was devoid of sleep spindles and K complexes. In general, Dement-Kleitman stage 1 corresponds to Loomis Stages A and B. Sleep *stage 2* was classified when sleep spindles and/or K complexes were

intermingled with a low-voltage, mixed-frequency background EEG. *Stage 3* was characterized by appearance of slow waves (100 μV or more at a frequency ≤2 cycles/sec), and finally *stage 4* was assigned to epochs composed of 50% or more of these high-amplitude, slow waves. When REMs occurred during stage 1 sleep, the stage was designated *REM sleep*.

Williams and Karacan (1959)

Recording Montage. Robert L. Williams is one of the unsung pioneers of sleep medicine. In June of 1959, the sleep laboratories at the University of Florida College of Medicine in Gainesville began making continuous all-night sleep recordings in normal, healthy individuals.[16] With the rationale that, to understand sleep disorders, one must first characterize normal human sleep, "normative" data were collected over the next decade from both male and female children, adolescents, teenagers, young adults, adults, and seniors. In 1974, the compilation of normal values for sleep were published in book form, stratified by sex and age group (3–5 years, 6–9 years, 10–12 years, 13–15 years, 16–19 years, 20–29 years, 30–39 years, 40–49 years, 50–59 years, 60–69 years, and 70–79 years). The recording technique used by Williams and colleagues employed three channels of EEG derivations (F1-F7, C3-A2, and O3-OzPz) and two channels of electro-oculogram (EOG) derivations (Left Eye–A2 and A2–Right Eye). Notably absent from this montage was a channel for assessing submentalis muscle tone to detect REM sleep–related atonia. This was not an oversight; by contrast, the developers of this system provide a strong argument against including submentalis electromyography (EMG). The authors wrote, "Since there are wide individual differences in tonus of the chin muscles which begin to undergo changes during adulthood, this measure becomes less reliable with age starting as early as age 40 and is useless with elderly subjects."

The selection of three EEG channels stemmed from recognition that EEG from particular derivations had differential usefulness for visualizing specific waveforms. A monopolar channel near the vertex (C3-A2) is generally reliable for recording most waveforms, including vertex sharp waves, K complexes, sleep spindles, theta activity, and slow waves. This is why most recording systems use a central lobe channel or even rely totally on this channel for all brainwave activity. Recording a single all-purpose EEG signal was advantageous back when amplifiers were expensive and the number of channels limited. Nonetheless, it was well known among sleep researchers and neurologists that EEG alpha alterations associated with wakefulness and sleep were most prominent in occipital leads. Therefore, Williams and colleagues incorporated O3-OzPz into the montage to facilitate and improve scoring reliability of sleep onset, awakenings, and central nervous system (CNS) arousals. The inclusion of a third

EEG channel (recorded over the frontal lobe [F1-F7]) was designed to enhance delta (and slow-wave) activity detection and visualization. With their focus on sleep changes over the life span, Williams and colleagues were keen to obtain high-quality data for delta bandwidth activity because it was often the primary outcome measure in studies of sleep and aging.

Sleep Staging. Polygraph chart speed at the University of Florida College of Medicine in Gainesville was 15 mm/sec rather than the 10 mm/sec commonly used elsewhere. Consequently, each page contained 20 seconds of data and each set of 3 pages constituted a 1-minute epoch. In the Williams-Karacan scoring system, wakefulness is designated *stage 0*. An epoch is classified as stage 0 if it contained "at least 30 seconds of 8 to 12 Hz occipital activity, with a minimum amplitude of 40 microvolts peak-to-peak." *Stage 1* criteria were (1) less than 30 seconds of occipital alpha activity and (2) no more than one well-defined spindle or K complex. It was permissible to use muscle artifact and eye movements to facilitate staging in alpha nonproducers. *Stage 2* required at least two well-defined sleep spindles or K complexes, or one of each. Additionally, the epoch could contain no more than 12 seconds of 40-µV (or greater), 1–3-cycles/sec slow waves. Between 13 and 30 seconds of 1–3-cycle/sec slow waves was obligatory for scoring *Stage 3*, and 30 seconds or more were necessary to classify an epoch as *Stage 4*. Eye movements were scored independently from the EEG activity. Epochs of stage 1 sleep that also contained REMs were designated as *Stage 1-REM*. On occasion, usually in connection with polysomnograms recorded from study subjects taking sedative-hypnotics (e.g., flurazepam), *Stage 2-REM* would also occur.

The Standardized Manual (1968)

As sleep research progressed, a problem began mounting. Technique and terminology could differ radically from one sleep center to the next; for example, REM sleep was also called paradoxical sleep, desynchronized sleep, active sleep, D sleep, and even unorthodox sleep. To alleviate this difficulty, an ad-hoc committee was formed by members of the sleep research society to develop *A Manual of Standardized Terminology, Techniques and Scoring System for Sleep Stages of Human Subjects.*[17] This committee, chaired by Drs. Allan Rechtschaffen and Anthony Kales (thus the manual is consequently often called the *R&K*) was composed of a veritable pantheon of sleep luminaries, including William C. Dement, Michel Jouvet, Bedrich Roth, Laverne C. Johnson, Howard P. Roffwarg, Ralph J. Berger, Allan Jacobson, Lawrence J. Monroe, Ian Oswald, and Richard D. Walter. This group developed a standardized set of examples and rules for scoring sleep stages.

Recording Montage. The R&K specifies that sleep is scored from a monopolar centrally derived (either C3-A2

or C4-A1) EEG tracing and EOGs recorded from the outer canthus of each eye (also referenced to A2). A fourth channel, EMG from the submentalis (chin), is also specified for detecting changes in the level of muscle tone. Using these four channels, rules are provided for classifying each epoch into wakefulness or one of five possible sleep stages.

Sleep Staging. According to the R&K, *stage W* (wakefulness) is scored when the EEG for more than 50% of an epoch contains alpha activity (while eyes are closed). For the small percentage of individuals who do not produce EEG alpha activity, blinking, high EMG, fast activity (EEG beta activity), and the absence of theta activity or vertex sharp waves may aid differentiation between wakefulness and sleep. *Stage 1* is scored when alpha comprises less than 50% of an epoch and the low-voltage, mixed-frequency EEG-EOG tracings do not contain K complexes, spindles, or REMs. Vertex sharp waves and slow rolling eye movements may be present. *Stage 2* is scored when there are sleep spindles and/or K complexes but high-amplitude delta and slow waves (≥ 75 µV) comprise less than 20% of the epoch's duration. *Stage 3* is scored when an epoch contains 20–50% delta or slow waves that are 75 µV or greater. *Stage 4* is scored when an epoch contains more than 50% delta or slow waves that are 75 µV or greater. *REM sleep* is scored when REMs and muscle atonia accompanying a stage 1 EEG pattern. Epochs could also be scored as *movement time* (MT) when artifact obscured the majority of the tracing and the preceding and following stage differed. In general, MT could be invoked when it was not possible to classify the epoch as W, 1, 2, 3, 4, or REM.

These stage scoring rules were not very different from existing systems of the day. Most laboratories were using some variant of the Dement-Kleitman system or the Williams-Karacan system. The real key to the success of this project was consensus. This is not to say that participants did not disagree, argue, debate, shout, and mutter epithets—they did. In fact, legend has it (and Allan Rechtschaffen corroborates it) that, in the heat of one particularly vehement argument, one of the chairmen barred the doors, decreeing that no one could leave until consensus was reached. The genius of the group was that they understood *consensus* had to be attained. If each participant had returned to his laboratory and ignored R&K recommendations in favor of continuing their existing practice, the project would have failed.

Smoothing Rules. Perhaps the most difficult, and most poorly understood, feature of the R&K system were the 3-minute rules. These were a special set of rules used to determine the beginning and ending of an episode of REM sleep or stage 2 sleep. At first blush, one might wonder why such rules should even be needed; however, when one begins considering the multitude of scenarios that actually occur, the necessity of specific rules becomes obvious. For example, consider an epoch of REM sleep that is followed immediately by another epoch that has no eye movements or sleep spindles but has a K complex and increased muscle tone at the 21st second of the epoch. Is the epoch scored as REM sleep or as stage 2 sleep? Furthermore, suppose there were 2 epochs with stage 1 EEG (without REMs) intervening the two epochs described previously. Would they be scored as REM sleep, stage 1, or stage 2? It is for these decisions that the 3-minute rules are invoked. The rationale for scoring these epochs as REM sleep is twofold. First, the central notion about sleep stages is that there are underlying neurophysiologic "state" generators. The REM state persists "tonically" even when eye movements are not present. Therefore, REM sleep continues until there is evidence that a new set of state generators have become activated, in this case producing a sleep spindle and ending REM-related muscle atonia. The second rationale for the 3-minute rules was that they smoothed over the irregularities that often accompany state-to-state transitions. This tends to minimize some of the individual differences between subjects and thereby highlights commonalities of sleep within and between individuals. Remember, early researchers were looking to characterize *normal* human sleep and consequently focused on how similar sleep was from night to night and from subject to subject.

Interestingly, this final issue—the R&K system's tendency to maximize polysomnographic similarities and to minimize, underplay, or even obscure differences between records—became a key point of criticism and contention. The 3-minute rules systematically reduce variability, as does the intrinsic nature of time domain classification. For example, an epoch in the middle of a continuing series of stage 2 sleep epochs that had a 5-second alpha burst related to an arousal would not be represented in sleep staging. Thus, a system designed to characterized normal sleep might not perform optimally when characterizing abnormal sleep. Indeed, the authors would wager that the vast majority of sleep studies conducted around the world tonight will be performed for clinical purposes. When these recordings are interpreted, their differences from normal sleep will be emphasized. Therefore, a recording and scoring system maximizing differences, rather than commonality, would be advantageous.

However, most of the differences observable on the multitude of polysomnograms recorded tonight for clinical purposes will be detected using channel tracings that were never even part of the R&K system. That is, arousals will be detected using occipitally derived EEGs; apneas, hypopneas, oxygen desaturations, and abnormal breathing patterns will be detected using airflow, effort, and oximetry channels; leg movements will be scored from anterior tibialis EMGs; and cardiac arrythmias will be noted from electrocardiographic recording. These all represent *extensions to* and not *modifications of* the R&K system. Thus, the main flaw, if it is a flaw, in the R&K system is omission of terminology, recording technique, and scoring systems for things other than "...Sleep Stages of Human Subjects," the stated purpose.

The American Academy of Sleep Medicine Scoring Manual (2007)

In their preface, the American Academy of Sleep Medicine (AASM) Scoring Manual Steering Committee writes with reference to the R&K system, "...the rapidly emerging field of sleep medicine requires a more comprehensive system of standardized metrics that considers events occurring outside of normal brain activity."[18] In the almost 4 decades between these two publications, there certainly had been attempts to bridge the gaps. These include specific scoring guidelines developed by independent research groups and by fully sanctioned clinical society task forces. Terminology, technique, and scoring criteria have been published for CNS arousals, respiratory events, periodic limb movements, teeth grinding, middle ear muscle activity, sleep-related erections, and cyclic alternating patterns in the EEG. The AASM, however, reasoned that it would be helpful to bring the most relevant elements of clinical sleep methodology under one roof and into a single source book. This also offered an opportunity to apply principles of "evidence-based medicine" and the Rand/UCLA Appropriateness Method to decision making about recommended and optional guidelines. The project also offered the possibility for comprehensiveness, simplifications, and long-overdue minimum specification regarding computerization. In this section (to maintain the chapter's organization), we only review changes related to sleep staging. Other AASM recommendations follow in their appropriate sections.

Recording Montage. When it comes to recording methods for sleep staging, the expression *plus ca change, plus ca meme chose* couldn't be more appropriate. The "new" AASM recommended recording montage for sleep stage scoring includes frontal, central, and occipital EEG (see the section describing the Williams and Karacan [1959] system)—specifically, F4-M1, C4-M1, and O2-M1 with backup electrodes placed at F3, C3, O1, and M2. An alternative to this fully monopolar-based montage is also sanctioned: Fz-Cz, Cz-Oz, and C4-M1. Backup electrodes include placements at Fpz, C3, O1, and M2. The recommended eye movement recording remained the same as in R&K (with the designation "E" for "eye" rather than ROC and LOC [right outer canthus and left outer canthus] and the more accurate "M" designating mastoid reference behind the ear rather than the older designation "A"). Thus, the recommended eye movement recording montage is E1-M2 and E2-M1, with E1 placed 1 cm below the LOC and E2 placed 1 cm above the ROC (or vice versa). The 1-cm vertical displacement of LOC and ROC is to provide some ability to detect nonhorizontal eye movements. An alternative montage is offered for better detection of vertical eye movements (E1-Fpz and E2-Fpz, where both E1 and E2 are placed 1 cm below the outer canthus of each eye).

Sleep Staging. The AASM's updated scoring system firmly establishes epoch length at 30 seconds and has the scorer assign a stage to each epoch. In general, when an epoch contains features of more than one stage, the classification represents the stage characterizing the majority of that epoch. Consistent with previous systems, *stage W* is scored when alpha activity comprises more than 50% of the epoch. In the absence of clear alpha activity, wakefulness can be identified by eye blinks, saccadic eye movements (consistent with reading), or conjugated saccadic eye movements associated with high muscle tone. *Stage N1* predominately concords with R&K and Williams-Karacan stage 1 sleep. It is marked by theta activity, alpha slowing, vertex sharp waves, and slow eye movements. None of these features are required; however, one or more usually occur. The low-voltage, mixed-frequency background with theta activity in the absence of slow waves, sleep spindles, K complexes, and REMs is scored as stage N1 (Fig. 18–9). *Stage N2* epochs are recognized by the presence of a sleep spindle or K complex and the absence of significant delta activity. Significant delta activity is when 75 μV or more of frontally recorded delta activity lasts for more than 20% (6 seconds) of an epoch (Fig. 18–10). Epochs containing significant delta activity should be scored as *stage N3* (Fig. 18–11). Since stage N3 encompasses both stage 3 and stage 4, stage 4 has been eliminated. The AASM manual allows for using a bipolar montage (Fz-Cz) but does not indicate how amplitude criteria should be adjusted (if amplitude criteria are not adjusted, less N3 would be scored from the tracing of Fz-Cz activity). *Stage R* represents REM sleep (and will

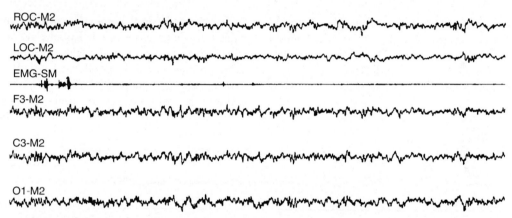

FIGURE 18–9 Sleep stage N1—a 30-second epoch of sleep classified as stage N1 that was recorded and scored according to the AASM scoring manual. (C3, left central; EMG-SM, electromyogram-submentalis; F3, left frontal; LOC, left outer canthus; M2, right mastoid; O1, left occipital; ROC, right outer canthus.)

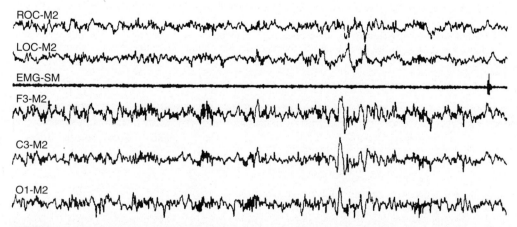

FIGURE 18–10 Sleep stage N2—a 30-second epoch of sleep classified as stage N2 that was recorded and scored according to the AASM scoring manual. (C3, left central; EMG-SM, electromyogram-submentalis; F3, left frontal; LOC, left outer canthus; M2, right mastoid; O1, left occipital; ROC, right outer canthus.)

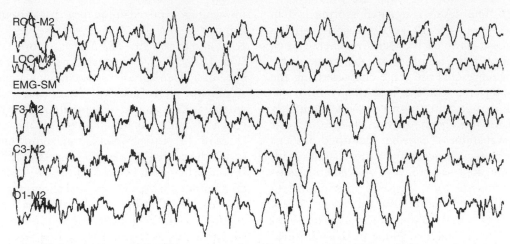

FIGURE 18-11 Sleep stage N3—a 30-second epoch of sleep classified as stage N3 that was recorded and scored according to the AASM scoring manual. (C3, left central; EMG-SM, electromyogram-submentalis; F3, left frontal; LOC, left outer canthus; M2, right mastoid; O1, left occipital; ROC, right outer canthus.)

likely still be called REM sleep by most people). Stage R is scored when there is low-voltage, mixed-frequency EEG, low chin EMG levels, and REMs (Fig. 18–12). Finally, stage MT has been eliminated. Table 18–1 summarizes the EEG-EOG-EMG characteristics of each sleep stage.

Smoothing Rules. Generally speaking, most smoothing rules have been eliminated. Epochs are scored according to the characteristics that make up their majority. However, because not all epochs in stage R have associated eye movements, stage R continues to be scored until a spindle, K complex, or arousal occurs or when chin

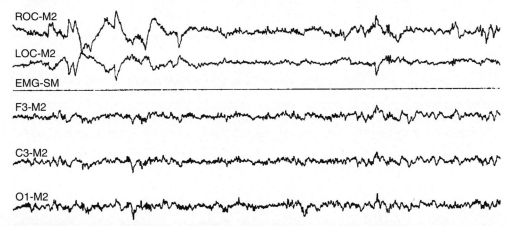

FIGURE 18-12 Sleep stage R—a 30-second epoch of sleep classified as stage R that was recorded and scored according to the AASM scoring manual. (C3, left central; EMG-SM, electromyogram-submentalis; F3, left frontal; LOC, left outer canthus; M2, right mastoid; O1, left occipital; ROC, right outer canthus.)

TABLE 18–1 Electroencephalographic, Electro-oculographic, and Electromyographic (EMG) Characteristics of Each Sleep Stage

Stage*	Brain Wave Activity	EMs†	EMG	Delta	Spindle	Alpha	Beta	Mentation
W	Predominant alpha activity; ≥15 sec alpha activity in epoch	S & R	++	−	−	++	+	Thoughts
N1	Alpha activity replaced by low-voltage, mixed-frequency activity; vertex sharp waves	S	↓	−	−	+	−	Hypnagogic
N2	Sleep spindles and K complexes in background EEG; overall <6 sec delta activity in epoch	−	↓	+	++	−	−	−
N3	General EEG synchrony and ≥6 sec delta activity in epoch	−	↓	++	+	−	−	−
R	Low-voltage, mixed-frequency activity; sawtooth theta activity	R	−	−	−	+	+	Dreams

*R, rapid eye movement sleep; W, wakefulness.
†EMs, eye movements: R, rapid; S slow.
++, prominent defining feature; +, increased level often seen; −, absent under normal circumstances; ↓, decreased from awake state.

EMG increases. If the majority of the final epoch containing stage R meets criteria, it is scored as stage R; otherwise it is categorized as the predominating stage. Stage R terminates with a transition to stage W or N3, an increase in chin EMG level, or an arousal that is followed by low-voltage, mixed-frequency EEG and slow eye movements. Similarly, a body movement followed by slow eye movements will terminate a stage R episode. Finally, spindles or K complexes occurring in the first half of an epoch terminates stage R. The scoring manual has a detailed set of examples to guide scoring.

Sleep Stage Changes across the Night

Regardless of which system is used for staging, the overall normal sleep stage pattern (sometimes called sleep macroarchitecture) across the night is fairly consistent. A healthy young adult good sleeper will spend 7–8 hours in bed and sleep 85–90% of that time. It may take such sleepers 5–15 minutes to fall asleep, and normal entry into sleep for an adult is through stage N1, which quickly evolves into N2. N3 usually follows and persists for some time before giving way to an episode of stage R. Usually the duration of the first stage R episode is brief (5–15 minutes) and the sleeper then goes back into N2 and possibly N3 for the next hour and a half. Stage R re-occurs at this point and is usually longer in duration than the first episode. Succeeding N-R cycles usually have less stage N3, more N2, and longer stage R duration as the sleep period progresses. Thus, one could generalize a prototypical night's sleep as having most of the stage N3 in the first third of the night and most of the stage R in the second half of the night. The stage R comes in 4–6 discrete episodes occurring approximately 90–100 minute apart (Fig. 18–13). Overall, stage N2 will account for approximately half of the night's sleep and stage R will account for another fifth to quarter.[19] Stage N1 should encompass less than 5% of total sleep time, distributed mainly at sleep-wake transitions. The remainder of sleep time will consist of stage N3. Men and women will not differ much in sleep stage percentages; however, women may have slightly more stage N3 than men as age advances.

Sleep Stage Changes as a Function of Age

Over the life span, total sleep time gradually decreases. Stage N3 begins decreasing after adolescence. This trend continues as a function of age, and stage N3 may completely disappear in elderly individuals. REM sleep duration declines spectacularly at life's beginning, decreasing from more than 50% at birth to 20–25% at adolescence.[19] For the next 50 years, stage R percentage remains stable. However, after 65 years stage R may begin to decline again (Fig. 18–14).

The overall decline in total sleep time is also associated with increasing sleep fragmentation by CNS arousals and awakenings. Some of the sleep disturbances are produced by accumulated pathologies that adversely affect sleep (e.g., arousals and awakenings from nocturnal pain). However, some sleep disturbances are nonspecific or of unknown etiology and may relate to a age-related deterioration of the underlying physiologic sleep mechanism. Regardless of cause, many elderly will spend more time in bed but less time sleeping.

SLEEP DISTURBANCES AND INSTABILITY

Sleep Stage Measures

Polysomnography offers the opportunity to objectively assess sleep disturbances and instability. While it is well known that sleeping in the laboratory can produce sleep disruption, this "first night effect" quickly dissipates and successive nights can be used to evaluate sleep integrity. One approach is to calculate parameters from sleep stages. Some of the parameters proven useful in clinical trials and investigative sleep studies include latency to sleep, latency to persistent sleep, sleep efficiency, total sleep time, number of awakenings, wake time after sleep onset, the number of ascending stage 1 occurrences, and the total number of sleep stage shifts. When comparing recordings of different durations (total recording times), indexed measures are needed on parameters other than latencies to sleep. For example, awakenings per hour can be used as a indexed value for number of awakenings. By contrast, when clinical trials fix the time in bed as a constant, untransformed measures can be used directly (e.g., wake after sleep onset).

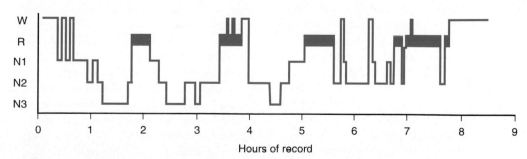

FIGURE 18–13 Sleep stage histogram for a normal, young adult subject. (N1, sleep stage 1; N2, sleep stage 2; N3, sleep stages 3+4; R, rapid eye movement sleep; W, wakefulness.)

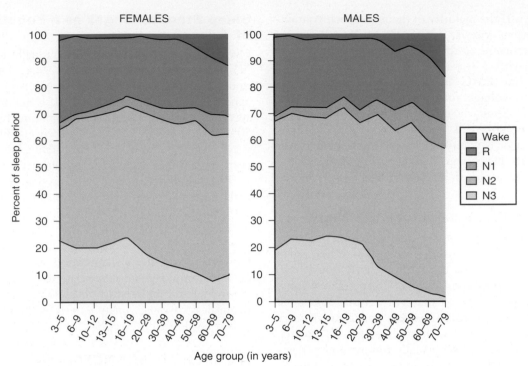

FIGURE 18–14 Sleep stage changes as a function of age. (N1, sleep stage 1; N2, sleep stage 2; N3, sleep stages 3+4; R, rapid eye movement sleep.) Data points extrapolated from Williams et al.[16]

ASDA and AASM Arousal Scoring

The need for a technique to score brief CNS arousals became apparent when polysomnography began to be used clinically. A patient might have several hundred obvious sleep disturbances; however, they were not reflected in sleep stage scoring because their duration was insufficient to alter sleep stage. To qualify as an awaking, alpha activity must present for half the duration of an epoch—that is, be 15 seconds or longer in duration. Thus, the 5-second alpha intrusion routinely occurring at the termination of a breathing event or leg movement falls under the radar of sleep stage scoring systems, and therefore goes unnoticed. To correct this situation, an AASM (at that time called the American Sleep Disorders Association [ASDA]) task force was formed to develop criteria for scoring CNS arousals.[20] Derived largely from the work at Henry Ford Hospital, arousals were defined in terms of "EEG speeding." This encompassed abrupt shifts from sleep (of at least 10 seconds' duration) to faster EEG activities (including theta, alpha, and beta). In REM sleep, the "EEG speeding" also had to be accompanied by increased activity in the submentalis EMG recording (Fig. 18–15). The minimum duration of "EEG speeding" was set at 3 seconds. This duration was based on what the members of the task force could reliably score by hand. It was recognized that computerized signal processing systems might well be able to reliably score shorter events; however, the rules being developed at that time were for visual scoring.

The overall scoring rules for CNS arousals were not changed by the AASM Manual Arousal Scoring task force. However, the original 11 rules that defined what *did* and *did not* qualify as an arousal were simplified. This simplification was expressed as a single statement of what an arousal *is*, with two explanatory notes.

Cyclic Alternating Pattern

The cyclic alternating pattern (CAP) is a dynamic alternation of EEG bursts and quiescence that can be visualized during polysomnography.[21] As a technique to investigate sleep, CAP has been championed by Drs. Terzano and Parrino, whose steadfast interest and scholarly work with CAP has drawn other researchers' attention to this EEG activity. CAP consists of an active *A phase* that can be a vertex sharp wave; a K complex; a K-alpha; a burst of high-amplitude, low-frequency waves; a burst of polymorphic waves; or a burst of high-amplitude theta or alpha activity. These *A phases* are followed by quiescent *B phases*. These transient electrocortical events are distinguishable from background activity and repeat in a cycle, usually every 20–40 seconds (Fig. 18–16). There are three types of A phases. The first does not meet AASM criteria for arousal (A1). The second includes enough alpha activity to sometimes qualify as an arousal (A2); however, classification is determined by alpha percentage of the overall A-phase duration (i.e., desynchronized portion must be between 20% and 50%). Thus, whether an A2 meets AASM arousal criteria depends on whether the alpha-

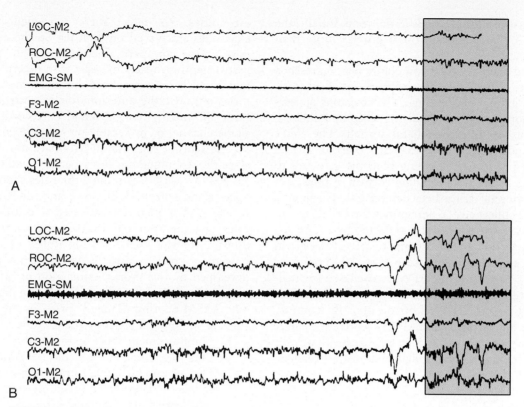

FIGURE 18–15 Examples of CNS arousals from REM sleep **(A)** and NREM sleep **(B).** (C3, left central; EMG-SM, electromyogram-submentalis; F3, left frontal; LOC, left outer canthus; M2, right mastoid; O1, left occipital; ROC, right outer canthus.)

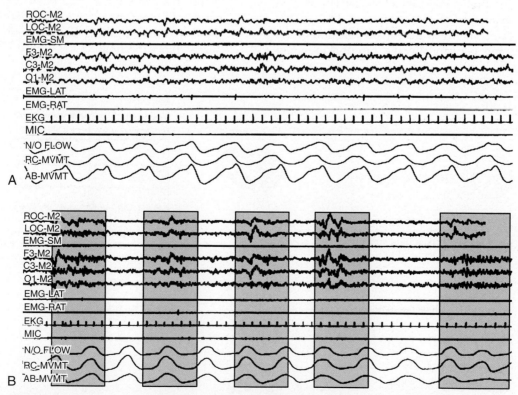

FIGURE 18–16 Samples of non-CAP activity **(A)** and CAP activity **(B).** (AB-MVMT, abdominal movement; C3, left central; CAP, cyclic alternating pattern; EKG, electrocardiogram; EMG-LAT, electromyogram–left anterior tibialis; EMG-RAT, electromyogram–right anterior tibialis; EMG-SM, electromyogram-submentalis; F3, left frontal; LOC, left outer canthus; M2, right mastoid; MIC, microphone for snoring; N/O FLOW, nasal-oral airflow; O1, left occipital; RC-MVMT, rib cage movement; ROC, right outer canthus.)

wave portion is 3 or more seconds in duration. Finally, the third type of A phase meets arousal criteria more than 95% of the time.[22]

It is theorized that the CAP's slow component represent a human correlate of higher brain reinforcement of subcortical antiarousal gating mechanisms. The thalamus appears to play an important role in preserving sleep by inhibiting transmission of incoming peripheral stimuli. The Wake Inhibition Sleep Preservation (WISP) hypothesis postulates that, when the protective ascending thalamic gate fails to block incoming activity, a descending cortical response can help reinforce the gate (as has been demonstrated in animals by Steriade and colleagues[23]). Sometimes the WISP system succeeds in preserving sleep and is reflected by a CAP A1. By contrast, the WISP system's attempt to preserve sleep will sometimes fail, and this process is seen as a CAP A2 or A3 (or AASM arousal). Sequences of CAP A1 in such a conceptualization would represent sleep instability (as often seen during sleep right before REM sleep occurs). By contrast, many CAP A2s and virtually all CAP A3s represent a failure of the system to preserve sleep (which would explain why the CAP rate is higher among individuals with insomnia) (Figs. 18–17, 18–18, and 18–19).

MOVEMENT

Leg and Limb Movement

In its simplest form, the movement that occurs in individuals with periodic limb movement disorder (PLMD) is a Babinski-like extension of the great toe. This movement, however, can sometimes also involve flexion of the ankle, the knee, and occasionally the hip and/or upper extremities. To detect these movements, two surface electrodes are placed on each leg on the anterior tibialis muscle (2–4 cm apart). Electrodes can be placed on the gastrocnemius muscle to assist with determining whether movement is artifact related; however, most sleep laboratories only use the anterior tibialis electrode placement. Both left and right legs should be recorded either on a single channel or preferably on separate channels.

The scoring rules for PLMD have not changed much since the technique was described in detail by Coleman.[24] An ASDA Task Force refined the rules slightly and developed standardized definitions and illustrations.[25] The recent AASM manual reasserted a distilled list of the rules and incorporated PLMD scoring into the larger domain of "Movement Scoring Rules." These recent leg movement rules are partly derived from the guidelines developed by the World Association of Sleep Medicine–International Restless Legs Syndrome Study Group.[26] The AASM Scoring Manual[18] provides the following five rules for defining a leg movement event:

1. The movement must be one-half second or longer. This rule is unchanged from the ASDA guidelines.
2. The movement's total duration must be 10 seconds or less. This criterion is increased from a 5-second cutoff previously stipulated.
3. The minimum amplitude to score a leg movement must be at least an 8-μV increase over resting EMG level. This differs from the previous rule specifying that the burst had to be at least 25% greater than calibrated movements recorded during behavioral maneuvers during the polysomnographic presleep "biocalibration."

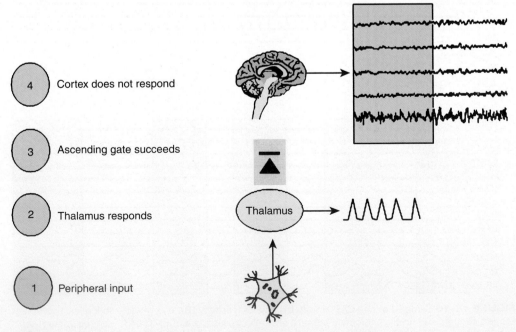

4. Cortex does not respond

3. Ascending gate succeeds

2. Thalamus responds

1. Peripheral input

Thalamus

FIGURE 18–17 Dynamics of the Wake Inhibition Sleep Preservation (WISP) system during stable sleep.

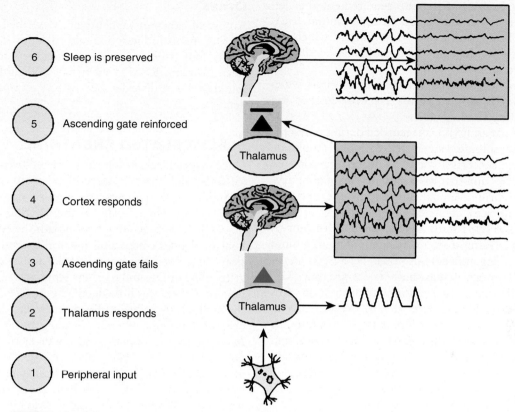

FIGURE 18–18 Dynamics of the Wake Inhibition Sleep Preservation (WISP) system during unstable but preserved sleep.

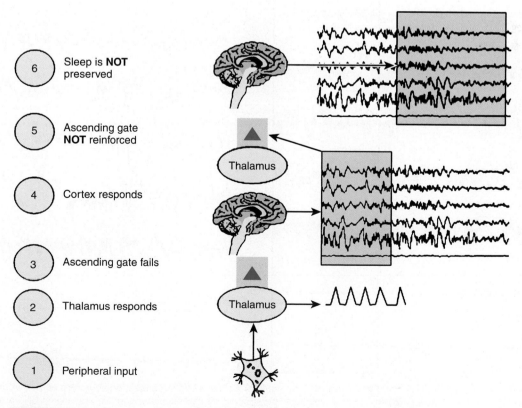

FIGURE 18–19 Dynamics of the Wake Inhibition Sleep Preservation (WISP) system leading to disturbed sleep.

4. Following logically from the requirement that leg movement detection hinges on a minimum 8-μV increase above resting level, the point at which the EMG exceeds the 8-μV threshold marks the leg movement onset.

5. Finally, the leg movement's end point occurs when EMG level drops to within 2 μV or less of the EMG resting level.

While it is true that an EMG, as recorded during polysomnography, is an uncalibrated signal, these adopted amplitude criteria have been successfully used to program automated leg movement detection that has a high degree of accuracy.

The AASM Scoring Manual continues with criteria for a periodic leg movement series or episode. A series of periodic leg movements must have a sequence of four or more movements (criteria are unchanged). The minimum interval between leg movements must be 5 seconds or more, while the interval maximum is 90 seconds. Leg movements can occur in association with arousal or without any sleep disturbance (Fig. 18–20). Movements of both of a person's legs (if recorded) that are separated by less than 5 seconds are considered a single movement (occurring in both legs). Alternating leg muscle activation must come in four groupings or more, have a minimum frequency of 0.5 cycles/sec and a maximum frequency of the alternating EMG bursts is 3.0 cycles/sec.

Other

A host of other movements are described in the AASM scoring manual. These include rules for defining hypnagogic foot tremor, excessive fragmentary myoclonus, sleep bruxism, REM sleep behavior disorder, and rhythmic movement disorder (see AASM scoring manual[18] for details).

SLEEP-RELATED BREATHING

Once it became clear that sleep-related breathing disorders (SRBDs) did not exclusively occur in hypoventilating morbidly obese patients, respiratory monitoring during polysomnography quickly became routine. The American Thoracic Society in conjunction with the ASDA published joint guidelines concerning medical outcomes research on sleep-disordered breathing but did not address the nitty-gritty of recording and scoring technique.[27] Thus, for a very long time there was little detailed guidance in this area, and the methods described in Bornstein's (aka, Sharon Keenan) chapter[28] in Guilleminault's *Sleeping and Waking Disorders: Indications and Techniques* became a de facto standard. It was not until many years later, and well after the book had gone out of print, that the Chicago Group's recommendations were published.[29] Even with that, their recommendations were principally for research rather than for standard clinical

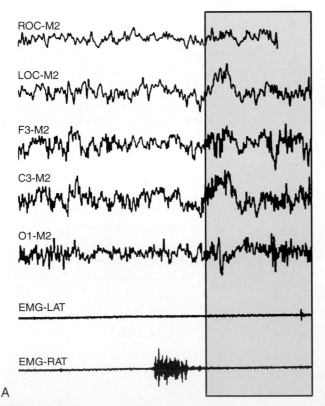
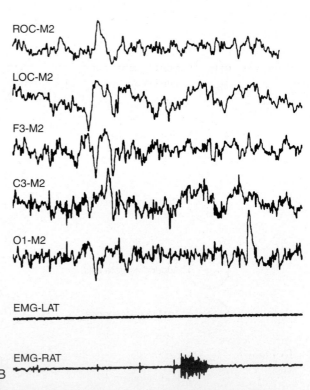

FIGURE 18–20 Leg movements with and without a CNS arousal. **(A)** A burst of right leg electromyographic activity immediately followed by an arousal (*shaded area*). **(B)** An electromyographic burst of similar magnitude without accompanying CNS arousal. (C3, left central; EMG-LAT, electromyogram–left anterior tibialis; EMG-RAT, electromyogram–right anterior tibialis; F3, left frontal; LOC, left outer canthus; M2, right mastoid; O1, left occipital; ROC, right outer canthus.)

routine. In the meantime, all manner of controversy surrounding recording technique, nomenclature, and interpretation had surfaced.

Currently, the vast majority of patients evaluated in clinical sleep laboratories are referred for assessment of SRBDs. Ironically, the recording, scoring, and interpretation of sleep-related breathing data is probably the least standardized part of polysomnography. For years, Medicare used to consider 30 episodes of sleep apnea as the sole cutting score for sleep-disordered breathing; hypopnea and oxygen desaturation events were not even considered. In 2001, Medicare recognized hypopnea as a clinically significant sleep-related breathing event if it was associated with 4%, or greater, oxygen desaturations.[30] Unfortunately, Medicare did not recognize hypopneas that produce CNS arousals and sleep fragmentation. In the sleep and respiration methodologic arena, the AASM scoring manual was long overdue. Even though it leaves several issues unresolved, this professional organization–sanctioned guideline is a welcome and critically needed document.

Recording Technique

Four key aspects of breathing are measured during polysomnography: airflow, respiratory effort, blood oxygenation, and CNS arousal or awakening. Airflow can be measured using thermistors, thermocouples, nasal pressure transducers, capnographs, microphones, calibrated inductance plethysmography, or with a pneumotachometer. Respiratory effort can be measured with piezo-electric respiratory belts, inductance plethysmography, esophageal pressure devices, strain gauges, or intercostals EMG electrodes. Blood oxygenation is measured with oximetry, and CNS arousals and awakenings are scored from occipital and central EEG.[31]

From this array of transducers, devices, apparatus, and approaches, the AASM scoring manual[18] recommends the following methods as primary. Alternative sensors are for use when the recommended signal is not reliable; however, they are not recommended as alternatives for primary use. The AASM scoring manual recommendations are summarized as follows:

1. To identify apnea, use a thermal sensor placed at the nose and mouth (alternative sensor is the nasal pressure tranducer).
2. To identify hypopnea, use a nasal pressure transducer (alternative is inductance plethysmograph or oronasal thermal sensor).
3. To identify effort, use either an esophageal manometer or inductance plethysmograph (alternative sensor is intercostals EMG).
4. To identify O_2 desaturations, use a pulse oximeter with its signal averaged over 3 seconds or less.

To identify CNS arousal or awakening, no recommendation is made. However, it is probably safe to assume that staging and arousal scoring standard techniques would be recommended.

Terminology (Types and Classification of Events)

Apnea

In essence, apnea is a cessation of airflow for 2 or more respiratory cycles. The AASM scoring manual's operational definition is a 90% or greater drop in the peak-to-trough amplitude on the nasal/oral airflow channel for 10 seconds or more. Furthermore, the amplitude reduction must persist for at least 90% of the event's duration. Apneas can be classified as central, obstructive, or mixed. A *central apnea* is scored when inspiratory effort is absent throughout the duration of the event. An *obstructive apnea* is scored when there is continued or increasing inspiratory effort throughout the duration of the event. Finally, *a mixed apnea* is scored when there is a lack of inspiratory effort initially followed by a resumption of an unsuccessful attempt to breathe during the later portion of the event (Fig. 18–21).

Hypopnea and Respiratory Effort–Related Arousals

In essence, a hypopnea is a shallow breath in which there is decreased tidal volume. Furthermore, there is nothing intrinsically pathophysiologic about a hypopnea. However, a hypopnea associated with flow limitation that ultimately produces an arousal so that the sleeper can dilate his or her airway and resume ventilation is a significant respiratory event. Additionally, a hypopnea associated with significant oxygen desaturations is medically noteworthy. Thus, it is not the hypopnea itself that is pathophysiologic but rather its consequence.

As straightforward and logical as this may seem, the operational definition for hypopnea remains controversial. One problem stems from recording technique; that is, most sleep laboratories measure flow qualitatively, and such measures do not proportionally estimate tidal volume. Therefore, couching airflow changes in terms of percentage decrease from baseline is problematic. Guilleminault et al.'s[32] original definition of hypopnea as a reduction in airflow without complete cessation of breathing adhered closely to the general principle but left open the question of how much decrease in airflow was minimally required to score a hypopnea. A wide assortment of definitions were developed using different cutting scores for percentage of airflow decrease. Then in 2001, the AASM Clinical Practice Review Committee[33] defined hypopnea largely based on the definition used in the Sleep Heart Health epidemiologic studies.[34] This definition was subsequently adopted by Medicare. Hypopnea was suddenly redefined as a 10-second or longer 30% reduction from baseline in thoracoabdominal effort or airflow accompanied by a 4% oxygen desaturation. This definition completely disregarded the consequence of a hypopnea on the sleeping brain. As a result, the respiratory events (formerly call hypopnea) that were associated with CNS arousal but less than 4% desaturation were reassigned to

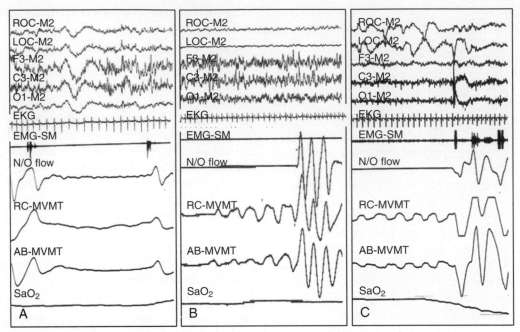

FIGURE 18–21 Episodes of sleep apnea. **(A)** A central-type episode during which the cessation of breathing is accompanied by no movement of the rib cage and abdomen (no respiratory effort). **(B)** A mixed-type episode that begins with a pause in respiratory effort (and airflow) but continues to have flow cessation even as respiratory effort begins and continues. **(C)** An obstructive-type episode in which there is a complete cessation of airflow notwithstanding an uninterrupted effort to breath. (AB-MVMT, abdominal movement; C3, left central; EKG, electrocardiogram; EMG-SM, electromyogram-submentalis; F3, left frontal; LOC, left outer canthus; M2, right mastoid; N/O FLOW, nasal-oral airflow; O1, left occipital; RC-MVMT, rib cage movement; ROC, right outer canthus.)

a category of events known as respiratory effort–related arousals (RERAs). RERAs originally were a category of events that were so subtle they might not even be detectable without esophageal manometry.

The AASM scoring manual[18] provides two sets of scoring rules for hypopnea. The first is an operationalized refinement of the Medicare definition and is recommended for clinical practice. The *recommended criteria* for scoring hypopnea are met when

1. the nasal pressure signal amplitude drops by 30% or more compared to baseline,
2. the event lasts 10 seconds or more,
3. at least 90% of the event duration maintains the 30% amplitude drop, and
4. a 4% or greater O_2 desaturation occurs as a result.

The AASM scoring manual's *alternative criteria* for scoring hypopnea represent a return to the scoring used before the Medicare redefinition came about. These better operationalized criteria specify that a hypopnea is scored when

1. the nasal pressure signal amplitude drops by 50% or more compared to baseline,
2. the event lasts 10 seconds or more,
3. at least 90% of the event duration maintains the 50% amplitude drop, and
4. a 3% or greater O_2 desaturation occurs "or the event is associated with arousal."

Although the alternative criteria provide a welcome rediscovery of the *brain's* importance to sleep-disordered breathing, there is a rub! The U.S. Government prohibits treating Medicare patients differently than other patients in one's practice. Therefore, if your sleep program provides services for Medicare, you are constrained to always use the first set of criteria. However, if Medicare is irrelevant to your practice (e.g., you practice in Tasmania), you may choose whichever rule you prefer. Another problem created by having two definitions for the same term is ambiguity, and hypopnea now has two official definitions. It would have been preferable to either add a distinguishing modifier to the word *hypopnea* or to flat out create two new words. Perhaps *desaturating hypopnea* could be used for the first definition and *traditional hypopnea* for the latter. It really does not matter what names are chosen as long as they differ. One could call the first one George and the other Gracie; at least we would understand what each means without having to read the footnotes (Fig. 18–22).

Apnea, Hypopnea, and RERA Summary Statistics

Traditionally, expression of nightly totals for sleep-related respiratory events included calculation of an apnea index (AI) and apnea-hypopnea index (AHI). The AI is the number of apnea episodes per hour of sleep, and the

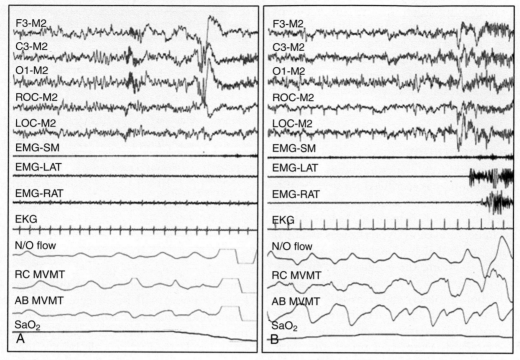

FIGURE 18–22 Episodes of sleep hypopnea. The AASM scoring manual defines two sets of rules for scoring hypopnea. **(A)** A hypopnea episode that meets criteria of the Recommended rule that requires a 4% drop in oxygen saturation. **(B)** An episode that would not be scored as a hypopnea using the Recommended rule but would qualify according to the Alternative rule (note the prominent CNS arousal terminating the event and disrupting sleep). (AB-MVMT, abdominal movement; C3, left central; EKG, electrocardiogram; EMG-LAT, electromyogram–left anterior tibialis; EMG-RAT, electromyogram–right anterior tibialis; EMG-SM, electromyogram-submentalis; F3, left frontal; LOC, left outer canthus; M2, right mastoid; N/O FLOW, nasal-oral airflow; O1, left occipital; RC-MVMT, rib cage movement; ROC, right outer canthus; Sao2, arterial oxygen saturation.)

AHI is the number of apnea plus hypopnea episodes per hour of sleep. After the Medicarization of hypopnea took place, another summary statistic was added to include those hypopneas that were now tabulated as RERAs. Thus, a respiratory disturbance index (RDI) is routinely reported and is the number of apnea, hypopnea, and RERA episodes per hour of sleep. The irony here is that the acronym RDI originally stood for "respiratory desaturations index," which was created to be distinct from the AHI. At some point, clinicians began using RDI synonymously with AHI. In the end, with the Medicare definition requiring 4% desaturations, the AHI actually became a desaturations index and the RDI is now used to indicate that non-desaturating events are also included. Therefore, if the first set of hypopnea criteria are used for scoring, the AI, AHI, and RDI should be reported. If the second definition is used, reporting the AI and AHI should be sufficient. Note that the AASM scoring manual does not discuss tabulating the RDI. Why is this important? When one attempts to titrate positive airway pressure and the first (Medicare-type) definition is used, the AI and AHI are insufficient to determine optimal pressure; the RDI must be calculated for each pressure to compare outcomes.

RECORDING EQUIPMENT AND ADVANCING TECHNOLOGIES

As is often the case with new technology, what we envision and what evolves travel two separate paths. Take, for example, the videophone, a device always right at home in our conception of what the future will look like. However, even though we've long had the technical capability to make videophones, and notwithstanding several attempts to market such devices, videophones are absent from the landscape. By contrast, the forerunner of our modern-day FAX machine was judged by Xerox to be not worth developing because no one would want one. Despite this prediction, the FAX machine became an integral component of business communication and has remained so for more than 2 decades.

Our expectations with respect to computerized sleep recording were similarly misguided. When thinking about digital polysomnography, we were mainly focused on the computer's potential for effortlessly detecting waveforms, tabulating sleep-disordered breathing events, and automatically scoring sleep stages. However, these systems found their way into our laboratories for other reasons entirely. As mundane as it may seem, the principal driving force behind sleep laboratory automation was the elimination of paper tracings. The paper polysomnograph is all but extinct. The last major polysomnographic paper manufacturer has closed its doors. Nonetheless, computerized sleep systems have yet to extract and organize the seemingly boundless wealth of physiologic information in new, clinically useful ways or provide reliable automatic sleep staging.

Digital Polysomnography

Technology constantly evolves, and sometimes the elegance of the older technology is sacrificed for greater efficiency and/or reduced cost. When sailing vessels declined in favor of motorized ships, many bemoaned the loss of such graceful vessels as clippers and caravels on the seas and their replacement by noisy, smoke-belching machinery. Much like that switch from sails to steam, the evolution from traditional paper polysomnographs to today's digital systems has been marked by both progress and regression. One of the serious hurdles facing early digital sleep system developers was the absence of guidance from scientific and clinical organizations. No standards were set a priori; therefore, developers had to rely on advice from individuals who appeared to have expertise in both engineering and sleep medicine. Sometimes the advice was good and sometimes not. To complicate matters, until this past decade, the computational and storage resources of microcomputers were only marginally up to the task. Video display resolution and speed were problematic unless nonstandard devices were integrated. Removable mass storage was expensive and finicky.

All that has changed. Today, CPUs are lightning fast, gigabytes of memory are standard, high-definition screens are affordable, and super-high-capacity DVD writers are ubiquitous. Free from technological limitations that shackle development, manufacturers have developed and marketed a dazzling array of digital polysomnographic systems. The market, however, is now being driven more by cost than quality, and decisions about purchase are being made by administrators rather than sleep specialists. The result is an ever greater need for guidance from the scientific and clinical community, and the AASM has responded. A digital polysomnography task force was appointed, co-chaired by the senior author (M.H.) and Thomas Penzel, and the process began. One of the AASM scoring manual's goals was to provide recommendations for digital polysomnography. Important progress was made on this front even though we were not able to address all of the relevant topics.

Sorely needed were recommendations concerning signal quality and resolution. It was easy to agree that at least 12 bits were needed to represent amplitude (this provides a number line from 0 to 4095 or, if 2s-complement is used to represent positive and negative values, from −2048 to +2047). This resolution is enough to adequately cover the plus or minus (approximately) 2.5-V range with regulated current (I_{REG}). Moreover, it makes it likely that

TABLE 18–2 AASM Digital Task Force Recommendations for Polysomnographic Signal Sampling Rates

Polysomnographic Signal Being Recorded	Desirable (Hz)	Minimal (Hz)
Electroencephalogram	500	200
Electro-oculogram	500	200
Electromyogram	500	200
Electrocardiogram	500	200
Airflow—thermistors and thermocouples	100	25
Airflow—nasal pressure	100	25
Respiratory effort—esophageal pressure	100	25
Respiratory effort—rib cage and abdominal movement	100	25
Snoring sounds	500	200
Oximetry	25	10
Body position	1	1

minimum discernable voltage differences (exceeding the level of noise) will be detected. The recommendations concerning temporal resolution were more difficult to formulate, but after much discussion and significant compromise, we decided to provide both minimal and desirable sampling rates for each recording channel (Table 18–2). Sampling rates were set high enough to accurately reconstruct waveforms and provide enough data to potentially overcome frequency aliasing (if printed in high resolution). Additionally, frequencies appropriate for actual or digitally simulated high- and low-pass filter settings for each type of bioelectrical signal were determined (Table 18–3).

What Was Gained?

As already mentioned, sleep recordings became paperless (and inkless). Most of us do not miss lugging heavy boxes of paper around or the 5-foot-high piles of recordings leaned against the walls in corridors and hallways. Storage space was reduced from rooms to file drawers and record disposal became a trifle. There were no more pens and ink wells to clean, unclog, replace, stain carpets, and ruin clothing. Consumable supply costs plummeted. The machinery itself shrank, weighed less, and even became portable.

Digital polysomnography made data display dynamically scalable. With paper, the recording speed dictated

TABLE 18–3 AASM Digital Task Force Recommendations for Polysomnographic Signal Filter Settings for Routine Recording

Polysomnographic Signal Being Recorded	Setting (Hz) Low Frequency	Setting (Hz) High Frequency
Electroencephalogram	0.3	35
Electro-oculogram	0.3	35
Electromyogram	10	100
Electrocardiogram	0.3	70
Respiration—airflow effort channels	0.1	15
Snoring	10	100

the viewable product. There was no opportunity to expand or compress the recording (except to look at and flare the edge of the paper recording). What was recorded was what we got to see. This did mean, however, that we knew what the night technologist was seeing during the recording process. We also knew what the scorer was seeing when he or she scored each event and classified each epoch as a sleep stage.

The computerized systems also allow us to rapidly jump to any place in the recording. Some systems allow the user to split the screen and have two different time bases displayed simultaneously. Digital polysomnography makes data display ultimately manipulatable, after the fact. Channels can be moved, deleted, recolored, rescaled, inverted, and massaged with filters. With all of this transformational power, it becomes critically important for an audit trail to be kept so that the sleep specialist can see what the night technologist or scorer was seeing when he or she changed continuous positive airway pressures or scored a particular event or sleep stage. Finally, digital video (if properly implemented) allows the night technologist, scoring technologist, or interpreting clinician to see and hear the sleeping patient synchronized with the polysomnographic activity.

What Was Lost?

Casualties of the switch to computerized polysomnography include the disappearance of the selector panel, high-quality amplifiers, and in some cases calibration signals. The sounds associated with making an overnight recording have also vanished. The fact that one used to be able to actually audibly recognize REM sleep, periodic leg movements, and awakenings as distinctive sound patterns of pen chattering is no longer appreciated.

More importantly, amplifier quality and flexibility have seriously eroded. Many current systems provide signals that look "choppy." Somehow, the inertial damping of the mechanical pen and the attenuating roll-off of analog filters created EEG, EOG, and EMG signals of a quality that has not been matched by digital systems. The sharp-edged, steep roll-off and notch filters mainly used today produce spikier waveforms that are more difficult to read. However, maybe that is a bias from having learned using paper tracings. The next generation may come to like the spiky, choppy display. One thing, however, that is not a matter of preference is the loss of flexibility to re-montage records on-the-fly. A simulated selector panel would solve many problems faced during recording.

The task force developed a wish list for manufactures. Content experts participated in a series of polls conducted according to the Rand/UCLA Appropriateness Method. As a result, some items on the list were elevated to the status of recommendations, others became options, and some were dropped (Table 18–4).

TABLE 18–4 AASM Digital Task Force List of Recommended and Optional Features for Computerized Polysomnographic Systems	
Final Designation	**Digital Polysomnography Feature Being Considered**
Recommended	1600×1200 display resolution
	Video must be synchronized and be recorded at 1 frame/sec or more
	Independent 50/60-Hz filters for each channel
	Ability to independently set sampling rate for each channel
	Ability to check impedance for each channel against a selected reference
	Histogram with stage, breathing events, PLMs, Sao_2, and arousals.
	Histogram should have a cursor position page jump feature.
	Control key to toggle *biocalibration* section on/off, machine calibration section on/off
	Improved filter design that can functionally simulate analog-type roll-offs rather than removing all activity and harmonics within a bandwidth
	Recallable "see what tech was seeing" when the recording was made. Should include a complete audit trail of filter settings, resolutions, and other adjustments
	Recallable "see what tech was seeing" when the recording was scored. Should include a complete audit trail of filter settings, resolutions, and other adjustments
	Ability to time-scale on a single page ranging from 5 sec to the entire night
Optional	FFT or spectral analysis on window (omitting data artifact–marked segments)
	"Channel off" control key
	"Channel invert" control key
	Channel repositioning by click and drag
	Recallable display setup profiles (including colors) activated by control key sequences
	Page autoturning and autoscrolling
No Designation Provided	Channel control bar with display/nondisplay toggle
	Multiple window display with different time bases
	No toggle or key needed to display data
	Position cursor over channel and use up/down keys to rescale amplitude on-the-fly
	Page autoturning and autoscrolling speed control on mouse wheel
	Page autoturning and autoscrolling continuation during static lookback viewing
	Surround window for stages $\pm$ 4 with current in center
	Surround or simple window for body position, PAP setting
	Sounds accompanying autoscrolling (with volume control)

FFT, fast Fourier transform; PAP, positive airway pressure; PLMs, periodic leg movements; Sao_2, arterial oxygen saturation.

Attended and Unattended Sleep Recordings

In 1994, the AASM differentiated among four levels of sleep recordings.[35] The classification is based on the number and type of signals recorded. *Level I* is standard polysomnography—that is, the type of overnight sleep study that is routinely recorded in laboratories for clinical purposes with a sleep technologist present. It is sometimes called comprehensive polysomnography, attended laboratory polysomnography, CPT 95810, or CPT95811 (if positive airway pressure is administered). Regardless of the name, level I recordings include measures of EEG, EOG, submentalis EMG, heart rhythm, respiratory effort, oxygen saturation, body position, and anterior tibialis EMG (Table 18–5). *Level II* is equivalent to level I in all respects in terms of recording channels (i.e., it is comprehensive); however, the recording is made without an attendant present. *Level III* recordings are also known as *cardiopulmonary sleep studies*. These sleep studies include 4 or more channels. The recordings usually include measures of airflow, respiratory effort, oxygen saturation, and heart rhythm. Level III devices are recorders typically designed for home use, and seldom display the physiologic activity on a screen for monitoring purposes. Data are cached into memory and subsequently downloaded to a personal computer for display, scoring, editing, and generating a report of sleep study results. The recorders are compact, portable, and sometimes worn like Holter monitors. Finally, *level IV* devices are similar but record only one or two channels (e.g., pulse oximeters used to document the need for supplemental oxygen).

The AASM recommends that level I studies be used when laboratory facilities are readily available. The level I study provides the best sensitivity and specificity for the full range of sleep disorders and does not generate "errors of omission" when the pathophysiology is something other than a breathing disorder (a key issue with level III studies). Level III device use for diagnosis is rapidly evolving. By the time this is published, the Center for Medicare & Medicaid Services will have approved reimbursement for level III devices. AASM guidelines at the time of this writing provide for limited level III device use when there are extenuating circumstances.[36] AASM guidelines stipulate that (1) evaluations should be supervised by a practitioner who is board eligible or certified in sleep medicine, (2) evaluations should be performed only on patients having a high pretest probability of moderate to severe obstructive sleep apnea, and (3) evaluations may be performed on patients with immobility and safety issues that preclude in-laboratory study. These guidelines also indicate that portable studys should not be used for general screening in asymptomatic individuals, individuals who have concomitant sleep disorders, or individuals with comorbid illnesses that may compromise the testing system's accuracy.

Level III (cardiopulmonary) studies can diagnose SRBD in patients with high prestudy probabilities (i.e., those exceeding 70%). A variety of validated techniques can be used to calculate prestudy probability (we use the Multivariate Apnea Prediction Test[37] in conjunction with Epworth Sleepiness Scale[38] scores). AASM guidelines specify that level III studies can be performed when patients have severe symptoms and attended standard polysomnography is not readily available. The guidelines also allow level III studies for patients who cannot be studied in the sleep laboratory. Finally, level III studies can be used for follow-up after SRBD is diagnosed with attended standard polysomnography and therapy is initiated.

As useful as cardiopulmonary studies may be to confirm a positive diagnosis for SRBD, a negative cardiopulmonary study does not rule out all forms of SRBD (especially upper airway resistance syndrome) or non-SRBD sleep problems. Thus, a negative study using a level III device provides very little diagnostic information and requires follow-up evaluation, usually with level I, attended polysomnography.

TABLE 18–5 AASM Classification System for Recording Techniques and Devices Designed to Evaluate Sleep and/or Sleep-Disordered Breathing

Level	Original Designation	Current Designation	Description
I	Standard polysomnography	Attended laboratory polysomnography	This is the type of study usually conducted in a sleep laboratory. It includes recordings of EEG, EOG, submentalis EMG, airflow, respiratory effort, ECG, Sao$_2$, and usually leg movement. A technologist is present throughout the study.
II	Comprehensive portable polysomnography	Unattended polysomnography	Recordings are similar or same as level I; however, the study is not continuously monitored by a technologist.
III	Modified portable sleep-apnea testing	Unattended cardiopulmonary recording	This is a recording specifically designed to detect sleep-disordered breathing. It usually consists of 4 or more channels that include measures of airflow, respiratory effort, electrocardiogram, and oximetry. Snoring sounds and body position are also sometimes recorded.
IV	Continuous (single- or dual-) bioparameter recording	Unattended single- or dual-channel recording	A portable unit that records and stores one or two data channels (e.g., a pulse oximeter)
Unclassified	None	Other	There are several devices that do not fit into the level I–IV categories; however, they can be used to test for sleep-disordered breathing (e.g., WatchPAT)

ECG, electrocardiogram; EEG, electroencephalogram; EMG, electromyogram; EOG, electro-oculogram; Sao$_2$, arterial oxygen saturation.

Integrating New Technologies into a Sleep Disorders Program

A formidable array of level III and yet-to-be-classified devices are currently available. Most of these technologies are competent when placed in the right hands. Like any other form of new technology, the authors submit that the challenge is to determine how they best fit into our overall sleep programs. To make this determination, the goals of the program must be examined. If the goal is to provide sleep services in an optimal manner, there is likely a place for cardiopulmonary recording. If the goal is to maximize the number of laboratory studies performed, there may still be a place (as a case finding tool), but it is less likely. The time is long past for debating whether we should or should not used nonlaboratory assessment to diagnose SRBDs. *It is precisely that debate that has slowed our progress in determining how best to use the new technology.* Each technology has its own particular strengths and weaknesses. When properly combined, the unique properties of each can complement one another to a program's advantage.

Sleep programs that integrate home monitoring have been described in the literature.[39–41] Success seems to hinge on several factors, including (1) proper patient selection, (2) use of an appropriate portable recorder, (3) interpretation of the portable recording by a qualified sleep specialist, (4) readily available access to laboratory polysomnography (when needed), and (5) systematic follow-up.

Proper patient selection involves estimating prestudy probability for SRBD. An assortment of symptom checklists, questionnaires, and composite scales that use anthropometric and self-reported data exist. The patient can be referred for portable study when clinical suspicion is high. If prestudy probability is low, the patient is not sleepy, or overall symptom presentation is mixed, the patient should be referred for full laboratory assessment. Determining the competency of a portable recorder can be difficult. Relying on published literature is problematic because the technology advances so rapidly. For example, the particular model of instruments is often obsolete and unavailable by the time its validation study is published. Unfortunately, there is no "consumer report" or review clearing house for such products. Selection is based on collegial advice (word-of-mouth), experience during a rental period or manufacturer-arranged test trial period, device demonstrations, and aggressiveness of the sales representative.

Once the cardiopulmonary recording is made, it should first be technically validated by reviewing for signal quality and second be interpreted clinically (if it is technically adequate). Technical validation of the

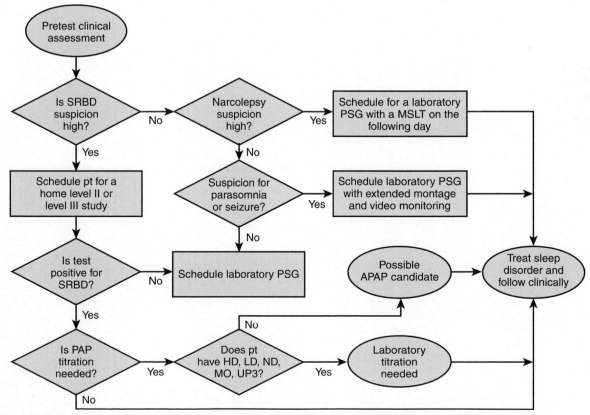

FIGURE 18–23 Integrating level II and III sleep recording devices into a clinical sleep program. (APAP, autotitrating positive airway pressure; HD, heart disease; LD, lung disease; MO, morbid obesity; MSLT, Multiple Sleep Latency Test; ND, neurologic disease; PAP, positive airway pressure; PSG, polysomnography; Pt, patient; SRBD, sleep-related breathing disorder; UP3, uvulopalatopharyngeoplasty.)

recording is much more crucial for level III studies than for laboratory polysomnography. After all, the technologist's primary function in attended, level I studies is to assure recording quality by reattaching transducers, re-referencing electrodes, minimizing electrical interference, and even replacing recording devices, if needed. Monitoring transducers are appropriately attached, placed, and operationally checked by the technician. Finally, the recording is continuously monitored for whether intervention is required. By contrast, in home recordings, when a transducer falls off, it usually stays off; when a wire gets unplugged, it usually stays unplugged. Consequently, home studies, even though they have many fewer data channels than full polysomnograms, can be more challenging to read and interpret. An experienced sleep specialist familiar with cardiopulmonary recorder recordings should review the data and refer the patient for attended polysomnography if the test is negative. When the portable study is positive for obstructive sleep apnea, the patient is referred for either laboratory positive airway pressure titration or home self-adjusting autotitration positive airway pressure (APAP) (if such a procedure is used in the sleep program). Using APAP for unattended titration is beyond the scope of this chapter; the interested reader should see the AASM guidelines for more information.[42] Follow-up after the home recording is crucial to determine if anything unusual happened during recording. It is also important to explain treatment choices, provide cautions about the use of sedative-hypnotics and alcohol, emphasize the cardio- and cerebrovascular risk factors, and counsel patients about sleepiness-related dangers of driving and operating heavy equipment. Follow-up is key after therapy has been initiated to check for persistent signs or symptoms of sleep problems that were potentially missed by cardiopulmonary monitoring (Fig. 18–23).

Level III recorders are another tool available for practicing sleep medicine. These devices do not replace polysomnography but rather complement it when appropriate. Properly integrated nonlaboratory assessment techniques can facilitate diagnosis of patients with more severe sleep-disordered breathing. In oversubscribed and/or capitated programs, home monitoring can free up laboratory resources for the more difficult cases.

REFERENCES

A full list of references are available at www.expertconsult.com

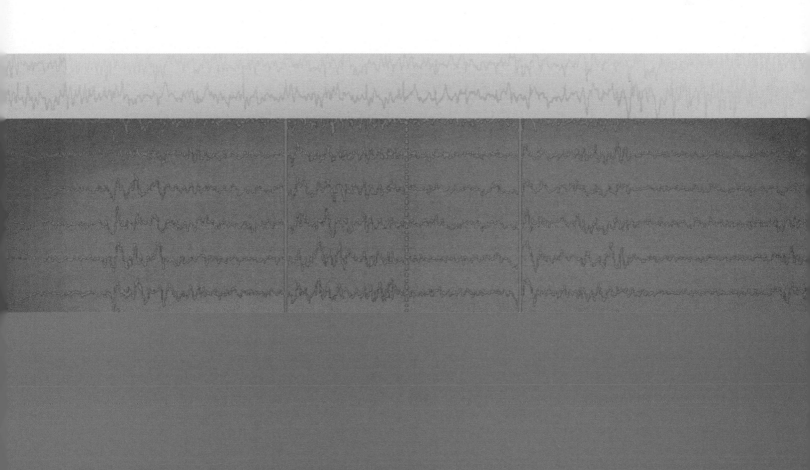

PART III

Clinical Aspects

CHAPTER 19

Approach to the Patient with Sleep Complaints

Sudhansu Chokroverty

INTRODUCTION

Several epidemiologic studies have clearly shown that sleep complaints are very common in the general population.[1–14] Two important multiple-center studies were conducted by Coleman and his colleagues.[8,9] The first study,[8] conducted over a 2-year period (1978–1980), included 4698 patients, each of whom underwent a polysomnographic (PSG) study. The proportions of diagnostic categories in those patients with sleep complaints, after those evaluated for impotency are excluded, are 51% with hypersomnia, 31% with insomnia, 15% with parasomnia, and 3% with sleep-wake schedule disorders. A subsequent report by Coleman[9] on 3085 patients over a 1-year period (1981–1982) showed remarkable consistency with the results of the first study. The most frequent disease categories included in these surveys were sleep apnea, narcolepsy, and insomnia related to psychiatric or psychophysiologic disorders.

The 1979 Institute of Medicine[7] study concluded that about one-third of all adults in the United States experienced some sleep disturbances. Surveys conducted more recently[11–14] confirmed these findings. Approximately 35% of adults ages 18–79 years reported difficulty in the preceding year falling asleep, staying asleep, or both.[11] In the Gallup survey of 1991,[12] 36% of adults reported some sleep problem (9% considered the problem chronic and 27% occasional). In the survey conducted between 1981 and 1985 by the U.S. National Institute of Mental Health Epidemiologic Catchment Area Study,[11] 10% reported difficulty sleeping for 2 weeks or longer in the preceding

6 months, for which no medical or psychiatric cause could be found. In a recent telephone interview survey[1] of 25,500 individuals (ages 15–100 years) using the sleep-EVAL system covering 7 European countries (France, United Kingdom, Germany, Italy, Portugal, Spain, and Finland), nonrestorative sleep was prevalent in 10.8% of this sample. The prevalence was higher in women than men and was the highest in the United Kingdom and Germany, and lowest in Spain. The author concluded that nonrestorative sleep was associated with daytime impairment of function and the author identified several factors, such as young age, stress, anxiety, depression or a physical disease as well as dissatisfaction with sleep. A state-of-the-art consensus conference conducted by specialists at the National Institutes of Health suggested the term "comorbid insomnia" rather than secondary insomnia for conditions associated with insomnia because of the absence of a definite cause-and-effect relationship between the condition and insomnia.[15] A high prevalence of insomnia was also noted by Morin et al.[2]

Doghramji[5] mentioned the importance of recognizing sleep disorders in a primary care setting. In this setting, few patients present with overt sleep complaints but rather generally present with symptoms of fatigue, excessive sleepiness, and impaired waking function. Physicians must maintain a high index of suspicion for sleep disorders and ask appropriate sleep-related questions as insomnia may lead to potentially life-threatening automobile crashes and industrial accidents in addition to negatively impacting a patient's quality of life. Primary care physicians should also ask about occupations and sleeping habits in order to diagnose sleep disorders. Ohayon and Paiva[16] directed our attention to assessment of global sleep dissatisfaction as an indicator of insomnia severity in a general population survey in Portugal. Using the sleep-EVAL system, the authors interviewed by telephone 1858 participants ages 18 years or older who were representative of the general population of Portugal. The authors gave a figure of 28.1% of the sample having insomnia symptoms for at least 3 nights a week, and global sleep dissatisfaction was noted in 10.1% of the sample. The most frequent symptom was difficulty maintaining sleep (21%). Global sleep dissatisfaction was noted in 29.4% of the subjects with insomnia symptoms. They noted daytime consequences more frequently among subjects with insomnia symptoms and global sleep dissatisfaction.

Two important international surveys were conducted by Soldatos et al.[2] and by Leger and Poursain.[4] Leger and Poursain investigated the prevalence of insomnia in the general population in France, Italy, Japan, and the United States. This survey included telephone interviews by professional interviewers of a representative sample of the general population ages 18 years and older in each of the four countries. Insomnia was reported by 37.2% of respondents in France and Italy, 6.6% in Japan, and 27.1% in the United States. The most prominent symptom was sleep maintenance insomnia (73%), followed by difficulty initiating sleep (61%) and poor sleep quality (48%). The most commonly reported next-day symptoms included daytime fatigue and impairment of concentration and attention. The authors noted that the rate of reporting insomnia symptoms to physicians was generally low and, of those individuals who did consult a physician, only a few were prescribed any medications. Thus, the results of the survey suggested an under-recognition and undertreatment of insomnia. In a later paper, Leger et al.[17] reported the results of an international survey of sleep problems in the general population of the United States, France, Germany, Italy, Spain, and the United Kingdom. The sleeping problems imposed considerable burden but were under-reported and undertreated. The survey by Soldatos et al.[2] on International Sleep Well Day (March 21) in 2002 showed that 24% of subjects did not sleep well and 31.6% had insomnia.

These self-reported sleep problems could be underestimated in the general population. In all of these studies, there is a prevalence of sleep complaints in about one-third of the adult population, and in about 10% insomnia is a persistent complaint associated with impairment of daytime function. In a report by Ancoli-Israel and Roth,[18] the percentage of individuals with insomnia symptoms is as follows: waking up feeling drowsy or tired, 72%; waking up in the middle of the night, 67%; difficulty going back to sleep after waking up, 57%; difficulty falling asleep, 56%;

and waking up too early, 44%. Martikainen et al.[19] described the adverse impact of insomnia on somatic health problems in middle-aged individuals. In a population-based study, Young[20] reported excessive daytime sleepiness in 1 in 5 adults. Some important epidemiologic factors identified in various studies include old age, female gender, poor education and lower socioeconomic status, recent stress, depression, anxiety, alcohol, drug abuse, and a physical disease. It is important for physicians to be aware of this high prevalence of sleep disturbances, which cause considerable physical and psychological stress.

Categories of Sleep Disorders

An approach to a patient with sleep complaints must begin with a comprehensive knowledge of the disorders listed in the second edition of the International Classification of Sleep Disorders (ICSD-2)[21] so that the patient can be evaluated in a proper manner, paying particular attention to the history and physical findings before ordering laboratory tests. The ICSD-2 lists eight broad categories of disorders of sleep along with several subcategories under each category, as well as additional sleep-related disorders in Appendices A and B (see Chapter 20). The eight broad categories consist of (1) insomnia; (2) sleep-related breathing disorders; (3) hypersomnia of central origin not due to a circadian rhythm sleep disorder; (4) circadian rhythm sleep disorders; (5) parasomnias; (6) sleep-related movement disorders; (7) isolated symptoms, apparently normal variants, and unresolved issues; and (8) other sleep disorders.

The category of *insomnia* includes acute insomnia; psychophysiologic insomnia; paradoxical insomnia (sleep state misperception); idiopathic insomnia; insomnia due to a mental disorder; inadequate sleep hygiene; behavioral insomnia of childhood; insomnia due to a drug or substance; insomnia due to a medical condition; insomnia not due to a substance, sleep-related breathing disorder, or other nonphysiologic condition, unspecified (nonorganic); and physiologic insomnia, unspecified (organic).

The category of *sleep-related breathing disorders* includes central sleep apnea syndromes, including primary central sleep apnea, central sleep apnea due to Cheyne-Stokes breathing pattern, central sleep apnea due to high-altitude periodic breathing, central sleep apnea due to a medical condition not Cheyne-Stokes breathing pattern, central sleep apnea due to a drug or substance, and primary sleep apnea of infancy (formerly primary sleep apnea of newborns). Also included in this category are obstructive sleep apnea syndromes (OSASs), including adult obstructive and pediatric obstructive sleep apnea; sleep-related hypoventilation/hypoxemia syndrome; sleep-related hypoventilation/hypoxemia due to a medical condition; and other sleep-related breathing disorders (sleep apnea/sleep-related breathing disorders, unspecified).

Hypersomnias of central origin not due to a circadian rhythm sleep disorder, sleep-related breathing disorder, or other causes of disturbed nocturnal sleep include narcolepsy with cataplexy, narcolepsy without cataplexy, narcolepsy due to a medical condition, narcolepsy unspecified, recurrent hypersomnia, Kleine-Levin syndrome, menstrual-related hypersomnia, idiopathic hypersomnia with long sleep time, idiopathic hypersomnia without long sleep time, behaviorally induced insufficient sleep syndrome, hypersomnia due to a medical condition, hypersomnia due to a drug or substance, hypersomnia not due to a substance or known physiologic condition (nonorganic hypersomnia, not otherwise specified [NOS]), and physiologic (organic) hypersomnia, unspecified (organic hypersomnia, NOS).

Circadian rhythm sleep disorders include delayed sleep phase type, advanced sleep phase type, irregular sleep-wake type, free-running type, jet lag type, shift work type, circadian rhythm sleep disorder due to a medical condition, other circadian rhythm sleep disorder, circadian rhythm disorder (NOS), and other circadian rhythm due to a drug or substance.

Parasomnias are characterized by abnormal movements and behavior during sleep but do not necessarily disrupt sleep architecture. Parasomnias include disorders of arousal from non–rapid eye movement (NREM) sleep (confusional arousals, sleepwalking, and sleep terrors); parasomnias usually associated with rapid eye movement (REM) sleep (REM sleep behavior disorder, including parasomnia overlap disorder and status dissociatus; recurrent isolated sleep paralysis; and nightmare disorder); and other parasomnias (sleep-related dissociative disorders, sleep enuresis, sleep-related groaning or catathrenia, exploding head syndrome, sleep-related hallucinations, sleep-related eating disorders, parasomnia unspecified, parasomnia due to a drug or substance, and parasomnia due to a medical conditions).

Sleep-related movement disorders include restless legs syndrome (RLS), periodic limb movement disorder, sleep-related leg cramps, sleep-related bruxism, sleep-related rhythmic movement disorder, sleep-related movement disorder unspecified, sleep-related movement disorder due to a drug or substance, and sleep-related movement disorder due to a medical condition.

Isolated symptoms, apparently normal variants, and unresolved issues include long sleeper, short sleeper, snoring, sleep talking, sleep starts (hypnic jerks), benign sleep myoclonus of infancy, hypnagogic foot tremor and alternating leg muscle activation during sleep, propriospinal myoclonus at sleep onset, and excessive fragmentary myoclonus.

The *other sleep disorders* category includes other physiologic (organic) sleep disorders, other sleep disorders not due to a substance or known physiologic condition, and environmental sleep disorder.

Appendix A includes sleep disorders associated with conditions classifiable elsewhere: fatal familial insomnia, fibromyalgia, sleep-related epilepsy, sleep-related headaches, sleep-related gastroesophageal reflux disease, sleep-related coronary artery ischemia, and sleep-related abnormal swallowing, choking, and laryngospasm.

Appendix B includes other psychiatric and behavioral disorders frequently encountered in the differential diagnosis of sleep disorders (mood disorders, anxiety disorders, somatoform disorders, schizophrenia and other psychotic disorders); disorders usually first diagnosed in infancy, childhood, or adolescence; and personality disorders.

CLINICAL CHARACTERISTICS OF COMMON SLEEP COMPLAINTS

More detailed discussion of common sleep complaints is provided in several chapters (Chapters 20, 24, 26–29, and 32–37) of this volume. The following sections summarize these complaints.

Some common sleep complaints are trouble falling asleep and staying asleep (insomnia); falling asleep during the day (daytime hypersomnolence); inability to sleep at the right time (circadian rhythm sleep disorders); and complaints of thrashing or moving about in bed with repeated leg jerking (parasomnias and other abnormal movements, including nocturnal seizures and RLS). Table 19–1 lists the common sleep complaints.

Cardinal manifestations in a patient complaining of insomnia include all or some of the following:

- Difficulty falling sleep
- Frequent awakenings, including early morning awakening
- Insufficient or total lack of sleep
- Nonrestorative sleep
- Daytime fatigue, tiredness, or sleepiness
- Lack of concentration or irritability
- Anxiety and sometimes depression
- Forgetfulness
- Preoccupation with psychosomatic symptoms such as aches and pains

Cardinal manifestations of hypersomnia include the following:

- Excessive daytime somnolence (EDS)
- Falling asleep in inappropriate places and other inappropriate circumstances
- Lack of relief of symptoms after additional sleep at night
- Daytime fatigue and inability to concentrate
- Impairment of motor skills and cognition

TABLE 19–1 Common Sleep Complaints

- Cannot sleep (trouble falling asleep and staying asleep, with nonrestorative sleep)
- Cannot stay awake (falling asleep during the day)
- Cannot sleep at the right time
- Thrashing and moving about in bed and experiencing repeated leg jerking

Additional symptoms of hypersomnia depend on the nature of the underlying sleep disorder (e.g., snoring and apneas during sleep witnessed by a bed partner in patients with OSAS; attacks of cataplexy, hypnogogic hallucinations, sleep paralysis, automatic behavior, and disturbed night sleep in patients with narcolepsy).

ETIOLOGIC DIAGNOSIS

Insomnia and hypersomnia are symptoms and do not constitute a specific diagnosis. Every attempt should be made to find a cause for these complaints. The causes are described in several chapters in this book (Chapters 20, 24–30, 32–34, 36, and 37) and are briefly enumerated here.

Insomnia is defined as an inability to obtain an adequate amount of sleep to feel restored and refreshed in the morning, and to function adequately in the daytime.[21] The insomnia complaint does not necessarily depend on the total hours of sleep. There is considerable individual variation in sleep requirement. The category of adjustment insomnia is the only class of acute insomnia resulting from an identifiable stressful situation. This lasts from a few days to a few weeks, 3 months at most. Once the stressful event is removed and the patient adjusts to the event, the sleep disturbance resolves. Causes of acute insomnia include a change of sleeping environment (the most common cause of transient insomnia, the so-called first-night effect; jet lag; unpleasant room temperature); stressful life events (e.g., loss of a loved one, divorce, loss of employment, preparing to take an examination); acute medical or surgical illnesses (including intensive care unit stays); and use of stimulant medications (e.g., theophylline, β blockers, corticosteroids, digoxin, bronchodilators) or withdrawal of central nervous system (CNS) depressant medications. Causes of chronic insomnia are listed earlier in the section describing categories of the ICSD-2.[21]

Etiologic differential diagnosis of EDS includes both physiologic and pathologic causes (see Chapter 3). Briefly, physiologic causes include sleep deprivation and sleepiness related to lifestyle and irregular sleep-wake causes. Pathologic causes of EDS include primary sleep disorders (obstructive sleep apnea and central sleep apnea syndromes, narcolepsy or idiopathic hypersomnia, circadian rhythm sleep disorders, recurrent or periodic hypersomnia, occasional complaints in patients with RLS or periodic limb movements in sleep [PLMS], behaviorally induced insufficient sleep syndrome, and inadequate sleep hygiene); general medical, psychiatric, and neurologic causes; and medication- and toxin/alcohol-related hypersomnia.

For patients complaining of abnormal movements and behavior during sleep, the differential diagnosis should include disorders of arousal from NREM sleep (confusional arousals, sleepwalking and sleep terror); REM sleep parasomnias (REM sleep behavior disorder [RBD], recurrent isolated sleep paralysis, and nightmare disorder); and other parasomnias that were listed earlier. The differential diagnosis for patients complaining about abnormal movements and behaviors should also include the sleep-related movement disorders listed previously. In addition, sleep-related epilepsy, including nocturnal frontal lobe epilepsy must be considered in the differential diagnosis of abnormal movements and behaviors during sleep.

METHOD OF CLINICAL EVALUATION

A physician equipped with this background knowledge should attempt to make a clinical diagnosis based on the history and physical examination of a patient who complains of sleep disturbance. Polysomnographic study, the Multiple Sleep Latency Test (MSLT), and other laboratory tests must be confirmatory and secondary to the clinical diagnosis, which depends on a multifactorial analysis of many facets of a sleep complaint.

History

The first step in the diagnosis and assessment of a sleep/wakefulness disturbance is a careful evaluation of the sleep complaints. The history should seek information on sleep habits; drug and alcohol consumption; psychiatric, medical, and neurologic illnesses; history of previous illness; and family history[22–25] (Table 19–2).

Sleep History

The sleep history[22–25] is fundamentally important and is the first step in identifying the nature of the sleep disorder. Symptoms during the entire 24 hours should be evaluated, not just those that occur at sleep onset or during sleep at night. In addition to intrinsic and extrinsic dyssomnias, 24-hour symptomatic evaluation helps diagnose and manage circadian rhythm sleep disorders. The clinician should pay attention to symptoms that occur in the early evening or at sleep onset (e.g., paresthesias and uncontrollable limb movements of RLS), during sleep at night (e.g., repeated awakenings, snoring, and cessation of breathing in OSAS), on awakening in the morning

---

TABLE 19–2 Clinical Evaluation by History of a Patient with Sleep Complaints

- Sleep history
- Sleep questionnaire
- Sleep log or diary
- Drug and alcohol history
- Psychiatric history
- General medical history
- Neurologic history
- History of previous illnesses
- Family history

(e.g., feeling exhausted and sleepy in OSAS), or in the late morning and afternoon (e.g., daytime fatigue and excessive somnolence in OSAS and irresistible desire to have brief sleep in narcolepsy). Early morning awakening may be noted in insomnia due to depression. Abnormal motor activities may be associated with RBD and other parasomnias and found in patients with seizures.

In evaluating sleep history, Kales and coworkers[22–24] enumerated six important principles: (1) define the specific sleep problem, (2) assess the clinical course, (3) differentiate between various sleep disorders, (4) evaluate sleep/wakefulness patterns, (5) question the bed partner, and (6) evaluate the impact of the disorder on the patient.

One should analyze the onset, frequency, duration, and severity of the sleep complaint; its progression, evolution, and fluctuation over time; and any events that could have initiated it.[21] An analysis of these factors may differentiate transient disorders from persistent ones. The physician should inquire about the patient's functional status and mood during the day, any medicines and their effects on the sleep complaint, and sleep hygiene.

Finally, psychological, social, medical, and biological factors and their interactions should be considered to understand the patient's problem.[26] An interview with the bed partner, caregiver, and, in the case of a child, a parent, is important for diagnosis of abnormal movements (PLMS or other body movements), abnormal behavior (parasomnias, nocturnal seizures), and breathing disorders during sleep. The bed partner may also be able to answer questions about the patient's sleeping habits, history of drug use, psychosocial problems (e.g., stress at home, work, or school), and changes in sleep habits.

Sleep Questionnaire

A sleep questionnaire containing a list of pertinent questions relating to sleep complaints; sleep hygiene; sleep patterns; medical, psychiatric, and neurologic disorders; and drug or alcohol use may be filled out by the patient to save time in obtaining the history.

Sleep Log or Sleep Diary

A sleep log kept over a 2-week period is a valuable indicator of sleep hygiene and can also be used to monitor progression following therapeutic intervention. Such a log should include notations of bedtime, arising time, daytime naps, amount of time needed to go to sleep, number of nighttime awakenings, total sleep time, and feelings on arousal (e.g., refreshed or drowsy).

Drug and Alcohol History

The physician should inquire about drugs that could cause insomnia (e.g., CNS stimulants, bronchodilators, β blockers, corticosteroids, sedative-hypnotics) or hypersomnolence. In addition, the physician should have information about alcohol consumption and dependence as well as about insomnia related to drug withdrawal (e.g., intermediate- or short-acting benzodiazepines, nonbenzodiazepine hypnotics).[22–24] Caffeine consumption and smoking should also be considered as contributing factors to insomnia.

Psychiatric History

Attention should be paid to signs of possible psychiatric or psychophysiologic disorders (e.g., depression, anxiety, psychosis, obsession, life stress, personality traits).[22–25] If sleep disorders are secondary to a psychiatric illness, treating it alleviates the sleep disturbance in most cases. If the sleep complaint persists after such treatment, an additional cause or a primary sleep disorder should be suspected.

Medical and Neurologic History

The physician should question the patient about any reported symptom that has been associated with a variety of medical and neurologic illnesses (see Chapters 29 and 33). These symptoms direct attention to secondary sleep disorders.

History of Illnesses

The patient history might contain information about past medical, psychiatric, or neurologic disorders that could be responsible for the present sleep disturbance. It is also important to learn about and evaluate the premorbid personality of the patient. Finally, a history of a drug or alcohol habit or use of street drugs may reveal the role of these agents in the sleep complaint.

Family History

In certain sleep disorders, family history is very important.[22] A family history is found in about one-third of patients with narcolepsy and RLS. OSAS, with or without obesity, has also been described in family members. There is a high prevalence of sleepwalking, sleep terrors, and primary enuresis in family members. Many neurologic disorders, including fatal familial insomnia, have a family history. Currently, an intensive search is ongoing for a gene specific for narcolepsy and RLS.

Physical Examination

It is essential to conduct a thorough physical examination of every patient with a sleep complaint. It may uncover clues to important medical disorders, such as those involving respiratory, cardiovascular, gastrointestinal, or endocrine systems, or to a neurologic disease, especially one affecting the neuromuscular system, cervical spinal cord, or brain stem region, which may cause sleep-related breathing disorders as well as insomnias. In OSAS,

TABLE 19–3 Physical Findings in Patients with Obstructive Sleep Apnea Syndrome

- Obesity in the majority of patients (70%)
- Increased body mass index (body weight in kg/height in m²)
  - Overweight: ≥ 25 to 29
  - Obese: ≥ 30
- Increased neck circumference (>17 inches in men and >16 inches in women)
- In some patients, the following may be observed:
  - Large edematous uvula
  - Low-hanging soft palate
  - Large tonsils and adenoids (especially in children)
  - Retrognathia
  - Micrognathia
  - Polycythemia
  - Hypertension
  - Cardiac arrhythmias
  - Evidence of congestive heart failure

TABLE 19–5 Epworth Sleepiness Scale*

Eight Situations

1. Sitting and reading
2. Watching television
3. Sitting in a public place (e.g., a theater or a meeting)
4. Sitting in car as a passenger for an hour without a break
5. Lying down to rest in the afternoon
6. Sitting and talking to someone
7. Sitting quietly after a lunch without alcohol
8. In a car, while stopped for a few minutes in traffic

*Scale to determine the individual scores: 0 = would never doze; 1 = slight chance of dozing; 2 = moderate chance of dozing; 3 = high chance of dozing. Total score is the sum of the individual scores. Modified from Johns MW. A new method for measuring daytime sleepiness: the Epworth Sleepiness Scale. Sleep 1991;14:540.

physical examination may uncover upper airway anatomic abnormalities, which may need surgical correction if medical and continuous positive airway pressure (CPAP) treatments fail to relieve the symptoms. Examination may reveal systemic hypertension, which is a risk factor for sleep apnea. Table 19–3 lists physical findings which may be noted in patients with OSAS.

Subjective Measures of Sleepiness

A variety of scales have been developed to assist the subjective degree of sleepiness. The Stanford Sleepiness Scale (Table 19–4) is a 7-point scale that measures subjective sleepiness but may not be reliable with persistent sleepiness.

Another scale is the visual analog scale of alertness and well-being. In this scale, subjects are asked to indicate their feelings on an arbitrary line measuring from 0 mm on the left side to 100 mm on the right side. This scale has been used successfully in circadian rhythm disorders. The Epworth Sleepiness Scale evaluates general level of sleepiness.[27,28] The patient is rated on eight situations each of which is scored as 0 to 3 (with 3 being the highest chance of dozing off). The maximum score is 24, and a score greater than 10 suggests the presence of excessive sleepiness (Table 19–5). This scale has been weakly correlated with MSLT scores.

CLINICAL PHENOMENOLOGY

Clinical characteristics of some common sleep disorders are briefly described in the following sections. More detailed discussion can be found in several chapters of this volume (Chapters 24–28).

Obstructive Sleep Apnea Syndrome

Based on the definition of at least five apneas or hypopneas per hour of sleep accompanied by EDS,[27] the prevalence of OSAS is 4% in men and 2% in women between ages 30 and 60. There is a strong association between OSAS and male gender, increasing age, and obesity. The condition is common in men older than age 40, and among women the incidence of OSAS is greater after menopause. Approximately 85% of patients with OSAS are men, and obesity is present in about 70% of OSAS patients. Several risk factors are associated with OSAS (Table 19–6).

The symptoms of OSAS can be divided into two groups (see Chapter 24): those occurring during sleep and those occurring during waking hours (Table 19–7). Nocturnal symptoms include habitual loud snoring, choking during sleep, and cessation of breathing and abnormal motor activities during sleep (e.g., shaking and jerking movements, confusional arousals or sleepwalking), severe sleep disruption, heartburn as a result of gastroesophageal reflux, nocturnal enuresis (noted mostly in children), and profuse sweating at night. The daytime symptoms include

TABLE 19–4 Stanford Sleepiness Scale

Score	State Before Testing
1	Wide awake, active, and alert
2	Awake and able to concentrate but not functioning at peak
3	Relaxed, awake, and responsive but not fully alert
4	Feeling a little foggy
5	Difficulty staying awake
6	Sleepy, prefer to lie down
7	Cannot stay awake; sleep onset is imminent

Modified from Hoddes E, Zarcone V, Smythe H, et al. Quantification of sleepiness: a new approach. Psychophysiology 1973;10:431.

TABLE 19–6 Risk Factors for Sleep Apnea

- Male sex
- Menopause
- Increasing age
- Obesity
- Increasing neck size (>17 inches in men and >16 inches in women)
- Alcohol consumption
- Smoking
- Racial factors (e.g., increasing prevalence in United States among African Americans, Mexican Americans, and Pacific Islanders)

TABLE 19–7 Signs and Symptoms in Obstructive Sleep Apnea Syndrome

Nocturnal Symptoms During Sleep

- Loud snoring (often with a long history)
- Choking during sleep
- Cessation of breathing (apneas witnessed by bed partner)
- Sitting up or fighting for breath
- Abnormal motor activities (e.g., thrashing about in bed)
- Severe sleep disruption
- Gastroesophageal reflux causing heartburn
- Nocturia and nocturnal enuresis (mostly in children)
- Insomnia (in some patients)
- Excessive nocturnal sweating (in some patients)

Daytime Symptoms

- Excessive daytime somnolence
- Forgetfulness
- Personality changes
- Decreased libido and impotence in men
- Dryness of mouth on awakening
- Morning headache (in some patients)
- Automatic behavior with retrograde amnesia
- Hyperactivity in children
- Hearing impairment (in some patients)

EDS, which is characterized by sleep attacks lasting 0.5–2 hours and occurring mostly when the patient is relaxing (e.g., sitting down or watching television). The prolonged duration and the nonrefreshing nature of the sleep attacks differentiates them from narcoleptic sleep attacks. Other diurnal events include personality changes such as impairment of memory, irritability, impairment of motor skills, morning headache, sometimes hypnagogic hallucinations, automatic behavior with retrograde amnesia, and hyperactivity (in children). In men, impotence is often associated with severe and long-standing cases of OSAS.[30] Physical examination may reveal obesity in approximately 70% of cases, in addition to anatomic abnormalities in the upper airway. In severe cases, polycythemia and evidence of cardiac failure, pulmonary hypertension, and cardiac arrhythmias may be noted (see Table 19–3).

OSAS is associated with increased morbidity and mortality as a result of both short-term consequences (impairment of quality of life and increasing traffic- and work-related accidents), and long-term consequences resulting from comorbid conditions such as hypertension, heart failure, myocardial infarction, cardiac arrhythmia, and stroke due to both supratentorial and infratentorial infarctions and transient ischemic attacks, as well as cognitive dysfunction, depression, and insomnia.[31] Several prospective longitudinal studies have shown a clear association between OSAS and systemic hypertension, which may be noted in approximately 45% of patients with OSAS. In contrast, in about 30% of cases of essential hypertension OSAS is noted. Several studies have shown improvement of hypertension or reduction of need for antihypertensive medications after effective treatment of OSAS with CPAP titration (see Chapter 25). Pulmonary

hypertension is noted in approximately 15–20% of cases. Cardiac arrhythmias in the form of premature ventricular contractions, ventricular tachycardia, sinus pauses, and third-degree heart block as well as sudden cardiac death have been attributed to OSAS. Heart failure, mostly systolic but also diastolic (in which the studies are limited), is associated with both obstructive and central sleep apneas but mostly central sleep apneas (including Cheyne-Stokes breathing).[32,33] The presence of central apnea including Cheyne-Stokes breathing increases the mortality of patients with heart failure.[32] Cognitive dysfunction is noted in moderately severe to severe OSAS patients, but this shows improvement after satisfactory treatment with CPAP titration (see Chapter 25). There is an increasing awareness about the presence of depression and insomnia in patients with OSAS but, in the absence of adequate studies, the exact prevalence and impact of these conditions on OSAS cannot be determined. There is also an increased association between OSAS and metabolic syndrome (a combination of hypertension, increased insulin resistance with type 2 diabetes mellitus, hypertriglyceridemia, and obesity).[34]

Narcolepsy-Cataplexy Syndrome

The onset of narcolepsy-cataplexy in most cases is in adolescents and young adults, with a peak incidence between the ages of 15 and 30. The ICSD-2[21] divides narcolepsy into three types: narcolepsy with cataplexy, narcolepsy without cataplexy, and secondary narcolepsy. The major clinical manifestations of narcolepsy include narcoleptic sleep attacks (100%), cataplexy (70%), sleep paralysis (25–50%), hypnagogic hallucinations (20–40%), disturbed night sleep (70–80%), and automatic behavior (20–40%). In addition to the major manifestations, patients with narcolepsy may have four important comorbid conditions (Table 19–8): sleep apnea, PLMS, RBD, and nocturnal eating disorder. The classic sleep attack is an irresistible desire to fall asleep in inappropriate circumstances and at inappropriate places (e.g., while talking, driving, eating, playing, walking,

TABLE 19–8 Major Manifestations of Narcolepsy and Comorbid Conditions

	Percentage Occurrence
Major Manifestations	
Narcoleptic sleep attacks	100%
Cataplexy	70%
Sleep paralysis	25–50%
Hypnagogic hallucinations	20–40%
Disturbed night sleep	70–80%
Automatic behavior	20–40%
Comorbid Conditions	
Sleep apnea	Up to 30%
Periodic limb movements in sleep	10–60%
REM sleep behavior disorder	Up to 12%
Sleep-related eating disorder	

running, working, sitting, listening to lectures, or watching television or movies; during sexual intercourse; or when involved in boring or monotonous circumstances). These spells last from a few minutes to as long as 20–30 minutes and the patient generally feels refreshed upon waking. There are wide variations in frequency of attacks, anywhere from daily, weekly, or monthly to every few weeks to months. Attacks generally persist throughout the patient's lifetime, although fluctuations and rare temporary remissions may occur. Patients often show a decline in performance at school and work and encounter psychosocial and socioeconomic difficulties as a result of sleep attacks and EDS.

These sleep attacks are often accompanied by cataplexy, characterized by sudden loss of tone in all voluntary muscles except respiratory and ocular muscles. The attacks are triggered by emotional factors such as laughter, rage, or anger more than 95% of the time. The attacks may become partial and are rarely unilateral. Most commonly, patients may momentarily have head nodding, sagging of the jaw, buckling of the knees, dropping of objects from hands, or dysarthria or loss of voice, but sometimes they may slump or fall forward to the ground for a few seconds. The duration is usually a few seconds to minutes, and consciousness is retained completely during the attack. Generally, cataplectic spells begin to occur months to years after the onset of sleep attacks, but occasionally cataplexy is the initial manifestation. Cataplexy is a lifelong condition, but it generally is less severe and may even disappear in old age. Rarely, status cataplecticus occurs particularly after withdrawal of anticataplectic medications. Sleep paralysis, hypnagogic hallucinations, disturbed night sleep, and automatic behavior are the other manifestations of narcolepsy-cataplexy syndrome.

Symptomatic or secondary narcolepsy-cataplexy may result from dyencephalic and midbrain tumors, multiple sclerosis, strokes, vascular malformations, encephalitis, cerebral trauma, and paraneoplastic syndrome, in which anti-Ma2 antibodies may present with narcoleptic-like sleep attacks and other manifestations. Symptomatic narcolepsy is associated with cataplexy and develops in children affected with type C Niemann-Pick disease.

Idiopathic Hypersomnia with or Without Long Sleep Time

Idiopathic hypersomnia closely resembles narcolepsy syndrome. This disorder is characterized by EDS that has a presumed but not proven CNS cause and is associated with either normal (6–10 hours) or prolonged (>10 hours) nocturnal sleep documented by history, actigraphy, sleep logs, or PSG.[21] The onset of the disease is generally around the same age as narcolepsy (15–30 years). The sleep pattern, however, is different from that of narcolepsy. The patient generally sleeps for hours but the sleep is not refreshing. Because of EDS, the condition may be mistaken for sleep apnea. However, the patient does not give a history of cataplexy, snoring, or repeated awakenings throughout the night. Some patients may have automatic behavior with amnesia for the events. Physical examination uncovers no abnormal neurologic findings. This disabling and lifelong condition should be differentiated from other causes of EDS (see Chapter 3). There is no clear association between idiopathic hypersomnia and human leukocyte antigens (HLAs). The MSLT shows evidence of pathologic sleepiness without sleep-onset REMs.

Insomnia

Insomnia is the most common sleep disorder affecting the population and is the most common disease encountered in the practice of sleep medicine. Insomniacs complain of difficulty initiating and maintaining sleep, including early morning awakening and nonrestorative sleep occurring three or four times per week persisting for more than a month and associated with an impairment of daytime function. Acute insomnia may be associated with an identifiable stressful situation. Most cases of insomnia are chronic and comorbid with other conditions, which include psychiatric, medical, and neurologic disorders or drug and alcohol abuse. In some cases, no cause is found and the condition is labeled idiopathic or primary insomnia or psychophysiologic insomnia.

Restless Legs Syndrome

RLS is the most common movement disorder but is uncommonly recognized and treated despite a lucid description of the entity in the middle of the last century. There is not a single diagnostic test for RLS, hence the diagnosis rests entirely on clinical features and is based on the International Restless Legs Syndrome Study Group criteria first established in 1995 and modified slightly in 2003. These criteria include essential criteria and supportive and associative features as listed in Table 19–9. RLS is a lifelong sensorimotor neurologic disorder that often begins at a very young age but is mostly diagnosed in the middle or later years. Prevalence increases with age and plateaus for some unknown reason around age 85–90. All four essential diagnostic criteria (see Table 19–9) are needed to establish the diagnosis of RLS. The overall prevalence has been estimated at about 10% for adult populations, but the prevalence of most severe cases is approximately 2.5%. In most surveys, the prevalence is greater in women than in men and the disease is chronic and progressive. Family studies of RLS suggest an increased incidence (around 40–50%) in first-degree relatives of idiopathic cases. A high concordance (83%) in monozygotic twins and complex segregation analysis suggests an autosomal dominant mode of inheritance. Linkage analysis documented significant linkage to at least five different chromosomes (12Q, 14Q, 9P, 2P, and 22P). A recent genome-wide association study of RLS has identified common variants in certain genomic

TABLE 19–9 Essential Diagnostic Criteria and Supportive and Associated Features of Idiopathic RLS
Essential Diagnostic Criteria
• An urge to move the legs usually accompanied or caused by uncomfortable sensations in the legs
• The urge to move or unpleasant sensations beginning or worsening during periods of rest or inactivity such as lying or sitting
• The urge to move or unpleasant sensations are partially or totally relieved by movements, such as walking or stretching, at least as long as the activity continues
• The urge to move or unpleasant sensations are worse in the evening or night than during the day or only occur in the evening or night
Supportive Features
• Dopaminergic responsiveness
• Presence of periodic limb movements in sleep or in wakefulness
• Positive family history
Associated Features
• Usually progressive clinical course
• Normal neurologic examination in the idiopathic form
• Sleep disturbance

regions conferring more than 50% increase in risks to RLS. These recent results linking certain genes to RLS suggest a biological basis for the condition.

The sensory manifestations of RLS include intense disagreeable feelings that are described as creeping, crawling, tingling, burning, aching, cramping, knife-like, or itching sensations. These sensations occur mostly between the knees and ankles, causing an intense urge to move the limbs to relieve the feelings. Sometimes similar symptoms occur in the arms or other parts of the body, particularly in advanced stages of the disease or when the patient develops augmentation (a hypermotor syndrome with symptoms occurring at least 2 hours earlier than the initial period with intensification and spreading to other body parts) resulting from long-standing use of dopaminergic medications. Most of the movements, especially in the early stages, are noted in the evening when the patient is resting in bed. In severe cases, movements may be noted in the daytime when the patient is sitting or lying down. At least 80% of RLS patients have PLMS and may also have periodic limb movement in wakefulness. The condition generally has a profound impact on sleep; often the patient seeks medical attention because of sleep disturbance, which is a problem of initiation, although difficulty maintaining sleep also occurs because of associated PLMS. Neurologic examination is generally normal in the idiopathic form.

Parasomnias

Parasomnias can be defined as abnormal movements or behaviors, including those that occur into sleep or during arousals from sleep, intermittent or episodic, or

without disturbing the sleep architecture.[21] The ICSD-2 lists 15 items, and some of these entities are rare. Several parasomnias may be mistaken for seizures, especially complex partial seizures and nocturnal frontal lobe epilepsy. Somnambulism, night terror, confusional arousals, sleep enuresis, RBD, and nightmares are some of the parasomnias that can be mistaken for seizures. Characteristic clinical features combined with electroencephalographic (EEG) and PSG recordings are essential to differentiate these conditions.

Sleepwalking (Somnambulism)

Sleepwalking is common in children between the ages of 5 and 12 (Table 19–10). Sometimes it persists into adulthood or, rarely, begins in adults. Sleepwalking begins with an abrupt onset of motor activity arising out of slow-wave sleep during the first third of sleep. Episodes generally last less than 10 minutes. There is a high incidence of positive family history. Injuries and violent activities have been reported during sleepwalking episodes, but generally individuals can negotiate their way around the room. Rarely, the occurrence of homicide has been reported and sometimes abnormal sexual behavior occurs; sleep deprivation, fatigue, concurrent illness, and sedative-hypnotics are precipitating factors.

Sleep Terror (Pavor Nocturnus)

Sleep terror also occurs during slow-wave sleep (Table 19–11). Peak onset is between the ages of 5 and 7 years. As with sleepwalking, there is a high incidence of family history of sleep terror. Episodes of sleep terror are characterized by intense autonomic and motor symptoms, including a loud, piercing scream. Patients

TABLE 19–10 Features of Sleepwalking (Somnambulism)
• Onset: common between ages 5 and 12 yr
• High incidence of positive family history
• Abrupt onset of motor activity arising out of slow-wave sleep during the first third of the night
• Duration: <10 min
• Injuries and violent activity reported occasionally
• Precipitating factors: sleep deprivation, fatigue, concurrent illness, sedatives
• Treatment: precaution, benzodiazepines, imipramine

TABLE 19–11 Features of Sleep Terrors
• Onset: peak is between ages 5 and 7 yr
• High incidence of familial occurrences
• Abrupt arousal from slow-wave sleep during the first third of the night with a loud, piercing scream
• Intense autonomic and motor components
• Sleepwalking also seen in many patients
• Precipitating factors: stress, sleep deprivation, fever
• Treatment: psychotherapy, benzodiazepines, tricyclic antidepressants

appear highly confused and fearful. Many patients also have a history of sleepwalking episodes. Precipitating factors are similar to those described in sleepwalking.

Confusional Arousals

These occur mostly before age 5 years. As in sleepwalking and sleep terror, there is a high incidence of familial cases and the episodes arise out of slow-wave sleep but occasionally may occur out of stage 2 NREM sleep. The patient may have some automatic and inappropriate behavior, including abnormal sexual behavior (sex-somnia or sleep sex) when the episodes occur in adults. The majority of spells are benign, but sometimes violent and homicidal episodes in adults have been described. Precipitating factors are the same as in sleepwalking or sleep terror.

REM Sleep Behavior Disorder

RBD is an important REM sleep parasomnia commonly seen in elderly individuals (Table 19–12). A characteristic feature of RBD is intermittent loss of REM sleep–related muscle hypotonia or atonia and the appearance of various abnormal motor activities during sleep. The patient experiences violent and dream-enacting behavior during REM sleep, often causing self-injury or injury to the bed partner. RBD may be idiopathic or secondary; most cases are now thought to be secondary and thought to be associated with neurodegenerative diseases. It is seen with increasing prevalence in patients with Parkinson's disease (PD), multiple system atrophy (MSA), diffuse Lewy body disease with dementia (DLBD), corticobasal degeneration, olivopontocerebellar atrophy, and progressive supranuclear palsy. Many patients with narcolepsy, a probable degenerative disease of the hypocretin-containing neurons in the lateral hypothalamus, may also present with RBD. Some authors have proposed that RBD may be an α-synucleinopathy disorder because α-synuclein inclusions have been observed in many of the associated neurodegenerative diseases (e.g., PD, MSA, DLBD). RBD may precede many of these degenerative diseases. RBD may sometimes be drug induced (e.g., sedative-hypnotics, tricyclic antidepressants, anticholinergics, selective serotonin reuptake inhibitors) or associated with alcoholism and structural brain stem lesions. RBD has been linked to dopamine dysfunction based on positron emission tomography scan findings of reduced striatal presynaptic dopamine transporter and single-photon emission computed tomography scan findings of reduced postsynaptic dopamine D_2 receptors. REM sleep without muscle atonia is the most important PSG finding. Experimentally similar behavior has been noted after bilateral peri–locus ceruleus lesions in cats.

Nightmares

Nightmares—intense, frightening dreams followed by awakening and vivid recall—occur during REM sleep. The most common time of occurrence, therefore, is from the middle to the late part of the night. Nightmares are typically normal phenomena. Approximately 50% of children have nightmares beginning at 3–5 years of age. The incidence of nightmares continues to decrease as one grows older, and the elderly have very few or no nightmares. Nightmares are common after sudden withdrawal of REM-suppressant drugs and can also occur as side effects of certain medications, such as antiparkinsonian drugs, anticholinergics, and β blockers.

Sleep-Related Eating Disorders

Sleep-related eating disorders are common in women between the ages of 20 and 30 and consist of recurrent episodes of involuntary eating and drinking during partial arousals from sleep. Sometimes the patient displays strange eating behavior (e.g., consumption of inedible or toxic substances such as frozen pizza, raw bacon, and cat food). The episodes cause sleep disruption with weight gain; occasionally injury has been reported. The condition can be either idiopathic or comorbid with other sleep disorders (e.g., sleepwalking, RLS-PLMS, OSAS, narcolepsy, irregular sleep-wake circadian rhythm disorder) and with use of medications such as triazolam, zolpidem, and other psychotropic agents. The most common PSG findings are multiple confusional arousals with or without eating, arising predominantly from slow-wave sleep but also from other stages of NREM sleep and occasionally from REM sleep.

Catathrenia (Expiratory Groaning)

This parasomnia is characterized by recurrent episodes of expiratory groaning (high-pitched, loud humming or roaring sounds) that occur in clusters predominantly during REM sleep but may also occur during NREM sleep.[35–37] Polysomnographic findings resemble central apnea with protracted expiratory bradypnea without oxygen desaturation. Simultaneous audio recordings will bring out the characteristic groaning. The clinical relevance and pathophysiology of this condition remain unknown.

TABLE 19–12 Features of REM Sleep Behavior Disorder

- Onset: middle-aged or elderly men
- Presents with violent dream-enacting behavior during sleep, causing injury to self or bed partner
- Often misdiagnosed as a psychiatric disorder or nocturnal seizure (partial complex seizure)
- Etiology:
  - 40% idiopathic
  - 60% causal association with neurodegenerative disorders, structural central nervous system lesion, or use of alcohol or drugs (sedative-hypnotics, tricyclic antidepressants, anticholinergics, selective serotonin reuptake inhibitors)
- Polysomnography: REM sleep without muscle atonia
- Experimental model: bilateral peri–locus ceruleus lesions
- Treatment: 90% response to clonazepam

Sleep-Related Movement Disorders

The new category of sleep-related movement disorders is included in the ICSD-2.[21] These movements consist of relatively simple stereotyped movements disturbing sleep. RLS, PLMS, rhythmic movement disorder, bruxism, and nocturnal leg cramps are included in this category.

Rhythmic Movement Disorder

Rhythmic movement disorder is noted mostly in those younger than age 18 months and is occasionally associated with mental retardation. It is a sleep-wake transition disorder with three characteristic movements: head banging, head rolling, and body rocking. Rhythmic movement disorder is a benign condition and the patient outgrows the episodes.

Nocturnal Leg Cramps

These are intensely painful conditions accompanied by muscle tightness that occurs during sleep. The spasms usually last for a few seconds but sometimes persist for several minutes. Cramps during sleep are generally associated with awakening. Many normal individuals have nocturnal leg cramps; the cause remains unknown. Local massage or movement of the limbs usually relieves the cramps.

Bruxism (Tooth Grinding)

Bruxism often presents between ages 10 and 20, but it may persist throughout life, often leading to secondary problems such as temporomandibular joint dysfunction. Both diurnal and nocturnal bruxism may be also associated with various movement and degenerative disorders such as oromandibular dystonia and Huntington's disease. It is also commonly noted in children with mental retardation or cerebral palsy. Nocturnal bruxism is noted most prominently during stages 1 and 2 NREM sleep and REM sleep. The episode is characterized by stereotypical tooth grinding and is precipitated by anxiety, stress, and dental disease. Occasionally, familial cases have been described. Local injections of botulinum toxin into the masseter muscle may be used to prevent dental and temporomandibular joint complications.

LABORATORY INVESTIGATIONS

Laboratory investigations for sleep disorders should be considered an extension of the history and physical examination. First and foremost in the diagnosis of sleep disorders is a detailed history including sleep and other conditions as outlined earlier. This should be followed by careful physical examination to uncover any underlying medical, neurologic, or other causes of sleep dysfunction. Laboratory tests should include a diagnostic workup for the primary condition causing secondary or comorbid sleep disturbance and a workup for the sleep disturbance itself. The two most important laboratory tests for diagnosing sleep disturbance are PSG and the MSLT. Various

---

TABLE 19–13 Laboratory Tests to Assess Sleep Disorder

- Diagnostic workup for the primary or comorbid condition causing sleep disturbance
- Laboratory tests for the diagnosis and monitoring of sleep disorders
  - Overnight polysomnography (PSG)
  - Multiple Sleep Latency Test (MSLT)
  - Maintenance of Wakefulness Test
  - Actigraphy
  - Video-PSG
  - Standard electroencephalography (EEG) and video-EEG monitoring for suspected seizure disorders
- Imaging studies
  - Upper airway imaging for obstructive sleep apnea syndrome
  - Neuroimaging studies (e.g., computed tomography, magnetic resonance imaging) and cerebral angiography in cases of suspected neurologic illness causing sleep disorder
  - Positron emission tomography and single-photon emission computed tomography in special situations
- Miscellaneous tests
  - Pulmonary function tests in cases of suspected bronchopulmonary and neuromuscular disorders causing sleep-disordered breathing
  - Human leukocyte antigen for suspected narcolepsy
  - Cerebrospinal fluid hypocretin 1 level in suspected narcolepsy
  - Serum iron and ferritin levels for patients with restless legs syndrome
  - Electromyography and nerve conduction studies to exclude comorbid or secondary restless legs syndrome

---

other tests are also important for assessment of a patient with sleep dysfunction (Table 19–13).

Polysomnographic Study

An overnight PSG study is the single most important laboratory test for the diagnosis and treatment of patients with sleep disorders, particularly those associated with EDS. An all-night PSG study is required rather than a single-day nap study. The single-day nap study generally misses REM sleep, and the most severe apneic episodes are noted during REM sleep. Maximum oxygen desaturation also occurs at this stage; therefore, a daytime study cannot assess severity of symptoms. For CPAP titration, an all-night sleep study is essential. To determine the optimum level of pressure during CPAP titration, both REM and NREM sleep are required, including titration in supine position.

Indications for Polysomnography

Table 19–14 lists indications for overnight PSG in a sleep laboratory as proposed by the American Academy of Sleep Medicine (AASM). These include diagnosis of sleep-related breathing disorders, CPAP titration in patients with sleep-related breathing disorders, follow-up to assess effectiveness of treatment in OSAS patients, preoperative procedure in patients undergoing upper airway surgery for OSAS, evaluation of suspected narcolepsy, evaluation of atypical or violent parasomnias, and diagnosis of RBD and periodic limb movement disorder.

For parasomnias, the AASM[38] made the following recommendations: PSG is indicated for evaluating sleep-related behaviors that are violent or otherwise potentially

TABLE 19–14 Indications for Overnight Polysomnography

- A PSG study is routinely indicated:
  - For the diagnosis of sleep-related breathing disorders
  - For continuous positive airway pressure (CPAP) titration in patients with sleep-related breathing disorders
  - Before undergoing uvulopalatopharyngoplasty
  - For assessment of results after an oral appliance treatment for obstructive sleep apnea syndrome
  - For parasomnias if these are unusual or atypical or if the behaviors are violent or otherwise potentially injurious to the patient or others
  - For diagnosis of REM sleep behavior disorder
  - In patients suspected of having nocturnal seizures
  - A PSG study may be indicated for patients whose insomnia has not responded satisfactorily to a comprehensive behavioral or pharmacologic treatment program for the management of insomnia. If a sleep-related breathing disorder or associated periodic limb movements in sleep (PLMS) is strongly suspected in a patient with insomnia, a PSG study is indicated.
- A follow-up PSG is indicated:
  - When the clinical response is inadequate or when symptoms reappear despite a good initial treatment with CPAP
  - After substantial weight loss or weight gain, which may have occurred in patients previously treated successfully with CPAP
- An overnight PSG followed by a Multiple Sleep Latency Test the next day is routinely indicated in patients with suspected narcolepsy.
- An overnight PSG is required in persons with suspected PLMS but is not routinely performed to diagnose restless legs syndrome.
- An overnight PSG, preferably video-PSG with multiple channels of EEG, is indicated in patients suspected of having nocturnal seizures.

TABLE 19–15 Guidelines for Unattended Portable (Ambulatory) PSG Monitoring

- Unattended portable PSG monitoring is indicated:
  - As an alternative to in-laboratory PSG in patients with a high pretest probability of moderate to severe obstructive sleep apnea syndrome (OSAS)
  - For the diagnosis of OSAS in patients for whom in-laboratory PSG is not possible because of immobility, safety concerns, or critical illness
  - To monitor the therapeutic response to treatment other than continuous positive airway pressure for sleep apnea
- Unattended portable PSG monitoring is not indicated for:
  - The diagnosis of OSAS in those with significant comorbid medical disorders
  - The diagnostic evaluation of patients with suspected comorbid sleep disorders
  - General screening of asymptomatic individuals
- The recording must be supervised by a physician who is either board certified in sleep medicine or eligible for such certification, who must review the raw data and edit if needed.
- An experienced technologist must apply the sensors.
- At a minimum, the recording must include airflow, respiratory effort, and blood oxygen saturation.
- A follow-up visit to review the results should be performed.
- A negative or technically inadequate recording in a patient with a high degree of clinical suspicion for OSAS should require an in-laboratory PSG.

injurious to the patient or others, as well as for patients who have unusual or atypical behaviors during sleep. PSG may also be indicated in situations with forensic considerations. However, PSG is not routinely indicated for typical and uncomplicated parasomnias.

PSG is not routinely indicated to diagnose or treat RLS. PSG is indicated when a diagnosis of PLMS is considered as a result of a complaint by the patient or bed partner of repetitive limb movements during sleep, frequent awakenings, difficulty maintaining sleep, or excessive daytime somnolence.

PSG is not routinely indicated for diagnosis of circadian rhythm sleep disorders or depression. Indications for PSG in patients with insomnia are somewhat controversial. The diagnosis of insomnia is basically clinical. The AASM guidelines[38] do not list PSG for routine evaluation of transient or chronic insomnia. PSG may be useful, however, when the cause of insomnia is uncertain or when behavioral or pharmacologic treatment is unsuccessful. If a patient with insomnia is suspected of having a sleep-related breathing disorder or PLMS, PSG is indicated as outlined earlier.

Indications for Ambulatory PSG

Table 19–15 lists indications and guidelines for unattended portable (ambulatory) PSG monitoring as proposed by the Task Force of the AASM.[39]

Polysomnographic Findings in Sleep Disorders[40]

Characteristic PSG findings in OSAS include recurrent episodes of apneas and hypopneas (Fig. 19–1) that are mostly obstructive or mixed and a few episodes of central apnea accompanied by oxygen desaturation and followed by arousals with resumption of breathing. An apnea-hypopnea index (AHI, the number of apneas/hypopneas per hour of sleep) of 5 or below is considered normal, and an AHI index of 5–15 may be considered evidence of mild OSAS, 16–29 as evidence of moderate OSAS, and 30 or more as evidence of severe OSAS. Similarly, oxygen saturation of 85–89% may be found in mild OSAS, whereas in moderate OSAS 80–84% is typical and in severe OSAS 79% and below is the usual finding. An arousal index of up to 10 is considered normal, and 10–15 can be considered borderline; an arousal index above 15 is definitely abnormal. There are some sleep architectural changes in OSAS (reduction of slow-wave and REM sleep); most of the sleep is spent in stage 2 NREM sleep. Other findings include short latency, increased time spent awake after sleep onset, and excessive snoring. In patients with central sleep apnea syndrome, the apneas are all central for at least 50% of apneas. PSG findings in patients with Cheyne-Stokes breathing consist of a characteristic crescendo-decrescendo pattern of breathing followed by apneas or hypopneas (Fig. 19–2) for at least 3 consecutive cycles and five or more central apneas or hypopneas per hour of sleep or at least 10 consecutive minutes of cycle duration.

Overnight PSG findings in patients with narcolepsy include short sleep latency, excessive disruption of sleep with frequent arousal, reduced total sleep time, excessive

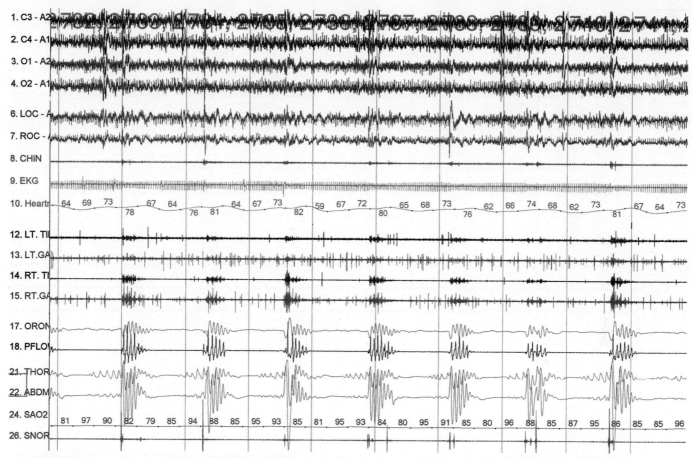

FIGURE 19–1 Overnight polysomnographic (PSG) recording in a patient with upper airway obstructive sleep apnea syndrome (OSAS) showing recurrent episodes of mixed apneas (initial control followed by obstructive events) during stage 2 NREM (N2) sleep. Top 4 channels show electroencephalograms (international nomenclature). (A1, left ear; A2, right ear; ABDM, abdominal respiratory effort; CHIN, submental electromyogram [EMG]; EKG, electrocardiogram; GA, gastrocnemius EMG; LOC, left electro-oculogram; LT, left; ORON, oronasal airflow; PFLO, nasal pressure transducer recording airflow; ROC, right electro-oculogram; RT, right; SAO2, oxygen saturation [%] by finger oximetry; SNOR, snoring sound recording; THOR, chest respiratory effort; TI, tibialis anterior EMG.)

body movements, reduced slow-wave sleep, and sleep-onset REM (seen in 40–50% of patients). Some narcoleptic patients may have associated sleep apnea, particularly central apnea. In approximately 9–59% of patients PLMS has been noted, and in up to 36% of narcoleptic patients RBD has been described.

The characteristic PSG findings in RBD consist of absence of muscle atonia and presence of increased phasic electromyographic (EMG) activities in the upper and lower limbs during REM sleep. It is important to record EMGs from both upper and lower limbs because, in some patients with RBD, EMG activities are present in the upper limbs but not in the lower limbs.

In RLS, PSG findings document sleep disturbance and PLMS (see Fig. 12–9), which is found in at least 80% of patients. Diagnosis of periodic limb movement disorder is based on the PLMS index (number of periodic limb movements per hour of sleep) of 15 and over plus symptoms of sleep disturbance. A high PLMS index with arousal is more significant than an index without arousal.

Pitfalls of PSG

PSG is the single most important laboratory test for assessment of sleep disorders, particularly in patients presenting with EDS and those suspected of nocturnal seizures, parasomnias, or other abnormal motor activities. However, PSG has considerable limitations. There is no standardized uniform protocol used consistently in all sleep laboratories, making the comparison of the data from one laboratory to another somewhat misleading. The most severe limitations are that an overnight in-laboratory PSG is labor intensive, time consuming, and expensive. A single-night PSG may miss the diagnosis of mild OSAS, PLMS, parasomnias, and nocturnal seizures. PSG data and the patient's clinical findings may not be concordant. Standard PSG study cannot diagnose upper airway resistance syndrome definitively. PSG cannot determine the etiology of apnea-hypopnea syndrome. PSG is not helpful in the diagnosis of insomnia, the most common sleep disorder in the general population. PSG is not helpful in the diagnosis

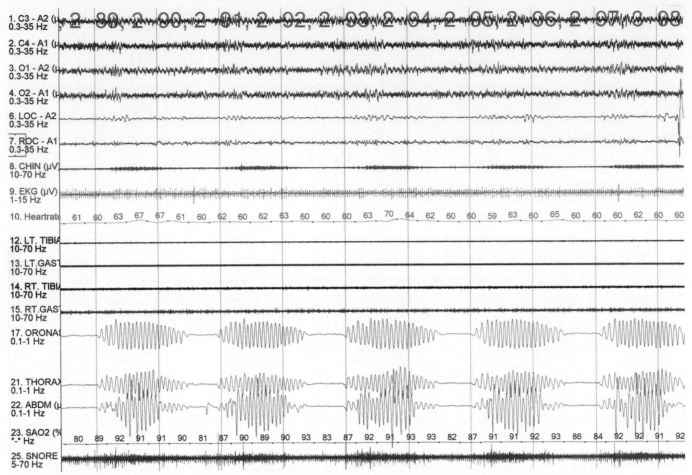

FIGURE 19–2 PSG recording from a 70-year-old woman showing the classic crescendo-decrescendo pattern of Cheyne-Stokes breathing (CSB) during stage 2 NREM sleep. The presence of CSB throughout most of the NREM sleep (with marked decrement or absence during REM sleep) in this patient with a history of hypertension and excessive daytime sleepiness suggests occult left ventricular failure. The PSG montage is similar to that in Figure 19–1.

or treatment of circadian rhythm sleep disorders. PSG data may be confounded by first-night effects (e.g., increased wakefulness and stage 1 NREM sleep, and decreased slow-wave and REM sleep). Standard PSG does not measure arterial partial pressure of CO_2 and thus may miss hypoventilation, which is an early abnormality (particularly REM hypoventilation) in neuromuscular disorders. Standard PSG does not adequately measure cardiac function (1 channel of electrocardiography [ECG] is inadequate), which may affect the prognosis of OSAS. Furthermore, cardiorespiratory sleep studies, which do not include EEG, may produce false-negative findings in mild to moderate OSAS patients. Standard PSG does not include autonomic monitoring, which may be important for assessment of autonomic activation as well as for assessing autonomic changes that are intense during sleep.

Video-Polysomnographic Study

A video-PSG study is important for documenting abnormal movements and behavior during sleep at night in patients with parasomnias, including RBD, nocturnal seizures, and other unusual movements occurring during sleep. Parasomnias are generally diagnosed on the basis of a clinical history, but sometimes a video-PSG study is required to document the condition. For suspected nocturnal epilepsy, a video-PSG study using additional electrodes to include multiple-channel EEG and multiple montages covering both parasagittal and temporal regions bilaterally is required for optimal detection of epileptiform activities. Ideally, if sleep epilepsy is suspected, video-PSG recordings should be capable of EEG analysis at the standard EEG speed of 30 mm/sec to identify epileptiform discharges. Multiple EMG channels to record from additional muscles (e.g., forearm flexor and extensor muscles, masseter and other muscles) for patients with suspected RBD and bruxism are recommended.

Video-PSG may help characterize the movements, differentiate one jerk from another, identify a specific entity, and most importantly differentiate abnormal motor activities from nocturnal seizures. Video-PSG may aid in the diagnosis of other coexisting sleep disorders (e.g., OSAS,

RBD, narcolepsy). Video-PSG does help us classify abnormal motor activities during sleep into several identifiable entities (e.g., motor parasomnias, nocturnal seizures, involuntary diurnal movements persisting during sleep, PLMS, excessive fragmentary myoclonus seen in a variety of sleep disorders, dissociative disorders, nocturnal jerks and body movements seen in patients with OSAS). Many parasomnias may be mistaken for nocturnal seizures (e.g., confusional arousals, sleepwalking, sleep terror, sleep talking, bruxism, rhythmic movement disorder, RBD, nightmares, and dissociative disorders). RBD and nightmares occur during REM sleep. These conditions can be diagnosed and differentiated from one another based on characteristic clinical features combined with EEG and video-PSG findings. Table 19–16 lists indications for video-PSG.

Multiple Sleep Latency Test

The MSLT is an important test to effectively document EDS (see Chapter 16). Narcolepsy is the single most important indication for performing MSLT. The presence of two or more sleep-onset REM periods from four or five nap studies and sleep-onset latency of less than 8 minutes strongly suggest a diagnosis of narcolepsy[21] (Fig. 19–3). Abnormalities of REM sleep regulatory mechanisms (e.g., OSAS, behaviorally induced insufficient sleep syndrome, use of REM-suppressant medications) or circadian rhythm sleep disturbance may also lead to REM sleep abnormalities during an MSLT.

Maintenance of Wakefulness Test

The Maintenance of Wakefulness Test (MWT) is a variant of the MSLT, measuring a subject's ability to stay awake. It also consists of four to five trials of remaining awake occurring every 2 hours. Each trial is terminated if no sleep occurs after 40 minutes or immediately after

---

TABLE 19–16 Indications for Video-PSG

- Unusual and complex arousal disorders
- Complex behaviors suspicious of RBD but not absolutely certain based on the history
- Behavior and motor events at night suggesting possible nocturnal seizure disorder
- EDS in patients with epilepsy, to determine if excessive sleepiness is due to repeated nocturnal seizures, an undesirable side effect of antiepileptic medications, or an associative sleep disorder (e.g., sleep apnea).
- Suspected psychogenic dissociative disorder
- Sleep-related movement disorders (e.g., rhythmic movement disorders, bruxism), which may be mistaken for nocturnal seizures
- Involuntary diurnal movement disorder persisting during sleep
- Coexisting secondary sleep disorder (e.g., narcolepsy and RBD; OSAS and sleepwalking; narcolepsy and sleep apnea)
- For medicolegal purpose when the patient presents with violent behavior during sleep; video-PSG studies are mandatory to evaluate suspicions for correct diagnosis of parasomnias or seizure disorders.

---

the first 3 consecutive epochs of stage 1 NREM sleep or the first epoch of any other stage of sleep.[20] If the mean sleep latency is less than 8 minutes, it is then considered an abnormal test. The MWT is less sensitive than the MSLT as a diagnostic test for narcolepsy but is more sensitive in assessing the effect of treatment (e.g., CPAP titration in OSAS and stimulant therapy in narcolepsy).

Standard Electroencephalographic Study

An EEG is necessary to investigate suspected epilepsy (see Chapter 30).

Ambulatory Electroencephalography or Polysomnography

Ambulatory EEG or PSG is sometimes useful for patients with suspected sleep epilepsy, for understanding circadian variation, and for studying circadian rhythm sleep disorders. However, technical problems associated with unattended recording are serious limitations.

Actigraphy

This is another laboratory test for assessing sleep disorders that uses an actigraph (also known as an actometer) worn on the wrist or ankle to record acceleration or deceleration of body movements (Fig. 19–4), which indirectly indicates the state of sleep or wakefulness. The actigraph can be worn for days or weeks, and this test complements a sleep log or diary in diagnosing circadian rhythm sleep disorders (Fig. 19–5) and in assessing patients with insomnia (Fig. 19–6), including paradoxical insomnia or sleep state misperception; inadequate sleep hygiene; and prolonged daytime sleepiness. Actigraphy is useful to document rest-activity patterns over days and weeks when a sleep log is not able to provide such data. Advantages of actigraphy over PSG include the following: easy accessibility; inexpensive recording over extended periods of days, weeks, or months; recording of 24-hour activities at all sites (home, work, laboratory); usefulness in uncooperative and demented patients when laboratory PSG study is not possible; ability to conduct longitudinal studies during therapeutic intervention (e.g., cognitive behavioral therapy or pharmacologic treatment) in patients with insomnia; usefulness in paradoxical insomnia; and ability to document delayed or advanced sleep phase state or circadian rhythm sleep disorder, free-running type. Although not adequately standardized, actigraphy may have a role in patients with RLS and PLMS.

Neuroimaging Studies

Neuroimaging studies include anatomic and functional (physiologic) studies. These studies are essential when a neurologic illness is suspected of causing a sleep disturbance (see Chapter 29).

Pulmonary Function Tests

Pulmonary function tests are important for excluding intrinsic bronchopulmonary disease, which may affect sleep-related breathing disorders (see Chapter 29).

Electrodiagnosis of the Respiratory Muscles

Electromyographic recordings of the upper airway and diaphragmatic and intercostal muscles may detect changes in these muscles in various neurologic diseases (see Chapter 29).

Other Laboratory Tests

Appropriate laboratory tests should always be performed to exclude any suspected medical disorder that may be the cause of a patient's insomnia or hypersomnia. These tests may include blood and urinalysis, ECG, Holter monitor ECG, chest radiography, and other investigations to rule out gastrointestinal, pulmonary, cardiovascular, endocrine, and renal disorders. In rare patients, when autonomic failure causes a sleep disturbance or sleep-related breathing disorder, autonomic function tests may be required for the diagnosis of the primary condition.

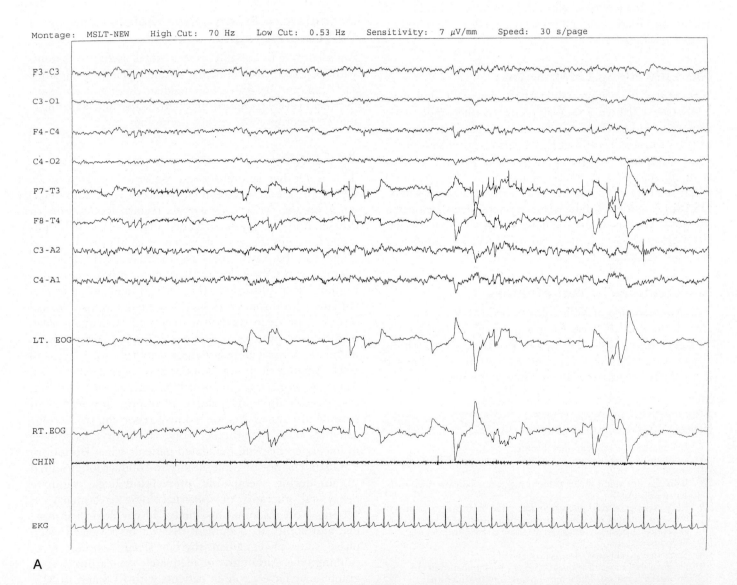

A

FIGURE 19–3 A case of narcolepsy in a 60-year-old woman with new onset of intermittent episodes of sudden transient bilateral leg weakness, excessive daytime sleepiness, and intermittent periods of transient confusion. A daytime EEG was normal. Overnight PSG was significant for sleep architecture changes with an immediate sleep onset latency, presence of only 1 REM cycle, with a decreased REM sleep percentage (7%), an increased arousal index of 23 without associated apnea or periodic limb movements, and excessive fragmentary myoclonus in NREM and REM sleep. The MSLT showed a mean sleep latency of 1.6 minutes, consistent with pathologic sleepiness, and the presence of 2 (of 4) sleep-onset REM naps suggestive of REM sleep dysregulation as seen in narcolepsy. **(A)** A 30-second epoch from the MSLT showing the presence of sleep-onset REM occurring 7 minutes after sleep onset. Prominent REMs are seen in the EOG channels and anterior temporal EEG electrodes.

Continued

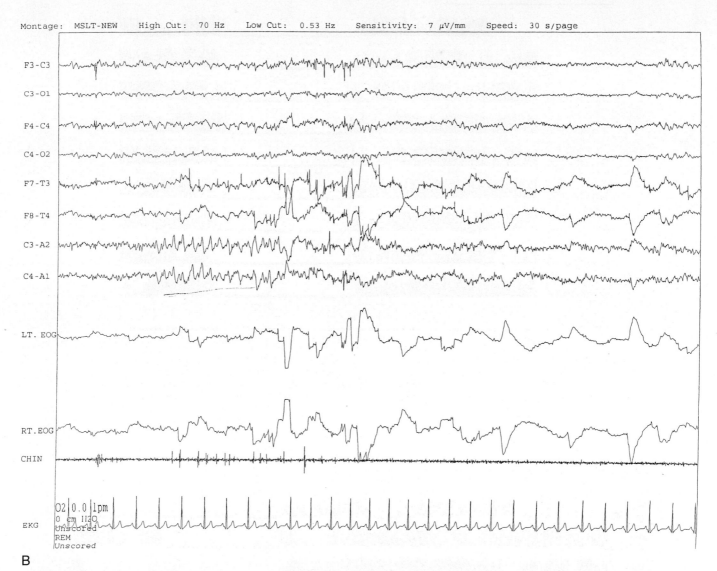

Montage: MSLT-NEW   High Cut: 70 Hz   Low Cut: 0.53 Hz   Sensitivity: 7 μV/mm   Speed: 30 s/page

B

FIGURE 19–3—Cont'd (B) A 30-second epoch taken from the same sleep nap as in **A,** showing the presence of prominent sawtooth waves (*underlined*) in C3 and C4 electrode channel references to contralateral ears. Eye movements characteristic of REM sleep are noted as described. (chin, electromyography of chin; EEG, top eight channels; EKG, electrocardiography; Lt. and Rt. EOG, left and right electro-oculograms.) *(Reproduced with permission from Chokroverty S, Thomas RJ, Bhatt M [eds]. Atlas of Sleep Medicine. Philadelphia: Elsevier Saunders, 2005.)*

In patients with narcolepsy, HLA typing may be performed because most patients with narcolepsy show positivity for HLA DR2 DQ1 and DQB1*0602 antigens. Another important test is measurement of cerebrospinal fluid hypocretin 1 levels, which are found to be low (<110 pg/ml) in patients with narcolepsy-cataplexy who are HLA DQB1*0602 positive. In patients with narcolepsy without cataplexy and in some other neurologic conditions, cerebrospinal fluid hypocretin may be low normal. In selected patients suspected of having a psychiatric cause of EDS, neuropsychiatric testing (e.g., the Minnesota Multiphasic Personality Inventory) may be helpful.

In patients with RLS, EMG and nerve conduction studies are important to exclude polyneuropathies or lumbosacral radiculopathies and other lower motor neuron disorders that may be associated with RLS or cause symptoms resembling idiopathic RLS. Other important laboratory tests in patients with RLS include those necessary to exclude diabetes mellitus, uremia, anemia, and other associated conditions. It is particularly important to obtain levels of serum iron (including serum ferritin and transferrin), serum folate, fasting blood glucose, blood urea nitrogen, and creatinine. In a subgroup of patients with RLS, serum iron and ferritin levels are found to be low; it is important to measure these because correction of these abnormalities may improve the condition. The role of nerve biopsy remains controversial. In the vast majority of patients, a nerve biopsy is not

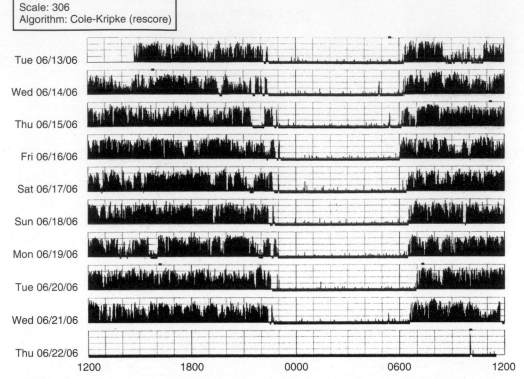

Scale: 306
Algorithm: Cole-Kripke (rescore)

Tue 06/13/06
Wed 06/14/06
Thu 06/15/06
Fri 06/16/06
Sat 06/17/06
Sun 06/18/06
Mon 06/19/06
Tue 06/20/06
Wed 06/21/06
Thu 06/22/06

1200   1800   0000   0600   1200

FIGURE 19–4 Normal sleep-wake schedule. This wrist actigraphic recording from a 50-year-old healthy woman without sleep complaints shows a fairly regular sleep-wake schedule. She goes to bed between 10:30 PM and 11:00 PM and wakes up around 6:30 AM except on the fourth and eighth day. Physiologic body shifts and movements during sleep are indicated by a few *black bars* in the *white areas*. The waking period is indicated by *black bars*.

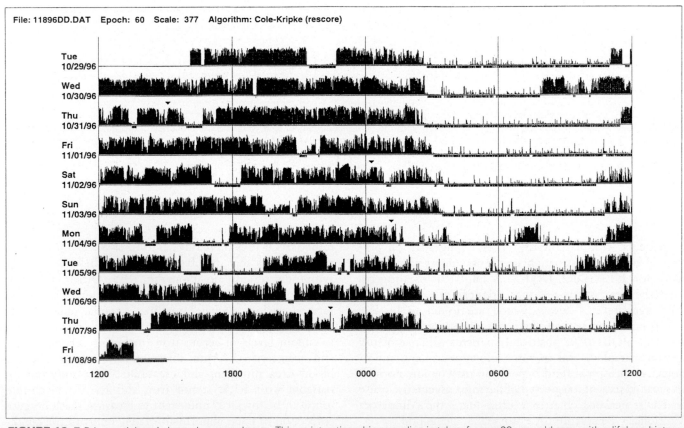

File: 11896DD.DAT   Epoch: 60   Scale: 377   Algorithm: Cole-Kripke (rescore)

Tue 10/29/96
Wed 10/30/96
Thu 10/31/96
Fri 11/01/96
Sat 11/02/96
Sun 11/03/96
Mon 11/04/96
Tue 11/05/96
Wed 11/06/96
Thu 11/07/96
Fri 11/08/96

1200   1800   0000   0600   1200

FIGURE 19–5 Primary delayed sleep phase syndrome. This wrist actigraphic recording is taken from a 29-year-old man with a lifelong history of delayed sleep onset and delayed wake-up time. The actigram shows his typical sleep period from 3:00 AM to 4:00 AM to 9:00 AM to noon (*white areas*). If he has to wake up early in the morning, he feels exhausted and sleepy all day. He feels fine if he is allowed to follow his own schedule. Melatonin at night did not help him. Morning bright light therapy was suggested but the patient declined. *(Reproduced with permission from Chokroverty S, Thomas RJ, Bhatt M [eds]. Atlas of Sleep Medicine. Philadelphia: Elsevier Saunders, 2005.)*

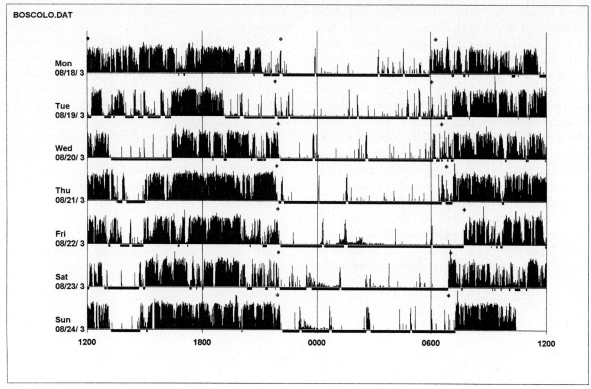

FIGURE 19–6 Actigraphy in insomnia (sleep state misperception). A 59-year-old man complaining of insomnia since the age of 12 years was diagnosed to have an Axis 2 personality disorder (dependent personality) according to the *Diagnostic and Statistical Manual of Mental Disorders, Fourth Edition,* as well as panic attacks, and is being treated with benzodiazepines (diazepam 3 mg, flurazepam 30 mg) and zolpidem 10 mg. He denies any symptoms of restless legs syndrome (RLS), excessive daytime sleepiness, or daytime sleep attacks. Subjective sleep duration is 3–4 hours per night. In the past he had used numerous drugs for sleep amelioration, but no clear and stable subjective improvement was noted. Actigraphic monitoring (during drug dosage reduction: diazepam 2 mg, flurazepam 15 mg, and no zolpidem) shows a clear misperception of sleep duration and quality. The recording shows normal nocturnal motor activity and sleep efficiency and duration; note sleep period during the afternoon. He complained of sleeping not more than 3 hours each night. PSG on the third night revealed the following: TST, 387 minutes; SE, 73.5; WASO, 122 minutes; number of awakenings, 17; SWS %, 1.3; PLMS index, 1.9. (PLMS, periodic limb movements in sleep; PSG, polysomnography; SE, sleep efficiency; SWS, slow-wave sleep; TST, total sleep time; WASO, wake after sleep onset.) *(Reproduced with permission from Chokroverty S, Thomas RJ, Bhatt M [eds]. Atlas of Sleep Medicine. Philadelphia: Elsevier Saunders, 2005.)*

necessary, but it may be obtained for research purposes and when there is strong suspicion of polyneuropathy.

PRINCIPLES OF MANAGEMENT OF SLEEP DISORDERS

The first principle of treatment of sleep disorders is to find the cause of the sleep disturbance and vigorously treat the primary or comorbid condition causing the sleep disturbance. If a satisfactory treatment is not available for the primary condition or does not resolve the problem, then treatment should be directed at a specific sleep disturbance. It is beyond the scope of this chapter to discuss the management of various neurologic and medical disorders causing sleep disturbances, and the reader is referred to several chapters (Chapters 24, 26–30, 32, and 33) in this volume. Some general sleep hygiene measures (Table 19–17) should apply to all sleep disorder patients.

TABLE 19–17 Sleep Hygiene Measures

- Keep a regular sleep-wake schedule, including weekends.
- Avoid caffeinated beverages after lunch.
- Avoid smoking, especially in the evening.
- Avoid alcohol near bedtime.
- Restrict sleep to amount needed to feel rested.
- Do not go to bed hungry.
- Adjust bedroom environment.
- Do not engage in planning the next day's activities at bedtime.
- Exercise regularly for about 20 to 30 minutes, preferably 4 to 5 hours before bedtime and not immediately before bedtime.

SUMMARY AND CONCLUSIONS

This chapter outlines the approach to a patient with a sleep complaint. The approach should begin with a careful clinical analysis of the patient's symptoms, keeping in mind the International Classification of Sleep Disorders and its pertinent manifestations along with the underlying basic science foundations of such disorders. The detailed history should consist of a sleep history (including night sleep complaints and daytime sleepiness), as well as family, psychiatric, medical (including neurologic), drug, and alcohol histories. Physical examination should include neurologic and general medical and other organ system examination. A sleep diary or log is often very useful. The patient history and physical examination should provide information about the patient's quality of life and how sleep disturbances are affecting daily activities, including those associated with the patient's professional, family, and social lives. An occasional sleep complaint (insomnia or sleepiness) is common, but if the symptoms are persistent or frequent and are interfering with daily life, professional advice should be sought. In most cases, diagnosis can be made on clinical grounds with minimal laboratory investigation, minimizing the patient's suffering and expenses. In this way, we honor the Hippocratic Oath by comforting patients and causing no harm.

Most of the time, patients with sleep complaints seek the advice of their primary care physician, who may decide, based on the patient history and physical examination, that a patient's sleep complaints are due to a medical, psychiatric, or neurologic condition. The next step would be for the primary care physician either to treat the condition causing the sleep disturbance, or to refer the patient to an appropriate specialist. For primary sleep disorders, it is advisable to refer the patient to a sleep specialist, who may then decide to conduct further laboratory tests (e.g., PSG, MSLT, actigraphy, video-PSG) and provide treatment.

⊙ REFERENCES

A full list of references are available at www.expertconsult.com

CHAPTER 20

Classification of Sleep Disorders

Michael J. Thorpy

INTRODUCTION

The classification of sleep disorders has been of particular interest to physicians since sleep disorders were first recognized. The first major classification, the Diagnostic Classification of Sleep and Arousal Disorders that was published in 1979,[1] organized the sleep disorders into categories that formed the basis of the current classification systems. In 1990, the International Classification of Sleep Disorders (ICSD) was produced after a 5-year process initiated by the American Sleep Disorders Association. The ICSD development process involved the three major international sleep societies at that time—the European Sleep Research Society, the Japanese Society of Sleep Research, and the Latin American Sleep Society—and resulted in the production of a diagnostic and coding manual, the *International Classification of Sleep Disorders: Diagnostic and Coding Manual.*[2] The ICSD classification, developed primarily for diagnostic, epidemiologic, and research purposes, was widely used and allowed better international communication in sleep disorder research. In 2003, the American Academy of Sleep Medicine initiated the process of a complete revision and update of the ICSD. The resulting text, the ICSD-2, was published in 2005[3] (Table 20–1).

The ICSD-2 classification lists approximately 77 sleep disorders, each presented in detail and with a descriptive diagnostic text that includes specific diagnostic criteria. The ICSD-2 has eight major categories: (1) insomnia; (2) sleep-related breathing disorder; (3) hypersomnia not due to a sleep-related breathing disorder; (4) circadian rhythm sleep disorder; (5) parasomnia; (6) sleep-related movement disorder; (7) isolated symptoms, apparently normal variants, and unresolved issues; and (8) other sleep disorders. Additional sleep-related disorders are categorized in two appendices: (A) sleep disorders associated with conditions classifiable elsewhere; and (B) other psychiatric/behavioral disorders frequently encountered in the differential diagnosis of sleep disorders.

ICSD-2 CLASSIFICATION CATEGORIES

Insomnia

The insomnias are defined by a repeated difficulty with sleep initiation, duration, consolidation, or quality that occurs despite adequate time and opportunity for sleep and results in some form of daytime impairment. Insomnia complaints typically include reported difficulties initiating and/or maintaining sleep. Extended periods of nocturnal wakefulness and/or insufficient amounts of nocturnal sleep usually accompany these complaints. Occasionally, insomnia complaints are characterized by the perception of poor-quality or "nonrestorative" sleep, even when the amount and quality of the usual sleep episode is perceived to be "normal" or adequate. Chronic insomnia can be divided into two subtypes: primary or secondary. Primary insomnia is insomnia that can have both intrinsic and extrinsic factors involved in the etiology, but primary insomnia is not regarded as being secondary to other disorders. Secondary forms of insomnia can occur when insomnia is a symptom of a medical or psychiatric illness, other sleep disorders, or substance abuse. A new term, *comorbid insomnia*, has been recommended.[4] This term has been introduced because of the inability to draw firm conclusions about the nature of the secondary associations

TABLE 20–1   Classification of Sleep Disorders According to ICSD-2, International Classification of Diseases (ICD), and *Diagnostic and Statistical Manual of Mental Disorders, Fourth Edition, Text Revision* (DSM-IV-TR)

ICD-9-CM	ICD-10	DSM-IV-TR*	Classification
Insomnia			
307.42	F51.04	307.42	Psychophysiological Insomnia
307.42	F51.03	307.42	Paradoxical Insomnia
307.41	F51.02	307.42	Adjustment Insomnia
V69.4	Z72.821	307.42	Inadequate Sleep Hygiene
307.42	F51.01	307.42	Idiopathic Insomnia
327.02	F51.05	327.02	Insomnia due to Mental Disorder
V69.5	Z73.81	307.42	Behavioral Insomnia of Childhood
327.01	G47.09	327.01	Insomnia due to a Medical Condition
292.85	F10-19	291.85	Insomnia due to a Drug or Substance
291.82	F10-19	291.82	Insomnia due to Alcohol
327.00	G47.00		Physiologic (Organic) Insomnia, Unspecified
780.52	F51.09		Insomnia Not due to a Substance or Known Physiological Condition, Unspecified
Sleep-Related Breathing Disorder			
327.21	G47.31	780.57	Primary Central Sleep Apnea
786.04	G47.39	780.57 or 327.xx	Central Sleep Apnea including Cheyne-Stokes Breathing Pattern
327.22	G47.37	780.57 or 327.xx	Central Sleep Apnea including High-Altitude Periodic Breathing
327.27		327.xx	Central Sleep Apnea due to a Medical Condition Not Cheyne-Stokes Breathing Pattern
327.29	F10-19		Central Sleep Apnea due to a Drug or Substance
770.81	P28.3		Primary Sleep Apnea of Infancy
327.23	G47.33	780.57	Obstructive Sleep Apnea, Adult
327.23	G47.33	780.57	Obstructive Sleep Apnea, Pediatric
327.24	G47.34	780.57	Sleep-Related Nonobstructive Alveolar Hypoventilation, Idiopathic
327.26	G47.36		Sleep-Related Hypoventilation/Hypoxemia due to Lower Airways Obstruction
327.26	G47.36		Sleep-Related Hypoventilation/Hypoxemia due to Neuromuscular and Chest Wall Disorders
327.26	G47.36		Sleep-Related Hypoventilation/Hypoxemia due to Pulmonary Parenchymal or Vascular Pathology
327.25	G47.35		Congenital Central Alveolar Hypoventilation Syndrome
327.20	G47.30	780.57	Sleep Apnea/Sleep-Related Breathing Disorder, Unspecified
Hypersomnia Not due to a Sleep-Related Breathing Disorder			
347.01	G47.41		Narcolepsy with Cataplexy
347.00	G47.419		Narcolepsy without Cataplexy
347.11	G47.42		Narcolepsy due to Medical Condition with Cataplexy
347.10	G47.42		Narcolepsy due to Medical Condition without Cataplexy
347.00		347.00	Narcolepsy, Unspecified
327.13	G47.13	307.44	Recurrent Hypersomnia
327.11	G47.11	307.44	Idiopathic Hypersomnia with Long Sleep Time
327.12	G47.12	307.44	Idiopathic Hypersomnia without Long Sleep Time
307.44	F51.12		Behaviorally Induced Insufficient Sleep Syndrome
327.14	G47.14	327.14	Hypersomnia due to a Medical Condition
292.85	F10-19	292.85	Hypersomnia due to a Drug or Substance
291.82	F10-19	292.82	Hypersomnia due to Alcohol
327.15	F51.19	327.15	Hypersomnia Not due to a Substance or Known Physiological Condition
327.10	G47.10		Physiological (Organic) Hypersomnia, Unspecified
Circadian Rhythm Sleep Disorder			
327.31	G47.21	327.31	Delayed Sleep Phase Type
327.32	G47.22		Advanced Sleep Phase Type
327.33	G47.23		Irregular Sleep-Wake Type
327.34	G47.24		Non-entrained Type (Free Running)
327.37	G47.20		Circadian Rhythm Sleep Disorder due to a Medical Condition
327.39	G47.20		Other Circadian Rhythm Sleep Disorder
327.35	F51.21	327.35	Jet Lag Type
327.36	F51.22	327.36	Shift Work Type
292.85	F10-19	292.85	Circadian Rhythm Sleep Disorder due to a Drug or Substance
291.82	F10-19	291.82	Circadian Rhythm Sleep Disorder due to Alcohol
Parasomnia			
327.41	G47.51		Confusional Arousals
307.46	F51.3	307.46	Sleepwalking
307.46	F51.4	307.46	Sleep Terrors

Continued

TABLE 20–1 Classification of Sleep Disorders According to ICSD-2, International Classification of Diseases (ICD), and *Diagnostic and Statistical Manual of Mental Disorders, Fourth Edition, Text Revision* (DSM-IV-TR)—**Cont'd**

ICD-9-CM	ICD-10	DSM-IV-TR*	Classification
327.42	G47.52	307.47[†]	REM Sleep Behavior Disorder
327.43	G47.53		Recurrent Isolated Sleep Paralysis
307.47	F51.5	307.47[†]	Nightmare Disorder
300.15	F44.9	300.15	Sleep-Related Dissociative Disorders
788.36	N39.44	307.6	Sleep Enuresis
327.49	G47.59		Catathrenia (Sleep-Related Groaning)
327.49	G47.59		Exploding Head Syndrome
368.16	R29.81		Sleep-Related Hallucinations
327.49	G47.59	307.50	Sleep-Related Eating Disorder
327.40	G47.50	307.47[†]	Parasomnia, Unspecified
292.85	F10-19	292.85	Parasomnia due to a Drug or Substance
291.82	F10-19	291.82	Parasomnia due to Alcohol
327.44	G47.54	327.44	Parasomnias due to a Medical Condition

Sleep-Related Movement Disorder

ICD-9-CM	ICD-10	DSM-IV-TR*	Classification
333.99	G25.81		Restless Legs Syndrome
327.51	G47.61		Periodic Limb Movement Disorder
327.52	G47.62		Sleep-Related Leg Cramps
327.53	G47.63		Sleep-Related Bruxism
327.59	G47.69		Sleep-Related Rhythmic Movement Disorder
327.59	G47.60		Other Sleep-Related Movement Disorder, Unspecified
327.59 or 292.85	F10-19	292.85	Sleep-Related Rhythmic Movement Disorder due to a Drug or Substance
327.59			Sleep-Related Rhythmic Movement Disorder due to a Medical Condition

Isolated Symptoms, Apparently Normal Variants, and Unresolved Issues

ICD-9-CM	ICD-10	DSM-IV-TR*	Classification
307.49	R29.81	307.47[†]	Long Sleeper
307.49	R29.81	307.47[†]	Short Sleeper
786.09	R06.5		Snoring
307.49	R29.81		Sleep Talking
307.47	R25.8		Sleep Starts, Hypnic Jerks
781.01	R25.8		Benign Sleep Myoclonus of Infancy
781.01	R25.8		Hypnagogic Foot Tremor and Alternating Leg Muscle Activation
781.01	R25.8	307.47[†]	Propriospinal Myoclonus at Sleep Onset
781.01	R25.8	307.47[†]	Excessive Fragmentary Myoclonus

Other Sleep Disorder

ICD-9-CM	ICD-10	DSM-IV-TR*	Classification
307.48	F51.8		Environmental Sleep Disorder
327.8	G47.9		Other Physiological (Organic) Sleep Disorder, Unspecified
327.8	G47.9		Other Sleep Disorder not due to Substance or known Physiological Condition

Appendix A: Sleep Disorders Associated with Conditions Classifiable Elsewhere

ICD-9-CM	ICD-10	DSM-IV-TR*	Classification
046.8	A81.8		Fatal Familial Insomnia
729.1	M79.0		Fibromyalgia
345	G40.5		Sleep-Related Epilepsy
784.0	R51		Sleep-Related Headaches
530.1	K21.9		Sleep-Related Gastroesophageal Reflux
411.8	I25.6		Sleep-Related Coronary Artery Ischemia
787.2	R13.1		Sleep-Related Abnormal Swallowing, Choking, and Laryngospasm

Appendix B: Other Psychiatric/Behavioral Disorders Frequently Encountered in the Differential Diagnosis of Sleep Disorders[‡]

Mood Disorders
Anxiety Disorders
Selected Somatoform Disorders
Schizophrenia and Other Psychotic Disorders
Selected Disorders Usually Diagnosed in Infancy, Childhood, or Adolescence
Personality Disorders

*The codes used for the DSM-IV-TR are for the most part interchangeable with the codes used for ICD-9-CM. A blank entry indicates that there was no specific DSM-IV-TR code; however, a more general code may be used.

[†]The "307.47" code is a nonspecific code for dyssomnias (which are primary disorders that disturb nighttime sleep or impair wakefulness) and parasomnias, as well as for nightmare disorder.

[‡]DSM-IV-TR codes are utilized here.

or the direction of causality in secondary insomnia. In addition, the use of the term *secondary* was believed to trivialize the importance of comorbid insomnia and potentially promote undertreatment. Comorbid insomnia is the most prevalent form of chronic insomnia. Both insomnia and secondary insomnia may be comorbid with another medical or psychiatric disorder.

There are six major types of insomnia. *Adjustment sleep disorder*[5,6] is insomnia that is associated with a specific stressor. The stressor can be psychological, physiologic, environmental, or physical. This disorder exists for a short period of time, usually days to weeks, and usually resolves when the stressor is no longer present. *Psychophysiological insomnia*[7,8] is a common form of insomnia that is present for at least 1 month and characterized by a heightened level of arousal with learned sleep-preventing associations. There is an overconcern with the inability to sleep. Negative conditioning of sleep plays a major part in the etiology of this form of insomnia. *Paradoxical insomnia*[9,10] is a complaint of severe insomnia that occurs without evidence of objective sleep disturbance and without daytime impairment of the extent that would be suggested by the amount of sleep disturbance reported. The patient often reports little or no sleep on most nights. It is thought to occur in up to 5% of insomniac patients. *Idiopathic insomnia*[11,12] is a long-standing form of insomnia that appears to date from childhood and has an insidious onset. Typically there are no factors associated with the onset of the insomnia, which is persistent without periods of remission. *Insomnia due to a mental disorder*[13,14] is insomnia caused by an underlying mental disorder. *Inadequate sleep hygiene*[15,16] is a disorder associated with common daily activities that are inconsistent with good-quality sleep and full daytime alertness. Such activities include irregular sleep onset and wake times; stimulating and alerting activities before bedtime; substances ingested around sleep, including alcohol or caffeine; and smoking cigarettes. These practices do not necessarily cause sleep disturbance in other people. For example, an irregular bedtime or wake time that might be instrumental in producing insomnia in one person may not be important in another.

Behavioral insomnia of childhood[17,18] includes the subtypes *limit-setting sleep disorder* and *sleep-onset association disorder*. Limit-setting sleep disorder is stalling or refusing to go to sleep that is eliminated once a caregiver enforces limits on sleep times and other sleep-related behaviors. Sleep-onset association disorder occurs when there is reliance on inappropriate sleep associations such as rocking, watching television, holding a bottle or other object, or requiring environmental conditions such as a lighted room or an alternative place to sleep.

Several secondary insomnias are listed. *Insomnia due to a drug or substance*[19,20] is diagnosed when there is dependence on or excessive use of a substance such as alcohol, a recreational drug, or caffeine that is associated with the occurrence of the insomnia. The insomnia may be associated with the ingestion or discontinuation of the substance.

Insomnia due to a medical condition[19,21] is diagnosed when a medical or neurologic disorder gives rise to the insomnia. *Insomnia not due to a substance or known physiological condition, unspecified* (nonorganic insomnia), is the diagnosis applied when the insomnia cannot be classified elsewhere and is suspected to be due to an underlying mental disorder, psychological factor, or sleep-disruptive practice.

Differentiation between the use of the diagnoses *inadequate sleep hygiene* and *insomnia due to a drug or substance* requires some explanation. Caffeine ingestion in the form of coffee or soda can produce a disorder of inadequate sleep hygiene if the intake is normal and within the limits of common use but the timing of ingestion is inappropriate, whereas caffeine ingestion that is considered excessive or abnormal by normal standards can lead to a diagnosis of insomnia due to a drug or substance.

Sleep-Related Breathing Disorder

The disorders in this subgroup are characterized by disordered respiration during sleep. *Central apnea syndromes*[22,23] include those in which respiratory effort is diminished or absent in an intermittent or cyclical fashion due to central nervous system dysfunction. Two major forms of central sleep apnea are associated with underlying pathologic or environmental causes, such as *Cheyne-Stokes breathing pattern*[24,25] or *high-altitude periodic breathing*.[26,27]

Primary central sleep apnea[22,23] is a disorder of unknown cause characterized by recurrent episodes of cessation of breathing during sleep without associated ventilatory effort. A complaint of excessive daytime sleepiness, insomnia, or difficulty breathing during sleep is reported. The patient must not have hypercapnia (partial pressure of CO_2 >45 mm Hg). Five or more apneic episodes per hour of sleep are required by polysomnography. *Central sleep apnea including Cheyne-Stokes breathing pattern*[24,25] is characterized by recurrent apneas and/or hypopneas alternating with prolonged hyperpnea in which tidal volume waxes and wanes in a crescendo-decrescendo pattern. This pattern is characteristically seen in non–rapid eye movement (NREM) sleep and does not occur in rapid eye movement (REM) sleep. This pattern is typically seen in medical disorders such as heart failure, cerebrovascular disorders, and renal failure. *Central sleep apnea including high-altitude periodic breathing*[26,27] is characterized by cycling periods of apnea and hyperpnea with the apnea being associated with no ventilatory effort. The cycle length is typically between 12 and 34 seconds. Five or more central apneas per hour of sleep are required to make the diagnosis. Most people will have this ventilatory pattern at elevations greater than 7600 m, and some at lower altitudes. *Central sleep apnea due to a medical condition not Cheyne-Stokes breathing pattern* is the diagnosis applied to patients who have brain stem lesions of vascular, neoplastic, degenerative, demyelinating, or traumatic origin.

A secondary form of *central sleep apnea due to a drug or substance*[28,29] is most commonly associated with long-term opioid use. This substance causes respiratory depression by acting on the μ-receptors of the ventral medulla. A central apnea index of greater than 5 is required for the diagnosis. *Primary sleep apnea of infancy*[30,31] is a disorder of respiratory control most often seen in preterm infants (apnea of prematurity), but it can occur in predisposed infants (apnea of infancy). This may be a developmental pattern, or secondary to other medical disorders. Respiratory pauses of 20 seconds or longer are required for the diagnosis.

The *obstructive sleep apnea syndromes* include those in which there is an obstruction in the airway resulting in increased breathing effort and inadequate ventilation. Upper airway resistance syndrome has been recognized as a manifestation of obstructive sleep apnea syndrome and therefore is not included as a separate diagnosis. Adult and pediatric forms of obstructive sleep apnea syndrome are discussed separately because the disorders have different methods of diagnosis and treatment.

Obstructive sleep apnea, adult[32,33] is characterized by repetitive episodes of cessation of breathing (apneas) or partial upper airway obstruction (hypopneas). These events are often associated with reduced blood oxygen saturation. Snoring and sleep disruption are typical and common. Excessive daytime sleepiness or insomnia can result. Five or more respiratory events (apneas, hypopneas, or respiratory effort–related arousals) per hour of sleep are required for diagnosis. Increased respiratory effort occurs during the respiratory event. *Obstructive sleep apnea, pediatric*[34,35] is characterized by features similar to those seen in adults, but cortical arousals may not occur, possibly because of a higher arousal threshold. At least one obstructive event, of at least two respiratory cycles in duration, per hour of sleep is required for diagnosis.

Sleep-related hypoventilation/hypoxemic syndromes is a group heading for disorders that produce hypoventilation with hypoxemia during sleep. The disorder *sleep-related nonobstructive alveolar hypoventilation, idiopathic*[36,37] is characterized by reduced alveolar ventilation resulting in oxygen desaturation in patients with normal mechanical properties of the lungs. *Congenital central alveolar hypoventilation syndrome*[38,39] is a failure of automatic central control of breathing in infants who do not breathe spontaneously or breath shallowly and erratically. *Sleep-related hypoventilation/hypoxemia due to a medical condition* is a group heading that applies to abnormalities in lung or vascular pathology, including lower airways obstruction and neuromuscular or chest wall disorders. *Sleep-related hypoventilation/hypoxemia due to pulmonary parenchymal or vascular pathology*[40,41] is due to lung disease with significant oxygen desaturation such as that seen in chronic obstructive pulmonary disease, cystic fibrosis, and interstitial lung disease, as documented by pulmonary function testing or imaging studies. *Sleep-related hypoventilation/hypoxemia due to lower airways obstruction*[42,43] is seen in patients with lower airways disease such as chronic obstructive lung disease. *Sleep-related hypoventilation/hypoxemia due to neuromuscular and chest wall disorders*[44,45] is seen in patients with neuromuscular disease or kyphoscoliosis.

A final category is *sleep apnea/sleep-related breathing disorder, unspecified*. This category is for sleep-related breathing disorders that cannot be classified elsewhere but are believed to be a function of respiratory disturbance in sleep.

Hypersomnia Not due to a Sleep-Related Breathing Disorder

The hypersomnia disorders are those in which the primary complaint is daytime sleepiness and the cause of the primary symptom is not disturbed nocturnal sleep or misaligned circadian rhythms. Daytime sleepiness is defined as the inability to stay alert and awake during the major waking episodes of the day, resulting in unintended lapses into sleep. Other sleep disorders may be present, but they must first be effectively treated.

Narcolepsy with cataplexy[46,47] requires the documentation of a definite history of cataplexy. This diagnosis may be confirmed by sleep studies with a mean sleep latency of ≤8 minutes and 2 or more sleep-onset REM periods, or cerebrospinal fluid hypocretin levels of less than 110 pg/ml. A diagnosis of *narcolepsy without cataplexy*[48,49] is made when cataplexy is not present but when there is sleep paralysis, hypnagogic hallucinations, or supportive evidence in the form of a positive Multiple Sleep Latency Test. *Narcolepsy due to a medical condition (with or without cataplexy)*[50,51] is the diagnosis applied to a patient with sleepiness who has a significant neurologic or medical disorder that accounts for the daytime sleepiness.

Recurrent hypersomnia[52,53] consists of two subtypes: *Kleine-Levin syndrome* and *menstrual-related hypersomnia*. Kleine-Levin syndrome is associated with episodes of sleepiness with binge eating, hypersexuality, or mood changes. Menstrual-related hypersomnia usually occurs within a few months of menarche.

Idiopathic hypersomnia with long sleep time[54,55] is the classic form of idiopathic hypersomnia that is characterized by a major sleep episode that is at least 10 hours in duration. In contrast, *idiopathic hypersomnia without long sleep time*[56,57] is the commonly seen disorder of excessive sleepiness with unintended naps that are typically unrefreshing. *Behaviorally induced insufficient sleep syndrome*[58,59] occurs in patients who have a habitual short sleep episode and who sleep considerably longer when the habitual sleep episode is not maintained.

Hypersomnia due to a medical condition[60,61] is hypersomnia that is caused by a medical or neurologic disorder. Cataplexy or other diagnostic features of narcolepsy are not present. *Hypersomnia due to a drug or substance*[62,63] is diagnosed when the complaint is believed to be secondary to current or past use of drugs. *Hypersomnia not due to a substance or known physiological condition*[64,65] is excessive sleepiness that is associated with a psychiatric diagnosis.

Circadian Rhythm Sleep Disorder

The circadian rhythm sleep disorders share a common underlying chronophysiologic basis. The major feature of these disorders is a persistent or recurrent misalignment between the patient's sleep pattern and the pattern that is desired or regarded as the societal norm. Maladaptive behaviors influence the presentation and severity of the circadian rhythm sleep disorders. The underlying problem in the majority of the circadian rhythm sleep disorders is that the patient cannot sleep when sleep is desired, needed, or expected. The wake episodes can occur at undesired times as a result of sleep episodes that occur at inappropriate times; therefore, the patient may complain of insomnia or excessive sleepiness. For several of the circadian rhythm sleep disorders, once sleep is initiated, the major sleep episode is of normal duration with normal REM-NREM cycling.

Circadian rhythm sleep disorder, delayed sleep phase type,[66,67] which is more commonly seen in adolescents, is characterized by a delay in the phase of the major sleep period in relation to the desired sleep time and wake time, whereas *circadian rhythm sleep disorder, advanced sleep phase type,*[68,69] which is more commonly seen in the elderly, is characterized by an advance in the phase of the major sleep period in relation to the desired sleep time and wake time. *Circadian rhythm sleep disorder, irregular sleep-wake type,*[70,71] a disorder that has a lack of a clearly defined circadian rhythm of sleep and wakefulness, is most often seen in the institutionalized elderly and is associated with a lack of synchronizing agents such as light, activity, and social activities. *Circadian rhythm sleep disorder, non-entrained type (free-running)*[72,73] occurs because there is a lack of entrainment to the 24-hour period and the sleep pattern often follows that of the underlying free-running pacemaker with a sequential shift in the daily sleep pattern.

Circadian rhythm sleep disorder, jet lag type (jet lag disorder)[74,75] is related to a temporal mismatch between the timing of the sleep-wake cycle generated by the endogenous circadian clock produced by a rapid change in time zones. The severity of the disorder is influenced by the number of time zones crossed and the direction of travel, with eastward travel usually being more disruptive. *Circadian rhythm sleep disorder, shift work type (shift work disorder),*[76,77] is characterized by complaints of insomnia or excessive sleepiness that occur in relation to work hours that are scheduled during the usual sleep period. *Circadian rhythm sleep disorder due to a medical condition*[78,79] is related to an underlying primary medical or neurologic disorder. A disrupted sleep-wake pattern leads to complaints of insomnia or excessive daytime sleepiness.

Other circadian rhythm sleep disorder is an irregular or unconventional sleep-wake pattern that can be due to social, behavioral, or environmental factors. Noise, lighting, or other factors can predispose someone to developing this disorder.

The appropriate timing of sleep within the 24-hour day can be disturbed in many other sleep disorders, particularly disorders associated with the complaint of insomnia. Patients with narcolepsy can have a pattern of sleepiness that is identical to that described as due to an irregular sleep-wake type. However, because the primary sleep diagnosis is narcolepsy, the patient should not receive a second diagnosis of a circadian rhythm sleep disorder unless the disorder is unrelated to the narcolepsy. For example, a diagnosis of jet lag type could be stated along with a diagnosis of narcolepsy, if appropriate. Similarly, patients with mood disorders or psychoses can, at times, have a sleep pattern similar to that of delayed sleep phase type. A diagnosis of delayed sleep phase type would be coded only if the disorder is not directly associated with the psychiatric disorder.

Some disturbance of sleep timing is a common feature in patients who have a diagnosis of inadequate sleep hygiene. Only if the timing of sleep is the predominant cause of the sleep disturbance and is outside the societal norm would the patient be given a diagnosis of a circadian rhythm sleep disorder. Limit-setting sleep disorder is also associated with an altered time of sleep within the 24-hour day. If the setting of limits is a function of the caregiver, then the sleep disorder is more appropriately diagnosed as a limit-setting sleep disorder.

Parasomnia

The parasomnias are undesirable physical or experiential events that accompany sleep. These disorders consist of sleep disorders that are not abnormalities of the processes responsible for sleep and awake states per se but are undesirable phenomena that occur predominantly during sleep. The parasomnias consist of abnormal sleep-related movements, behaviors, emotions, perceptions, dreaming, and autonomic nervous system functioning. They are disorders of arousal, partial arousal, and sleep stage transition. Many of the parasomnias are manifestations of central nervous system activation. Autonomic nervous system changes and skeletal muscle activity are the predominant features. The parasomnias often occur in conjunction with other sleep disorders such as obstructive sleep apnea syndrome. It is not uncommon for several parasomnias to occur in a single patient.

Three parasomnias, called *disorders of arousal*, have typically been associated with arousal from non-REM sleep. *Confusional arousals*[80,81] are characterized by mental confusion or confusional behavior that occurs during or following arousal from sleep. These arousals are common in children and can occur not only from nocturnal sleep but also from daytime naps. They sometimes can occur in association with obstructive sleep apnea syndrome. *Sleepwalking*[82,83] is a series of complex behaviors that occur with sudden arousals from slow-wave sleep and result in walking behavior during a state of altered consciousness. Sleep terrors[84,85] also occur from slow-wave sleep and are associated with a cry or piercing scream accompanied by autonomic nervous system activation and behavioral manifestation of intense fear. Individuals may be difficult to arouse from the episode and when aroused can be confused and subsequently amnestic for the episode. These two disorders can often coexist together and sometimes one form may blend into the other or be difficult to distinguish from the other.

Several parasomnias are typically associated with the REM sleep stage. Some common underlying pathophysiologic mechanism related to REM sleep may underlie these disorders. REM sleep behavior disorder[86,87] (RBD) has abnormal behaviors that occur from REM sleep that can cause injury or sleep disruption. The behaviors are often violent, with dream enactment that is action filled. The disorder can occur in narcolepsy, and many patients with Parkinson's disease have RBD. The delayed emergence of a neurodegenerative disorder can occur, especially in men over the age of 50 years. There are two subtypes: parasomnia overlap syndrome and status dissociatus. Parasomnia overlap syndrome is RBD associated with a disorder of arousal. Status dissociatus is RBD in an extreme form with unidentifiable sleep stages.

Recurrent isolated sleep paralysis[88,89] can occur at sleep onset or upon awakening and is characterized by an inability to perform voluntary movements. Ventilation is usually unaffected. Hallucinatory experiences often accompany the paralysis. Nightmare disorder[90,91] is characterized by recurrent nightmares that occur from REM sleep, and result in an awakening with intense anxiety, fear, or other negative feelings.

Sleep-related dissociative disorders[92,93] are disorders that involve a disruption of the integrative features of consciousness, memory, identity, or perception of the environment. These disorders can occur in the transition from wakefulness to sleep or after an awakening from stage 1 or 2 sleep. A history of physical or sexual abuse is common in such patients. These patients fulfill the DSM-IV criteria for dissociative disorder. Sleep enuresis[94,95] is recurrent involuntary voiding that occurs during sleep. Enuresis is considered primary in a child who has never been dry for 6 months or longer; otherwise it is called secondary. Catathrenia (sleep-related groaning)[96,97] is an unusual disorder in which there is a chronic, often nightly, expiratory groaning that occurs during sleep. The affected person is often unaware of the groaning. The disorder is rare and the pathophysiology unknown. Exploding head syndrome[98,99] is characterized by a loud imagined noise or sense of a violent explosion that occurs in the head as the patient is falling asleep or during waking in the night. Sleep-related hallucinations[100,101] are predominantly visual hallucinations that occur prior to sleep onset or upon awakening from sleep. Sleep-related eating disorder[102,103] involves recurrent eating and

drinking episodes during arousals from nocturnal sleep. The eating behavior is uncontrollable, and often the patient is unaware of the behavior until the next morning. It can be associated with sleepwalking and can be medication induced.

Parasomnia, unspecified is usually a temporary diagnosis until a definitive diagnosis is made. Parasomnia due to a drug or substance is a parasomnia that has a close temporal relationship with exposure to a drug, medication, or biological substance. Parasomnia due to a medical condition is the manifestation of a parasomnia associated with an underlying medical or neurologic disorder.

Sleep-Related Movement Disorder

The sleep-related movement disorders are characterized by relatively simple, usually stereotyped, movements that disturb sleep. Disorders such as periodic limb movement disorder and restless legs syndrome are classified in this section of th ICSD-2.

Restless legs syndrome[104,105] is characterized by a complaint of a strong, nearly irresistible urge to move the legs. The sensations are worse at rest and occur more frequently in the evening or during the night. Walking or moving the legs relieves the sensation. Periodic limb movement disorder[106,107] is often associated with restless legs syndrome but can occur as an independent disorder. In this condition repetitive, highly stereotyped limb movements occur during sleep. Sleep-related leg cramps[108,109] are painful sensations that cause sudden intense muscle contractions usually of the calves or small muscles of the feet. Episodes commonly occur during the sleep period and can lead to disrupted sleep. Relief is usually obtained by stretching the affected muscle. Sleep-related bruxism[110,111] is characterize by clenching of the teeth during sleep that can result in arousals. Often the activity is severe or frequent enough to result in symptoms of temporomandibular joint pain or wearing down of the teeth. Sleep-related rhythmic movement disorder[112,113] is a stereotyped, repetitive rhythmic motor behavior that occurs during drowsiness or light sleep and results in large movements of the head, body, or limbs. Typically seen in children, the disorder can also be seen in adults. Head and limb injuries can result from violent movements. Rhythmic movement disorder can also occur during full wakefulness and alertness, particularly in individuals who are mentally retarded.

Other sleep-related movement disorder, unspecifed is a temporary diagnosis of a movement disorder until a more definitive diagnosis can be made. Sleep-related movement disorder due to a drug or substance is a movement disorder not specified elsewhere that appears to have a substance as the basis. Sleep-related movement disorder due to a medical condition is a movement disorder that occurs during sleep that is diagnosed before a psychiatric disorder can be ascertained.

Isolated Symptoms, Apparently Normal Variants, and Unresolved Issues

This section of the ICSD-2 lists sleep-related symptoms that are on the borderline between normal and abnormal sleep. Sleep length and snoring are two examples.

A *long sleeper*[114,115] is a person who sleeps more in the 24-hour day than the typical person. Sleep is normal in architecture and quality. Usually sleep lengths of 10 hours or greater qualify for this diagnosis. Symptoms of excessive sleepiness occur if the person does not get that amount of sleep. A *short sleeper*[114,115] is a person with a routine pattern of obtaining 5 hours or less of sleep in a 24-hour day. In children, this sleep length can be 3 hours or less than the norm for age group. *Snoring*[116,117] is diagnosed when a respiratory sound is disturbing to the patient, a bed partner, or others. This diagnosis is made when the snoring is not associated with either insomnia or excessive sleepiness. Snoring not only can lead to impaired health but may be a cause of social embarrassment and can disturb the sleep of a bed partner. Snoring associated with obstructive sleep apnea syndrome is not diagnosed as snoring. *Sleep* talking[118,119] can be either idiopathic or associated with other disorders such as RBD or sleep-related eating disorder.

Sleep starts (hypnic jerks)[120,121] are sudden brief contractions of the body that occur at sleep onset. These movements are associated either with a sensation of falling, a sensory flash, or a sleep-onset dream. *Benign sleep myoclonus of infancy*[122,123] is a disorder of myoclonic jerks that occur during sleep in infants. It typically occurs from birth to age 6 months and is benign and resolves spontaneously. *Hypnagogic foot tremor and alternating leg muscle activation*[124,125] occurs at the transition between wake and sleep or during light NREM sleep. It is demonstrated by recurrent electromyographic potentials in one or both feet that are longer than the myoclonic range (greater than 250 msec). *Propriospinal myoclonus at sleep onset*[126,127] is a disorder of recurrent sudden muscular jerks in the transition from wakefulness to sleep. The disorder may be associated with severe sleep-onset insomnia. *Excessive fragmentary myoclonus*[128,129] is small muscle twitches in the fingers, toes, or corner of the mouth that do not cause actual movements across a joint. The myoclonus is often a finding during polysomnography that is often asymptomatic or can be associated with daytime sleepiness or fatigue.

Other Sleep Disorders

These disorders are difficult to fit into any other classification section. *Other physiological (organic) sleep disorder* is a temporary diagnosis until a definitive diagnosis can be made. *Other sleep disorder not due to substance or known physiological condition* is a disorder that cannot be classified elsewhere that is suspected of having a psychiatric or behavioral basis. *Environmental sleep disorder*[130,131] is a sleep disturbance that is caused by a disturbing environmental factor that disrupts sleep and leads to a complaint of either insomnia or excessive sleepiness.

Appendix A: Sleep Disorders Associated with Conditions Classifiable Elsewhere

Fatal familial insomnia[132–134] is a progressive disorder characterized by difficulty in falling asleep and maintaining sleep that develops into enacted dreams and stupor. Autonomic hyperactivity with pyrexia, excessive salivation, and hyperhidrosis leads to cardiac and respiratory failure. It is a prion disease that leads eventually to death. *Fibromyalgia*[135,136] is characterized by widespread pain of at least 3 months' duration and muscle tenderness, as determined by palpation. *Sleep-related epilepsy*[137,138] is diagnosed when epilepsy occurs during sleep. Several epilepsy types are associated with sleep, including nocturnal frontal lobe epilepsy, benign epilepsy of childhood with centrotemporal spikes, and juvenile myoclonic epilepsy. *Sleep-related headaches*[139,140] are headaches that occur during sleep or upon awakening from sleep. Chronic paroxysmal hemicrania, hypnic headache, or cluster headaches can all occur during sleep. *Sleep-related gastroesophageal reflux*[141,142] is characterized by regurgitation of stomach contents into the esophagus during sleep. Shortness of breath or heartburn can result, but occasionally the disorder can be asymptomatic. *Sleep-related coronary artery ischemia*[143,144] is ischemia of the myocardium that occurs at night. *Sleep-related abnormal swallowing, choking, and laryngospasm*[145,146] is a disorder in which dysfunction of the muscles of deglutition lead to pooling of saliva in the upper airway with coughing and choking and arousal from sleep.

Appendix B: Other Psychiatric/Behavioral Disorders Frequently Encountered in the Differential Diagnosis of Sleep Disorders

This final section of the ICSD-2 lists the psychiatric diagnoses that are often encountered during an evaluation of sleep complaints. Many psychiatric disorders are associated with disturbances of sleep and wakefulness. The main sleep-related features are presented. Psychiatric diagnoses that are discussed include mood disorders; anxiety disorders; somatoform disorders; schizophrenia and other psychotic disorders; disorders first diagnosed in infancy, childhood, or adolescence; and personality disorders.[147,148]

SUMMARY AND CONCLUSION

The classification of sleep disorders, preferably done on a pathophysiologic basis, is necessary to discriminate among disorders in order to facilitate an understanding of the symptoms, etiology, pathophysiology, and treatment. The earliest classification systems were largely organized according to the major symptoms, as the pathophysiologic basis for many of the sleep disorders was unknown. The main symptoms in sleep medicine are insomnia, excessive sleepiness, and abnormal events that occur during sleep. These three categories allow for a classification system that is easily understood by physicians and is useful for developing a differential diagnosis. With the development of modern sleep research, some categories now can be based on pathophysiology. The International Classification of Sleep Disorders, edition 2 (ICSD-2), published in 2005, combines a symptomatic presentation (insomnia) with one organized in part on pathophysiology (circadian rhythms) and in part on body systems (breathing disorders). This organization is necessary because of the varied nature of the sleep disorders and the fact that the pathophysiology for many of the disorders is unknown. The ICSD-2 is not just a listing of the sleep disorders but is a text manual that lists relevant information on the diagnostic features and epidemiology to help the reader more easily differentiate among the disorders.

✪ REFERENCES

A full list of references are available at www.expertconsult.com

CHAPTER 21

Epidemiology of Sleep Disorders

Maurice Moyses Ohayon and **Christian Guilleminault**

INTRODUCTION

The epidemiology of sleep disorders is still a fledgling discipline encompassing a broad range of phenomena, such as insomnia, hypersomnia, sleep apnea, and parasomnias. Surveys in the field remain scarce, and existing figures are difficult to compare owing primarily to the considerable shift undergone by sleep disorder classifications over the years. This in itself may account in large part for the wide variance in prevalence rates between the earliest and the most recent studies. Methodologic differences and sample size are other factors warranting scrutiny. Also, the interpretation of results is limited by the near-exclusive reliance on self-reported data. Consequently, the picture of sleep disorders in the general population remains hazy, but a sharper resolution is in the offing as the literature steadily grows and improves.

This chapter provides a general review of the epidemiologic surveys into sleep disorders over the past 20 years. It is divided into four main sections covering the phenomena most commonly investigated in the general population: (1) insomnia and associated syndromes; (2) excessive sleepiness; (3) sleep-disordered breathing; and (4) parasomnias.

THE HAZARDS OF SLEEP CLASSIFICATIONS

Classifications represent the advancement of our knowledge and understanding of sleep disorders. They are attempts to provide operationalized criteria to delineate abnormal sleep in all its forms. Abnormality, however, exists relative to a norm. This would imply that we know

what constitutes normal sleep, but not abnormal sleep. Yet, the contrary is true. At this point in time, we can only say what does *not* constitute normal sleep. The International Classification of Sleep Disorders (ICSD)[1] was the first exhaustive attempt to classify abnormal sleep.

The difficulty in distinguishing between normal and abnormal sleep is reflected in the evolution of the classifications and definitions of symptomatology. For example, insomnia was defined by the American Institute of Medicine in 1979 as unsatisfactory sleep.[2] In the same year, the Association of Sleep Disorders Centers published its first classification,[3] in which insomnia was referred to as a "heterogeneous group of conditions... considered to be responsible for inducing disturbed sleep or diminished sleep" (p. 21).

In 1987, the American Psychiatric Association for the first time devoted a section in the *Diagnostic and Statistical Manual of Mental Disorders, Third Edition, Revised* to sleep disorders.[4] The section was essentially divided into dyssomnias (insomnia, hypersomnia, and sleep-wake disorders) and parasomnias (sleepwalking, sleep terrors, and nightmares). Insomnia was defined as difficulty initiating sleep (DIS), difficulty maintaining sleep (DMS)—be it in the form of disrupted sleep (DS) or early morning awakening (s)— or nonrestorative sleep lasting at least 1 month, occurring at least three times a week, and causing either distress or daytime repercussions.

In 1990, efforts by an international group of sleep researchers and sleep specialists produced the ICSD,[1] which listed nearly 80 sleep disorder diagnoses. In this classification, insomnia was more stringently defined by taking into account severity, frequency of symptoms, and impact on social and occupational functioning. Two updates of this classification have been published since that time.[5,6]

In the *Diagnostic and Statistical Manual of Mental Disorders, Fourth Edition*, the latest edition of the classification published in 1994,[7] the American Psychiatric Association decided to harmonize its sleep disorder criteria and diagnoses with those of the ICSD-90. Insomnia was defined as a complaint of DIS, DMS, or nonrestorative sleep lasting at least 1 month and causing either distress or daytime consequences.

This evolution in classifications is also reflected in the epidemiologic studies of sleep disorders. This has rendered comparisons between earlier and more recent surveys problematic for three principal reasons: (1) symptomatology is defined differently across studies; (2) time frames are also different; and (3) different methodologies have been used to collect data.

INSOMNIA AND ASSOCIATED SYNDROMES

Since the end of 1970s, more than 50 epidemiologic studies have assessed the prevalence of insomnia symptomatology in the general population. Methodologies have included face-to-face interviews, postal questionnaires, telephone interviews, or a combination of two of these.

The definition of insomnia has also varied considerably from one survey to another. Earlier studies evaluated insomnia based on the presence of DIS or DMS regardless of the frequency or severity of the symptoms or daytime consequences. These studies were done simply by asking about the presence of these symptoms. Subsequently, DIS or DMS were assessed using the frequency of the symptom, an occurrence of 3 nights or more per week being necessary for the symptom to be present. Other studies asked about the severity of the symptoms, for example, being bothered "a lot" or "not at all" by the symptom.

Other studies, in addition to assessing the presence of insomnia symptoms, inquired about daytime repercussions of these symptoms such as daytime sleepiness, irritability, depressive or anxious mood, or needing to seek help. Finally, other studies inquired about dissatisfaction with sleep quantity or quality.

Epidemiology of Insomnia Complaints

In epidemiologic studies, the binary query about the presence of insomnia symptoms gave high prevalence rates, with an average around 33%. One of the earliest epidemiologic surveys on insomnia symptoms was carried out by Bixler et al.[8] in the metropolitan area of Los Angeles with 1006 respondents age 18 years or older. The overall prevalence of insomnia symptoms was 32.2% (DIS: 14.4%; DS: 22.9%; EMA: 13.8%). Subsequent studies[9–13] found a similar prevalence in the general population when inquiries were made about the presence of insomnia symptoms.

Epidemiologic studies using frequency to determine the prevalence of insomnia symptoms are the most common.[14–23] In some studies, the subjects had to make a subjective assessment of the frequency of the symptom on a 4- or 5-point scale[14,19,22,24]—for example, "never," "sometimes," "often," or "always," with "often" or "always" being the cut-off point to determine the presence of insomnia. Mostly, however, frequency of the symptom is assessed on a weekly basis[13–19]: for example, never, one or two nights, three or four nights, five nights or more per week; a frequency of three nights or more per week being the cutoff used to conclude the presence of insomnia. The prevalence of insomnia symptoms drops to around 16–21% when frequency is used to determine the presence of insomnia, and has similar rates among countries.

Epidemiologic studies using severity of the symptoms (e.g., being bothered a lot; having great or very great DIS or DMS or a major complaint) gave prevalences of insomnia between 10% and 28% of the general population.[25–29]

In most of the studies that assessed the prevalence of insomnia symptoms accompanied with daytime consequences, the prevalence was much lower, about 10%.[16,17,20,30–32] One study provided a higher prevalence than the other studies mainly because the rate was based on lifetime estimation.[30]

Dissatisfaction with the quantity of sleep can be expressed as a complaint of not sleeping enough or sleeping too much. Not sleeping enough has been reported with prevalences ranging from 20% to 41.7% in the general population.[26,33–35] Sleeping too much is far less frequent, with prevalences ranging between 2.8% and 9.5%.[8,31,36]

Dissatisfaction with quality of sleep had various definitions. In some studies, participants were asked to assess their level of satisfaction with their sleep. The prevalence of individuals reporting being dissatisfied with their sleep ranged from 8% to 18.5%.[37–41] Other studies have inquired about perception of sleep as being poor or subjects considering themselves as being insomniac. Between 10% and 18.1% of the population reported being poor sleepers or being insomniacs.[23,42–44]

Unfortunately, most of these studies did not provide any information about the chronicity of these symptoms. Studies that did measure chronicity showed that insomnia is mostly chronic. Only 4% of subjects with insomnia symptoms reported a duration of 1 month or less. About 6% of these subjects evaluated the duration as between 1 and 6 months; 5% said the duration wa between 6 and 12 months, and 85% mentioned a duration of 1 year or more (68% said it had lasted 5 years or more).[45]

Insomnia in the Elderly

Almost all epidemiologic studies have reported an increased prevalence of insomnia symptoms with age, reaching close to 50% in elderly individuals (≥65 years old). However, reports of the prevalence of insomnia with daytime consequences and the prevalence of sleep dissatisfaction have been mixed.

Insomnia in the elderly noninstitutionalized population has been the subject of several epidemiologic studies.[40,46–56] Most of these studies were limited to insomnia symptoms; only two studies assessed sleep dissatisfaction.[49,56] Prevalence based on presence/absence of insomnia symptoms had a very high rate (up to 65%). In elderly community-based samples, the prevalence of insomnia symptoms and sleep dissatisfaction did not significantly increase with age but were higher in women than in men. Some studies found that insomnia symptoms without sleep dissatisfaction have a weak association with physical diseases and mental disorders.

Summary

The definition of insomnia symptoms varies considerably across studies, as do the time frame and the wording of questions (Table 21–1). Most investigations assessed DMS, DIS, and EMA but defined these differently. Few specifically addressed the daytime consequences or distress accompanying insomnia symptomatology.[20,27,31–34] The mental health status of insomnia complainers was rarely explored,[28,31–34] despite it being the most frequently associated factor observed in sleep clinics.[64–66]

EXCESSIVE SLEEPINESS

Until recently, excessive sleepiness had received less attention than insomnia, though its consequences can be severe. For instance, sleepiness is involved in approximately 16% of motor vehicle accidents in England.[67] Moreover, it has been suggested that half the work-related accidents and a quarter of household accidents are caused by sleepiness.[68]

Existing studies (Table 21–2) can be divided into two main categories: those measuring hypersomnia symptoms and those assessing excessive daytime sleepiness (EDS). In the former, participants are generally queried regarding perceived sleep excess or daytime naps. In the latter, "daytime sleepiness" refers to sleep propensity in situations of diminished attention. However, the terms *hypersomnia* and *excessive daytime sleepiness* are often used interchangeably, and EDS is defined differently across surveys.

Epidemiology of Excessive Sleepiness Symptoms

Hypersomnia rates have been reported in four U.S. studies. Karacan et al.[19] found a rate of 0.3%, Bixler et al.[8] found 4.2%, and Ford and Kamerow[31] reported a 6-month prevalence of 3.2%. In this last study, subjects were asked whether they had gone a period of 2 weeks or more in which they slept too much (hypersomnia). No gender difference was observed and the rate was highest in the youngest age group (18- to 24-year-olds). Using the same criteria as Ford and Kamerow, Breslau et al.[30] found a lifetime prevalence of hypersomnia of 16.3% in

their young adult sample (21-30 years of age). Klink and Quan[9] measured EDS by asking participants whether they fell asleep during the day. They found an overall prevalence of 12%. The rate increased with age but was not gender related. In their study, Téllez-Lòpez et al.[29] found a rate of hypersomnia of 9.5% (defined as "getting too much sleep") and a rate of EDS of 21.5% (defined as "a strong need to sleep in the day"). In both cases, rates decreased with age for women.

Hays et al.[79] assessed the mortality risk associated with EDS in an elderly sample of 3962 subjects living in the community. Measuring EDS on the basis of self-reported napping, they reported a rate of 25.2%. They found that elderly persons who napped most of the time and made two or more errors on a cognitive status test had a higher mortality rate by a factor of 1.73. Frequent daytime nappers were more likely to be men, to be overweight, and to report insomnia complaints and depressive symptoms. They were also more limited in their physical activity and had more functional impairment. The study by Kripke et al.[80] revealed that long sleep (>9 hours per night) and short sleep (<4 hours per night) were associated with a mortality risk 1.8 times higher at a 6-year follow-up, compared with the rest of the population. A similar study performed in California by Wingard and Berkman[81] found that, among people who slept either more than 9 hours or less than 6 hours per night, the mortality risk for men and women, respectively, was 1.7 and 1.6 times as high as for the general population.

Most of the epidemiologic surveys focusing on the phenomenon of excessive sleepiness in the general population have been conducted in the Nordic countries (Iceland, Finland, Sweden). Gislason and Almqvist[25] reported a moderate EDS prevalence of 16.7% and a major EDS prevalence of 5.7% in their male sample. Both significantly decreased with age. Another study was performed by Janson et al.[82] on a young adult population from three countries (20–44 years of age). They found a prevalence of daytime sleepiness, occurring at least 1 day per week, of about 40%; daily daytime sleepiness was observed in about 5% of the sample.

Martikainen et al.,[69] who used a more restrictive definition of EDS, found that 9.8% of their 1190 Finnish respondents ages 36–50 years reported being "clearly more tired than others," experiencing a "daily desire to sleep in the course of normal activities," or feeling "very tired daily." Hublin et al.[70] found a prevalence of daytime sleepiness occurring daily or almost daily of 9% in their Finnish twin cohort. Finally, Ohayon et al.[36] assessed daytime sleepiness on a severity scale in their U.K. sample. Severe daytime sleepiness was observed in 5.5% of their sample, and moderate daytime sleepiness in 15.2%.

Unlike insomnia symptoms, EDS is generally not gender related. Whether its prevalence increases or decreases with age is not clear, as both trends have been observed.[9,25]

TABLE 21-1 Definition and Prevalence of Insomnia in the General Population

Authors	Year	Location	N	Age	Definition	Prevalence (%) Male/Female
Karacan et al.[19]	1976	Alachua County, FL (USA)	1645	≥18	Trouble with sleep often or all the time	10.9/15.4
Bixler et al.[8]	1979	Los Angeles, CA (USA)	1006	≥18	Presence of DIS, DMS, or EMA	28.9/34.8
Welstein et al.[13]	1983	San Francisco, CA (USA)	6340	≥6	Presence of DIS, DMS, or EMA	31.0
Karacan et al.[24]	1983	Houston, TX (USA)	2347	≥18	Often or always has DIS or DMS	18.6/28.6
Lugaresi et al.[42]	1983	San Marino, Italy	5713	≥3	Always or almost always has a bad sleep	9.9/16.8
Mellinger et al.[28]	1985	USA	3161	≥18	Being bothered a lot by DIS, DMS, or EMA	14.0/20.0
Klink and Quan[9]	1987	Tucson, AZ (USA)	2187	≥18	Presence of DIS, DMS, or EMA	37.8
Gislason and Almqvist[25]	1987	Uppsala, Sweden	3201 men	30–69	Major complaints of DIS or DMS	DIS: 6.9 DMS: 7.5
Liljenberg et al.[27]	1988	Gävleborg & Kopparberg counties, Sweden	3557	30–65	Great or very great DIS or DMS	DIS: 5.1/7.1 DMS: 7.7/8.9
Ford and Kamerow[31]	1989	Baltimore, MD; Durham, NC; Los Angeles, CA (USA)	7954	≥18	Presence of DIS, DMS, or EMA lasting ≥2 wk, and seeking professional help for the problem, or using sleep-promoting medication, or interfering a lot with daily life	7.9/12.1
Husby and Lingjærde[26]	1990	Tromsø, Norway	14,667	20–54	Being bothered by sleeplessness	29.9/41.7
Quera-Salva et al.[12]	1991	France	1003	≥16	Presence of DIS, DMS, or EMA	48.0
Weyerer and Dilling[57]	1991	Upper Bavarian area, Germany	1536	≥15	• Mild insomnia • Moderate/severe insomnia	15.0 13.5
Klink et al.[10]	1992	Tucson, AZ (USA)	2187	≥18	Presence of DIS, DMS, or EMA	34.1
Brabbins et al.[48]	1993	Liverpool, UK	1070	≥65	DIS, DMSs or EMA; 1-mo prevalence	35.0
Janson et al.[18]	1995	Reykjavik, Iceland; Uppsala & Göteborg, Sweden; Antwerp, Belgium	2202	20–45	Having DIS or EMA at least 3 times/wk	DIS: 6–9 EMAs: 5–6
Téllez-López et al.[29]	1995	Monterrey, Mexico	1000	≥18	Being bothered a lot by DIS, DMS, or EMA	16.4
Blazer et al.[47]	1995	North Carolina (USA)	3976	≥65	DIS, DMS, or EMA, most of the time	DIS:14.8 DMS: 26.6 EMAs: 14.3
Foley et al.[50]	1995	East Boston, MA; New Haven, CT; Iowa & Washington counties (USA)	9282	≥65	DIS or EMA, most of the time	19.5–29.4/25.4–36.4
Henderson et al.[52]	1995	Canberra and Queanbeyan, Australia	874	≥70	DIS or EMA, nearly every night in the past 2 wk	12.6/18.0
Olson[22]	1996	Newcastle, Australia	535	≥16	Difficulty sleeping often or always	17.3/24.9
Breslau et al.[30]	1996	Southeast Michigan (USA)	1007	21–30	Presence of DIS, DMS, or EMA lasting ≥2 wk, and seeking professional help for the problem, or using sleep-promoting medication, or interfering a lot with daily life	21.4/26.7 (lifetime)
Yeo et al.[41]	1996	Singapore	2418	15–55	Dissatisfaction with sleep	12.9/17.5
Ganguli et al.[51]	1996	Mid-Monongahela Valley, PA (USA)	1050	66–97	• DIS sometimes or usually • DS sometimes or usually • EMA sometimes or usually	26.7/44.1 19.2/35.8 8.7/23.3
Ohayon[32]	1997	France	5622	≥15	• DIS, DMS, EMA, or NRS + daytime consequences • Dissatisfaction with sleep • DSM-IV insomnia diagnoses	12.7 15.6/24.4 5.6
Ohayon et al.[33]	1997	UK	4972	≥15	• DIS, DMS, EMA, or NRS + daytime consequences • Dissatisfaction with sleep • DSM-IV insomnia diagnoses • DSM-IV insomnia diagnoses	9.1 6.8/10.6 6.4 4.4

Continued

TABLE 21–1   Definition and Prevalence of Insomnia in the General Population—Cont'd

Authors	Year	Location	N	Age	Definition	Prevalence (%) Male/Female
Ohayon et al.[34]	1997	Montreal, Canada	1722	≥15	• Dissatisfaction with sleep	8.7/13.2
Kageyama et al.[43]	1997	Tokyo, Maebashi, Nagasaki, Naha, and Kawasaki, Japan	3600 women	≥20	• DSM-IV insomnia diagnoses • Dissatisfaction with sleep	4.4 11.2
Mallon and Hetta[53]	1997	Sweden	876	65–79	Moderate or major complaints of DIS, DS, or EMA	DIS: 14/30 DS: 31.4 EMAs: 33.4
Newman et al.[55]	1997	Forsyth, NC; Sacramento, CA; Washington County, MD; Pittsburgh, PA (USA)	5201	≥65	Presence of DIS, DS, or EMA	DIS: 14/30 DS: 65/65 EMAs: 17/15
Asplund and Aberg[44]	1998	Jamtland county, Sweden	3669 women	40–64	Bad night's sleep	18.1%
Maggi et al.[58]	1998	Veneto region, Italy	2398	≥65	Often or always having DIS or EMA	35.6/54.0
Ancoli-Israel and Roth[14]	1999	USA	1000	≥18	Difficulty sleeping on a frequent basis	9.0
Hetta et al.[16]	1999	Sweden	1996	≥18	• DIS, DMS, or EMA + daytime consequences • Having DIS, DMS, or EMA at least 3 times/wk	9.0 22.0
Hoffmann[17]	1999	Belgium	1618	≥18	• DIS, DMS, or EMA + daytime consequences • Having DIS, DMS, or EMA at least 3 times/wk	13.0 22.0
Vela-Bueno et al.[23]	1999	Madrid, Spain	1131	≥18	• Having DIS, DMS, or EMA at least 4 times/wk • Considered themselves insomniacs	17.7/27.4 7.8/14.4
Chiu et al.[49]	1999	Hong Kong, China	1034	≥70	Consider themselves as having insomnia	8.6/17.5
Yamaguchi et al.[59]	1999	Kanazawa, Japan	236	>60	Insomnia ≥3 nights/wk	14.0/19.7
Mallon et al.[11]	2000	Sweden	1870	45–65	Presence of DIS, DMS, or EMA	25.4/36.0
Doi et al.[15]	2000	Japan	3030	≥20	Often or always DIS, DMS or EMA	17.3
Léger et al.[20]	2000	France	12778	≥16	• Having DIS, DMS, or EMA at least 3 times/wk • DIS, DMS, or EMA + daytime consequences	25.0/34.0 14.0/23.0
Barbar et al.[46]	2000	Hawaii (USA)	3845 men	71–93	DIS, DS, EMA	32.6
Ohayon and Zulley[38]	2001	Germany	4115	≥15	• DIS, DMS, EMA, or NRS + daytime consequences • Dissatisfaction with sleep • DSM-IV insomnia diagnoses	8.5 5.6/8.2 6.0
Ohayon et al.[40]	2001	UK, Germany, Italy	2429	≥65	DIS, DS, EMA, NRS ≥3 nights/wk	DIS: 16.0 DS: 33.0 EMA: 16.0 NRS: 11.0
Pallesen et al.[61]	2001	Norway	2001	≥18	DIS or DMS ≥3 nights/wk + daytime consequences	11.7
Ohayon and Partinen[21]	2002	Finland	982	≥18	• DIS, DMS, EMA, or NRS + daytime consequences • Dissatisfaction with sleep • DSM-IV insomnia diagnoses	37.6 11.9 11.7
Ohayon and Smirne[39]	2002	Italy	3970	≥15	• Dissatisfaction with sleep • DSM-IV insomnia diagnoses	10.1 6.0
Ohayon and Vechierrini[56]	2002	Paris, France	1026	≥60	Dissatisfied with sleep quality or quantity	11.5/16.0
Ohayon and Hong[60]	2002	South Korea	3719	≥15	• DIS, DS, EMA, NRS ≥3 nights/wk • Insomnia diagnoses	14.8/19.1 4.7/5.1
Bixler et al.[62]	2002	Pennsylvania (USA)	1741	≥20	• Mild to severe DIS, DMS or NRS • Having insomnia for at least 1 yr	21.7/23.1 5.9/9.0
Kiejna et al.[63]	2003	Poland	47,924	≥15	Having insomnia	18.1/28.1

DIS, difficulty initiating sleep; DMS, difficulty maintaining sleep; DS, disrupted sleep; DSM-IV, *Diagnostic and Statistical Manual of Mental Disorders, Fourth Edition*; EMA, early morning awakening; NRS, nonrestorative sleep.

TABLE 21–2 Prevalence of Excessive Sleepiness in the General Population of America and Western Europe Countries

Authors	Year	Location	N	Age	Prevalence (%)
Frequency					
Liljenberg et al.[27]*	1988	Sweden	3557	30–65	5.3
Martikainen et al.[69†]	1992	Tampere, Finland	1190	36–50	9.8
Janson et al.[18†]	1995	4 cities in Iceland, Sweden, Belgium	2202	20–45	20.6
Hublin et al.[70†]	1996	Finland	11,354	33–60	9
Zielinski et al.[71]*	1999	Warsaw district, Poland	1186	38–67	26.1 + pb: 2.5
Liu et al.[72]*	2000	Japan	3030	≥20	15
Ohayon et al.[73†]	2002	UK, Germany, Italy, Spain, Portugal	18,980	≥15	4
Hara et al.[74†]	2004	Bambui, Brazil	1066	≥18	16.8
Severity					
Gislason and Almqvist[25]	1987	Uppsala, Sweden	3201 men	30–69	M:16.7 S: 5.7
Ohayon et al.[33]	1997	UK	4972	≥15	M:15.2 S: 5.5
Zielinski et al.[71‡]	1999	Warsaw district, Poland	1186	38–67	22.3 0.7
Nugent et al.[75]	2001	North Ireland	2364 men	≥18	M: 8.8 S: 11.8
Ohayon et al.[73]	2002	UK, Germany, Italy, Spain, and Portugal	18,980	≥15	M: 8.7 S: 3.8
Souza et al.[76‡]	2002	Campo Grande, Brazil	408	≥18	18.9
Ohayon and Vechierrini[56]	2002	Paris, France	1026	60–101	M: 6 S: 5.2
Takegami et al.[77‡]	2005	Hokkaido region, Japan	4412	≥20	8.9
Bixler et al.[78]	2005	Dauphin and Lebanon, PA (USA)	16,583	≥20	8.7

*Frequency assessed using adjective ("very often," "often," "rarely," "never").
†Frequency assessed using frequency during the week.
‡Severity assessed using the Epworth Scale.
M, moderate; pb, problems in functioning; S, severe.

Epidemiologic surveys have confirmed, however, that EDS can be the primary symptom of idiopathic hypersomnia or narcolepsy. In addition, EDS can be caused by various factors such as poor sleep hygiene,[33,70] work conditions,[33] and psychotropic medication use.[33,70] EDS has been found to be associated also with sleep-disordered breathing,[33,70,82] psychiatric disorders (especially depression),[31,33,70,79] and physical illnesses.[33,82]

Narcolepsy

Numerous attempts have been made to estimate the prevalence of narcolepsy in different parts of the world. Findings have varied, but it is it is now generally accepted that the overall prevalence is 50 in 100,000 or lower.[73,83–98] Table 21–3 summarizes the studies of the prevalence of narcolepsy in Europe and other countries.

SLEEP-DISORDERED BREATHING

Sleep-disordered breathing, especially snoring, has been studied mostly in the European general population. Prevalence rates for snoring indicate that this phenomenon is very common and increases with age, particularly among men, in whom the prevalence of occasional snoring can reach up to 60%.

Snoring

The Italian study by Lugaresi et al.[99] set the prevalence of habitual snoring at 19% in the general population, which, however, translated into lopsided gender rates of 24.1% for men and 13.8% for women. Using the criterion of snoring occurring at least 4 nights per week, Fitzpatrick

et al.[100] reported a prevalence of 11% in a sample of 1478 British subjects age 18 years or older; here, too, the rate was markedly higher for men (16%) than for women (7%). A study conducted in Denmark[101] yielded rates for nightly snoring of 19.1% for men and 7.9% for women in a sample of 1504 subjects 30–60 years old. Another Danish study[102] involving 2937 men 54–74 years of age reported a rate of 49.9% for snoring "always" or "often." An Icelandic study[103] carried out with 1505 women ages 40–59 years found a prevalence of 21.7% for intermittent snoring (1–5 nights per week) and 11.2% for habitual snoring (6 or 7 nights per week).

Another study[104] surveyed 3750 men ages 40–59 years from a Finnish twin cohort. Here, 8.8% of the sample reported snoring "almost always," and 20.4% snoring "often." Using home monitoring with 294 men ages 40–65 years, the Busselton health survey[105] found that 81% of subjects snored more than 10% of the night, and 22% more than half the night. The study undertaken by Ohayon et al.[106] in the United Kingdom with 4972 subjects age 15 years or older reported prevalence rates for regular snoring of 47.7% among men and 33.6% among women.

Follow-up surveys are essential to identify the potential long-term consequences of diseases and symptoms. Two studies have explored the course of snoring and the mortality risks for snorers. A prospective Danish survey spanning a 6-year period was conducted by Jennum et al.[102] with 2937 men ages 54–74 years. Of these, 49.9% reported snoring "always" or "often." The authors did not find a higher mortality in snorers than in non-snorers, and both groups had the same risk of suffering from

TABLE 21–3 Prevalence of Narcolepsy

Authors	Year	Population/ Location	N	Age Range	Methods	Prevalence Per 100,000
Solomon[83]	1945	Black Americans	10,000	16–34	Navy recruits (men)	20
Dement et al.[84]	1972	Northern California (USA)	Unknown	Unknown	Population sample; newspaper advertisement, telephone interview	50*
Dement et al.[85]	1973	Southern California (USA)	Unknown	Unknown	Population sample; TV advertisement, telephone interview	67*
Honda[86]	1979	Japan	12,469	12–16	School sample; questionnaire	160
Roth[87]	1980	Czech Caucasians	Unknown	Unknown	Patient material; polysomnography	20*
Franceschi et al.[88]	1982	Italy	2518	6–92	Unselected inpatients; questionnaire, polysomnography	40
Lavie and Peled[89]	1987	Israeli Jews and Arabs	1526	30–57	Patient material; polysomnography, HLA typing	0.23*
Ondzé et al.[95]	1987	France	14,195	>15	Patients of all physicians of "Le Gard" region; questionnaire + follow-up by phone interview and more detailed questionnaire	21
Tashiro et al.[92]	1992	Japan	4559	17–59	Sample of employees; questionnaire, personal interview	180
al Rajeh et al.[90]	1993	South Arabia	23,227	≥1	Subjects with abnormal responses evaluated by a neurologist; face-to-face interviews	40
Hublin et al.[91]	1994	Finland	12,504	33–60	Twin cohort; postal questionnaire, telephone interview, polysomnography, HLA typing	26
Wing et al.[93]	1994	China	342	≥18	Patient material; polysomnography, HLA typing	1–40*
Billiard[94]	1996	France	Unknown	Unknown	Male military recruits, "Le Gard" region	50
Han et al.[96]	2001	China	70,000	5–17	Consecutive patients attending a pediatric neurology clinic; screening questionnaire + polysomnography, MSLT, HLA typing	40
Ohayon et al.[73]	2001	UK, Germany, Italy, Portugal, and Spain	18,980	15–100	Representative sample of general population; telephone interview with Sleep-EVAL system	47
Silber et al.[97]	2002	Olmsted County, MN (USA)	Unknown	0–109	Patient material between 1960 and 1985	57*
Wing et al.[98]	2002	Hong Kong, China	9851	18–65	Representative sample of general population; Echelle Ullanlinna Narcolepsy Scale, polysomnography, MSLT, HLA typing	34

*Prevalence was extrapolated.
HLA, human leukocyte antigen; MSLT, Multiple Sleep Latency Test.

ischemic heart disease. A Finnish 5-year follow-up study was performed with 1190 participants at year 1 and 626 at year 5.[104] Subjects were 36–50 years of age at the start. At both assessments, the prevalence of habitual snoring increased with age and was higher in men. At follow-up, the highest increase in snoring (up 10%) was reported by the younger age group of men (36 years). In year 1, they found a higher incidence of "doze-offs" at the wheel among habitual snorers (22%), compared with non-snorers (14.8%). In 1990, they found a slightly higher rate of snorers involved in traffic accidents due to sleepiness.

Sleep Apnea

Sleep apnea is characterized by repeated breathing cessations lasting at least 10 seconds during sleep. The number of apnea and hypopnea events per hour, called the apnea-hypopnea index (AHI), is used to determine whether breathing patterns are abnormal. Usually, an AHI of 5 or more is considered an indicator of an inordinate number of sleep respiratory disturbances. When a sleep apnea syndrome is suspected, polysomnographic recordings are

necessary to confirm the diagnosis. Obstructive sleep apnea syndrome is associated with a high number of obstructive and mixed events. However, this criterion can be misleading in the general population as the severity of this sort of sleep-disordered breathing tends to be unimodally distributed.[107] It is not surprising, then, that few surveys have attempted to estimate the prevalence of sleep apnea syndrome or obstructive sleep apnea syndrome in community-based samples (Table 21–4).

One of the oldest studies of obstructive sleep apnea was performed in Israel by Lavie[108] with 300 working men, of which 78 were examined polysomnographically. He found that 2.7% of the sample had an AHI ≥10 and that 0.7% had an AHI ≥20. In the Finnish twin cohort study, Telakivi et al.[120] did polysomnographic recordings on 25 snorers and 27 non-snorers selected from among 278 men ages 41–50 years. They estimated that 0.4% of this population had an AHI ≥20 and that 1.4% had an AHI ≥10, with an oxygenation desaturation index (ODI) of at least 4%.

Gislason et al.[109] assessed 3201 Swedish men ages 30–60 years and carried out polysomnographic recordings on

TABLE 21-4 Prevalence of Sleep Apnea Syndrome in Selected Samples

Authors/Location and Year	N (n Recorded)	Age	Target Population	Method	Criteria	Prevalence (%)
Lavie[108] Israel, 1983	1502 (78)	32–67	Male workers	1. Questionnaire 2. Polysomnography	AI ≥10	0.89
Gislason et al.[109] Uppsale, Sweden, 1988	3201 (61)	30–69	Men, general population	1. Postal questionnaire 2. Polysomnography, sleepy snorers	AHI ≥30 + daytime sleepiness	1.3
Cirignotta et al.[110] Bologna, Italy, 1989	1170 (40)	30–69	Men, general population	1. Postal questionnaire 2. Polysomnography, every-night snorers	AHI ≥10	2.7
Martikainen et al.[1C4] Tempere, Finland, 1994	1985: 1190	36–50	General population	1. Postal questionnaire	ODI ≥4% >5/hr	1.8
	1990: 626 (22)			2. Polysomnography, habitual male snorers	ODI ≥4% >10/hr	1.1
Ancoli-Israel et al.[111] San Diego, CA (USA), 1991	615 (427)	65–95	General population	Home	AI ≥5	24.0
Stradling and Cosby[112] Oxford, UK, 1991	1001 (893)	35–65	Men, age-sex register of one group general practice	Polysomnography	RDI ≥10	62.0
Gislason et al.[103] Reykjavik, Iceland, 1993	1505 (35)	40–59	Women, general population	Oximetry	ODI ≥4% >5/hr	5.0
					ODI ≥4% >10/hr	1.0
					ODI ≥3% >10/hr + symptoms	0.8
					AHI ≥30 + daytime sleepiness	2.5
Young et al.[113] USA, 1993	3513 (625)	30–60	State employees	1. Postal questionnaire 2. Polysomnography, sleepy snorers	AHI ≥5	4.0 (M) 2.0 (W)
Olson et al.[114] Australia, 1995	2202 (441)	35–69	General population	1. Questionnaire 2. Polysomnography, snorers	AHI ≥10	5.7 (M) 1.2 (W)
Bearpark et al.[105] Busselton, Australia, 1995	486 (294)	40–65	Men, general population	1. Questionnaire 2. Respiratory measurment, overrepresentation of snorers and sleep complainers	RDI ≥5 + at least occasional daytime sleepiness	12.2
					RDI ≥5 + at least often daytime sleepiness	3.1
Bixler et al.[115] Pennsylvania (USA), 1998	4364 (741)	20–100	Men, general population	1. Telephone interview 2. Polysomnography	AHI ≥10 + daytime symptoms	3.3
Bixler et al.[116] Pennsylvania (USA), 2001	12,219 (1000)	20–100	Women, general population	1. Telephone interview 2. Polysomnography	AHI ≥10 + daytime symptoms	1.2
Duran et al.[117] Vitoria-Gasteiz, Spain, 2001	2148 (555)	30–70	Men and women, general population	1. Home interview 2. Portable respiratory recording 3. Polysomnography	AHI ≥10	19.0 (M) 14.9 (W)
Ip et al[118] Hong Kong, 2004	1532 (106)	30–60	Women, general population	1. Questionnaire 2. Polysomnography	AHI ≥5	3.7
					AHI ≥5 + excessive daytime sleepiness	2.1
Udwadia et al.[119] Bombay, India, 2004	658 (250)	35–65	Men, general population	1. Questionnaire 2. Polysomnography	AHI ≥5	19.5
					AHI ≥5 + excessive daytime sleepiness	7.5

AI, Apnea index; AHI, Apnea/hypopnea index; ODI, Oxygen desaturation index; RDI, Respiratory disturbance index.

61 sleepy snorers. Based on their polysomnographic findings, these authors estimated that 0.9% of this population had an AHI ≥10 and that 1.4% had an AHI ≥20. Gislason et al.[103] conducted a similar survey with 1505 Icelandic women 40–59 years of age, performing polysomnographic recordings on 35 snorers with EDS. They estimated that about 2.5% of this population was affected with a sleep apnea syndrome (daytime sleepiness accompanied by an AHI ≥30).

Cirignotta et al.[110] recorded 156 men recruited from a sample of 1510 Italian men ages 30–69 years. They estimated that 4.8% of this population had an AHI greater than 5 and 3.2% an AHI greater than 10. In Spain, Duran et al.[117] interviewed 2148 individuals from the general population and performed polysomography on 555 of them. The prevalence of AHI ≥10 was 19% among men and 14.9% among women.

The Busselton health survey[105] found that 12.2% of men ages 40–65 years had at least five respiratory disturbances per hour of sleep (respiratory disturbance index [RDI] ≥5) along with "at least occasional" daytime sleepiness, and that 3.1% had an RDI ≥5 along with "at least often" daytime sleepiness. Another Australian survey[114,121] involved 2202 subjects ages 35–69 years, of whom 441 subjects who complained about their sleep or snored were monitored polysomnographically. It was estimated that the rate of obstructive sleep apnea syndrome (based on an AHI ≥15) was 3.6% in the sampled population (5.7% among men vs. 1.2% among women).

The Wisconsin Sleep Cohort study[113] surveyed 3513 workers ages 30–60 years. They invited all habitual snorers and 25% of the nonhabitual snorers to a one-night polysomnographic recording. In all, 625 subjects accepted. For women, 18.9% of the habitual snorers and 5% of the nonhabitual snorers had an AHI of 5 or greater. For men, the corresponding figures were 34% and 16.1%, respectively. Based on these findings, the prevalence of sleep apnea syndrome (daytime sleepiness and/or nonrestorative sleep and an AHI ≥5) was estimated at 4% among men and 2% among women.

Two studies performed using large community-based samples[115,116] screened for possible sleep-related breathing disorders and recorded 1741 participants. The prevalence of sleep apnea, defined as an AHI ≥10 accompanied by daytime symptoms was estimated at 3.3% among men[115] and 1.2% among women.[116]

The 5-year follow-up survey by Martikainen et al.[104] found that the prevalence of symptoms indicating possible sleep apnea rose to 2.3% over the study period (combination of snoring and breathing pauses during sleep: 4.7% in 1985 vs. 7% in 1990). They also found that being overweight and weight gain were the best predictors of an AHI greater than 5 and an ODI ≥4%, and self-reported snoring and breathing pauses the best predictors of an AHI greater than 10 and an ODI ≥4%.

Unlike snoring and other sleep disorder symptoms, obstructive sleep apnea syndrome has not been the subject of any sound epidemiologic survey in the general population. None of the studies to date have used a true random sample of subjects to be monitored polysomnographically. Most were cohort studies. This is a major flaw in this field of research, despite many claims to the contrary.

RESTLESS LEGS SYNDROME

Restless legs syndrome (RLS), initially reported by Ekbom,[122] is a neurologic disorder characterized by disagreeable leg sensations occurring most often at sleep onset that provoke an irresistible urge to move the legs. Patients with RLS mostly complain of itching, creeping, tingling sensations in their legs, mostly between the ankle and the knee. These unpleasant sensations occur when the subject is at rest and are more pronounced in the evening or at night. The unpleasant sensations are relieved temporarily with leg movements.

RLS may begin at any age, but most patients suffering from RLS are over age 40. About 40% of patients diagnosed with RLS during adulthood reported having experienced symptoms before the age of 20 years. Some studies reported that as many as 80% of RLS sufferers have also periodic limb movements in sleep.[123] The etiology of RLS is not well known, but several pathophysiologic mechanisms have been proposed. The disorder appears to have a familial component in many cases. Montplaisir et al.[123] reported that 63% of the 127 RLS patients they studied said there is at least one family member with similar symptoms. Another study found that 42.3% of patients with idiopathic RLS and 11.7% of those with RLS due to uremia had a definitive positive hereditary RLS.[124]

RLS has seldom been investigated in the general population (Table 21–5). Using a limited set of one or two questions, the prevalence of RLS symptoms was estimated to be around 10%.[125,126] Three European studies used a set of criteria to assess the prevalence of RLS in the general population. One was done only with men,[127] another was conducted with elderly subjects,[128] and the last was performed with subjects 15 years of age or older.[129] Rothdach et al.'s study[128] with elderly people found a prevalence of 9.8%. Ohayon et al.,[129] in the same age group, found a prevalence of 8.6%. The study in Swedish men[127] reported a prevalence of 5.8%. Ohayon et al.[129] found a prevalence of 5.4% in the men of their sample.

In two studies RLS was not gender related,[126,129] and in two others the prevalence of RLS was about two times higher in women than in men.[125,128] Three studies showed that RLS increased with age.[125,126,129] The prevalence of RLS symptoms is close to 20% in elderly people and around 5% for subjects younger than age 30.[125,126] In the Ohayon et al. study, prevalence of RLS diagnosis ranged from 2.7% in the 15- to 18-year-old group to 8.3% in the group of subjects age 60 and older.[129]

TABLE 21-5 Prevalence for Restless Leg Syndrome or Symptoms

Authors	Year	Location	N	Age	Criteria	Prevalence (%)	Comments
Lavigne and Montplaisir[125]	1994	Canada	2019	≥18	None	10.0	Household interviews, prevalence based on a single question
Phillips et al.[126]	2000	Kentucky (USA)	1803	≥18	None	9.4	Telephone interviews, prevalence based on a single question
Ulfberg et al.[127]	2000	Sweden	2608 men	18–64	IRLSSG	5.8	Postal questionnaire, 4 questions based on criteria described by the IRLSSG (need positive answers to all questions)
Rothdach et al.[128]	2000	Augsburg, Germany	385	65–83	IRLSSG	9.8	Face-to-face interview, 3 questions based on criteria described by the IRLSSG (need positive answers to all questions)
Ohayon and Roth[129]	2002	5 European countries	18,980	15–100	ICSD	5.5	Telephone interviews, prevalence based on ICSD criteria evaluated by an expert system
Sevim et al.[130]	2003	Mersin, Turkey	3234	≥18	IRLSSG	3.2	Face-to-face interview, 4 questions based on criteria described by the IRLSSG (need positive answers to all questions) + the IRLSSG severity scale
Berger et al.[131]	2004	Pomerania, Germany	4310	20–79	IRLSSG	10.6	Face-to-face interview, 3 questions based on criteria described by the IRLSSG (need positive answers to all questions)
Allen et al.[132]	2005	USA + 5 European countries	15,391	≥18	IRLSSG	7.2	Face-to-face and telephone interview, 4 screening questions + the IRLSSG severity scale
Phillips et al.[133]	2006	USA	1506	≥18	None	9.7	2005 National Sleep Foundation poll, telephone interview, 3 questions based on criteria described by the IRLSSG

ICSD, International Classification of Sleep Disorders; IRLSSG, International Restless Legs Syndrome Study Group.

PARASOMNIAS

Parasomnias include a group of sleep disorders characterized by abnormal behavioral or physiologic events occurring at different sleep stages or during sleep/wake transitions. The most recent edition of the ICSD[6] divides parasomnias into three subgroups: arousal (confusional arousals, sleepwalking, and sleep terrors), rapid eye movement (REM) sleep disorders (nightmares, sleep paralysis, REM sleep behavior disorder), and other parasomnias. In the first ICSD,[1] sleep/wake transition (rhythmic movement disorder, sleep starts, sleep talking, and nocturnal leg cramps) was included under parasomnias.

Parasomnias have seldom been investigated in the adult general population. Arousal parasomnias (confusional arousals, sleepwalking, and sleep terrors) occur primarily in childhood and normally cease by adolescence. In the adult general population, a study by Bixler et al.[8] set the prevalence of sleepwalking at 3%. Téllez-Lòpez et al.[29] reported a prevalence of 1.9% in their Mexican survey. In the Finnish twin cohort study, Hublin et al.[134] obtained a prevalence of 0.7% among adult men and 0.5% among adult women (with at least 1 episode per month). Infrequent episodes (less than monthly) were reported by 3.2% of men and 2.6% of women. Ohayon et al.[135] reported a prevalence of 2% in their U.K. sample.

These studies showed that sleepwalking is not gender related but is more common among younger subjects (<25 years) and almost never reported by elderly persons. The most dramatic consequence of this parasomnia is the harm that sleepwalkers can inflict on themselves or others. Cases of murder during sleepwalking episodes have been documented.[136]

The prevalence of sleep terrors and confusional arousals in adulthood have seldom been investigated. In children, studies have reported prevalence rates for sleep terrors ranging from 1% to 6.5%.[137–139] A British epidemiologic study[135] with 4972 subjects between 15 and 99 years of age reported a 2.2% prevalence of night terrors. As for confusional arousals, a study conducted with 13,057 subjects age 15 years or older found a prevalence of 2.9%.[140]

Epidemiologic data on the sleep/wake transition parasomnias[1] are scarce. Téllez-Lòpez et al.[29] reported a prevalence rate of 21.3% for sleep talking and 3% for frequent sleep talking. Again, this phenomenon is more frequent in the younger age group (≤30 years). The prevalence of nocturnal leg cramps is not well documented, but certain studies have suggested they are quite frequent among the elderly.[141] Ohayon et al.[36] in their U.K. study reported that nocturnal leg cramps were more frequently observed in subjects with severe daytime sleepiness (4.7%), compared with nonsleepy subjects (0.5%).

Regarding the group of REM sleep disorder parasomnias, nightmares have been reported to occur at least once a week in 5% of the adult population.[142] Sleep paralysis is one of the symptoms mainly associated with narcolepsy, but it can also occur individually (i.e., isolated sleep paralysis). Těllez-Lòpez et al.[29] found a sleep paralysis prevalence of 11.3% (occurring at least sometimes). Where more narrowly defined populations are concerned, Goode[143] and Everett[144] observed rates of 4.7% and 15.4%, respectively, for self-reported sleep paralysis in medical students, and Bell et al.[145] noted a prevalence of 41% in black Americans. In a study of adults living on the northeast coast of Newfoundland, Ness[146] reported a rate of 62% for "old hag" attacks, as sleep paralysis is popularly known in that part of Canada. An epidemiologic study[147] performed with 8085 subjects between 15 and 99 years of age found that 6.2% had at least 1 episode of sleep paralysis in their lifetime; 0.8% experienced severe sleep paralysis (at least 1 episode per week) and 1.4% moderate sleep paralysis (at least 1 episode per month). Another study performed with 158 subjects age 70 years or older reported that 17.7% of them already had experience of "ghost oppression."[148]

REM sleep behavior disorder was first described in the late 1970s by Japanese researchers[149] and labeled as such by Schenck et al.[150] This disorder is characterized by "injurious or disruptive behaviours emerging during REM sleep, which ordinarily exhibits a generalized skeletal muscle atonia." Its prevalence in the general population is not well documented. Ohayon et al.[151] estimated it at 0.5% based on the minimal criteria proposed by the ICSD.[1,5,6]

CHALLENGES FOR THE EPIDEMIOLOGY OF SLEEP DISORDERS

Insomnia and Associated Syndromes

In the past decade, research into insomnia symptomatology has established that sleep complaints are common in the general population and affect primarily women and the elderly. Epidemiologists must now distinguish between the various subtypes of insomnia. Few surveys present insomnia complaints as a whole when assessing their causes and consequences. Moreover, epidemiologic data on transient and seasonal patterns of insomnia are nonexistent. Longitudinal epidemiologic data on the evolution and consequences of insomnia complaints are still lacking. To date, only two surveys have addressed this specific subject in the general population.[30,31]

Excessive Sleepiness

A uniform operational definition of excessive sleepiness is still missing. Although many surveys have been undertaken on the topic, differences in definition and the variance in results do not make it possible to reach any definite conclusions. As is the case for insomnia complaints, the causes and consequences of excessive sleepiness are rarely presented as a whole. The prevalence of transient or seasonal patterns of this symptoms are not known, nor is its longitudinal evolution in the general population.

Sleep-Disordered Breathing

The study of obstructive sleep apnea syndrome in the general population suffers primarily from a subsample selection bias. Few studies have drawn subjects for polysomnographic recordings in true random fashion. Most of these surveys used a sleep questionnaire to screen potential subjects with obstructive sleep apnea. Consequently, certain categories are likely to be underrepresented, such as individuals unaware of their symptoms. In addition, many of these studies did not record enough cases to reach a 95% level of precision, thus undermining the validity of results. Prevalences, therefore, have likely been underestimated.

◔ REFERENCES

A full list of references are available at www.expertconsult.com

CHAPTER 22

Human and Animal Genetics of Sleep and Sleep Disorders

Stéphanie Maret, Yves Dauvilliers and Mehdi Tafti

INTRODUCTION

After more than a century of modern scientific study of sleep, its biological function remains an enigma. In all mammals and birds and in some invertebrates such as drosophila, a substantial portion of life is spent in this behavioral state, and we know that lack of sleep or disturbed sleep has strong negative consequences on health and performance. Because of the conservation of this behavior during evolution (since its appearance) and the fact that long-term sleep deprivation may lead to death in animal models, we think that sleep fulfills a fundamental and vital biological need. Substantial progress has been achieved in our understanding of the neurobiology underlying the expression and regulation of sleep, but little is known about the molecular basis of sleep. As a complex behavior, sleep is influenced by both genetic and environmental factors as was demonstrated early on in familial and twin studies that assessed the role of genes in sleep and sleep disorders. The current progress in sequencing the genomes of species as different as human, mouse, zebrafish, and drosophila brought great expectation that genes related to sleep and sleep disorders could be identified. The discovery of a point mutation in the prion protein gene as the cause of fatal familial insomnia, followed by the discovery of the role of hypocretins in human narcolepsy, proved that through genetic approaches unexpected molecular pathways or new sleep-related genes remain to be discovered. In this chapter, we review the various approaches that can be used to identify and isolate sleep-related genes, and we then present a general overview of the different sleep disorders for which a genetic component has been described.

GENETICS OF NORMAL SLEEP AND THE ELECTROENCEPHALOGRAM

Sleep and wakefulness are complex behaviors and thus are influenced by many genetic and environmental factors. Twin studies are of interest to determine the respective contribution of genetic and environmental factors to a given phenotype. The first study of genetics of sleep can be dated to a publication by Geyer in 1937.[1] He reported a higher concordance between sleep habits of monozygotic (MZ) than dizygotic (DZ) twins. In 1951, Gedda reported rare cases of concordant long sleepers (up to 15 hours) in MZ twins.[2] Gedda and Brenci first estimated that the heritability of sleep duration is over 30%.[3] These authors later confirmed that sleep duration is highly similar even in twins living apart, discounting the influence of environmental effects.[4] Results from twin studies also showed that the waking electroencephalographic (EEG) patterns of MZ twins have a much higher resemblance than those of DZ twins or unrelated subjects, again confirming that this highly complex phenotype might be tightly controlled by genes and little affected by environment. In 1966, Zung and Wilson[5] performed the first polysomnographic sleep recordings in twins and found the temporal sequence of sleep stages to be almost completely concordant between MZ twins. More recent observations indicate that even the pattern of rapid eye movements (REMs) presents higher concordance between MZ than DZ twins[6] and that between 40% and 50% of the variance in sleep duration and the presence of a sleep disorder can be accounted for by genetic effects.[7,8] These and other studies have shown that a number of sleep aspects are strongly determined by genes (Table 22–1).

Animal studies (mainly in mice and rats) show the presence of considerable interindividual variations in the different aspects of sleep even when animals are kept under identical environmental conditions from birth. Nevertheless, when several inbred strains of mice or rats are recorded, a far greater interstrain than intrastrain variability is reported for non-REM (NREM) and REM sleep, again indicating that environmental factors play a secondary role.[22–29] As every aspect of sleep needs to be considered as a separate complex trait, a systematic approach is necessary to identify the genetic factors underlying each of these traits.[30,31] In the early 1970s, Valatx[22] pioneered the experimental genetics of sleep by studying inbred, recombinant inbred, and hybrid mice. He reported that several aspects of sleep, including the amount of paradoxical sleep, are controlled by genetic factors.[23,25,26] These studies, complemented with a diallelic study by Friedmann,[24] clearly suggested that, although some aspects of sleep can follow a simple segregation, most other sleep traits cannot be predicted by classic genetic laws. Among many animal models,[32] the fruit fly *Drosophila melanogaster* is a highly valuable one for dissecting the molecular mechanisms underlying sleep. This invertebrate shows all the features of sleep: it has a consolidated, circadian period of inactivity, which is characterized by increased arousal thresholds as well as a specific posture and resting place, and its rest is homeostatically regulated.[33,34] Thus rest in *Drosophila* is a sleeplike state. Moreover, this model organism is small, economical,

and rapidly reproducing, and has fewer genes, constituting an excellent tool for genetic analyses.[35]

One of the major advantages of animal models is the possibility of genetic manipulation by loss or gain of function of key genes. Based on the available knowledge in physiology and pharmacology, candidate genes can be identified and experimentally manipulated to assess their role in sleep. The first transgenic investigations in the field of sleep research included the cytokine pathway,[36] with *Il1a, Il10, Tnf,* and *Tnf* receptors-1 and -2; the neurotransmitter pathway,[37] with dopamine, histamine, and serotonin; and the clock genes.[38] Table 22–2 summarizes the effects of transgenic manipulations on sleep in mice, and in almost all cases some significant effects are observed confirming the involvement of the underlying gene. Therefore, the candidate gene approach is only valuable in verifying whether a gene of interest has any detectable effect and cannot help identifying new genes.

Since sleep and wakefulness are very different in terms of brain activity, physiology, and behavior, it is reasonable to expect that there are differences also at the level of gene expression. Moreover, the temporal dynamics of sleep homeostasis, indexed as EEG delta power in NREM sleep, are compatible with the dynamics of gene expression, and sleep deprivation could thus lead to changes in gene expression. This should help to find genes functionally relevant to the homeostatic regulation of sleep, although it cannot be ruled out that the changes in expression of some of these genes are merely driven by the sleep-wake distribution instead of being functionally relevant.

In 1990, by using the substractive hybridization techniques in rats sleep deprived for 24 hours, Rhyner and colleagues[101] were the first to isolate several messenger RNA (mRNA) clones with increased or decreased relative expression in the brain. Analysis of the structure of two

TABLE 22–1 Twin Studies of Sleep and the Waking EEG

Sleep and EEG Phenotype	Results	References
Sleep habits	Higher concordance in MZ	Geyer[1]
Long sleepers	Concordant in MZ	Gedda[2]
Sleep duration	Correlated in MZ	Gedda and Brenci[3]
Sleep length, quality	Significant heritability	Partinen et al.[8]
Rare waking EEG variants	Single autosomal dominant gene	Vogel[9–11]
EEG patterns	Higher resemblance	Young et al.,[12] Juel-Nielsen and Harvald[13]
Temporal sequence of sleep stages	Concordant in MZ	Zung and Wilson[5]
REM sleep percentage	Higher concordance in MZ	Gould et al.[14]
Sleep latency	Correlated in MZ	Webb and Campbell[15]
Awakening measures	Correlated in MZ	Webb and Campbell[15]
Stage changes	Correlated in MZ	Webb and Campbell[15]
REM amount	Correlated in MZ	Webb and Campbell[15]
Temporal pattern of REMs	Correlated in MZ	Chouvet et al.[6]
REM period length–spindle density	Correlated in MZ	Hori[16]
Amount of stage 2 and 4 sleep	Correlated in MZ	Linkowski et al.[17]
Waking alpha rhythms	Correlated in MZ	Davis and Davis[18]
Waking alpha EEG	85% similarity in MZ, 5% in DZ	Lennox et al.[19,20]
Waking delta, theta, alpha, and beta EEG	76–89% heritability	van Beijsterveldt et al.[21]

DZ, dizygotic; EEG, electroencephalogram; MZ, monozygotic; REM, rapid eye movement.

TABLE 22–2 Effects of Transgenic Manipulations on Sleep

Gene for:	Mouse Model	Main Effects
5-HT$_{1a}$	Knock-out	↑ REMS, no REMS increase after SD[39]
5-HT$_{1b}$	Knock-out	↑ REMS, no REMS increase after SD[40] ↓ SWS
5-HT$_{2a}$	Knock-out	↓ NREMS in baseline[41] No increase in EEG power density after SD
5-HT$_{2c}$	Knock-out	↑ W[42] ↓ NREMS in baseline ↑ Rebound in NREMS and EEG delta power Altered REMS
Serotonin transporter	Knock-out	↑ REMS[43] ↑ REMS bouts lasting longer
Dopamine transporter	Knock-out	No response to amphetamine/modafinil[44]
Dopamine β-hydroxylase	Knock-out	↑ 2 hr sleep every day[45] ↑ Delta power[45] More difficult to wake up[46] ↓ Latency to sleep[47]
Histamine H$_1$ receptor	Knock-out	No response to orexin A (hypocretin-1)[48]
Histamine H$_3$ receptor	Knock-out	Insensitive to thioperamide[49] ↓ Stereotypic response to methamphetamine Insensitive to scopolamine
Histidine decarboxylase	Knock-out	↑ REMS[50] ↓ W at dark onset ↓ Cortical EEG theta during W
Prepro-orexin	Knock-out	Narcolepsy[51] ↑ Response to modafinil
Orexin/ataxin3	Transgenic	Narcolepsy[52]
Ox2R	Knock-out	Dysregulation of W and NREMS[53] ↓ Sleep continuity Longer lasting EEG delta after SD
Ox1R/Ox2R	Knock-out	Narcolepsy, similar to prepro-orexin knock-out[54]
Leptin	Knock-out	↑ Numbers of arousal[55] ↑ Stage shifts Impaired sleep consolidation ↓ Diurnal rhythm of sleep/wake, NREMS delta power ↓ NREMS, REMS after sleep deprivation in magnitude and duration
GABA$_A$-α1	Point mutation	No effect on diazepam-induced sleep changes[56]
GABA$_A$-α2	Knock-out	↓ Suppression of delta activity induced by diazepam[57]
GABA$_A$-α3	Point mutation	↓ Slow-wave activity in NREMS[58] ↑ Frequencies above 15 Hz
GABA$_A$-β3	Point mutation	↓ REMS during light period[59] ↑ EEG delta power during NREMS[58]
Adenosine A1 receptor	Knock-out	No effect[60]
Adenosine A2a receptor	Knock-out	No wake-promoting effect of caffeine[61]
β2 Nicotinic receptor	Knock-out	↑ REMS episodes[62] ↓ NREMS fragmentation[62] ↓ Arousal from sleep[63]
α4 Nicotinic receptor	Knock-in	↑ Brief awakenings[64]
Inducible NOS	Knock-out	↑ REMS[65] ↓ NREMS during dark period
N-type Ca^{2+} channel α1 β subunit	Knock-out	↑ Consolidation of REMS[66] ↑ EEG spectral power during W and REMS ↓ EEG spectral power during NREMS
Thalamic Cav3.1 T-type Ca^{2+} channel	Knock-out	↑ W frequency and duration[67]
Potassium channel subunit Kv3.1	Knock-out	↑ Ambulatory and stereotypic activity in conjunction with sleep loss[68]
Potassium channel subunit Kv3.2	Knock-out	↓ EEG power density between 3.25 and 6 Hz in NREMS[69] ↓ EEG power density between 3.25 and 5 Hz in REMS
Potassium channel subunit Kv3.3	Knock-out	No effect[68]
Kv3.1/Kv3.3	Double knock-out	Ataxia, myotonus, tremor, hyperactivity[68] ↓ TST
Cbeta4	Knock-out	2 Hz faster EEG peak frequency during REMS[70]
Fatty acid amide hydrolase	Knock-out	↑ NREMS[71] ↑ Intense episodes of NREMS
Ube3a	Deletion	↓ NREMS[72] ↑ W ↑ W and NREMS episodes number Altered REMS No rebound in delta power Slight rebound in REMS

Continued

TABLE 22–2 Effects of Transgenic Manipulations on Sleep—Cont'd

Gene for:	Mouse Model	Main Effects
Rim1a	Knock-out	↓ Baseline dark period NREMS[73]
Rab3a	Mutagenesis	↑ NREMS[74]
		↓ Response to SD in REMS
mPer1	Knock-out	↓ Response to SD in frontal EEG power[75]
mPer2	Knock-out	↓ Response to SD in frontal EEG power[75]
mPer3	Knock-out	No effect[76]
mPer1,2	Double knock-out	No effect[76]
NPAS2	Knock-out	↓ Baseline dark period NREMS[77]
Clock	Mutagenesis	↓ TST, NREMS; no REMS increase after SD[78]
BMAL1/Mop3	Knock-out	↓ Daily amplitude of sleep-wake[79]
		↑ TST
		↑ Sleep fragmentation
		↑ Delta power at baseline
		↓ Compensatory response to SD
Cry1,2	Double knock-out	↑ NREMS, consolidation, EEG delta power during NREMS[80]
Dbp	Knock-out	↓ Sleep continuity, no increase in REMS after SD[81]
		↓ Daily amplitude in EEG delta power
c-Fos	Knock-out	↓ NREMS[82]
		↑ W
Fos-B	Knock-out	↓ REMS[82]
CREB αδ	Double knock-out	↓ W over 24 hr[83]
		↑ NREMS over 24 hr[83]
Prion protein	Knock-out	↓ Sleep continuity, longer lasting EEG delta after SD[84,85]
PGD synthase	Transgenic	↑ NREMS after tail clipping[86]
PGD receptor	Knock-out	No NREMS increase after lateral ventricle PGD$_2$ infusion[87]
GH	Transgenic	↑ NREMS moderately[88]
		↑ REMS greatly during the light period
GHRH	Knock-out	↓ Spontaneous NREMS[89]
		↓ REMS during light period
		↓ Deprivation-induced enhancement in EEG slow-wave activity
GHRH receptor	Knock-out	↓ Spontaneous REMS and NREM
		↓ NREMS response to 4 hr SD
GH and insulin-like GF-I	Knock-out	↓ NREMS[91]
Insulin	Transgenic	Genetic background effect[92]
β-Amyloid precursor protein	Transgenic	↓ REMS[93]
		↑ REMS fragmentation
TNF-R1	Knock-out	↓ TST[94]
TNF-R2	Knock-out	↓ REMS at baseline light period[95]
		↑ Slow wave activity after SD
TNF and lymphotoxin α	Double knock-out	↓ REMS at baseline light period[95]
		↑ Slow-wave activity (2.75–4 Hz)
IFN-R1	Knock-out	↓ REMS[96]
IL-10		↑ NREMS during dark period[97]
IL-6	Knock-out	LPS-induced profound hypothermia[98]
		↑ REMS[99]
IL1-type 1R	Knock-out	↓ TST during dark period[100]

↑, increase; ↓, decrease; EEG, electroencephalography; GABA, γ-aminobutyric acid; GF, growth factor; GH, growth hormone; GHRH, growth hormone-releasing hormone; 5-HT, 5-hydroxytryptamine; IFN, interferon; IL, interleukin; LPS, lipopolysaccharide; NOS, nitric oxide synthetase; NREMS, non–rapid eye movement (REM) sleep; PGD, prostaglandin D; REMS, REM sleep; SD, sleep deprivation; TNF, tumor necrosis factor; TST, total sleep time; W, wakefulness.

of these clones identified neurogranin and dendrin.[102,103] Neuner-Jehle et al.[103] demonstrated that mRNA and protein for neurogranin and dendrin were differentially modulated in different regions of the rat brain by prolonged wakefulness. The laboratory of Cirelli and Tononi has continued this work to include changes in gene expression after spontaneous periods of sleep and wakefulness and long-term sleep deprivation in rats.[104] They have used several techniques such as mRNA differential display and complementary DNA microarrays to systematically screen brain gene expression. These authors have screened 10,000 of the 30,000 genes estimated to be

expressed in the rat cerebral cortex, and their results indicate that only approximately 5% seem to be modulated by sleep and wakefulness.[105] The majority of genes are up-regulated during sleep deprivation/spontaneous wakefulness relative to sleep. The same genes changed their expression during spontaneous wakefulness and sleep deprivation, but in the latter condition the changes were more pronounced. A few genes are up-regulated during sleep, but so far their function remains mostly unknown (e.g., membrane protein E25).

Modulated genes include a few functional categories[105] such as immediate early genes, transcription factors, growth factors, adhesion molecules, heat shock proteins, neurotransmitters, hormone receptors, metabolism and energy proteins, transporters, and enzymes.

Two major classes of genes are rapidly induced after only 3 hours of wakefulness or sleep deprivation: the immediate early genes/transcriptional factors (*Arc*, *Fos*, and *NGF1-A*) and the mitochondrial genes. The immediate early genes are a specific class of genes that are rapidly induced by a variety of extracellular stimuli. Interestingly, the expression of *Fos* is increased in the ventrolateral preoptic area during sleep, suggesting a sustained cellular activity in this area during sleep.[106] The mitochondrial genes include those for subunit 1 of cytochrome C oxidase, subunit 2 of NADH dehydrogenase, and 12S ribosomal RNA and are encoded by the mitochondrial genome only.[105]

After 8 hours of wakefulness, there is an up-regulation of genes related to energy metabolism such as those for glucose transporter (*Glut1*), glycogen synthase, and glycogen phosphorylase. The genes for several heat shock proteins and chaperones, such as *HSP60*, *HSP70*, and *BiP*, are also up-regulated. The components of the presynaptic and postsynaptic neurotransmission machinery show also higher mRNA levels after 8 hours of wakefulness probably in relation with neuronal plasticity.[105]

An interesting fact is that genes induced by short periods of wakefulness are no longer up-regulated if the deprivation is prolonged. One exception is the aryl sulfotransferase gene (*AST*), which is induced proportionally to the time spent awake: that is, greater than twofold after 8 hours of spontaneous or enforced wakefulness and greater than fourfold after long-term sleep deprivations (4–14 days). This enzyme is responsible for the breakdown of the wakefulness-related catecholamines by sulfonation of norepinephrine, serotonin, and dopamine. It is therefore suggested to play a role in counteracting the waking-related monoaminergic release.[104,105] These findings illustrate that the molecular genetics approach, complemented with other genetic techniques, is powerful in identifying new genes that are implicated in sleep homeostasis and that the mouse, rat, and drosophila models are appropriate models, especially when used in parallel.

Although these data demonstrate that the molecular approach is a valuable tool to find sleep genes, a gene that does not show transcriptional modification may nonetheless play an important role. New techniques are emerging to profile gene expression at the cellular level, such as laser capture microdissection[107] combined with high-throughput linear amplification of RNA.[108] Nevertheless, these techniques are not suitable for the identification of constitutively expressed sleep genes, which can only be discovered by forward genetics.

Conceptually the forward genetic approach is the most powerful strategy for the isolation of genes involved in any biological process, since it is the only approach that does not make biased assumptions. In the genome-wide search for genes affecting a particular phenotype, no a priori assumptions on the gene systems involved are made. Although this approach may lead to already known physiologic mechanisms, its strength is that systems previously unknown to be involved in sleep may be uncovered. Therefore, a genome-wide search is the method of choice if we are to discover new "sleep" genes.

Mutagenesis

Whereas the quantitative trait loci (QTL) analysis (see later) aims at identifying "naturally" occurring allelic variants or gene mutations that modify sleep, mutagenesis is based on a randomly induced mutation approach. A strong mutagen such as ethylnitrosourea (ENU) is used to mutate spermatogonia. Assuming a mutation frequency of 0.0015 per locus per gamete,[109] there is approximately a 50% probability of finding a dominant mutation by screening a first generation of 650 offspring. With high-throughput screening for either dominant or recessive mutations, a major effect on a given trait can be identified. The individual mouse or fruit fly for which an aberrant phenotype has been identified has then to be crossed to establish the mode of inheritance of that trait. The isolation of *Clock* is an excellent example of the feasibility of this technique.[110,111] After the treatment of mice with ENU, Vitaterna and colleagues observed a mouse exhibiting a longer circadian period of approximately 25 hours when kept in constant darkness.[110] This mouse was crossed with a wild-type mouse to establish the mode of inheritance of the trait. The mutated animal carried a semi-dominant mutation in a locus required for the maintenance of normal circadian rhythmicity. Linkage analysis mapped this trait onto chromosome 5, and a positional cloning was undertaken and the mutated gene *Clock* (Circadian Locomotor Output Cycle Kaput) was identified.[111] More recently, this technique allowed the discovery of *Rab3a*, with a mutation that altered both circadian period and homeostatic response to sleep loss, in the mouse.[74] The choice and success of each of the approaches is determined by the gene effect. Although some mutations can induce remarkable phenotypic changes, others produce only subtle effects that, in addition, can be confounded by gene-gene interactions (epistasis) and genetic background (modifier gene).[112] Mutagenesis is therefore more successful for fully penetrant dominant or recessive mutations, whereas QTL analysis is more powerful in detecting natural allelic variations controlling complex traits.[113]

QTL Analysis

QTL has been proposed as a powerful approach in the genetics of complex traits. A quantitative trait is a phenotype showing continuous variations in a population.

Generally complex phenotypes such as sleep are regulated by multiple genes, each of them having a small effect. The QTL technique is based on DNA natural polymorphisms, which are nonlethal mutations preserved in a population because of their neutral, subtle, or advantageous effect. As discussed in this section, QTL analysis can be successfully applied to the genetic dissection of both sleep amount and the sleep EEG.

QTLs for Sleep Amount

The 24-hour amount of sleep also shows highly significant differences between inbred mouse strains.[23,24,29] The two extremes regarding the amount of sleep over a 24-hour period are AKR/J (AK) and DBA/2J (D2) strains. AK mice sleep ~3 hours more than D2 mice.[29] Multiple genes may be found to be responsible for this difference, and therefore a QTL analysis is appropriate. A first QTL analysis was performed in 7 CXB (BALB/cByJ × C57BL/6ByJ) recombinant inbred lines for the amount of REM sleep, and four QTLs were identified on chromosomes 5, 7, 12, and 17.[114] Toth and Williams[115] studied sleep in a larger CXB recombinant inbred panel and found QTLs on chromosomes 4, 16, and 17. Interestingly, both QTL studies reported different loci for the duration of diurnal and nocturnal and for total REM sleep time during 24 hours, suggesting that different genes are involved in the expression and regulation of REM sleep. In both studies, none of the QTLs could satisfy a stringent statistical significance level certainly due to the small number of recombinant inbred strains (7 to 13).

A significant QTL was identified in 25 BXD recombinant inbred lines (C57BL/6 and DBA/2) on chromosome 1 for the amount of REM sleep in the 12-hour light period.[116] Overall, between 40% and 60% of the variance in sleep amounts and distribution can be explained by the additive effects of 6–15 genes in BXD recombinant inbreds, indicating, as for other complex traits, a polygenic basis for sleep. So far no significant QTL has been found for the amount of NREM sleep.[114–116]

QTLs for Sleep EEG

In 1996, van Beijsterveldt et al.[21] recorded the waking EEGs of 91 MZ and 122 DZ twins during quiet resting with eyes closed. Spectral powers were calculated for the frequency bands alpha, beta, delta, and theta. The average heritabilities for all these frequencies bands were 76% for delta, 89% for theta and alpha, and 86% for beta. In other words, the rhythmic brain electrical activity is one of the most heritable traits in humans.[21,117,118] This important finding in humans was extended by us to the EEG activity during sleep in mice by using quantitative genetic analysis.

Quantitative analysis of the spectral EEG activity during sleep demonstrates an important variation between different inbred strains for both REM and NREM sleep.[119] The theta peak frequency (TPF) was found to vary greatly with genotype.[119,120] The TPF was significantly different between C57BL/6J (B) and BALB/cByJ (C) mice during REM sleep, the first being slow (5.75–6.25) and the second fast (6.75–7.75). Over 80% of the interstrain variability could be explained by genetic effects. In BXC F1 mice, the TPF was similar to that of B and significantly faster than C mice, suggesting that the C allele was recessive. By using 89 polymorphic markers QTL analysis in 47 F2 mice identified a single highly significant locus on mouse chromosome 5, suggesting the presence of an autosomal recessive phenotype under the control of a single gene. This single locus could explain more than 65% of the variance. After genotyping a backcross population, a strong linkage was found with the polymorphic marker D5Mit240. By genotyping 200 additional backcross mice and recording sleep in 31 selective recombinant mice, the region of interest was narrowed down to 2.4 cM. Different candidate genes were analyzed, and the short-chain acyl-coenzyme A dehydrogenase gene (Acads) within the region showed a spontaneous mutation in C mice. This finding suggests a major role for mitochondrial β-oxidation during sleep, which is fatty acid chain-length specific because long-chain acyl-coenzyme A dehydrogenase (Acadl) deficiency does not affect theta frequency. This finding constitutes the first identification of a sleep QTL.[120]

It was also noticed that, during NREM sleep, DBA/2J (D2) mice show a reduced delta activity and have their EEG dominated by theta activity compared to most other inbred strains. The theta-delta ratio (TDR) on relative power spectra was determined for B6 and D2 mice and differed by more than 5 standard deviations.[121] The TDR of the F1 mice was similar to that of B6 mice and significantly different from D2 mice, suggesting that the D2 allele is recessive. A panel of 25 BXD recombinant inbred lines was recorded and QTL analysis was performed with more than 800 polymorphic markers on the whole genome. A single significant QTL was identified in the centromeric region of chromosome 14 that was responsible for more than 55% of the total variance, clearly indicating the presence of an autosomal recessive gene. Fine mapping revealed a single nucleotide polymorphism in the second untranslated exon of the retinoic acid receptor beta gene (Rarb). The different transcripts of this gene were amplified by reverse transcriptase–polymerase chain reaction and sequenced. Seven polymorphisms including the biallelic marker were found between B6 and D2, one silent in the coding region and five in the untranslated 5′ regions. To test this candidate gene, we recorded different transcript knock-out mice and their D2 hemizygotes. While the Rarb knockout had increased delta activity, a complete recovery of delta power was observed in Rarb1,3/D2, confirming the implication of this gene. Rarb transcripts were expressed at significantly higher levels in the brains of D2 compared to B6 mice, indicating that the polymorphisms in the gene had an effect on the transcription in vivo. By testing six other inbred strains, we noticed that only *Rarb1* varied with delta power. Retinoic acid, the active derivative of vitamin A, plays a major role during ontogenesis and particularly during the development of the brain through dopaminergic pathways. Sleep and the sleep EEG are also developmentally regulated. Whether it is through brain development and plasticity or through dopaminergic pathways that *Rarb* regulates the contribution of delta activity during slow-wave sleep (SWS) remains to be documented.[121]

QTLs for Sleep Homeostasis

Two main processes regulate sleep: a circadian and a homeostatic process.[122] Delta power, a measure of EEG activity in the 1- to 4-Hz range, in SWS is in a quantitative and predictive relationship with prior wakefulness. Delta power is negatively correlated with the response to arousing stimuli[123] and SWS fragmentation[124] and therefore can be seen as a measure of SWS intensity. Sleep loss evokes an increase in delta power during subsequent SWS that is proportional to the loss,[125–127] whereas excess sleep results in an attenuation of delta power.[128] The time constant for the accumulation of a need for NREM sleep (increase in delta power), but not for its decline, varies greatly between inbred mouse strains.[127] QTL analysis was performed in 25 BXD recombinant inbred strains for the segregation of the rebound of delta power after 6 hours of sleep deprivation. Results showed that additive genetic factors accounted for more than 67% of the total variance.[127] By analyzing 788 polymorphic markers for a genome-wide scan, a significant QTL was identified on chromosome 13 and a suggestive one on chromosome 2. The QTL on chromosome 13 explained 49% of the total variance in delta power rebound, suggesting the presence of a major gene. Confirmation of the chromosome 13 QTL was obtained in baseline recordings of the same animals. This result suggests that sleep need is under strong genetic control and genes can be identified underlying NREM sleep homeostasis.[127]

By using gene profiling in three mouse inbred strains differing in their sleep need, we have identified *Homer1a* as the best transcriptional marker of sleep need.[129] Interestingly, *Homer1a* maps exactly to the same chromosome 13 QTL that we had already identified for sleep need.[127] We have also generated transgenic mice to investigate the transcriptional changes occurring in *Homer1a*-expressing neurons in the brain after sleep deprivation. Again, *Homer1a* was identified together with four other activity-induced genes, all up-regulated by glutamate. Homer1 proteins are postsynaptic density proteins linking metabotropic glutamate receptors to other intracellular effectors mediating the effects of N-methyl-D-aspartate and aminohydroxymethyl isoxazole propionate receptors as well as the intracellular calcium stores. Activation of Homer1a

disrupts this signaling pathway and buffers the intracellular calcium. Our findings suggest a role for sleep in intracellular calcium homeostasis for protecting and recovering from the neuronal activation imposed by wakefulness. Since *Homer1a* is also induced by electroconvulsive therapy and antidepressants, we propose that its induction by sleep deprivation might correlate with the well-documented antidepressant effects of sleep deprivation.

GENETICS OF SLEEP DISORDERS

Normal sleep is a highly complex behavior in its regulation and physiology, and a single defect at the molecular level of one of its component can cause a dysregulation and lead to a very disabling sleep disorder. As the molecular mechanisms of normal sleep are just beginning to be elucidated, the study of sleep disorders might be an alternative approach to understand the sleep function and to find new drug targets. With the recent discovery of the hypocretin deficiency in canine and human narcolepsy, the genetics of sleep and sleep disorders appears as a very promising avenue in our understanding of sleep disorders. Familial and twins studies indicate an important influence of genetic factors on sleep disorders, and the recent linkage analysis and candidate gene analysis on multiplex families resulted in the discovery of gene mutations, susceptibility factors, or linkage evidence in several sleep disorders. Three diseases are reported to result from a single gene mutation: fatal familial insomnia, familial advanced sleep phase syndrome, and primary insomnia. A unique narcolepsy case has also been observed to be caused by a single gene mutation. Most other sleep disorders have complex genetics with susceptibility genetic factors and environmental effects.

Disorders Caused by a Single Gene

Fatal Familial Insomnia

In 1986, Lugaresi and colleagues described a 53-year-old man who suffered from progressive insomnia, dysautonomia (pyrexia, diaphoresis, myosis, and sphincter disturbances), dysarthria, tremor, and later myoclonus and coma, identifying the first sleep disorder for which a gene mutation has been identified: fatal familial insomnia (FFI).[130] Two sisters of the patient and several relatives had the same symptoms leading to coma and death after 9 months. The major features of FFI include a progressive reduction of sleep duration, an early disappearance of sleep spindles, a loss of SWS, and the disintegration of the NREM-REM sleep cycle.[131] This autosomal dominant disease affects both sexes equally, with high penetrance, and leads uniformly to death. Parchi et al. observed on postmortem tissues a massive neuronal loss and astrogliosis in the mediodorsal thalamic nuclei in association with relatively modest amounts of abnormal prion protein.[132] Selective atrophy, loss of neurons, and astrogliosis of the anteroventral thalamic nucleus cause behavioral changes, whereas impairment of the mediodorsal thalamic nucleus disrupts sleep and wakefulness and is associated with the loss of EEG spindle activity.[133] The damage of serotonergic and γ-aminobutyric acid (GABA) ergic neurons leads to sleep-wake disturbance.[130,133] The degenerations of the thalamic nuclei are caused by a point mutation at codon 178 of the prion protein gene (PrP) on chromosome 20.[134]

Familial Creutzfeldt-Jacob disease (CJD) is also associated with codon 178 mutation (substitution of asparagine for aspartate) and spongiform degeneration leading to dementia, but the two conditions differ at codon 129, with all FFI patients having a methionine and CJD patients a valine at this position. Furthermore, homozygosity at codon 129 seems to have a clinical course of less than 1 year, severe insomnia, continuous motor overactivity, and severe dysautonomia.[135] The prion protein becomes protease resistant in the brain and is implicated in a group of disorders of the central nervous system termed *spongiform encephalopathies*, but the mechanism by which the mutant prion protein exerts its toxic effects remains unknown.

In 1999, Mastraianni et al.[136] described a patient with symptoms and lesions very similar to those of FFI but lacking the mutation at codon 178, suggesting a sporadic form of fatal insomnia. Parchi et al.[137] reached the same conclusion by studying five new patients. Mastraianni inoculated mice with brain homogenates from subjects having FFI or sporadic fatal insomnia and observed the same type and distribution of cerebral lesions.[136] Therefore, fatal insomnia can occur in the absence of the D178N mutation.

Familial Advanced Sleep Phase Syndrome

Familial advanced sleep phase syndrome (FASPS) is an abnormality of human circadian behavior that segregates in a highly penetrant autosomal dominant manner. Polysomnographic measurements of sleep and plasma melatonin and body temperature rhythms indicate that all measures are phase advanced by ~4 hours.[138] Genetic studies in drosophila, fungi, plants, and animals led to the identification and characterization of clock genes responsible for circadian behavior.[139–141] In mammals, several genes are determinant for circadian oscillation: *clock, bmal1, per,* and *cry.* Toh et al. found in a four-generation family linkage between FASPS and the marker D2S395 on chromosome 2qter where the *PER2* gene maps. *hPer2,* a human homolog of the *Drosophila period* gene, was found to be mutated in affected members of one family with FASPS.[142] A mutation at position 2106 (A to G) of the hPer2 complementary DNA leading to a substitution of a serine at amino acid 662 for a glycine (S662G) is therefore responsible for FASPS in this family. The mutation affects the casein kinase I epsilon (CKIε)

binding domain of hPER2 protein and causes hypophosphorylation of CKIε in vitro. In a mammalian clock model, mPer2 is a positive regulator of the Bmal1 feedback loop, raising the possibility that phase advance of hPer2 could phase advance the feedback loop.[143] However, not all the families tested, and not all members of the same family, are linked with the hPer2 locus, suggesting a genetic heterogeneity in FASPS.

A recent study identified a missense mutation (T44A) in the human CKIδ gene in a three-generation family affected by FASPS.[144] An A-to-G mutation was identified to be responsible for a threonine-to-alanine alteration at amino acid 44 in the CKIδ protein. This mutant kinase also decreases the enzymatic activity in vitro. When this mutated gene was introduced into *Drosophila,* it was found to lengthen the circadian period. Transgenic mice were also created with a human BAC clone containing the entire wild-type CKIδ gene with the T44A variant, and an opposite effect was observed: free-running periods were significantly shorter in these mutant mice. This suggests that the interactions of the clock components as part of the circadian network may be different or species dependent.[144]

Primary Insomnia

Molecular studies of primary insomnias are very rare, but a recent study reported a missense mutation in a single patient with chronic insomnia. This mutation is a substitution of the amino acid arginine for histidine at position 192 (R192H) in exon 6 of the gene coding the GABA$_A$ β3 subunit, altering GABA$_A$ receptor function in vitro.[145] The β3 subunit is suggested to be implicated in sleep processes by the observation that β3 knock-out mice are not responsive to the hypnotic action of oleamide.[146]

Narcolepsy

In 2000, Peyron and colleagues reported the only known case of human narcolepsy caused by a point mutation, impairing hypocretin trafficking and processing.[147] A patient with severe symptoms and a very early age at onset (6 months) had a T-to-G transversion in the preprohypocretin gene, resulting in a leucine-to-arginine substitution in the signal peptide.

Disorders with Human Leukocyte Antigen Association

REM Sleep Behavior Disorder

REM sleep behavior disorder (RBD) is a parasomnia that mainly affects middle-aged or older men. It occurs only during REM sleep and is characterized by the loss of skeletal muscle atonia related to REM, resulting in complex and vigorous dream-enacting behaviors.[148] An association with drug use, toxic exposure, and neurologic disorders is reported.[149] Gagnon and colleagues reported that RBD was detected using polysomnographic recordings in about

33% of patients with Parkinson's disease.[150] RBD-type behaviors may be seen in up to 25% of Parkinson's disease patients[151] and may appear before the onset of motor symptoms of this disorder in approximately 40% of older-onset RBD patients.[152] RBD is also associated with dementia with Lewy bodies.[153] These two associations reflect an underlying synucleinopathy. Genetically, RBD seems associated with the human leukocyte antigen (HLA) DQw1 allele, more precisely with DQB1*05 and DQB1*06.[154] Replication studies are needed and should be facilitated by the increasing number of patients diagnosed with this disorder.

Sleepwalking

Sleepwalking is a frequent childhood parasomnia, affecting up to 20% of children,[155] but generally disappears at adulthood.[156] Sleepwalking is a parasomnia explained as a disorder of arousal occurring during SWS,[157] generally 1–3 hours after sleep onset, and resulting in walking during sleep with a partial or complete amnesia the next day. It is considered to be a dissociative reaction between motor and cortical activity. Epidemiologic surveys, including familial and twins studies, suggest a strong genetic component in sleepwalking,[158–161] with over 50% of concordance for MZ compared to 10–15% for DZ twins.[158,159,162] Furthermore, the prevalence of sleepwalking in first-degree relatives of an affected subject is estimated to be at least 10 times greater than in the normal population.[158] Two modes of inheritance have been proposed, multifactorial[162] and autosomal recessive with incomplete penetrance.[163] In a recent study in 60 white subjects and their families, we have reported a positive association between the HLA DQB1*05 subtype.[164] The frequency of DQB1*05 was increased in sleepwalking patients, while DQB1*0602 (associated with narcolepsy) was slightly decreased. Detailed analysis in families indicated that the polymorphic amino acid Ser74, shared by all DQB1*04 and *05 alleles, is the HLA DQB1 polymorphism most tightly associated with this parasomnia. DQB1*05 has also been implicated in RBD.[154] A common genetic predisposition to sleepwalking and RBD may explain the coexistence of both disorders in some patients. A close relationship between the immune system and sleep can be proposed and might involve some immune-related regulation of motor control during sleep.[164] Further replication and family studies are needed to confirm this association.

Kleine-Levin Syndrome

Kleine-Levin syndrome is a rare and sporadic disorder mainly affecting adolescent men, characterized by periodic hypersomnia and different behavioral abnormalities such as cognitive and mood disturbances, compulsive hyperphagia, hypersexuality, and signs of dysautonomia.[165–168] The etiology of Kleine-Levin syndrome remains unknown, although an intermittent dysfunction

at the diencephalic-hypothalamic interface is suggested.[169,170] Another hypothesis is an imbalance in serotonergic or dopaminergic systems or an abnormality in the metabolism of these two neurotransmitters.[171,172] Katz and Ropper reported the first familial case with two affected siblings.[173] The sister and brother shared the HLA DR2 and DQ1 antigens. In a study in 30 unrelated patients and their families, we have observed an increased frequency of the HLA DQB1*0201 allele (28.3% vs. 12.5% in controls).[174] Three of the patients but none of the controls were homozygous for this allele. In 17 heterozygous parents, 11 (64.7%) had transmitted this allele, suggesting a preferential transmission. The recurrence of the episodes, the frequent infectious precipitating factors at onset, young age at onset, and the association with HLA DQB*0201 are in favor of an autoimmune etiology for this disorder.[174]

Delayed Sleep Phase Syndrome

Despite normal sleep architecture, delayed sleep phase syndrome (DSPS) is characterized by a persistently delayed sleep onset and offset. Shibui and colleagues found that the melatonin rhythms of these patients were delayed compared to controls.[175] However, the mechanism underlying this disease is still unknown, although different hypothesizes have been proposed: a prolonged intrinsic period beyond the range of entrainment to the 24-hour day, a reduced sensitivity of the oscillator to photic entrainment, or an abnormal coupling of the sleep-wake cycle to the circadian rhythm.[176–178] Although DSPS seems to have a heterogeneous etiology, associations with HLA DR1[179] and PER3 gene polymorphisms[180,181] have been reported. The exact role of PER3 is not clearly established, but this protein heterodimerizes with PER1 and -2 and CRY1 and -2 before entering the nucleus to inhibit the transcriptional CLOCK/BMAL1 complex.[182,183] An alteration of PER3 phosphorylation could change its function and alter the cellular circadian machinery.

Narcolepsy

Narcolepsy is a rare and disabling disorder characterized by a tetrad of symptoms: cataplexy, excessive daytime sleepiness, sleep paralysis, and hypnagogic hallucinations.[184,185] In Western countries the prevalence is 0.03–0.1% of the general population[186,187]; in Japan the prevalence is the highest,[188] and in Israel the lowest.[189] The onset of the disease occurs between 15 and 30 years of age,[190] generally with both sexes equally affected. The major abnormality in narcolepsy is an intrusion of REM sleep–like features during wakefulness, such as hypnagogic hallucinations, sleep paralysis, and cataplexy, and an inability to stay awake during the daytime. Up to 10% of narcolepsies are familial, and the risk for first-degree relatives is 20–40 times higher than for the general population.[191] This indicates a strong genetic influence on the development of the disease. However, twin studies reported only 25–31% concordance, clearly indicating a major importance of environmental factors.[192]

Numerous studies have demonstrated that narcolepsy has one of the tightest associations with a specific HLA allele. First an association with HLA class I Bw35 was reported in Japanese patients, whereas in whites HLA Bw7 was associated.[193,194] In the early 1980s, a 100% association with HLA DR2/DQw1 was shown in Japanese patients[193] and 85–95% in whites.[195–197] Four alleles corresponding to DRB1*1501, DRB5*0101, DQA1*0102, and DQB1*602 are associated with the disease. Eighty-eight percent to 98% of patients affected by narcolepsy with clear cataplexy are HLA DQB1*0602 positive, versus 40–60% of narcolepsy patients with mild or atypical or no cataplexy.[198]

Although HLA DQB1*0602 remains the best genetic marker for narcolepsy, other genetic factors contribute to its susceptibility. Several studies have sought associations with non-HLA gene polymorphisms. A significant association between narcolepsy and the monoaminergic pathway involving monoamine oxidase A (MAO-A) and the catechol-O-methyltransferase (COMT) gene was reported.[199–201] A sexual dimorphism in the activity of the COMT gene as well as an effect on the severity of daytime sleepiness suggest a more critical alteration of the dopaminergic/noradrenergic than the serotonergic pathways in the pathophysiology of narcolepsy.[200] COMT genotype seems to influence sleep-onset REM periods together with sleep paralysis. Another study reported an involvement of tumor necrosis factor (TNF)-α promoter polymorphism in narcolepsy.[202] *TNFA* may be another susceptibility gene, particularly in association with HLA DRB1*1501.[203] Another association with TNF receptor 2 has been reported in Japanese patients, indicating the possibility of an additive effect.[204]

Narcolepsy is also found in dogs and is clinically and electrophysiologically similar to the human disease. Through linkage analysis and positional cloning, mutations in the hypocretin-2 receptor were identified as the cause of canine narcolepsy.[205] Simultaneously, a similar phenotype in mice was observed after a targeted deletion of the pre-prohypocretin gene.[206] The human 131–amino acid pre-prohypocretin is encoded by a gene on chromosome 17q21 and is synthesized by neurons located exclusively in the lateral, posterior, and perifornical hypothalamus.[207] A mutation in the pre-prohypocretin gene was identified in an atypical case of narcolepsy, but so far no mutation has been found in hypocretin receptors genes.[147] In a few postmortem narcoleptic brains, an 85–95% reduction in the number of hypocretin neurons has been reported, strongly suggesting that a selective destruction of hypocretin neurons in the hypothalamus is the most probable etiology for narcolepsy.[147,208] Since 90% of human cases of narcolepsy are sporadic and monozygotic twins show only partial concordance (25–31%), the

development of the disease should involve environmental factors directly interacting with genetic susceptibility factors. Therefore, because of the tight association with HLA, an autoimmune process could be the cause of an acute or progressive and selective degeneration of hypocretin-containing neurons in the hypothalamus. Environmental factors might trigger narcolepsy by inducing an autoimmune reaction that targets hypocretin-containing neurons.

In familial forms, several subjects affected over several generations are rare, making mapping studies through linkage analysis very difficult. Nevertheless, two studies are available; the first included eight small Japanese families and found only a suggestive linkage (logarithm of the odds [lod] score = 3.09) to 4p13-q2[209]; the second one, from our laboratory, included a single extended French family with 4 individuals with narcolepsy with clear-cut cataplexy and 10 others affected with the minor form of narcolepsy (excessive daytime sleepiness with questionable cataplexy or without cataplexy). In this study, a single significant (multipoint lod score = 4.00) locus was identified in a 5-Mb region on chromosome 21q.[210] A recent study in Japanese sporadic narcolepsy patients identified a narcolepsy resistance gene on chromosome 21.[211] However, this locus does not map to the adjacent region identified by us in a Franch family[210]; nevertheless it has been shown that the expression of MX2, which maps to our chromosome 21 locus, is down-regulated in peripheral blood cells of Japanese narcolepsy patients.[212]

Disorders with Other Gene Associations

Obstructive Sleep Apnea Syndrome

Obstructive sleep apnea syndrome (OSAS) is a common, chronic, and complex disorder characterized by repetitive episodes of upper airway obstruction that occur during sleep, usually associated with a reduction in blood oxygen saturation. OSAS typically leads to excessive daytime sleepiness, an increased risk of high blood pressure, and cardiovascular complications. Snoring is one of the main symptoms of OSAS, but while 30–50% of the general population snores, only 4–5% are affected by OSAS.[213] The concordance rates for snoring and OSAS are higher in MZ than DZ twins, with heritabilities of about 50%.[213,214] Numerous families of patients have been reported to be at significantly higher risk. The segregation is explained by the fact that most of the risk factors involved in the pathophysiology of this condition are largely genetically determined. Body fat distribution and metabolism (especially upper body obesity), craniofacial dysmorphism, central regulation of breathing, and neural ventilatory control abnormalities predispose to the obstruction of the upper airways. Palmer et al.[215] performed a 9-cM genome scan on 66 white pedigrees and found linkage between the apnea-hypopnea index and chromosome 1p (lod score = 1.39), 2p (1.64), 12p (1.43), and 19p (1.4). Body mass index was linked to significant markers on 2p (lod score = 3.08), 7p (2.53), and 12p (3.41). After adjustment for body mass index, suggestive lod scores for OSAS persisted only on chromosome 2p (1.33) and 19p (1.45).[215]

Three recent studies reported a possible link between apolipoprotein E ε4 and OSAS.[216–218] Apolipoprotein E is a polymorphic protein encode by three alleles at a single gene locus on chromosome 19q13. The same allele has been associated with Alzheimer's disease and cardiovascular disease in the general population. The probability of moderate to severe sleep-disordered breathing is significantly higher in patients with apolipoprotein E ε4, independently of age, sex, body mass index, and ethnicity. This potential association is not, however, confirmed in older patients (>79 years old). A polymorphism in angiotensin-converting enzyme was also reported in moderate OSAS and was found to be tightly associated in hypertensive patients.[219] Finally, another study indicated an association between haptoglobulin polymorphism and OSAS complicated with cardiovascular disease, suggesting that hyptoglobulin phenotype is an important susceptibility factor.[220]

Restless Legs Syndrome

Restless legs syndrome (RLS) is one of the most common sleep and movement disorders, affecting 2–5% of the general population.[221] According to the diagnostic criteria, RLS is characterized by an irresistible desire to move the limbs, usually associated with paresthesias and/or dysesthesias and motor restlessness, and results in nocturnal insomnia and chronic sleep deprivation.[221] RLS affects both sexes equally and the age at onset is variable, although early onset and anticipation phenomena have been reported in familial cases.[222,223] Several studies reported that more than 50% of patients with RLS had a positive family history and that an affected person is three to six times more likely to have a family history than an unaffected person.[221] The symptoms start or worsen at rest and improve with activity. In over 87% of cases RLS is associated with periodic limb movements in sleep (PLMS).[224] The pathophysiology of RLS is still unknown, although dopaminergic dysfunction and brain iron metabolism abnormalities may be implicated.[225]

Pedigree analysis in families of 12 pairs of monozygotic twins suggested an autosomal dominant mode of inheritance and 83% concordance in monozygotic twins.[226] A genetic basis of this syndrome is supported by studies reporting a positive family history in 63–92% of patients, strongly suggesting that a significant portion of the familial aggregation is due to genetic factors, proposed to be transmitted with an autosomal dominant mode of inheritance with incomplete penetrance and probable anticipation effect.[227,228] An RLS susceptibility locus has been mapped on the short arm of chromosome

12 in a large French-Canadian family (lod score = 3.59).[229] Two main candidates in the region are the neurotensin gene (12q21), an important modulator of dopaminergic transmission, and the homolog of the *Drosophila* clock gene *timeless* (12q12-q13). However, another study could not confirm the susceptibility locus in either of the families studied.[230] Other mapping studies in different ethnic groups are needed because the RLS locus on chromosome 12 has been mapped based on a recessive mode of inheritance, while in most familial cases a dominant mode of inheritance and variable expressivity is evident. This could suggest a genetic heterogeneity for the disease. Accordingly, in a large Italian family with RLS and PLMS, evidence for linkage was obtained on chromosome 14q based on an autosomal dominant mode of inheritance.[231] Another study identified 9p24-22a as a new susceptibility region in two American families, again with the assumption of an autosomal dominant mode of inheritance.[232] Finally, a recent linkage analysis in a large Italian family reported a suggestive locus on chromosome 19p13.[233] A putative association between a polymorphism of MAO-A and RLS was reported,[234] while a more recent study indicated that a polymorphism of neuronal nitric oxide synthase, which maps to the RLS locus on chromosome 12q, is associated with RLS in whites.[235] Two very recent genome-wide association studies reported three new RLS susceptibility genes.[236,237]

Primary Nocturnal Enuresis

Primary nocturnal enuresis is another common type of parasomnia in children, affecting 10% of 7-year-old children and even 1–2% of adolescents. Nocturnal enuresis is bed-wetting beyond the age of 5 years, when nocturnal bladder control would normally be expected. Enuresis is referred to as primary if the patient has not had at least 6 months of nocturnal continence. Familial and twins studies have suggested a genetic background for enuresis, although psychosocial environmental factors have a major modulatory effect.[238] Backwin showed that the incidence of the illness is highest in families in which both parents have been enuretic (77%).[239] In most cases, enuresis has an autosomal dominant mode of transmission with high penetrance (90%).[240] Four gene loci on chromosomes 8q, 13q, 12q, and 22q11 have been identified to be involved in primary nocturnal enuresis, suggesting its heterogeneity and the involvement of different pathways, including the bladder, the kidney, or the central control.[238,240,241] A Finnish study in twins reported a concordance rate of 0.43 for MZ versus 0.19 for DZ twins in childhood, whereas it was 0.25 versus 0, respectively, in adulthood.[242] A recent linkage analysis reported a 2-point lod score of 4.2 in six families with dominant primary nocturnal enuresis around the aquaporin-2 (*AQP2*) water channel locus (12q).[243] However, no mutation in the coding sequence was detected, excluding this gene in families in which the disease co-segregates with chromosome 12q.

CONCLUSIONS

Sleep disorders are among the most common health problems encountered in medicine and have important social and economic impacts. New technologies as well as the current progress in genome sequencing projects of different species raise new hopes to understand the molecular basis of sleep and its disorders. The number of sleep disorders for which a genetic contribution can be established is expanding rapidly, and both genetic linkage and genome-wide association studies of large number of families and cases affected by a well-defined sleep disorder should be systematically undertaken to lead to the discovery of the genetic basis of the disorders and finally to their eventual evidence-based treatment. An interesting and striking feature of an important number of sleep disorders is that they are strongly associated with HLA, suggesting a hypothetical interrelationship between sleep and the immune system that still needs to be discovered. We know that microbial products and cytokines strongly influence sleep-wake behavior and the architecture of sleep, and we know that in humans the primary response to antigens following viral infections is associated with acute enhanced sleep amount, and also that growth hormone–releasing hormone and interleukin-1 have a sleep-promoting effect. However, no direct molecular mechanism has been identified that could link these observations. The relationship between the immune system and sleep-wake behavior may arise at different levels: immune-related molecules could play a role in the development of certain disorders, as hypothesized in narcolepsy, or sleep and brain immunity could be related through stress factors or may even have a regulatory effect on each other.

Finally, two new fields will need special attention in the near future: pharmacogenomics and pharmacogenetics. Pharmacogenomics involves genome-wide analysis of the genetic determinants of drug efficacy and toxicity, while pharmacogenetics is the study of genetic causes of individual variations in drug response. Because evidence-based treatments for sleep disorders are rare, investigating the molecular bases of drug response might reveal new pathways where future drugs can be targeted.

◉ REFERENCES

A full list of references are available at www.expertconsult.com

CHAPTER 23

Nutrition and Sleep

Markku Partinen

INTRODUCTION

New information about effects of nutrition in psychiatric and neurologic diseases has been published during the past 10–20 years. In clinical practice, many narcoleptics complain of excessive afternoon sleepiness after heavy lunches and especially if they had been eating meals with high contents of carbohydrates. Effects of different types of meals on sleep have been investigated, particularly in the 1960s and 1970s, but amazingly little is still known about effects of food on sleep and alertness. The worldwide epidemic of obesity is currently one of the greatest public health problems.[1,2] Obesity is a strong risk factor for cardiovascular diseases, and it is also an important risk factor for obstructive sleep apnea. Dietary factors most likely play a much more important role in the regulation of daytime vigilance than what is recognized. As early as the 1960s, Roberts and his collaborators[3] found that, especially in African Americans, there was an association between diabetes and narcolepsy. They also found that eating carbohydrates during the daytime worsened sleepiness of narcoleptic subjects.[3] More recently, restless legs syndrome (RLS) has been associated with low ferritin levels, suggesting a possible dysfunction in iron metabolism.[4,5] Starting from revolutionary theories by Magistretti and Pellerin,[6] there is increasing evidence that glial cells have a crucial role in brain metabolism.[6–11] Much new information has also been published about the important role of the enteric nervous system (ENS) and the brain-gut relationship.[12–17] It is possible that nutrition is much more important in sleep-wake regulation, sleep disorders, and the global well-being of our brains than what is currently known.

The most important factors regulating sleep duration and vigilance levels are length and quality of sleep, duration of waking time, and different social and biological *Zeitgebers*. Also, various medications and nutritional factors have effects on sleep-wake regulation. The direct effect of foods on the central nervous system (CNS) may occur by different routes: direct nervous connections through the vagus nerve and nucleus tractus solitarius (NTS), cognitive processes, and humoral effects.

ENTERIC NERVOUS SYSTEM AND SLEEP

Signals from different receptors in the gut are transmitted to the CNS by neural connections and humoral effects. The afferent fibers of the gut-brain neural connection run through afferent vagal and sympathetic nerves. The different sensors respond to mechanical stimuli (distention of the stomach, contractions of the intestine) and to chemical stimuli from nutrients in the lumen of the gut and from gut hormones, neurotransmitters, neuromodulators, cytokines, and inflammatory mediators produced by the bacterial flora in the gut (Table 23–1). The neural stimuli travel from sensory neurons to interneurons. Different motor, secretory, and vascular reflex activities exist in the body. Information from different parts of the gut also passes to the brain stem for vasovagal reflexes and to the spinal cord for different spinal reflexes. In the brain stem, most afferent vagal fibers terminate on the NTS. There is a viscerotopic representation of different parts of the

TABLE 23–1 Neuromediators in the Enteric Nervous System

Acetylcholine
Amino Acids
- **γ-Aminobutyric acid**
- **Glutamate**

Gases
- Carbon monoxide
- **Nitric oxide**

Monoamines
- **Dopamine**
- **Histamine**
- **Noradrenaline (norepinephrine)**
- **Serotonin** (5-HT), especially 5-HT$_3$, 5-HT$_4$, and 5-HT$_{1p}$ receptors

Peptides and Hormones
- *Agouti-related peptide*
- Angiotensin II
- Calbindin
- Calcitonin gene–related peptide
- **Cholecystokinin**
- *Cocaine- and amphetamine-regulating transcript peptide*
- **Corticotropin-releasing hormone**
- Cortisol
- **Delta Sleep-Inducing Peptide**
- *Galanin*
- Gastrin-releasing peptide
- **Ghrelin**
- **Growth hormone–releasing hormone**
- Incretins
  - Gastric inhibitory polypeptide
  - Glucagon-like peptide-1
- **Insulin**
- **Leptin**
- **α-Melanocyte-stimulating hormone**
- Neuromedin B
- *Neuromedin U and neuromedin S (in the SCN)*
- Neuropeptide Y
- Neurotensin
- Opioid peptides
  - Dynorphin
  - Endorphins
  - Enkephalins
- **Orexins** (hypocretin), especially orexin A
- Peptide YY (peptide tyrosine tyrosine)
- *Pituitary adenyl cyclase activating peptide*
- **Somatostatin**
- **Substance P**
- **Thyrotropin-releasing hormone**
- **Vasoactive intestinal peptide**

Prostaglandins (in the gut, especially E and F)
Purines
- **Adenosine**
- *ATP*

Almost all if not all neuromediators of the enteric nervous system are involved also in sleep/wake regulation or regulation of circadian rhythms. The most studied transmitters are printed in **boldface** and some new transmitters with increased recent interest in sleep research are printed in *italics*.
SCN, suprachiasmatic nucleus.

enteric system in the NTS. From the NTS, information goes up to the hypothalamus and the amygdala; this probably plays a role in satiety and emotional aspects of eating and may be important in the regulation of alertness, sleepiness, and sleep-wake regulation.

Cholecystokinin and many other humoral factors have a role in the CNS-ENS network. The regulation of the sleep-wake cycle is complex, and there are different theories. The important brain transmitters in sleep-wake regulation include norepinephrine, acetylcholine, 5-hydroxytryptamine (5-HT), dopamine, glutamate, histamine, adenosine, γ-aminobutyric acid (GABA), and hypocretin. Also, prostaglandins and different peptides have an effect on regulation of alertness/sleepiness. In the past, the focus was on norepinephrine, acetylcholine, and 5-HT. They all play important roles, but do not explain "why we sleep." The role of adenosine and regulation of brain energetics is probably central. During wakefulness, extracellular adenosine increases; this increase of adenosine decreases wakefulness and causes sleepiness. Caffeine, the most common stimulant, is an adenosine receptor antagonist.

Role of Neuromediators

Peptides and Hormones

Cholecystokinin is a mixture of peptides, of which octapeptide is the most effective. It is secreted by duodenal and jejunal cells after eating food. Cholecystokinin acts on the gall bladder and the pancreas, stimulating bile production and the release of pancreatic digestive enzymes. It also acts on vagal neurons projecting to the brain stem, giving a signal of satiety that inhibits further need for eating.

Ghrelin is a peptide containing 28 amino acids. It is secreted mainly by endocrine cells in the mucosa of the stomach, especially when a person is hungry, increasing appetite. It acts on the hypothalamus to stimulate feeding, counteracting the inhibitory effects of leptin and peptide YY$_{3-36}$ (PYY$_{3-36}$; see later).

Leptin is a protein of 167 amino acids and is manufactured mainly in fat cells in adipose tissue. The amount of circulating leptin correlates positively with the amount of fat in the body. Leptin has many CNS effects. It counteracts the effects of neuropeptide Y (NPY) and inhibits secretion of α-melanocyte-stimulating hormone. As a consequence, leptin decreases appetite and inhibits food intake, contrary to ghrelin. A decrease of leptin is associated with an increase of hunger and appetite.

Neuropeptide Y is a potent feeding stimulant secreted by cells in both the gut and hypothalamic neurons. It causes increased storage of ingested food as fat. NPY inhibits transmission of pain signals to the brain.

Peptide YY$_{3-36}$ is close in structure to NPY but, contrary to NPY, is a potent inhibitor of feeding. PYY$_{3-36}$ is released by cells in the intestine after meals. The secretion increases with the amount of calories eaten, especially when these derive from proteins rather than from carbohydrates or fats. This may explain partly why people who eat a lot of carbohydrates are often hungry, developing obesity.

α-Melanocyte-stimulating hormone is responsible for tannin in humans. It is found in the brain, where it acts to suppress appetite.

Orexins (hypocretins)[18,19] were originally considered to be important particularly in central control of food intake. It is now evident that they have a much larger spectrum of action, including energy homeostasis, sleep-wake behavior, nociception, reward-seeking behavior, and drug addiction.[15,21–23] Orexins are also widely present in the gastrointestinal (GI) tract.[15] In the ENS, they have a role in regulation of GI motility, and also in gastric, intestinal, and pancreatic secretions.[15,24] The relationships among enteric regulation, eating behavior, regulation of arousal, narcolepsy,[25–27] and the orexin-hypocretin system remain to be further clarified. It is most probable that there are important interactions that explain many of the symptoms, including the effects of fasting and carbohydrate intake on the vigilance of narcoleptic subjects versus normal people.

The inhibitory effects of leptin last a long time, in contrast to the rapid inhibition of eating behavior produced by cholecystokinin and the slow suppression of hunger between meals mediated by PPY_{3-36}. Both leptin and ghrelin have been investigated in several studies attempting to find a relationship between obesity, sleep apnea, and weight loss, but leptin has not been found to have any potential use for weight-loss therapy. Leptin is low among subjects with anorexia nervosa[28] and high among obese subjects.[29,30] Low levels of leptin are also associated with hyperactivity, and it has been hypothesized that leptin could have a role in the treatment of severely hyperactive patients.[28]

Serotonin

Serotonin (5-HT) is an important neurotransmitter in the CNS with important effects on sleep-wake regulation. It also has an important role in regulation of GI function through an interaction with the ENS. The ENS can be considered the body's second brain, with more than 100 million neurons of different types. Up to 60–90% of the total body amount of 5-HT is in the GI tract, and 2–20% of all enteric neurons express 5-HT. The control of 5-HT's release from enterochromaffin cells is complex. Stimulatory receptors include β-adrenergic receptors, muscarinic and nicotinic acetylcholine receptors, and $5\text{-}HT_3$ receptors. Inhibitory receptors include α_2-adrenergic, histamine H_3, $GABA_B$, adenosine A2, and $5\text{-}HT_4$ receptors. In the GI tract, 5-HT is eliminated mainly by monoamine oxidase metabolism.[13,16]

An interesting element from the point of view of sleep and movement disorders is the $5\text{-}HT_{1p}$ receptor. This receptor is probably involved in the secretory and peristaltic reflexes of the GI tract. The molecular identification of this receptor is not yet clear. Lui and Gershon suggested that this receptor is a heterodimer of the $5\text{-}HT_{1B/1D}$ receptor and the dopamine D_2 receptor.[31] Other studies have also shown that dopamine is involved in GI tract regulation. Gershon's group has also shown

in knock-out mice that intestinal motility is abnormal when D_2 is absent.[14] A dysfunction of the intestinal dopamine system probably explains many of the GI symptoms, especially problems of constipation that are usually present very early among patients with Parkinson's disease. It remains to be seen whether there are some associations with symptoms of RLS, lack of iron, and dysfunction of the 5-HT–dopamine system of the GI tract.

Irritable bowel syndrome (IBS) is one of the most common GI disorders. It is twice as frequent among women as among men. IBS is related to dysfunction of the enteral serotonin system. There are no published epidemiologic studies about the occurrence of IBS among patients with RLS. In our own clinical database, GI symptoms had been tabulated from 141 RLS patients (unpublished observations). Of these patients, 17 (12%) had GI symptoms that could be diagnosed as IBS type. Because we had not tabulated this history systematically, the true prevalence might be higher. Also, the diagnosis of IBS had not been verified, so all we can say is that GI symptoms are quite common in patients with RLS and may be related to dysfunction of the enteral 5-HT–dopamine system. In one study, 10 of 13 patients with RLS and IBS had marked improvement in their RLS symptoms after treatment of small intestine bacterial overgrowth (SIBO). Five patients also remained symptom free during the follow-up of 54–450 days. The therapy of SIBO was based on rifaximin, which is a rifamycin-based nonsystemic antibiotic, meaning that the drug will not pass the GI wall into the circulation.[32]

Case Example

A 53-year-old male biochemist developed severe insomnia 3 weeks after returning from a congress in South America. He had difficulty falling asleep and he woke up repeatedly, sleeping only 2–3 hours. After 3 weeks of insomnia, he became exhausted and consulted our sleep clinic. He was lean. One week before consultation he had started zopiclone and fluoxetine because he was diagnosed to have depression, which he denied. There was no previous history of insomnia. The polysomnography at the laboratory was consistent with his history. Total sleep time was only 2.3 hours and there was no slow-wave sleep. No apnea or periodic limb movements were found.

In the clinical interview at the sleep clinic, it was found that he had had diarrhea with a fever during his travel. He took ciprofloxacin for 5 days but, because he continued to have diarrhea, he consulted an internist. A variety of laboratory tests were done to exclude all potential bacterial, viral, and tropical diseases. Nothing specific was found, but he was given two more antibiotics, including metronidazole. The diarrhea became much better, and his body temperature was between 37.0° and 37.3° C. Insomnia developed 1 week after the last antibiotics had been taken. The problem was discussed with the patient. The internists concluded that he had had either bacterial or viral enteritis but no serious disease had been found. He speculated that the strong antibiotics had destroyed the entire bacterial flora, including healthy saprophyte bacteria.

Because his general condition was quite good, we decided to stop further laboratory examinations and start down-titrating zopiclone and fluoxetine. He also started to take ω-3 fatty acids, and *Lactobacillus casei/Enterococcus faecium* to normalize his intestinal flora. We encouraged him to restart exercise. After 3 weeks, he began to sleep normally as he had done before. His insomnia was of a psychophysiologic type, and anxiety (fear of some severe disease) probably also played a role. It is possible that his insomnia could have been caused by a change in the intestinal flora and hence changes in the ENS-CNS regulation. The amelioration of his insomnia by reintroducing bacteria in the diet, without any other treatment, is in favor of this theory but without any clear proof.

Role of Neurosteroids

Neurosteroids are synthesized in astrocytes, oligodendrocytes, Schwann cells, Purkinje cells, hippocampal neurons, and retinal amacrine and ganglion cells.[33–36] Cholesterol is transported to glial mitochondria, where it is converted to pregnenolone. In the cytosol, pregnenolone is then converted to different neurosteroids such as allopregnanolone and dehydroepiandrosterone (DHEA). DHEA is a precursor of testosterone, which is converted to estradiol by an aromatase.[34,36] Vitamin D is also an important neurosteroid.[37] Synthesis of neurosteroids is regulated by interactions between neurons and glial cells.

Neurosteroids have many important actions. Allopregnanolone activates neuronal $GABA_A$ receptors having anxiolytic, sedative, sleep-inducing, and anticonvulsant effects. Benzodiazepines, alcohol, and γ-hydroxybutyrate increase brain levels of allopregnanolone. Thus these drugs may potentiate GABAergic transmission directly and also by increasing allopregnanolone. Pregnenolone sulfate, DHEA, and DHEA sulfate (DHEA-S) are inhibitory, noncompetitive modulators of $GABA_A$ and positive modulators of *N*-methyl-D-aspartate (NMDA) receptors by facilitating calcium influx. Estradiol inhibits NMDA receptors. Neurosteroids acting on NMDA are implicated in cognition, neuroprotection, and neurotoxicity. While pregnenolone sulfate is excitotoxic to cortical and retinal cells, DHEA and DHEA-S have neuroprotective effects against glutamate toxicity. However, the exact mechanisms of such neuroprotective effects are not clear.

Neurosteroids have been implicated in many neurologic and psychiatric disorders, including epilepsy, neurodegenerative diseases, schizophrenia, and depression. For example, depression is associated with reduced levels of allopregnanolone in cerebrospinal fluid. Antidepressant treatment with fluoxetine increases allopregnanolone levels.[38] There is also some evidence that DHEA helps in the treatment of depression. The beneficial effect of DHEA correlates with a decrease of glucocorticoids, which are increased in depression.

There is increasing evidence about many important roles of neurosteroids in regulation of vigilance as well. It remains to be studied whether nutritional factors could also play some role in this. DHEA is marketed in pharmacies and health shops. Little is known about possible positive (and, perhaps, also negative) long-term neuropsychiatric effects of nutritional factors that may cause changes in brain neurosteroids.

Role of Neurohormetic Phytochemicals

Several lines of evidence have shown that diets rich in fibers, vegetables, and fruits are associated with reduced risk of cardiovascular disease and many neurologic diseases.[39,40] There is also evidence that a vegetarian diet helps in weight control, and in this way prevents obesity and occurrence of obstructive sleep apnea. As stated previously, rapidly absorbed low-fiber carbohydrates induce sleepiness. Therefore, a vegetarian diet with a lot of fiber and slowly absorbing "good" carbohydrates is better for staying alert during waking time. Some of the positive effects are explained by antioxidant effects of different phytochemicals, but there is also evidence that some effects may be due to subtoxic effects of some neurotoxic molecules in the gut. *Hormesis* refers to a process in which low doses of a given toxic substance induce beneficial effects while larger doses of the same substance are toxic to cells and organisms.[41,42] Examples of endogenous molecules with neurohormetic actions are nitric oxide, carbon monoxide, glutamate, and calcium.

Many articles have been published about neuroprotective and other beneficial effects of natural substances. These include α-tocopherol, lycopene, resveratrol (in red grapes, red wine, peanuts, and soy), sulforaphanes (in broccoli), catechins (in green tea), allicin and allium (in garlic), curcumin (in turmeric), hypericin (in St. John's wort), and many others. In randomized clinical trials, hypericin (*Hypericum* extracts) has shown clinical efficacy comparable with the efficacy of some commonly used antidepressants, including citalopram, paroxetine, and fluoxetine.[43–49] This is of interest to sleep specialists because antidepressants are also used in treating insomnia, especially if it is thought to be associated with underlying depression. Much more research is needed to find out if natural substances affect sleep-wake behavior.

Spices may also affect sleep, perhaps by a neurohormetic action. In one study on six young men, tabasco and mustard in the evening reduced slow-wave and stage 2 sleep, reduced total time awake, and prolonged sleep onset. The spicy food in the evening elevated body temperature during the first sleep cycle. It is possible that capsaicin affects sleep by its effects on body temperature.[50]

Caffeine, Adenosine, and Sleep

Caffeine, used mainly in the form of coffee, is the world's most common psychoactive drug. Caffeine is present in coffee, tea, cola, energy drinks, and chocolate, and it induces wakefulness. Its stimulant properties depend on its ability to reduce adenosine transmission in the brain. Caffeine acts as an antagonist to adenosine A1 and especially to adenosine A2 receptors.[51] Huang and collaborators found in knock-out mice that caffeine increased wakefulness in both wild-type mice and A1 receptor knock-out mice, but not in A2a receptor knock-out mice. Thus, caffeine-induced wakefulness may be due mainly to its effects on adenosine A2a receptors.[52]

Porkka-Heiskanen and her collaborators[53] have also recorded human sleep electroencephalograms (EEGs). The longer the previous wakefulness period is, the longer and deeper is the following sleep. The inhibitory neuromodulator adenosine is one promising candidate for a sleep-inducing factor. Its concentration is higher during wakefulness than during sleep, it accumulates in the brain during prolonged wakefulness, and local perfusions as well as systemic administration of adenosine and its agonists induce sleep and decrease wakefulness. The hypothesis is that adenosine accumulates in the extracellular space of the basal forebrain during wakefulness, increasing the sleep propensity. The increase in extracellular adenosine concentration decreases the activity of the wakefulness-promoting cell groups, especially the cholinergic cells in the basal forebrain. When the activity of the wakefulness-active cells decreases sufficiently, sleep is initiated. During sleep, the extracellular adenosine concentrations decrease, and thus the inhibition of the wakefulness-active cells decreases, allowing awakening and a new wakefulness period.[53]

In addition to coffee, caffeine is found in tea, cola drinks, energy drinks, and chocolate. Theobromine is also present in large quantities in chocolate. Dark chocolate is stimulating; 100 g of 70% chocolate corresponds to 1–2 cups of coffee depending on strength of the coffee and size of the cup. Caffeine is a CNS stimulant. Its actions are variable among different people. Caffeine is absorbed rapidly, and peak activity is achieved in 30–60 minutes. The duration of action is usually 4–6 hours, but in elderly subjects with slower metabolism the duration may be up to 16–20 hours. Insomniacs are usually advised to avoid coffee after 6:00 PM, but in some sensitive persons with insomnia, coffee at noon may disturb falling asleep in the evening.

One cup of coffee contains 75–125 mg of caffeine. A large amount of caffeine, usually over 300–500 mg (depending on individual sensitivity), causes restlessness, anxiety, trembling, tinnitus, and feelings of euphoria/delirium. Everyday use of more than 500 mg of caffeine leads to caffeinism with insomnia, fatigue, and different psychosomatic symptoms. It has been estimated that perhaps 10–20% of coffee drinkers have caffeinism. Chronic coffee drinkers have often developed tolerance to caffeine, and some people may drink more than 10 cups of coffee daily. They have withdrawal symptoms if they do not have their coffee. Coffee is a well-known factor disturbing sleep.[54-57] Two or three cups of coffee (or in sensitive persons just one cup) before bedtime is followed by difficulty falling asleep and restless sleep.

Landolt et al.[58] administered 200 mg of caffeine in the morning and analyzed the sleep stages and EEG power spectra during the subsequent night in nine healthy men. They also measured caffeine levels in saliva, which decreased from a maximum of 17 μmol/L 1 hour after intake to 3 μmol/L at 23:00 in the evening. Compared to placebo, sleep efficiency and total sleep time were significantly reduced after the morning intake of caffeine.[58] Slow-wave sleep decreases and amount of stage 1 sleep usually increases after drinking coffee. Insomnia and RLS are more frequent among habitual coffee drinkers than among others. Paradoxically, in some persons one or two cups of coffee may ameliorate quality of sleep. The reason can be behavioral conditioning, but it is also known that caffeine has a stimulating effect on both breathing and cardiac function. In patients with RLS, symptoms worsen by drinking a lot of coffee. Missak postulated that the human body—in cases of iron deficiency and chronic renal failure—may produce a substance similar to caffeine.[59]

Epidemiologic studies in Turku, Finland, and elsewhere have provided evidence that caffeine, an adenosine receptor antagonist, reduces the risk for Parkinson's disease. There are indications of specific interactions between striatal adenosine A2a and dopamine D_2 receptors. In one study, the dopaminergic effects of caffeine were examined with [^{11}C]raclopride positron emission tomography in eight healthy habitual coffee drinkers after 24 hours of caffeine abstinence. Compared to oral placebo, 200 mg of oral caffeine induced a 12% decrease in midline thalamic binding potential ($p < 0.001$). A trend-level increase in ventral striatal [^{11}C]raclopride binding potential was seen, with a correlation between caffeine-related arousal and putaminal dopamine D_2 receptor binding ($r = -.81$, $p = 0.03$). These findings indicate that caffeine has effects on dopaminergic neurotransmission in the human brain, which may be different in the striatum and the thalamus.[60]

GLUCOSE, LACTATE, AND GLIAL CELLS

The main sources of energy for the brain are glucose and lactate. According to Magistretti's theory, lactate may be the most important source of neuronal energy.[61] Most of the glucose from brain capillaries enters glial cells through the blood-brain barrier. In astrocytes, glucose is metabolized into lactate by glycolysis. The rate of lactate metabolism depends on brain activity and use of oxygen. Mitochondrial function should be intact for proper functioning.

Besides the heart, the CNS is the only part of the body that may have both functional and structural changes after hypoglycemia. However, the brain resists fasting better than other organs. The brain uses glucose at a rate of about 70 mg/min and contains about 1–2 g of glucose, which is sufficient for about 90 minutes if no more glucose is obtained from circulation. There are no strong associations between behavioral symptoms and plasma glucose levels, but fatigue and other symptoms usually occur when glucose levels are below 1.5–2 mmol/L. Common reasons for hypoglycemia are overdose of diabetic medications, high insulin levels, and severe malnutrition.

Glutamate, adenosine, and GABA have crucial roles in controlling brain energetics and lactate formation in the glia. The role of lactate as a source of energy needs to be studied in more detail.

Interestingly, these theories also fit some other findings about the importance of glial cells in control of synaptic transmission and neuronal activity. Newman,[11] Montana et al.,[62] and Zhang et al.[63] pointed out the role of astrocytes in regulation of synaptic activity, and, as Hertz and Zielke have written, astrocytes may be the "stars of the show."[10] All functions of glutamate are regulated by astrocytes. Glutamate is the most important excitatory brain transmitter, and all is dependent on the ability of astrocytes to produce glutamate and glutamine.[10] The studies by Aubert and his collaborators of CNS lactate kinetics support these findings, indicating that neurons are lactate-consuming cells, whereas astrocytes are lactate producers. Lactate production by glial cells (mostly astrocytes) increases with enhanced glutamatergic activation, and consumption of lactate by neurons also increases as a result of glutamatergic activity.[64] It may well be that many neurologic and psychiatric diseases will turn out to be mainly glial diseases. This may also be true for fatigue and sleepiness. Do we sleep to ensure having sufficient energy for waking brain activity? In this case, the solution for the basic mechanisms of sleep-wake regulation may also be found by investigating the glial-neuronal network, rather than concentrating our research efforts only on neuronal synaptic relationships. If neurons do not have enough food (energy) of proper quality, they may starve and will not function normally.

MEALS AND SLEEP

Rapidly Absorbing Carbohydrates and Large Meals

Clinicians treating narcoleptics know that rapidly absorbing carbohydrates induce sleepiness in the afternoon among their patients. What about the effect of carbohydrates in normal subjects? Most studies in which different foods have been compared with each other show that carbohydrates at lunch induce afternoon sleepiness more than proteins. In a study by Spring et al.,[65] normal adults consumed either a high-protein or high-carbohydrate meal. Two hours later their mood and performance were tested. Women, but not men, reported greater sleepiness after a carbohydrate as opposed to a protein meal. Men, but not women, reported greater calmness after a carbohydrate as opposed to a protein meal. Age of subjects

had an effect on the response to meals. When meals were eaten for breakfast, persons older than 40 years felt more tense and less calm after a protein-rich than after a carbohydrate-rich meal. Older subjects did not like a morning protein meal as much as a carbohydrate meal, but objective performance was impaired more after a carbohydrate-rich lunch than after a protein-rich lunch. Sustained selective attention, as measured by dichotic shadowing, was impaired in the afternoon after consuming a high-carbohydrate lunch. In sum, these findings suggest negative effects on concentration after a high-carbohydrate, low-protein lunch.[65]

In another study,[66] fatiguing effects of lunch after carbohydrate-rich meals were compared to other types of meals. Observed behavioral changes were correlated with changes in plasma glucose, insulin, and amino acids. Only the carbohydrate meal significantly increased fatigue, which could not be attributed to hypoglycemia because plasma glucose remained elevated. The afternoon fatigue began when the carbohydrate meal elevated plasma tryptophan but ended even though the ratio remained elevated. Fatigue after a high-carbohydrate lunch could not be explained by reactive hypoglycemia or sweet taste, and could partially be explained by the hypothesis that fatigue parallels an elevation of tryptophan.[66] Associations among a carbohydrate-rich meal, an increase of tryptophan, and feelings of fatigue have also been confirmed in other studies.[67,68]

Rapid increase of insulin and its effect on tryptophan are related to symptoms of fatigue. As early as the late 1970s and early 1980s, Närvänen and colleagues studied extensively mechanisms of the relationship among glucose, increase of insulin, sleepiness, and increased levels of tryptophan and serotonin. Especially after rapidly absorbing carbohydrates as well as after a glucose intolerance test, insulin is rapidly increased. This rapid increase of insulin is associated with an increase in the ratio of tryptophan to large neutral amino acids (LNAAs) causing abnormal neuroglycopenic symptoms. In practice this may be seen as "sugar drunkenness."[68] These findings have been confirmed by Cunliffe et al., who found that subjects consuming a pure carbohydrate meal were more tired with feelings of fatigue and had had slower reaction times.[69] A general feeling of mental or central fatigue was noticed after a pure isocaloric fat meal. The ratio of tryptophan to LNAAs was decreased after a pure fat or mixed meal and rose after a pure carbohydrate meal. The authors concluded that central and subjective fatigue after carbohydrate intake may be related to an increase in tryptophan relative to other competitive amino acids. Pure fat intake may also have a negative influence on CNS arousal.[69]

The amount of food eaten is also related to feelings of sleepiness. Solid foods cause more sleepiness than liquid foods. Valuable studies have also shown that the larger the meal, the sleepier the person is afterward.[70] It may be that filling the stomach with plenty of food might have a stronger effect than different constituents of food per se.[71]

Sleepiness and fatigue after lunch are usually unwanted. For this reason, people wanting to avoid post-lunch sleepiness should avoid rapidly absorbing carbohydrates and large meals. Needless to say, alcohol during lunch increases sleepiness. In the evening the sleep-facilitating effects of carbohydrates may be beneficial. Recently Afaghi et al.[72] explored the effect of the glycemic index (GI) on sleep in 12 healthy men. Their subjects were administered standard, isocaloric (3212 kJ; 8% of energy as protein, 1.6% of energy as fat, and 90.4% of energy as carbohydrate) meals of either Mahatma (GI = 50 [low]) or Jasmine (GI = 109 [high]) rice 4 hours before their usual bedtime. On another occasion, the same high-GI meal was given 1 hour before bedtime. Sleep onset latency shortened significantly after a high-GI meal compared with a low-GI meal. The high-GI meal given 4 hours before bedtime had better action on sleep latency than the same meal given just 1 hour before bedtime (9.0 ± 6.2 vs. 14.6 ± 9.9 minutes; $p = 0.01$).[72] This finding confirms earlier studies showing that a (light) carbohydrate-rich diet during dinner may be beneficial for sleep.

Postlunch Fatigue

A siesta after lunch is still common in some parts of the world, although it has disappeared from most developed countries. Even in developed countries a feeling of tiredness in the afternoon is common. According to Bell,[73] 71% of narcoleptics and 9% of healthy adults suffer often or always from postprandial sleepiness. The vigilance level has a bimodal pattern: alertness is at its lowest level after midnight, and there is another dip in alertness occurring during the afternoon independent of whether one has been eating or not. The effects of different types of meals have been studied. There is evidence that heavy meals cause more fatigue than light meals. There is also agreement that alcohol during lunch causes sleepiness in the afternoon. In clinical settings, there is some evidence that rapidly absorbing carbohydrates in particular cause more sleepiness and fatigue after lunch than slowly absorbing carbohydrates and proteins, but we need more studies to know the truth. Subjects also tended to feel more sleepy and fatigued 2–3 hours after a high-fat, low-carbohydrate meal than after low-fat, high-carbohydrate breakfast.[74]

Obesity and Sleep

Obesity is an epidemic, especially in Western countries. It is believed that the epidemic is a consequence of eating too much food with energetic value combined with a decrease of physical activity. This is probably true, but it does not explain everything. In the medical world, research on cardiovascular diseases has been one of the primary foci. High cholesterol levels are associated with an increase in cardiovascular morbidity. Therefore, the food industry has been developing foods with no cholesterol, and people are advised to avoid butter and fats. However, the food industry has also been developing more and more foods and soft drinks with high sugar content (e.g., Coca-Cola, Pepsi-Cola). Despite eating less, fat people become more and more obese, suggesting that other factors must be involved.

From a physiologic standpoint, body fat is deposited in excess amounts when caloric intake exceeds caloric expenditure.[75] Most of our calories are expended in a resting state. We know that obese patients with sleep apnea have difficulty losing weight. It has been questioned whether obese people have a lower resting metabolism than lean people. Are obese people like diesel motors? Using whole-body direct calorimetry and other methods that enable measurement of basic metabolism, researchers have shown that obese subjects often have lower resting metabolic rates that persist after weight reduction, that people with a high genetic propensity for obesity often show this decreased resting metabolism before they become obese, and that these people are more likely to regain their weight after weight reduction. The mechanism of the low resting metabolic rate in many obese people is not known.[75] Eating less food with high energy content is needed to lose weight. Also, avoiding rapidly absorbing carbohydrates should be an element in weight reduction. Avoiding fats and increasing exercise do not help if an obese subject continues to drink sweet soft drinks and eat a lot of potatoes, white bread, or sweets. It is important to note that, with excess caloric intake, carbohydrates convert to fat. Citrate from the citric acid cycle diverts from mitochondria into cytosol for fatty acid synthesis. After a meal rich in carbohydrates, insulin release from the pancreas causes a 30-fold increase in glucose transport into adipocytes.

DIETARY PATTERNS AND SLEEP

Effect of Fasting on Sleep

Effects of fasting on sleep length differ depending on the study. Fasting was associated with shorter sleep in some human studies and with increased sleep in others. Results of studies on the effect of fasting on sleep architecture are somewhat divergent. Fasting, resulting in decreased energy intake, seems to be associated with an increase of slow-wave sleep, and a decrease of rapid eye movement (REM) sleep and sleep stages 1 and 2. In the earlier studies this was explained by the restorative function of slow-wave sleep.[76,77] In the 1980s it was thought that sleep was mainly for the brain and had little restorative value.[78] It is now known that sleep not only is important for the brain, but also has a restorative function.[79,80] The relationship is complex. In experimental studies, caloric restriction protects the brain against aging and disease. Markers of oxidative stress were lower in cultured neuronal cells treated with caloric restriction serum compared with those treated with ad libitum serum.[81]

The effects of the intermittent type of fasting during Ramadan differ from those of continuous fasting. In one study, the main finding was that during Ramadan sleep latency was increased and sleep architecture was modified. Slow-wave sleep and REM sleep decreased during Ramadan. The effects of Ramadan fasting on nocturnal sleep have been explained by changes in drinking and meal schedule, rather than an altered energy intake, which may be preserved.[82]

Ketogenic Diet and Sleep

The ketogenic diet has been used for a long time in the treatment of severe epilepsy. It is efficient but it is usually only a temporary solution. Some efforts have been made to develop other diets that are based mainly on lowering amounts of carbohydrates in order to lower blood sugar levels without inducing marked metabolic ketosis. Early results have been promising. Again, these diets are based on Magistretti's theories and on theories about the role of astrocytes[10,11,62,63,83]; the mechanisms of action are poorly known. It is possible that in fact brain cells, especially glial cells, perform better when glucose levels are lower. This is followed by better synaptic function and less paroxysmal activity.

According to theories on brain energetics, the ketogenic diet could help people to sleep better and have better alertness during the daytime. Hallbook et al. have recently published first results supporting this idea.[84] They examined 18 children with treatment-resistant epilepsy. All children had polysomnography studies before starting a ketogenic diet and after 3 months on the diet. Eleven children were evaluated after staying on the diet for 1 year. Seizures were controlled with the diet, and it was associated with decreased total sleep and total night sleep. There was no change in amount of slow-wave sleep, and REM sleep was increased. Stage 2 sleep was decreased ($p = 0.004$), and sleep stage 1 was unchanged. There was a significant correlation between increased REM sleep and improvement in quality of life.

Brown has formed an interesting hypothesis to explain the positive mental effects of a low-carbohydrate diet.[85] Better vigilance, feelings of well-being, and feelings of mild euphoria have been attributed to increased production of ketone bodies, which can replace glucose as an energy source for the brain, as Magistretti has postulated.[6,83] Brown noted that one of these ketone bodies, β-hydroxybutyrate (BHB), is an isomer of γ-hydroxybutyrate, which is used as treatment for alcohol and opiate dependence and also for narcolepsy with cataplexy. Brown hypothesized that the positive mental effects with fasting and a low-carbohydrate diet may be due to shared actions of BHB and GHB on the brain. BHB, like GHB, is a weak partial agonist for GABA_B receptors.[85]

Power Naps

Short alerting naps or "power naps" have shown to be an efficient way of increasing alertness in the workplace or when driving a car. First, 100–150 mg of caffeine is taken in the form of coffee or an energy drink. This is followed by a 15- to 30-minute-long nap. During short naps, caffeine is absorbed and postnap drowsiness (sleep drunkenness) may be avoided. Alertness is increased for 3–6 hours.[86–88] Some physicians advise elderly people to avoid daytime naps. There is, however, no good evidence showing that a nap in the afternoon would be harmful for night sleep, providing that the nap has been short enough (<1 hour).[89] Long daily naps may be related to some underlying medical pathology, but according to Naska et al.,[90] naps of any duration seem to be healthy.

ALCOHOL AND SLEEP

Excessive use of alcohol is associated with complaints of insomnia. Alcohol shortens sleep latency, but it may also disturb sleep later at night. Two or more drinks of whisky or other liquors increase snoring and are a strong risk factor for obstructive sleep apnea.[91–95] There is evidence that heavy drinking of alcohol is associated with smoking, obesity, poor physical condition, ill health behavior, and insomnia.[96–108] One or 2 glasses of alcohol may help a person to fall asleep, but more than 2 glasses worsen the quality and architecture of night sleep,[109–114] in addition to causing snoring and sleep apnea. Larger amounts of alcohol (0.5–1 g/kg body weight) diminish REM sleep during the first third of the night, but there is often a rebound of REM sleep later at night. This correlates with awakenings early in the morning. If alcohol is used in larger quantities, REM sleep is diminished during the whole night. The blood alcohol level at the time of going to sleep correlates with a decrease of REM sleep.[115] According to many studies, alcohol decreases slow-wave sleep, but according to other studies slow-wave sleep, especially during the first third of the night, may increase. In any case, the normal sleep architecture is easily disturbed with larger doses of alcohol.[116,117] Alcoholics sleep poorly. Even worse, the sleep of alcoholics may be disturbed for many years after drinking has stopped.[118] This must be taken into account when treating insomniacs with a history of alcoholism since they may need psychological support for many years.

Could alcohol be used as an alternative to hypnotics? There is evidence that one glass of wine or spirits in the evening may help in falling asleep both among working adults and elderly people. There have been some studies in residential facilities for the elderly, where use of hypnotics has been compared with use of wine or sherry. In a randomized study, 1 glass of alcohol was better than 1 tablet of a hypnotic.[119] Use of hypnotics is a problem in geriatric institutions, because use of hypnotics among elderly people is associated with increased mortality.

No studies have shown any benefits for every-night use of hypnotics, but many studies have shown risks of routine hypnotic use.[120–126] Alternatives to hypnotics are needed, especially for elderly people. One of them is a social hour. In some residential facilities for the elderly, 1 glass of wine or sherry, served in a day room/living room, is offered during a social hour in the evening. It is possible that most of the beneficial effects are explained by behavioral factors.[119,127] The elderly people who are given a glass of sherry do not usually drink it immediately, but stay in the day room/living room for some time. This results in a delay in going to bed, which is associated with fewer awakenings during early morning hours after midnight.

ESSENTIAL FATTY ACIDS AND SLEEP

The polyunsaturated fatty acids (PUFAs) linoleic acid, α-linolenic acid (α-LA), eicosapentaenoic acid (EPA), and docosahexaenoic acid (DHA) are essential fatty acids in many mammals, including humans (see *Nutrition and Development of the Central Nervous System* later). α-LA is a precursor of DHA, and EPA is converted to DHA in the body. A sufficient amount of PUFAs from food is necessary for health and well-being. Both DHA and EPA are ω-3 acids, and both may be obtained by eating fish oils. The American Heart Association has recommended that the amount of long-chain ω-3 fatty acids should exceed 650 mg/day. In Britain, more than 1000 mg/day is recommended by the British Heart Association.[132] Fatty fish is the best source of ω-3 fatty acids. One hundred grams of salmon contains about 1000 mg of ω-3 fatty acids and 100 g of herring contains about 2000 mg. White fish meat contains much less of these essential fatty acids than fish with fatty meat. There is increasing evidence that a reduced amount of ingested ω-3 fatty acids is associated with fatigue, depression, and problems of attention.[128–131] ω-3 Fatty acids have been tested in the treatment of subjects with attention deficit disorder and in subjects with depression, female subjects with borderline personality disorder, fatigue in multiple sclerosis, memory disturbances, dementia, and some other neuropsychiatric diseases.[129,130,133–145] Randomized controlled studies have shown that ω-3 acids help, but there are still some conflicting results and more well-conducted randomized studies are needed.[130,133–135,137–141,146–149]

Decreased DHA and decreased brain-derived neurotrophic factor (BDNF) have been implicated in bipolar disorder. In a study by Rao et al., the authors show that dietary deprivation of ω-3 PUFAs for 15 weeks in rats increased their depression and aggression. The dietary ω-3 PUFA deprivation for 15 weeks decreased the frontal cortex DHA level and reduced frontal cortex BDNF expression, cyclic AMP response element binding protein (CREB) transcription factor activity, and p38 mitogen-activated protein kinase (MAPK) activity. Activities of other CREB-activating protein kinases were not significantly changed. The addition of DHA to rat primary cortical astrocytes in vitro reversed most of the effects caused by dietary fatty acid deprivation. DHA is able to regulate BDNF via a p38 MAPK–dependent mechanism. That may explain some of its therapeutic effects in brain diseases characterized by disordered cell survival and neuroplasticity.[150]

There is some evidence showing that essential fatty acids may modulate sleep. Fagioli from Italy studied eight children who were fed by total parenteral nutrition without essential lipids and seven other children who received a daily supplement of essential lipids in their parenteral nutrition. Slow-wave sleep was significantly decreased in the group of children who did not receive fatty acids as compared to those who did.[151] ω-3 Fatty acids are also necessary for early brain development and infant sleep. Cheruku et al. measured plasma DHA from 17 women at parturition.[152] They found a significant positive correlation with concentration of DHA and quality of the newborn infants' sleeping patterns as measured by a sleep mattress method. This is thought to relate to more mature brains of the newborn infants.

NARCOLEPSY AND MEALS

In the 1960s, Roberts and his collaborators studied 326 narcoleptic patients. They reported that, of 40 African Americans in their narcolepsy population, 70% had recurrent hypoglycemia without diabetes mellitus.[3] In routine clinical practice, many patients with narcolepsy often complain of excessive sleepiness in the afternoon, particularly if they have eaten a lunch rich in carbohydrates and especially if they have eaten a sweet dessert. Avoiding a heavy, carbohydrate-rich lunch and desserts helps them to be more alert in the daytime. Based on this experience, patients with narcolepsy should be routinely advised to avoid rapidly absorbing carbohydrates, especially at lunchtime.

In spite of clinical experience, there is very little scientific knowledge about the effects of different types of meals on symptoms of narcolepsy. Bruck et al. studied 12 narcoleptics and 12 matched controls in a double-blind crossover study.[153] They measured behavior after a light lunch supplemented with a drink of either 50 g of glucose or placebo (in the form of an artificially sweetened drink). In the narcoleptic subjects, glucose was associated with decreased wake duration, reduced latency to sleep onset, and more spontaneous and induced sleep stage changes during a Wilkinson auditory vigilance task. The subjects also had a sleep EEG during a 45-minute nap. In a polygraphic score of sleepiness,[154] more slow-wave sleep stages were observed after glucose than after placebo. Eleven of the 12 narcoleptics had significantly more REM sleep after glucose as compared to the placebo drink.[153] The authors discussed their results in relation to serotonin synthesis and an increase of insulin after glucose.

Sodium oxybate, a pharmacologic compound related to GHB, is considered today as one of the best treatments for narcolepsy with cataplexy. Sodium oxybate also ameliorates nocturnal sleep. The mechanisms of action are not fully understood. Its effect on the GABA system is considered to be important, but it is tempting to think that some of the effects may be similar to the effects of a ketogenic diet. Brown noted that BHB, a ketone, is an isomer of GHB; both are also partial agonists of $GABA_B$ receptors.[85]

In a study by Husain et al., the effects of a low-carbohydrate, ketogenic diet on sleepiness and other narcolepsy symptoms were studied among nine patients with narcolepsy.[155] The patients with narcolepsy were asked to adhere to the Atkins diet plan, and their symptoms were assessed using the Narcolepsy Symptom Status Questionnaire (NSSQ). The NSSQ-Total score decreased by 18% from 161.9 to 133.5 ($p = 0.0019$) over 8 weeks. Subjectively, patients with narcolepsy experienced modest improvements in daytime sleepiness when they were on a low-carbohydrate, ketogenic diet.[155]

Obesity among narcoleptics is an interesting issue, because hypocretin is also associated with feeding behavior. One could assume that lack of hypocretin in narcoleptics could be associated with increased feeding behavior, overeating, and obesity. Arnulf and her collaborators studied 13 narcoleptics and 9 healthy age/sex/ethnicity-matched controls.[156] Their patients with narcolepsy (both typical narcolepsy-cataplexy syndrome and narcolepsy without cataplexy) tended to be overweight. There was no significant difference in the basic metabolic balance. Overweight narcoleptics had lower resting energy expenditure and food intake than patients with normal weight and controls, indicating calorie restriction. Plasma glucose, cortisol, thyroxine, thyroid-stimulating hormone, prolactin, and sex hormone levels did not differ between groups. Narcoleptic patients had more problems in eating behavior, and they also had more signs of bulimia compared to controls. In sum, in this study low hypocretin values were not associated with obesity per se, but the narcoleptic subjects tended to eat more than needed, causing them to be overweight. The overweight narcoleptics tended to have lower energy consumption at rest, as do many other overweight people compared to people of normal weight.[75] This makes weight loss more difficult.

DIETARY MINERALS AND SLEEP

Iron

Iron has an important role in many enzymatic processes. Sufficient iron in the CNS is necessary for normal functioning of dopamine receptors. Tyrosine hydroxlase regulates dopamine synthesis. Iron and tetrahydrobiopterin are cofactors of tyrosine hydroxylase. Iron is also linked to functions of GABA, serotonin, and opioid peptides. In experimental cell cultures, dopaminergic cells of the substantia nigra can be destroyed by chelation of iron by desferoxamine. Adding opioids in these cell cultures is protective. Iron also has a catalytic effect in oxidative mechanisms of the CNS. Measuring serum ferritin and soluble transferring receptor from a venous blood sample allows estimation of tissue iron levels. In RLS, S-ferritin is often low, in which case giving iron per os, or intravenously in more severe cases, should be part of the treatment.

In patients with RLS, 45 µg/L is usually used as the lower limit at which one should consider giving iron supplementation, even if hemoglobin is normal. Usually the soluble transferrin receptor values are also low. Iron should be given as Fe^{2+} (bivalent iron) together with vitamin C to increase absorption of iron from the gut. If ferritin levels do not rise and the symptoms are bothersome, intravenous iron might be considered. Iron dextran should be avoided because of potential risks, but safe formulations exist, such as Venofer. Several studies have already shown the benefits of intravenous iron, beginning with the early experiences from Sweden in the 1950s.[157–161] The issue of iron and RLS is discussed in more detail elsewhere in this book (see Chapter 28).

Yehuda and Yehuda noted that in young children sleep disturbances, fatigue, and possible learning disturbances may be related to iron deficiency early in life.[162] These findings require further study. To determine if there is a relationship between low serum ferritin and sleep disturbance in children with autism spectrum disorder, an 8-week open-label treatment trial on 33 children with oral iron supplementation was done. Seventy-seven percent had restless sleep at baseline, which improved significantly with iron therapy, suggesting a relationship between sleep disturbance and iron deficiency in children with autism spectrum disorder. Sixty-nine percent of preschoolers and 35% of school-age children had insufficient dietary iron intake. Mean ferritin increased significantly (16–29 µg/L). It may be that children with autism spectrum disorder should be screened for iron deficiency.[163]

Kuhn and Brodan[164] studied the effects of 5 days of sleep deprivation on the circadian rhythm of serum iron in a group of six healthy male volunteers. The results were compared with a control group of five individuals whose normal sleep cycle was preserved, but whose daily regimen was otherwise identical with that of the sleep deprivation group. Their biorhythms were analyzed using cosinor analysis. Sleep deprivation markedly reduced the mean level of iron, diminished the absolute and relative amplitude of oscillations, disturbed the shape of the daily course of serum iron, and gradually decreased the computative acrophase (i.e., shortened the period of rhythm). Forty-eight hours of recovery resulted in only a partial normalization of all the observed changes. The potential mechanisms of the observed changes are discussed by the authors.[164]

Copper, Zinc, and Other Minerals

Copper acts as a cofactor in many enzymatic processes, including those mediated by ceruloplasmin, monoamine oxidases, cytochrome oxidase, and superoxide dismutase. The largest part of dietary copper (96%) is bonded into ceruloplasmin and ferroxidase, which are needed in many phases of iron metabolism. Lack of copper can manifest as neutropenia, microcytic anemia, growth disturbances, or slowing of erythropoiesis. Copper deficiency also may present as myeloneuropathy resembling vitamin B_{12} deficiency. Menkes' syndrome is an example of a genetic disturbance of copper metabolism causing deficiency of copper. Wilson's disease is an autosomal recessive disease that causes accumulation of copper in the liver and brain. It is practically impossible to take in too much copper from a normal diet. Intake of large amounts of vitamin C, zinc, iron, and cysteine worsen the absorption of copper from the gut. Lack of copper may also occur after poor diet, excessive consumption of zinc tablets, and bariatric surgery.

Zinc is also required in many enzymatic processes (carbonic anhydrase, alkaline phosphatases, many different dehydrogenases, etc.). In the CNS, zinc is abundant in the so-called zinc-containing synapses of glutamatergic neurons. Such neurons are located mainly in the prefrontal lobe; frontal dysfunction may result from lack of zinc. Conversely, bivalent zinc may cause excitotoxic damage. Other minerals (e.g., magnesium, manganese) are also important for proper functioning of the CNS.

NUTRITION AND DEVELOPMENT OF THE CENTRAL NERVOUS SYSTEM

Malnutrition affects development of the brain. One of the pioneers in this field has been Myron Winick, a pediatrician specializing in embryology and growth development.[165] In the 1960s, he spent several months in Chile, where he noticed at the time of autopsy that malnourished children had a reduced number of brain cells. Later his group published similar results from Jamaica. Studies among Korean orphans less than 1 year old with adequate nutrition or malnourishment have shown that malnourishment is associated with poor functional outcome at the age of 12 years. In developed countries, the most important nutritional factor for early disturbance of brain development is alcohol (i.e., fetal alcohol syndrome). Children with fetal alcohol syndrome have low birth weight, retarded growth, dysmorphic facial features, and learning deficits. In developing countries, many other types of significant intrauterine and early postnatal malnutrition may affect brain development. In these countries, malnutrition is usually associated with poor living conditions, poor hygiene, and poor socioeconomic status.

Nutrition plays an important role in the development of the human CNS. Prenatal malnutrition affects the developing brain in many ways. Adequate intake of proteins, minerals, and vitamins is necessary for proper brain development, including brain growth, neurogenesis, cell migration, and cell differentiation. Are some nutrients more important than others? Folate deficiency is associated with disturbances of neural tube development during early gestation. There is evidence that malnutrition may result in various types of minimal brain dysfunction, disorders of attention, and learning disabilities.[165] There is also evidence that malnutrition during pregnancy is associated with an increased incidence of some behavioral and psychiatric problems, including mental retardation and schizophrenia. Studies have shown that malnutrition may cause diffuse lesions and functional disturbances in connections between neurons and glia, axonal and dendritic circuits, and the development of various neurotransmitter systems.[166,167] Fortunately, the human brain is plastic, and the effects of malnutrition may be at least partly reversed by proper nutrition later in childhood.[165] In addition, genetic effects, living environment, possible infections, and many other factors are important. Pascual and collaborators have published their results on neuroglycopenia, a syndrome caused by insufficient glucose availability during brain development in the early years of life.[8] The cause of neuroglycopenia may be nutritional energy deficiency or a genetic mutation of the cerebral glucose transporter type 1 (*GLUT1*). In the latter case, children with neuroglycopenia may suffer from a combination of epilepsy, motor dysfunction, and neuropsychological abnormalities.

During gestation and early postnatal life, the PUFAs linoleic acid, α-LA, EPA, and DHA are necessary for proper development and functioning of cell membranes. DHA is present in high concentrations in retinal and cerebral cortical brain lipids. It is particularly necessary for development of the brain and retina, and is normally supplied via the placenta and milk. By which mechanism do ω-3 fatty acids act in the CNS? Neuronal cell membranes contain phospholipids, and dietary ω-3 fatty acids are needed for proper constitution and functioning of these membranes. There is evidence that a sufficient amount of dietary ω-3 relative to ω-6 fatty acids is needed for proper CNS function. Too much ω-6 relative to ω-3 fatty acids may be harmful. ω-6 Fatty acids are metabolized to prostaglandins with higher inflammatory potential compared with those generated from ω-3 fatty acids. Sufficient tryptophan and tyrosine intake are needed for production of the serotonin and catecholamines.[168] The ω-3/ω-6 ratio is also linked to proper functioning of serotoninergic and catecholaminergic neurotransmission. Several studies have shown that the ideal ratio of ω-3/ω-6 fatty acids is about 1:4. In many countries this ratio is close to 1:30, which means that people have much more ω-6 acids relative to the important ω-3 acids. The ratio of membrane ω-3 to ω-6 PUFAs can be modulated by nutrition.[168] This is also probably true for proper sleep-wake regulation, but more studies are needed to prove this. These results do not directly prove that malnutrion during early childhood causes problems in the development of the sleep-wake cycle. It is, however, very possible.

SUMMARY

Sleepiness during the afternoon and poor sleep after a heavy evening meal and heavy alcohol consumption are very familiar to most people. Despite this, little is known about the effects of different constituents of meals on sleep. There is evidence that a heavy lunch and rapidly absorbing carbohydrates enhance sleepiness in the afternoon. This may add to daytime sleepiness, and for that reason they should be avoided when one wants to avoid fatigue. On the contrary, a light evening meal rich in carbohydrates may help one to fall asleep. The relationships between the ENS and CNS need to be studied much more in the future. There is already evidence that chronic sleep deprivation increases risk of obesity and adult-onset diabetes. Better information about nutritional issues must be taken into consideration in future studies.

⊘ REFERENCES

A full list of references are available at www.expertconsult.com

CHAPTER 24

Obstructive Sleep Apnea Syndrome

Christian Guilleminault and Michael Zupancic

INTRODUCTION

Obstructive sleep apnea syndrome (OSAS) is a condition characterized by repeated episodes of upper airway closure during sleep. It is associated with a constellation of symptoms and objective findings.[1] The most common presenting complaints are loud, disruptive, interrupted snoring, associated with unrefreshing sleep and excessive daytime sleepiness (EDS) or fatigue. OSAS may long remain undetected because the breathing disturbances occur at night, but the consequences are reflected in impairment of daytime function. Amazingly, many patients with even severe sleep apnea of many decades' duration remain unaware of the cause of their difficulties. Bed partners are invaluable informants, describing frightening cessations of breathing, choking sounds, and stridorous gasps when breathing resumes. The course is a slowly progressive one. Thus, the patient's daytime performance becomes insidiously more impaired, until the patient eventually decompensates and presents to the health care system, either volitionally or as a result of one of the complications of sleep apnea. Sleepiness is typically misperceived as a natural consequence of aging. There is a disparity between the prevalence of OSAS in the community and recognition among medical professionals of the frequency and impact of OSAS; this disparity is particularly sizable among primary care providers and health system managers.[2]

Complete obstruction of the upper airway is termed *obstructive apnea* and partial closure is referred to as *hypopnea*. When measured by polysomnographic (PSG) recording, obstructive apneas are defined as total cessation of airflow at the nose and mouth, lasting at least 10 seconds, associated with ongoing thoracic and abdominal efforts to inspire. Hypopneas are seen as greater than 30% decreases in airflow, lasting at least 10 seconds, associated with continued respiratory efforts.[3] Hypopneas are usually associated with a drop in blood oxygen saturation.[1,3,4] Gould and coworkers[5] have suggested defining hypopnea differently by focusing more on thoracoabdominal effort. If inductive plethysmography is used, hypopnea is defined as a decrease in thoracoabdominal effort of at least 50%.[5] More advanced technology has shown that a small decrease in tidal volume (V_T) may involve only one breath (or respiratory cycle), and lead to a transient, electroencephalography (EEG)–defined arousal, when associated with increased respiratory efforts while asleep. The current, noninvasive means of measuring oxygen saturation in arterial blood (Sao_2) do not indicate a recognizable drop in Sao_2 in association with this V_T decrease. If repeated, however, the short arousal will have an impact on sleep continuity—that is, lead to sleep fragmentation. In the strictest sense of the term, a reduction of airflow with a short arousal is a hypopnea, and some sleep specialists do not limit the term *hypopnea* to the definitions outlined earlier. This may be appropriate, given that very short events can have pathophysiologic consequences and impair well-being, as with upper airway resistance syndrome (UARS).[6–9] Both apneas and hypopneas are terminated with a large inspiratory breath.

Central apneas are seen on PSG as episodes of cessation of thoracic and abdominal respiratory efforts as well as nasal-oral airflow, lasting at least 10 seconds. Long-standing obstructive apnea may result in disturbances of central and peripheral respiratory reflexes, in turn causing central apneas. Moreover, the increase in inspiratory effort associated with obstructive events may be detectable only with esophageal manometry. Because this diagnostic tool is not in common use in sleep laboratories, these events are often interpreted as central apneas. Mixed apneas are composed of central and obstructive components.

The number of apneas and hypopneas are separately totaled, then divided by the hours of total sleep time to yield an apnea index (AI) and hypopnea index (HI). The AI and HI are summed to determine the apnea-hypopnea index (AHI), which is the average number of apneas and hypopneas per hour of sleep.[10]

The minimum AHI and AI required to constitute a mild disorder is debated.[11] The symptomatology that is produced by a given objective amount of respiratory disturbance varies from individual to individual. As the AI or AHI increases, however, so does the severity of symptoms. The correlation between AHI severity and long-term morbidity is not precisely delineated. This complex relationship is confounded by nightly fluctuations in the AHI, the amount of oxygen desaturation, and the percentage of time spent with reduced oxygen saturation. For clinical purposes, an AHI higher than 5 events/hr is most commonly considered to be in the pathologic range.[12,13] The term *sleep-disordered breathing* (SDB) has been given multiple definitions that render usage of this term difficult. It was initially created to report on the presence of abnormal breathing events that did not qualify for the definition of "hypopnea" that requires SaO_2 drop or visual EEG arousal and a set decrease in airflow. It became obvious over time that patients may have an impairment without having the required SaO_2 drop, or that the visually score EEG arousal was difficult to recognize. Also, introduction of the nasal cannula pressure transducer mode of recording led to recognition of flow limitation, and usage of an esophageal pressure (P_{es}) sensor to detect the presence of abnormal respiratory effort has changed the way breathing events are scored. Tabulation of these extra events led to calculation of a respiratory disturbance index (RDI) that added apneas, hypopneas, and these extra events that also impact on a patient's well-being. Others used "sleep-disordered breathing" as an equivalent of AHI, rendering the value of the term at that time very questionable.

OSAS lies along a continuum of SDB. There are controversies about the linearity of this continuum: it appears from recent data that there could be a point of "no return" where lesions in the upper airway leave permanent traces that may continuously impact on upper airway motor control during inspiration. Some, and we are part of this group, want to subdivide this reported "continuum" in two segments: chronic snoring and upper airway resistance (and there is no clear demonstration that chronic snorers do not always present some degree of

upper airway resistance) with limited symptoms and usually no daytime sleepiness, through an increasing clinical severity, with progressive degrees of obstructive apnea based on RDI and oxyhemoglobin desaturations. (This second stage has for some been always associated with a variable degree of upper airway neurologic lesions that may leave permanent sequelae.) UARS may be present without associated snoring but with associated daytime sleepiness or fatigue.[6,7]

The specific pathophysiology of these syndromes is discussed later in this chapter. As the incidence and prevalence of UARS have not been characterized, most of the presentation focuses on the well-known OSAS.

EPIDEMIOLOGY

The risk of developing OSAS increases with age, and the PSG pattern of obstructive apnea is strongly correlated with abdominal and neck obesity and male gender (however, when android obesity is present, subjects present with a combined syndrome: upper airway impairment and restrictive chest bellows impairment due to obesity).[14–17] Prevalence of OSA reaches a maximum between the fifth and seventh decades.[18] Menopausal women develop OSAS at a rate similar to that of men. The Wisconsin Sleep Cohort Study evaluated the association between premenopause, perimenopause, and postmenopause and SDB in a group of 589 women. Using multivariate regression analysis adjusted for age, body habitus, smoking, and other potential confounding factors, Young et al. calculated the odds ratios for an AHI greater than 5 events/hr of sleep to be 1.2 for perimenopause, and 2.6 (range 1.4–4.8) for postmenopause.[19] These results suggest that the menopausal transition in significantly associated with an increased risk of SDB independent of known confounding factors.

Some minority populations appear to have a higher prevalence of SDB, indicating that race may be a risk factor. Two such populations are Pacific Islanders[20] and Hispanic Americans,[21] although there have been no studies that control for comorbid conditions found more frequently in these populations than in whites. As data from the Cleveland Family Study indicate, blacks may be at increased risk for sleep apnea.[22] In this study, the increased prevalence was not accounted for by differences in exposure to alcohol or tobacco or differences in body mass index (BMI). Moreover, this effect was most apparent in individuals younger than 25 years of age. Variable age of puberty, speed of development of secondary sexual characteristics, and mucosal enlargement associated with hormonal surge may have biased these findings. In contrast, a study in New Zealand comparing sleep apnea severity among Maoris, Pacific Islanders, and Europeans reported that race was not an important predictor of severity when adjusted for factors such as neck size, BMI, and age.[23] Familial aggregates of OSAS clearly indicate that risk factors for the development of this condition may exist very early in life.[24–26]

Initial studies that attempted to define rates of OSAS were limited by biases that tended to underestimate actual prevalence. Early studies by Lavie[27] in Israel and Gislason et al.[28] in Sweden assessed the prevalence of OSAS in the adult male population to be 7% and 1.3%, respectively. More recent studies of large, comprehensive population samples suggest a prevalence rate of OSAS at least two times higher than those early estimates.[29,30] In 1993, Young and colleagues published a large community-based study of adults 30–60 years of age that calculated, if OSA was defined as having an AHI greater than 5 events/hr, a prevalence of 9% in women and 24% in men.[13] If the AHI of greater than 5 events/hr was associated with symptoms of excessive sleepiness, however, the prevalence was 2% and 4% in women and men, respectively.[13] These studies are limited as they looked mainly at whites.

OSAS has been associated with mortality both from vascular complications and from highway and industrial accidents. Two retrospective studies by Partinen et al.[31] and by He and colleagues[32] found an increased mortality rate for patients with OSAS, particularly in those younger than 50 years of age. As previously stated, OSAS is underdiagnosed. Untreated OSAS is a cause of death, as already shown by the study of Partinen et al.,[31] and serious injury on the road and in the workplace.[33–36] Work by Findley et al.[36] suggests that the accident rate for OSAS patients is seven times that of the general population. Other studies have shown similar findings.[37,38]

MORBIDITY: CARDIOVASCULAR SYSTEM

Over the past several decades, obstructive sleep apnea (OSA) has been shown to play a central role in hypertension, cardiovascular and cerebrovascular risk, metabolic syndrome, and longevity.

Hypertension

Systemic and pulmonary hemodynamics undergo acute and chronic changes as a consequence of obstructive apnea, most of which reverse on successful treatment of the upper airway obstruction. During normal sleep, blood pressure dips as compared to that during wakefulness. In subjects with OSA, nocturnal blood pressure remains elevated during sleep, with significant fluctuations in systemic arterial pressure occurring cyclically with episodes of apnea. During obstructive apneic events, there is an initial decline of blood pressure followed by an elevation that becomes maximal after ventilation resumes. In a study of 10 moderate to severe apneics, systolic and diastolic pressures rose approximately 25% from their baseline values during apneas (i.e., from 126 to 159 mm Hg systolic and from 65 to 83 mm Hg diastolic).[39] When apneas occur continually throughout the night, and are associated with very severe oxygen desaturations, elevations may be extreme, exceeding 200 mm Hg systolic and 120 mm Hg diastolic.[40]

Evidence implicates several mechanisms that contribute to cyclic increases in blood pressure. A fall in partial pressure of arterial oxygen and an increase in acidosis signal the carotid chemoreceptors to trigger vasomotor center–mediated arteriolar constriction, which leads to increased systemic vascular resistance. Increased ventilatory effort against a closed upper airway in the face of air trapping leads to significant right-to-left bowing of the interventricular septum and decreased cardiac output.[41,42] Left ventricular collapse can occur with very negative inspiratory pressures.[43] With resumption of ventilation, and the abrupt shift from sleep to wake, there is a release of vagal parasympathetic predominance and heightened sympathetic tone. Pulmonary stretch reflexes induce tachycardia, which increases cardiac output. Changes in preload and afterload due to repetitive Müller's and, at times, Valsalva maneuvers also contribute to the changes in cardiac output. Evidence of elevated sympathetic nervous system activity can be measured by increased urinary catecholamine levels, which return to normal after treatment of apnea.[43,44]

Investigation of OSA subjects using microneurography on the peroneal nerve in the popliteal fossa during wake and sleep has further enhanced our knowledge about sympathetic activity in people with OSA. In healthy individuals, muscle sympathetic nerve activity (MSNA) at the popliteal level shows low sympathetic activity, particularly at rest during daytime wakefulness in experimental conditions. OSA patients have elevated MSNA during wakefulness, with a very significant increase in discharge rate.[45–47] It is believed that the repetitive hypoxemia associated with apnea and hypopneic events leads to important changes in the autonomic nervous system neuronal network, with a resetting of the sympathetic receptors.[47] This resetting leads to the continuous discharges that persist during the daytime when hypoxemic events are not present. The abnormal waking sympathetic activity is thought to lead to vascular changes, including progressive endothelium impairment involving the nitric oxide system,[48,49] which has been strongly implicated in the development of plaques and atherosclerosis.[50,51] These are some of the mechanisms believed to be responsible for developing hypertension with OSA.

Independent of the associated mechanisms, OSA is a risk factor for hypertension[52]; other factors are difficult to tease out as, unfortunately many studies have been performed on obese OSA patients and it is impossible to completely dissociate the role of obesity from the role of upper airway obstruction during sleep. Hypertension is also a frequent comorbid condition with sleep apnea.[52–55] Approximately 30% of patients with systemic hypertension have sleep apnea, whereas 50% or more of patients with sleep apnea have systemic hypertension, and the percentage of those with refractory hypertension is even higher. The Sleep Heart Health Study, a cross-sectional analysis of over 6000 subjects, showed an independent association between OSA and hypertension. The most compelling evidence that OSA is an independent risk factor for hypertension comes from the Wisconsin cohort group. This population study involved over 700 government employees and collected medical and sleep data via detailed questionnaires, physical examinations, and PSG. Peppard et al. found that having OSA (diagnosed by PSG) significantly increased the risk of developing hypertension 4 years later compared to the risk in subjects without SDB, independent of known confounding factors.[55] This increased risk was greater in those subjects with more severe disease. Subjects with mild obstructive sleep apnea (AHI of 5–14.9 events/hr) were 2.03 times (95% confidence interval [CI], 1.29–3.17) more likely to have OSA than normals, and subjects with an AHI of 15 events/hr or more were 2.89 times (95% CI, 1.46–5.64) more likely to have OSA. Even those with mild SDB (AHI of 0.01–4.9 events/hr) were not immune from the negative effects of disorded sleep and were more likely to develop hypertension 4 years later, with an odds ratio of 1.42 (95% CI, 1.13–1.78) compared to subjects without SDB.[55]

Hypertension may be generated by sympathetic overactivity triggered by intermittent hypoxemia, large negative fluctuations in intrathoracic pressure, and repetitive arousals from sleep.[54,56,57] Hypertension may improve after treatment of apnea.[58] The ameliorative effect of treatment has been found after upper airway surgery[59] and nasal continuous positive airway pressure (CPAP).[60] Moller et al.[61] performed 24-hour blood pressure monitoring and measured plasma levels of vasoactive hormones in 24 OSA patients and 18 control subjects. Compared with the controls, OSA patients had significantly higher blood pressure and heart rate, and the sleep-related nocturnal blood pressure drop was reduced.[61] Thirteen OSA patients re-examined after 14 months of CPAP therapy demonstrated reduction in blood pressure, which correlated with a decrease in both plasma renin and plasma angiotensin II concentrations.[61] However, many patients with hypertension and OSA do not go back to normal blood pressure.

Sin et al. reported that 40% of 301 patients with congestive heart failure had OSA and systemic hypertension. After controlling for other risk factors, OSA patients were 2.89 times (95% CI, 1.25–6.73) more likely to have systolic hypertension than those without OSA. The degree of systolic blood pressure elevation was directly related to the frequency of hypopneas and apneas.[62]

In OSA patients there is evidence the body tries to compensate for hypertension. Increased release of atrial natriuretic peptide (ANP) during sleep has been found in sleep apnea, with concomitant increases in urine and sodium output.[63] ANP suppresses the renin-angiotensin-aldosterone system, and plasma renin activity curves have been found to be abnormally flattened in apneics during sleep.[64] These changes lower blood volume and blood pressure and may play a protective or compensatory role against blood pressure elevations in OSA. Treatment of apnea normalizes ANP, thereby diminishing diuresis and natriuresis, and increases renin and aldosterone release.

Heart Failure

Heart failure also appears to occur as a consequence of OSA. The Sleep Heart Health Study reported that OSA is associated with a relative odds ratio of 2.38 for heart failure, independent of other known risk factors.[65] OSA is also prevalent in patients with heart failure. Javaheri et al.[66] performed PSG in 81 ambulatory men with stable, treated systolic heart failure. Fifty-one percent of the patients had moderate to severe sleep apnea with an AHI $\geq$ 15 events/hr, and the group had an average of AHI of 44 events/hr.[66] Chan et al. reported in a series that about 50% of patients with isolated diastolic heart failure had an AHI of at least 10 events/hr.[67]

Whether heart failure patients with SDB benefit from CPAP treatment is unclear. Several studies have shown that short-term use of CPAP in patients with heart failure and obstructive sleep apnea improved left ventricular ejection fraction, blood pressure, and ventricular systolic volume.[68,69] CPAP is recommended for heart failure patients with clear-cut OSA.[68,69] However, in addition to obstructive events, heart failure patients may present with a variety of abnormal respiratory activities while sleeping. They may have central events; mixed events, Cheyne-Stokes respirations, and repetitive diaphragmatic pauses; or a combination of mixed, obstructive, and rare central events. This last subgroup may derive some benefit from nasal or bilevel CPAP. However, a careful analysis of the PSG pattern is needed, and an in-laboratory titration for pressure is mandatory, evaluating the appearance of dyspnea reported during the titration night. Bradley et al. reported the first studies and concluded that nasal CPAP is not a recommended treatment for heart failure patients who suffer from central sleep apnea (defined as >50% of apnea episodes central in etiology) as treatment did not improve quality of life, number of hospitalizations, or survival.[70] Kasai et al. reported that CPAP therapy in patients with heart failure and moderate to severe OSA were less likely to die or be hospitalized than untreated patients, though those who were poorly compliant CPAP were most likely to reach these unwanted end points.[71]

Pulmonary Hypertension

Moderate to severe increases in pulmonary arterial pressure occur with each apneic episode. Maximal pulmonary pressures are generated during rapid eye movement (REM) sleep. They coincide with maximal hypoxemic and hypercapnic values[58] and probably reflect hypoxic pulmonary vasoconstriction. When pressure gradients between the pulmonary artery lumen and thoracic cavity are evaluated, transpulmonary arterial pressure decreases during the first 25 seconds of apnea, then increases until breathing returns and transiently rises more rapidly.[72] Another homodynamic change consists of reductions in cardiac output of up to one third of baseline values in apneas longer than 35 seconds.[41]

The development of persistent pulmonary hypertension during wakefulness and cor pulmonale may be caused by severe hypoxemia during sleep,[73,74] but is more likely in daytime hypoxemia.[75] There has again been controversy regarding the persistence of daytime pulmonary hypertension. Earlier studies estimated the prevalence of pulmonary hypertension in OSA patients to be as high as 20–41%.[76–78] However, these studies were small and did not control for other risk factors for pulmonary hypertension. There is, however, agreement that a subgroup of OSA patients present with pulmonary hypertension, usually moderate, during the day associated with their sleep-related problem. The American College of Chest Physicians recommends that evaluation for OSA should be part of the initial workup in patients with pulmonary hypertension.[79] Possible mechanisms thought to cause pulmonary hypertension include hypoxemia-induced endothelial cell dysfunction and pulmonary artery remodeling.[80] The reversal of pulmonary hypertension in OSA patients is reported to be poor after treatment.[81]

Cardiac Arrhythmias

Cardiac arrhythmias that occur exclusively during sleep are common in apneics. Sinus arrhythmia accompanies each obstructive respiratory cycle, in which rate diminishes with the cessation of airflow and accelerates when breathing resumes. These changes can be mild or severe, resulting in repetitive cycles of bradycardia and tachycardia fluctuating from fewer than 30 to more than 120 bpm.[82] Severe sinus bradycardia (fewer than 30 bpm) affects approximately 10% of sleep apneics and is usually seen with severe hypoxemia.[83–85] These aberrations of rate combined with hypoxemia predispose to conduction defects, malignant arrhythmias, and perhaps sudden death. Asystoles of up to 13 seconds, second-degree atrioventricular (AV) block, premature ventricular contractions (PVCs), and runs of ventricular tachycardia are among documented apnea-related abnormalities.[84] A prospective study of 147 consecutive patients demonstrated significantly higher prevalence of nocturnal paroxysmal asystole in OSA patients and increased episodes of bradycardia and pauses that correlated with the severity of the sleep apnea.[86]

Proposed mechanisms for bradycardia, Mobitz type I AV block, and asystole involve vagal nerve activation due to both Müller's maneuver and hypoxemic carotid body stimulation. Electroencephalographic arousal with airway reopening and lung expansion triggers cardiac acceleration. Increased sympathetic tone due to hypoxemia and acidosis may be expressed after vagal influence is withdrawn, leading to PVCs, sinus tachycardia, and ventricular tachycardia. PVC frequency and other ventricular arrhythmias have been shown to correlate with severity of oxygen desaturation, increasing threefold with desaturations lower than 60% (as compared to 90%).[87]

From a global perspective, many of these physiologic changes in response to asphyxia may be viewed as an attempt to preserve perfusion to the critical cerebral and coronary systems. Increased systemic pressure selectively perfuses these critical central vessels, whereas bradycardia decreases myocardial oxygen consumption. As bradycardia becomes more profound, however, myocardial perfusion may become more impaired, because the perfusion gradient drops as diastole is prolonged. Coronary ischemia may result in ventricular arrhythmia. On return of ventilation, cardiac rate and output rise in the setting of sympathetic dominance and decreased systemic resistance. The demand for myocardial oxygen to accomplish this work outweighs the supply of reperfused blood, rendering the myocardium vulnerable to malignant arrhythmias.[88]

OSA may increase one's risk of developing atrial fibrillation (AF) and its recurrence after cardioversion. In one study, consecutive patients who underwent cardioversion for AF were compared to patients without AF who were referred for management of cardiovascular disease at a tertiary medical facility. The prevalence of OSA was statistically higher in patients with AF (49%) compared to those without AF (32%).[89] Kanagala et al. showed that the recurrence rate of AF at 12 months after cardioversion in patients with untreated OSA was nearly twice that of untreated OSA patients (82% vs. 42%, respectively).[90]

Coronary Artery Disease, Myocardial Infarction, Stroke, and Early Death

Sleep apnea and even snoring have been epidemiologically linked to increased incidences of myocardial infarction and stroke.[91,92] Spriggs and coworkers[93] looked at risk factors for stroke in approximately 400 individuals with OSAS who had been matched with controls for sex and age and found an odds ratio of 3.2 for symptoms of snoring. Another study found an increased odds ratio even after adjustment for ethanol use, hypertension, and heart disease. The ratio increased approximately fourfold if obesity, observed apneas, and a subjective sense of EDS were present.[91] A study of over 1000 patients showed an increased hazard ratio in OSA patients of 2.24 of stroke or death from any cause over a several-year period.[94] After adjustment for multiple risk factors (age, sex, race, obesity, hypertension, etc.), the hazard ratio remained significant at 1.97 (95% CI, 1.12–3.48). Furthermore, analysis indicated that those with more severe OSA were more likely to reach these end points. Though this study strongly suggests OSA increases the risk of stroke or death, it may statistically underestimate its risk in the development of these end points as many of the OSA patients were treated surgically or with CPAP during the study period.[94]

The increased incidence of stroke is likely secondary to multiple reasons. During apneic events there is a greater chance of hypoxemia, hypercapnia, increased frequency of cardiac arrythmias, increased coagulation, and para-doxical embolism through a patent foramen ovale. Cere-bral blood flow may be variable during apneic events as evidenced by transcranial Doppler studies. However, Yaggi et al.[94] presented convincing data indicating that OSA is an independent risk factor for stroke.

Stroke and transient ischemic attacks are also a risk factor for OSA. Over half of patients with acute strokes or transient ischemic attacks have OSA.[95,96] Stroke patients who have OSA appear to have higher mortality as well.[96] One study has shown that successfully treating stroke patients who have OSA with CPAP significantly decreased the risk of subsequent vascular events.[97] How-ever, larger studies suggest that only a minority of stroke patients with OSA are able to tolerate CPAP.[98]

OSA may be a predisposing factor to atherosclerosis and plaque formation, as discussed earlier, due to its action on the arterial endothelium and the nitric oxide system. Kaynak et al.[99] preformed ultrasonographic examination of both carotid arteries to evaluate intima-media thickness and the presence of plaque in 114 male patients referred for evaluation of SDB. Patients with OSA had significantly increased intima-media thickness compared with habitual snorers. Age and BMI were sig-nificantly associated with intima-media thickness, whereas age and RDI were most predictive for plaque.[99]

OSA has been linked to other risk markers for cardio-vascular disease, including increased levels of leptin, C-reactive protein, and homocysteine, and insulin resistance syndrome.[100] However, some of the abnormalities observed have been determined not to be related to OSA but to the frequently associated obesity; as an exam-ple, C-reactive protein is not elevated in OSA patients with a maximum BMI of 25 kg/m^2 despite a mean AHI of 30 events/hr.[101] Abnormal levels of leptin and ghrelin seen in these subjects seems to be related more to the severity of the sleep fragmentation (or total sleep loss) induced by the syndrome that directly results from apnea and hypopnea.[102] Leptin and ghrelin levels can normalize in patients once their sleep apnea has been treated.[103]

Several studies have shown decreased mortality asso-ciated with OSA patients treated with tracheostomy or CPAP.[31,104] He et al.,[32] comparing cumulative survival after 5 years of untreated versus treated patients with an AI greater than 20 events/hr, showing that cumulative survival was approximately 75% in the untreated group as compared to almost 100% for the treated group, was criticized due to the large number of subjects lost at fol-low-up. A study by Partinen et al. comparing mortality

in OSA subjects 5 and 8 years following tracheostomy or no treatment showed decreased mortality in treated subjects.[31] A large study from Spain involving over 800 patients showed that OSA patients compliant with CPAP, compared to those who were not treated, were more likely to survive over a several-year period. The survival rate was positively associated with increased CPAP usage.[104] Marin et al.[105] published a study involving several hun-dred Spanish men and showed that fatal and nonfatal car-diovascular events occurred more frequently in untreated OSA patients compared to treated OSA patients. Further-more, treated patients with sleep apnea had a frequency of fatal and non-fatal cardiovascular events similar to that of simple snorers.[105]

Earlier studies showed an increased incidence of pro-teinuria in OSA patients.[106,107] However, more recent studies have not shown this correlation.[108,109]

PATHOPHYSIOLOGY

SDB is caused by increased resistance while breathing secondary to narrowing at one or more sites of the upper airway. Locations of narrowing include the nose, retropa-latal region, retroglossal region, or, less commonly, the hypoglossal region.

The size of the pharyngeal upper airway is dependent on a balance of forces between the upper airway dilators, which maintain upper airway patency, and the negative pharyngeal intraluminal pressure created during thoracic expansion as a result of inspiration. Skeletal factors also play a role. Bernoulli's principle dictates that narrowing of any segment while airflow is maintained causes an increased velocity of airflow in that segment. This decreases intraluminal pressure and further narrows the segment, favoring upper airway collapse. In sleep, the stage (REM vs. non-REM [NREM]) also influences upper airway patency as REM sleep is associated with ato-nia. Lack of coordination between inspiratory muscles and upper airway dilators leads to upper airway occlusion during sleep. This was reported as early as 1978 by Guil-leminault and Motta[110] in an investigation of patients with postpoliomyelitis syndrome who had been treated with a cuirass ventilator. These patients developed a neg-ative intrathoracic pressure that could not be counter-acted by the upper airway dilators and that led to the development of OSAS. These findings were later confirmed by Hyland et al.[111] and by Simmonds and Branthwaite.[112]

More recent studies have shown abnormal activity of the dilatory pharyngeal muscles (genioglossus and tensor palatine) in OSA patients. During the waking state, the activity of these muscles is increased compared to con-trols.[113] With sleep onset, there is normally an increase in resistance due to a decrease in upper airway muscle tone. In OSA patients, there is a greater diminishment in muscle tone compared to controls as measured by electromyography (EMG).[114] A working model for OSA may be that, in the presence of a susceptible airway (one that is already narrowed by obesity, a small chin, enlarged tonsils, etc.), the factors that act to maintain upper airway patency and minimize increases in upper airway resistance during sleep are inadequate, with consequent SDB. Recent studies have suggested that a potential upper airway stabilizing mechanism may be initiated by the flow of air into the pharynx during inspiration. Although the complete details of this reflex have not been described, it appears that a reflex loop is activated once inspiration start the flow of air into the upper airway, with the following sequence of events: (1) sensory neurons in the upper airway are activated; (2) sensory afferents travel to the brain stem, which subsequently activates the efferent hypoglossal nerve that innervates the genioglossus and geniohyoid; and (3) genioglossus and geniohyoid contraction keeps the pharynx open during inspiration. This reflex may be altered in OSA patients because of damage to the muscle and nerves from the vibratory trauma of snoring. This theory is supported by the findings of abnormal sensory nerves and nerve function seen in both histologic preparations and neurophysiologic studies of upper airway muscles in OSA patients.[115–117]

As mentioned previously, with sleep onset there is an increase in resistance due to a decrease in upper airway muscle tone.[118] This increase in upper airway resistance has no known consequences in normal subjects. In snorers, however, there is a further increase with each snore. In response to this increased resistance, many subjects are able to increase their inspiratory effort and maintain normal V_T. Increased effort is demonstrated by P_{es} monitoring, which may reach peak inspiratory nadirs of -12 to -15 cm H_2O. The effort is constant over time, and in some patients does not negatively impact sleep architecture or oxygen saturation. However, in other cases, the upper airway dilators are unable to oppose the negative pharyngeal intraluminal pressure sufficiently to maintain minute ventilation and normal gas exchange.[119] In these cases, inspiratory effort is increased as reflected by an increase in P_{es} nadir. With increasing inspiratory efforts, there is a decrease in the width of the upper airway, as upper airway dilators are unable to exactly match the inspiratory negative pressure. At some point an abnormally negative P_{es} pressure is reached, V_T is reduced for one to three breaths due to the further narrowing of the upper airway passage, and an arousal response is triggered. This response is transient and short lived (as short as 2 seconds with visual EEG scoring).

It is interesting to note that a large percentage of OSAS patients have subtle craniofacial abnormalities, such as a highly arched hard palate, a long soft palate with low placement and redundant tissues, and a moderately retroplaced mandible.[120,121] It has been suggested that these abnormalities are responsible for obstructive apnea during the first weeks of life in certain subjects.[122] These abnormalities are related to genetic factors, and we have investigated several families in which a small upper airway has been passed down for generations.[123]

As stated previously, the upper airway begins at the nares and includes the nasal vestibule, nasopharynx, oropharynx, and hypopharynx. The pharynx is an especially vulnerable portion of the upper airway because it serves both digestive and respiratory functions. It must be sufficiently floppy to contract and guide food into the esophagus, while alternately maintaining sufficient muscle dilation to keep from being sucked closed.

Nasal obstruction from any cause, including allergic congestion, inflamed lymphoid tissue, or septal deviation, can initiate obstructive nocturnal respiratory pathology by converting breathing from the nasal to the oral route. Oral breathing predisposes to abnormal airway dynamics favoring pharyngeal collapse and backward displacement of the base of the tongue. The dilating genioglossus and geniohyoid muscles become mechanically disadvantaged and airway resistance is increased.

The next potential level of obstruction arises at the nasal and oropharynx due to enlarged adenoidal, tonsillar, and soft palate tissues. Enlargement of these tissues is secondary to hereditary and acquired factors. Allergies and recurrent upper respiratory infections can cause hyperplasia and scarring of lymphoid tissue. Snoring renders the uvula more edematous due to suction and trauma, which further compromises the small oropharyngeal space. Macroglossia may be due in part to obesity and is implicated in OSAS.[119]

As mentioned earlier, a constellation of jaw malformations are associated with OSAS, including a highly arched hard palate and class II dental occlusion (overjet). The position of the mandible relative to the maxilla determines the posterior extension of the tongue. Because the genioglossus muscle inserts on the mandible, with retrognathia or micrognathia the genioglossus originates on a backwardly displaced mandible and thus extends further posterior, predisposing to hypopharyngeal obstruction. During sleep in the supine position, gravity pulls the tongue further into the pharyngeal lumen, and varying degrees of decreased muscle tone additionally relax the tongue dorsally.

Chronic nasal obstruction during childhood that results in oral breathing may induce craniofacial changes predisposing to sleep apnea later in life. This has been shown in rhesus monkeys with experimentally partially occluded nostrils that developed mandibular deficiency relative to paired controls. Oral breathing changed EMG activity in facial muscle groups, leading to altered forces on the developing facial skeleton.[124–126] Partial improvement in these changes occurred if the obstruction was relieved early enough. Upper airway obstruction from enlarged adenoids in children has been shown to lead to decreased mandibular size and retrognathia, among other craniofacial changes.[127–131]

Adiposity compromises the upper airway not only because the "double chin" externally compresses the pharynx in the supine position, but also through internal infiltration of parapharyngeal structures (i.e., the adipose tissue alters and reduces airway space). Pharyngeal dilator muscle mechanics may be compromised by this loading.[132] Additionally, upper airway imaging studies have shown that patients with OSA have narrow airways due to adipose tissue in the lateral walls of the pharynx.

Testosterone may contribute to obstruction by inducing more parapharyngeal muscle bulk and more centripetal fat distribution. This might explain the fact that snoring often begins at puberty or during the immediate postpubertal period. Even a few kilograms of excessive weight can tip the balance toward upper airway obstruction in anatomically vulnerable patients.

Morbid obesity degrades waking and sleeping ventilation in addition to its impact on upper airway dynamics. Adipose deposition around the abdomen, diaphragm, and ribs reduces thoracic cage compliance, requiring increased work to breathe.[133] Functional residual capacity is decreased, and atelectasis of dependent airways may create ventilation-perfusion mismatch with hypoxemia.[134] In the supine position, the abdominal weight creates additional load, which increases hypoxemia.[135] During REM sleep, muscle atonia renders accessory respiratory muscles such as the intercostals and upper airway dilators functionally paralyzed. Thus, the diaphragm contributes mostly to inspiration against the load created by the heavy chest mass, leading to the profound oxygen desaturations seen during REM sleep in some obese patients.

Summary

Partial or complete upper airway occlusion is related to the development of greater subatmospheric intrathoracic pressure during inspiration. This subatmospheric pressure is transmitted to the pharyngeal region, creating "suction" on the soft tissues, which are the major constituents of the pharyngeal airway. To prevent closure, reflexes are normally activated at least 500 msec before the beginning of inspiration to activate the contraction of upper airway dilator muscles in opposition to this subatmospheric intrathoracic pressure.

During sleep, many of the upper airway dilator muscles have much less contractile power than the diaphragm. The genioglossus and geniohyoid muscles are particularly affected. The motor activity of these muscles is abnormal in OSA patients, with heightened contraction during the daytime and decreased contraction at sleep onset. This physiologic change allows the development of abnormal inspiratory upper airway resistance, which may result in partial or complete occlusion. If abnormalities of the upper airway due to anatomic, physiologic, or neurologic causes reduce size to a level lower than critical or limit the capabilities of upper airway dilator muscles, a more or less pronounced collapse will occur during sleep in this very flexible region. The obesity hypoventilation syndrome with increased arterial partial pressure of carbon dioxide (PCO_2) has been described during the awake state. It is thought to result from reduced hypoxic and hypercapnic ventilatory drives and is not attributed to weight-related mechanical factors.[136]

Neural factors that relate to state changes from wakefulness to sleep, as well as changes across sleep stages, play an adjunctive role in the anatomic considerations of the genesis of OSAS. During sleep, the wake-related contribution to ventilatory drive is lost. This wakefulness stimulus[137] consists of factors that are independent of metabolic and voluntary components. With sleep onset, autonomic integration of acid-base and oxygen homeostasis is believed to occur in the medulla. Inputs to this regulator include peripheral chemoreceptors for PCO_2 and partial pressure of oxygen (PO_2); central chemoreceptors for pH and PCO_2; and stretch receptors in the lung, thoracic wall, and upper airway. Ventilatory responses to both hypercapnia and hypoxia are decreased in all stages of sleep,[138,139] with more profound decrements usually occurring during phasic REM than in NREM sleep states. REM sleep–related decrements in muscle tone leading to changes in thoracoabdominal mechanics with distortion of the thoracoabdominal wall will be further increased in obesity. During sleep, PO_2, V_T, and minute ventilation are decreased, whereas PCO_2 increases by 2–6 mm Hg. These changes are attributed to a resetting of the CO_2 set point and a depressed ventilatory drive per given level of PCO_2 compared to wakefulness. For unknown reasons, males have a reduced ventilatory response to CO_2 compared to females.[140]

With sleep onset, sensitivity of the central CO_2 set point to the peripheral chemoreceptors is reduced. This results in a central apnea or a reduction in diaphragmatic effort and a decrease in tidal volume (central hypopnea), which allows PCO_2 to rise. If resumption of breathing induces obstruction by the mismatched timing mechanism discussed earlier, or if the dilatory muscles of the oropharynx have decreased tonicity, then a brief arousal may be triggered. Arousal resets the PCO_2 to the awake set point and increases ventilation. With the resumption of sleep, a cycling of central apnea, obstructive apnea, and arousal will occur.[141] This is commonly observed in the mixed apneas typically seen in obstructive sleep apneics. Any cause of sleep fragmentation, such as periodic limb movements, may bring about the unstable respiratory state in predisposed individuals that produces this common type of sleep-onset apneas.

In addition to the chemoreceptor influences described earlier, pressure-sensitive reflexes exert a more rapid influence on upper airway patency. Located throughout the upper airway,[141] pressure-sensitive reflexes coordinate the interplay of forces between inspiratory pump muscles and dilator muscles in a breath-to-breath fashion. When suction pressure produced by the diaphragm is registered, these reflexes increase genioglossus muscle activity, moving the tongue anteriorly and prolonging the duration of inspiration. Longer inspiratory times reduce the peak suction pressure, facilitating patency of the airway.

These reflexes are normally reduced during sleep but may be defective or ineffective in patients with sleep apnea. Issa and Sullivan[142] found upper airway closure to occur at abnormally low inspiratory pressures in patients with sleep apnea during a study in which the nasal airway was occluded. Even when peripheral chemoreceptor drive was added, which should facilitate patency, there was no augmentation in activation of the dilator muscles, as measured by closing pressure.

The degree of hypercapnia in sleep apnea is influenced by input from the peripheral chemoreceptors on upper airway dilators and the inspiratory pump as well as the ability of these reflexes to trigger arousal with resumption of ventilation. Most OSAS patients are normocapnic while awake. However, a limited population of severe sleep apneics display hypercapnia while awake that is not attributable to pulmonary disease or obesity. The hypercapnia in these patients indicates hypoventilation due to downward resetting of chemoreceptor reflex sensitivity. Sullivan's group[143] showed that these patients had decreased carotid body responses to hypoxemia and failed to develop normal augmentation of response to superimposed arterial hypercarbia. Elevated levels of CO_2 were required to produce a ventilatory response. These patients demonstrated long periods of obstructive apnea or hypopnea, concomitant with sustained arterial oxygen desaturations and arterial CO_2 elevations.

Resetting of chemoreceptors may allow the endurance of longer apneic events while asleep without producing arousals. Because the chemoreceptor responses are depressed, they do not lead to increased inspiratory efforts—as would normally occur with sensitive reflexes—thereby preventing the partially occluded upper airway from being sucked entirely closed. Diminished inspiratory efforts through a narrow upper airway cause reduced total ventilation, with oxyhemoglobin desaturation and CO_2 elevation. Tracheostomy or nightly treatment with nasal CPAP normalizes awake hypercapnia, suggesting that sleep apnea is a major factor in its development.

SNORING

Snoring is a noise produced when vibration occurs at several levels of the upper airway. It may be associated with various degrees of upper airway resistance. It may be heard after a complete airway obstruction; with a significant hypopnea; or with hypoventilation, leading to a cohort of symptoms. It may be associated with a limited and intermittent drop in V_T and be associated with isolated sleepiness. It may cause sleep fragmentation or present with no other clinical symptoms. The notion that snoring itself may engender cardiovascular risk is in

question. Studies that suggested this probably failed to separate out subpopulations with UARS (discussed later), or situational apneics based on such behavior elicitors as alcohol or sedative use. Although more research is required, it is likely that chronic heavy snorers eventually become patients with clinically significant syndromes of obstruction. The diagnosis of "benign snoring" may not truly exist, as data from the Wisconsin cohort study showed that people who snored and did not have obstructive sleep apnea (an AHI below 5 events/hr) had an elevated risk of developing hypertension over several years.[55]

Vibration from snoring may damage the tissue and nerves of the upper airway, decreasing compensatory mechanisms that maintain airway patency. As already mentioned, however, snoring is not a prerequisite for partial upper airway occlusion leading to clinical symptoms.

Upper Airway Resistance Syndrome

UARS[6-9] (Fig. 22–1) may cause a chronic complaint of EDS that is objectively confirmed by abnormal scores on the Multiple Sleep Latency Test (MSLT). It was first described in patients who suffered from EDS. A retrospective study selected 54 patients previously diagnosed at Stanford University with idiopathic hypersomnolence based on pathologic MSLT scores, who were also snorers.[8] The mean group MSLT score was 6.1 minutes, with abnormal scores defined as less than 8 minutes. These patients did not fit standard criteria for OSAS in terms of RDI, significant oxygen desaturations, or both.

In 14 patients (9 women, 5 men), nocturnal sleep showed fragmentation with repetitive 3- to 14-second alpha rhythm EEG arousals, with a mean of 49 ± 11 arousals per hour of sleep. When studied by esophageal balloon manometry (a technique reflecting intrathoracic inspiratory efforts as negative "suction" pressure) and a pneumotachometer with face mask to quantify airflow, a pattern emerged. Increasing inspiratory efforts were demonstrated by excessively negative P_{es} nadirs between −13 and −51 cm H_2O (normal is greater than −8), accompanied by decreasing peak flows and V_Ts one to three breaths before the arousals. These sequences were punctuated by repetitive arousals. Because the arousals and snoring would have been the only abnormalities identifiable by standard PSG recordings, these patients would not have met standard criteria for OSAS based on oxygen desaturation or apneas and hypopneas as measured by nasal-oral thermistor.

These 14 patients underwent CPAP titration to eliminate the snoring and alpha arousals. At a 3-week follow-up, subjective complaints of EDS were eliminated in all 14 patients, MSLT scores normalized to a group mean of 13 ± 3 minutes, and arousals were reduced to eight per hour of sleep.

In a series of 93 UARS patients, Guilleminault and Chowdhuri[9] reported that 56% were women, 32% were

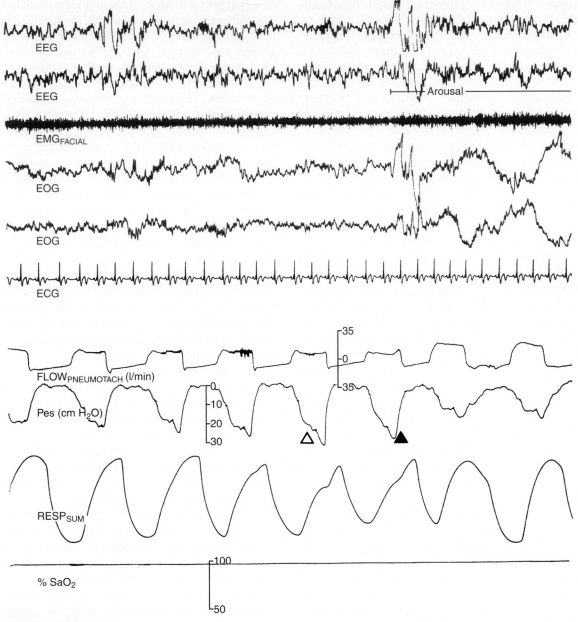

FIGURE 24–1 Polysomnographic recording showing an example of upper airway resistance syndrome. Note that peak increase in effort (indicated by the *solid arrowhead*) is associated with a small drop in peak flow and tidal volume triggering a transient electroencephalographic arousal. (ECG, electrocardiogram; EMGFACIAL, facial muscle electromyogram; EOG, electro-oculogram (right and left); FLOWPNEUMOTACH, pneumotachometer to quantify airflow; Pes, esophageal manometry to record esophageal pressure; RESPSUM, respiratory effort; SaO2, saturation with oxygen.)

of East Asian origin, and the mean age was 38 ± 14. Thus sex, race, and age distribution differs from the typical OSA patient demographics. UARS patients frequently complain of insomnia, sleep fragmentation, and fatigue. Their psychological profile often reveals high anxiety. Other clinical features of UARS patients include cold extremities, postural hypotension, history of fainting, a low systemic arterial blood pressure (below 105 mm Hg), orthostasis on tilt-table testing, myalgias, and functional somatic complaints.[9] During sleep, UARS patients demonstrate an increase in alpha rhythm and a relative increase in delta sleep, unlike OSA patients, who show a predominance of stage 1 and 2 NREM sleep with a decrease in delta sleep. Additionally, NREM sleep has been shown to be more disturbed in UARS patients than controls, with an increase in EEG cyclic alternating pattern (CAP) rate that correlates to symptoms of fatigue and sleepiness.[144]

Despite the recognition of UARS as a distinct disorder, many patients remain untreated and experience worsened symptoms of insomnia, fatigue, and depressed mood over time.[145]

The difference between UARS and OSA patients is hypothesized to be caused by genetically predetermined and environmentally altered pharyngeal receptors, particularly mechanoreceptors. Patients with UARS may have intact, sensitive, peripheral pharyngeal function or hyperfunction, whereas OSA patients may have primary pharyngeal receptor dysfunction. Patients with UARS awaken in response to relatively small increases in respiratory effort compared to OSA patients, whose arousal threshold requires much higher inspiratory pressures (up to −40 to −80 cm H_2O).

Secondary Apnea

A variety of medical conditions and craniofacial malformations are commonly associated with OSAS. Patients with congenital conditions including micrognathia, such as Pierre Robin, Hunter's, and Treacher-Collins syndromes and Crouzon's disease, present in childhood; children with cleft palates repaired by a pharyngeal flap have developed iatrogenic obstruction. Cranial base abnormalities associated with OSAS include achondroplasia and Klippel-Feil syndrome malformations. Down syndrome patients have large tongues and retrognathia, predisposing to upper airway obstruction. Children with Prader-Willi syndrome may suffer OSAS due to morbid obesity. Treatment of Prader-Willi syndrome with growth hormone may worsen OSA, which may even lead to death.[146] Endocrine abnormalities causing OSAS include hypothyroidism with myxedema, which causes macroglossia and parapharyngeal tissue infiltration. Acromegaly is a known cause of macroglossia.

Neurologic disorders associated with OSAS include the Shy-Drager syndrome of multisystem degeneration (central and obstructive apnea) and neuromuscular diseases involving facial and thoracoabdominal musculature such as poliomyelitis and myotonic and muscular dystrophies. Patients with acquired or hereditary neuropathies (such as amyotrophic lateral sclerosis and Charcot-Marie-Tooth disease) are also at a higher risk of developing OSA. History of stroke or transient ischemic attacks significantly increases risk of OSA. Secondary kyphoscoliosis will worsen nocturnal respiratory function. Lesions of the temporomandibular condyle leading to retrognathia may be developmental or acquired due to rheumatoid arthritis, osteomyelitis, or trauma.

EVALUATION

History: Nighttime Symptoms

Pertinent symptoms of OSAS fall into daytime and nocturnal categories. Loud guttural snoring, at its worst in the supine position, punctuated by choking sounds and followed by cessation of breathing, is virtually pathognomonic. Although snoring commonly starts around the time of puberty, presentation to a physician is typically prompted by a recent increase in snoring intensity associated with weight gain. The sleep of the bed partner is compromised by the patient's high-amplitude snoring and restless sleep. The volume may be so loud as to exceed standards set by the Occupational Safety and Health Administration for workplace safety.[147] The apneic phase can last from seconds to more than a minute. These respiratory cessations may frighten bed partners, who often remain vigilant to wake the patient to resume breathing. Commonly, partners begin sleeping in separate rooms, which may create stress in the relationship.

Restless sleep in large part stems from sleep fragmentation caused by airway obstruction. Repetitive EEG arousals lasting seconds may terminate apneic episodes, thereby causing a regain of "wakeful" muscle tone observed on the chin EMG. This facilitates a restorative breath, allowing the cycle to repeat. Behavioral arousals accompany some of these EEG arousals, resulting in position changes, abrupt rising of the upper torso from the bed, and large flailing limb movements. Some of these movements appear to be agitated, with concomitant groaning or crying out of short dysphoric phrases. The vast majority of brief arousals are not consciously recalled on awakening, although the patient may appreciate that the quality of sleep has been poor. Clues to restless sleep are obtained by asking the patient how disturbed are bedcovers by morning, and how many times he or she awoke during the night.

It is surprisingly infrequent for the patient to awaken with actual awareness of an asphyxial sensation such as choking or gasping. When this does occur, it may be accompanied by a "feeling of dying," and the patient may run to the window or sit up at the edge of the bed. Rarely, patients are still unable to draw an inspiratory breath upon awakening, but usually can do so after coughing. It is believed that this may be due to adhesion of the uvula to the posterior pharynx.

There appears to be a subpopulation of sleep apneics in whom the presenting complaint is sleep maintenance insomnia. Some of their arousals trigger full awakenings that last at least several minutes. Because they remain unaware of the respiratory antecedents of these awakenings, OSAS should be considered among the differential diagnoses in evaluating patients with chronic difficulties maintaining sleep.

The clinician should ask about symptoms related to snoring, such as the presence of a dry mouth or sore throat on awakening. Asking the patient if he or she drinks water overnight may also elicit information on a dry upper airway. Morning headaches that resolve within an hour of awakening should also be asked about, as they may be clues to nocturnal hypercarbia and increased intracranial pressure. These headaches are typically generalized or bifrontal in nature. The occurrence of nocturnal confusional spells, such as watering the houseplants with milk, may be due to either hypoxemia or slow-wave sleep (SWS) parasomnias triggered by respiratory-induced arousal.

Multiple episodes of nocturia have been related to elevated plasma levels of ANP and catecholamines.[148,149] After the first night of treatment with nasal CPAP, a return to normal levels with concomitant decrease in urinary volume to approximately 50% of pretreatment amounts has been reported. This helps explain why enuresis is more common in children with OSAS and was reported in 7% of 120 apneic adults seen successively at Stanford in 1992.[149a] Confusion and increased intraabdominal pressure from inspiratory attempts against a closed upper airway may also contribute to enuresis.

Symptoms of nocturnal esophageal acid reflux and heartburn are facilitated when excessively negative intrathoracic pressure exerts upward suction on abdominal contents, and increased abdominal pressure expels the contents. The patient may also complain of nocturnal aspiration. Bruxism may be noted and may be a clue to dental malocclusion resulting from the common jaw misalignment etiologically related to OSA. A history of orthodontic treatment to correct an overjet is common. The patient may have a history of wisdom tooth extraction secondary to impaction. These individuals may also manifest morning headaches or dysfunction of the temporomandibular joint.

History of seasonal or environmental allergies should be sought, as these are common causes of nasal obstruction in adults and adenotonsillar enlargement in children. Studies of rhesus monkeys with chronic and temporary nasal obstruction suggest that nasal obstruction with mouth breathing during childhood is etiologically related to subsequent mandibular growth insufficiency.[125,126] We have documented craniofacial abnormalities with cephalometric radiography that were not appreciated on clinical examination.[127]

Nocturnal diaphoresis of the face and chest may be seen in association with the increased effort required to inspire against resistance during the night. Increased caloric expenditures to breathe may also account for a subpopulation of sleep apneics who have difficulty gaining weight.

Ethanol or other sedatives used before bedtime worsen OSAS by at least two mechanisms. They greatly diminish the contraction of the upper airway dilators, as well as interfering with the organization of reflexes coordinating upper airway dilators with the contraction of inspiratory muscles.[150] They may also increase the cortical arousal threshold, allowing more prolonged apneas and severe oxygen desaturations. A history of increased snoring or development of any of the symptoms discussed earlier in association with sedating substances should raise the index of suspicion for OSAS. In elderly patients with AI greater than 5 events/hr, sedative use or sleep deprivation may escalate the AI into the pathologic range.[151]

History: Daytime Symptoms

The cardinal daytime symptom of OSAS is EDS, which manifests as a tendency to inadvertently fall asleep during quiet or passive activities, to take intentional naps, or to experience short but repetitive attention lapses while doing monotonous tasks. Such sleepiness is the consequence of sleep fragmentation. Patients usually misperceive the act of dozing off as being caused by the characteristics of the situation (i.e., boredom), rather than by their abnormal intrinsic degree of somnolence. It helps to inform patients that quiet settings do not produce sleepiness, but merely unmask it. Patients often forget or deny episodes of daytime sleepiness, which may better be elicited from household members who frequently observe the patient dozing while watching television or reading. Momentary lapses into sleep while driving are a potentially lethal consequence of somnolence, and history of these lapses should always be sought by inquiring about motor vehicle accidents due to sleepiness or inadvertently dozing at the wheel or swerving into another lane. Such incidents are particularly likely on long or monotonous trips. Affirmative answers require rapid treatment interventions.

Symptoms of fatigue, tiredness, and lack of energy are frequently reported by patients with OSA and must be enquired about during the clinical interview. These symptoms are more frequently reported and emphasized by OSA patients than sleepiness.[152]

Cognitive complaints resulting from EDS are common, and may be the only clue to OSA in those who misperceive their sleepiness. Automatic behavior, when an action is performed without subsequent recall, is an extreme manifestation of such cognitive impairment. Increased errors and poor judgment may place patients at risk of losing their jobs.[12] Severe morning confusion and disorientation, termed *sleep drunkenness*, may be a sequela of preceding hypoxemia. Studies have shown OSA patients have problems with attention, executive behavior, visuospatial learning, motor performance, and constructional ability.[153] A meta-analysis showed a trend for improved performance of cognitive outcomes in OSA patients treated with CPAP compared to placebo.[154] Larger studies are currently underway evaluating the impact CPAP has on cognitive performance.

Sleep fragmentation may produce personality changes that are often first noted by family members. These include moodiness, irritability, anxiety, aggression, and depression. More marked personality changes involving irrational behavior, jealousy, and paranoia have been reported. Sleepy patients report less enjoyment from previously engaging activities. They are typically misperceived as unmotivated or lazy, descriptors they come to believe if the underlying etiology remains undiscovered.

Diminished libido or impotence is not an uncommon complaint, even in nonelderly OSA patients. Fanfulla et al.

reported abnormal bulbocavernosus reflex in 68% of 25 male OSA patients with AHI greater than 10 events/hr.[155] These abnormalities correlated significantly with the severity of OSA and the severity of gas exchange alterations, but did not vary with age. With treatment of OSA, sexual function may improve.[156]

In taking the medical history, inquiries regarding systemic sequelae must be sought. These include the existence and duration of borderline or elevated blood pressure; angina; symptoms of right heart failure, including peripheral edema; and transient cerebrovascular ischemic symptoms.

Physical Examination

Patient evaluation begins with observing the patient in the waiting room for sleeping or snoring. Obesity (BMI > 28 kg/m^2) and neck circumference greater than 40 cm have shown a sensitivity of 61% and specificity of 93% for OSA regardless of gender.[157] The distribution of weight should be noted, as more midline depositions favor nocturnal respiratory pathology. In particular, adiposity or muscularity of the neck predisposes to upper airway obstruction, and severe abdominal obesity may also predispose to alveolar hypoventilation. A nasal voice is a clue to nasal obstruction, and mild hoarseness is often noted in heavy snorers. The lateral facial profile should be inspected for retrognathia or micrognathia, keeping in mind that the relevant site is the indentation below the lip that identifies the genial tubercle, where the tongue makes insertion on the mandible. The patient should bite down to demonstrate dental occlusion. Overjet is recorded in millimeters, and underbite should be noted as well. Palpate the temporomandibular joint while the patient opens the jaw widely for subluxation or a click as evidence of jaw misalignment. The oral cavity is inspected for dental prostheses, size of tongue, and soft palate tissue size and appearance. Soft palate edema and erythema may be due to snoring. A soft palate inferiorly positioned behind the tongue may be due to stretching from chronic excessive suction as a result of snoring. Tonsillar hypertrophy is noted. The hard palate is checked for a high arch, which has been found to correlate with OSAS.

Evidence of upper airway obstruction is obtained by evaluating breathing in the supine position with the jaw slackened slightly open and the nares occluded, to simulate oral breathing during sleep. If snoring or labored breathing results, this is good evidence that even greater difficulties will occur during sleep. The nose should be assessed for septal deviation, polyps, flaring of the nostrils, collapse of the internal valves, and patency of either vestibule with the opposite naris occluded. The thyroid should be examined for evidence of enlargement.

Blood pressure and pulse are measured and a general physical examination is performed, bearing in mind signs of dysrhythmia or heart failure. Lung auscultation provides clues of pulmonary pathology that would exacerbate oxygen desaturation caused by upper airway obstruction. A complete neurologic evaluation may uncover neuromuscular disorders impacting on upper airway patency and respiratory muscle function. A complete physical examination can eliminate the presence of generalized diseases, particularly those causing lymph node enlargement or mucosal infiltration, which may reduce the upper airway lumen.

The history and examination should reveal secondary causes of OSAS, including searching for a local tumor in the upper airway. Suspicion is raised in the presence of rapid emergence of obstructive symptoms not associated with weight gain, throat pain, constant hoarseness or other vocal cord dysfunction, prominent difficulties swallowing, or nasal regurgitation. Such symptoms should prompt otolaryngologic evaluation.

Laboratory Evaluation

Polysomnography

A full-night PSG study in the sleep laboratory is the main method of evaluation (level 1 study). The study devotes various channels to the recording of the EEG (i.e., F3–M1, C4–M1, C3–M1, 01–02), electro-oculogram (EOG), chin and limb (usually anterior tibialis) noninvasive EMG, qualitative measurements of oral-nasal airflow, thoracic and abdominal respiratory efforts, electrocardiogram (ECG), and pulse oximetry. An entire night of study is generally recommended, as opposed to a partial night, because substantial changes in respiratory disturbance typically occur from one sleep cycle to another across the night. Because REM sleep predominates toward the end of the night, REM sleep–related respiratory disturbances might easily be missed without a full night of study.

However, in some circumstances a split-night study can be considered. The split-night study requires the recording and analysis of the same parameters as a standard diagnostic full-night PSG. Recent guidelines from the American Association of Sleep Medicine (AASM) state that a split night study may be considered in patients if four criteria are met.[158] The first is that an AHI of at least 40 events/hr be documented during a minimum 2-hour diagnostic PSG. Split-night studies may be considered at an AHI of 20–40 events/hr, based on clinical judgment (e.g., if there are also repetitive long obstructions and major desaturations). The second criterion is that CPAP titration be carried out for more than 3 hours as respiratory events can worsen as the night progresses. The third criterion is that PSG documents that CPAP eliminates or nearly eliminates respiratory events during REM and non-REM sleep, including REM sleep with the patient in the supine position. The last criterion is that a second full-night PSG with CPAP titration be performed if the diagnosis of a sleep-related breathing disorder is confirmed but the second and third criteria are not met.[158]

A monitored level 1 PSG allows quantification of various factors that are disturbed in sleep apneics, including the RDI, oxygen desaturation, sleep-stage percentages, and sleep efficiency. Sleep fragmentation can be assessed as variable-length awakenings or EEG arousals lasting only several seconds. CAP can be sought in non-REM sleep as a subtle indication of cortical arousals.[159] PSG helps determine whether the arousals are due to apnea or unsuspected factors such as periodic limb movements or primary insomnia. Associations between sleep stage and positional influences on respiratory disturbance can be made. Cardiac arrythmias and their relationship to oxygen desaturation and sleep stage can be identified. Relatively invasive techniques to measure upper airway pressure may have circumscribed clinical usefulness. UARS (discussed earlier) may only be suspected based on transient alpha rhythm EEG arousals on the standard PSG, warranting additional investigation using esophageal manometry. Catheter systems allowing measurement of differential pressures at different levels of the upper airway may also help in determining the level of collapse at which surgical intervention should be addressed.[160–162]

Pulse transit time measures the transmission time for the arterial pulse pressure wave to travel from the aortic valve to the periphery; it increases during arousal-induced increases in blood pressure. Pulse transit time has a high sensitivity and specificity in distinguishing between central and obstructive apnea-hypopnea and may be used if P_{es} monitoring is not available on attended PSG.[163]

Technologies that allow in-home sleep monitoring are rapidly emerging. Portable units range from study level 2 to 4. Level 2 units contain a minimum of seven channels, including EEG, EOG, chin EMG, ECG or heart rate, airflow, respiratory effort, and oxygen saturation. Level 3 units contain a minimum of four channels, including ventilation or airflow (with at least two channels of respiratory movement, or respiratory movement with airflow), heart rate or ECG, and oxygen saturation. Level 4 units measure a single parameter or two parameters, such as oxygenation and heart rate.

Although portable studies are a more convenient and less expensive alternative to standard PSG, there are significant limitations. The absence of trained personnel to intervene in the event of technical difficulty or medical emergency is one of the primary shortcomings. Concern has also been raised about the precision and accuracy of some portable units for the evaluation of more subtle cases of SDB, such as those with a predominance of hypopneas or UARS.[164] The most recent practice parameters published by the AASM approve the use of level 3 unattended portable monitoring units for the diagnosis of OSA in a limited setting.[165] The guidelines state that these unattended studies can be performed only in conjunction with a comprehensive sleep evaluation by a board-eligible or board-certified sleep medicine specialist. A sleep medicine specialist must also interpret the study. Portable testing should only be preformed on adult, nonelderly patients with a high pretest probability of having moderate to severe OSA without other sleep disorders, including central sleep apnea, periodic limb movement disorder, insomnia, parasomnias, circadian rhythm disorders, or narcolepsy. Furthermore, patients are not eligible for portable testing if they have comorbid medical conditions that may degrade the test accuracy, such as chronic obstructive pulmonary disease (COPD) or peripheral vascular disease. These recommendations further state there is insufficient evidence to use level 2 or 4 devices in an unattended setting.[166]

Multiple Sleep Latency Test

The MSLT[167] is considered to be an objective measure of EDS. A series of daytime naps (usually five) of 20 minutes' duration at 2-hour intervals is performed to determine time to sleep onset. These sleep latencies are averaged. Scores under 8 minutes in the absence of confounding factors (e.g., insufficient preceding nocturnal total sleep time, use of hypnotic medication) are generally regarded as abnormal. REM occurrences during naps are also noted.

Because the demonstration of EDS is not required for the diagnosis of OSAS, MSLTs are not mandatory in the evaluation of OSAS. If a PSG for suspected OSAS is negative, however, MSLT performed the subsequent day may help diagnose a different sleep disorder of excessive somnolence, though 5–15% of OSA subjects can have MSLT findings consistent with narcolepsy. When complaints of sleepiness persist after adequate treatment is instituted, an MSLT may reveal an unsuspected second sleep disorder requiring a separate treatment approach.

In large clinical populations, the severity of OSA based on AHI was not particularly predictive of sleepiness as objectively measured by the MSLT.[168]

Imaging Studies

As an adjunct to clinical evaluation, particularly when surgical treatment is contemplated, various imaging procedures can help identify the site(s) of upper airway obstruction. For a comprehensive review, the interested reader is referred to papers by Shepard et al.[169] or Faber and Grymer.[170] Imaging is also imperative when the history raises suspicion of a mass lesion as the cause of upper airway obstruction. It should be kept in mind that procedures performed on an awake patient do not reveal the actual anatomy during sleep, when postural and state-related changes in muscle tone alter the awake relationships.

Cephalometric radiographs provide a midline view of relevant cranial base and facial bones with their soft tissue appendages. Maxillary or mandibular deficiency can be calculated, and awake posterior airway space measured as the distance between the base of the tongue and posterior pharyngeal wall. Soft palate and lymphoid tissue extent is identified.

Fiberoptic endoscopy of the upper airway down to the vocal cords performed in the seated and supine positions provides further assessment of the possible sites of collapse. The patient can perform Valsalva and Müller's maneuvers to elicit collapse, although the predictive value for identifying candidates for surgical success after uvulo-palatopharyngoplasty (UPPP) is limited.[171–173] Fiberoptic endoscopy should be systematically performed to eliminate secondary causes of upper airway obstruction if signs and symptoms are consistent with them.

Computed tomography (CT) scanning provides detailed surveys of cross-sectional levels of the upper airway, and magnetic resonance imaging (MRI) can be used to image multiple planes. CT and MRI have mainly been used as research tools due to their expense. Newer techniques such as fast CT scanning may prove to have prognostic clinical usefulness in selecting candidates for successful surgical outcomes. The 50-msec scan time, as compared to 2–5 seconds for conventional CT, is sufficiently rapid to show dynamic dimensional changes across various levels of the upper airway during the respiratory cycle. It can potentially be used in a sleeping patient.

Videofluoroscopy of the pharynx in anteroposterior and lateral directions offers another means for observing dynamic anatomic changes in the upper airway during ventilation. It is of limited clinical usefulness in view of its significant radiation exposure.

Other Studies

Pulmonary function tests, including spirometry and arterial blood gases, are a useful adjunct in investigation. Diminished vital capacity has been identified as a risk factor for SDB both in the Cleveland Family Study and in the elderly.[22,174] Although associated with excess cardiovascular morbidity, a lowered vital capacity may be a marker for central obesity or an indicator of the presence of OSAS.[175,176] Patients with daytime hypoxemia or CO_2 retention due to intrinsic lung disease might be expected to show severe oxygen desaturations with the addition of obstructive sleep pathology, and may require cautious addition of low-flow oxygen to nasal CPAP. Those with restrictive pulmonary dynamics based on morbid obesity might require special treatment with bilevel positive airway pressure (BIPAP) or intermittent positive pressure ventilation delivered by nasal mask. Arterial blood gases provide the most relevant information for a sleep evaluation if obtained after the patient remains supine for 20 minutes. This aids in detection of insufficient ventilation associated with the supine position.

Thyroid function screening will exclude hypothyroidism as a cause of apnea and daytime somnolence. Polycythemia without known lung disease should lead to a consideration of sleep apnea.

TREATMENT

Behavioral Recommendations

Once OSAS is diagnosed, treatments can be suggested based on evaluation of contributing factors and disease severity. It has long been known that weight loss in obese patients is effective in the reduction of the number of apneas, sleep fragmentation, and the extent and number of desaturations. In overweight patients without obvious fixed anatomic considerations such as retrognathia, weight loss may result in eventual cure. For most patients, nasal CPAP should be instituted along with weight loss measures. These measures include weight reduction surgery, diet with or without pharmacologic intervention, and exercise. When applicable, a program of exercise may be facilitated after daytime somnolence is ameliorated by CPAP. For those who are not completely cured by weight loss, the significant reduction in weight often allows a lower CPAP pressure requirement or increases the likelihood of a surgical cure. Patients with large losses should be re-titrated to the lowest effective pressure.

Elimination of central nervous system depressants such as ethanol or sedatives from the bloodstream at bedtime decreases the severity of OSAS. If a strong positional relationship is discovered, with obstruction limited to the supine position, recommendation to remain in a lateral or prone position can be made. A sock filled with a golf or tennis ball and sewn onto the back of the pajamas or T-shirt may help patients learn to avoid the supine position. A full-length wedge pillow may also be helpful in this respect. In mild cases, attention to position may suffice.

Pharmacologic Treatment

Currently there are no U.S. Food and Drug Administration (FDA)–approved medications that treat OSA. Tricyclic antidepressants such as protriptyline have been used to increase muscle tone and diminish REM sleep time in cases of mild or REM sleep–related OSAS. Progesterone acts as a respiratory stimulant in obese patients but has no impact on an obstructed airway. Paroxetine has been shown to mildly decrease apneas during NREM sleep.[177] Provigil has an FDA approval to treat residual daytime sleepiness of treated OSA patients, with statistical improvements in Maintenance of Wakefulness Test, Epworth Sleepiness Scale, and quality-of-life scores compared to controls.[178] Unfortunately, to date, pharmacologic approaches designed specifically to treat SDB have been largely unsuccessful.

Continuous and Bilevel Positive Airway Pressure

An enormous advance in the treatment of OSAS began in the early 1980s with the first commercially available continuous positive pressure generators. These bedside machines compress room air and channel it through a soft vinyl or silicone nasal mask, a full-face (nasal-oral) mask, or endonasal cushions at a given pressure. CPAP serves as a pneumatic splint to keep the upper airway patent. Pressure requirements must be established during sleep for each patient. Optimum pressure is the lowest one that completely eliminates obstructive apneas, hypopneas, snoring, and mask flow limitation and normalizes arterial Po_2. Patients who routinely consume ethanol in the evening are most accurately titrated to CPAP after consuming their usual intake, which raises the pressure requirement.

BIPAP differs from CPAP by using separate inspiratory and expiratory pressures. BIPAP machines time themselves to patient-initiated breathing. By reducing the pressure on expiration, BIPAP lowers the resistance against which the patient must exhale. This is advantageous for patients with severely restrictive pulmonary dynamics, such as those with emphysema, the morbidly obese, and those with neuromuscular weakness. Patients with normal lungs who could not tolerate CPAP might feel more comfortable on BIPAP, especially those requiring higher CPAP pressures (approximately 13 cm H_2O). Those with severe discomfort due to drying of the mucosa could benefit from BIPAP because of the overall decrease in airflow relative to CPAP. BIPAP also offers a higher range of inspiratory pressures than CPAP, with maximum pressures of 40 cm H_2O. The newer devices with extended pressure range also have the ability to control inspiratory time (flow) and are therefore more appropriate for patients with isolated neuromuscular disease. Intermittent positive pressure ventilation may be more useful in some patients with sleep-related hypoventilation who cannot be maintained on bilevel units.

A PSG study to titrate CPAP or BIPAP pressure should be performed for 1 entire night to allow adequate assessment. A second titration night can be done if an adequate pressure was not identified the first night. Ideally the optimum pressure is checked for adequacy throughout all stages and positions. It is especially critical to evaluate the patient in the supine position, when the maximum pressure requirement occurs. Unfortunately, financial constraints increasingly dictate that split-night studies be performed. This method of diagnosis and treatment tends to underestimate the severity of disease because treatment takes place in the latter half of the night when apnea is usually at its worst. In severe apneics, a rebound of unusually long REM sleep and SWS that may be out of circadian phase occurs once adequate airway patency is attained. REM sleep rebound shows unusually prominent phasic activity, whereas the SWS episodes may show exceptionally high voltages. Rare but dangerous sequelae of REM rebound have been seen in severe apneics with CO_2 retention under slightly suboptimal pressure. Arousal is suppressed during a long rebound, and if partial upper airway closure persists, dangerous hypoxemia may result.[171]

Autotitrating positive airway pressure (APAP) devices offer a theoretical advantage of foregoing a traditional CPAP titration study by delivering the lowest pressure needed to prevent respiratory disturbances. These devices may decrease side effects of traditional CPAP such as air swallowing and abdominal bloating and are theoretically able to accurately record flow leaks, hypopneas, and apneas. They detect snoring, apneas, hypopneas, flow limitation, and changes in airway resistance or impedance, which are then interpreted by a central processing unit based on specific diagnostic algorithms to determine the resultant voltage for the APAP blower in response to these signals.[179] Studies have shown significant variability between different APAP devices, with undertreatment of 13–60% of patients using the devices (residual RDI > 5 during treatment).[180] There is insufficient evidence to use these devices to diagnose OSA.[181]

The 2007 AASM practice parameters on APAP devices give sleep specialists the option to use these devices in an unattended setting to treat uncomplicated OSA patients.[181] Potential patients include those with moderate to severe OSA without significant comorbidities such as congestive heart failure, COPD, central sleep apnea syndromes, or hypoventilation syndromes. Sleep specialists have the option of treating these OSA patients with APAP devices either left in the self-adjusting mode or set at the prescribed 90th or 95th percentile pressure and utilized during a several-week trial period. Patients prescribed APAP devices should be closely followed by a sleep medicine specialist to ensure adequate treatment. A standard CPAP titration should be preformed in patients whose symptoms do not resolve with APAP.[181]

A severe limitation of APAP devices is that they determine pressures differently, and there are few studies comparing various APAP devices to each other and to set CPAP devices. APAP is not superior (and many would argue not even equivalent) to a fixed CPAP pressure determined by an attended titration. Therefore, AASM guidelines state that "polysomnography directed CPAP titration is still the standard method for determination of effective CPAP pressure."[181] With improvements in technology, greater clinical experience, and growing literature on the subject, APAP devices will likely be more widely used in the future.

Treatment with nasal CPAP or BIPAP offers advantages of safety and assured efficacy over surgical approaches. They offer immediate and complete treatment for OSAS and are less costly than extensive surgical approaches. They can be used temporarily while weight loss is pursued or surgery is contemplated. Positive pressure eliminates risk factors for associated morbidity along with daytime somnolence. Modern CPAP units are small, portable, and quiet. Most gradually adjust the pressure upward to the preset pressure, allowing sleep onset to occur at more comfortable lower pressures.

Disadvantages of CPAP lie in psychological resistance to ongoing nightly reliance on a machine. Poor compliance is the main obstacle to this treatment modality. Patients may feel claustrophobic and intolerant of the restriction of their movement and may perceive the treatment as an obstacle to intimacy with their bed partner and as a reminder of their mortality. The devices are annoying to some patients, although they are continually improved. Those traveling frequently may find it inconvenient. Generally, young adults and patients who are dating find this treatment to have an unacceptable social impact.

Common physical difficulties encountered include reactive nasal congestion or rhinitis, sinusitis and epistasis or drying of the nasal-oral mucosa, discomfort or skin trauma from a poorly fitting mask, and allergic reaction to (or contact dermatitis with) the mask. Nasal symptoms usually subside after the first few months and can be ameliorated with heated humidification, daily nasal rinses, and a nasal steroid inhaler. Comfort issues and dermatitis should be closely supervised and addressed with trials of various mask adaptors and styles or by altering the mode of delivery via nasal pillows or other mask types. Psychological distress is minimized by support from the entire sleep laboratory team, with reassurance and understanding at the time of initiation and close follow-up. Sleep apnea support groups exist in many areas to help with coping and compliance. Occasionally, a brief course of bedtime hypnotics is required, with the patient's full understanding that the severity of apnea will worsen if the medication is used without the CPAP device. Flow leaks through an open mouth can be minimized by use of a chin strap.

Long-term compliance has been only fair, with an estimate of 60–85% of patients using their machines regularly after 1 year.[182,183] Compliance has been associated with the severity of daytime hypersomnolence before CPAP, but not with pretreatment disease severity as indicated by the RDI or oxygen saturation nadir. Intellectual understanding of the benefits of nightly use (i.e., to decrease cardiovascular risk factors) appears insufficient to motivate long-term compliance. Cognitive behavioral interventions may improve compliance.[184] In one study, use of a C-flex device was shown to significantly increase patient compliance.[185]

In patients who do not wish to undergo the extensive surgeries that might be required to produce a complete cure, selective surgery to relieve nasal obstruction can reduce pressure requirements and improve CPAP tolerance. In patients with more than mild oxygen desaturation on diagnostic testing (i.e., <85%) who choose surgical treatment, CPAP initiation may be contemplated preoperatively to decrease the postoperative risk of further desaturation due to edema. Preoperative CPAP also reduces soft palate edema due to snoring and improves overall health status. Weight loss before surgery while using CPAP increases the chance of successful cure by creating more airway space through parapharyngeal tissue reduction.

Surgical Approaches

The first surgical treatment for OSAS was tracheostomy. This intervention is rarely needed now, because of the pervasive use of positive pressure therapy. Although used infrequently, tracheostomy provides immediate profound improvement for some individuals with severe OSAS. Maintenance of a tracheostomy is associated with some morbidity and psychosocial implications.

Surgery is individually tailored to overcome upper airway obstruction after a thorough analysis of the three main levels of potential obstruction: the nose, soft palate, and base of the tongue or hypopharynx. Often, more than one level must be treated, either sequentially or simultaneously. Patients must understand that surgical treatment is an extensive and more costly process with greater risks than medical treatment. In addition, surgery carries no guarantee of cure in an individual patient, with only statistical cure rates available.

Nasal obstruction can be corrected with septoplasty, polypectomy, or radiofrequency turbinate reduction. Though these procedures can improve nasal breathing and SDB, nasal surgery alone successfully treats only a minority of OSA patients.

Soft palate resection via UPPP or uvuloflap surgery has an approximately 40% response rate in individuals but is much less successful in obese patients.[186–188] However, the success rate can be as high as 80% in properly selected patients.[189] Depending on how "success" is defined, these rates may be altered considerably. Most surgeons consider OSA surgery as success if a 50% reduction of the AHI achieved. The most common postoperative adverse sequelae include severe pain for approximately 2 weeks, transient nasal reflux and nasal speech due to palatal incompetence, minor loss of taste, and tongue numbness. Major complications involve permanent nasal reflux or nasal speech due to permanent velopharyngeal incompetence and scarring with retraction leading to palatal stenosis.

Because UPPP ameliorates snoring due to vibration of the uvula without addressing potential obstruction behind the base of the tongue, a major sign of ongoing residual obstruction may be masked. It is therefore imperative to follow up all surgeries with a postoperative sleep study. Ideally, this study should be delayed at least 4 months after surgery to allow thorough resolution of edema and readjustment of respiratory reflexes. Those patients with moderate to severe apnea can be maintained on CPAP in the interim and withdrawn 2 weeks before study to allow expression of airway changes from potential residual obstruction.

Genioglossus advancement via inferior sagittal osteotomy is a technique pioneered at Stanford University[190] that addresses the retroposition of the tongue by advancing the insertion point of the genioglossus, the geniotubercle. The surgeon makes a small mandibular incision at the geniotubercle, pulls the bone segment through the jaw, and allows the fracture to heal. This is usually performed in conjunction with UPPP. The success rates have been variable, ranging from 23% to 77%.[191–194] Common complications are minor and consist of transient dental nerve anesthesia. Mandibular fracture may occur if the incision extends into the alveolus.

Hyoid advancement can expand the airway by moving the tongue base and pharyngeal musculature forward. This is achieved by attaching it to the thyroid cartilage. This procedure is usually performed in conjunction with genioglossus advancement to improve OSA, but some surgeons will combine it with UPPP alone.[193–197] The success rate of hyoid advancement is variable and ranges from 17% to 65%.[193–197] This surgery requires an external incision on the neck.

Maxillomandibular advancement (MMA) is another surgical option to improve OSA. It is generally reserved for patients for whom other treatments have failed and who do not want to be treated with nasal CPAP. This procedure expands the entire airway, including the nasopharyngeal and hypopharyngeal airway. Patients undergoing MMA who have previously undergone the earlier discussed surgeries can have excellent improvement of OSA. Generally the jaws must be advanced 8–14 mm for adequate treatment of OSA. MMA is currently the most effective sleep apnea surgical procedure, with success rates generally between 75% and 100%.[187,191–193,198,199] MMA shows promising cure rates long term, but weight gain is associated with the recurrence of OSA.[200]

Tongue base suspension suture is thought to reduce the collapsibility of the tongue during sleep. It is often performed in conjunction with UPPP, with variable success rates reported.[201,202] Radiofrequency reduction of the base of the tongue may also improve OSA by increasing the retropharyngeal airway space. Though this procedure does improve OSA when performed alone, it does not appear to be as successful in the long run.[203] Many surgeons perform this procedure in conjunction with UPPP or MMA.

Bariatric surgery with significant weight loss has been shown to improve and even cure OSA in morbidly obese patients.[204,205]

Oral Appliances

Various types of dental devices have been used to treat OSA. They work by increasing airway space, providing a stable anterior position of the mandible, and advancing the tongue or soft palate, and possibly by changing genioglossus muscle activity.[206] The devices are worn only during sleep. There are a variety of oral appliances; some are prefabricated and are relatively inexpensive, while others are custom made by dentists. The advantage over surgery is that there is no permanent change of anatomy and no surgical risk involved.

The most effective devices are those that cause the mandible to protrude forward. A recent meta-analysis concluded that oral appliances mildly improved subjective daytime sleepiness and SDB compared with controls, but less well than CPAP.[207] Though patients tend to be more compliant with wearing oral appliances than using CPAP, these devices tend not to be as effective in treating OSA.[184] Patients are more likely to achieve success with an oral appliance if they have less severe OSA, are nonobese, have positional OSA, and are able to significantly protrude their jaw from baseline.[208]

According to recent AASM guidelines, oral appliances can be used in patients with mild to moderate OSA who prefer them to CPAP therapy, or who do not respond to, are not appropriate candidates for, or fail treatment attempts with CPAP.[209] As mentioned, the success rate of oral appliances often mirrors the severity of OSA, with patients with mild OSA more likely to achieve success than those with severe OSA. Referral to a dentist who is adequately trained and has understanding of SDB is paramount. Minor tooth movement and small changes in occlusion can develop in some patients after prolonged use.

OBSTRUCTIVE SLEEP APNEA IN CHILDREN

OSA occurs in premature and full-term infants as well as in children (see also Chapter 38). Though this disorder was relatively recently described, it is a common disorder affecting 3% of children 2–8 years of age.[210,211] In very young patients, the apnea usually becomes apparent as a result of color change and bradycardia. In most children, a constellation of daytime and nighttime clinical symptoms signals the condition. At different ages, different symptoms are more common. Postpubertal teenagers do not differ from young adults, but younger children often present a different clinical picture.

Clinical Features

OSAS can be associated with a series of daytime and nighttime signs and symptoms that may not be obvious at an initial evaluation.[212,213] The daytime symptoms include EDS so severe that school authorities suggest medical consultation, and abnormal daytime behavior ranging from aggressiveness and hyperactivity to pathologic shyness and social withdrawal. Children may exhibit more subtle symptoms including inattention, daytime fatigue, learning problems, morning headaches, frequent upper airway infections, failure to thrive, and obesity. Nocturnal symptoms seen at all ages include difficulty breathing while asleep, heavy snoring, apneic episodes, restless sleep, nocturnal sweating, nightmares, and SWS parasomnias. Absence of normal growth or failure to thrive can be seen at most ages.

Reasons for seeking consultation vary with age. Before 12 months of age, children may present with noisy nocturnal breathing, disturbed nocturnal sleep, and repetitive crying, or a poorly established day-night cycle may be the presenting features of OSA. OSA may also contribute to the occurrence of an apparent life-threatening event due to abnormal autonomic cardiovascular control and an increased arousal threshold.[214,215]

In toddlers, nocturnal crying spells or sleep terrors may prompt an evaluation for OSA. Grouchy or aggressive behavior, daytime mouth breathing, and difficulty waking up may be seen. Difficulty breathing while asleep, heavy snoring, apneic episodes observed by parents, restless sleep, nightmares, and night terrors are the most frequent reasons for consultation. This may be partly due to the parents' ability to evaluate a young child's sleep often and the fact that young children fall asleep early, allowing parents to note abnormal sleep behavior.

In children older than 5 years, EDS (associated with complaints of tiredness and daytime fatigue), abnormal daytime behavior, learning disabilities, frequent morning headaches, nocturnal enuresis, and major discipline problems are common reasons for consultation. A few children are referred at a late stage of the syndrome. These children not only present significant failure to thrive but also may have been hospitalized for unexplained acute cardiac failure or unexplained development of systemic hypertension. The cardiac failure often will have occurred after the child had contracted a cold or bronchopneumopathy, which may not have been severe but, in combination with the chronic nocturnal problem, nevertheless led to the acute failure.

Symptoms of attention-deficit/hyperactivity disorder (ADHD) have been positively associated with SDB in children. Chervin et al. showed that children diagnosed with ADHD had a threefold increase in snoring compared with controls.[216] Other studies have shown similar findings.[217-219] What is even more interesting is that snoring on its own has been shown to be a strong risk factor for future emergence or aggravation of ADHD symptoms.[219]

Classically the pediatric patient presenting with OSA has large tonsils and is underweight and having difficulty increasing his or her weight, despite a normal appetite. He or she also may be shorter than expected. Nocturnal secretion of growth hormone in children with repetitive apneas has been shown to be abnormally low. We have noted a similar decrease with heavy snoring, due to decreased growth hormone levels released during sleep and elevated caloric expenditure from increased work of breathing. As childhood obesity is becoming an epidemic, more obese patients are presenting with OSA and the incidence of pediatric OSA will likely rise. It is estimated that up to one third of obese children have OSA.[211,220]

The clinical evaluation of children should be as thorough as for adults, and suspicion of OSAS should lead to PSG monitoring during sleep.

Polysomnographic Testing

Although repetitive apneas may be seen in children with equal frequency as in adults, most commonly the PSG indicates only intermittent apneas. Sometimes no apneas are monitored, even when a florid symptomatology exists.[221] A pediatric sleep study is evaluated differently than an adult record. The criterion for an apnea or hypopnea duration is equal to two breaths for the patient or 10 seconds, whatever is shorter. An RDI greater than 1/hr is considered abnormal in the pediatric population.[222] Pediatric OSA patients have fewer cortical arousals with breathing events and their sleep architecture tends to be better preserved compared to adult OSA patients.

Prepubescent children have a greater tendency to present complete apneas during REM sleep. During NREM sleep, prepubescent children with OSAS present as loud snorers. Documented by a sonogram, snoring is commonly associated with an increase in respiratory rate. The degree of tachypnea is variable within a given age group and sometimes within a given subject during the night. The increase in breathing frequency compensates for the decrease in V_T and allows maintenance of normal minute ventilation with an appropriate level of oxygen saturation. However, partial upper airway obstruction leads to great enhancement of respiratory efforts, which is obvious when one observes the laborious, noisy mouth breathing during sleep. P_{es} measures demonstrate the increase in respiratory efforts. P_{es} nadir may reach -35 to -40 cm H_2O without induction of a complete collapse of the upper airway in children 5–6 years old. Increased efforts may also be demonstrated by monitoring of intercostal-diaphragmatic EMG. Surface electrodes placed 10 mm apart near the eighth right intercostal space, between the axillary and maxillary lines, permit collection of the EMG activity of the inspiratory muscles. The signal can be integrated, and, depending on the calibration procedures used, semi-quantitative or quantitative measurements may be obtained. Measurement with surface electrodes and integration of abdominal muscle activity during expiration may demonstrate the degree of active expiratory effort that some of these children have to perform.

Despite the increase in respiratory efforts associated with snoring and increased upper airway resistance, children may not present with very fragmented sleep. The short alpha rhythm EEG arousals seen with increased upper airway resistance in adults may be much more uncommon here. Breathing may appear laborious, however, and increased efforts are often demonstrated by perspiration (at the head and neck or generalized). This suggests that the daytime sleepiness observed in these children despite near-normal sleep structure and absence of microarousals cannot be explained by sleep fragmentation alone. Polygraphic monitoring must thus focus not only on the presence or absence of apnea (with the knowledge that absence of apnea may be very misleading) but also on increase in respiratory effort and breathing frequency, as well as the importance of thoracoabdominal mechanical changes.

The repetitive inspiratory efforts expended during complete or, more often, partial upper airway obstruction lead to abnormal septal motion with leftward shift of the interventricular septum and the development of pulsus paradoxus.[139] Cardiac arrhythmias, particularly asystole and secondary AV block, may be seen, and intermittent increase in systolic blood pressure may be noted. Finally, systemic hypertension has been observed in association with OSAS. Systemic hypertension in prepubertal children completely disappears with tracheostomy. The only cases of systemic hypertension found to be clearly idiopathic and for which treatment of OSAS led to complete and long-term normalization of blood pressure were in prepubertal or pubertal children.[223]

Asthma and Upper Airway Obstruction During Sleep

In children, a relationship exists between asthma and upper airway obstruction. Allergic reactions very early in life lead to mucosal swelling and enlargement of the pharyngeal region. There is a well-known interaction between the size of the upper airway and craniofacial development, particularly development of the mandible, during early childhood. Presence of upper airway allergies will thus limit maxillomandibular growth and cause a decrease in the size of the upper airway. Small upper airways are often associated with increased upper airway resistance during sleep, leading to increased respiratory efforts and the development of snoring during sleep. Increased upper airway resistance and nocturnal snoring worsen asthma, causing increased risk of a nocturnal asthma attack.

Orthodontic Complications and Upper Airway Obstruction During Sleep

Children with partial or complete upper airway obstruction during sleep frequently have maxillomandibular growth retardation. Abnormal orthodontic features are common. Class II malocclusion is frequently seen but is not the only orthodontic problem. As 60% of facial development is complete by 4 years of age and 90% by 11 years of age, it is important to recognize orthodontic involvement. It is also important to understand that inappropriate orthodontic treatment that further impairs maxillomandibular growth may catalyze the appearance of snoring and significantly increase upper airway resistance during sleep. Abnormal maxillomandibular development may be responsible for the nocturnal occurrence of snoring and bruxism.

Treatment

Nasal obstruction is rarely the only factor in the development of apnea in children, but it can be a contributing factor. In rare cases, correcting the obstruction can alleviate, if not cure, the OSAS.

Tonsillectomy and Adenoidectomy

Tonsillectomy alone or tonsillectomy with adenoidectomy is standard treatment of pediatric OSA. Early studies showed that this procedure can cure over 80% of pediatric OSA cases and improves the vast majority. However, more recent studies suggest that OSA may persist in 45% of postoperative patients.[224] Too often, however, not enough attention is paid to problems that may be associated with enlarged tonsils and adenoids (i.e., abnormally long soft palate, reposition of the mandible, or soft tissue infiltration behind the base of the tongue), which may explain residual apnea after tonsillectomy. Furthermore, if tonsillectomy and adenoidectomy are performed during the prepubertal years in boys, there is a chance that the extensive soft tissue growth that occurs during puberty may cause a reappearance of OSAS in those whose airway space is already compromised by a malocclusion (a mild to moderate retroposition of the lower mandible). Fiberoptic endoscopy must be performed systematically in association with one imaging test to determine the extent of soft tissue surgery needed, but the classic UPPP is not recommended in children.

Orthodontic and Maxillomandibular Surgery

As previously indicated, children with OSAS often have a retroposition of the mandible, a steep mandibular plane, or an abnormally narrow, high-arched palate. These abnormalities are not always obvious. No one can overlook Pierre Robin syndrome, but specialists do not always appreciate a mandibular problem, and orthodontists may not be aware of the impact on the upper airway of a moderately abnormal mandible. Relatively noninvasive orthodontic approaches using rapid maxillary expansion in conjunction with traditional orthodontic treatments have been shown to effectively treat sleep apnea in children with lasting positive results.[225–227] Maxillary distraction results in widening of the palate and the nose; therefore, this procedure improves nasal occlusion. Rapid maxillary distraction is usually preformed in pediatric patients whose OSA persists despite tonsillectomy and adenoidectomy.

When maxillofacial abnormalities are clearly related to the presence of OSAS in children, maxillofacial surgery may be considered. Piecuch[228] reported a child treated with maxillofacial surgery for OSAS. Kuo et al.[229] have reported two cases and Bear and Priest[230] three cases of OSAS that were resolved by maxillofacial surgery. Bell et al. reported eight cases of OSA treated with maxillomandibular advancement with a 50% success rate.[231] The most extensive series of patients (teenagers and adults) treated with maxillofacial surgery was reported by Riley et al.[198] Mandibular distraction osteogenesis, used in conjunction with orthodontics, has been used to successfully treat six pediatric OSA patients.[232] Although positive results have been reported with surgery in pubertal children, we recommend investigating orthodontic approaches before considering maxillomandibular surgery.

Tracheostomy

In the past, tracheostomy was a frequent treatment when tonsillectomy and adenoidectomy were insufficient. Tracheostomy resolves the OSAS, but it may cause secondary problems such as depression in children after surgery, and families commonly have difficulty accepting the surgery and caring for the stoma. Nevertheless, tracheostomy is clearly beneficial in many cases. The need for tracheostomy can be alleviated by the use of other treatment modalities.

Nasal Continuous Positive Airway Pressure

Prepubertal children as young as 6 months old have been treated with nasal CPAP at Stanford since 1984, and long-term treatment has been successful.[233] Several manufacturers currently supply nasal CPAP for young children, and Respironics provides masks for infants and very young children.

The complications and problems associated with this treatment have been related to (1) the fact that the children (many of whom were mentally retarded) had difficulty understanding how the mask and CPAP equipment functioned; (2) problems with the parents' collaboration with the medical team to train the child to keep the nasal mask on his or her face; (3) air leaks at the edge of the mask causing reappearance of apnea and eye irritation; and (4) skin allergy to the masks in small children. The first two problems resulted in some children abandoning nasal CPAP treatment; the other problems, although occasionally bothersome, never led to interruption of therapy. The theoretical risk of stomach dilation due to incorrect administration or other problems has never been reported. One issue to consider is that no system has an alarm to indicate complete displacement of the mask. In very young children, hand restraint during sleep may be necessary to adapt the child to the apparatus.

Pediatric patients using CPAP should be re-evaluated for mask fit every 6 months because of rapid craniofacial growth. An annual visit with a craniofacial specialist should occur to affirm that the headgear and mask do not worsen a maxillary growth deficiency.[234]

SUMMARY

OSAS is common and must be considered a disease with diverse, adverse systemic consequences, including cardiovascular risk. As such, inquiries into the existence of snoring and EDS should be part of a physician's general examination. Because daytime somnolence appears in many guises, such as fatigue and cognitive difficulties, a high index of suspicion for this condition must be maintained. Sleep apnea diminishes the restorative capacity of sleep, thereby degrading quality of life. Obstructive sleep apnea appears to be a risk factor for several medical diseases; the strongest association is with hypertension. Evaluation and treatment are now readily available at sleep disorders centers. Treatment recommendations can be tailored to the patient's problems, taking into consideration individual preference, age, personality, lifestyle, and objective findings with PSG.

◎ REFERENCES

A full list of references are available at www.expertconsult. com

CHAPTER 25

Positive Airway Pressure in the Treatment of Sleep Apnea-Hypopnea*

Mark H. Sanders[†], **Patrick J. Strollo Jr., Charles W. Atwood Jr., Ronald A. Stiller** and **Christopher P. O'Donnell**

INTRODUCTION

The application of nasal continuous positive airway pressure (CPAP) for the treatment of obstructive sleep apnea in adults was first described in 1981.[1] Since then, it has become the medical therapy of choice for obstructive sleep apnea/hypopnea (OSA/H). Fundamentally, conventional positive airway pressure (PAP) systems that are employed to treat OSA/H patients consist of a generator that directs airflow downstream to the patient via tubing and an interface (e.g., nasal mask, oral-nasal mask, nasal cannula or prongs, or oral interface; discussed later in this chapter). Air, under the clinician-prescribed degree of positive pressure, is then introduced into the upper airway. This pressure pneumatically splints the upper airway, thereby maintaining patency of this conduit and minimizing resistance to airflow. The splinting effect constitutes the primary mechanism of therapeutic action.[2,3] Note has been made that the direct relationship between lung volume and upper airway patency may be related to

traction on mediastinal and upper airway structures created during lung inflation,[4,5] and it has been postulated that at least part of the effect of CPAP in maintaining upper airway patency is mediated through augmentation of lung volume. Studies have shown that augmentation of lung volume by CPAP contributes to its effectiveness, but the effect is relatively small.[2,3,6]

Regardless of the mechanism, nasal CPAP has documented effectiveness in eliminating obstructive and mixed apneas.[7] Some "central" apneas, particularly those observed in patients with predominantly obstructive events, are also eliminated by nasal CPAP.[7,8] This finding supports the contention that the central portion of mixed apneas and many central apneas may actually represent delayed inspiratory effort due to prolongation of the preceding expiration related to expiratory upper airway instability with augmented upper airway resistance and slowing of expiratory airflow.[9,10] It is also consistent with stabilization of oscillating ventilatory control during CPAP administration.[11–14]

POSITIVE PRESSURE MODALITIES USED TO TREAT OBSTRUCTIVE SLEEP APNEA/HYPOPNEA

Continuous Positive Airway Pressure

The first PAP modality described to treat adults with OSA/H was CPAP.[1] CPAP may also be conceptualized as *constant* PAP, reflecting the fact that, by conventional

*Supported in part by NIH RO1 AG023977, M01-RR000056.

†Mark H. Sanders, MD, is a scientific consultant for Philips-Respironics, Inc. and a co-inventor of BiPAP® with a financial interest in that brand and related technologies by Respironics, Inc. Dr. Sanders had given lectures supported by Respironics, Inc. Dr. Sanders has been on advisory panels for Sanofi and Cephalon. Patrick J. Strollo Jr., MD, has received research grants from ResMed, Philips-Respironics, Inc., and the National Football League. Charles W. Atwood Jr., MD, has received research grants from ResMed, Philips-Respironics and Medcare. He is an advisor to Cephalon and Itamar Medical. Christopher O'Donnell, PhD, has given a talk at Fisher and Paykel.

definition, this modality delivers the same magnitude of pressure to the patient during inspiration and expiration (i.e., the pressure delivered during the patient's exhalation equals that delivered during inhalation). Fixed-pressure CPAP (i.e., the same pressure is delivered throughout the sleep period) is the standard to which all other modalities are compared.

Bilevel Positive Pressure

Studies of the pathogenesis of OSA/H have indicated that upper airway resistance increases during expiration despite the absence of negative intrapharyngeal pressure during this phase of the breathing cycle.[9,15,16] Sanders and coworkers speculated that instability of the upper airway during expiration is the initial event in the sequence leading to obstructive apnea.[10] Moreover, it was conceptualized that the splinting action of positive pressure in the upper airway, during both inspiration and expiration, was necessary to eliminate obstructive events, *but* less pressure is required to maintain adequate upper airway patency during expiration than during inspiration. This was based on the hypothesis that, during expiration, inherent upper airway instability represents the primary factor that favors airway closure, whereas during inspiration inadequate upper airway patency is related to two factors: the collapsing influence of negative intraluminal pressure and the inherent instability of the airway. The importance of expiratory events was subsequently demonstrated by computed tomography and magnetic resonance imaging to observe expiratory narrowing of the upper airway.[17–20] Application of expiratory positive airway pressure by Mahadevia and colleagues[21] was associated with a reduction in apnea frequency, although these investigators postulated that the improved upper airway function was related to increased oxyhemoglobin saturation secondary to increased functional residual capacity.

Bilevel positive pressure (bilevel PP) provides the ability to independently adjust the inspiratory and expiratory pressure such that the pressure delivered during exhalation need not be as high as that delivered during inhalation.[22–26] By allowing independent adjustment of the inspiratory positive airway pressure (IPAP) and expiratory positive airway pressure (EPAP), bilevel PP provides the potential to treat OSA/H patients with expiratory pressure that is lower than inspiratory pressure.[22] Setting the EPAP at a level that prevents upper airway occlusion during or at end-expiration permits the patient to generate inspiratory airflow or volume at the initiation of inspiratory effort, and this triggers delivery of IPAP, which supports upper airway patency during the inspiratory phase of the breathing cycle. Over and above preventing complete upper airway occlusion, delivery of a sufficient level of IPAP augments upper airway patency, and eliminates partial obstructions (hypopneas) as well as upper airway obstruction-related desaturations and arousals from sleep. If the airway were to become occluded

during expiration (e.g., EPAP not set sufficiently high), IPAP would not be triggered and the apnea would become apparent.

In an investigation of 13 patients with OSA/H in which optimal settings of nasal CPAP and bilevel PP were compared, Sanders and Kern[22] observed that the EPAP delivered during bilevel PP was significantly lower than the level of CPAP, and the mean value of EPAP for the group was 37% lower than the required level of CPAP ($p < 0.001$). In contrast, there was no difference between the level of IPAP during bilevel PP administration and the level of CPAP. There was comparable relief of OSA/H using both modalities. Several subsequent studies have confirmed the effectiveness of bilevel PP in the treatment of OSA/H in adults.[24–27]

Most bilevel PP devices can be used in three modes. In the "spontaneous" mode, IPAP is delivered in response to a patient "trigger." In the "spontaneous-timed" mode, the patient may trigger the delivery of IPAP, but in addition, the physician may set the device so that IPAP is delivered at prescribed intervals if a spontaneously triggered delivery does not occur within that interval. This backup feature is infrequently needed in treating patients with OSA/H, although it has been helpful in providing nocturnal ventilatory assistance to other patient groups such as those with ventilatory muscle dysfunction resulting from neuromuscular disease and those with nocturnal hypoventilation due to chest wall deformities such as kyphoscoliosis. The spontaneous-timed mode may be beneficial in patients with Cheyne-Stokes breathing (CSB) and those who develop problematic Central Sleep Apnea on CPAP in the context of Complex Central Sleep Apnea (see later in this chapter). In these patients, the capability for spontaneous triggering facilitates tolerance of the device by the awake patient, whereas during sleep the timed bilevel PP "breaths" delivered at prescribed intervals prevent the long breathing pauses between lung inflations that are characteristic of central sleep apnea. Additionally, it is now recognized that, at least in some patients, central sleep apnea events may be associated with a closed upper airway.[28–30] Thus, it may be necessary to provide a critical level of EPAP to facilitate delivery of IPAP to the patient. CPAP and bilevel PP are discussed in the context of complex central sleep apnea, CSB, and cardiovascular disease later in this chapter. There is also a "timed" mode for bilevel PP devices in which IPAP is delivered with a clinician-set frequency and the patient cannot initiate delivery. In general, we have not found this mode to offer benefit over the "spontaneous-timed" mode.

Autotitrating CPAP and Bilevel PP

Autotitrating CPAP (APAP) and bilevel PP devices employ proprietary algorithms to detect impending collapse or instability of the upper airway and adjust the amount of pressure that is delivered in order to maintain patency. Following a period of upper airway stability, the pressure gradually decreases (according to each manufacturer's algorithm) until impending collapse or instability is again detected. The delivered pressure is then increased per the algorithm. Thus, the pressure "floats" throughout the night with the intention of meeting the patient's requirements in real time (Fig. 25–1).

At least in part, the putative advantages of the autotitrating devices (APAP and auto-titrating bilevel PP) are to reduce the pressure to which patients are exposed and thereby to increase comfort, satisfaction, and adherence to therapy. Bilevel PP also is capable of assisting or augmenting ventilation by virtue of the gradient between end-expiratory and inspiratory pressures. The autotitrating devices attempt to respond to concern that the optimal therapeutic PAP prescription may vary across the night (e.g., across various body positions) and across nights. Indeed, investigators recently reported that a notable proportion of patients receiving a prescription of fixed-pressure CPAP were subsequently found to have an apnea-hypopnea index (AHI) >10 on the same prescription.[31] However, the patients with AHI >10 did not differ significantly from those without persistent OSA/H with regard to quality of life, mood, vitality, or Epworth Sleepiness Scale score.

A review and a meta-analysis of APAP reveals that these devices may provide comparable alleviation of OSA/H and perceived daytime sleepiness, compared with fixed-pressure CPAP with a mean pressure that is about 2 cm H_2O lower. This does not appear to translate into improved adherence to therapy, however.[32,33] It is important to note that studies that examined APAP efficacy excluded patients with underlying cardiopulmonary disease as well as other comorbidities. Further studies are needed before recommending routine use of this modality in patients with these comorbidities. Issues related to CPAP, bilevel PP, and APAP modalities are discussed later in the chapter.

"Pressure-Relief" CPAP and Bilevel PP

"Pressure-relief" CPAP and bilevel PP have recently been introduced.[34,35] These provide expiratory pressure relief that is proportional to expiratory airflow, while pressure increases rising to the prescribed EPAP level at end-expiration. In expiratory pressure relief, the pressure-relief bilevel PP device provides relief of pressure at end-inspiration.[34] Plausibly, this is facilitated by the high lung volume at end-inspiration that contributes to upper airway patency as well as the fact that, as inspiration reaches its end, airflow diminishes with consequent reduction in collapse-promoting negative intrapharyngeal pressure. Pressure-relief CPAP was as effective in reducing sleep-disordered breathing events and improving sleep continuity as conventional CPAP.[35] Gay and coworkers[34] demonstrated comparability between pressure-relief and convention bilevel PP in alleviating OSA/H; however, there are too few studies of these modalities on which to base conclusions.

Adaptive Servo-ventilation

Although CPAP and bilevel PP therapy may be associated with improvement in CSB and Central Sleep Apnea, sometimes there is no improvement or worsening.[36,37] Adaptive servo-ventilation (ASV) has recently been introduced into clinical practice primarily to address CSB in the context of heart failure as well as idiopathic and Complex Central Sleep Apnea or Treatment-Emergent Central Sleep Apnea (central sleep apnea that becomes clinically problematic during application of conventional CPAP or bilevel PP during treatment of OSA/H). In general, these devices provide a variable degree of inspiratory pressure support that stabilizes the patient's ventilation over time. Thus, if there is a reduction in the patient's spontaneous ventilation, the degree of

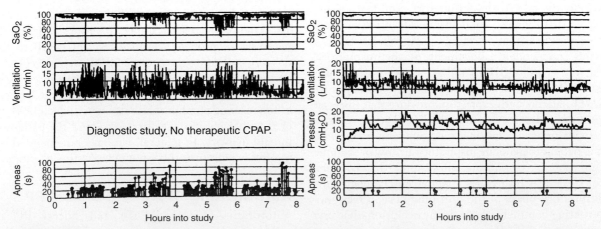

FIGURE 25–1 Arterial oxyhemoglobin saturation (SaO_2), minute ventilation, CPAP mask pressure, and apneic events recorded with an oximeter and a prototype of an intelligent CPAP machine in a patient with sleep apnea. **Left,** Diagnostic study with repeated episodes of obstructive apnea. **Right,** Autotitrating CPAP with pressure levels that vary across the recording. *(Reproduced with permission from Polo O, Berthon-Jones M, Douglas NJ, et al. Management of obstructive sleep apnoea/hypopnoea syndrome. Lancet 1994;344:656.)*

inspiratory positive pressure support will increase proportionately to minimize a decrement in ventilation.[38] A backup rate of IPAP delivery may also be set by the clinician.

Teschler et al.[38] evaluated the effects of supplemental oxygen, CPAP, bilevel PP, and ASV in patients with CSB (with primarily central sleep apnea) due to heart failure and reported that ASV provided the greatest reduction in AHI, slightly but statistically significantly lower than on bilevel PP. Sleep continuity, sleep efficiency, percent slow-wave sleep, and percent rapid eye movement (REM) sleep were comparable on ASV and bilevel PP. Of note, however, the ASV settings in this investigation included a backup rate of 15 breaths/min, and the backup rate on the bilevel PP was set at the patient's awake spontaneous breathing rate, less 2 breaths/min (for the study group, the range of backup rate was 13–18 breaths/min). It is not possible to determine how much improvement in CSB was specifically due to the ASV or bilevel PP algorithm as opposed to the presence of a backup rate on both modes in this study. A subsequent case series by Banno et al.[36] reported improved CSB on ASV that had failed to improve on CPAP. These authors indicated that they employed the same default settings as Teschler et al.,[38] and therefore a backup rate may also have been used.

A small case series of heart failure patients with CSB who failed CPAP and bilevel PP (with a backup rate) reported a beneficial effect of ASV.[39] The ASV employed in this study included a default backup mode. A randomized 4-week crossover trial of ASV prescribed at therapeutic settings (including a backup rate) versus ASV prescribed at subtherapeutic settings (with a backup rate of 15 breaths/min) was performed on patients with heart failure and CSB.[40] The results demonstrated significantly greater improvement of the AHI during the intervention with ASV at therapeutic settings. Although the active intervention resulted in a substantial reduction in objectively assessed sleepiness compared with subtherapeutic ASV, there were no statistically significant changes in the secondary outcome measures of the study, including subjective sleepiness, questionnaire assessment of health status, and performance using a driving simulator with either therapeutic ASV or subtherapeutic ASV. However, plasma brain natriuretic peptide and urinary metadrenaline excretion fell on the active intervention, suggesting a favorable physiologic impact of ASV. These results suggest that ASV results in physiologic improvements, but the absence of subjective improvement in sleepiness is disappointing.

The general features of various PAP modalities are summarized in Table 25–1. It is important to note that

TABLE 25–1 General Features of Positive Pressure Delivery Modalities*

Positive Pressure Modality	General Features
Continuous positive airway pressure (CPAP)	• The clinician may prescribe the CPAP level. • Positive pressure delivered during inspiration equals that delivered during expiration.
"Pressure-relief" CPAP	• The clinician may prescribe the CPAP level. • Positive pressure delivered during expiration decreases in proportion to the increasing expiratory airflow early in expiration and increases back to the prescribed CPAP level as the patient's expiratory airflow decreases with the approaching end of exhalation. • The clinician can set the degree of pressure relief.
Bilevel positive pressure	• The clinician may prescribe the level of inspiratory positive airway pressure (IPAP) and expiratory positive airway pressure (EPAP). • EPAP may be set independent of IPAP, but EPAP may not be higher than IPAP. • Some models permit prescribing a timed backup rate.
Pressure-relief bilevel positive pressure	• Same as for bilevel positive pressure except the clinician may also prescribe inspiratory and expiratory pressure relief.
Autotitrating CPAP	• CPAP level fluctuates over the period of use according to a manufacturer-designed algorithm. • The clinician may prescribe the minimum-maximum range within which the pressure may fluctuate.
Autotitrating bilevel positive pressure	• IPAP and EPAP levels fluctuate over the period of use according to a manufacturer-designed algorithm. • The clinician may prescribe the minimum EPAP and maximum IPAP within which the pressure may fluctuate. • The clinician may prescribe the maximum IPAP-EPAP gradient ("pressure support") up to a manufacturer-designed limit.
Adaptive servo-ventilation	• The clinician prescribes an EPAP level. • Different brands have different algorithms for establishing the minimum and maximum IPAP level and minimum level of pressure support. • In general, the pressure support varies to maintain a target ventilation or a target airflow; there is a default timed backup rate.

*Algorithms and modes of operation vary across manufacturers and models. This table is not intended to represent definitive features of specific brands and models but rather to describe general features.

algorithms and modes of operation vary across manufacturers and models. This table is not intended to represent definitive features of specific brands and models but rather to describe general features.

Effectiveness of PAP in Treating Patients with OSA/H

There is abundant evidence that, when applied in sufficient pressure, PAP effectively eliminates OSA/H events as well as respiratory effort–related arousals. Following initiation of CPAP therapy during sleep, most OSA/H patients with daytime sleepiness at baseline report increased subjective alertness.[41–43] There is, however, variability across studies. In a meta-analysis of randomized trials, Marshall and coworkers[44] reported that, after controlling for placebo effects, the Epworth Sleepiness Scale score[45] increased significantly, but only by 1.2 points in patients with mild to moderate OSA/H. The effect of CPAP on objective metrics of sleep propensity during the day (e.g., Multiple Sleep Latency Test [MSLT] or Maintenance of Wakefulness Test) is less clear, with only some studies showing an effect and a less compelling impact in patients with mild OSA/H.[42,43,46,47] The meta-analysis by Marshall et al. examined the ability to remain awake under soporific conditions, assessed by the Maintenance of Wakefulness Test and observed that, over the three randomized trials in which this assessment was performed, sleep latency increased significantly but only by 2.1 minutes, and there was no significant change in the sleep latency during the MSLT in the four trials in which it was assessed.[44] The investigators called into question the clinical significance of their changes. Another meta-analysis[48] reported a significant reduction in the Epworth Sleepiness Scale score by an average of approximately 3

points, with relatively greater reductions in patients with severe OSA/H. These investigators also observed only a marginal improvement in the MSLT after introduction of CPAP therapy.

In the context of vigilance and alertness, a critically important functional outcome to examine is the effect of OSA/H and subsequent therapy on motor vehicle crashes.[49] In this regard, a number of studies employing driving simulators have demonstrated improved performance following initiation of CPAP therapy.[50–53] Similarly, a comparison of the number of accidents per driver per year over the 3 years before and following CPAP therapy in OSA/H patients demonstrated a notable reduction, reaching levels that were comparable to those in individuals without OSA/H[54] (Fig. 25–2).

Turkington and coworkers[52] reported that benefits on driving performance, assessed using a simulator, may be evident within 7 days of initiating therapy, while, more recently, Orth et al. observed improvement after only 2 days.[53] This is consistent with earlier data indicating that there may be a reduction in subjective daytime sleepiness after just 1 night of nasal CPAP therapy,[55] and that progressive reduction in objective daytime alertness (assessed by the MSLT) may occur over 2 weeks following initiation of therapy.[56] The progressive nature of the improvement in symptoms and the apparent variability in response, as reflected in the previous discussion of the meta-analyses of CPAP effectiveness, highlights the importance of recognizing that patients may not be sufficiently alert to resume full activities (especially those that require vigilance, such as operating vehicles or potentially dangerous tasks) within the first several days of treatment. In addition, although studies have concluded that driving simulators may provide insight into on-the-road driving

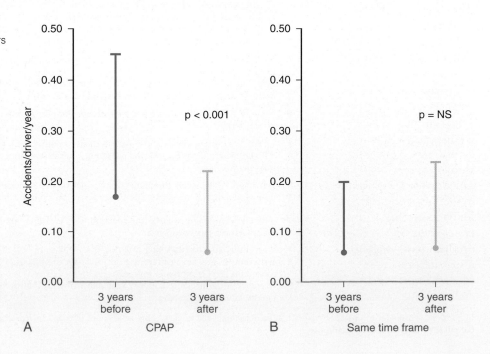

FIGURE 25–2 A, Accident rates (mean ± SD) for patients with OSA/H over the 3 years before and after initiation of CPAP therapy. **B,** Accident rates (mean ± SD) for control subjects over the same time interval. *(Reproduced with permission from George CFP. Reduction in motor vehicle collisions following treatment of sleep apnoea with nasal CPAP. Thorax 2001;56;508.)*

performance, differences do exist.[53,57] It is important for the clinician to recognize that in general, studies examining treatment effect on motor vehicle crashes have been uncontrolled. To better assess the improvement in symptoms of daytime sleepiness, it is essential that the health care team make follow-up contact with the patient soon after the initiation of therapy. Close follow-up will facilitate evaluation of the patient's ability to perform activities that require alertness as well as to assess therapeutic adherence (see discussion below).

PAP often has a beneficial impact on other symptoms of OSA/H. Studies have reported relief of tiredness, reduced snoring, decreased nocturnal awakenings with perceived choking or gasping, and a reduction in nocturia.[46,58 64] It is appropriate to note at this point, however, that nocturia—at least in conjunction with benign prostatic hypertrophy—has been reported to negatively influence adherence to PAP therapy,[65] probably due to the inconvenience of removing and replacing the interface. It may be possible to extrapolate this finding to OSA/H patients with nocturia that is unassociated with prostatic hypertrophy. In light of the potentially beneficial effect of PAP use on nocturia, patients should be counseled to persevere with adherence to achieve a favorable outcome, and the etiology of residual nocturia should be investigated and treated.

The impact of PAP on quality-of-life measures and neurocognition has also been assessed. Engleman and co-investigators reported the results of a placebo-controlled trial of CPAP in patients with mild OSA/H; use of CPAP for >2.5 hr/night was associated with improved visuomotor skill, social function, and vitality (using the Medical Outcomes Short Form-36 [SF-36]). In addition, the Hospital Anxiety and Depression Scale Depression Score was reduced. In a non–placebo-controlled study comparing "conservative" management and CPAP for moderate to severe OSA/H, McFayden and colleagues[66] examined the results of the disease-specific Functional Outcomes of Sleep Questionnaire (FOSQ) as well as the SF-36 and found that CPAP was associated with improved psychosocial function and the patient's (but not the spouse's) marital satisfaction. Conversely, Barnes et al. found no effect on neurobehavioral function or quality-of-life metrics on the SF-36 or the FOSQ.[46] These investigators speculated that differences in the study population, particularly related to gender, may explain the disparate results. Studies of patients with moderate to severe OSA/H (e.g., the most symptomatic individuals prior to treatment) indicate the largest effect sizes are in the contexts of sleepiness and vitality. Studies have suggested that patients with moderately impaired pretreatment cognitive performance experience modest improvements.[42,43,67] Moreover, data suggest that daily use of PAP for at least 6 hours over 3 months is associated with clinically relevant improvement in verbal memory in some, but not all, OSA/H patients.[68]

Although encouraging, further investigation is required to assess the generalizability of these observations to a more representative sample of OSA/H patients, including those with comorbidities (such patients were excluded from the study of Zimmerman and coworkers[68]).

SIDE EFFECTS OF PAP THERAPY

Like most treatment interventions, PAP is often associated with a variety of generally minor, but troublesome side effects (Table 25–2).[16,19,25,45–50,58,61,69–80] Side effects may be attributable to either the patient-device interface or the sensation of high airflow or pressure. Some patients simply perceive the lifestyle and other challenges associated with nasal PAP to be unacceptable.[3,46,48,61,72,79,81,82] Such individuals are often, but not invariably, younger patients who are unable to envision indefinite nasal PAP therapy. Although some studies have concluded that side effects do not impact on adherence to therapy,[61,73] others have concluded the converse, citing side effects as a reason for nonadherence.[83]

Claustrophobia

Not uncommonly, patients complain of claustrophobia in conjunction with enforced breathing through a nasal mask or nasal prongs system, or with CPAP in general.[47,48,51,71,72,80,84] For those patients who are uncomfortable breathing exclusively via the nasal route, an oral-nasal mask that permits breathing through either the oral or nasal route may be a useful alternative[85,86] (see later). Clinicians should be aware of one study demonstrating that, when patients were randomly assigned to either nasal or oral-nasal interface, adherence was lower while using the latter.[87] This study did not examine adherence to CPAP when an oral-nasal mask was prescribed as a "salvage" intervention for patients with complaints regarding a nasal interface. A desensitization program to promote acclimatization to nasal CPAP may be useful in some patients,[84] and a study found that the sensation of claustrophobia diminishes over time with perseverance of treatment.[80] The investigators suggested that early identification of patients who are likely to be claustrophobic and institution of interventions targeted to address this issue (e.g., desensitization, education, and support) may be of considerable value.[80,88]

Problems Related to Nasal Route of Breathing

Problems with skin abrasion or leakage of air directed into the eyes, with or without consequent conjunctivitis,[61,89] may result from a suboptimal mask fit. Other complaints related to the nasal route of breathing include nasal dryness, congestion, and rhinorrhea. The reported prevalence of such effects varies from 25% to 65%. One study observed that use of nasal prongs or pillows was associated with better adherence to therapy than a nasal mask.[90]

TABLE 25–2 Side Effects of Nasal CPAP

Side Effect	Management Measures
Mask Related Skin abrasion or rash Conjunctivitis from air leak	• Optimize mask fit from wide selection of commercially available types of masks, select nonallergenic material • Protective skin covering • Customized mask • Reinforce hygienic care of device • Eye patch
Pressure or Airflow Related Chest discomfort Aerophagia Sinus discomfort Smothering sensation Difficulty exhaling Difficulty initiating and/or maintaining sleep Pneumothorax or pneumomediastinum Pneumoencephalus	• Pressure ramp • Reduce pressure with bilevel positive airway pressure • Try to reduce requisite pressure using oral appliance + CPAP (no published data)
Problems Related to the Nasal Route Rhinorrhea Nasal congestion, nasal and/or oral dryness Epistaxis (may be massive, especially in anticoagulated patients)	• Heated humidification • Saline nasal spray • Topical nasal steroid preparation • Consider trial of nasal aerosol of ipratropium bromide solution • Chin strap for oral dryness • Oral-nasal mask interface • Desensitization over time
Other Noise Cumbersomeness or inconvenience Spousal intolerance	• Longer tubing to move device further from bedside (consult device manufacturer for permissible lengths) • Intensify education of patient and spouse • Recommend attending a patient support group (A.W.A.K.E Network of the American Sleep Apnea Association)

Although the percentage of days during which patients used CPAP was slightly greater when using the nasal pillows (94% vs. 86%), the time of CPAP use per night across all nights as well as specifically on those nights during which patients used CPAP was not statistically different between the two interfaces. There was no difference between the interfaces with regard to relief of sleep-disordered breathing and functional outcome assessed by the FOSQ. The authors reported that overall satisfaction was greater with use of the nasal pillows. In our experience, we have found that interface preference varies across patients. Moreover, preferences vary over time in individual patients, with many switching back and forth across interfaces. It may be reasonable to provide patients with several interfaces from which they may choose on any given night. Of course, follow-up is important to ensure ongoing success in alleviation of OSA/H and symptoms.

Nasal Dryness and Congestion

Nasal dryness and congestion can occasionally be treated simply with either administration of saline nasal spray at bedtime or a room humidifier. For some patients, a topical nasal steroid may be effective. Addition of a low-resistance humidifier to the PAP system may also be extremely helpful in certain patients, and heated humidification systems have attracted increasing use in recent years. Richards et al. documented increased nasal resistance in the presence of high nasal flow, such as occurs when there is a mouth leak during nasal CPAP application.[75] Incorporation of a heated, but not an unheated, humidifier into the CPAP system minimized the increase in nasal resistance, presumably by increasing the relative humidity of the inspired gas and reducing release of inflammatory mediators. The superiority of heated humidifiers to nonheated humidifiers in restoring relative humidity to inhaled air was confirmed in a more recent study by Fleury et al.[91] The issue of routine prescription of a heated humidifier at the time of the initial PAP prescription has been the focus of several investigations, often yielding conflicting results. In a setting more clinically relevant to OSA/H patients than that employed by Richards et al., Duong and coworkers[92] measured nasal airway resistance before and after a night of CPAP in patients randomized to receive heated humidification or placebo. There was no significant difference between the groups with regard to total nasal airway resistance in the evening before CPAP use or in the morning following

CPAP use. There was also no difference between the groups with regard to the overnight percent change in nasal airway resistance.

Massie et al.[93] reported that, compared with a cold humidifier, heated humidification of CPAP-delivered air resulted in a statistically significant improvement in adherence, albeit by only an average of 0.6 hours. While there were less frequent reports of dry mouth, throat, and nose during application of heated humidification, the global adverse side effect score did not differ by heated versus cold humidification. Three quarters of the patients preferred heated humidification, reflecting that a measurable minority did not. In a more recent study, Mador et al.[94] compared adherence and quality of life in a group of 49 OSA/H patients prescribed to receive CPAP with heated humidification versus 49 control patients who were not initially prescribed heated humidification but did receive it only if nasal symptoms occurred that were unresponsive to other measures. Six control patients crossed over to heated humidification. There was no difference in adherence or Calgary Sleep Quality of Life Index between the groups over 12 months. There was no improvement in adherence in control patients who crossed over to heated humidification, although nasal symptoms diminished. Similarly, in a randomized crossover trial, Neill et al.[95] observed that, compared with placebo humidification, heated humidification of CPAP was associated with fewer upper airway symptoms and a slightly greater degree of use initially following setup. However, at the end of week 3 there was no difference in adherence or in satisfaction with therapy. The authors concluded that heated humidification may be useful in addressing side effects but is not appropriate for routine prescription to all patients. Nevertheless, it appears that heated humdification may provide benefit to at least some patients. Rakotonanahary et al.[96] observed that chronic nasal mucosal disease, nasal septum deformity, and a history of uvulopalatopharyngoplasty predicted need for heated humidification of PAP.

Thus, there is considerable literature that does not support benefit to the *routine* prescription of heated humidification to all OSA/H patients at the time of initial setup, although there are selected subsets who benefit from such a prescription. It is reasonable to approach the issue of heated humidification from the perspective expressed by Brown in commenting, "If it's dry, wet it."[97] In this context, the data indicate that patterns of adherence (or nonadherence) are established early on,[98] so there is considerable wisdom in obtaining follow-up very soon after the patient receives the PAP unit in order to detect and address factors that may diminish the enthusiasm to be adherent to treatment.

Although routine use is to be discouraged, occasional administration of a vasoconstrictive nasal spray may be helpful when nasal congestion is related to a self-limited condition such as an upper respiratory tract infection.

Whereas nasal dryness is rarely a serious problem, massive epistaxis has been reported.[99] Mucosal dryness may be a contributory factor to the epistaxis, which did not recur after placement of a humidifier in the CPAP system. In light of this report, it seems prudent to follow patients with a history of bleeding tendencies, epistaxis, or coagulopathy who are on PAP with particular care, and to consider humidifying the delivered air from the outset of therapy.

Rhinorrhea

Rhinorrhea after initiation of PAP therapy, present in approximately 35% of patients,[61] is often a difficult problem to control. The cause of this untoward effect is likely to be related to inflammation, as in nasal congestion. Similarly, Pépin et al. did not observe a beneficial effect from humidification, although it is uncertain if a heated humidifier was employed.[61] Therefore, it may be worth trying a heated humidifier, as described previously, for the treatment of rhinorrhea. Although we are unaware of published, systematically conducted research studies, we have found the administration of chromoglycate or anticholinergic nasal sprays such as ipratropium bromide or Azelastine nasal spray (if used, care must be taken due to sedating potential) may be only variably effective among patients with rhinorrhea. However, as noted previously, nasal steroids have been observed to provide more consistent benefit.

When evaluating a patient with rhinorrhea, it is essential to consider the possibility of a cerebrospinal fluid leak. Kuzniar et al.[100] described two patients who developed rhinorrhea after initiation of CPAP therapy, which subsequently proved to reflect a cerebrospinal fluid leak that in one patient was complicated by meningitis. Clinicians should keep this uncommon but real possibility in mind when assessing rhinorrhea in CPAP users.

Barotrauma and Chest Discomfort

When providing positive pressure therapy, the clinician must always consider the potential for barotrauma. Although clinicians should be vigilant for pneumomediastinum and pneumothorax, these are uncommon in OSA/H patients receiving CPAP, at least as assessed by review of the literature. Pneumocephalus has been reported in a sleep apnea patient with a cerebrospinal fluid leak who was placed on nasal CPAP[101] and in a patient on nasal CPAP who presented with headache.[102] Pneumocephalus should be considered when any patient using CPAP therapy develops a nasal discharge, or neurologic signs and symptoms including headache, seizures, dizziness, or cranial nerve palsy.

A small number of patients complain of chest discomfort on nasal CPAP therapy.[74,103,104] This is probably related to the positive end-expiratory pressure and consequent elevation of resting lung volume,[105] which stretches the chest wall muscles and cartilaginous structures, creating a sensation of chest wall pressure that may persist after awakening.

Although the complaint of chest discomfort should be completely evaluated in any patient, if a cardiopulmonary workup in an OSA/H patient on CPAP is nondiagnostic, efforts should be made to reduce the expiratory pressure, if necessary by using bilevel PP (discussed later). Similarly, a certain proportion of patients perceive discomfort when exhaling against positive expiratory pressure.[58,104] If the level of CPAP cannot be satisfactorily reduced, a trial of bilevel PP may be considered[106] (see later).

Effects on Arterial Blood Gases and Oxyhemoglobin Saturation

While it is usually beneficial to patients with OSA/H, administration of nasal CPAP may be associated with untoward effects on arterial blood gases and oxyhemoglobin saturation. Pépin et al.[61] reported severe oxyhemoglobin desaturation during nasal CPAP therapy in a hypercapnic sleep apnea patient with cor pulmonale. Similarly, Krieger et al.[107] reported persistent and notable desaturation despite CPAP administration *with* supplemental oxygen to hypercapnic OSA/H patients. Although the cause of this desaturation is not certain, it may be due to one or more of the following: (1) worsening hypoventilation related to the added mechanical impedance to ventilation associated with exhalation against increased pressure; (2) increased dead-space ventilation[108]; and (3) that venous return and cardiac output decrease due to increased intrathoracic pressure during CPAP administration in patients with impaired right or left ventricular function and inadequate filling pressure. With regard to the potential contribution of alveolar hypoventilation to nocturnal oxyhemoglobin desaturation during CPAP therapy, Fukui et al.[109] noted that nasal CPAP failed to reduce sleep-related hypercapnia during non-REM sleep in OSA/H patients, and Piper and Sullivan[110] observed persistent sleep desaturation on CPAP in severe OSA/H and hypercapnia. Similarly, Resta et al.[18] reported that hypoventilation during sleep on CPAP was more likely to occur in more obese patients and those with higher arterial partial pressure of carbon dioxide ($PaCO_2$). This highlights the prudence of conducting CPAP trials under monitored conditions in patients at high risk for nocturnal hypoventilation, including individuals with chronic ventilatory failure (awake hypercapnia) and morbidly obese individuals.

Despite these caveats and troublesome experiences, CPAP administration has also been reported to improve awake arterial blood gases in OSA/H patients with hypercapnia and cor pulmonale.[111–113] A study has demonstrated that CPAP therapy for OSA/H reduces pulmonary artery pressure in patients with mild pulmonary artery hypertension.[114] In this study, the pulmonary systolic pressure was related to both the AHI and diastolic dysfunction.

The mechanism responsible for augmented alveolar ventilation during wakefulness in hypercapnic persons has not been clearly defined. The literature is not consistent with regard to the effect of CPAP on the slope of the hypercapnic ventilatory response curve in OSA/H patients, with some of the differences related to measuring different parameters of ventilatory control and others perhaps related to differences in subject populations. Some investigations observed no change in the slope of the carbon dioxide/ventilation relationship in normocapnic patients.[115,116] Recently, Mateika and Ellythy observed an elevation in the ventilatory recruitment threshold to CO_2 in normocapnic OSA/H patients compared with normal subjects, with no difference in ventilatory response above this threshold.[117] This may provide insight into the earlier observation by Berthon-Jones et al., who reported a leftward shift in the ventilatory response to carbon dioxide following initiation of CPAP therapy without a change in the slope of the line representing the relationship between carbon dioxide tension and ventilation.[116] These data are consistent with a reduction in the chemoreceptor (s) set point to $PaCO_2$ following initiation of therapy.

Although the issue has not been systematically explored specifically in hypercapnic OSA/H patients, it is possible that alleviation of sleep-related hypercapnia with alleviation of apneas and hypopnea alters the hypercapnic threshold by reducing serum buffering capacity. Alternatively, enhanced chemosensitivity to carbon dioxide during wakefulness may be due to relief of hypoxic depression of central nervous system respiratory centers. While it had been previously believed that sleep deprivation reduces hypercapnic ventilatory responsivity,[118] more recent data, collected over 24 hours of sleep deprivation with electroencephalographic documentation of wakefulness, refuted the earlier study.[119] These issues notwithstanding, studies indicate that CPAP often does not reduce $PaCO_2$ during sleep and wakefulness in hypercapnic patients,[18,108,109] and reliance on this modality to reduce awake hypercapnia may be problematic[110]; augmentation of ventilation after maintenance of upper airway patency may facilitate improvement in diurnal hypercapnia.[106]

ACCEPTANCE OF AND ADHERENCE TO PAP THERAPY

The most significant disadvantage to PAP therapy is its volitional nature, such that patients must actively participate in their own treatment both in terms of the number of nights used as well as the number of hours used per night. Although the optimal duration of nightly PAP use—or for that matter, the minimal amount of use that confers benefit—are unknown, recent studies suggest that use of at least 6 hr/night confers greater cardiovascular mortality risk reduction compared with fewer hours of use per night[120] (Fig. 25-3). In addition, PAP use for >6 hr/night over 3 months has been associated with a greater likelihood of normalized memory performance.[68] Viewed from the opposite perspective, sleeping for as little as 1 night without CPAP is associated with increased sleepiness.[55,121] These data highlight the need for clinicians to facilitate maximal PAP use by patients.

Before adherence to a therapeutic PAP prescription can be considered, the patient must accept the opportunity to receive this therapy. The acceptance rate of CPAP varies across a number of studies, ranging from 62% to 92%.[70,71,122–127] Among the reasons for nonacceptance are difficulty falling asleep, frequent nocturnal awakenings, and mask discomfort. In addition, those who accept CPAP therapy are generally more likely to complain of greater tiredness as well as episodes of falling asleep at undesirable times.[123]

In recent years, there has been increasing interest in "split-night" polysomnography in which the initial portion of the night is spent in performing a diagnostic evaluation for OSA/H and the remainder of the night is devoted to establishing a PAP prescription.[106,126–133] If the diagnosis of OSA/H is established during the initial portion of the night, a therapeutic titration of CPAP is undertaken. The impact of this paradigm has been explored and, in general, split-night studies provide an acceptable strategy for laboratory evaluation and initial PAP prescription without negatively impacting acceptance and adherence in patients with severe OSA/H.[126,127,132–134] Some data suggest, however, that long-term adherence may not be as high in patients with mild to moderate OSA/H as in patients with more severe OSA/H, thereby mandating particularly close follow-up in the former group.[132] Current recommendations of the American Academy of Sleep Medicine include that a CPAP titration may be conducted after observing an AHI of ≥40 (or AHIs of 20–40, based on clinical judgment) over at least 2 hours of diagnostic polysomnography, and a CPAP prescription may be established based on a titration over at least 3 hours of sleep that documents that CPAP eliminates or nearly eliminates the respiratory events during non-REM and REM sleep (including REM sleep in the supine position).[134] Although a number of investigations have included bilevel PP devices in assessing acceptance as well as adherence to therapy following split-night studies,

neither these devices nor APAP modalities have been the specific subject of these studies.

Once a patient has "accepted" CPAP therapy, he or she must be adherent to it. In the last several years, investigators and clinicians have been able to objectively monitor daily use and patterns of use over time with meters and software that have been incorporated into the PAP devices. Such objective metrics are particularly important in assisting clinicians with management since subjective patient reports overestimate time of use.[70,72,125,135] Objective adherence monitoring is now the standard of care, with its utility highlighted by the observation that suboptimal patterns of usage are established shortly after initiation of therapy, so that the clinician needs to recognize and address the contributory factors early on.[79–82,98] Moreover, information regarding the degree to which a patient is adherent to PAP is essential for assessment of a suboptimal clinical response. If a patient's symptoms are inadequately resolved after the initiation of PAP treatment, possible reasons other than poor adherence include delivery of insufficient pressure to maintain upper airway patency during sleep (perhaps due to an incorrect prescription or because of technical issues such as air leaks through the mouth or skin-mask interface that impair delivery of the prescribed pressure), misdiagnosis of the etiology of the individual's symptoms, the contribution of comorbid elements to the patient's symptoms, or failure to use the device for a sufficient duration on a regular basis. Currently available software within PAP devices provides information regarding delivered pressure and the magnitude of leaks, as well as an estimate of the AHI on PAP therapy. This constellation of information can provide the clinician with important management insights.

Despite the availability of software providing objective adherence information to clinicians, there remain gaps in our knowledge in this regard. For example, although the clinician may know the average duration of daily PAP, the *total sleep time* is not known. This information is highly desirable for optimal interpretation of the

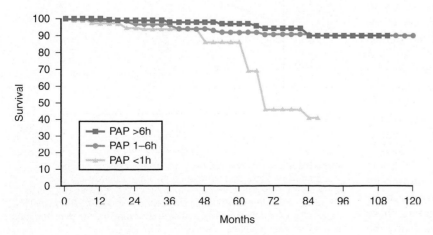

FIGURE 25–3 Kaplan-Meier cumulative survival rates according to categories of PAP compliance. Survival rates in the patients using PAP >6 hr/night were significantly higher than in the patients using PAP <1 hr/night. Cumulative survival rates in patients using PAP 1–6 hr/night were significantly greater than in patients using PAP <1 hr/night. Cumulative survival rates were not different in the patients using PAP >6 hr/night compared with patients using PAP 1–6 hr/night. *(Reproduced with permission from Campos-Rodriguez F, Pena-Grinan N, Reyes-Nunez N, et al. Mortality in obstructive sleep apnea-hypopnea patients treated with positive airway pressure. Chest 2005;128:624.)*

machine-use data. For example, 4 hours of PAP use may reflect acceptable adherence if the patient is asleep or at least in bed with intention to sleep for 4.5 hours (e.g., a late night at work with an early appointment in the morning). On the other hand, 4 hours of PAP use may reflect inadequate adherence if the patient is asleep for 8 hours. It is evident that it is highly desirable for the clinician to have objective information about a patient's usual bed and sleep time during follow-up subsequent to initiation of PAP therapy.

In general, utilization of PAP ranges from 4 to 6 hr/day, with considerable interindividual variability and a measurable proportion of patients with <2 hr/night or complete nonadherence. As discussed earlier, >6 hours of use per night is associated with reduced cardiovascular mortality and increased likelihood of normalizing memory function.[68,120] The relative value of <6 hours of use per night is unclear, as if there is a threshold of nightly use above which no further benefit is obtained in this regard as well as with respect to cardiovascular and cerebrovascular morbidities. Existing data suggests that optimal relief of daytime sleepiness requires nightly use of PAP. As also noted earlier, sleeping for as little as one night without PAP results in increased sleepiness[55,121]—but is it necessary to use PAP during *all* sleep time? Hers et al. observed persistent benefit in oxyhemoglobin saturation and sleep continuity for the remainder of the night after CPAP was discontinued following 4 hours of use.[136] The investigators postulated that the persistent improvement is related to greater sleep continuity while on CPAP, with increased upper airway stability during the latter portion of the night after CPAP was removed. This hypothesis is based on earlier data demonstrating increased upper airway collapsibility following a period of sleep fragmentation.[137] These investigators as well as others[138] speculated that duration of nightly use of CPAP by at least some OSA/H patients is determined by their perception of the amount of use required to obtain a satisfactory degree of symptomatic benefit.

It is intuitively evident that greater insight regarding the determinants of adherence would facilitate treatment modifications that would promote more universal and optimal utilization by patients. Unfortunately, our understanding remains incomplete. Some reports suggest that adherence improves as the patient's perception of sleep propensity increases.[70,83,139,140] Importantly, the patient's perception of daytime sleepiness, assessed using specific questionnaires such as the "hypersomnia score"[70] or the Epworth Sleepiness Scale,[45] predicts adherence with CPAP more reliably than the MSLT, which is an objective measure of sleepiness.[58,72,141] Some studies have noted that, after adjusting for confounding factors, lower AHI is an independent risk factor for non-adherence.[83,139] Conversely, several investigators have observed that adherent patients cannot consistently be differentiated from nonadherent patients by the frequency or variety of side effects of CPAP therapy, initial AHI, gender, weight, or the prescribed level of CPAP.[58,72,74,125,141–143] More recently, the contribution of "self-efficacy," including the patient's perception of the consequences of untreated OSA/H and expectations of treatment outcome,[79] as well as psychological factors such as coping strategies and willingness to modify behavior,[81,82] have been examined in the context of adherence. Stepnowski et al. observed that adherence to CPAP was uninfluenced by baseline depression, stress, or anxiety but was significantly related to the patient's score on a Ways of Coping Questionnaire[81] (Fig. 25–4). Additional important contributions to adherence include the response to therapy with regard to sleepiness, performance and mood, home/family environment/support, encumbrance on lifestyle (e.g., ease of travel, intimacy), and interface comfort.

As discussed earlier, patients commonly experience side effects in conjunction with PAP therapy. Although evidence regarding the impact of side effects on acceptance and adherence varies, it is reasonable and prudent for the clinician to make every effort to minimize if not eliminate them (see Table 25–2). It is likely that the perception of a given side effect varies across individuals and therefore may have a different degree of impact. Thus, a simple comparison of prevalence in compliant and noncompliant patients may be misleading and obscure the impact of a particular side effect on the compliance of individual patients. Several practices may enhance patient acceptance and compliance with CPAP

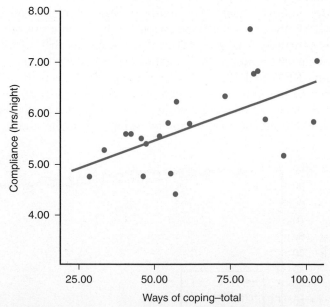

FIGURE 25–4 Relation between the total Ways of Coping Questionnaire score and adherence (average number of hours of CPAP use per night). Adherence = 4.38 + 0.02 * Ways of Coping. *(Reproduced with permission from Stepnowsky CJ Jr, Bardwell WA, Moore PJ, et al. Psychologic correlates of compliance with continuous positive airway pressure. Sleep 2002;25:758.)*

therapy. These are outlined in Table 25–2 as well as later in this chapter. Appropriate patient selection for chronic PAP therapy is an important factor, and educating the patient, utilizing discussion and educational literature addressing the nature of OSA/H, the consequences of untreated OSA/H, and a detailed discussion of therapeutic options and implications, is essential.[144] It is intuitively obvious that patients who require "arm-twisting" to take a PAP unit home, even after efforts have been made to explain the need for the device and the manner in which it operates, are unlikely to use it conscientiously on a long-term basis. Therefore, PAP should be provided only to patients who are reasonably receptive to using it or who are sufficiently open minded to give it a reasonable home trial.

Patient–PP Device Interface Options

Since the initial report in 1981 of CPAP therapy for adults with OSA/H, which described use of a customized nasal mask,[1] there has been an appropriate and ever-growing cornucopia of interfaces from which patients and clinicians may choose in an effort to enhance comfort and convenience. These interfaces include commercially available nasal prongs/pillows or cannula systems, commercial and custom-made nasal masks, commercially available oral-nasal masks,[85,86] and an oral interface.[145] In a 3-week randomized crossover design study comparing nasal pillows and a nasal mask, Massie and coworkers[90] reported that, when using the nasal pillows, there were less frequent adverse effects and less air leak reported as well as less trouble initiating and maintaining sleep. However, there was no difference between the two types of interfaces with regard to the time of PAP use per night, Epworth Sleepiness Scale score, or FOSQ score.

Clinicians also have the option to prescribe an oral-nasal mask or oral interface for patients who are unwilling or unable to use an exclusively nasal interface or who are unable to keep their mouth sufficiently closed during sleep to permit maintenance of adequate positive intrapharyngeal pressure. In our experience, a chin strap is only variably helpful, and when necessary, the delivery of positive pressure via an oral-nasal mask should be considered. These interfaces also have the advantage of increasing humidity in the inspired air, independent of an external humidifier.[95] Oral-nasal interfaces have successfully reduced the AHI in a substantial majority of the patients in whom they have been applied.[85,86] However, oral-nasal interfaces may be less acceptable than nasal interfaces to patients who have had an unsuccessful uvulopalatopharyngoplasty.[87]

Particular care must be taken when employing an oral-nasal mask, owing to the potential risk of aspiration of gastric contents if the patient vomits. Although to our knowledge this complication has not been encountered in patients with OSA/H, it remains a concern. Accordingly, patients using an oral-nasal mask for nocturnal PAP should be instructed not to take anything by mouth to allow gastric emptying before applying the positive pressure. Furthermore, before initiating PP therapy via an oral-nasal mask, patients should be routinely instructed to notify their physician if they are experiencing nausea or vomiting from any cause. They should also be provided with a nasal interface as a temporizing, if not long-term, option and counseled to sleep with the head of the bed elevated.

Coverage of both the nose and mouth by an oral-nasal mask also raises theoretical concerns regarding the potential consequences of machine failure, when airflow that can be entrained by the patient through a nonfunctional or dysfunctional device is limited or nonexistent. Safety valves should be incorporated in the circuit, close to the patient, to facilitate inhalation of fresh air and/or to minimize dead space in the event of machine malfunction. Optimally, an alarm should also be present to signal power failure.

There does not appear to be a significant effect of interface on the requisite positive pressure required to stabilize the upper airway during sleep.[86,90,145] Since patients may change their interface preference over time, they should be made aware that a choice remains open to them at all times during their treatment.

Variations and Modalities of PAP Therapy for OSA/H: Implications for Acceptance and Adherence

Clinical experience indicates that nasal CPAP maintains upper airway patency and acceptable oxygenation during sleep in the overwhelming majority of patients with OSA/H. Some patients find the administration of CPAP sufficiently bothersome to precipitate complete intolerance of therapy or at least result in unsatisfactory adherence. Use of variations of CPAP and other PAP modalities have been explored to address patient complaints that appear to be specific to CPAP.

Pressure Ramping

For some patients, the sensation of positive pressure is sufficiently unpleasant to cause difficulty with initiating sleep. Pressure ramping of CPAP allows adjustment of the rate of rise in delivered pressure over time, from a clinician-specified level to the target therapeutic pressure. Thus, a window of time is created during which the delivered pressure is lower than the target pressure and the patient may find it easier to fall asleep. Because the level of positive pressure may be transiently below that required to maintain upper airway patency during sleep, pressure ramping may allow apnea, hypopnea, and oxyhemoglobin desaturation to occur for a variable period of time, until the pressure reaches the prescribed, optimal value. We are unaware of published studies that address the level of risk that the delay in optimal pressure delivery may present to patients, nor are any data available regarding the effectiveness of pressure ramping on patient adherence to CPAP therapy. In fact, Pressman et al. described a case of "ramp abuse" in which a patient repeatedly awoke to reactivate the ramp.[146] Although the published recordings may have been influenced by movement artifact, failure of sleep continuity and probable repetitive episodes of oxyhemoglobin desaturation (because the pressure was subtherapeutic during the time that the patient was asleep) were evident. As Pressman et al. pointed out, such abuse will not be detected if only CPAP machine run time is monitored as a reflection of adherence. Conversely, monitoring run time at the prescribed pressure gives the clinician insight into this activity.

Thus, although pressure ramping is a conceptually attractive feature, its degree of effectiveness and safety remain to be documented, and the specific patient populations for which it might provide maximal benefit have yet to be identified. Whether or not it should be routinely prescribed for all patients has not been systematically evaluated, but since it is available on most commercially available CPAP machines, clinicians may consider pressure ramping should a patient encounter difficulty in initiating sleep due to CPAP. A careful subsequent follow-up is essential.

Bilevel PP Therapy

This modality has been discussed above. Because in many patients it permits PAP treatment of OSA/H using expiratory pressures that are not mandated to be as high as inspiratory pressures,[22–25] bilevel PP has been prescribed with the intent to reduce complaints or likelihood of complaints related to some side effects, including a smothering sensation, chest wall discomfort, and bothersome nasal or sinus pressure related to the sensation associated with breathing against a positive pressure. Additionally, some patients may be at increased risk for barotrauma by virtue of emphysema or bullous lung disease (though a review of the literature suggests that this is not a prevalent complication of CPAP therapy for OSA/H), while in others, elevated expiratory pressure may be associated with a tendency toward alveolar hypoventilation.[24,25,27,110]

The existing literature does not support routine prescription of bilevel PP rather than CPAP with the intent to improve adherence.[125] There may be a subset of OSA/H patients who prefer the bilevel PP, including but not limited to the very obese, those with higher Pa_{CO_2}, and those with underlying pulmonary or neuromuscular disease.[133] Bilevel PP may be a therapeutic alternative for patients who find nasal CPAP uncomfortable[106] or for those in whom the delivery of PAP represents an unacceptable degree of risk (i.e., patients with bullous lung disease). Prospective, controlled studies are required to determine if and to what degree bilevel PP is successful as salvage therapy for OSA/H populations who are nonadherent to CPAP.

APAP and Auto-titrating Bilevel PP

APAP devices have been previously described in this chapter. The capacity to provide a pressure that "floats" across the sleep period and varies in response to the physiologic requirements to maintain upper airway patency led to the assumption that this mode would improve adherence. To our knowledge, there have not been published, systematic trials of autotitrating bilevel PP in this regard, but there has been a recent meta-analysis examining studies of APAP.[33] Although APAP was comparable to fixed-pressure CPAP in reducing the AHI and did so with a 2-cm H_2O reduction in mean pressure, this modality did not confer a benefit in adherence over fixed-pressure CPAP (Fig. 25–5). Thus, routine prescription of APAP rather than fixed-pressure CPAP cannot be recommended at this time. However, it may be beneficial in improving

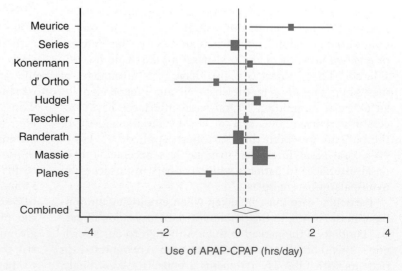

FIGURE 25–5 Comparison of nightly adherence to autotitrating CPAP (APAP) versus fixed-pressure CPAP. A positive score indicates a better adherence to APAP than CPAP. *X axis,* Nightly adherence with APAP minus adherence on CPAP. *Y axis,* Investigations reporting adherence data. The *dashed line with the diamond* at the bottom represents the pooled effect though the mean of the estimate. *(Reproduced with permission from Ayas NT, Patel SR, Malhotra A, et al. Auto-titrating versus standard continuous positive airway pressure for the treatment of obstructive sleep apnea: results of a meta-analysis. Sleep 2004;27:249.)*

comfort and tolerance in selected patients. Systematic studies are required to assess the impact of autotitrating bilevel PP.

Pressure-Relief CPAP and Bilevel PP

There are few studies addressing the effect of pressure-relief CPAP on adherence. One nonrandomized study demonstrated that adherence to pressure-relief CPAP over 3 months was significantly better than adherence to conventional CPAP.[147] There was no difference between pressure-relief and conventional CPAP with regard to the degree of change in subjective sleepiness and FOSQ score. Another study, utilizing a randomized, 7-week crossover design comparing pressure-relief CPAP and conventional CPAP, confirmed the comparability between pressure-relief CPAP and conventional CPAP in alleviating sleep-disordered breathing but found no difference in adherence over 7 weeks.[148] Similarly, there was no significant difference with regard to complaints. To our knowledge there are no published systematic studies examining the impact of routinely prescribed pressure-relief bilevel PP on adherence. However, a recent study suggested that pressure-relief bilevel PP may provide some benefit as a salvage therapy for patients who are sub-optimally adherent to CPAP despite intensive education and interventions to maximize comfort.[148a] Thus, there are too few data on which to make conclusions about the role of pressure-relief CPAP and bilevel PP. While these modalities may be useful in specific patients, there are no data to indicate benefit from routine prescription to all patients at initial setup.

Follow-Up of CPAP Patients and Its Role in Enhancing Adherence

As noted above, it appears that an individual's pattern of CPAP use (or nonuse) is established very shortly after initiating home therapy.[71,72,124,149] It is therefore reasonable to consider that enhanced adherence would result from early and consistent contact between the patient and the care provider in an effort to identify and resolve problems with therapy, provide encouragement, and give support. While this may be a reasonable line of thought, the literature provides conflicting information on this subject. One study indicated that positive reinforcement by periodic telephone contact does not favorably influence therapeutic compliance.[73] In contrast, considerably larger investigations have demonstrated improved adherence in conjunction with intensive educational and support measures after initiation of home treatment.[88,150] Chervin and coworkers[144] reported that patients who had received educational literature regarding sleep-disordered breathing and CPAP or bilevel PP use and patients who received follow-up telephone calls from health care personnel were more adherent than patients who had received neither of these interventions. In contrast, intensive follow-up of PAP patients in Hong Kong did not improve adherence when compared to standard care.[151]

It is also essential that a physician and staff who are experienced in the care of OSA/H patients and the difficulties they encounter act as continuing support and educational resources to answer questions and provide reassurance when uncertainties arise. At our center and others, patient support groups serve a very important function in fostering a climate of openness and sharing of information as well as providing a forum for discussion of issues relevant to all types of sleep-disordered breathing (OSA/H, nocturnal ventilatory failure associated with neuromuscular and chest wall disorders, etc.) and overall health. Group meetings provide patients with the realization that they are not and should not be isolated by their disorder. This is crucial, since many OSA/H patients have been labeled by society as lazy or malingerers, resulting in social ostracism and low self-esteem. Many of the consequences of OSA/H are reversible by PAP therapy, with remarkable and gratifying results for all concerned. In our experience, there is no doubt that important benefits are obtained from support groups, judging from the excellent long-term attendance and favorable patient comments.

Summary

When all things are considered, adherence to PAP, which entails the presence of a relatively cumbersome box at or near the bedside and an equally cumbersome (if not unappealing) interface over the nose, is surprisingly good. Adherence to PAP compares favorably to therapies that most would consider substantially less noxious, such as metered-dose inhalers for treating asthma.[152] Without doubt, this relates to the remarkable symptomatic improvement experienced by the majority of users.

TRADITIONAL AND EVOLVING METHODS OF INITIATING PAP THERAPY

Traditionally, patients have undergone an attended (by a technologist), monitored (by polysomnography) trial of PAP to establish therapeutic levels of pressure prior to initiating long-term therapy. Because the requisite level of PAP may vary according to body position and sleep stage, clinicians should be certain that the delivered pressure is effective in maintaining adequate upper airway patency and oxygenation during sleep in all positions, including and especially the supine position (and when possible during supine REM sleep). It also provides an opportunity for the patient to examine the PAP unit and various interfaces before home use. The most comfortable and leak-free interface with the device (i.e., nasal mask, prongs, or oral-nasal mask) can be selected. Then, while the patient is still awake, he or she may be provided with an opportunity to experience PAP across a wide range of pressures, to permit familiarization with the associated sensations. Another advantage of attended evaluation of the patient on PAP is the immediate availability of knowledgeable and caring health care professionals who can respond to questions and allay concerns. When wearing a PAP device for the first time, patients have been anecdotally reported to awaken in the middle of the night disoriented and perhaps frightened by the apparatus. Under these circumstances, albeit rare, reassurance is readily supplied by the laboratory personnel conducting the trial.

Several other benefits have also been attributed to polysomnographically monitored trials of CPAP therapy. Fry and coworkers[153] observed an increased frequency of periodic leg movements in sleep (PLMS), with and without accompanying arousals during nasal CPAP therapy. These investigators hypothesized that the improved sleep quality and architecture associated with relief of OSA/H by nasal CPAP "unmasks" PLMS. However, several subsequent studies observed that the Periodic Limb Movement Index was not appreciably different during a diagnostic polysomnogram and during CPAP therapy,[154,155] although arousals may diminish in conjunction with PLMS during CPAP therapy, at least acutely.[154] Nonetheless, periodic limb movement disorder may coexist with OSA/H and may persist after alleviation of OSA/H on CPAP, and a patient may not obtain symptomatic abatement of daytime sleepiness or fatigue. Thus, a monitored initial trial of CPAP addresses many issues and concerns that, if not considered, may lead to dismissal of this form of therapy as a viable therapeutic option. Attention to these factors at the outset of therapy will maximize the opportunity for a successful outcome.

Split-Night Diagnostic and CPAP Titrations

This paradigm for initiating PAP therapy has been discussed above in the context of acceptance and adherence. The current health care environment has fostered exploration of alternative means of establishing PAP therapy for OSA/H in order to facilitate access to limited diagnostic and therapeutic resources.[156] As noted earlier in this chapter, some clinicians are requesting that diagnostic and PAP titrations be conducted in single, split-night studies. Although this may lead to a satisfactory CPAP prescription for many patients,[122,126–132] there are a number of patients for whom the duration of time available for CPAP titration is too limited in the context of a split-night study to achieve a satisfactory prescription.[131] In particular, patients with milder degrees of OSA/H in whom the titration is initiated later in the night (because more prolonged monitoring was needed to establish the diagnosis of OSA/H) are more likely to have unsuccessful split-night titrations.

An American Academy of Sleep Medicine statement of practice parameters indicates that a split-night paradigm is an alternative to the 2-night diagnostic and therapeutic titration PAP strategy to develop a PAP prescription if the AHI is ≥40 over a diagnostic study duration of at least 2 hours. A split-night study also may be warranted when the AHI is 20–40 in an appropriate clinical context and when PAP titration is conducted over more than 3 hours, with elimination or near-elimination of disordered breathing events, including during REM sleep in the supine position.[134] It should be noted that some reimbursement guidelines mandate that the diagnostic study duration be at least 2 hours *of sleep*. Clinicians should take care to check on local and current guidelines in this regard. Recent studies have also indicated that the split-night-PSG strategy and the traditional 2-night paradigm provide similar benefits, but the former is associated with lower cost.[157,158] In addition, split-night studies may reduce the waiting time for initiation of therapy.[159]

Home CPAP Titration

Some investigators have advocated in-home initiation of CPAP therapy employing both attended monitoring and unattended/unmonitored titrations.[160,161] Waldhorn and Wood described titration of CPAP by a technologist in the patient's home using a portable 4-channel monitor recording heart rate, chest wall movement, CPAP pressure in the mask, and oxyhemoglobin saturation to guide CPAP adjustment.[161] The authors reported elimination of apneas, hypopneas, and snoring, but this was assessed by the 4-channel monitor and not polysomnography. Self-reported adherence to CPAP therapy in this group of 17 patients was an average of 7.23 ± 1 hours (mean ± standard deviation [SD]) per night, which is at least comparable to values obtained by conventional in-laboratory titration. Coppola and Lawee[160] reported their experience with unattended home CPAP titration in which 11 patients had increases in CPAP level in response to telephone interviews between the clinician, patient, and bed partner that revealed persistent snoring, apnea observed by the bed partner, and/or symptoms consistent with OSA/H. Good subjective outcome was reported in these studies, but the absence of objectively assessed adherence (which was unavailable at the time of these studies) is a significant limitation of these data.

Whether or not attended, in-home titration provides a cost-effective and efficient alternative to in-laboratory methodology remains to be determined, but clearly, committing a technician to spend a night monitoring one titration constitutes a measurable utilization of resources. In addition, the applicability of this paradigm across all home environments and social conditions, as well as for patients without bed partners, remains to be determined.

Use of Predictive Formulas to Estimate or Establish the CPAP Pressure Prescription

A CPAP prescription consists of the pressure that maintains satisfactory upper airway patency and oxyhemoglobin saturation during sleep, while providing satisfactory sleep continuity using a interface that is well-tolerated by the patient.

Several investigators have suggested that the requisite level of CPAP can be estimated with sufficient clinical accuracy to obviate the need for monitored titration, thus providing a starting point at which titration may begin either in the monitored environment, in order to maximize the time available to "fine-tune" the final pressure prescription, or in the home setting, with further adjustments made on the basis of clinical guidelines or the results of home diagnostic evaluation.[162–164] Miljeteig and Hoffstein[162] reported that the three variables that best predicted the minimal therapeutic CPAP level (defined as that which reduced the AHI to <10) were body mass index (BMI), AHI, and neck circumference. This combination accounted for approximately 67% of the variability in minimal CPAP level in a group of 38 patients, using the following formula:

$$CPAP_{min} = -5.12 + (0.13 \times BMI \, [kg/m^2]) + (0.16 \times neck \; circumference \, [cm]) + (0.04 \times AHI)$$

In a subsequent data set from 129 patients, reported in the same paper, the minimal CPAP predicted from this equation was 8 ± 2.1 cm H_2O and the value obtained during laboratory titration was 8.1 ± 3 cm H_2O (mean $\pm$ SD). Seventy-one percent of patients had predicted values within 2.5 cm H_2O of the measured values, and 95% had predicted CPAP levels within 5 cm H_2O of the measured values. The investigators indicated that their predictive equation may not be applicable to all patients due to variability in individual responses to a given level of CPAP.

In a subsequent study of 26 patients, Hoffstein and Mateika prospectively tested the predictive value of the previous equation.[163] For the group as a whole, there was no significant difference between the predicted and the polysomnographically titrated optimal CPAP levels defined as the lowest titrated pressure at which the AHI was less than 10. In 38% of patients $CPAP_{predicted} = CPAP_{optimal}$; in 38% of patients, $CPAP_{predicted}$ was within 1 cm H_2O of $CPAP_{optimal}$; in 15% of patients, $CPAP_{predicted}$ was within 2 cm H_2O of $CPAP_{optimal}$; and in 8% of patients, $CPAP_{predicted}$ was >2 cm H_2O of $CPAP_{optimal}$. In general, $CPAP_{predicted}$ underestimated $CPAP_{optimal}$, although $CPAP_{predicted}$ was grossly inaccurate in 8% of the patients, being too high in one and too low in the other. It is important to recognize that the criteria for defining effective CPAP level did not include elimination of respiratory effort–related arousals, as may be seen in the upper airway resistance syndrome.[165]

In an open randomized trial, Hukins examined prescription of a CPAP level based on the patient's BMI with that established during a polysomnographic titration.[164] In the formulaic group, CPAP was initially prescribed at 8 cm H_2O if the BMI was <30, 10 cm H_2O if the BMI was between 30 and 35, and 12 cm H_2O was prescribed if the BMI was 35 or more. If the patient could not tolerate the prescribed pressure, it was decreased. The pressure was increased if there was persistent sleepiness or snoring. The formulaic pressure was slightly but significantly higher than that established by polysomnographic titration (13 ± 2 vs. 11.8 ± 2.4 cm H_2O, $p = 0.04$). A sleep study was done after 3 months. Sleep efficiency was greater in the formulaic group, with comparable AHI and Arousal Index as well as percent slow-wave sleep and REM sleep. After 3 months, the polysomnographically prescribed pressure group tended to have a lower Epworth Sleepiness Scale score than the formulaically prescribed group (6.9 ± 3.6 vs. 9.2 ± 5.6, $p = 0.07$), but there was no difference in discontinuation of therapy, adherence, or quality of life as reflected by the SF-36. The average time to initiation of therapy was notably shorter in the formulaically prescribed group. Hukins concluded that the formulaic prescription strategy could be used when there would be an untoward delay in initiating CPAP treatment were the prescription to be developed through in-laboratory polysomnographic titration. Assessment of comparability of the two prescription strategies past the 3-month milestone remains to be done.

Along similar lines, a randomized, single-blind 5-week crossover trial compared a CPAP prescription based on an in-laboratory polysomnographic titration, determining a CPAP level that remained unchanged, and a prescription that was initially based on the formula described by Hoffstein et al.,[163] with subsequent patient self-titration according to perception of effectiveness and comfort.[166] Participants were provided with information regarding the indication for and how to adjust CPAP as well as interfaces. There was no difference between the two prescription strategies with regard to adherence, quality of life using disease-specific instruments, perceived sleepiness, and objective ability to maintain wakefulness under soporific conditions. The CPAP that was identified by patients to be optimal during the self-adjusting study arm was 10.1 ± 2.0 cm H_2O (mean $\pm$ SD) compared with the 9.7 ± 2 cm H_2O that was determined during the polysomnographic titration arm. On average, over the 5 weeks in the self-titrating arm of the study, patients made 5.7 changes in the CPAP level from the initial level determined according to formula. The investigators concluded that establishing an initial CPAP prescription using a formula with subsequent patient adjustment is as effective as more conventional methods and may enhance the efficiency with which limited resources are utilized. It should be noted that the duration of this study was only 5 weeks in each arm. Moreover, as the investigators indicated, this strategy may only be applicable in patients with an understanding of the self-titrating instructions and the ability to adjust their own CPAP devices. Clearly, regardless of the method employed to establish the PAP prescription, patient education and follow-up remains an essential element.

Use of APAP Devices

The general principles and use of APAP in the context of adherence have been previously discussed in this chapter.

One potential venue for APAP is application in the sleep laboratory with subsequent examination of the data to identify a single "best" level of CPAP to prescribe for chronic therapy with a "fixed" CPAP device (e.g., the value at or below which the pressure is during 90% of the study, or CPAP$_{90\%ile}$). This would enable titration in an attended environment but without obligating the technologist to manually adjust the level of CPAP. Thus, the technologist's responsibility would de-intensified, perhaps permitting a lower technologist-to-patient ratio (with resultant reduction in cost). Alternatively, in-laboratory titration may be bypassed and the patient sent home on an autotitrating device for a short period to establish the CPAP$_{90\%ile}$ on which a fixed-pressure CPAP device may be prescribed. Finally, the patient may simply be provided with an autotitrating device to use at home in the autotitrating mode.

In a randomized controlled study of 360 OSA/H patients, Masa et al.[167] compared standard polysomnographic titration with a formula-based prescription[162] and APAP. The evaluative period was 12 weeks. In the formula-based prescription group, the pressure could be increased by 1–2 cm H_2O if the patient's bed partner noted snoring or apnea, after which an "optimal" pressure was deemed to have been identified. There was no difference across the groups with regard to withdrawals. The autotitrating group had a lower response on the SF-36 physical and the EuroQuality of Life Scale than the standard titration group, but there was no difference between the improvement in the formula-based group and the standard titration group. There were no differences among the groups with regard to adherence, side effects, and complaints. The investigators concluded that titration of CPAP can be accomplished with an APAP device or in a paradigm using a predictive formula to establish an initial pressure prescription. It should be noted that this study excluded patients with chronic illnesses or conditions such as cancer, chronic pain, renal failure, moderate or greater chronic obstructive pulmonary disease, substance addiction, and CSB; individuals who had a previous uvulopalatopharyngoplasty; those without a partner; patients with "important" chronic nasal obstruction; and those who lacked sufficient skill in adjusting a nasal mask. Whereas the observations of Masa et al.[167] are of considerable interest, the numerous clinical exclusions reduce generalizability to a measurable proportion of OSA/H patients seen in sleep disorders centers at this time.

More recently, in a study similar to that of Masa et al., West and coworkers[168] compared 6 months of APAP; initial application of APAP to identify the CPAP$_{90\%ile}$, which was used to provide a fixed-pressure CPAP prescription; and a CPAP prescription based on neck circumference and the frequency of dips in oxyhemoglobin saturation during baseline sleep. Individuals were not excluded from this study based on comorbidities. At 6 months, data were available in 86 of the 98 randomized patients. The investigators observed that, after 6 months, there was no difference among the groups with regard to the hours used per night, Epworth Sleepiness Scale score, objective ability to maintain wakefulness, 24-hour ambulatory blood pressure, health assessed using the SF-36, and the Sleep Apnea Quality of Life Index. The investigators concluded that more complicated treatment initiation and maintenance strategies using APAP offered no benefit to patients over a simpler, formula-based prescription strategy.

In summary, APAP has evolved as a technology, but its place in establishing and maintaining the PAP prescription over a prolonged duration, across the wide spectrum of OSA/H patients, remains to be clearly defined. At the present time, it appears that utilizing APAP to establish the CPAP$_{90\%ile}$ on which to base a fixed-pressure CPAP prescription is neither better nor worse than standard strategies or formula-based strategies. Perhaps the most important determinant will be the availability of resources as well as the circumstances and wishes of individual patients.

EFFECT OF POSITIVE AIRWAY PRESSURE THERAPY OF OSA/H ON SYSTEMIC DISORDERS

Effect of PAP Therapy on Cardiovascular Mortality in OSA/H Patients

As noted earlier in this chapter, several studies have documented increased cardiovascular mortality in OSA/H patients, with reduction following initiation of and subsequent adherence to PAP therapy.[120,169,170] Although these studies were not randomized controlled trials comparing the effects of PAP therapy with sham-PAP, the results are reasonably compelling. In this light, Peker and colleagues[171] assessed incident cardiovascular events in middle-aged men with OSA/H over 7 years and noted that the incidence of cardiovascular events in patients who were adequately treated (by PAP, uvulopalatopharyngoplasty, or oral appliances) was about 7% in contrast to about 57% in patients who were inadequately treated.

Observations regarding the effect of PAP in patients with OSA/H should not be generalized to patients with central sleep apnea or CSB in conjunction with heart failure. A multicenter, randomized controlled trial of CPAP versus no CPAP in patients with central sleep apnea and heart failure associated with reduced left ventricular (LV) function was stopped early due to relatively higher mortality in the group receiving CPAP compared with the group not receiving CPAP, over the first 18 months of participation in the study.[172] It should be noted that after the initial 18 months, survival was better in the group receiving CPAP. Over the entire duration that the study was being conducted, there was no difference in transplant-free survival between the groups. The authors speculated that the early mortality in the group receiving CPAP may have been attributable to the effects of PAP in the clinical context of relative intravascular volume depletion. They concluded that CPAP is not indicated to improve transplant-free survival in heart failure patients with central sleep apnea.

Effect of PAP Therapy on Cardiac Rhythm Disturbances in OSA/H Patients

Cardiac rhythm disturbances are common in OSA/H patients.[173–180] There are several potential mechanisms through which OSA/H predisposes to rhythm disturbances, including sleep-related changes in sympathovagal balance as well as alteration in sympathetic nervous system activity in conjunction with sleep-disordered breathing events, changes in QT interval, hypoxemia, and the influence of carotid chemosensitivity.[181–185] The favorable response of arrhythmias to CPAP therapy, especially in the absence of structural heart disease, reinforces the linkage between OSA/H and rhythm disturbances.[175,177,186–188] A recent randomized controlled trial reported that, after 1 month, CPAP therapy reduces the frequency of premature ventricular beats by nearly 60% in OSA/H patients with heart failure compared to patients who are not receiving CPAP, in whom there was no significant change.[188] The authors acknowledged that, despite randomization, the group receiving CPAP had less severe OSA/H at baseline. The importance of this study is highlighted by recognition that sleep[181–183] and OSA/H have been associated with increased QT interval and increased dispersion, which may predispose to serious and potentially fatal arrhythmias especially in the setting of ventricular irritability. In contrast to these studies, one study reported bradyarrhythmias (pauses >3 seconds and episodes during which heart rate was <40 beats/min) were more responsive to CPAP therapy than supraventricular arrhythmias.[177] The effect on ventricular tachyarrhythmias was not reported.

In summary, it is evident that nocturnal cardiac rhythm abnormalities are prevalent in patients with OSA/H and treatment with PAP often has an ameliorative effect on them. Clinical judgment is necessary to determine if other immediate interventions (e.g., reduction or elimination of β blockade in the case of bradyarrhythmias, antiarrhythmic medication, pacemaker) is indicated. Moreover, careful follow-up assessment is essential to determine if additional interventions are required.

Effect of PAP Therapy in OSA/H Patients with Heart Failure

A number of studies support the improvement in LV function after initiation of PAP therapy for patients with OSA/H and heart failure.[169,189 193] The mechanisms by which PAP may improve LV function in OSA/H patients with heart failure include relief of sleep-related hypoxemia, elimination of cyclic increases in LV afterload, reduction in sympathetic nervous system activation,[190,194,195] and reduced inflammation. Kaneko and colleagues observed that OSA/H patients with a notably reduced LV ejection fraction at baseline experienced a significant improvement after 1 month of CPAP therapy (an average increase of approximately 8% for the group).[192] These observations were reinforced by Mansfield et al.,[193] who conducted a randomized trial comparing a group of OSA/H patients with heart failure who were treated with CPAP for 3 months and a group who did not receive CPAP therapy. The group receiving CPAP experienced an improvement in LV ejection fraction by about 5%, while the group who did not receive CPAP had an increase of approximately 1.5% (Fig. 25–6). There was no change in systemic blood pressure during CPAP application to explain the beneficial effects, but there was a reduction in overnight urinary norepinephrine excretion, consistent with reduced sympathetic activity in the group receiving CPAP. Although this trial did not apply a placebo or sham CPAP control, the consistent results with other studies as well as other aspects of the design support the credibility of the results.

In summary, LV dysfunction in OSA/H patients may be improved by PAP therapy of sleep-disordered breathing.

Effect of PAP Therapy in OSA/H Patients with Hypertension

Epidemiologic studies have provided compelling evidence that OSA/H is associated with increased risk for systemic hypertension (HTN).[196–202] Sleep apnea has been identified by the Joint National Committee on Prevention, Detection, Evaluation and Treatment of High Blood Pressure as a risk factor for HTN.[203] Although it is plausible that PAP therapy would ameliorate diurnal HTN by eliminating intermittent hypoxic exposure and sympathetic nervous system activation, improved sleep continuity,[194,204–212] the literature provides conflicting data in this regard.

Using a randomized, placebo-controlled design to compare ambulatory blood pressure on CPAP and sham CPAP in subjectively sleepy (Epworth Sleepiness Scale score >9) OSA/H patients, Pepperell et al.[213] observed a small but significantly greater reduction in mean blood pressure during sleep in the active CPAP–treated group (93.7 ± 1.6 and 90.3 ± 1.4 mm Hg before and after 1 month of active CPAP, respectively; 96.2 ± 1.6 and 95.8 ± 1.5 mm Hg before and after 1 month of sham CPAP) and during wakefulness in the active treatment group (104.3 ± 1.3 and 101.9 ± 1.3 mm Hg before and after 1 month of active CPAP, respectively; 104.2 ± 1.4 and 106.1 ± 1.4 mm Hg before and after 1 month of sham CPAP). Although small, the reduction in blood pressure in the active CPAP group would have a notable public health impact on cardiovascular risk. A post-hoc analysis however suggested that individuals in who CPAP use reduced the AHI below 15 may

FIGURE 25–6 Change in left ventricular ejection fraction over 3 months in OSA/H patients who were not **(left)** and who were **(right)** treated with CPAP. The *asterisk* indicates patients who were in atrial fibrillation at the indicated point in time. *(Reproduced with permission from Mansfield DR, Gollogly NC, Kaye DM, et al. Controlled trial of continuous positive airway pressure in obstructive sleep apnea and heart failure. Am J Respir Crit Care Med 2004;169:361.)*

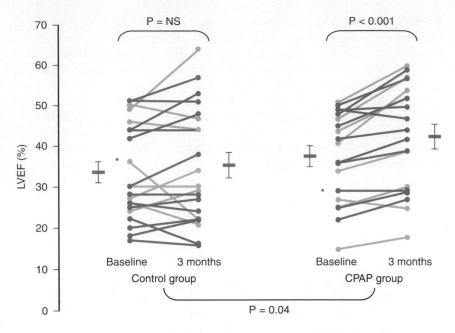

experience improved left ventricular function and heart transplant free survival time.[213a]

Similarly, in a randomized sham-CPAP controlled trial in individuals with moderate to severe OSA/H, including notable oxyhemoglobin desaturation, Becker and coworkers[214] observed a reduction in mean blood pressure by approximately 10 mm Hg after about 9 weeks of active CPAP therapy, while no change was observed in the group receiving sham CPAP (Fig. 25–7). The observation of Becker et al. may be the more noteworthy since the sham CPAP was associated with some improvement in OSA/H. Conversely, there are a number of well-designed studies of groups of OSA/H patients either with or without subjective sleepiness, and with HTN, that have failed to demonstrate a significant reduction in blood pressure with PAP therapy[215–217] (Fig. 25–8).

In summary, it is evident that further research is required to define the effect of PAP on HTN in OSA/H patients. For example, a small case series of OSA/H patients with medically refractory HTN received benefit from CPAP in this regard.[218] Perhaps the heterogeneity of the data with respect to the effect of PAP on HTN should not be surprising. Hypertension is probably heterogeneous in etiology and duration, with varying degrees of vascular remodeling also potentially influencing therapeutic responsiveness. There may be subsets of hypertensive OSA/H patients with greater likelihood of deriving blood pressure improvement from PAP therapy, and identifying these patients is a challenge for the future.

PAP Therapy and Stroke

The association between sleep-disordered breathing, including OSA/H, and increased risk for stroke is increasingly

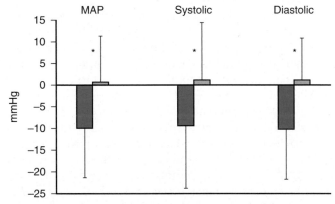

FIGURE 25–7 Change in blood pressure in OSA/H patients receiving active CPAP (*closed bars*) and sham CPAP (*open bars*). Difference in mean arterial pressure (MAP) $p = 0.01$; systolic pressure, $p = 0.04$; diastolic pressure, $p < 0.005$. *(Reproduced with permission from Becker HF, Jerrentrup A, Ploch T, et al. Effect of nasal continuous positive airway pressure treatment on blood pressure in patients with obstructive sleep apnea. Circulation 2003;107:68.)*

recognized. Data from the Wisconsin Sleep Cohort indicate that, even after adjusting for age, gender, smoking, HTN, alcohol use, and BMI, sleep-disordered breathing is associated with increased risk for prevalent stroke.[219] There was also a suggestion of an association between sleep-disordered breathing and incident stroke, but this did not reach statistical significance, perhaps due to the study being underpowered to address this issue. Of comparable importance, sleep-disordered breathing following a stroke is a poor prognostic indicator of survival and function.[220–225]

In a longitudinal observational cohort study, Yaggi and coworkers[223] reported the risk of first time incident stroke or death from any cause over a median follow-up period of 3.4 years in OSA/H patients (mean AHI = 35)

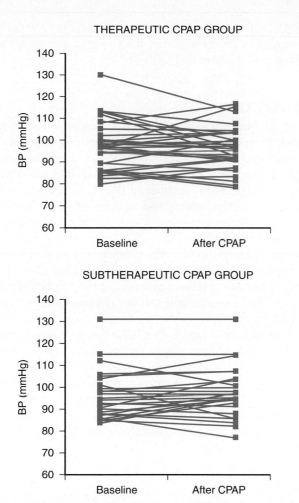

THERAPEUTIC CPAP GROUP

SUBTHERAPEUTIC CPAP GROUP

FIGURE 25–8 Change in blood pressure in OSA/H patients receiving therapeutic CPAP **(top)** and sham CPAP **(bottom).** *(Reproduced with permission from Campos-Rodriguez F, Grilo-Reina A, Perez-Ronchel J, et al. Effect of continuous positive airway pressure on ambulatory BP in patients with sleep apnea and hypertension: a placebo-controlled trial. Chest 2006;129:1459.)*

>50 years old compared with non-OSA/H patients (mean AHI = 2). There were 22 strokes in the OSA/H group and 2 strokes in the non-OSA/H group during the study interval. For the composite event of stroke or death, the probability of event-free survival was significantly less in the OSA/H group. These investigators observed a significant trend for increasing risk of stroke or death from any cause as the AHI increased, with the risk being threefold greater in OSA/H patients with AHI >36 compared with the non-OSA/H group. OSA/H remained significantly associated with first-time incident stroke and death from any cause, even after adjusting for gender, race, age, smoking status, alcohol ingestion, BMI, and the presence of diabetes mellitus, hyperlipidemia, atrial fibrillation, and HTN. There are several limitations of this study. The study population was substantially male and Caucasian, an analysis of the probability of incident stroke alone in individuals with and without OSA/H was not performed, and the degree to which OSA/H was independently associated with

first-time incident stroke (not combined with death from any cause) was not assessed. In addition, many of the participants in this study were prescribed treatment for OSA/H, and this factor, as well as adherence, was not assessed. It is therefore possible that first-time incident stroke and death from any cause were underestimated. The data are consistent with previous cross-sectional studies independently associating OSA/H with cardiovascular disease and death and therefore add to the concern regarding adverse outcomes from this disorder.

Consequently, the outcome of PAP therapy for sleep-disordered breathing following stroke is of substantial interest. This is a difficult issue to address, and the results of randomized placebo-controlled trials have not, to our knowledge been published. Martinez-Garcia et al.[226] observed that patients noted to have OSA/H following a first stroke and who were adherent to CPAP therapy had a significantly lower incidence of a second event compared to patients who were intolerant of CPAP. Of course, the possibility that the intolerant group were burdened by an unidentified additional risk for another cerebrovascular event cannot be excluded. Two randomized trials of CPAP versus no-CPAP therapy observed no benefit from CPAP therapy for severe OSA/H following stroke,[227,228] with the exception of improved depressive symptoms in the CPAP group in one of these studies.[228] Thus, to date studies provide conflicting data regarding the outcome of PAP therapy following stroke. However, a common theme is that there is a greater degree of nonadherence in these patients.[151,227,228] Altered cognitive function is probably at least partially responsible for the notable nonadherence in this population.[228] Further studies are required to determine if PAP therapy of OSA/H reduces risk for incident stroke and to define patient groups who may benefit from PAP. If there are stroke patients who will benefit from PAP therapy, research is required to define specific measures and programs that will promote adherence.

PAP Therapy of Abnormal Glycemic Control and Type 2 Diabetes Mellitus

There is increasing awareness of the association between OSA/H, abnormal glycemic control, type 2 diabetes mellitus, and other features of the metabolic syndrome.[229–236] Since insulin resistance, the metabolic syndrome, and diabetes are known risk factors for cardiovascular disease, if causation is established between OSA/H and these metabolic perturbations, the former would provide an attractive interventional target through which the burden of cardiovascular disorders could be reduced. Interventional studies provide one avenue to determine if OSA/H contributes to abnormal glycemic control. Only limited data are currently available. Utilizing a hyperinsulinemic euglycemic clamp to assess insulin sensitivity, Brooks et al.[237] demonstrated that 4 months of CPAP therapy increased insulin sensitivity in very obese OSA/H patients with non–insulin dependent diabetes. This did not translate into improved fasting glucose, and the authors speculated that the effect of the substantial obesity in the subject population and residual severe insulin resistance masked translation of increased sensitivity to improved glycemic control. Along these lines, Harsch and colleagues demonstrated that insulin sensitivity increased in nondiabetic OSA/H patients following 3 months of CPAP therapy, with the greatest response occurring in individuals with BMI <30.[238] More recently, Babu et al.[239] reported that diabetic patients with generally moderate or severe OSA/H who are adherent to CPAP, with use for >4 hr/day, have a progressive reduction in hemoglobin A_{1c} (HbA_{1c}) over time after initiation of PAP therapy. No such effect was observed in patients who used CPAP <4 hr/day. Furthermore, the reduction in HbA_{1c} was greatest in those patients with baseline values >7%. A strength of the study was that no adjustment of medication was permitted during the study interval. However, this was not a randomized trial, and data regarding weight at baseline at the end of the study interval were not described. Thus, the results should be taken in light of these limitations.

In summary, the data are far too limited to permit conclusions regarding the likelihood that PAP therapy of OSA/H will improve insulin sensitivity and glycemic control, independent of other factors. However, existing information provides cautious encouragement that, at least in less obese patients, treatment of OSA/H will confer metabolic benefit and perhaps downstream reduced cardiovascular risk. Moreover, a recent randomized controlled trial reported no difference between 3 months of active versus placebo CPAP with regard to insulin resistance or glycosylated hemoglobin in obese (mean BMI approximately 36) men with type 2 diabetes and OSA/H.[240]

SUMMARY

PAP constitutes a safe and effective treatment for OSA/H. There have been substantial modifications and developments over the last 25 years in an effort to provide greater patient comfort with regard to interface and modality. In addition, different modalities of PAP have been developed to better address subsets and nuances of sleep-disordered breathing. Importantly, randomized controlled trials have demonstrated efficacy of PAP therapy in improving patients' perception of daytime function, and other studies have provided compelling evidence for improved outcomes with respect to systemic disorders, including but not limited to LV function and cardiac rhythm disturbances in OSA/H patients. Nonetheless, further work is required to identify the best target threshold for patient adherence, identify and address those factors that impede optimal adherence, and identify those subsets of patients who are most likely to obtain benefits from this form of treatment.

Sleep medicine has come a long way since the days when tracheotomy or no therapy was the only treatment options that caregivers could offer their OSA/H patients.

⊘ REFERENCES

A full list of references are available at www.expertconsult.com

CHAPTER 26

Nature and Treatment of Insomnia

Charles M. Morin and **Ruth M. Benca**

INTRODUCTION

Insomnia is a prevalent health complaint in the general population and in clinical practice. It is often associated with daytime fatigue, mood disturbances, and functional impairments. Despite its high prevalence and burden, insomnia often goes undiagnosed and remains untreated. The conceptualization of insomnia and its treatment has evolved over the last 2 decades.[1,2] Whereas it was initially conceptualized exclusively as a symptom of other psychiatric or medical disorders, current classifications of sleep disorders make a distinction between the symptom and the syndrome of insomnia.[3,4] In addition, there have been significant advances in the therapeutics of insomnia, from a predominantly symptomatic approach to more focused interventions for perpetuating factors with cognitive behavioral therapy and for more targeted/selective brain receptors with pharmacotherapy.

PREVALENCE AND SIGNIFICANCE OF INSOMNIA

Population-based estimates indicate that about one-third of adults report insomnia symptoms, 9–12% experience additional daytime symptoms, 15% are dissatisfied with their sleep, and approximately 6–10% meet diagnostic criteria for an insomnia syndrome.[5,6] In primary care medicine, approximately 30% of patients report significant sleep disturbances.[7] Insomnia is more prevalent among women, middle-aged and older adults, shift workers, and patients with medical or psychiatric disorders.[5,8] Difficulties initiating sleep are more common among young adults, and problems maintaining sleep are more

frequent among middle-aged and elderly adults. The incidence of insomnia is higher among first-degree family members (daughter, mother) than in the general population,[9] although it is unclear whether this link is inherited through a genetic predisposition, is learned by observations of parental models, or is simply a by-product of another psychopathology.

Persistent insomnia can produce an important burden for the individual and for society, as evidenced by reduced quality of life, more functional impairments, and higher health care costs.[5,8,10] Individuals with chronic sleep disturbances report more psychological distress and reduced productivity relative to good sleepers; they take more sick leaves and utilize health care resources more often than good sleepers.[8] Persistent insomnia is also associated with prolonged use of hypnotic medications and with increased risk of major depression.[5,8,11,12]

NATURE OF INSOMNIA

Clinical Presentation and Findings

Subjective Sleep Complaint

Insomnia entails a spectrum of complaints reflecting dissatisfaction with the quality, duration, or continuity of sleep. These complaints may involve problems with falling asleep initially at bedtime, waking up in the middle of the night and having difficulty going back to sleep, waking up too early in the morning with an inability to return to sleep, and nonrestorative or unrefreshing sleep.[3,4] These difficulties are not mutually exclusive, as a person may experience mixed problems initiating and maintaining sleep. In addition, daytime fatigue, cognitive impairments, and mood disturbances (e.g., irritability, dysphoria) are extremely frequent and often the primary concerns prompting patients with insomnia to seek treatment.

In addition to clinical diagnostic criteria (Table 26–1), several quantitative indicators are useful to evaluate the severity and significance of insomnia. These include the intensity, frequency, and duration of sleep difficulties and their associated daytime consequences. For example, sleep-onset and sleep-maintenance insomnia are often defined by a latency to sleep onset and/or time awake after sleep onset greater than 30 or 45 minutes, with corresponding sleep time of less than 6.5 hours. Such criteria, while arbitrary, are useful to operationalize the definition of insomnia. Total sleep time alone is not a good index to define insomnia because there are individual differences in sleep needs. Some people may function well with as little as 5–6 hours of sleep and would not necessarily complain of insomnia, while others needing 9–10 hours may still complain of inadequate sleep. It is also important to distinguish the occasional insomnia that everyone experiences at one time or another in life from the more recurrent insomnia, usually defined by the presence of sleep difficulty 3 nights or more per week. A distinction is also made between situational/acute insomnia, a condition lasting a few days and often associated with life events or jet lag; short-term insomnia (lasting between 1 and 4 weeks); and chronic insomnia, lasting more than 1 month. Finally, it is necessary to consider the impact of insomnia on a person's psychosocial and occupational functioning to judge its clinical significance. As such, insomnia must be associated with marked distress or significant impairments of daytime functioning to make the diagnosis.[3,4,13]

Polysomnographic Findings

Polysomnographic (PSG) evaluation of self-defined insomniacs reveal more impairments of sleep continuity parameters (i.e., longer sleep latencies, more time awake after sleep onset, lower sleep efficiency) and reduced total sleep time compared to self-defined good sleepers. Sleep architecture shows increased amount of stage 1, reduced

---

TABLE 26–1 DSM-IV-TR Diagnostic Criteria for Primary Insomnia

- A subjective complaint of difficulties initiating or maintaining sleep, or nonrestorative sleep.
- Duration of insomnia is longer than 1 month.
- The sleep disturbance (or associated daytime fatigue) causes clinically significant distress or impairment in social, occupational, or other important areas of functioning.
- The sleep disturbance does not occur exclusively in the context of another mental or sleep disorder, and is not the direct physiologic effect of a substance or a general medical condition.

DSM-IV-TR, Diagnostic and Statistical Manual of Mental Disorders, Fourth Edition, Text Revision.

---

stages 3 and 4, and more frequent stage shifts through the night. Interestingly, sleep disturbances recorded in primary insomniacs are similar to those observed in patients with generalized anxiety disorder or some affective disorders such as dysthymia,[14–16] perhaps suggesting a common underlying thread to these conditions. In addition, there is a significant overlap in the sleep patterns of subjectively defined insomniacs and good sleepers such that some insomniacs may show better objective sleep than good sleepers and some good sleepers more sleep impairments than insomniacs. Investigations of the microstructure of sleep reveal increased beta activity in primary insomniacs relative to healthy controls, both around the sleep onset period and during non–rapid eye movement (NREM) sleep.[17–19] These data are consistent with the presumed role of attentional processes and information processing,[20–22] as well as with psychological findings of hypervigilance and a ruminative, worry-prone cognitive style among insomniacs.

Daytime Complaints and Findings

Along with subjective complaints of poor sleep, most patients with insomnia also report significant impairments of their daytime functioning, involving fatigue and difficulties with attention and concentration, memory, and completion of tasks.[23] Patients may initially report excessive daytime sleepiness, but a closer investigation usually reveals mental and physical fatigue rather than true physiologic sleepiness, which is more likely among patients with insomnia comorbid with another medical (e.g., pain) or sleep (e.g., sleep-related breathing disorders) disorder. Insomniacs have trouble sleeping at night, in part because of a chronic state of hyperarousal, which may also interfere with the ability or propensity for sleep during the day.

Objective evaluation of daytime performance with neurobehavioral measures usually reveals fairly mild and selective performance deficits (e.g., attention).[24] In general, performance impairments on these measures are more strongly associated with subjective than with objective sleep disturbances. Individuals with insomnia tend to have lower expectations and to perceive their performance as significantly impaired relative to what they should be able to accomplish, and as more impaired than that of normal controls. Discrepancies between actual and expected performance, and between subjective and objective performance, are similar to those observed between subjective and objective measures of sleep. Such divergence may reflect a generalized faulty appraisal of sleep and daytime functioning among individuals with insomnia.[25]

Collectively, these findings suggest that the subjective appraisal/perception of sleep and daytime functioning are partly modulated by psychological and cognitive factors that, in turn, are important determinants of insomnia complaints. These paradoxical findings illustrate the complexity of insomnia and why some individuals with insomnia symptoms do not complain about it, whereas others are dissatisfied with their sleep in the absence of significant evidence of sleep disturbances.

Comorbidity and Subtypes of Insomnia

There is extensive comorbidity between insomnia and psychiatric disorders, most notably with major depression and generalized anxiety disorder.[5,11,14,26,27] Comorbidity rates vary from 40% in population-based samples to nearly 50% in clinical samples from sleep disorders centers. Although current classifications of sleep disorders (ICSD and DSM-IV) make an essential distinction between primary and comorbid (secondary) insomnia, such distinction is not always easily made given the bidirectional relationship between insomnia and psychological symptoms and psychiatric syndromes.

The *Diagnostic and Statistical Manual of Mental Disorders, Fourth Edition* (DSM-IV) recognizes only one form of primary insomnia,[3] while the International Classification of Sleep Disorders (ICSD) distinguishes among three different subtypes: psychophysiologic, paradoxical, and idiopathic insomnia.[4] Psychophysiologic insomnia is presumed to result from the repeated pairings of situational (bed/bedroom) and temporal (bedtime) stimuli, normally associated with sleep, with conditioned arousal and insomnia. Such conditioning is more likely to develop among individuals with an increased psychological (worry-prone) and biological (hyperarousability) predisposition to insomnia. The sleep of individuals with psychophysiologic insomnia is more sensitive to daily stressors and is characterized by extensive night-to-night variability.[28] Sometimes, sleep is unexpectedly improved in a novel environment because the conditioned cues that keep a person awake at home are not present in that environment. For example, while the sleep of otherwise good sleepers is more disrupted during their first night of recording in the sleep laboratory (i.e., first-night effect), insomniacs may actually sleep better during their first night in the laboratory (i.e., reverse first-night effect).

Paradoxical insomnia involves a genuine complaint of poor sleep that is not corroborated by objective findings. A patient may perceive very little sleep (e.g., 2–3 hr/night), whereas PSG recordings show normal or near-normal sleep duration and quality. This condition is not the result of an underlying psychiatric disorder or of malingering. To some degree, all insomniacs tend to overestimate the time it takes them to fall asleep and to underestimate the time they actually sleep. In paradoxical insomnia, however, the subjective complaint of poor sleep is disproportionate to available objective findings. This condition is probably due to several factors, including the lack of sensitivity of electroencephalographic (EEG) measures and the influence of cognitive (information processing) and psychological variables during sleep. It may also represent the far end of a continuum of individual differences in sleep perception. Paradoxical insomnia may also be a prodromal phase for more objectively verifiable insomnia.[29]

Idiopathic (childhood) insomnia presents with an insidious onset during childhood, unrelated to psychological trauma or medical disorders, and is very persistent throughout adult life. It does not show the variability observed with other forms of primary insomnia. A mild defect of the basic neurologic sleep/wake mechanisms may be a predisposing factor—a hypothesis that comes from the observations that patients with this condition often have a history of learning disabilities, attention-deficit/hyperactivity disorder, or similar conditions associated with minimal brain dysfunctions. Despite the presence of daytime sequelae (e.g., concentration and motivational difficulties), and the evidence that sleep disturbance is more severe than in psychophysiologic insomnia, individuals with idiopathic insomnia often report less emotional distress than those with the psychophysiologic subtype, perhaps due to coping mechanisms they have developed over their lifetime.

Course and Prognosis

Insomnia can begin at any time during the course of the life span, but onset of the first episode is more common in young adulthood. It is often precipitated by stressful life events, such as marital separation, occupational or family stress, and interpersonal conflicts.[30,31] In a small subset of cases, insomnia begins in childhood, in the absence of psychological or medical problems, and persists throughout adulthood.[32] Insomnia is a frequent problem among women during menopause and often persists even after other symptoms (e.g., hot flashes) have resolved. Insomnia may also have a late-life onset, but this needs to be distinguished from "normal" age-related changes in sleep and from sleep disturbances due to health-related problems.

Potential risk factors for insomnia include female gender, advancing age, a worry-prone cognitive style, hyperarousal, and a past history of insomnia.[33,34] For most individuals, insomnia is transient in nature, lasting a few days and resolving itself once the initial precipitating event has subsided (Fig. 26–1). For others, perhaps those more vulnerable to sleep disturbances, insomnia may persist long after the initial triggering event has disappeared; other factors would then perpetuate sleep disturbances.[35] The course of insomnia may also be intermittent, with repeated brief episodes of sleep difficulties following a close association with the occurrence of stressful events.[36] Even when insomnia has developed a chronic course, there is typically extensive night-to-night variability in sleep patterns, with an occasional restful night's sleep intertwined with several nights of poor sleep.[28] The subtype of insomnia (i.e., sleep-onset or sleep-maintenance insomnia) may also change over time.[37] Although there is

THE COURSE OF INSOMNIA

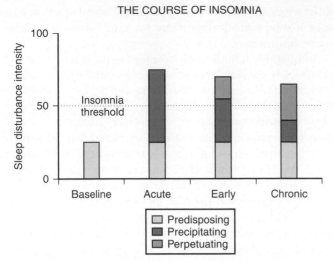

FIGURE 26–1 Illustration of a conceptual model of insomnia showing that three types of factors are involved during the course of insomnia. *(Reprinted with permission from Spielman AJ, Glovinsky PB. The varied nature of insomnia. In PJ Hauri [ed], Case Studies in Insomnia. New York: Plenum Press, 1991:1.)*

little information about its natural history, the prognosis for insomnia varies across individuals and is probably mediated by a combination of biologically related predisposing factors and psychological and behavioral perpetuating factors. It may also be complicated by the presence of comorbid psychiatric or medical disorders.

Etiology and Pathophysiology

Hyperarousal is considered the central feature of insomnia. Hyperarousal can be a state that is conditioned to sleep-related stimuli or a more enduring feature present throughout the 24-hour period. It is likely that both biological and psychological factors contribute to increase arousal and interfere with normal initiation and maintenance of sleep.

Biological Basis

Evidence of hyperarousal in insomnia is derived primarily from cross-sectional studies using different physiologic, hormonal, and EEG markers (see Perlis et al.[38]). For instance, numerous studies have reported increased body temperature, galvanic skin response, heart rate, and metabolic rate, both near sleep onset and during sleep, among individuals with insomnia relative to healthy good sleepers.[39] Studies using quantitative EEG techniques and evoked potential studies have also shown increased high-frequency (beta) activity during NREM sleep and higher amplitude of P300 responses in insomnia.[18,19,21,22] Neuroendocrine studies have yielded more mixed results, with some findings suggesting increased cortisol and adrenocorticotropic hormone levels during sleep and throughout the 24-hour period,[40,41] and other findings failing to reveal significant differences between insomniacs and good sleepers.[42] A recent neuroimaging study revealed increased cerebral glucose metabolic rates during wakefulness and NREM sleep in insomniacs compared to healthy controls.[43] Insomnia patients also exhibited smaller declines in glucose metabolism from wakefulness to sleep in wake-promoting brain areas such as the ascending reticular activating system. Another small magnetic resonance imaging study has shown reduced hippocampal volumes in primary insomniacs relative to health controls.[44]

Psychological Basis

Psychological and behavioral factors also play an important role in the development and maintenance of insomnia, as evidenced by higher levels of presleep cognitive arousal (e.g., intrusive thoughts, worries) and general psychological reactivity among individuals with insomnia relative to good sleepers. Insomniacs also tend to present an anxiety-prone personality style that may predispose them to worry more about sleep. Life events contribute to trigger insomnia, but it is often the reduced ability to cope with daily stressors, combined with increased cognitive arousal at bedtime, that leads to sleep disturbances.[45]

Learning and conditioning are also involved in the maintenance or exacerbation of sleep disturbances. While insomnia may initially be precipitated by stressful life events, a negative association often develops between sleeplessness and temporal (bedtime) and environmental (bed/bedroom) stimuli previously associated with sleep. This conditioned arousal may develop more rapidly among individuals already more vulnerable to insomnia. Over time, the combination of maladaptive sleep habits (e.g., napping, excessive amounts of time spent in bed) and sleep-related cognitions (e.g., unrealistic sleep expectations, worry about the consequences of insomnia, sleep-related monitoring) may exacerbate or perpetuate what might otherwise have been a transient sleep problem[33,45,46] (see Fig. 26–1). This process may contribute to heighten physiologic arousal at bedtime.

Although it remains unclear whether hyperarousal is a direct cause, a covariation, or even a consequence of insomnia, it remains a central feature in the pathophysiology of insomnia. Along with a reduced homeostatic sleep drive,[47] it is likely to arise from the interaction of biologically based predisposing factors and psychologically based exacerbating factors.

EVALUATION AND DIFFERENTIAL DIAGNOSIS

The diagnosis of insomnia is derived primarily from a detailed clinical evaluation of the patient's subjective complaint. The sleep history should cover the type of complaint (initial, middle, late insomnia), its duration (acute vs. chronic) and course (recurrent, persistent), typical sleep schedule, exacerbating and alleviating factors, perceived consequences and functional impairments, and the presence of medical, psychiatric, or environmental contributing factors. A complete history of alcohol and drug use and prescribed and over-the-counter medications is also essential.[33,48,49] Although PSG is not indicated for the routine evaluation of insomnia, it is often necessary to rule out other sleep disorders that might contribute to the insomnia complaint (e.g., periodic movements during sleep; sleep apnea).[50] Polysomnography can also be particularly useful in suspected case of paradoxical insomnia or when a patient is unresponsive to treatment.

The use of a sleep diary is essential in the evaluation of insomnia. The patient should keep a daily sleep diary for at least 1 week before initiating and throughout the course of treatment. The diary is useful to document initial insomnia severity, identify behavioral and scheduling factors that may perpetuate insomnia, and monitor treatment compliance and progress. Several additional patient-reported measures of insomnia symptoms, fatigue, anxiety, and depressive symptomatology may also provide useful complementary information in the evaluation of insomnia.[48] A more comprehensive psychological evaluation may be necessary for patients with suspected psychiatric disorders.

The role of actigraphy in insomnia evaluation and treatment monitoring is not well established. In the clinical context, actigraphy is not indicated for routine assessment, diagnosis, or management of insomnia, although it may represent a useful adjunct.[48,51] In the research environment, actigraphy is useful for examining night-to-night variability and for identifying individuals with circadian rhythm disorders. It has also been used to document treatment adherence and outcome in clinical trials of behavioral therapies for insomnia.[52] Although actigraphy is a potentially useful objective measure to complement self-report and PSG measures, not all actigraphy devices or algorithms are equivalent, and there may be significant variability in the reliability and validity of sleep/wake data derived from different devices.

Primary insomnia is a diagnosis made by exclusion. Thus, the differential diagnosis of primary insomnia requires the ruling out of several other conditions, including psychiatric (depression and anxiety), medical (pain), circadian (phase-delay syndrome), or other sleep-related (restless legs syndrome/periodic limb movement disorder, sleep-related breathing disorder) disorders. While the essential clinical features of insomnia are often similar for primary and comorbid insomnia, in primary insomnia, the sleep disturbance does not occur exclusively during the course of another sleep disorder or mental disorder and is not due to the direct physiologic effects of a substance or a general medical condition (see Table 26–1). A diagnosis of comorbid insomnia is made when the sleep disturbance is judged to be related temporally and causally to another psychiatric, medical, or sleep disorder,[3,4] although this judgment may sometimes be challenging.[53]

In clinical practice, the main differential diagnosis is usually between primary insomnia and insomnia comorbid with anxiety (generalized anxiety disorder [GAD]) or depression (dysthymia or major depression). This distinction is not always clear as several symptoms (e.g., sleep disturbance, fatigue, mood and cognitive problems) overlap among those conditions. Excessive worrying is the predominant feature of GAD; this characteristic is also present in primary insomnia, but its main focus is limited to insomnia and its potential consequences, whereas in GAD worrying is about multiple sources (e.g., health, family, work). In depression, the predominant clinical feature is sadness and a significant loss of interest. In primary insomnia, the interest is present but there is a lack of energy or fatigue, presumably resulting from sleep disturbances, preventing the individual from engaging in potentially pleasurable activities or social interactions. In addition to the nature of the symptoms, the history should also identify relative onset and course of each condition in order to determine whether insomnia is primary or secondary in nature.

TREATMENT

The first step in treating symptomatic insomnia is to identify and remove the contributing factors. General sleep hygiene recommendations are also useful as preventative strategies. Then, insomnia-specific therapies include psychological and behavioral interventions, medications, and a variety of complementary and alternative therapies (e.g., acupuncture, yoga, herbal therapies). This section focuses on psychological/behavioral and pharmacologic therapies; despite their increased popularity, most of the alternative therapies have not received adequate research evaluation in the management of insomnia.

Psychological and Behavioral Therapies

Treatment Goals and Indications

Psychological and behavioral therapies for insomnia include sleep restriction, stimulus control therapy, relaxation-based interventions, cognitive strategies, sleep hygiene education, and combined cognitive-behavioral therapy. A summary of those interventions is provided below and in Table 26–2; more extensive descriptions are available in other sources.[33] The main objectives of psychological and behavioral approaches are to alter those factors that perpetuate or exacerbate sleep disturbances. Such features may include hyperarousal, poor sleep habits, irregular sleep-wake schedules, and misconceptions about sleep and the consequences of insomnia. Although numerous factors can precipitate insomnia, when it becomes a persistent problem, psychological and behavioral factors are almost always involved in perpetuating it over time, hence the need to target those factors directly in treatment.[35] Another implicit goal of psychological treatment is to teach

TABLE 26–2 Psychological and Behavioral Treatments for Primary Insomnias

Therapy	Description
Stimulus control therapy	A set of instructions designed to strengthen the association between the bed/bedroom and sleep and to re-establish a consistent sleep/wake schedule: 1. Go to bed only when sleepy. 2. Get out of bed when unable to sleep. 3. Use the bed/bedroom for sleep only (no reading, watching TV, etc.). 4. Arise at the same time every morning. 5. No napping.
Sleep restriction therapy	A method designed to restrict time spent in bed as close as possible to the actual sleep time, thereby producing mild sleep deprivation. Time in bed is then gradually increased over a period of a few days/weeks until optimal sleep duration is achieved.
Relaxation training	Clinical procedures aimed at reducing somatic tension (e.g., progressive muscle relaxation, autogenic training) or intrusive thoughts (e.g., imagery training, meditation) interfering with sleep. Most relaxation requires some professional guidance initially and daily practice over a period of a few weeks.
Cognitive therapy	Psychotherapeutic method aimed at reducing worry and changing faulty beliefs and misconceptions about sleep, insomnia, and daytime consequences. Other cognitive strategies can also be used to control intrusive thoughts at bedtime and reduce excessive monitoring of the daytime consequences of insomnia.
Sleep hygiene education	General guidelines about health practices (e.g., diet, exercise, substance use) and environmental factors (e.g., light, noise, temperature) that may promote or interfere with sleep. This may also include some basic information about normal sleep and changes in sleep patterns with aging.
Cognitive behavioral therapy	A combination of any of the above-listed behavioral (e.g., stimulus control, sleep restriction, relaxation) and cognitive procedures.

patients self-management skills to cope more adaptively with residual sleep disturbances that may persist after therapy. The primary indication for behavioral treatment is in the management of persistent insomnia, with evidence available for both primary and comorbid insomnia.

Description of Therapies

Sleep Restriction. Poor sleepers often increase their time in bed in a misguided effort to provide more opportunity for sleep, a strategy that is more likely to result in fragmented and poor-quality sleep. Sleep restriction consists of curtailing the amount of time spent in bed to the actual amount of sleep.[54] For example, if a person reports sleeping an average of 6 hours per night out of 8 hours spent in bed, the initial "sleep window" (i.e., from initial bedtime to final arising time) would be set at 6 hours.

Subsequent adjustments to this sleep window are based on sleep efficiency (SE) for a given period of time (usually the preceding week); time in bed is increased by about 20 minutes for a given week when SE exceeds 85%, decreased by the same amount of time when SE is lower than 80%, and kept stable when SE falls between 80% and 85%. Periodic (weekly) adjustments are made until optimal sleep duration is achieved. Changes to the prescribed sleep window can be made at the beginning of the night (i.e., postponing bedtime), at the end of the sleep period (i.e., advancing arising time), or at both ends. To prevent excessive daytime sleepiness, time in bed should not be reduced to less than 5 hours per night. This procedure leads to improvements of sleep continuity through a mild sleep deprivation and reduction of sleep anticipatory anxiety. Caution is needed when using sleep restriction with patients operating heavy equipments or required to drive long distances (e.g., truck drivers).

Stimulus Control Therapy. Individuals with insomnia often become apprehensive around bedtime and come to associate the bedroom with frustration and arousal rather than with sleep. Stimulus control therapy[55] consists of a set of instructions designed to reassociate temporal (bedtime) and environmental (bed and bedroom) stimuli with rapid sleep onset and to establish a regular circadian sleep-wake rhythm. These instructions are (1) go to bed only when sleepy; (2) get out of bed when unable to sleep (e.g., after 20 min), go to another room, and return to bed only when sleep is imminent; (3) curtail all sleep-incompatible activities (i.e., no TV watching, problem solving in bed); (4) arise at a regular time every morning regardless of the amount of sleep the night before; and (5) avoid daytime napping. Despite the straightforward nature of these behavioral recommendations, the main challenge for most patients is to comply with all of them, which is essential to reverse the conditioning processes perpetuating insomnia.

Relaxation-Based Interventions. Relaxation is the most commonly used nondrug therapy for insomnia. Among the available relaxation-based interventions, some methods (e.g., progressive muscle relaxation) focus primarily on reducing somatic arousal (e.g., muscle tension), whereas attention-focusing procedures (e.g., imagery training, meditation) target mental arousal in the form of worries, intrusive thoughts, or a racing mind. Most of these methods are equally effective for treating insomnia. The most critical issue is to practice diligently and daily the selected method for at least 2–4 weeks. Professional guidance is often necessary in the initial phase of training.

Cognitive Therapy. Cognitive therapy is a psychotherapeutic method that seeks to alter dysfunctional sleep cognitions (e.g., beliefs, expectations, attributions) and maladaptive cognitive processes (e.g., excessive self-monitoring) through Socratic questioning and behavioral experiments. The basic premise of this approach is that appraisal of a given situation (sleeplessness) and excessive monitoring of sleep-related cues (e.g., fatigue, heart rate, time) can trigger an emotional response (fear, anxiety) that is incompatible with sleep. For example, when a person is unable to sleep at night and worries about the possible consequences of sleep loss on the next day's performance, this can set off a spiral reaction and feed into the vicious cycle of insomnia, emotional distress, and more sleep disturbances. Cognitive therapy is designed to identify dysfunctional cognitions and reframe them into more adaptive substitutes in order to short-circuit the self-fulfilling nature of this vicious cycle. Treatment targets may include unrealistic expectations ("I must get my 8 hours of sleep every night"), faulty causal attributions ("my insomnia is entirely due to a biochemical imbalance"), and amplification of the consequences of insomnia ("Insomnia may have serious consequences on my health").[33] Cognitive therapy is particularly useful to modify these maladaptive cognitions and to teach patients more adaptive skills to cope with insomnia.

Sleep Hygiene Education. Sleep hygiene education is intended to provide information about lifestyle (diet, exercise, substance use) and environmental (light, noise, temperature) factors that may either interfere with or promote better sleep. General sleep hygiene guidelines include (1) avoiding stimulants (e.g., caffeine) several hours before bedtime; (2) avoiding alcohol around bedtime, as it fragments sleep; (3) exercising regularly (especially in the late afternoon or early evening), as it may deepen sleep; (4) allowing at least a 1-hour period to unwind before bedtime; and (5) keeping the bedroom environment quiet, dark, and comfortable.[56] In addition to these guidelines, it is useful to provide basic information about normal sleep, individual differences in sleep needs, and changes in sleep physiology over the course of the life span. This information is particularly useful to help some patients distinguish clinical insomnia from short-sleep or normal (age-related) sleep disturbances. Although inadequate sleep hygiene is rarely the primary cause of insomnia, it may potentiate sleep difficulties caused by other factors or interfere with treatment progress. Addressing these factors should be an integral part of insomnia management, even though it is rarely sufficient for more severe insomnia, which often requires more directive and potent behavioral interventions.

Outcome Evidence

Evidence for Efficacy. Several meta-analyses[57–59] and systematic reviews commissioned by the American Academy of Sleep Medicine[52,60] have summarized the findings from clinical trials evaluating the efficacy of psychological and behavioral therapies for persistent insomnia. Evidence from these different sources shows that treatment produces reliable changes in several sleep parameters, including sleep-onset latency (effect sizes ranging from 0.41 to 1.05), number of awakenings (0.25–0.83), duration of awakenings (0.61–1.03), total sleep time (0.15–0.49), and sleep quality ratings (0.94–1.14). Based on Cohen's criteria, the magnitude of those therapeutic effects is large (i.e., $d > 0.8$) for sleep latency and sleep quality and moderate (i.e., $d > 0.5$) for other sleep parameters. When transformed into a percentile rank, these data indicate that approximately 70–80% of patients with insomnia benefit from psychological and behavioral treatments.

In terms of absolute changes, treatment reduces subjective sleep-onset latency and time awake after sleep onset from averages of 60–70 minutes at baseline to about 35 minutes post-treatment, and total sleep time is increased by 30 minutes, from 6 to 6.5 hours, after treatment. Thus, for the average insomnia patient, treatment effects may be expected to reduce sleep latency and time awake after sleep onset by about 50% and to bring the absolute values of those sleep parameters below or near the 30-minute cutoff criterion initially used to define insomnia. Treatment effects are similar for sleep-onset and sleep-maintenance problems, although fewer studies have targeted the latter type, and particularly early morning awakening problems. Overall, findings from meta-analyses represent fairly conservative estimates of treatment effects as they are based on averages computed across all nonpharmacologic interventions and insomnia diagnoses (i.e., primary and secondary). However, although the majority of patients benefit from treatment, only a small proportion (20–30%) of them achieves full remission, and a significant proportion of patients continue experiencing residual sleep disturbances.[60]

Treatment outcome has been documented primarily with prospective daily sleep diaries, although several studies have also complemented those findings with data from PSG[61–63] and with wrist actigraphy.[62,64,65] In general, the magnitude of improvements is smaller on PSG measures, but those changes tend to parallel sleep improvements reported on daily sleep diaries. Polysomnographic findings indicate that treatment does not only alter sleep perception, as measured by patient-reported outcomes, but also produces objective changes on EEG sleep continuity measures. Except for a modest increase in stages 3 and 4 following sleep restriction, there is little evidence of changes in sleep architecture with psychological and behavioral treatment.

Long-Term Outcomes. A fairly robust finding across behavioral treatment studies is that sleep improvements are well maintained over time, with data available up to 24 and even 36 months after treatment completion.[60,66] Although interventions that restrict the amount of time spent in bed may yield only modest increases (and even a reduction) of sleep time during the initial treatment period, this parameter is usually improved at follow-ups, with total sleep time often exceeding 6.5 hours. Long-term outcome must be interpreted cautiously, however, as few studies report long-term follow-ups and, among those that do, attrition rates increase over time. In addition, a substantial proportion of those patients with chronic insomnia who benefit from short-term therapy may remain vulnerable to recurrent episodes of insomnia in the long term. As such, there is a need to develop and evaluate the effects of long-term, maintenance therapies to prevent or minimize the occurrence of those episodes.[67]

Treatment of Comorbid Insomnia. Insomnia is often a pervasive problem among patients suffering from other medical and psychiatric conditions. Although the comorbid condition may subside with appropriate treatment, sleep disturbances often persist. Until recently, most treatment studies had focused on primary insomnia in otherwise healthy, young, and medication-free patients. Evidence from clinical case series,[68–70] suggests that patients with medical and psychiatric conditions can also benefit from insomnia-specific treatment, even though the outcome with those patients is more modest than with those who suffer from primary insomnia.[71] Controlled studies have also shown that cognitive behavioral therapy (CBT) is effective for treating insomnia associated with chronic pain,[72] fibromyalgia,[73] cancer,[74] and various medical conditions in older adults.[75,76] In general, insomnia symptoms are more severe among patients with comorbid disorders, but the absolute changes on those outcomes during treatment are comparable to those obtained by patients with primary insomnia.

Studies have also shown that older adults respond to insomnia treatment, particularly when they are screened for other sleep disorders that may increase in incidence in older age (e.g., restless legs syndrome, sleep apnea). A meta-analysis[77] suggested that effect sizes were comparable (moderate to large) for middle-aged and older adults on subjective measures of sleep latency, wake after sleep onset, and sleep quality. There is also increasing evidence that older adults with comorbid medical or psychological conditions can benefit from sleep-specific treatment.[75,76,78–80] Three clinical trials have shown that a supervised, structured, and time-limited withdrawal program, with or without psychological treatment, can facilitate discontinuation of hypnotic medications among older adults with insomnia who are prolonged users.[78,81,82]

Combined Therapies. Although there are several distinct psychological and behavioral therapies for insomnia, these interventions can be effectively combined together. An update of the evidence-based literature revealed a clear trend among investigators and clinicians for combining multiple interventions, with CBT becoming the standard approach in the field.[52] The most common combination involves a behavioral (stimulus control, sleep restriction, and, sometimes, relaxation), a cognitive, and an educational (sleep hygiene) component, usually referred to as CBT. Although there has been no complete dismantling of CBT to isolate the relative efficacy of each component, direct comparisons of some of those components indicate that sleep restriction, alone or combined with stimulus control therapy, is more effective than relaxation, which, in turn, is more effective than sleep hygiene education alone.[52,57,58] Sleep restriction tends to produce better outcome than stimulus control for improving sleep efficiency and sleep continuity, but it also decreases total sleep time during the initial intervention. Although some basic education about sleep hygiene is incorporated in most insomnia treatments, sleep hygiene education produces little impact on sleep when used as the only intervention. A study has shown that cognitive therapy alone can be effective in the management of insomnia.[83]

There is no strong evidence that a multicomponent approach is more effective than any of its single components. However, the appeal for this multimodal approach may come from the fact that it addresses different facets presumed to perpetuate sleep disturbances.[33,35,45] While little information is available about the active treatment mechanisms of CBT, some evidence suggest that stimulus control and sleep restriction are particularly effective for improving sleep continuity, whereas changes in sleep-related cognitions are associated with better maintenance of sleep changes over time.[84] With increasing evidence that hyperarousal is implicated in primary insomnia, there is a need for greater attention to identify the biological, as well as the psychological, mechanisms responsible for sleep changes.

Combined Behavioral and Pharmacologic Approaches

Behavioral and pharmacologic therapies can play a complementary role in the management of insomnia. There are some practical and clinical reasons for considering combining therapies. For example, no single treatment is effective with all forms of insomnia or acceptable to all patients. Even among treatment responders, few patients reach complete remission and some residual sleep disturbances often persist even after treatment. Thus, combined approaches should theoretically optimize outcome by capitalizing on the more immediate and potent effects of hypnotics and the more sustained effects of behavioral interventions.

Only a few studies have directly compared the effects of behavioral and pharmacologic therapies for insomnia. Three studies compared triazolam to relaxation[85,86] or sleep hygiene,[64] and four other investigations compared CBT to temazepam,[61] zolpidem,[87] or zopiclone.[88,89] Collectively, findings from these studies indicate that both therapies are effective in the short term (4–8 weeks), with medication producing faster results in the acute phase (first week) of treatment. Combined interventions appear to have a slight advantage over single-treatment modalities during the initial course of treatment, but it is unclear whether this advantage persists over time. Long-term effects are consistent for the single-treatment modalities; patients treated with CBT maintain their improvements, whereas therapeutic effects are typically lost after discontinuation of medication. Long-term effects of combined interventions are more equivocal. Some studies indicate that a combined intervention (i.e., triazolam plus relaxation) produces more sustained benefits than medication alone,[85,86] whereas others report more variable long-term outcomes.[61,64] Some patients retain their initial sleep improvements but others return to their baseline values. As behavioral and attitudinal changes are often essential to sustain sleep improvements, patients' attributions of the initial benefits may be critical in determining long-term outcomes. Attribution of therapeutic benefits to the hypnotic alone, without integration of self-management skills, may place a patient at greater risk for recurrence of insomnia once medication is discontinued. Thus, despite the intuitive appeal of combining behavioral and medication therapies, it is not entirely clear when, how, and for whom it is indicated to combine these treatment modalities for insomnia. Additional research is needed to evaluate the effects of combined treatments and to examine optimal methods for integrating these therapies.

Comparisons of effect sizes from meta-analyses[57,59,90] on different sleep variables indicate that behavioral therapy may have a slight advantage on measures of sleep-onset latency and sleep quality and pharmacotherapy (benzodiazepine receptor agonists) a more favorable outcome on total sleep time. One study examined different sequences of CBT and medication therapies.[89] The best results were obtained when CBT was introduced first in the sequence, but medication was found helpful to improve total sleep time, which may be an important advantage given that one component of CBT (i.e., sleep restriction) reduces total sleep time during the initial course of therapy and could lead some patients to premature therapy discontinuation.

Until more evidence-based treatment guidelines become available, several strategies can be considered for selecting the most appropriate treatment in the clinical management of insomnia. The use of hypnotic medication may be particularly indicated in the initial stage of therapy to break the vicious cycle of insomnia and to provide some rapid relief. However, CBT is essential to alter perpetuating factors and to teach coping skills. As such, it is a crucial treatment component to maximize durability of sleep improvements. Ideally, hypnotic medications should be discontinued, under supervision, after an initial treatment course of a few weeks. However, given that insomnia may be a recurrent problem, even among those who benefit from treatment initially, it may be necessary to use medications intermittently after the initial acute treatment phase.

Pharmacotherapy

Several different classes of medications are used for insomnia (Table 26–3), including both over-the-counter (OTC) and prescription agents; however, many of these

TABLE 26–3 Drugs Used to Promote Sleep

Drug	Dose Range (Dose Range in Elderly)*	Half-life (hr)	Effects on Sleep	Adverse Effects
Benzodiazepine Receptor Agonists				
Benzodiazepines				
Triazolam	0.25–0.5 mg (0.125–0.25 mg)	1.5–5.5	All: increased total sleep time, % stage 2, REM latency.	Dizziness, drowsiness, hypokinesia, dyskinesia, abnormal or impaired coordination, slurred speech, ataxia, amnesia, GI symptoms.
Temazepam	7.5–30 mg (7.5 mg)	6–16	All: decreased sleep latency, WASO, % stage 1, % SWS, % REM	
Estazolam	1–2 mg (0.5 mg)	10–24		Rebound/withdrawal effects more pronounced with shorter acting agents.
Quazepam	7.5–15 mg (7.5 mg)	For quazepam and 2-oxoquazepam, 25–41; *N*-desakyl-1-oxoquazepam, 70–75		
Flurazepam	15–30 mg (15 mg)	47–100		
Nonbenzodiazepines				
Zaleplon	10–20 mg (5–10 mg)	1	All: decreased sleep latency	All: dizziness, drowsiness, amnesia, GI symptoms. Zaleplon: myalgia and headache.
Zolpidem	10 mg (5 mg)	1.4–4.5		
Zolpidem CR	6.25–12.5 mg (6.25 mg)	2.8	Zolpidem CR: decreased WASO during first 6 hr.	
Eszopiclone	2–3 mg (1–2 mg)	5–5.8	Eszopiclone: decreased WASO.	Eszopiclone: unpleasant taste, dry mouth.

Continued

TABLE 26–3 Drugs Used to Promote Sleep—Cont'd

Drug	Dose Range (Dose Range in Elderly)*	Half-life (hr)	Effects on Sleep	Adverse Effects
Melatonin Receptor Agonist				
Ramelteon	8 mg (8 mg)	2.6	Sleep latency: ↓	Drowsiness, dizziness, fatigue. Do not use with fluvoxamine, ketoconazole, or fluconazole.
Antidepressants				
Amitriptyline	50–100 mg (20 mg)	10–28, including the metabolite nortriptyline	Total sleep time: ↑ Sleep latency: ↓ % Stage 2: ↑	Drowsiness, dizziness, confusion, blurred vision, dry mouth, constipation, urinary retention, arrhythmias, orthostatic hypotension, weight gain. Exacerbation of restless legs syndrome, periodic limb movement disorder, or REM sleep behavior disorder.
Doxepin	75–100 mg (25–50 mg)	8–24	% REM: ↓ REM latency: ↑	
Mirtazapine	15–45 mg (7.5–15 mg)	20–40	Total sleep time: ↑ Sleep latency: ↓ WASO: ↓	Drowsiness, dizziness, increased appetite, constipation, weight gain, agranulocytosis (rare).
Trazodone	150–400 mg (150 mg)	7	Sleep latency: ↓ WASO: ↓ % SWS: ↑	Drowsiness, dizziness, headache, blurred vision, dry mouth, arrhythmias, orthostatic hypotension, priapism.
Anticonvulsants				
Gabapentin	300–600 mg (300 mg)	5–7	WASO: ↔ to ↓ % SWS: ↑	Drowsiness, dizziness, emotional lability, ataxia, tremor, blurred vision, diplopia, nystagmus, myalgia, peripheral edema.
Tiagabine	4–8 mg (4 mg)	7–9	WASO: ↓ % SWS: ↑	Drowsiness, dizziness, ataxia, tremor, new-onset seizures in patients without epilepsy, difficulty with concentration or attention, nervousness, asthenia, abdominal pain, diarrhea, nausea.
Pregabalin	50–100 mg (25–50 mg)	6	Sleep latency: ↓ % SWS: ↑	Drowsiness, dizziness, ataxia, confusion, peripheral edema.
Antipsychotics				
Olanzapine	5–10 mg (5 mg)	21–54	Sleep latency: ↔ to ↓ WASO: ↓ % SWS: ↑ % REM: ↔ to ↓	Drowsiness, dizziness, tremor, agitation, asthenia, extrapyramidal symptoms, dry mouth, dyspepsia, constipation, orthostatic hypotension, weight gain, new-onset diabetes mellitus, tardive dyskinesia, neuroleptic malignant syndrome.
Quetiapine	25–200 mg (25 mg)	6	Insufficient data	
Over-the-Counter Agents				
Diphenhydramine	50 mg diphenhydramine chloride 76 mg diphenhydramine citrate (25 mg)	2.4–9.3	Sleep latency: ↓ WASO: ↔ to ↓ % SWS: ↔ to ↑ % REM: ↓	Drowsiness, dizziness, dyskinesias, dry mouth, epigastric distress, constipation. Tachycardia, risk of delirium, and falls in elderly.
Melatonin	Dosages not empirically determined.	0.5	Sleep latency: ↓	Concentration difficulty, dizziness, fatigue, headache, irritability.

*Doses listed are recommended maximum amounts for a single dose.

GI, gastrointestinal; REM, rapid eye movement; SWS, slow-wave sleep; WASO, wake after sleep onset; ↔, no change; ↑, increase; ↓, decrease.

are not approved by the U.S. Food and Drug Administration (FDA) for the treatment of insomnia. Current FDA-approved insomnia medications include a group of benzodiazepine receptor agonists (BZRAs) and one melatonin receptor agonist. Although not FDA approved for treatment of insomnia, sedating antidepressants have been prescribed widely; from 1987 to 1996, their use as sleep-inducing agents increased by almost 150%, whereas the use of FDA-approved hypnotics fell by over 50%.[91] As recently as 2002, three of the top four most commonly prescribed medications for insomnia were sedating antidepressants.[92] Other classes of prescription medications used with increasing frequency for their potential sleep-inducing side effects include anticonvulsants and atypical antipsychotics.

There are a number of likely reasons for the widespread use of nonapproved medications for insomnia. Until the introduction of eszopiclone in 2005, FDA labeling for all BZRA hypnotics stated that they were indicated for the short-term treatment of insomnia, preferably not for more than a few weeks, and it was recommended that patients be re-evaluated if drugs were to be used longer. Since chronic insomnia typically lasts for years,[93] this meant that those with chronic insomnia could only receive short-term treatment. In addition, concerns about tolerance, dependence, and abuse made physicians as well as patients reluctant to use these agents long term. Until the introduction of ramelteon in 2005, no FDA-approved hypnotics were nonscheduled. Antidepressants, anticonvulsants, and antipsychotics, in contrast, are nonscheduled substances and can be used long term. Furthermore, with the recognition that many insomnia patients have comorbid depression and/or anxiety, the use of an antidepressant might be appealing to treat the mood problem as well as the insomnia; the doses of antidepressants that are prescribed for insomnia, however, are almost always subtherapeutic for the treatment of depression. There is a relative lack of data showing that treatment of insomnia reduces any of its comorbidities, which is another possible barrier to the prescription of hypnotics; physicians may be discouraged from prescribing drugs that are perceived to have potential adverse effects.

More individuals with insomnia self-medicate than take prescription medications, and the fact that many individuals self-medicate for insomnia suggests that the disorder may be undertreated. Population-based studies have found that, over 12- to 18-month periods, 10–13% of people have used only alcohol to help them fall asleep and 10% have used OTC agents alone, whereas only 5–8% have used only prescription medications.[94,95] Polls by the National Sleep Foundation have found that 16–28% of adults have used alcohol and 22–29% have used OTC agents for sleep at some point during their lives.[96,97] In general, patients who self-medicate with alcohol or OTC agents tend to do so for shorter periods of time and have less severe insomnia than those who take prescription medications.[94]

Benzodiazepine Receptor Agonists

The current FDA-approved BZRAs for insomnia include the older benzodiazepines (estazolam, flurazepam, quazepam, temazepam, triazolam) and the newer nonbenzodiazepines (eszopiclone, zaleplon, zolpidem) (see Table 26–3). These medications all bind to the γ-aminobutyric acid (GABA) type A receptor complex. $GABA_A$ receptors are the predominant inhibitory receptors in the brain, and the binding of a BZRA leads to increased flow of negatively charged chloride ions into a neuron, making it less likely to fire an action potential. Benzodiazepines bind to all subtypes of $GABA_A$ receptors, whereas some of the newer nonbenzodiazepines, particularly zaleplon and zolpidem bind preferentially to the type I $GABA_A$ receptor. This different pattern of receptor binding affinity may be associated with slight differences in clinical effects. The type I receptor is thought to mediate both the hypnotic and amnestic effects of BZRAs, but drugs acting selectively on this receptor may be less effective as muscle relaxants or anxiolytics. Clinically, it is important to remember that all BZRAs have the potential to produce amnesia.

Benzodiazepines. Benzodiazepine hypnotics, with the exception of triazolam, have relatively long half-lives. Estazolam, flurazepam, quazepam, and temazepam all reduce latency to sleep onset and tend to improve sleep maintenance, as indicated by decreased waking time after sleep onset, reduced number of awakenings, and/or increased total sleep time.[98–104] Triazolam also promotes sleep onset, but because of its short half-life, does not appear to be as helpful for sleep maintenance.[105–107] Benzodiazepines decrease time spent in stage 1 sleep and increase stage 2 sleep, but they also tend to suppress slow-wave sleep and, possibly, rapid eye movement (REM) sleep. Adverse effects of benzodiazepine hypnotics include daytime sedation, cognitive and psychomotor impairment, and memory impairment[101,107]; such effects are more common with higher doses and longer acting agents. Abrupt withdrawal may be associated with rebound insomnia with triazolam as well as the longer acting agents.[105,108]

As noted earlier, benzodiazepine hypnotics are indicated for the short-term treatment of insomnia. None has been studied in a randomized clinical trial for more than 12 weeks,[109] so that long-term efficacy data are not available.

Nonbenzodiazepines. The nonbenzodiazepine BZRAs include those with short half-lives (zaleplon and zolpidem) that are indicated primarily for promoting sleep onset, and those with either a longer half-life (eszopiclone) or a controlled-release formulation (zolpidem MR) that reduce sleep latency and improve sleep maintenance. Zaleplon, with the shortest half-life of currently available agents at about 1 hour, may be dosed as long as the patient has at least 4 hours remaining in bed; 4–6 hours after ingestion of 10 or 20 mg of zaleplon, healthy volunteers did not demonstrate next-day impairment in driving ability, memory, or psychomotor function.[110] Although 5- to 10-mg doses of zaleplon primarily promote sleep onset, a dose of 20 mg increases subjective total sleep time.[111,112]

Zolpidem is currently the most commonly prescribed sleep agent. It is effective in promoting sleep onset, and also increases total sleep time at doses of 10 mg or greater in both subjective and sleep laboratory studies.[113] The increase in sleep efficiency and/or total sleep is likely due to reduced sleep latency, since consistent effects on waking time after sleep onset have not been observed. A 12-week, placebo-controlled study demonstrated that intermittent use (three to five times per week) of zolpidem was associated with continued benefit on the nights the drug was taken and no obvious evidence of rebound insomnia on the nights it was not taken.[114] Zolpidem has also been shown to be effective in subjects with depression treated with selective serotonin reuptake inhibitors (SSRIs), resulting in subjective increased total sleep and improved sleep quality and daytime function.[115] Doses of 10 mg of zolpidem administered during the night did not lead to clinically significant effects on driving or psychomotor skills the next day, at least 4–6 hours after ingestion, in healthy subjects or insomnia patients,[110,116] but higher doses produced significant impairment.[110] Zolpidem MR consists of a dual-layer tablet: a shell containing 7.5 mg of immediate-release zolpidem and a core containing 5 mg of zolpidem that is released in a delayed fashion for a total of 12.5 mg. There is also a 6.25-mg tablet containing 3.75 mg immediate-release/2.5 mg delayed-release zolpidem. The half-life of zolpidem MR remains short, but the duration of action is longer than with zolpidem, as evidenced by decreased waking time during hours 3–6 post-ingestion, presumably related to the higher blood levels. A double-blind, placebo-controlled multicenter study showed clinical efficacy with zolpidem MR at a dose of 12.5 mg for up to 6 months when taken for 3–7 nights per week, without significant rebound insomnia upon discontinuation.[117] Subjects who took medication reported shorter sleep onset latencies, improved sleep maintenance, and evidence of better next-day function as indicated by subjective reports of improved concentration and decreased morning sleepiness.

Eszopiclone was the first hypnotic to be indicated for the treatment of insomnia without recommendations for restricted duration of use. It has a longer half-life than any of the other nonbenzodiazepines, which accounts for its effects on improving sleep maintenance. In a 6-month placebo-controlled clinical trial, it showed persistent efficacy in reducing latency to sleep onset, decreasing wakefulness during sleep, and increasing total sleep time, as subjectively reported.[118] In another 6-month double-blind study, eszopiclone was shown not only to reduce insomnia, but also to enhance quality-of-life measures and reduce reported work limitations.[119] It is also one of the first agents for which data suggest improved daytime function and/or decreased comorbidity from other disorders. Elderly insomnia patients taking 2 mg of eszopiclone reported reduced daytime napping,[120] and depressed patients given a combination of fluoxetine plus eszopiclone had better sleep and higher rates of response and remission 8 weeks later in comparison to depressed patients given fluoxetine plus placebo.[121]

Outcome Evidence

Efficacy of BZRAs. Several meta-analyses have assessed the efficacy of BZRA hypnotics in comparison to placebo in the treatment of chronic insomnia. In a review of studies done on adults less than 65 years old, benzodiazepines and zolpidem were shown to produce significant subjective improvement in sleep latency, total sleep, number of awakenings, and sleep quality, with moderate effect sizes ranging from 0.56 to 0.71.[90] A meta-analysis of studies performed on adults and elderly adults showed that benzodiazepines produced significant improvements in both subjective and objective sleep parameters; sleep latency was reduced by 4.2 minutes objectively and 14.3 minutes subjectively, and total sleep amount was increased by 61.8 minutes objectively and 48.4 minutes subjectively.[101,122] Another analysis of drug effects in elderly insomnia patients showed significant improvement in sleep quality (effect size 0.14), increased total sleep (25.2 minutes), and decreased awakenings (effect size 0.63) with sedative use as compared with placebo.[123] A comparison of benzodiazepine hypnotics with nonbenzodiazepines concluded that zolpidem may show benefits over temazepam in terms of reducing sleep latency and improving sleep quality, and over zaleplon in terms of increasing sleep duration and improving sleep quality.[124] Zaleplon, however, may produce less rebound insomnia than zolpidem. This analysis was limited, however, by the lack of directly comparative studies and short durations of the studies, which makes it difficult to assess longer term effects.

BZRA Side Effects. A number of adverse outcomes have been associated with drugs in this class, whether benzodiazepines or nonbenzodiazepines. Sedation/daytime sleep "hangover" and impaired cognitive and psychomotor performance can be seen at peak blood levels, and may occur the following day with longer acting agents.[125] Anterograde amnesia, or loss of memory for events that occur after taking a hypnotic, is more common with higher doses and with drugs with rapidly increasing plasma levels (e.g., triazolam and the nonbenzodiazepines) or when BZRAs are used in combination with alcohol; confusional arousals or sleepwalking episodes may be a related phenomenon. BZRAs should therefore always be taken immediately prior to bedtime to minimize the risk of amnesia or parasomnias, and discontinued in patients who report these side effects.

All medications used for sleep, including BZRAs but also antidepressants and anticonvulsants, can increase the risk of nighttime falls in elderly patients.[126–128] However, insomnia is an independent predictor of falls in the elderly,[129] and a study has suggested that insomnia, but not hypnotic use, was associated with a greater risk of falls.[130] Other side effects associated with BZRAs include tolerance, rebound insomnia, abuse, and withdrawal. Although concerns about tolerance are likely a factor for physicians and patients in avoiding or limiting use of these agents, in fact the few longer term studies that have been performed with eszopiclone, zolpidem, and zaleplon have not shown evidence of obvious tolerance.[114,115,119,131] Rebound insomnia, or the worsening of insomnia to a degree greater than baseline, is generally seen for not more than 1–2 days, and not in all studies. Abuse of and dependence on BZRAs may occur in patients with histories of substance abuse, but the risk is generally overestimated for those without such histories; insomnia patients tend to show therapy-seeking, not drug-seeking, behavior.[132] Nevertheless, BZRAs should be avoided in those with tendencies to abuse substances.

An attempt to assess risks and benefits for BZRAs in the treatment of insomnia concluded that, although these agents improved sleep, they also led to adverse effects in comparison to placebo[101,122]; daytime drowsiness was increased by an odds ratio of 2.4 and dizziness or lightheadedness was increased by an odds ratio of 2.6. However, the increase in adverse events did not lead to increased rates of discontinuation of hypnotics. A study regarding the use of BZRAs in elderly insomnia patients, however, raised concerns that there were significant risks with both benzodiazepines and nonbenzodiazepines, including adverse cognitive events (4.78 times more common), adverse psychomotor events (2.61 times more common), and daytime fatigue (3.82 times more common).[123] The authors concluded that, in elderly patients, the risks of BZRAs might outweigh the benefits in some cases.

Indications and Limitations. The benzodiazepines zolpidem and zaleplon are indicated for "the short-term treatment of insomnia," whereas eszopiclone and zolpidem MR are indicated for "the treatment of insomnia," without language limiting duration of use. BzRAs should not be used during pregnancy (all are in FDA Pregnancy Category C) or in patients with histories of substance abuse. They should be used with caution in patients who have pulmonary or liver disease and in the elderly; dosage reductions at least are recommended in these populations. No hypnotics are approved for use in children under 18 years of age.

Melatonin and Melatonin Receptor Agonist

Melatonin, a hormone produced by the pineal gland, is available as an OTC preparation and has been widely used for insomnia and related sleep problems. Currently ramelteon is the only melatonin receptor agonist approved by the FDA for the treatment of insomnia and is available

by prescription. These agents presumably act through their effects on melatonin receptors in the suprachiasmatic nucleus in the brain, although their exact mechanism has not been determined.

Melatonin. OTC melatonin preparations are rapidly absorbed and have a short half-life (up to 1 hour). They are not regulated by the FDA and are thus not approved for treatment of insomnia. The hypnotic effects of melatonin appear to be relatively smaller in comparison to BZRAs; a meta-analysis concluded that the average decrease in sleep latency was 4 minutes, total sleep time was increased by 12.8 minutes, and sleep efficiency increased by 2.2%.[133] A more recent study of melatonin for secondary insomnia and circadian rhythm disorders (i.e., jet lag and shift work) failed to find any significant differences in comparison to placebo, except for a slight increase (1.9%) in sleep efficiency. Several studies, however, have demonstrated that low doses of melatonin (300–500 µg) were effective in producing phase shifts in normal subjects and entraining circadian rhythms in blind individuals.[134–136] Melatonin does not appear to have obvious side effects other than sedation.

Ramelteon. Ramelteon, currently the only FDA-approved hypnotic that is not a BZRA, is an agonist of melatonin type 1 (MT_1) and type 2 (MT_2) receptors and is structurally unrelated to melatonin; it does not show affinity for the GABA receptor complex or other receptors thought to be involved in sleep or wakefulness. It has a relatively short half-life (2.6 hours), and its metabolite also acts as an MT_1/MT_2 agonist. The most robust effects of ramelteon on sleep are the reduction of latency to sleep onset, but it has also been reported to increase total sleep time in some studies[137]; it does not appear to decrease wakefulness after sleep onset. Ramelteon is indicated for the treatment of insomnia characterized by difficulty with sleep onset. Its main side effects are somnolence, dizziness, and fatigue. Important distinctions from the BZRA class include no evidence of tolerance, withdrawal, rebound insomnia, cognitive or psychomotor impairment, or daytime sedation, and it is therefore not classified as a controlled substance by the FDA.[138] There are no data at present regarding its efficacy in treating circadian rhythm disorders.

Ramelteon may not be as efficacious for insomnia as some of the BZRAs, but other factors make it an attractive alternative for many patients: its low toxicity and wide safety margin; lack of many of the adverse effects associated with BZRAs; and its ability to be used in patients with substance abuse histories and a variety of medical disorders, including mild to moderate pulmonary disease. It should not be used in combination with fluvoxamine or other potent inhibitors of cytochrome P450 isozyme 1A2, since this leads to dramatically increased levels of ramelteon. It is not recommended for use in pregnant women (FDA Pregnancy Category C).

New Warnings for Hypnotics

In 2007, the FDA introduced a change in labeling for hypnotics, including BZRAs and ramelteon, based on reports of rare but potentially serious adverse events following ingestion of hypnotics (www.fda.gov/bbs/topics/NEWS/2007/NEW01587.html).[139] These included severe allergic reactions and complex sleep-related behaviors, such as sleep-driving, sleep-eating, and sleep sex, in which individuals engaged in these activities without fully awakening. Such reactions are more likely to occur when hypnotics are combined with other sedatives, including alcohol, or taken at higher than recommended doses.

Sedating Antidepressants

Despite a relative lack of data and no FDA indication for insomnia, sedating antidepressants, such as the tricyclic antidepressants (TCAs), trazodone, and mirtazapine, are some of the most commonly used agents for treating chronic insomnia. In general, there are relatively few efficacy data regarding the use of these agents in primary insomnia.

Tricyclic Antidepressants. Amitriptyline and doxepin are some of the more commonly used TCAs in the treatment of insomnia.[10] Their therapeutic effects on depression are related to inhibition of serotonin (5-hydroxytryptamine [5-HT]) and norepinephrine reuptake, whereas their effects on sleep are probably mediated by their antagonistic effects on histamine type 1 (H_1), serotonin type 2 ($5HT_2$), and α-adrenergic type 1 receptors. Doxepin has the most potent antihistamine effects in this class. TCAs tend to have long half-lives, which often leads to daytime sedation and other adverse effects. In general, when used to promote sleep, they are prescribed at doses lower than those recommended for treating depression.

The effects of TCAs on sleep have been studied more frequently in patients with major depressive disorder, in whom they have been shown to reduce latency to sleep onset and increase sleep efficiency.[140,141] A PSG study in subjects with primary insomnia showed that low doses of doxepin (1, 3, or 6 mg) led to improvements in objective sleep and subjective sleep maintenance and duration in comparison to placebo, without evidence of side effects such as anticholinergic effects, hangover, or memory impairment.[142] TCAs at higher doses have profound effects on sleep architecture, most notably suppression of REM sleep.[143,144] REM sleep rebound and sleep disturbance may thus occur following abrupt discontinuation of TCAs, making them less attractive for intermittent dosing.

TCAs can also have adverse effects on sleep, including the exacerbation of restless legs syndrome or periodic limb movement disorder, or precipitation of REM sleep behavior disorder.[145] They can also induce hypomania or mania in patients with underlying bipolar disorder, which is generally associated with severe insomnia.

All tricyclics have significant anticholinergic effects, which lead to many of their side effects, including dry mouth, constipation, urinary retention, and sweating; amitriptyline has the strongest such effects. Orthostatic hypotension can result from α_1-adrenergic receptor antagonism, increasing the risk for falls. The TCAs also have quinidine-like effects on cardiac conduction, which can result in prolongation of the QT interval; cardiotoxicity is a major concern, and these drugs have a high degree of lethality in overdosage.

Trazodone. Trazodone has been one of the most frequently prescribed drugs for insomnia over at least the past decade, and is probably used almost exclusively for this purpose at present, usually in doses of up to 100 mg at bedtime. Its popularity is probably due to its low cost, low abuse potential, and lack of restrictions on long-term use. Its effects on sleep are probably due to its antihistaminergic effects at the H_1 receptor, α_1-adrenergic receptor antagonism, and $5HT_2$ receptor antagonism. Given its widespread use, there are surprisingly few studies documenting its effects on sleep. Most of the studies showing positive effects on sleep were performed in depressed subjects, although most of these were limited by problems such as small sample sizes and lack of placebo controls; trazodone resulted in reduced sleep latency, increased sleep efficiency, and total sleep in several studies in depressives.[146] Only one double-blind, placebo-controlled study has been performed in primary insomnia; in this study, trazodone 50 mg and zolpidem 10 mg were compared with placebo over a 2-week period.[147] During the first week, trazodone and zolpidem led to subjective reductions in sleep latency, increases in total sleep and sleep quality, and decreased wakefulness after sleep onset, but zolpidem produced a greater reduction in sleep latency than trazodone. During the second week, trazodone did not differ from placebo, whereas zolpidem still produced a significantly shorter sleep latency and more total sleep. In terms of trazodone's objective effects on sleep architecture, the most consistent finding has been an increase in slow-wave sleep. There are insufficient data to conclude that trazodone does not lead to tolerance or rebound insomnia.

Trazodone is associated with a number of frequent adverse effects, including daytime sedation/drowsiness, dizziness, dry mouth, gastrointestinal upset, blurred vision, and headache; these have led to fairly high discontinuation rates in clinical trials.[146] Although less common, trazodone may also have significant cardiovascular effects, such as orthostatic hypotension, prolonged QT interval, and cardiac arrhythmias. Priapism, although quite rare, is a medical emergency and can occur even with low doses. One of the major metabolites of trazodone, *meta*-chlorophenylpiperazine, has serotonergic effects and may contribute to serotonin syndrome (confusion/delirium, hyperreflexia, autonomic instability) when trazodone is used in combination with other serotonergic agents. These potential side effects raise concerns about using trazodone in elderly or medically ill populations.

Mirtazapine. Mirtazapine tends to be used at low doses (7.5–15 mg) as a sleep-inducing agent and probably affects sleep through antagonism of H_1, $5HT_2$, and $\alpha1$-adrenergic receptors. As with trazodone, there are relatively few data regarding its efficacy for insomnia. In normal subjects, mirtazapine increased sleep efficiency and slow-wave sleep on the first night of treatment as determined in a sleep laboratory setting.[148] In an uncontrolled PSG study of depressives treated with 30 mg of mirtazapine, slow-wave sleep increased, REM latency was prolonged, wakefulness after sleep onset decreased, and subjective ratings of sleep improved.[149] In a comparison with fluoxetine, depressed subjects who received mirtazapine showed significantly improved sleep by PSG criteria.[150] It is generally believed that lower doses of mirtazapine are more sedating than higher doses, but there are few objective clinical data in support of this. Common side effects of mirtazapine include drowsiness, daytime sedation, dry mouth, increased appetite, and weight gain. Its low toxicity is an advantage in comparison to some of the other sedating antidepressants.

Atypical Antipsychotics

Atypical antipsychotics, particularly quetiapine and olanzapine, are also used with increasing frequency for insomnia. In contrast to the older antipsychotics that act primarily through blockade of dopamine type 2 receptors, the newer agents also act on a variety of receptors in addition, including antagonism of $5HT_{2A}$ and $5HT_{2C}$ receptors, antihistaminergic effects, and antagonism of α_1-adrenergic receptors. Although they may have a role in treating comorbid insomnia in patients with primary indications for their use (e.g., psychotic disorders, bipolar disorder, treatment-refractory depression), their use in primary insomnia should be avoided if possible. One controlled study on the effects of quetiapine at 25 or 100 mg performed in healthy male volunteers[151] resulted in shorter sleep latency, increased total sleep and sleep efficiency, and improved subjective sleep quality. The 100-mg dose, however, caused a significant increase in periodic leg movements. In another study by the same group, ziprasidone produced effects similar to quetiapine, but also led to increased slow-wave sleep and REM sleep suppression.[152] One night of administration of olanzapine to healthy male volunteers produced effects similar to quetiapine in comparison to placebo.[153] In an open-label study in depressives, olanzapine added to SSRI treatment led to increased sleep efficiency and slow-wave sleep.[154]

In addition to the lack of efficacy data for insomnia, atypical antipsychotics are associated with adverse events. They have lower rates of extrapyramidal effects than the older antipsychotics, but these may still occur. Other concerns are risks for weight gain, glucose intolerance, dyslipidemia, daytime sedation, and cognitive impairment. These agents carry a "black box" warning for increased risk of sudden death in elderly patients with dementia.

Anticonvulsants

Several anticonvulsants acting on the GABA system to increase GABA effects in the brain have been used in the treatment of insomnia. There are few, if any, data regarding their use in insomnia, but they appear to have some sedating and/or sleep-promoting effects. Their advantages include low toxicity and that they are not controlled substances. Gabapentin is thought to increase synaptic levels of GABA, but its mechanism of action is not clearly understood.[155] There are no studies on the efficacy of gabapentin for insomnia, but it has been reported to increase slow-wave sleep in patients with epilepsy,[156] improve insomnia ratings in an open-label study of alcoholics with insomnia,[157] and increase slow-wave sleep in normal adults.[158] Gabapentin is generally well tolerated and has low toxicity, but can cause daytime sedation, dizziness, and leukopenia.

Tiagabine inhibits GABA reuptake through inhibition of the GABA transporter. It is one of the few anticonvulsants with data from placebo-controlled studies in insomnia. In a study of elderly subjects with insomnia, doses of 4–8 mg significantly increased slow-wave sleep, and doses of 6–8 mg led to decreased awakenings.[159] At the 8-mg dose, subjects reported subjective decreases in total sleep, less refreshing sleep, worse daytime functioning, and more adverse events. Similar effects were seen in a study of tiagabine in healthy elderly subjects.[160] A study in nonelderly adults with primary insomnia using tiagabine doses up to 16 mg also showed that the drug produced increased slow-wave sleep and decreased waking after sleep onset (at the 16-mg dose), but there was no significant effect on latency to persistent sleep.[161] Again, higher doses were associated with more adverse effects, including decreased next-day alertness and cognitive performance, dizziness, and nausea. Thus although potentially helpful for insomnia, the side effects of tiagabine may limit its utility.

Pregabalin, like gabapentin, was designed as a GABA analogue; like gabapentin, its mechanism is unclear. A comparison of alprazolam with pregabalin in healthy subjects showed that both drugs reduced sleep latency and decreased REM sleep amount[162]; however, pregabalin led to significant increases in slow-wave sleep, whereas alprazolam decreased it; only alprazolam prolonged REM sleep latency. The most common side effects of pregabalin are dizziness and somnolence.

Still an investigational agent, gaboxadol is a $GABA_A$ receptor agonist that has been shown to reduce sleep latency, decrease wakefulness after sleep onset and number of awakenings, and increase slow-wave sleep in normal elderly subjects without obvious next-day impairment.[163] Gaboxadol also improved objective and subjective parameters of nocturnal sleep in normal subjects who had napped during the daytime.[164]

Antihistamines

Antihistamines are the active ingredient in most OTC medications and act through antagonism of H_1 receptors. Diphenhydramine and doxylamine are found in virtually all OTC sleeping medications, but it is important to note that doxepin (described earlier), is a more potent antihistamine than any of the OTCs. Histamine$_1$ antagonists cause sedation in most individuals, but can lead to paradoxical excitation in some individuals, particularly with higher doses and/or in children and the elderly. Despite the widespread use of these agents, there are almost no data regarding their effects on sleep, and there are no rigorous, placebo-controlled studies in insomnia. A study of the subjective effects of diphenhydramine in psychiatric patients with insomnia showed that it led to global improvement in sleep in about two-thirds of subjects,[165] and another outpatient study found that mild to moderate insomnia patients in a family practice setting reported more restful sleep and shorter sleep latency with 50 mg diphenhydramine in comparison to those taking placebo.[166] An assessment of motor activity and subjective sleep parameters in normal adults showed minimal or no effects on sleep parameters, and a tendency for increased motor activity.[167] Finally, a study in normal men showed that diphenhydramine led to rapid tolerance of its sedative effects,[168] suggesting that these agents may not be useful for long-term treatment.

These agents are associated with significant adverse effects, such as daytime sedation, cognitive impairment, increased risk of accidents, dizziness, tinnitus, gastrointestinal symptoms, weight gain, and increased intraocular pressure in narrow-angle glaucoma; as a result, their use has been strongly discouraged for patients with allergic rhinitis in favor of antihistamines without central nervous system effects.[169]

Current Status of Pharmacotherapy for Insomnia

The National Institutes of Health held a State-of-the-Science Conference on Manifestations and Management of Chronic Insomnia in Adults in 2005 (http://consensus.nih. gov/2005/2005InsomniaSOS026html.htm). This nonpartisan review of currently available treatments came to several conclusions regarding pharmacotherapy for insomnia.

Benzodiazepine Receptor Agonists. BZRAs, including benzodiazepines and nonbenzodiazepines, are effective in the short-term treatment of insomnia, and most have not been studied long term using randomized clinical trials; eszopiclone has shown sustained efficacy for 6 months in primary insomnia patients. Adverse effects of BZRAs include residual daytime sedation, motor coordination and cognitive impairment, dependence, and rebound insomnia. Side effects are greater in elderly patients. Side effects related to the newer BZRAs are much lower, probably related to their shorter half-lives. Abuse liability of BZRAs does not appear to be a major problem, but data related to long-term use for insomnia require further study.

Sedating Antidepressants. Trazodone is the most commonly prescribed medication for insomnia in the United States. It is sedating and improves several sleep parameters, but there are no studies of long-term use for chronic insomnia. Doxepin has beneficial effects for insomnia for up to 4 weeks; there are insufficient data for other antidepressants such as amitriptyline and mirtazapine for the treatment of insomnia. All antidepressants have significant adverse effects.

Other Agents. There are no data regarding the use of antipsychotics for the treatment of insomnia; these agents have significant risks, and they are not recommended for use in insomnia. Antihistamines are commonly used, but there are no data regarding their efficacy for insomnia. Furthermore, they have significant adverse effects. Melatonin is not regulated by the FDA and there is significant variability in preparations. It appears to be effective for circadian rhythm disorders, but there is little evidence for efficacy in the treatment of insomnia. There are no data regarding safety in long-term use.[2]

SUMMARY AND CONCLUSIONS

Insomnia is a prevalent health complaint that may present as a primary disorder or as a condition comorbid to a medical or psychiatric disorder. Persistent insomnia is associated with significant morbidity and health care costs. Progress has been made to standardize research diagnostic criteria, but there is still little information about the psychological and biological bases of insomnia and about its natural history and long-term prognosis. Significant advances have also been made in developing and validating therapeutic approaches for the management of both acute and chronic insomnia. Despite these advances, insomnia remains under-recognized and undertreated in clinical practice. Additional research is needed to improve insomnia therapies and outcomes. A significant challenge for the future will be to disseminate more efficiently validated therapies and practice guidelines and increase their use in practice. Additional research is also needed to further document the etiology and natural history of insomnia, and to optimize therapeutic outcomes, not only in terms of reducing insomnia symptoms but also in terms of impact on other indicators of morbidity and cost-effectiveness.

ACKNOWLEDGMENT

Preparation of this chapter was facilitated by research grants from the National Institute of Mental Health (MH60413) and by the Canadian Institutes for Health Research (MT-42504).

⊘ REFERENCES

A full list of references are available at www.expertconsult. com

CHAPTER 27

Narcolepsy

Christian Guilleminault and **Vivien C. Abad**

HISTORICAL OVERVIEW

The term *narcolepsy* was first coined by Gelineau[1] in 1880 to designate a pathologic condition characterized by irresistible episodes of sleep of short duration recurring at close intervals, sometimes accompanied by falls or "astasias" (episodic weakness triggered by strong emotion), later called *cataplexy*.[2] In his 1881 monograph "De la Narcolepsie," Gelineau[3] described narcolepsy as an independent syndrome, as well as a symptom of other diseases. In 1934, Daniels[4] emphasized the association of daytime sleepiness, cataplexy, sleep paralysis, and hypnagogic hallucinations. Calling these symptoms the *clinical tetrad*, Yoss and Daly[5,6] and Vogel[7] described sleep-onset rapid eye movement periods (SOREMPs) in narcoleptic patients, a finding confirmed in subsequent years.[8,9] In 1975, participants in the First International Symposium on Narcolepsy defined the syndrome as follows:

The word narcolepsy refers to a syndrome of unknown origin that is characterized by abnormal sleep tendencies, including excessive daytime sleepiness (EDS) and, often, disturbed nocturnal sleep and pathologic manifestations of REM sleep. The REM sleep abnormalities include sleep-onset REM periods and the dissociated REM sleep inhibitory processes cataplexy and sleep paralysis. EDS, cataplexy, and, less often, sleep paralysis and hypnagogic hallucinations, are the major symptoms of the disease.[10]

This definition highlights rapid eye movement (REM) sleep dysfunction in narcolepsy, while more recent research focuses on the role of genetic and autoimmune factors in the development of narcolepsy. Although most cases occur sporadically, genetic factors probably form a susceptibility background upon which unknown environmental triggers act. In the early 1980s, Juji, Honda, and colleagues reported that virtually all Japanese narcoleptics tested were DR2 positive.[11,12] Molecular typing at the DNA level has identified DQB1*0602 as a marker for narcolepsy across ethnic groups.[13,14] In addition, the hypocretin system has been strongly implicated in the development of narcolepsy. Hypocretin deficiency is found in almost all cases of narcolepsy with cataplexy.[15,16] However, the second edition of the International Classification of Sleep Disorders (ICSD-2) does not require either human leukocyte antigen (HLA) abnormalities or hypocretin deficiency for diagnosis.[17]

CLINICAL FEATURES

The ICSD-2 classifies narcolepsy into three categories: narcolepsy with cataplexy, narcolepsy without cataplexy, and secondary narcolepsy[17] (Table 27–1). Clinical symptoms as described in the following sections and polysomnographic (PSG) abnormalities form the backdrop for diagnosis.

Daytime Naps and Excessive Daytime Sleepiness[4,6,18,19]

Superimposed on a background of frequent drowsiness in narcoleptics are episodes of a strong, sometimes overwhelming, desire for sleep that recur several times during the day. Conducive circumstances, such as monotonous, sedentary activities or a heavy meal, may facilitate this inclination, but it can also occur even when the patient is fully engrossed in a task. Episodes occur two to five

TABLE 27–1 Categories of Narcolepsy

Narcolepsy with Cataplexy (Gelineau Syndrome)	Narcolepsy Without Cataplexy (REM Hypersomnia, Essential Hypersomnia)	Secondary Narcolepsy
Essential Features		
Excessive daytime sleepiness, cataplexy	Excessive daytime sleepiness with or without SP, HH, automatic behavior; MSLT mean sleep latency ≤8 min and ≥2 SOREMPs	Direct cause is a coexisting medical or neurologic condition; excessive sleepiness of variable severity with or without SP, HH, insomnia, or automatic behavior. Associated disorders include tumors or sarcoidosis of the hypothalamus, multiple sclerosis plaques impairing the hypothalamus, paraneoplastic syndrome with anti-Ma2 antibodies, Neimann-Pick type C disease, Coffin-Lowry syndrome, head trauma, myotonic dystrophy, Prader-Willi syndrome, Parkinson's disease, and multisystem atrophy
Associated Features		
SP, HH, nocturnal sleep disruption, memory lapses, ptosis, blurred vision, diplopia, RBD, increased body mass index	Memory lapses, automatic behavior, ptosis, blurred vision, diplopia; sensation of muscle weakness triggered by stress, sex, or intense activity/exercise; nightmares; RBD; nocturnal sleep disruption with frequent awakenings	Not known
Demographics		
Prevalence of 0.02–0.18% in United States and Western Europe, 0.16–0.18% in Japan; both sexes affected, with slight male preponderance; can occur at any age, but seldom diagnosed before age 5	Unknown population prevalence; 0.02% of narcolepsy population has narcolepsy without cataplexy; both sexes can be affected at any age	Not known
Predisposing and Precipitating Factors		
Associated with HLA subtype DR2/DRB1*1501 and DQB1*0602 in whites and Asians; DQB1*0602 is more specifically associated in African Americans; DQB1*0302 increases susceptibility to narcolepsy, while DQB1*0501 and DQB1*0601 are protective in the presence of DQB1*0602. Reported triggers are head trauma, abrupt change in sleep-wake patterns, sustained sleep deprivation, or unspecified viral illness.	40% are HLA DQB1*0602 positive; a small percentage has low CSF hypocretin levels; triggers may be head trauma or unspecified viral illness	Not known
Familial Patterns		
Low prevalence; risk of first-degree relative is 1–2% (10- to 20-fold increase compared to general population); multiplex families (60–100%) are HLA DQB1*0602 positive; 29% concordance in monozygotic twin pairs	Relatives of patients with narcolepsy with cataplexy are more likely to experience this	Not known
Onset, Course, and Complications		
Onset usually after age 5 and commonly between ages 15 and 25 yr. Earliest symptom is usually sleepiness; cataplexy often occurs within a year of onset and rarely precedes it; HH, SP, and disturbed nocturnal sleep manifest later. If untreated, it can lead to isolation, disability, depression, weight gain, failure in school and at work. Higher incidence of type 2 diabetes.	Onset during adolescence; if untreated, it is socially disabling and isolating; failure in school and at work can result	Not known

Continued

TABLE 27–1 Categories of Narcolepsy—Cont'd

Narcolepsy with Cataplexy (Gelineau Syndrome)	Narcolepsy Without Cataplexy (REM Hypersomnia, Essential Hypersomnia)	Secondary Narcolepsy
Pathology and Pathophysiology		
Loss of approximately 50,000–100,000 hypocretin-containing hypothalamic neurons; CSF hypocretin levels are dramatically decreased	Unknown cause in most cases. In a minority, there is loss of hypocretin-containing hypothalamic neurons; 10–20% who are HLA DQB1*0602 positive have low CSF hypocretin levels	Not known
Polysomnographic and Other Objective Findings		
Overnight PSG shows short sleep latency (<10 min) and a SOREMP; MSLT demonstrates mean latency <8 min (typically <5 min) and ≥ 2 SOREMPs; CSF hypocretin <110 pg/ml in 90% of patients; HLA DQB1*0602 usually present (but not diagnostic)	Overnight PSG shows sleep latency <10 min and a SOREMP; stage 1 sleep may increase, and there are frequent awakenings	

CSF, cerebrospinal fluid; HH, hypnagogic hallucinations; HLA, human leukocyte antigen; MSLT, Multiple Sleep Latency Test; PSG, polysomnography; RBD, REM sleep behavior disorder; REM, rapid eye movement; SOREMP, sleep-onset REM period; SP, sleep paralysis.
Adapted from American Academy of Sleep Medicine. International Classification of Sleep Disorders, 2nd ed rev: Diagnostic and Coding Manual. Chicago: American Academy of Sleep Medicine, 2005.

times per day and vary from a few minutes (if the patient is in an uncomfortable position) to more than an hour (if the patient is reclining). Narcoleptics characteristically awaken refreshed, and a refractory period of 1 to several hours occurs before the next episode. In addition to the sleep episodes, patients function at a low level of alertness with poor concentration and error-prone performance at school and work. Memory lapses and even gestural, deambulatory, or speech automatisms also occur.

Cataplexy[19–25]

Cataplexy is an abrupt and reversible decrease in or loss of muscle tone most frequently elicited by emotion. It may involve a limited (commonly postural) number of muscles or the entire voluntary musculature. Most typically, the jaw sags, the head falls forward, the arms drop to the sides, and the knees unlock. The duration of a cataplectic attack, partial or total, is highly variable but is commonly from a few seconds to 5 minutes. Attacks may be elicited by emotion, stress, fatigue, or heavy meals. A review of 200 of our narcoleptic patients with cataplexy at the Stanford Sleep Disorders Clinic revealed the following triggers for cataplexy: laughter (100%), amusement (82%), surprise with joy (78%), elation (75%), attempt at repartee (69%), anger/frustration (57%), and sexual intercourse (38%). Cataplexy can also occur without clear precipitating acts or emotions. The frequency of cataplectic episodes widely varies from rare events during a year-long period in some patients to numerous attacks in a single day in others. However, episodes occur more frequently when patients avoid napping and feel sleepy or feel emotionally drained, or chronically stressed.

The severity and extent of a cataplexy attack can vary from a state of absolute powerlessness that seems to involve the entire voluntary musculature, to limited involvement of certain muscle groups, to no more than a fleeting sensation of weakness throughout the body. Although the extraocular muscles are probably not involved, eye weakness can occur, and the patient may complain of blurred vision. Complete paralysis of extraocular muscles has never been reported, but the palpebral muscle may be affected. Speech may be impaired and respiration may become irregular during an attack—symptoms that may be related to weakness of the abdominal muscles. Long diaphragmatic pauses have never been recorded, but short diaphragmatic pauses similar to those seen during nocturnal REM sleep have been noted. Complete loss of muscle tone may be experienced during a cataplectic attack, resulting in total collapse with risk of serious injuries, including skull and other fractures. Commonly, however, the attacks are not so dramatic, and they may even be unnoticed by nearby individuals. An attack may consist only of a slight buckling of the knees. Patients may perceive this abrupt and very short-lived weakness and stop moving or stand against a wall. The condition may be slightly more obvious when there is a combination of sagging jaw and inclined head. Speech may be broken because of intermittent weakness affecting the arytenoid muscles. As seen during nocturnal REM sleep, the abrupt muscle inhibition is interrupted by sudden bursts of returning muscle tone, which at times even seems enhanced. If the weakness involves only the jaw or speech, the subject may exhibit masticatory movement or an attack of stuttering. If it involves the upper limbs, the patient complains of clumsiness, reporting episodes such as dropping a cup or spilling liquids when surprised, laughing, and so forth.

Because these attacks of partial flaccidity are short and may not resemble a classic full-blown attack of cataplexy, they are often ignored by physicians, even though this is by far the most common way these attacks present. Without an electromyographic (EMG) recording, their transience may make them easy to miss, even by a skilled observer.

Cataplexy is associated with inhibition of the monosynaptic H and muscle stretch reflexes. Physiologically, H reflex activity is fully suppressed only during REM sleep, which points to the relationship between the motor inhibitory components of REM sleep and the sudden atonia and areflexia seen during a cataplectic attack.

Functional brain imaging has shown that the frequency of cataplectic attacks correlates with increased postsynaptic dopamine (D_2) receptor binding, suggesting an alteration of the striatal dopaminergic system.[23] Cerebral perfusion studies using ^{99m}Tc-ethylcysteinated dimer in 25 narcoleptic-cataplectic subjects during standard wakefulness demonstrated diffuse hyperperfusion of bilateral anterior hypothalami, basal ganglia (caudate nuclei, pulvinar), parahippocampal and cingulatge gyri, and subcortical white matter, when compared to normal subjects.[24] This suggests the presence of basal cerebral dysfunction in narcolepsy-cataplexy even outside cataplectic episodes.[24] Interestingly, during status cataplecticus in a narcoleptic-cataplectic subject, single-photon emission computed tomography indicated hyperactivity in the cingulate area, both orbitofrontal cortices, the right temporal cortex, and the right putamen.[25] During the cataplectic episode, hypothalamic perfusion did not change, nor was there any significant hypoperfusion in other areas.[25] Using these data, Chabas et al.[25] suggested that cataplexy is an overactive neuronal state, involving cortical and subcortical areas that are specific to the attacks and not activated between episodes, and postulated that cataplexy is an intermediate stage between normal REM sleep and normal wakefulness.

Sleep Paralysis[4,6,19,26,27] and Hallucinations[6,19,27]

Sleep paralysis is a terrifying experience that occurs when a narcoleptic falls asleep or awakens. Patients find themselves suddenly unable to move their extremities, speak, open their eyes, or even breathe deeply, although they are fully aware of their condition and able to recall the experience afterward. Some patients report that a touch or a call can release them from their paralysis. In many episodes of sleep paralysis, especially the first occurrence, the patient may be prey to extreme anxiety associated with the fear of dying. This anxiety is often greatly intensified by the hallucinations that can accompany the sleep paralysis. Up to one-third of all narcoleptic patients, and up to half of narcoleptic patients with cataplexy experience hallucinations more commonly at sleep onset, and to a lesser extent at sleep termination. The narcoleptic's hypnagogic hallucinations often involve vision, and the manifestations usually consist of simple forms (colored circles, parts of objects) that may be constant in size or changing. The image of an animal or a person may present itself abruptly in black and white or, more often, in color. Auditory hallucinations are also common, but other senses are seldom involved. The auditory hallucinations can range from a collection of sounds to an elaborate melody. The patient may also be menaced by threatening sentences or harsh invective. With more experience of the phenomenon, the patient usually learns that episodes are brief and benign, rarely lasting longer than 20 minutes and always ending spontaneously.

A common and interesting type of hallucination reported at sleep onset involves elementary cenesthopathic (abnormal) sensations (e.g., picking, rubbing, light touching), sensations of changes in location of body parts, or feelings of levitation or extracorporeal experiences, which may be quite elaborate. For example, the patient may say, "I am above my bed and I can also see my body below," or "I am a few feet up and people jump over my body." The association of sleep paralysis has led researchers to postulate gamma loop involvement in some of these hallucinations. The abrupt motor inhibition that involves the spinal cord motor neurons may lead to a significant decrease in feedback of information normally used by the central nervous system to gauge the position of the body and the relation of the limb segments to each other.

Disturbed Nocturnal Sleep and Associated Sleep Disorders

Patients with narcolepsy fall asleep readily at night, but their nocturnal sleep is fragmented.[4,19,27–31] Frequent awakenings with periods of wakefulness during the night are common, and may be interspersed with terrifying dreams. Periodic limb movements in sleep and parasomnias (sleep terrors, sleepwalking, sleeptalking, and REM sleep behavior disorder) are increased.[28,32–36] Narcolepsy patients have higher percentages of REM sleep without atonia, phasic EMG activity, and REM density compared to normal controls.[37]

Special Features in Children[38–45]

In at least 30% of cases, narcolepsy presents during childhood with symptoms occurring as early as 2 years of age. Cardinal symptoms in children are similar to those in adults, but presentation may vary due to maturational factors and significant impact of symptoms on behavior. Children and adolescents tend to conceal or deny symptoms. Frightening hypnagogic hallucinations in children may produce refusal to go to bed or mimic night terrors. Excessive sleepiness may present as prolonged overnight sleep in very young children; in adolescents, daytime sleepiness may be mistaken for laziness, depression, or hyperactivity.

Subtle forms of cataplexy may be misconstrued as syncope, seizures (absence, generalized with astatic seizures, or focal seizures),[43] or psychologically based phenomena.

The definitive diagnosis of narcolepsy is challenging in prepubertal children. Unfortunately, the Multiple Sleep Latency Test (MSLT) is not very useful in prepubertal children, because it has never been evaluated in children younger than 7 years of age.[44] In a study of Chinese-Taiwanese children by Huang et al., the presence of 2 SOREMPs in an MSLT did not differentiate narcoleptic-cataplectic children from those who had hypersomnia.[45] Nevertheless, the MSLT can still be helpful in supporting the diagnosis of narcolepsy in children and teenagers, as there is a predominance of patients who have narcolepsy-cataplexy in children who have 3 or more SOREMPs.[44,45] HLA testing for the HLA DQB1-0602 marker can be utilized to support the diagnosis. When the picture is still unclear, cerebrospinal fluid (CSF) hypocretin measurement can be useful.

Onset and Course of Clinical Symptoms

The first symptoms of narcolepsy often develop near puberty. The peak age of reported symptoms is between ages 15 and 25 years, but narcolepsy and other symptoms have been noted at 3–6 years and a second, smaller peak occurs between 35 and 45 years.

EDS and irresistible sleep episodes usually occur as the first symptoms, either independently or associated with one or more other symptoms. They are enhanced by idleness, indoor activity, and high temperature. Symptoms often abate with time, but they never phase out completely. Cataplexy attacks generally appear in conjunction with abnormal episodes of sleep but may occur as much as 20 years later. Uncommonly, they occur before the abnormal sleep episodes, in which case they are a major source of difficulty in diagnosis. Frequency can vary from a few episodes during the subject's entire lifetime to one or several episodes per day.

Hypnagogic hallucinations and sleep paralysis do not affect all subjects and often are transitory. Disturbed nocturnal sleep seldom occurs in the first stages and generally increases with age.[46] Once symptoms are established, the clinical course over the years remains relatively static, although both worsening and amelioration of symptoms can also occur.

PSYCHOSOCIAL ASPECTS

Narcolepsy profoundly affects quality of life. A group of 500 narcolepsy subjects in the United Kingdom had significantly lower median scores in all eight domains of the Medical Outcomes Short Form-36, a standardized health care–related quality-of-life scale, when compared to the general population.[47] Other studies have also demonstrated poor scores in the domains of physical and mental well-being, vitality, social functioning, and

role functioning.[48–50] Approximately 57% of narcolepsy subjects are depressed.[47] Narcoleptics perceive symptom-related restrictions on education, home, work, and social life, and personal and work relationships suffer.[50] Disrupted nocturnal sleep affects mood and behavior of children and interferes with their learning. Lack of understanding of symptoms by others fosters embarrassment, irritability, feelings of shame, depression, attention seeking, and other difficult behaviors in children and adolescents with narcolepsy.[51] Disputes with parents may arise if the parents either do not understand or have difficulty coping with the child's behavior. Work and home accidents and sleep-related driving accidents are common.[52–54] Forty percent to 48% of narcoleptics report falling asleep at the wheel, and 25–29% of narcoleptics describe accidents due to sleepiness compared to 6% of controls.[48,52,55] Driving issues in narcoleptics interfere with their capacity to work and contribute to disability. A survey performed on the Stanford Sleep Disorders Clinic narcoleptic population showed that 62% of its narcoleptics older than 47 years of age had no recourse other than to apply for Social Security disability benefits.

DIAGNOSTIC PROCEDURES: EVALUATION OF SLEEPINESS

Assessment Scales

Severity of daytime sleepiness may be assessed subjectively, using severity scales such as the Stanford Sleepiness Scale[56] or the Epworth Sleepiness Scale (ESS), and objectively, using the MSLT[57–59] and the Maintenance of Wakefulness Test (MWT). The American Academy of Sleep Medicine (AASM) recently updated the guidelines for the performance of the MSLT and MWT.[58] A low but statistically significant correlation between the MSLT and MWT ($r = .41$) accounts for less than 17% of the variability between the two tests.[59] Alertness and sleepiness are two factors that account for 91% of all variance between the MSLT and MWT.[59] Both measures are sensitive to circadian effects and sleep deprivation.

Multiple Sleep Latency Test

The MSLT was designed by Carskadon and Dement[57] to measure physiologic sleep tendencies in the absence of alerting factors. It is based on the assumption that sleep latency is reduced by physiologic sleepiness. To ensure accurate interpretation of the MSLT findings, the ICSD-2[17] requires that the MSLT be performed under the following conditions:

- The patient must be free of drugs that influence sleep for at least 15 days (or at least five times the half-life of the drug and longer acting metabolite).
- The sleep-wake schedule must have been standardized for at least 7 days before PSG testing (and documented by sleep log or actigraphy).

- Nocturnal PSG should be performed on the night immediately preceding the MSLT to rule out other sleep disorders that could mimic the diagnostic features of narcolepsy without cataplexy; a minimum of 6 hours of sleep is expected during the PSG.

Use of other usual medications (e.g., antihypertensives, insulin) should be planned so that undesired influences (stimulating or sedating) are minimized. Standardized procedures are followed. The MSLT consists of four or five scheduled naps, usually at 10:00 AM and 12:00, 2:00, 4:00, and 6:00 PM, during which the subject is polygraphically monitored in a comfortable, soundproof, dark bedroom.

The latency between lights-out time and sleep onset is calculated for each nap, and the number of SOREMPs, defined as REM sleep that occurs within 15 minutes of sleep onset, is noted. In normal populations, MSLT scores vary with age among pediatric,[60] adolescent,[61] and adult[62,63] populations, with young adults having the shortest latencies and prepubescent children having the longest latencies (18.5 ± 4.8 minutes).[64,65] In adults, mean sleep latency scores under 8 minutes are generally considered to be in the pathologic range, while those over 10 minutes are considered normal. The ICSD-2[17] criteria for narcolepsy utilize a mean sleep latency of ≤8 minutes. A meta-analysis calculated that the mean ± standard deviation (SD) sleep latency for 255 narcolepsy subjects was 3.1 ± 2.9 minutes, but also reported that 16% of narcolepsy subjects had mean sleep latency >5 minutes.[58] Caution in interpreting MSLT results is needed, because extrapolation based on studies of normal subjects suggests that approximately 16% of the normal population could have a mean sleep latency <5 minutes. Obtaining a psychiatric history is also important in interpretation of MSLT results, since depression may shorten sleep latency in some patients, while anxiety or tension may prolong sleep latency.

Within the context of objective marked sleepiness, the occurrence of 2 or more SOREMPs during the MSLT (in the absence of other causative factors, such as sleep deprivation, delayed sleep phase syndrome, obstructive sleep apnea, or REM-suppressant medication withdrawal with REM rebound) are suggestive of narcolepsy.[66] The presence of 2 or more SOREMPs yields a sensitivity of 0.78 and a specificity of 0.93 in the diagnosis of narcolepsy.[58] Bishop et al.[67] reported that 17% of 139 "normal" subjects exhibited 2 or more SOREMPs during their MSLT, and SOREMPs have also been reported in 2–7% of patients with other sleep disorders[68] and even more often in obstructive sleep apnea syndromes, where up to 25% of severely affected subjects may present with similar findings.[69,70] SOREMPs can also be seen in infancy, chronic sleep fragmentation or sleep deprivation, jet lag, delayed sleep phase syndrome, withdrawal from REM-suppressant medications, depression, schizophrenia, and Kleine-Levin syndrome.

Maintenance of Wakefulness Test[71–73]

The MWT measures the ability to remain awake under soporific conditions for a defined period of time. It is primarily used to follow the treatment of hypersomnia with stimulant medications to objectively document the ability to stay awake. The mean sleep latency for the MWT 40 test is 35.2 ± 7.9 min, with a lower limit of normal (−2 SD) of 19.4 minutes. For the MWT 20 test, the mean sleep latency is 18.1 ± 3.6 minutes, with a lower limit of normal of 10.9 minutes.[72] The latest AASM Standards of Practice Committee considered a mean sleep latency of <8 minutes on the 40-minute MWT protocol as abnormal, whereas values between 8 and 40 minutes were considered to be of uncertain significance.[58] In a group of 11 narcoleptic subjects and 11 control subjects tested with the MSLT and the MWT, both tests differentiated the narcoleptic from the control subjects on the frequency of daytime REM sleep episodes.[73] However, SOREMPs ranged from 0 to 5 on the MWT for narcoleptic subjects, while all narcolepsy subjects had a minimum of 2 SOREMPs on the MSLT.[73]

Polysomnography

In narcoleptics, sleep latency is short (<10 minutes) and sleep architecture is disturbed, with frequent awakenings and increased stage 1 NREM sleep. In about 25–50% of narcolepsy with cataplexy subjects, a SOREMP is observed. A SOREMP during nocturnal PSG is a highly specific finding for narcolepsy in the absence of any other sleep disorder.

Continuous 24- or 36-hour PSG monitoring provides information about the actual number, duration, time, and type of daytime sleep episodes and confirms disrupted nighttime sleep. In addition, this extended long PSG recording may identify the dissociated REM sleep inhibitory process that characterizes cataplexy. This dissociated REM process produces an awake electroencephalogram and electro-oculogram recording associated with complete absence of chin EMG recording and bursts of muscle twitches, which are typical of REM sleep. Microsleep episodes and microarousals can also be monitored. Due to the intensive labor involved, as well as costs not usually reimbursed by insurance, prolonged monitoring is not commonly performed except in a research setting.

The positive diagnosis of narcolepsy requires a minimum of two major symptoms: EDS and sleep attacks or attacks of narcolepsy associated with objectively documented SOREMPs. The clinical association of excessive daytime sleepiness and cataplexy, when observed by an experienced physician, is pathognomonic of the narcolepsy syndrome. If EDS and cataplectic attacks are sufficient to confirm narcolepsy, why require PSG in cases in which one or both are absent? The history of cataplexy can be difficult to affirm. Absolute cataplexy, which causes the subject to collapse on the floor, is uncommon. Subjects often have time to reach a chair or wall to prevent a complete collapse. Most commonly, cataplexy is only partial, involving the head and neck, upper limbs, mandibular and upper airway muscles, or knees. This partial cataplexy is often difficult to interpret, especially in cases in which the subject has only a positive history of cataplexy without current symptoms. It is in these cases that polygraphic monitoring with positive MSLT findings can confirm the diagnosis.

Additional Diagnostic Procedures

Actigraphy and Sleep Diary

These tests can be used to assess the duration and quality of sleep during the week prior to multiple sleep latency testing.

Blood or Urine Drug Screen

Blood or urine samples are collected on the day of the multiple sleep latency testing to exclude the use of drugs that can affect sleep latency. This is helpful particularly in factitious narcolepsy claims as part of drug-seeking behavior in requesting stimulant prescriptions.

Cerebrospinal Fluid Hypocretin Testing

Low CSF hypocretin-1 (Hcrt-1) levels ($\leq$110 pg/ml or one-third of mean normal control values) are found in more than 90% of patients with narcolepsy with cataplexy. It is a highly sensitive and specific marker for narcolepsy with cataplexy, but standardization of CSF hypocretin testing and sensitivity of the technique remains an issue. Clinical correlation is important, since other conditions such as multiple sclerotic plaques affecting the hypothalamus,[74] acute traumatic brain injury,[75] subarachnoid hemorrhage,[76] Prader-Willi syndrome,[77] Guillain-Barré syndrome,[78] and Hashimoto's encephalopathy with coma[79] can also be associated with low CSF hypocretin levels. Since up to 10% of narcoleptic subjects with cataplexy have normal CSF hypocretin levels,[17] a negative test does not exclude narcolepsy with cataplexy.

HLA Typing

Narcolepsy with cataplexy is very tightly linked with the HLA DQB1*0602 (and HLA-DR2 or DRB1*1501, DRB5*0101, and DQA1*0102) alleles in Asians and whites.[80–83] Depending on the series, 88–98% of patients with clear cataplexy are HLA DQB1*0602 positive, independent of ethnicity. Further studies on whites with cataplexy and EDS that address susceptibility to cataplexy and EDS have demonstrated the presence of both DQA1*0102 and DQB1*0602, suggesting complementation and indicating that these two alleles may be important for disease predisposition.

In contrast, only about 40% of patients with narcolepsy without cataplexy are HLA DQB1*0602 positive.[82]

However, the presence of HLA DQB1*0602 is not diagnostic for narcolepsy, as this is present in 38% of the normal African American population, 25% of the normal white population, and 12 % of the normal Japanese population.[17] Thus, HLA typing is never utilized to diagnose narcolepsy without cataplexy. HLA typing is best utilized as additional information in young patients who are at risk of developing narcolepsy with cataplexy later. (See additional discussion under *Can Human Leukocyte Antigen Aid in Diagnosis* later.)

Issues in Interpretation of Results

Can a Subject with EDS and a History of Cataplexy Have a Negative MSLT?

Van den Hoed and coworkers[84] and Moscovitch and colleagues[85] reviewed the issue of whether subjects who meet the criteria of having EDS and a history of cataplexy can receive a negative score (<2 SOREMPS) on the MSLT. Both groups analyzed patients seen at the Stanford Sleep Disorders Clinic. Moscovitch's group[85] had a larger population (306 narcoleptics). Seventy-seven percent of these patients had been seen by the same physician, who had a great deal of experience with narcolepsy. Based on clinical data, all were believed to have cataplexy, but only 83% of them presented with 2 or more SOREMPs at one PSG-MSLT period. Four successive days of MSLTs were necessary to observe 2 or more SOREMPs in every subject in the population. In another study of 106 narcolepsy subjects with cataplexy, Aldrich et al.[66] reported that only 71% have a mean sleep latency <8 minutes and 2 or more SOREMPs on the initial MSLT, and that repeated testing failed to raise this above 80%.

Can Someone Be Diagnosed as Narcoleptic Who Has No Cataplexy but Has Sleep-Onset REM periods?

In the Stanford database of 306 EDS subjects ages 32 years and older, 54 subjects had 2 SOREMPs on the MSLT without any history of cataplexy or family history of narcolepsy.[85] Investigations indicate that a small number of narcoleptics never develop cataplexy.[46,86]

The ICSD-2[17] classification of narcolepsy includes the category of narcolepsy without cataplexy (see Table 27–1). Although the true population prevalence of narcolepsy without cataplexy is unknown, among the narcoleptic population, 10–50% have narcolepsy without cataplexy.[17] Similar to narcolepsy with cataplexy, symptoms usually start during adolescence, nocturnal sleep is either normal or moderately disturbed, and daytime naps are refreshing. Accessory symptoms, such as sleep paralysis, hypnagogic hallucinations, or automatic behavior, may also be present. Although unambiguous cataplexy is absent, atypical sensations of muscle weakness triggered by stress, sex, or intense activity/exercise have been reported.[17] Nightmares and REM sleep behavior disorder may be observed. About 40% of these patients are HLA DQB1*0602 positive.[17]

Can MSLT Scores for EDS in Narcoleptics be Outside the Range Usually Reported?

From the Stanford University database of 500 narcoleptics with unequivocal cataplexy and complaints of mild sleepiness, two patients presented a mean MSLT score of 11 on two repeated investigations. Each of them had 2 SOREMPs during the MSLT. However 85% of the narcoleptics in Van den Hoed's and Moskovitch's groups had a mean sleep latency of <5 minutes.[84,85]

Can Human Leukocyte Antigen Aid in Diagnosis?

DQB1*0602 is a sensitive marker for narcolepsy with cataplexy across all ethnic groups, with a frequency of 76.1% in narcoleptics with cataplexy versus 40.9% in narcoleptics without cataplexy.[13] However, as indicated by Guilleminault and colleagues, the HLA-DR2 DQw6 DQB1*0602 haplotype is neither sufficient nor necessary for the diagnosis of narcolepsy.[80] (See HLA discussion in the section *Genetic Versus Environmental Factors* later for additional details.)

HLA typing plays a minor role in the diagnosis of narcolepsy and is not routinely necessary. Limitations to the use of HLA in the diagnosis of narcolepsy in clinical practice are that many patients with narcolepsy without cataplexy are HLA DQB1*0602 negative and a small number of narcolepsy with cataplexy subjects are also negative for this haplotype. Similarly, among non-narcoleptic controls, the prevalence of DQB1*0602 ranges from 18% to 35%.

However, HLA-DQ high-resolution typing (rather than DR2 or DR15 typing) may be useful in confirming the diagnosis of narcolepsy in certain cases. In patients with excessive daytime sleepiness without cataplexy, the presence of DQB1*0602 may support the diagnosis of narcolepsy, although its absence does not exclude it. In atypical cases or cases of narcolepsy without definite cataplexy, a negative DQB1*0602 result should trigger a more exhaustive search for other underlying sleep disorders.[82]

Can CSF Testing for Hypocretin-1 Aid in the Diagnosis?

A significant observation has been that CSF Hcrt-1 levels are decreased in patients with narcolepsy. CSF Hcrt-1 levels <110 pg/ml yield a 99% specificity and 87% sensitivity in the diagnosis of narcolepsy with cataplexy.[82] However, for narcoleptic patients with atypical or absent cataplexy, the specificity of this test remains high at 99%, but the sensitivity is low at 16%, as most cases have normal levels. Potential indications for CSF Hcrt-1 measurement are young children (<7 years of age) who may have difficulty following MSLT instructions; patients treated with psychotropic drugs who are unwilling/unable to interrupt treatment; patients with suspected narcolepsy with cataplexy but whose MSLT is negative; patients with other comorbid sleep disorders, such as sleep-disordered breathing or severe insomnia, in whom the MSLT is difficult to interpret; patients with secondary narcolepsy; and narcoleptic patients with cataplexy who do not appear to respond to high-dose stimulants.[82]

EPIDEMIOLOGY

The prevalence of narcolepsy varies across different populations.[87] The highest reported prevalence is in Japan at 160–590 per 100,000 population.[88–90] In five countries in Europe (the United Kingdom, Germany, Italy, Portugal, and Spain), Ohayon et al. reported a frequency of 47 per 100,000 population.[91] In the United States, the estimated prevalence is similar at 50–67 per 100,000.[92–94] However, in Finland, the estimated prevalence is 26 per 100,000.[95] The lowest frequency is among Israeli Jews at 0.23 per 100,000.[96]

There is no gender predominance in this disorder. Age of onset varies from childhood to the fifth decade. The mean age of onset is from 23.4 to 24.4 years, with bimodal peaks at 14.7 years and 35 years.[97] Early age of onset is associated with a family history of narcolepsy and increased severity manifested by a higher frequency of cataplexy and decreased mean sleep latency on the MSLT.[97] Month of birth is a proposed risk factor, with a peak incidence in March and trough in September.[98] Little has been reported about lifestyle and behavioral risk factors, such as exercise, tobacco use, or illicit drug use, with one study suggesting excessive alcohol use may be more common in narcoleptics.[99] There is increased association of obesity with narcolepsy,[99–101] but the role of leptin production, resistance, or a combination thereof is still not settled.[99] Taken together, these observations suggest that environmental factors in concert with genetic factors may trigger autoimmune processes targeting the hypocretin system.[98]

PATHOPHYSIOLOGY

Genetic Versus Environmental Factors

Human Narcolepsy and HLA

Westphal first described the familial occurrence of narcolepsy-cataplexy in 1877. Since then, the genetic aspect of narcolepsy has been investigated by several groups. Japanese researchers reported that 100% of the Japanese narcoleptic patients they studied expressed the haplotype known as DR15 DQw6.[11,12,102] British, French, Canadian, and U.S. investigators have also confirmed the association of narcolepsy with HLA-DR and HLA-DQ alleles, further supporting a genetic basis for susceptibility to narcolepsy.[86,103]

HLA testing techniques have evolved from serologic antibody-based technology to molecular typing at the DNA level. The HLA-DR and -DQ genes, both located on chromosome 6p21, encode HLA proteins composed of an α and a β chain. In the DQ locus, two polymorphic genes,

DQA1 and DQB1, encode both chains. Using serologic typing techniques at the DR2 level, investigations have identified two subtypes, DR15 and DR16. DR15 was identified in DR2 narcoleptic subjects.[104–106] Using DNA sequencing or oligotyping in DR2 narcoleptic subjects, DR15 has been sequenced into DRB1*1501-DRB1*1514.[82] At the DQ level, DQ1 has been serologically split into DQ5 and DQ6, and all narcoleptic patients have been found to possess DQ6. Molecular subtypes of DQ6 identified at the DQB1 level range from DQB1*0601 to DQB1*0618.[82,105] The DQ6 subtype in patients with narcolepsy is DQB1*0602, which is always associated with DQA1*0102.[14,39,81] In African Americans, either DRB1*1503 (a DNA-based subtype of DR2) or DRB1*1101 (a DNA-based subtype of DR5) is frequently observed together with DQB1*0602.[81,104,106,107] In whites and Asians, DRB1*1502 (a DNA-based DR2 subtype) is frequently observed with DQB1*0602 and DQA1*0102 in narcoleptic patients.[108] More rarely, DQB1*0602 is associated with other DRB1 alleles (DRB1*0301, DRB1*0806, DRB1*12022, and DRB1*1602). Across racial groups, DQB1*0602 is the most common haplotype associated with narcolepsy.

It has been proposed that the HLA-DQ alleles (especially DQB1*0602 and DQA1*0102) are the actual narcolepsy susceptibility genes. Evidence cited to bolster this hypothesis includes the following: (1) the narcolepsy susceptibility region within the DQA1-DQB1 interval has been mapped utilizing novel DNA markers without discovery of any new genes[106]; (2) in all narcolepsy susceptibility DR-DQ haplotypes, both DQA1*0102 and DQB1*0602 are present, suggesting that the active DQA1*0102/DQB1*0602 heterodimer is needed for disease predisposition; (3) there are multiplex families in which several members with narcolepsy have inherited DQB1*0602 from different branches of the family[80,109]; (4) subjects homozygous for DQB1*0602 subjects have a two- to fourfold increased risk for development of narcolepsy compared with DQB1*0602 heterozygous subjects[14,104]; and finally, (5) risk in DQB1*0602 heterozygous individuals is modulated by the other DQB1 allele, such that risk is increased in DQB1*0602/DQB1*0301 heterozygotes but is reduced in DQB1*0602/DQB1*0601 and DQB1*0602/DQB1*0501 heterozygotes.

Familial Occurrence and Environmental Factors

Among the first-degree relatives of 50 narcoleptic probands, Kessler and coworkers described 9 narcoleptic patients (18%) and 17 subjects (34%) with EDS.[110] Honda and associates found 14 narcoleptic patients (6%) and 56 subjects with EDS among the parents and siblings of 232 narcoleptic patients.[88] In a survey (interviews and questionnaires) published in 1988, Montplaisir and Poirier[111] reported that 23% of index cases had a family history of the disease and that 44% had at least one other relative who suffered from daytime sleepiness. In 1988, we[80] pooled 334 probands who met strict criteria for narcolepsy; using direct patient interviews, we found 18 patients (5%) who described a history of sleep attacks and cataplexy in a family member and 132 patients (40%) who reported EDS in another family member. We compared our results with our previous investigation[110] in 1972 and 1973. The 1972 study involved only 50 probands[110]; at that time, we had found a 5.5% family history of narcolepsy and cataplexy but a 34% prevalence of EDS. Thus, the first finding from these data was that a relationship does not necessarily exist between narcolepsy and EDS in other family members. Using objective criteria for sleepiness in 20 sleepy family members, we found that 1 family member had an abnormal sleep-wake schedule and only 2 qualified for the diagnosis of isolated idiopathic sleepiness. Although it is difficult to generalize from these findings, we believe that the published number of isolated EDS cases that can appropriately be related to narcolepsy (in questionnaire studies covering family members of narcoleptics) has been inflated. Determining the relationship between narcolepsy syndrome and EDS in family members requires systematic monitoring of all family members suspected of having EDS. This can be very expensive and difficult; in our population, most relatives live outside the area.

Our other finding from these data, echoed by the Japanese, Canadian, French, and German researchers, was that familial occurrence of narcolepsy is not a very frequent phenomenon.[102] More recent studies have determined that many of the earlier reports were confounded by unrecognized sleep apnea and that the risk for development of narcolepsy-cataplexy among first-degree relatives is much lower (1–2%), although the risk for isolated daytime sleepiness can be 4–5%.[109]

Several noteworthy findings have been obtained from a group of approximately 50 families with several affected members referred to Stanford from all over the world. In two families, one proband was HLA-DR2 DQw6 DQB1*0602 homozygous. In the German family studied by Mueller-Eckhardt and associates,[112] three siblings and one parent presented with narcolepsy. One affected sibling did not share the HLA haplotype (coming from the affected parent) with the two other affected siblings. This made the interpretation that the genetic transmission of the illness is purely through HLA-DR2 DQw6 unlikely. To explain the discrepancy, it has been suggested that there is a recombinant haplotype.[102,104,111–113] This notion is credible, but at best it is only one of many possibilities.

Probably the most damaging evidence against the genetic transmission of narcolepsy only through DQB1-0602 or a closely located gene is our report of a family in which six members presented all the clinical symptoms of narcolepsy and PSG-documented SOREMPs but had negative tests for HLA-DR15 DQw5 DQB1*0602. Not only were all family members DR15 DQw6 negative, but three-fourths of the patients with cataplexy did not share similar haplotypes. There was, however, a high familial incidence of both daytime sleepiness and cataplexy through several generations. The existence of a genetic element was therefore strongly supported. The first proband had two affected daughters born of two different fathers, making a recessive gene hypothesis unlikely for this family. The transmission of narcolepsy in this family can in some respects be compared with the canine model of narcolepsy, in which genetic transmission has been shown to be different from the dog leukocyte antigen complex, and is consistent with the classic mendelian mode of inheritance. A similar family was reported by Singh and colleagues.[114]

The percentage of narcoleptics who are positive for HLA DQB1*0602 is estimated at 88–98%. Well-documented cases of non–HLA-DR2 DQw6 DQB1*0602 narcoleptics prove that it is not necessary to be HLA-DR2 DQw6 DQB1*0602 positive to be narcoleptic. Moreover, family studies throughout the world have shown that many family members have shared the HLA haplotype for disease susceptibility with the proband and have never developed narcolepsy. For example, in one Japanese investigation of 17 families, 22 subjects had the same haplotype for disease susceptibility as the proband, but 13 subjects had no symptoms whatsoever, 8 exhibited EDS in non-PSG studies, and only 1 suffered from narcolepsy.[111,112] Our investigation showed similar results in the 18 families studied.[80]

Twin Studies. A final critical observation has been made by Montplaisir and Poirier[111] and our group at Stanford. We have observed monozygotic twin pairs who are discordant for narcolepsy. Twin studies are important in genetic investigations, and cases of monozygotic twins in whom narcolepsy was diagnosed are often cited as evidence for a genetic etiology of the disease. Many of the older cases, however, are unconvincing when judged by present standards. Before 1985, HLA typing was not widespread, and MSLTs often were not performed in the course of clinical evaluations of narcolepsy.

Three pairs of monozygotic twins discordant for narcolepsy have now been investigated in depth by Montplaisir and Poirier[111] (two pairs) and our team (one pair).[80] The two pairs of Canadian twins are over 50 years of age, and their monozygosity was established by HLA typing. The twins we studied were 42 years old, and monozygosity was established by HLA typing and DNA fingerprinting. Both expressed DR2 DQw6. In each case, the affected twin developed symptoms during the teenage years. Other twin studies have also been reported: Among 16 monozygotic twin pairs described in the literature, only 5 pairs were considered to be concordant.[115] Among these concordant pairs, Honda and colleagues reported a twin pair with marked difference in age of onset of narcolepsy.[115] The second-born twin demonstrated a typical course of narcolepsy, whereas the first-born twin had a very late onset of recurrent daytime sleep episodes at age 45 and cataplexy at age 50 years, apparently triggered by chronic emotional stresses and sleep insufficiency.[115]

The existence of discordant monozygotic twins indicates that nongenetic (i.e., environmental) factors participate in the development of narcolepsy. Different environmental precipitating factors have been cited, including head trauma (in six of nine patients who were either DR2 positive, DR4 positive, or DQW1 positive),[116] sudden change in sleep/wake habits,[117] infections, and stress.[115,118]

Other Genetic Factors. The issue of disease heterogeneity with possible involvement of other genes is raised by the increased risk of narcolepsy in first-degree relatives (10-fold in Japanese and 20- to 40-fold in whites, compared to the estimated risk of 2- to 3-fold based upon HLA-DR and -DQ subtypes) and the existence of narcolepsy in families without these HLA subtypes. In Japanese narcoleptic families, tumor necrosis factor-α gene polymorphism with thymine residue at position -857 (TNF-α [-857T]) in its promoter region has been linked with human narcolepsy independently of its strong association with HLA DRB1*1501.[119,120] In German narcoleptic families, the T allele of the C-857T polymorphism was strongly associated with narcolepsy in the subgroup of DRB1*15/16 (HLA-DR2 type)–negative patients, but not in DRB1*15/16-positive patients.[121] These results support genetic heterogeneity and differences in pathophysiology of HLA-DR2–positive and HLA-DR2–negative narcolepsy.[121] Meanwhile, a genome-wide linkage search in eight Japanese families with 21 DR2-positive patients (14 narcoleptic cases with cataplexy and 7 cases with an incomplete form of narcolepsy) suggested linkage to chromosome 4p13-q21, raising the suspicion that this might be a second locus for HLA-associated human narcolepsy.[122]

Dauvilliers and colleagues provided genetic evidence for the critical involvement of the dopaminergic and/or noradrenergic systems in human narcolepsy when they found sexual dimorphism and a strong effect of catechol-O-methyltransferase (COMT) genotype on narcolepsy disease severity and response to stimulant treatment.[123,124] Narcoleptic women with high COMT activity had much shorter mean sleep latencies on the MSLT compared to those with low COMT activity, while the opposite was true for men. COMT genotype also affected the presence of sleep paralysis and number of SOREMPs during the MSLT.[124] Sexual dimorphism in COMT activity affected the response to modafinil, such that the optimal daily dose of modafinil was lower in narcoleptic women compared to men and also lower in all narcoleptics with a low-COMT-activity genotype.[124]

Neuroanatomic, Neurochemical, and Immunologic Aspects

Animal models (canine and rodent) have provided a neurochemical and neuroanatomic model for human narcolepsy. Cataplexy is enhanced by cholinergic (M_2 or M_3

muscarinic receptor) sensitivity together with reduced monoaminergic (dopaminergic and/or adrenergic) tone, with involvement of the presynaptic α_2/D_2 (and/or D_3) autoreceptor and postsynaptic α_1-adrenergic receptor.[125] EDS results from hypoactivity of dopaminergic transmission and is alleviated through presynaptic modulation of dopamine.

The hypocretin (orexin) system plays an important role in the development of narcolepsy. Hypocretin-containing neurons are localized in the dorsolateral hypothalamus around the perifornical nucleus and project to the cerebral cortex, basal forebrain structures, amygdala, and brain stem structures (reticular formation, raphe nuclei, and locus ceruleus). Hypocretin-1 receptors are located in the ventromedial hypothalamic nucleus, dorsal raphe, and locus ceruleus, while Hcrt-2 receptors are located in the paraventricular nucleus and nucleus accumbens. Nishino et al. first described low to almost undetectable Hcrt-1 concentrations in the CSF in narcoleptics,[125] and this finding was subsequently confirmed in large series of CSF analyses.[126,127]

The role of autoimmune processes in producing narcolepsy has not been resolved. Investigations have shown that narcolepsy in Doberman pinschers is transmitted through a single autosomal recessive gene called *canarc I*. Gene markers for *canarc I* have indicated that it is not linked to the canine major histocompatiblity complex but is tightly linked to a mu-like gene. Mu is the switch region of the immunoglobulin heavy-chain gene. This finding in canine narcolepsy suggests involvement of the immune system in the pathophysiology of the disease.

In human narcolepsy, loss of hypocretin function has been postulated to be due to an immunologic process. Gliosis, a very important histopathologic indicator of central nervous system injury, is associated with increased glial fibrillary acidic protein (GFAP) staining of astrocytes. Thannickal et al. described reduced numbers of hypocretin-containing neurons and axons and an elevated level of hypothalamic gliosis in narcoleptic brains; the percentage loss of hypocretin cells and percentage elevation of GFAP staining were variable across forebrain and brain stem nuclei but were maximal in the posterior and tuberomammillary hypothalamic region.[128,129] These findings support the hypotheses that the loss of hypocretin function in narcolepsy results from a cytotoxic or immunologically mediated attack on the Hcrt-2 receptor or an antigen anatomically linked to this receptor, and that this process is intensified in regions of high axonal density.[128,129]

However, to date, no antibodies have been found supporting the autoimmune theory. Black and colleagues[130] tested for N-type and P/Q-type voltage-gated calcium channel antibodies, neuronal nicotinic acetylcholine receptor alpha 3 subunit, acetylcholine receptor–binding antibodies, striated muscle antibodies, type 1 Purkinje cell cytoplasmic antibodies, types 1 and 2 antineuronal

nuclear antibodies and amphiphysin antibodies, GAD-65 antibody, and thyroid microsomal and thyroglobulin antibodies in the serum of 43 patients with or without cataplexy, 41 with known HLA status.[130] No antibody test yielded significantly positive results for the group as a whole or for subgroups of patients with cataplexy or positive HLA DQB1*0602 status.[118] Similarly, screening for antiganglioside antibodies in hypocretin-deficient human narcolepsy has failed to demonstrate a correlation with increased titers of antiganglioside antibodies.[131]

Black and colleagues[132] tested the hypothesis that DQB1*0602-positive narcoleptic subjects with cataplexy have immunoglobulin G (IgG) reactive to human pre-prohypocretin and its cleavage products (including Hcrt-1 and -2). Using immunoprecipitation assays, immunofluorescence microscopy, and Western blots, no evidence was found for IgG reactive to pre-prohypocretin or its cleavage products in the CSF of these narcoleptic subjects.[132] Nonetheless, in support of the autoimmune theory are reports of narcoleptics with cataplexy responding to standard autoimmune therapies, such as intravenous immune globulin therapy,[133,134] plasmapheresis,[135] and prednisone.[136]

CURRENT TREATMENT (Table 27–2)

The goals of therapy listed in the 2000 and 2007 AASM practice parameters for the treatment of narcolepsy are to alleviate daytime sleepiness (thereby maximizing functionality for patients at work, school, and home and socially) and to control nocturnal symptoms of disrupted sleep, troublesome cataplexy, hypnagogic hallucinations, and sleep paralysis.[137,138] Behavior management is an important adjunct to optimal choice of medications. Because narcolepsy is a lifelong illness and patients require medications on a long-term basis, attention should be paid to potential side effects, risk of tolerance, and addiction potential.

Nonpharmacologic Management

Information

Narcolepsy has a profound impact on various aspects of the patient's life, and the patient needs to be adequately informed about the disorder at the time of diagnosis. Good sleep hygiene measures should be emphasized, including (1) maintaining a regular sleep-wake schedule; (2) avoiding smoking, especially at night; (3) avoiding alcohol and caffeinated beverages, particularly within 3–4 hours of bedtime; (4) optimizing the sleep environment so that it is comfortable and quiet; and (5) performing regular exercise for at least 20 min/day at least 4 hours prior to bedtime. Appropriate advice about scheduled daytime naps and avoidance of time-zone changes should also be given. The 2007 Practice Parameters indicate that a combination of regular bedtimes and two 15-minute regularly scheduled naps reduce unscheduled daytime sleep

TABLE 27–2 Treatment for Narcolepsy

Treatment for Cataplexy and Sleep Paralysis, with or Without Hypnagogic Hallucinations or Panic Reaction to Sleep Paralysis

Drug	Dosage	Comments
γ-Hydroxybutyrate (sodium oxybate)	6–9 g PO in 2 divided doses	First dose is at bedtime, second dose 2.5–4 hr later, both taken in bed (set alarm)
Antidepressants (without atropinic effects)		
Fluoxetine (20-mg tablets) PO	Normal dose: 20–60 mg given in the morning	
Venlafaxine (75-mg tablets) PO	Normal dose: 75–300 mg in the morning or 2 divided doses	
Viloxazine (50-mg tablets) PO	Normal dose: 150–200 mg daily	This dosage may be higher than usual dose ranges for depression
Antidepressants (with atropinic side effects)		
Clomipramine (25- or 50-mg tablets) PO	Normal dose: 75–125 mg daily at bedtime	
Protriptyline (5-mg tablets) PO	Normal dose: 10–15 mg in the morning or divided doses	Impotence is common with 15- to 20-mg dosages
Imipramine (25- or 30-mg tablets) PO	Normal dose: 75–125 mg daily (divided or in evening)	

Treatment for EDS

Behavioral Treatment	Scheduled short (15-min) daytime naps Best times: 10:30 AM, 1:00 PM, 4:00 PM Schedules most frequently used by patients: 1:00–2:00 PM and 4:30–6:00 PM
Nutrition	Avoid heavy lunches, alcohol, and foods or beverages that have paradoxical effects, such as chocolate
Medication	No medication completely alleviates daytime sleepiness, but some help to improve performance.

Best Medications

Drug	Dosage	Comments
Children and Adolescents		
Modafinil (first option)	100 mg in the morning and 100 mg at noon	If divided doses are difficult to administer, then 200 mg in the morning
Methylphenidate (if modafinil is not effective)	Maximum of 30 mg/day	15 mg in the morning and 15 mg at lunch in the best case or a 20- or 30-mg slow-release form in the morning
Adults		
Modafinil (100- or 200-mg tablets) PO	Normal dose: 100–400 mg/day, occasionally up to 600 mg/day	Single dose in the morning or divided doses with higher morning dose and smaller noon dose (e.g., 400 mg AM and 200 mg noon).
Sodium oxybate (GHB)	6–9 g/day	Given in divided doses, half at bedtime and half 2.5–4 hr later
Methylphenidate (5-mg tablets) PO	Usual dosage 20–40 mg/day; divided doses taken at least 30–45 min before or after a meal	Avoid one large dose due to short half-life. Avoid more than 50 mg/day—no clinical gain.
Dexedrine (5-mg tablets) PO	Usual dosage 10–40 mg/day	Divided doses or SR formula recommended to avoid other side effects. New patients should be tried on other drugs first.

Examples of Treatment Packages

Prepubertal Children

For sleepiness
- Contact school to alert teachers
- Nap at lunchtime
- Nap at 4:00–5:00 PM

Medications:
- Modafinil 100–200 mg. Start at 100 mg in the morning for 5 days, then add 100 mg at lunch if needed.
- Alternative: methylphenidate 10–20 mg. Usually 10 mg before meals on awakening, 5 mg at lunch, and 5 mg at 3:00 PM.

For cataplexy
- Fluoxetine 10–20 mg in the morning
- Venlafaxine 75–100 mg in the morning
- Clomipramine 50 mg at night

Pubertal Children

For sleepiness
- Contact school to alert teachers
- Emphasize need for regular nocturnal sleep schedule
- Try to obtain 9 hr nocturnal sleep
- Nap at lunch time and at 5:30 PM

Continued

TABLE 27–2 Treatment for Narcolepsy—Cont'd		
Treatment for Cataplexy and Sleep Paralysis, with or Without Hypnagogic Hallucinations or Panic Reaction to Sleep Paralysis		
Drug	**Dosage**	**Comments**
	Medications:	
	• Modafinil 100–400 mg. Start at 100 mg in the morning for 5 days, then add 100 mg at noon; if needed, after 5 days, 200 mg in the morning and 100 mg at noon, and if still sleepy, increase to 200 mg in the morning and 200 mg at noon.	
	• Methylphenidate 10–60 mg. Take 15 mg upon awakening before eating, then 10 mg at lunch and 10 mg at 3:00 PM; alternatively, 20 mg SR upon awakening before eating, then 10 mg at lunch and 10 mg at 3:00 PM.	
For cataplexy	• Fluoxetine 10–40 mg in the morning	
	• Venlafaxine 75–150 mg in the morning	
Adults		
For EDS	• Avoid shifting sleep schedule	
	• Avoid heavy meals and alcohol	
	• Regular timing of nocturnal sleep: 10:30 PM to 7:00 AM	
	• Naps: 15 min at lunchtime and at 5:30 PM	
	Medications:	
	For daytime sleepiness (stimulant effects vary on individual basis)	
	• Modafinil 100–400 mg/day. Use 100–200 mg on awakening and 100–200 mg at noon; *or*	
	• Methylphenidate 5 mg (3 or 4 tablets taken 30 min before meals); 10 mg when waking up; 5 mg before lunch; 5 mg at 3:00 PM or 20 mg SR in the morning.	
	If still sleepy:	
	• Modafinil 400 mg in the morning and 200 mg at noon; *or*	
	• Methylphenidate (SR) 20 mg in the morning plus 5 mg intermediate-release formulation after noon nap and 5 mg intermediate-release formulation at 4 PM; *or*	
	• Add GIIB (sodium oxybate) at bedtime: start with 1.5 g at bedtime and 1.5 g 2 hr later. Gradually increase to total dose of 4–4.5 g within 3–4 wk and keep increasing to at least 6 g (3 g at bedtime and 3 g 2 hr later). If needed, gradually increase to 4.5 g at bedtime and 4.5 g 2 hr later. Do not exceed 9 g/day because of risk of side effects during sleep. Cataplexy responds faster; EDS may take up to 4–6 wk to improve; slowly reduce other stimulants only after reaching therapeutic dose (i.e., 6 g or more/day).	
	If no response:	
	• Dextroamphetamine sulfate: Dexedrine spansule (SR): 15 mg at awakening; 5 mg after noon nap, 5 mg at 3:30 or 4:00 PM; *or* 15 mg at awakening and 15 mg after noon nap.	
For cataplexy	• Fluoxetine 20–60 mg *or*	
	• Venlafaxine 150–300 mg *or*	
	• GHB (as above) *or*	
	• Clomipramine 75–125 mg *or*	
	• Viloxazine 150–200 mg *or*	
	• Imipramine 75–125 mg	

Caveats: The use of antidepressants for cataplexy is not approved by the U.S. Food and Drug Administration (FDA). Also, the FDA has not approved any medication for narcolepsy in children less than 16 years of age.
EDS, excessive daytime sleepiness; GHB, γ-hydroxybutyrate; PO, oral; SR, sustained-release.

episodes and sleepiness, when compared to stimulant usage alone.[138] Patient information materials, such as the Narcolepsy Fact Sheet from the National Institute of Neurological Disorders and Stroke and materials from the National Sleep Foundation and the Narcolepsy Network, are useful in helping the patient, family members, and friends understand the illness. Referral to a patient support group is important.

Education and Employment

General information about narcolepsy should be made available to teachers, employers, and other health care professionals. Career counseling is important. Patients should avoid jobs that involve shift work, on-call schedules, professional driving, or any job that is monotonous and requires continued attention for long hours without breaks. The Americans with Disabilities Act requires employers to provide reasonable accommodations for all employees with disabilities. Narcoleptic patients can negotiate with employers to adjust their work schedules to allow naps when necessary and to perform their most demanding tasks when they are alert. Similarly, school personnel should be informed about any special needs, including medication requirements and scheduled naps, so that class schedules of children and adolescents with narcolepsy can be modified. Scheduled 15- to 20-minute naps every 4 hours during the daytime at school or work is helpful, since excessive daytime sleepiness can disrupt vigilance and concentration and impair performance.

Driving

The laws on driving that affect narcoleptics vary depending on the state the patient resides in. As of March 1994, six states in the United States had guidelines for narcolepsy: Maryland, North Carolina, Oregon, Utah, California, and Texas. The patient and physician should consult their specific state motor vehicle department for advice. State mandatory reporting requirements may apply to providers in the following states: California, Delaware, New Jersey, Nevada, Oregon, and Pennsylvania.

Patient Follow-up

Narcoleptic patients should be assessed promptly and followed up at regular intervals, preferably in 3 months from diagnosis, and then at least every 6 months.

Pharmacologic Treatment

Excessive daytime sleepiness, cataplexy, and disturbed nocturnal sleep are the major symptoms that warrant treatment with drugs. When troublesome, hypnagogic hallucinations and sleep paralysis also require treatment consideration. Medications are chosen based on targeted symptoms, and, at times, coadministration of two or more classes of medications may be needed to adequately address them. The AASM's 2000 and 2007 practice parameters for the treatment of narcolepsy indicate that modafinil effectively treats EDS due to narcolepsy and is considered standard therapy due to its favorable risk:benefit ratio.[137,138] Sodium oxybate (γ-hydroxybutyrate [GHB]) is effective for treatment of daytime sleepiness, cataplexy, and disrupted sleep, and may be effective for the treatment of hypnagogic hallucinations and sleep paralysis.[138,139] Amphetamine, methamphetamine, dextroamphetamine, and methylphenidate are effective treatment modalities for EDS.[137–139] Although they have a long record of efficacy, their risk:benefit ratios are not clearly established.[138,139] Selegiline may be an effective treatment for cataplexy and daytime sleepiness, but usage may be limited by potential drug interactions and diet-induced interactions.[138,139] Clinical experience with the use of selegeline in narcolepsy is limited, leading to concerns about utilizing selegeline as an initial agent for addressing sleepiness in narcolepsy.[138,139]

Ritanserin may be effective therapy for daytime sleepiness, but is not currently available in the United States.[138,139] A dose of 5 mg added to other medications improved subjective sleepiness in a group of narcolepsy patients ($n = 28$), but did not significantly improve mean sleep latency on the MSLT.[140] In another study, doses of 5 or 10 mg of ritanserin improved perception of sleep quality but did not significantly improve subjective sleepiness.[141] Pemoline is effective therapy for EDS, but rare and potentially lethal liver toxicity may be unpredictable; it is no longer available in the United States and is no longer recommended for the treatment of narcolepsy.[138,139]

For some patients, a combination of long- and short-acting stimulants (e.g., methylphenidate with modafinil) or sustained-release amphetamines may be effective.

Excessive Daytime Sleepiness

Stimulants commonly used for treatment of EDS are indirect sympathomimetic compounds—amphetamine-like drugs including methylphenidate, amphetamine, dextroamphetamine, and methamphetamine. Most of these drugs share a common molecular structure, a benzene ring with an ethylamine side chain. These compounds increase the release of dopamine, serotonin (5-hydroxytryptamine [5-HT]), and norepinephrine; inhibit reuptake of amines by the dopamine transporter; and produce higher synaptic concentrations of amines. Increased amine signaling may promote wakefulness through direct effects on the cortex or via activation of subcortical pathways.[142]

Mitler and Hajdukovic compared the relative efficacy of various drugs for treating EDS in narcolepsy, presenting them in terms of percentage of normal levels of sleepiness based on the MSLT or MWT.[143] Treatment sleep latencies as a percentage of normal were as follows: methylphenidate 60 mg (79.7%), dextroamphetamine 60 mg (70.3%), modafinil 300 mg (55.3%), ritanserin 5 mg (47%), and GHB 25 mg/kg (22.4%).[143] Using similar normalization techniques, Mitler et al. utilized modafinil 300 mg (MWT), dextroamphetamine 60 mg (MWT), methylphenidate 60 mg (MWT), and methamphetamine 40–60 mg (MSLT) in narcoleptic subjects.[144] Dextroamphetamine, methamphetamine, and methylphenidate brought measurements above 60% of normal levels, with the greatest change from baseline occurring with methamphetamine.[144]

Stimulants. Amphetamines and methylphenidate reduce sleepiness, increase sleep onset and REM sleep latency, and decrease the percentage of REM sleep. In standard stimulant doses (10–60 mg), amphetamines can enhance performance in simple motor and cognitive tasks; improve coordination; and increase strength, endurance, and mental and physical activation, even in situations of fatigue and boredom. Methylphenidate in standard doses of 20–80 mg/day is also effective for EDS. In adults, amphetamines or methylphenidate at dosages higher than 60 mg/day do not significantly improve EDS and result in long-term side effects, including sleep disruption. Optimal response to EDS is achieved using a combination of pharmacologic agents (intermediate-release formulations) and two short naps, with no stimulant drug taken after 3:00 PM. Stimulants (amphetamines and methylphenidate) are usually administered in three divided doses with a maximum of 20 mg in the morning, 20 mg at lunchtime, and 20 mg no later than 3:00 PM. The slow-release formulations may provide gradual and delayed responses during the day.

Common stimulant side effects include irritability (49%), headaches (48%), tremulousness and nervousness (35%), anorexia (22%), insomnia (11–17%), dyskinesias

(5%), palpitations (3%), hallucinations (3%), and psychosis (1.6%).[144] Rebound hypersomnia can occur at the end of transmitter availability for release and is well documented in the clinical setting. High doses of amphetamines can result in cognitive and behavioral pathology, including paranoid psychosis and repetitive thoughts. Amphetamines and related substances have high abuse potential. In children, transient side effects of stimulants include anorexia, insomnia, and weight loss, which remit with continued use.[144]

Mazindol is a weak stimulant with dopamine and adrenergic blocking properties that has not been as clinically effective as amphetamines and is currently not a commonly used drug. It has been used at daily doses ranging from 3 to 8 mg[146] with improvement in EDS but without effect on cataplexy, and at doses ranging from 0.5 to 4 mg/day with reduction in EDS and improvement in cataplexy in some subjects.[146]

Modafinil and Armodafinil. Modafinil is a novel wakefulness-promoting drug whose mechanism of action is unknown; armodafinil is the (R)-enantiomer of modafinil, with a longer half-life. Modafinil is hypothesized to selectively activate wake-generating sites in the hypothalamus (tuberomammillary nucleus and hypocretin neurons of the perifornical area).[147] Modafinil does not appear to be a direct or indirect α agonist, nor does it bind to norepinephrine, serotonin, dopamine, or γ-aminobutyric acid receptors. Blockade of reuptake of noradrenaline by the noradrenergic terminals on the sleep-promoting neurons from the ventrolateral preoptic nucleus may be a mechanism for modafinil's wake promotion.[147,148] Modafinil has a better safety profile, fewer side effects, and lower abuse risk potential compared to traditional stimulants, making it the current initial drug of choice for EDS, but it has no effect on cataplexy and other REM sleep–related symptoms. Dosages range from 100 to 600 mg/day (single dose or split dose) are shown in various studies to be associated with improvement in fatigue, mood, cognitive functioning, and health-related quality-of-life measures.[149–153] A split-dose strategy has been shown in three studies to provide better control of daytime sleepiness than a single daily dose.[138] Side effects are mild to moderate in 5–6% of patients and include headache, nausea, insomnia, emotional lability, nervousness, and dyspepsia. Headache, the most common complaint, can be reduced by a slow and gradual increase in dose.

Modafinil works best in stimulant-naive patients. Patients previously treated with traditional stimulants, such as dextroamphetamine or methylphenidate, can be successfully switched to modafinil.[154] However, patients requiring ≥45 mg/day of amphetamines complain of having less control over sleepiness compared to their prior medication. At the Stanford Sleep Disorders Clinic, approximately 20% of patients previously on amphetamines request discontinuation of modafinil (usually at doses of 400–600 mg/day) and resumption of their previous medications. Other inadvertent side effects of the switch from stimulants to modafinil are breakthrough cataplectic attacks and, more rarely, sleep paralysis. For patients with REM sleep–related symptoms previously controlled on amphetamines, an anticataplectic medication (e.g., venlafaxine 100 mg) may need to be added, or the dosage of the concurrent anticataplectic agent may be increased simultaneously with the prescription of modafinil. For patients experiencing late-day sleepiness even on 600 mg of modafinil (400 mg at 7:00 AM, 200 mg at noon), short-acting methylphenidate may be added as a rescue medication.

In a large, multicenter, randomized controlled trial of armodafinil, narcoleptic subjects who received 50 mg or 250 mg as a single-dose regimen experienced improvement in subjective sleepiness. The MWT also demonstrated efficacy, with improvement in mean sleep latencies compared to the placebo group.[139,155]

γ-Hydroxybutyrate (Sodium Oxybate). GHB (sodium oxybate) is a naturally occurring metabolite of the human nervous system that is highly concentrated in the hypothalamus and basal ganglia. At a dose of 30 mg/kg, it induces a normal sequence of non-REM and REM sleep lasting 2–3 hours in normal volunteers. Sodium oxybate is effective for the treatment of cataplexy, daytime sleepiness, and disrupted sleep.[138] It may also be effective for treatment of hypnagogic hallucinations and sleep paralysis.[138] The medication is usually given in two divided doses; both doses are prepared and at the bedside. The first dose is taken at bedtime, with the patient in bed to prevent falls; the second dose is taken 2.5–4 hours after the first dose, with the patient still in bed. The recommended starting dose is 4.5 g/day divided into two equal doses of 2.25 g. The dosage can then be increased at 2-week intervals in increments of 1.5 g/day (0.75 g/dose) to a maximum dose of 9 g/day. The usual effective dose ranges from 6 to 9 g/night; subjective sleepiness as measured by the ESS is reduced and the number of sleep attacks diminishes, with the greatest improvement at the 9-g dose.[138] Sodium oxybate (6 g/night × 4 weeks, then 9 g/night) improves objective alertness (as measured by the MWT) to a greater extent (average sleep latency of 11.97 minutes) compared to modafinil (200–600 mg/day; average sleep latency of 9.86 minutes).[156] The study also suggests an additive effect on alertness with a combination of sodium oxybate and modafinil. Adverse effects of sodium oxybate may include abnormal coordination, confusional arousals, amnesia, apathy, asthemia, respiratory complaints, hypesthesia, headache, metallic taste, nervousness, somnolence, weight loss, psychosis, episodes of enuresis, and transient worsening of nocturnal cataplexy. High dosages may be associated with nausea.

Selegiline. Selegiline is a monoamine oxidase type B inhibitor that is metabolized to amphetamine and methamphetamine. In a group of 17 narcolepsy patients, 40 mg of selegiline reduced the number of excessive sleepiness episodes by 36% and the duration of these episodes by 43%; the number of cataplectic attacks was also reduced by 89%.[157] Similar findings were reported in a study of 30 narcoleptic patients using selegiline 10–20 mg; dose-dependent REM suppression during nighttime sleep and daytime naps were found, and REM latency was increased.[158] Therapeutic concerns include limited experience with the high doses needed for narcolepsy, risk for diet-induced hypertension, and high cost of the medication.

Reboxitine. Reboxitine is a new selective noradrenaline reuptake inhibitor with antidepressant efficacy that is currently not available in the United States. In a small study ($n = 12$) of narcolepsy patients, reboxitine (10 mg) significantly improved daytime sleepiness (mean decrease of 48.6% on the ESS) and increased mean sleep latency on the MSLT by 54.7%.[159]

Ritanserin. Ritanserin is a 5-HT$_2$ antagonist that is used to treat sleepiness. In a study of 28 narcolepsy patients, the addition of 5 mg of ritanserin to usual medications improved subjective daytime sleepiness, but did not significantly change mean sleep latency on the MSLT.[140] In a study of 134 narcoleptics, adding ritanserin (5 or 10 mg) to usual treatment resulted in some improvement in subjective quality of sleep, but there was no significant improvement in daytime alertness.[141] Ritanserin significantly increased nocturnal slow-wave sleep (percentage of total sleep time) and significantly reduced non-REM stage 1 percentage during daytime sleep.[141] In contrast to the first study on narcoleptic patients, ritanserin improved only one subjective parameter, but did not improve objective sleep quality or number of "sleep attacks" or reduce "wake after sleep onset" during nighttime or daytime sleep.[141]

EDS in Children

We recommend modafinil for the treatment of EDS in children with narcolepsy, based upon our clinical experience with more than 1000 adults and children with narcolepsy. Modafinil is best administered in divided doses (morning and noon), but this may not be possible with children, so a single morning dose has been prescribed. However, single-dose administration may result in late-day sleepiness; a 5-mg tablet of methylphenidate may be added when the child returns from school, if needed. The methylphenidate must not be given too late, or sleep-onset insomnia may occur.

If modafinil cannot be prescribed, methylphenidate is the second best option. The intermediate-release (IR) forms of methylphenidate peak in 1–2 hours and wane after 3–5 hours. Methylphenidate is also available in extended-release formulations, which allow drug release over 8 hours. In children, the recommended dose is based on weight, and a maximum of 30 mg/day is administered in the slow-release formulation. Methylphenidate can be prescribed in divided doses (15 mg IR at 7:00 AM and 15 mg [maximum] IR at lunchtime) in the best case or as a 20- or 30-mg slow-release form in the morning. The sustained-release formulations can produce insomnia and anorexia in the evening.

Cataplexy and REM Sleep–Related Symptoms

REM sleep–associated muscle atonia occurs during wakefulness, resulting in cataplexy. The inhibitory pathways involving the lower motor neurons are affected by neurotransmitters, such as the muscarinic cholinergic and noradrenergic systems. Sodium oxybate administration in doses of 4.5, 6, and 9 g results in dose-dependent reductions in number of cataplectic attacks by 57%, 65%, and 87.7%, respectively.[139] In addition to sodium oxybate, tricyclic antidepressants, selective serotonin reuptake inhibitors (SSRIs), venlafaxine, and reboxetine may be effective therapy for cataplexy.[138] All antidepressants have an immediate effect on cataplexy. Tricyclic antidepressants were the earlier agents utilized for cataplexy, since they inhibit monoamine (serotonin, norepinephrine, epinephrine, and dopamine) reuptake and block cholinergic, histaminic, and α-adrenergic transmission. Among the tricyclic antidepressants, imipramine and desipramine are noradrenergic-specific uptake blockers and potent anticataplexy agents. Tricyclic antidepressants produce the following adverse effects: inhibition of fast sodium channels, resulting in potentially life-threatening adverse effects such as cardiac conduction disturbances and seizures; blockage of histamine receptors, resulting in sedation; and anticholinergic effects, producing constipation, impotence, and ejaculation problems. Thus, tricyclics are currently used only as a last resort.

The most commonly utilized drugs for cataplexy are drugs that have an active noradrenergic reuptake blocker metabolite, such as clomipramine and fluoxetine. Clomipramine and its metabolite desmethylclomipramine are potent inhibitors of the norepinephrine uptake pump and, to a lesser degree, inhibit the serotonin uptake pump and fast sodium channels. Fluoxetine and its metabolite norfluoxetine are potent inhibitors of the serotonin uptake pump. We recommend starting with 20 mg fluoxetine in the morning and increasing weekly to 60–80 mg each day in two divided doses, or starting with 50 mg of clomipramine at bedtime and increasing to a maximum of 200 mg/day in two divided doses. The usual doses for cataplexy are fluoxetine 40–60 mg given as a single dose or clomipramine 50 mg twice a day.

Alternatively, newer antidepressant medications, such as venlafaxine and atomoxetine, are highly effective anticataplexy agents that also improve sleep paralysis and hallucinations (hypnagogic or hypnapompic). Venlafaxine inhibits serotonin reuptake more than it inhibits norepinephrine reuptake, but has less effect on the dopamine systems. It is used in doses ranging from 75 to 300 mg/day, but has a high incidence of associated nausea and moderate insomnia, and a low incidence of anticholinergic side effects; sexual side effects are less than with other antidepressants. Venlafaxine's extended-release formulation may be preferred for cataplexy. Atomoxetine, a selective norepinephrine reuptake inhibitor, may be utilized in doses ranging from 18 to 100 mg/day, either as a single dose or in two divided doses for cataplexy unresponsive to fluoxetine or venlafaxine. Atomoxetine has a short half-life and reduces appetite.

Patients should be warned that abrupt discontinuation of antidepressants may lead to rebound cataplexy. In addition, abrupt discontinuation of SSRIs can lead to sensory abnormalities (including electric shock–like sensations), disequilibrium, insomnia, increased dreams, headache, lethargy, mood change, and, rarely, psychosis.

Special Issues in Women with Narcolepsy

Fertility/Contraception. Onset of puberty or the establishment of the menstrual cycle is not affected by either narcolepsy or the drugs utilized for treatment. Narcolepsy is not known to affect fertility.[160] Some narcoleptic women report a perimenstrual increase in daytime sleepiness and cataplexy episodes; these symptoms may require temporary increase in medication dosages during these periods. Methylphenidate, amphetamine, methamphetamine, dextroamphetamine, and mazindol do not reduce efficacy of oral contraceptives. However, modafinil modestly increases activity of the hepatic enzymes metabolizing oral contraceptive agents, thereby reducing their effectiveness. Women should be advised to switch to another form of contraception, or, for those who wish to continue using oral contraception, a product containing 50 mcg or higher ethinyl estradiol should be prescribed and continued for two cycles after stopping modafinil. Physicians should be aware that contraceptive pills can either enhance or inhibit the effects of tricyclic antidepressant drugs used to treat cataplexy.

Pregnancy. The U.S. Food and Drug Administration has established five categories of drugs based on potential for teratogenicity:

- Category A: controlled studies have shown risk to the human fetus in the first trimester and remote possibility of fetal harm

- Category B: animal studies indicate no fetal risk but no controlled studies have been performed in humans
- Category C: animal studies have shown teratogenic or embryocidal effects and there are no controlled human studies
- Category D: there is evidence of risk to human fetuses but benefits may make risk acceptable
- Category X: studies in animals or humans have demonstrated fetal abnormalities and the risks outweigh any possible benefit

The manufacturers of modafinil and stimulant drugs recommend that these be discontinued before conception and during pregnancy. With the cessation of sale of pemoline in the United States, only sodium oxybate remains as a Category B drug. Modafinil, fluoxetine, clomipramine, and venlafaxine are all Category C drugs. Although the tricyclic antidepressants and SSRIs are probably not teratogenic, cessation of the medication prior to conception and during pregnancy is probably warranted if the cataplexy is mild. When cataplexy is significant, the risk of injury during pregnancy with adverse effects on the fetus may be higher than the risk of teratogenicity. If medications for cataplexy are required during pregnancy, fluoxetine may be the preferred choice.

Full discussion and documentation of the discussion of risk:benefit ratio with the narcoleptic woman is important. Close coordination of care between the sleep specialist, the obstetrician, and the pharmacologist is important, particularly with issues of possible teratogenicity, increased risk of hypertension with stimulant medications, and potential drug interactions. The use of SSRIs and norepinephrine reuptake inhibitors during the last trimester of pregnancy may result in serious feeding and respiratory difficulties for neonates immediately after birth. Gradual tapering and slow withdrawal should be performed before the last trimester of pregnancy to minimize the risk of cataplexy rebound that usually occurs on the third or fourth day, with peak near day 10 following completion of withdrawal.

Breastfeeding and Other Precautions. Manufacturers of drugs utilized for EDS and cataplexy recommend avoidance of breastfeeding due to the medications appearing in breast milk. If breastfeeding is avoided, treatment for EDS and cataplexy can be restarted soon after delivery. In the immediate postnatal period, help from the partner/family may be needed, since the narcoleptic mother still needs her naps. Women with cataplexy should be advised regarding commonsense precautions, such as changing their baby on a mat on the floor rather than on the bed, and to avoid carrying the baby in their arms either indoors or outdoors, where hard surfaces are present.

CLINICAL VARIANTS AND ASSOCIATED ILLNESSES

There are clearly documented forms of "secondary" or "symptomatic" narcolepsy with EDS and cataplexy that are due to a coexisting medical or neurologic disorder. Insomnia, automatic behavior, sleep paralysis, or hypnagogic hallucinations may or may not be present. Cataplexy with EDS has been linked with other brain disorders since the early 1900s. Associated disorders include tumors, localized most frequently to the diencephalon or brain stem; large arteriovenous malformations, ischemic infarcts, or multiple sclerosis plaques in the diencephalon; head trauma; and limbic encephalitis. In young children, Niemann-Pick disease type C, characterized by hepatosplenomegaly, progressive ataxia, dystonia, dementia, and vertical supranuclear ophthalmoplegia, is often associated with early onset of cataplexy, as pointed out by Challamel et al.[161] In these children with Niemann-Pick disease, cataplexy was noted much earlier, with a mean age of onset of 6 years, compared to our group of prepubertal children with narcolepsy.[39,161–164]

The other cause of very-early-onset cataplexy is craniopharyngioma. This tumor, one of the most common brain tumors in children, accounts for 9% of all pediatric intracranial tumors (0.5–2.0 cases per 1 million population per year).[165] Craniopharyngioma often presents between ages 5 and 10 years and can invade the pituitary, optic chiasm, and hypothalamus. This neoplasm can lead to severe obesity, hypoventilation, and abrupt bilateral muscle weakness. With hypothalamic involvement, cataplexy and other symptoms may persist despite resection of the tumor. If the craniopharyngioma has not invaded the hypothalamus, surgical trauma related to tumor removal may result in transient cataplexy that will gradually subside[166]; however, if cataplexy is present before surgery, removal of the tumor is not associated with regression of cataplexy.

With the discovery of the hypocretin/orexin system and the ability to measure CSF Hcrt-1 levels, several case reports or short series have documented that lesions of the lateral and posterior hypothalamus, independent of cause (but mostly tumors), will lead to lesions of hypocretin-producing neurons associated with the development of EDS and cataplexy.[167–170] Some cases may be a diagnostic challenge. As an example, hypothalamic astrocytoma resulted in obesity, pseudo–Prader-Willi syndrome, and associated atypical cataplexy. In these cases of secondary cataplexy, the abrupt muscle weakness may not be triggered by laughter,[170] and depending on the onset of the neurologic syndrome, may be seen very early in life (such as in Niemann-Pick type C)[161–164] or late in life.

An interesting association has been reported between the development of cataplexy with very little sleepiness and clinical symptoms of limbic encephalitis[171]; an anti-Ma2 antibody test was positive, and a search for malignancy revealed testicular cancer. In limbic encephalitis, magnetic resonance imaging may demonstrate abnormalities in the limbic, diencephalic, or brain stem regions. These lesions are frequently associated with malignancy. In young males, the most common neoplasm is testicular cancer, while in other patients, the leading associated neoplasm is lung cancer.[172]

Neurologic symptoms precede the diagnosis of cancer in 50% of paraneoplastic syndromes. The development of cataplexy out of the usual age range, the presence of atypical cataplexy, and the lack of clear association with other symptoms of narcolepsy are warning flags that warrant further investigation (neurologic and otherwise) so as not to miss a rare paraneoplastic syndrome and to detect a primary cancer site. The existence of immunologic involvement in the narcolepsy syndrome and paraneoplastic syndromes is another interesting association.

In general, the secondary cataplexies are associated with specific lesions located in the lateral and posterior hypothalamus[173] involving the hypocretin/orexin neurons. These lesions can be detected by brain imaging. Less often, neurologic lesions will involve the brain stem, thereby interrupting the descending pathways that maintain active inhibition of the inhibitory reticular formation of Magoun and Rhines. Neoplasms in the brain stem can present in different ways. Isolated cataplexy has been seen with a pontomedullary pilocystic astrocytoma,[174] while cataplexy with variable EDS has been associated with brain stem glioblastoma[174] and subependymoma of the fourth ventricle.[175] Additionally, "status cataplecticus" has been reported with a midbrain glioblastoma involving the rostral brain stem and hypothalamus.[176]

Other sleep disorders may also coexist with narcolepsy. Obstructive sleep apnea may be seen more frequently with narcolepsy. A study of 100 sleep apnea patients found that 24% had 2 or more SOREMPs at MSLT (unpublished observation). The association of daytime sleepiness, cataplexy, and sleep apnea, however, can undoubtedly be noted, with cataplexy affirming the presence of the narcolepsy syndrome. Increased periodic limb movements in sleep (PLMS) have also been associated with narcolepsy.[31] However, aging, and the use of tricyclics, such as imipramine, clomipramine, and protriptyline, can also increase the number of PLMS. Montplaisir and Godbout do not believe from their own analysis that PMLS is an important factor in nocturnal sleep disruption in narcolepsy.[177]

DIFFERENTIAL DIAGNOSIS

The major considerations in the differential diagnosis of narcolepsy are idiopathic hypersomnia and the syndromes associating EDS with the presence of 1 or several SOREMPs. Idiopathic hypersomnia, which is characterized by EDS, should be considered a possible diagnosis only when obstructive sleep apnea and upper airway resistance syndrome have been ruled out. Unlike narcolepsy, the daytime somnolence associated with idiopathic hypersomnia is rarely relieved by short naps. In fact, naps may lead to sleep drunkenness and complaints of increased tiredness. Frequently reported with this syndrome are mild symptoms of autonomic nervous system dysfunction, such as cold hands and cold feet (Raynaud-type phenomena), light-headedness (rarely associated with a drop in systolic blood pressure sufficient to be called orthostatic hypotension), and frequent dull headaches similar to migraine headaches. In some instances, the syndrome develops immediately after infectious mononucleosis, Guillain-Barré syndrome, viral hepatitis, or atypical pneumonia, particularly that involving echoviruses, which suggests that a virus might participate in the appearance of idiopathic hypersomnia. Polysomnography and MSLTs in idiopathic hypersomnia show lack of SOREMPs and a mean sleep latency of approximately 6 minutes. Table 27–1 summarizes the categories of narcolepsy, including pertinent features, and Tables 27–3 and 27–4 list suggested approaches to diagnosis.

CONCLUSIONS

Despite the numerous advances made in narcolepsy research, narcolepsy remains a disabling neurologic illness that is poorly or incompletely controlled by treatment. Narcolepsy has profound effects on quality of life. It is a major employment problem for its victims and is often the source of job discrimination, job dismissal, early retirement, and depression due to these circumstances.

TABLE 27–3 How to Diagnose Narcolepsy

Symptom*	Assessment	Plan
Partial or complete cataplectic attacks, daytime sleepiness, and napping History of complete cataplectic attacks and current daytime sleepiness and napping Partial or complete cataplectic attacks and intermittent daytime drowsiness several times a week	Patient is narcoleptic	Confirm by nocturnal PSG followed the next day by MSLT. PSG shows presence or absence of sleep apnea, shows presence or absence of PLMs, and documents adequate amount of sleep. MSLT shows short sleep latencies and 2 SOREMPs. Risk of MSLT being negative with 1-day test is 3%.
Isolated cataplexy; no reports of EDS or napping Isolated EDS and daytime napping EDS, daytime napping, HH, SP	Patient has isolated cataplexy, is not narcoleptic, but ... Patient is not narcoleptic (see Table 27–4)	Confirm absence of EDS by PSG and MSLT Investigate family history for narcolepsy Perform HLA typing to search for DQB1*0602 Patient may be developing narcolepsy. Follow patient.

*By patient report.
EDS, excessive daytime sleepiness; HH, hypnagogic hallucinations; HLA, human leukocyte antigen; MSLT, Multiple Sleep Latency Test; PLMs, periodic limb movements; PSG, polysomnography; SOREMPs, sleep-onset REM periods; SP, sleep paralysis.

TABLE 27–4 What to Do When the Patient is Not a Bona Fide Narcoleptic*

If	Then

Patient presents with EDS, daytime napping, hypnagogic hallucinations, and sleep paralysis
• Patient is young.
• Sleep latencies in MSLT are short.
• More than 1 SOREMP.
• PSG shows no cause for EDS.
• There is family (first-degree relative) history of narcolepsy.
	1. Perform polygraphic recordings and daytime MSLT.
	2. Investigate first-degree relatives for narcolepsy.
	3. Consider patient's age.
	    Patient is probably developing narcolepsy.
	    Follow and treat as a narcoleptic. Do HLA typing and determine whether DQB1*0602 is expressed.

Patient presents with isolated EDS and daytime napping:
• Patient has no clinical symptoms for other causes of EDS.
• Tests produce a good, undisrupted nocturnal PSG without evidence of sleep-related problems.
• MSLT produces short latencies but ≤1 SOREMP.
• The family history includes narcolepsy.
• Patient is young.
• Patient has no clinical symptoms for other causes of EDS.
• Tests produce a good, undisrupted nocturnal PSG without evidence of sleep-related problems.
• MSLT produces short latencies but ≤1 SOREMP.
	1. Obtain good sleep history.
	2. Perform nocturnal PSG followed by next-day MSLT.
	3. Investigate family history for causes of EDS.
	4. Consider patient's age. Patient may be developing narcolepsy.
	    Follow and treat as a narcoleptic. Perform HLA typing.
	    Consider CSF examination for hypocretin.
	
	Patient is considered to have a disorder of daytime sleepiness (probably related to narcolepsy, but unproven to date). HLA typing may be considered. Treat as a narcoleptic.

Continued

TABLE 27–4 What to Do When the Patient is Not a Bona Fide Narcoleptic*—Cont'd

If	Then
• The family history includes narcolepsy. • The patient is middle-aged or older, with several years' history of sleepiness. • Patient has no clinical symptoms for other causes of EDS. • Tests produce good, undisrupted nocturnal PSG without evidence of sleep-related problems. • MSLT mean sleep latency ≤8 min and ≥2 SOREMPs.	Middle-aged or older patient has narcolepsy without cataplexy. Young patient may be developing narcolepsy. HLA typing may be considered. Treat with modafinil or other stimulants.
• Family history of narcolepsy. • Patient is young, middle-aged, or older with several years' history of sleepiness. • Patient has no clinical symptoms for other causes of EDS. • Tests produce good, undisrupted PSG without evidence of sleep-related problems. • MSLT produces short sleep latencies with ≤1 SOREMP. • There is no family history of narcolepsy.	Patient of any age is considered to have CNS hypersomnia (relation to narcolepsy unknown). Investigate for viral infection concomitant with syndrome onset, and possibly perform serologic studies for positive history. Investigate family for history of isolated daytime sleepiness. HLA typing is of scientific interest for better definition of the syndrome. Treat with stimulants.

*That is, if cataplexy is not currently and never has been present.
CNS, central nervous system; CSF, cerebrospinal fluid; EDS, excessive daytime sleepiness; HLA, human leukocyte antigen; MSLT, Multiple Sleep Latency Test; PSG, polysomnography; SOREMP, sleep-onset REM period.

Challenges for the future involve our ability to understand better its pathophysiology; identify environmental trigger(s) and how to avoid them; describe the interaction between genetic predisposition and environmental trigger(s); predict factors affecting individual response to specific therapeutic agents for EDS, cataplexy, and other REM sleep–related symptoms; and devise methods to prevent destruction of hypocretin neurons and/or ways to correct hypocretin deficiency. Future approaches may be directed toward further elucidation of genetic mutations leading to hypocretin neuronal destruction, correction of hypocretin deficiency through agonists, genetic engineering to replace deficient hypocretin, and immunologic therapy to prevent destruction of hypocretin-producing neurons through stem cell research or brain implants. Novel treatment strategies for EDS may include the use of histamine$_3$ antagonists and slow-wave sleep enhancers. New formulations of sodium oxybate may provide longer duration of action and more convenient solid preparations, and newer antidepressants may provide better control of cataplexy. Although the ultimate therapeutic goal is disease prevention, better control of disease symptoms with a view to normalizing quality of life is a more immediate objective.

REFERENCES

A full list of references are available at www.expertconsult.com

CHAPTER 28

Motor Functions and Dysfunctions of Sleep

Wayne A. Hening, Richard P. Allen, Arthur S. Walters
and **Sudhansu Chokroverty**

INTRODUCTION

The motor system is highly modulated by the changes in state from wakefulness to drowsiness to slow-wave sleep (SWS) and then to rapid eye movement (REM) sleep. Indeed, so significant are the changes in motor activity depending on state that various researchers have used quantitative recordings of motor activity, known as *actigraphy*, as a basis for determining sleep and wake states.[1] The importance of measuring such activity is growing and is reflected in a new section of this chapter that deals with the use of actigraphy in assessing sleep disorders.

This chapter is divided into four sections. The first briefly reviews normal motor activity and its changes during sleep, whereas the next two sections examine motor disturbances associated with sleep. These two sections are informally divided into two categories. On the one hand, there are motor disturbances present during the day (diurnal movement disorders) that may impact sleep, either directly through their motor effects or indirectly through a variety of other mechanisms. These are *movement disorders* that are seen by a neurologist or movement disorder specialist. On the other hand, there are the motor disturbances that are predominantly associated with sleep. They may be motor activity similar to what is normally found during waking hours that is abnormal and disruptive when it occurs during sleep (some parasomnias, such as sleep walking, are of this type) or abnormal motor activity that does not occur during the wake state, but is evoked by sleep. These are generally classified as *sleep disorders* and typically treated by a sleep disorders specialist. The second edition of the International Classification of Sleep Disorders (ICSD-2) has defined a specific category of sleep disorders called Movement Disorders of Sleep[2] and created rules for recognizing them during a sleep study (polysomnography [PSG]).[3] These two main categories of motor abnormalities are by no means completely distinct, and it is not unusual for a patient with a disorder in one category to be seen by a specialist in the other category. It is, therefore, useful to consider these two categories of sleep disturbances together in this chapter. Finally, the last section of the chapter contains information on specific investigative techniques that can be applied to diagnose and evaluate the sleep-associated motor dysfunctions.

This chapter has two major purposes: to describe and compare the various motor disturbances of sleep and to demonstrate a usable approach to the diagnosis and treatment of motor disturbances of sleep. Although this chapter touches briefly on the distinctions between the various movement disorders, it does not pretend to be a general review of movement disorders. Those in the sleep field who wish to refer to a general discussion of movement disorders can find a number of reviews that deal extensively with a wide spectrum of movement disorders.[4–6] There are also a number of excellent, more abbreviated treatments of this field in medical and neurologic textbooks.[7,8] The remaining chapters in this volume provide a suitable background for sleep-related issues for the neurologist or other individual whose primary field is movement disorders. Where issues have overlapped—such as those parasomnias that cause motor disturbances—we have referred to other chapters in this volume so as not to unnecessarily increase the length of this one.

THE MOTOR SYSTEM IN RELATION TO SLEEP

Before discussing specific motor disturbances of sleep, we review the normal physiology of the motor system during sleep and the patterns of normal motor activity that vary with the circadian rhythm, the different sleep stages, and human development and aging. Abnormal activity, in different cases, may follow this same background activity pattern or deviate from it in striking ways.

Circadian Activity Cycles

In many, if not most, animal species, the motor system's level of activity is dependent on the time of day. Even in the absence of a day-night light cycle (i.e., under constant conditions), such activity cycling persists in a *free-running state* with a circadian period. As discussed in Chapter 8, many other important physiologic variables, such as temperature, also show circadian periods. While there may be a number of supplementary oscillators that control these rhythms,[9–11] the suprachiasmatic nucleus (SCN) is thought to contain the most important oscillator[12] and to be the center that is responsible for the circadian variation of motor activity. The basic mechanism is a transcription-translation feedback loop,[13,14] elements of which are widely distributed in peripheral tissues.[15] In at least some species, a distinctive, localized subregion of the nucleus may be critically necessary to sustain locomotor rhythms,[16] while one report has found two distinguishable SCN motor controllers.[17] Another mediator may be an expression of clock genes, such as the period gene *rPer2*, which are widely distributed in different tissues and controlled by the SCN.[18] Studies indicate that a large amount of SCN output is channeled through the subparaventricular zone of the hypothalamus (SPZ), which contains a specific region specialized in modulating motor activity.[19] The SPZ also acts as an integrating center for various influences that can impact on circadian rhythm, such as food availability, ambient temperature, and social interactions. Some of the hypothalamic regulation of motor activity is via the hypocretin system, which stimulates activity at the end of the activity period (the evening for humans).[20,21]

In humans, of course, sleep is usually at night, so that activity is concentrated during the daytime hours. A number of studies have begun to suggest that the division of the 24-hour cycle into distinct single periods of waking with high levels of motor activity and of sleep with minimal motor activity is optimal. Indeed, the quality of sleep may be inversely related to the amount of motor activity: better sleep, less overall movement at night.[22] Movements are associated with autonomic activation.[23] The clear separation of these periods begins to break down in normal aging[23] and cases of poor sleep or sleep-related disorders, as well as in many movement disorders and degenerative conditions. Circadian treatment with morning bright light can sometimes restore sleep quality and reduce nocturnal movement.[24]

The Motor System and Sleep Stages

Changes in motor activity are dependent on the sleep state (i.e., wake, REM, non-REM [NREM] sleep stages). For example, one frequently used monitor of sleep-wake state, the chin electromyogram (EMG), is an indicator of branchial (brain stem) muscle tone. During wake, chin muscle tone is high and a tonically active chin EMG is interrupted by phasic contractions (facial expressions, tension, chewing, etc.). With relaxation and drowsiness, the level of EMG activity decreases. It further decreases as NREM sleep is achieved and deepens to SWS levels. Then, during REM sleep, EMG activity becomes minimal or even inapparent, although it may be occasionally interrupted with brief, irregular bursts of activity. These changes mirror, to a fair degree, the changes undergone by much of the motor system during sleep. As explained later, much of this variability can be understood on the basis of the altered activity of different levels of the motor system, as well as their interaction, during different sleep stages. In one interesting study, it was shown that another influence was the bed partner: partners tended to synchronize their movements during the night.[25]

It is important to note that the relationship between motor activities and sleep stages may need to be qualified in various contexts:

1. It should be remembered that, at a technical level, sleep scoring may not adequately reflect the underlying brain processes at the time of a given event such as a movement. Sleep is generally scored as arbitrary epochs of fixed length, usually 30 seconds, whereas physiologic processes may occur on a variety of time scales. This has led some investigators to examine microepochs of a few seconds for momentary state.[26]

2. It may not be possible to adequately score some sleep according to the traditional Rechtschaffen and Kales (R&K) scoring rules.[27] This has led to various proposals for revising the scoring system or even to use very different methods of scoring. The new American Academy of Sleep Medicine (AASM) scoring manual[28] (see Chapter 18) modifies R&K sleep scoring slightly. One important supplementary scoring system looks at periodic alternations in electroencephalographic (EEG) activity. In NREM sleep, especially stage 2, this periodicity is common and is designated the cyclic alternating pattern (CAP).[29] First described by Terzano and colleagues,[30] this pattern shows an alternation between bursts of both slow and fast activity

(A phase) alternating with a medium-frequency, lower amplitude activity (B phase). The burst-like activity (A phase) is associated with autonomic activation. The A phases can include greater or lesser amounts of faster frequencies: A1 has the least and A3 the most fast frequencies. A2 and A3 phases are often associated with arousals that can disrupt sleep.[31,32] A number of different abnormal sleep-related movements can be found to be associated with specific phases of the CAP cycle, especially the A phase.[33] These include periodic limb movements in sleep (PLMS),[34] parasomnias such as bruxism[35] or sleepwalking,[36,37] alternating leg movement activity during sleep (ALMA),[38] and nocturnal paroxysmal dystonia.[39] CAP, especially phases A1 and A2, occurs more in early childhood,[40] decreases during latency age,[41] may transiently increase during the adolescent period,[29,42] decreases in young adulthood,[29] and then increases again in older ages.[29] CAP is a normal pattern, but deviations from normal amounts, especially excessive CAP, can be abnormal.

3. The sleep stages themselves are not fully discrete or comprehensive. Fragments of a stage, such as REM-related atonia, may occur during other states, even in fully normal individuals. For example, Mahowald and Schenck[43] reported on six patients with marked admixture of features from the different sleep-wake states (i.e., wake, NREM sleep, REM sleep). These patients showed abnormal distribution of motor activity with relation to sleep features; similar findings have been reported after brain stem surgery[44] and in Guillain-Barré syndrome.[45]

4. Motor events, although typical of one sleep stage or state, may less commonly occur in other stages. PLMS occur primarily in NREM sleep, but may also occur in REM sleep,[46] especially in disorders of disturbed REM sleep such as narcolepsy and REM sleep behavior disorder (RBD).[47,48] These movements may also occur during arousals or periods of wakefulness after sleep onset (periodic limb movement in wakefulness [PLMW]), often as part of a periodic sequence of movements that span the sleep-wake divide.[49]

5. Many conditions are not completely pure but contain a combination of disorders related to different sleep stages. For example, narcolepsy is highly associated with PLMS,[50] and patients with somnambulism, which typically occurs in NREM sleep, may show REM sleep motor abnormalities suggestive of RBD.[51]

Table 28–1 provides a summary of the frequency of normal and abnormal motor activities that occur during the various phases of sleep and waking. Because many of these movements have not been fully and exhaustively studied, this table is a preliminary guide rather than a definitive pronouncement.

Drowsiness, Sleep Onset, and Arousals

In the period before sleep begins, humans, as well as other animals, enter a period of relative repose. This period has been called the pre-dormitum by MacDonald Critchley.[52] The subsequent transition to sleep is signaled by a variety of behavioral and EEG features.[53] Even before sleep onset, the motor system reduces its level of activity. It is during this period that the symptoms of restless legs syndrome (RLS) become prominent. RLS is relatively distinctive in that, unlike almost all other movement disorders, it is activated by rest. Another movement disorder activated in the transition to sleep is a form of propriospinal myoclonus.[54]

The transition to sleep features a very common sleep-related movement, the sleep start or hypnic jerk.[55] This is an abrupt, myoclonic flexion movement, generalized or partial, often asymmetric, that may be accompanied by a sensation. There is often an illusion of falling. Unless very frequent (which does rarely occur[56]), this is a benign movement that has little effect on sleep and carries no negative prognosis. While no formal epidemiology has been done, this movement likely occurs in the majority of people. When it occurs, it is usually a single event that causes a brief arousal. EMG records show relatively brief EMG complexes (<250 msec in duration) that may be simultaneous or sequential in various muscles.

Arousals—brief periods of interrupted, lighter sleep that may lead to full awakening—are often associated with movements. Arousals may both follow and lead movements such as body shifts. Abnormal movements, such as parkinsonian tremor,[26] may recur during arousals. Sleep-related movements, such as PLMS, may provoke frequent arousals or even awakenings, and may also continue during periods of arousal from sleep.

Transitions into and out of sleep may also be associated with sleep paralysis. In this condition, an individual is unable to move, although awake. Breathing and eye movements are usually preserved. This condition is thought to represent a variety of REM sleep tonic motor inhibition[57]; recordings of the state can show REMs together with a electrophysiologic pattern consistent with REM sleep.[58] Sleep paralysis may be associated with arousal from a REM period or, less commonly except in narcolepsy, progress into REM sleep from wake. Although most frequent in narcolepsy,[59] sleep paralysis also occurs in many non-narcoleptic individuals, sometimes with a familial pattern. Several studies suggest that, at least in some populations, sleep paralysis may be quite common.[60–62] In normal individuals it is generally infrequent, but may cause significant anxiety, especially the first time that it occurs. A similar condition, nocturnal alternating hemiplegia, involves paralysis limited to one side while awakening from sleep.[63] This may be a variant of hemiplegic migraine, a complicated headache disorder with paralysis due to suppressed activity in certain brain regions.

TABLE 28–1 Persistence of Movements During Sleep

Motor Activity	Awake/ Active	Drowsiness/ Sleep Onset	Arousal/ Awakening	Stage 1 NREM Sleep	Stage 2 NREM Sleep	Stages 3 and 4 NREM Sleep	REM Sleep
Normal Motor Activity							
Hypnic jerk	Unreported	Frequent	Occasional	Occasional	Rare	Rare	Unreported
Postural shifts	Very frequent	Frequent	Frequent	Common	Occasional	Rare	Occasional
Sleep myoclonus	Unreported	Rare	Rare	Common	Occasional	Rare	Frequent
Sleep paralysis*	N.A.	Common	Common	Rare	Unreported	Unreported	Frequent
Movement Disorders							
Bobble-headed doll syndrome	Frequent	Diminished	Diminished	None?	None?	None?	None?
Chorea	Very frequent	Frequent	Common	Occasional	Rare	Very rare	Rare
Dystonia	Very frequent	Common	Common	Occasional	Rare	Very rare	Rare
Fasciculations	Present	Present	Present	Present	Present	Present	Present
Hemiballismus	Very frequent	Common	Common	Occasional?	Occasional?	Very rare	Occasional?
Hemifacial spasm	Very frequent	Frequent	Frequent	Common	Common	Occasional?	Common
Hiccups (chronic)	Frequent	Frequent	Frequent	Common	Common	Common	Common
Myoclonus: cortical/ subcortical	Very frequent	Common?	Occasional?	Occasional?	Occasional?	Rare	Rare
Myoclonus: spinal	Very frequent	Frequent	Common	Common?	Common?	Occasional	Common?
Palatal tremor	Constant	Frequent	Frequent	Frequent	Frequent	Common?	Common?
Parkinsonian tremor	Very frequent	Common	Common	Occasional	Rare	Very rare	Occasional
Tics	Very frequent	Common	Common	Occasional	Occasional	Rare	Common
Sleep Disorders							
Benign infantile myoclonus	N.A.	Unreported	Unreported	Common	Common	Common	Common
Bruxism	Common	Occasional?	Occasional?	Frequent	Frequent	Occasional	Frequent
Fragmentary myoclonus	Unreported	Unreported	Unreported	Frequent	Frequent	Common	Occasional
Mandibular myoclonus	Unreported	Unreported	Occasional?	Frequent	Frequent	Uncommon	Common
NPD	N.A.	Unreported	Common?	Frequent	Frequent	Occasional	Rare
PLMS: isolated or with RLS	N.A.	Occasional	Occasional	Frequent	Common	Rare	Occasional
PLMS: narcolepsy, RBD	N.A.	Occasional?	Occasional?	Frequent	Common	Rare	Common
Propriospinal myoclonus at rest	N.A.	Frequent	Occasional	Rare	None	None	None
RBD	N.A.	Unreported	Occasional?	Rare	Rare	Rare	Frequent
Rhythmic movement disorder	Common	Very frequent	Common?	Common	Common	Rare	Occasional?
RLS: restlessness	Rare	Very frequent	Frequent	Occasional	N.A.	N.A.	N.A.
Sleep terrors	N.A.	Unreported	Common?†	Rare	Uncommon	Usual	Occasional?
Somnambulism	N.A.	Unreported	Common?	Occasional	Common	Frequent	Occasional
Somniloquy	N.A.	Occasional	Common	Common	Usual	Uncommon	Occasional?

*In narcolepsy, presents as cataplexy in wake state.

†Occurs together with incomplete, confusional state.

N.A., not applicable; ?, limited information; NPD, nocturnal paroxysmal dystonia; PLMS, periodic limb movements in sleep; RBD, REM sleep behavior disorder; RLS, restless legs syndrome.

NREM Motor Activity and Modulation

In NREM sleep, motor activity is less than in the waking or resting state. Postural shifts, which may signal stage changes (into or out from wakefulness or REM sleep), occur. There are also small flickering movements, called sleep myoclonus, that may cause no apparent movement and are associated with very brief, highly localized EMG potentials.[64,65] In some cases, these movements may have a greater amplitude and be of increased frequency, at which point they are called excessive fragmentary myoclonus, a possible sleep disorder.[66] The frequency of all movements decreases with depth of sleep, being least in SWS (NREM stages 3 and 4).[67–69] Postural shifts rarely occur before entrance into SWS. A number of abnormal motor activities, such as somnambulism or PLMS, occur predominantly during NREM sleep. In infants, who move more in sleep, most NREM movements are generalized, full-body movements or jerks, while REM movements tend to be more focal and uncoordinated.[70]

REM Motor Activity and Modulation

REM sleep is dramatically different from NREM. The motor system is dominated by central activation and peripheral inhibition. This opposition of forces has been colorfully characterized as a state in which the "underlying motor control landscape is actually ravished by storms of inhibition and brief whirlwinds of excitation" (Chase and Morales,[71] p. 560). In REM sleep muscle tone is tonically reduced, even below that of SWS, but bursts of small movements (sleep myoclonus), similar to those seen in NREM sleep but more clustered, occur phasically in association with bursts of REMs. During REM sleep, there is increased nervous system activity and a close balance between strong upper motor center excitation and inhibition at the level of the motor effecter. When the inhibitory influences break down, significant motor activity may be released. Infants lack this inhibition and have more movement during REM sleep. Inhibition can also be disrupted by lesions in the brain stem of animals that destroy the inhibitory centers,[72,73] or, it is believed, in human sleep disorders such as RBD.[74] The resulting movements may represent an "acting out" of dreams, which characteristically have a motoric component.[75]

Development and Aging

In addition to sleep stage, normal sleep movements are also affected by age: the number of movements during sleep is greatest in infants, then decreases with age.[67] For example, De Koninck and colleagues found that position shifts during sleep decreased from 4.7/hr in 8- to 12-year-old sleepers to 2.1/hr in those 65 to 80 years old.[76] But even within the first few months of life, movements decrease[77]; even infants with lower conceptual age at birth may have more motor activity.[70] Children are also thought to lack a fully "mature" sleep regulatory system.[78] For instance, in one study, Kohyama[79] found that younger infants appear to lack the profound motor inhibition during phasic REMs that is seen in older children and adults.[77] Perhaps as a result of such immaturity, parasomnias[80] such as bruxism, somnambulism,[81] or soliloquy are present with a greater prevalence during childhood, tending to decrease with age from early childhood on. Rhythmic movement disorder, formerly known as head banging or jactatio capitis, is also primarily a disorder of early childhood.[80,82] Similarly, toward the end of life, as neural and other bodily systems age and perhaps deteriorate, some forms of excessive motor activity may emerge again, including PLMS, RBD, and increased instability in NREM sleep manifest as an increase in CAP.[29] In at least one study, movements during sleep were increased in the elderly compared to younger adults.[83] In this population, greater activity during the day may be associated with lower levels of activity at night and better sleep quality.[84] The most "ideal" sleep, well organized and with few disturbing movements, is seen in latency-age preadolescents (ages 6–12). Sleep in younger children is less mature; beginning with adolescence, sleep starts to deteriorate,[85] although a major shift is not apparent until a considerably older age.

Physiology of the Motor System in Relation to Sleep

The motor system can be very roughly considered to have three main units or levels: higher centers, segmental centers, and the motor unit (motor neuron and related muscle fibers). The higher centers are located within the brain and brain stem, where they receive diverse information from other brain regions, including those involved with the senses. These centers include the motor, premotor, and supplementary motor cortices; the basal ganglia and cerebellum; and various brain stem nuclei, including the reticular nuclei of the pons and medulla. They provide descending control to segmental motor centers located at the brain stem and spinal cord levels, as well as some direct connections in the human to motor neurons. The segmental centers, in turn, channel and moderate descending and afferent inputs from somatosensory organs so as to control the "final common path," the motor neuron. In addition to serving as way or integrating stations, the segmental centers may generate their own activity. Many studies have shown that the brain stem and spinal cord, even in complete isolation, can produce patterned motor activity such as locomotion.[86–90] This indicates that they have endogenous oscillators that are based on organized neural networks. The motor neuron, with its associated set of muscle fibers within a specific muscle, collectively known as the *motor unit*, is the ultimate effector responsible for motor activity. Between the levels, there is continuous two-way communication. In addition, the motor system receives a continuous flow of inputs from the various afferent systems, including the different sensory systems. In later sections of the chapter, as we discuss different normal and abnormal sleep-related motor activity, we refer to this model of the motor system to suggest the levels likely to be involved or disturbed in a particular condition. Most motor disturbances of sleep originate at the level of the higher motor centers, although some arise at the segmental level and a few motor phenomena derive from the level of the motor unit.

Our understanding of the phenomena of normal and abnormal movements in sleep depends on our understanding of how the motor system functions and is controlled. In higher animals, such as humans, our understanding does not approach the precise mapping of identified, unique neurons and their subsequent manipulation that is possible in a lower animal such as the pleurobranch mollusk *Aplysia*[89,90] or the nematode worm *Caenorhabditis elegans*.[91,92] Several techniques, however, do allow us to begin to assemble a model of how the motor system changes during different states such as drowsiness, NREM, and REM sleep:

1. It is possible to record the activity and, with intracellular recordings, the underlying membrane events in single neurons. Most of these studies are performed in animals, including rats, cats, and monkeys, but such techniques can occasionally be used on humans in the course of surgery for cerebral disorders. This technique has been used to record a wide range of neurons during sleep. Most relevant for the motor system in sleep are studies of brain stem neurons, which control sleep states and their motoric concomitants, and the motor neurons themselves. This technique is the only one that allows us to uncover the role of specific neural elements in state-dependent function, although each study usually deals with only a limited set of neural elements. Lacking the full picture, the investigator must usually guess about the significance of any individual finding. With time and increasingly better techniques and analysis, it will be possible to put together a more complete picture of state-dependent motor behavior. In some experimental preparations, it is possible to record activity by using voltage-sensitive dyes that will change colors when a cell fires or fluoresce under specific states of the cell interior.[93–95]

2. It is possible to determine the motor output of the sleeping subject through the application of a variety of stimuli to elicit reflex responses or evoked potentials. By relating response to stimulus, this technique probes some of the lumped properties of the sensorimotor system. The information obtained is usually restricted to some measure of overall excitability, however, and the elucidation of what controls these excitability changes must be pursued by other techniques, such as single-neuron recording.

3. Information about the behavior of specific brain regions can be obtained by a variety of techniques that measure aggregate neural activity. Some of the most interesting results of probing human brain activity have come from the development of a variety of imaging techniques, including positron emission tomography (PET) and single-photon emission computed tomography (SPECT) scanning and functional magnetic resonance imaging (fMRI). Although never as precise as single-unit recording, imaging offers the possibility of noninvasively mapping the activity of many brain regions at once and re-examining them in a number of different sleep-wake states. In the following sections, some of the most important directions and findings that have been obtained with these techniques are summarized.

Modulation of Neuronal Firing

During waking, most brain cells tend to fire irregularly, at different frequencies in different brain regions. The general change during NREM sleep, and especially SWS, is for cells to fire more slowly (lower frequency), but with more of a tendency to fire bursts.[96] During SWS, for example, thalamic cells fire slowly and are less responsive to afferent activity. These changes are related to the greater synchronization of surface electrical activity (EEG) during sleep. In REM sleep, by contrast, cellular activity is increased in many regions. Motor areas of the brain, such as the primary motor cortex,[97] motor thalamus, red nucleus, and cerebellum,[96] often show these activity increases. This increased firing in the motor centers of the brain is presumably related to the increased descending drive that occurs during REM sleep.

Motor Neuronal Modulation

More focused studies have examined motor neurons in the brain stem and spinal cord and traced backward some of the descending influences that modulate them depending on state. Studies have begun to establish the brain stem centers whose altered activity is related to the various stages of sleep and wake and associated alterations in motor activity.[98] Particular information has been obtained about the control of REM sleep.[99] Neurons located near the border between the pons and midbrain, such as the pedunculopontine nucleus,[100] appear to release acetylcholine into the more central reticular formation of the pons and medulla. (These neurons can be divided into two classes: REM-on cells are selectively active during REM, while Wake/REM-on cells are also activated during wake. The REM-on cells are selectively inhibited by serotonin.[101]) Various, as of yet poorly defined, centers or cell groups in the reticular formation are then stimulated[102] to exert descending influences that act upon motor neurons. One current models suggests that cholinoceptive cells in a pontine inhibitor area project to the medulla, where they release glutamate to stimulate inhibitory neurons in the medullary reticular formation.[103] Some of this modulation may also occur through suppression of the orexinergic system, which appears to cause arousal and increased motor activity in wakefulness.[104]

Recordings from the motor neurons themselves have shown distinct sleep-dependent changes in their physiology. In relaxation and NREM sleep, motor neurons are slightly hyperpolarized (moved electrically away from their firing threshold) and less excitable.[71,105] This is due to inhibitory inputs known as inhibitory postsynaptic potentials (IPSPs). In REM sleep, the motor neurons are further hyperpolarized due to an increased frequency of small IPSPs as well as large IPSPs that occur only during phasic REMs,[106] but may represent the summation of simultaneously arriving small IPSPs.[107] At least the larger and perhaps both classes of IPSPs can be suppressed by perfusion of strychnine, suggesting that they are mediated by the neurotransmitter glycine.[71] The large IPSP may also be enhanced by endogenous opioids.[108] At least some of these IPSPs arise from the gigantocellular reticular nucleus of the medulla. IPSPs blocked by strychnine can be evoked by stimulating this nucleus, but only during a state similar to REM sleep (induced by carbachol stimulation of the pons in an animal model).[109] The axons from this nucleus descend, at least in part, in the reticulospinal tract.[110] Moreover, the same descending inhibitory input also depresses the Ia monosynaptic reflex, thereby decreasing the excitation of motor neurons by reflex input.[111] As a result of this inhibition of the motor neurons, the increased activity of the central motor system in REM sleep is generally not reflected in increased motor activity. Rather, muscles, such as the mentalis, show atonia while limb movements, either centrally or reflexly generated, are rare.

The bursts of myoclonic movements that sometimes accompany REMs apparently arise from a superimposed phasic excitation via excitatory postsynaptic potentials (EPSPs). This excitation does not depend on the major voluntary motor pathways, such as the corticospinal or rubrospinal tract, but presumably originates in the brain stem.[112] Pharmacologic studies suggest that these EPSPs are mediated by non–N-methyl-D-aspartate excitatory glutaminergic synapses.[113] Neuronal state has also been probed by measuring the level of c-Fos in cells; this protein is associated with active nuclear transcription and protein synthesis. While many interneuronal regions of the brain stem show increased activity in REM sleep, motor nuclei (masseter, facial, and hypoglossal nuclei) show depressed activity.[114] This is consistent with studies that have shown glycinergic inhibition of hypoglossal neurons in REM,[115] perhaps contributing to the difficulties with airway patency in this sleep stage.

Reflex Modulation

Since much of motor behavior is generated, at least in part, by reflexes, studying reflexes can be quite relevant to examining changes of the motor system with state. The most commonly studied reflex has been the tendon reflex or its electrical counterpart, the H reflex. This reflex is diminished in NREM sleep, especially SWS, and then almost completely abolished in REM sleep, especially during REMs.[112,116] Polysynaptic spinal reflexes are similarly depressed in NREM and REM sleep.[112] A somewhat related bulbar reflex, the response of the genioglossus muscle to negative pressure in the airway, is decreased in NREM sleep[117] and may be further reduced in REM sleep.[118,119] This reduced response has significant consequences, because reduced reflex gain may contribute to airway collapse and respiratory difficulties in sleep, especially obstructive apnea. It has been noted that some brain stem reflexes, such as vestibular

reflexes and the blink reflex, show decreased gain in NREM sleep, but may then recover partially in REM sleep.[120–122] This recovery of some brain stem reflexes during REM sleep parallels the relatively greater activity of the eye muscles, compared to trunk and limb muscles at that time, and reinforces the mixed picture of excitation and inhibition characteristic of REM sleep. Even drowsiness, short of actual sleep, can attenuate some reflexes, such as the vestibulo-ocular reflex, which has two outputs: quick restorative jerks to head rotation and slower smooth compensatory eye deviations.[123] The more polysynaptic quick jerks are more easily suppressed by even modest drowsiness. While all these various changes in reflex gain indicate altered excitability, they do not indicate where in the reflex arc the changes occur.

The basis for much of the reduced reflex gain during sleep is most likely inhibition of motor output, rather than decrease of sensory response. In one supportive study, Morrison and colleagues placed pontine tegmental lesions in cats that caused REM sleep without atonia.[124] They found that both orienting to tone stimuli and acoustic startle responses were evident in REM sleep in the lesioned cats, but rare or absent throughout sleep in intact cats. Since the same tones elicited brain stem–generated ponto-geniculo-occipital (PGO) waves in both normal and lesioned cats, it seems likely that the block to the further responses of orienting and startle reflexes is on the motor side of the reflex arc. PGO waves have also been identified in a human subject undergoing brain stem recording during placement of a pedunculopontine nucleus stimulator.[125] In contrast, sensory transmission may itself be altered by sleep. Studies have indicated that, in primary afferent neurons located both in the spinal cord[126] and in the brain stem,[127] there is a significant, presynaptically mediated decrease in responsiveness during REM sleep, but not NREM sleep.

Reflexes can also change their characteristic motor output in sleep,[128] indicating that sleep is not merely a general change in activity levels but a rearranged organization of responsiveness. Sensory stimulation, which would cause motor neuron excitation in waking, can cause additional inhibitory potentials in sleep.[129] In addition, certain reflexes that would be abnormal during waking, such as the Babinski sign, may be elicited in sleep (see Kleitman,[130] pp. 16–18; see also Fujiki et al.[131]).

Motor Evoked Responses

To more directly examine the impact of sleep on the motor system itself, motor evoked potentials (MEPs) can be studied. In one study of MEPs evoked by stimulating the motor cortex with a strong magnetic stimulus during sleep, it was noted that MEPs decreased during NREM sleep.[132] Results during REM sleep have shown a much greater degree of variability in amplitude of evoked responses. Hess and colleagues[132] found that responses were of normal or increased amplitude, while Fish and coworkers[133] found that average amplitude was decreased in three normal subjects despite some responses of higher amplitude than normal relaxed waking responses. The latter group also noted consistent prolonged latencies of the MEPs, consistent with inhibitory processes. In a group of narcoleptic patients, stimulation during cataplexy resulted in apparently normal MEPs.[134] While these results remain to be harmonized, the variability is consistent with the fluctuating balance between inhibitory and excitatory processes in REM. A finding of decreased mean amplitude, however, is more consistent with the general inhibitory balance of REM sleep in normal individuals. When sleep apneas are superimposed on sleep, MEP amplitude may decrease further.[135]

Imaging Studies

The development of new imaging techniques that permit assessment of activity in the waking brain provides an additional method of studying regional contributions to state-dependent motor activity. Studies of cerebral blood flow and metabolism have largely paralleled those of cellular activity. Blood flow and metabolism may be greater during REM sleep than in waking, but are widely depressed during NREM sleep, especially SWS.[136,137] Examining differential regional activities in relation to sleep states or features can provide insights into sleep mechanisms. In one study, Hofle and colleagues[138] correlated activity in different brain regions with power in different EEG frequency domains (e.g., delta, here 1.5–4.0 Hz). The greatest decrement associated with increased delta power (characteristic of SWS) was in the thalamus, consistent with the depressed thalamic activity of sleep. The presence of sleep spindles, most common in stage 2 NREM sleep, is associated with activation of the thalamus, paralimbic areas, and superior temporal gyrus.[139] Slow (11- to 13-Hz) and fast (13- to 15-Hz) spindles show this common activation, plus distinctive activations of the superior frontal gyrus (slow spindles) compared to sensorimotor cortical areas, medial frontal areas, and hippocampus (fast spindles).

During REM sleep, in contrast to NREM, there is activation of the brain stem core and thalamus as well as limbic areas of the brain and primary and secondary sensory areas,[136,140–142] including visual cortices.[143] Hong and colleagues[144] examined the association between REMs and blood flow and found associations both with the midline attentional system active in REM sleep and areas involved in generating waking saccadic eye movements and subserving visual attention. Higher cortical areas, including prefrontal cortex and multimodal sensory and associative cortex, remain suppressed during all sleep stages.[140,145] REM sleep can be divided into those baseline periods without REMs and the periods with REMs, during which sensory receptivity is decreased.[146] During actual REMs, fMRI studies have shown additional activation in the posterior thalamus and occipital visual cortex,[147] or within a thalamocortical network including limbic and parahippocampal areas.[146]

Additional studies have shown that the basal ganglia are suppressed in SWS, but very strongly activated in REM sleep.[140,148,149] The significance of these basal ganglia changes for the motor system and for movement disorders in sleep remains unclear, but is of great potential interest. These results in imaging studies suggest an evolving of sleep states in terms of the involved brain structures, including the motor system.

Imaging studies can also begin to assess potential deficits due to altered sleep conditions, such as sleep deprivation,[150] which can cause depression of frontal lobe activity that is only partially restored after a compensatory sleep.

DIURNAL MOVEMENT DISORDERS IN RELATION TO SLEEP

The relation between the diurnal movement disorders and sleep has become better known over the past several decades, in large part because of the major increase in the study of sleep. In some conditions, the level of symptoms may vary systematically with the sleep-wake cycle. For example, in dopa-responsive dystonia (DRD),[151] the patient feels best in the early morning, after sleep, and then deteriorates as the day continues. Furthermore, movement disorder specialists have become more aware of certain conditions primarily categorized as sleep disorders, such as RLS or RBD, that are more active during the night or during sleep. It has also become increasingly apparent that movement disorders are not absent during sleep and that they may cause or be associated with a variety of sleep disturbances. Surveys of patients with Parkinson's disease (PD) have shown that the majority report that they have some difficulties with sleep. Large numbers of patients complain of difficulty getting to sleep, inadequate time asleep, disrupted sleep, and daytime sleepiness.

Persistence of Diurnal Movements During Sleep

Different diurnal movement disorders show various degrees of persistence during sleep (see Table 28–1). In the past, it was almost universally believed that most movement disorders, such as the increased tonic spasms of dystonia or essential or parkinsonian tremor, are abolished by sleep. However, careful studies generally find that there are remnants of abnormal activity that persist during sleep or occur during brief transitions to light sleep or waking. As a rule, movement disorders are most likely to be present at transitions into and out of sleep or during the lighter stages of NREM sleep. Occasionally, they will be reactivated during REM sleep as well. Some movement disorders, while subsiding, have been reported to occur fairly commonly during sleep. Tics, especially in children, have been noted to occur during sleep. In children, this may reflect a relative immaturity of the mechanisms for suppressing unwanted movement during sleep.

In a thorough and careful study using EMG, accelerometry, and split-screen video recording, Fish and colleagues[26] examined the relation of motor activity not only to conventional sleep staging, but also to epochs with transitions (to lighter or deeper sleep stages or awake). They also monitored the 2-second periods before onset of dyskinesias in patients with PD, Huntington's disease, Tourette's syndrome, and torsion dystonia (both primary generalized and secondary) and scored them for presence of arousals, REMs, sleep spindles, and slow waves. They compared these dyskinesias to normal movements both in patients and in normal subjects; 41 of 43 patients had characteristic movements that persisted in sleep. Both normal movements and dyskinesias for every disorder followed the same general plan: most common in awakening epochs, followed by lightening, stage 1 sleep, REM sleep, and then stage 2 sleep, with no movements in pure stages 3 and 4 and deepening. Only Tourette's syndrome patients had dyskinesias during transition from wake to sleep. The 2-second period before both normal and abnormal movements showed arousals most commonly, followed by REMs, with spindles and slow waves both extremely unlikely to occur. These results support prior speculation[152] that both dyskinesias and normal movements are likely to be modulated by sleep in a similar fashion. The authors suggested this may be due either to the general suppression of centers for both normal and dyskinetic movements or suppression of some common descending pathway, such as the pyramidal tract.[26] It should be noted that all of these abnormal motor activities are thought to be generated in higher motor centers, most of them located above the brain stem.

Lower Motor Center Disorders

Movement disorders associated with abnormalities of the lower motor centers persist most commonly during sleep.[158] Most typical are the palatal myoclonus or palatal tremor family, in which there is low-frequency (typically, 1.5- to 2.5-Hz) oscillatory activity associated with brain stem damage within Mollaret's triangle (dentatorubro-olivary pathways, with damage most common in the central tegmental tract, which runs from the region of the red nucleus to the ipsilateral olive).[154] Essential[155] and psychogenic[156] forms have also been described.[157] While the frequency or persistence of these movements may vary with sleep stages,[158,159] palatal myoclonus still occurs during sleep. In addition, spinal myoclonus will often persist during sleep.[160] These can, in a general sense, be lumped together as segmental myoclonias. Similar persistence may be seen in hemifacial spasm,[161] which is thought to involve damage either in the brain stem facial nucleus or in the peripheral nerve (cross talk due to ephaptic transmission) or both.[162]

Also, fasciculations due to damage to the lower motor neuron may persist in sleep.[163]

Psychogenic Movement Disorders

It has been said that psychogenic movement disorders all subside during sleep or anesthesia and, in general, they can be expected to do so. However, in rare cases, there may be violations of this rule. These patients have not been studied systematically enough to reach a full conclusion, but it can be expected that they would be most likely to show persistent abnormalities at sleep onset, during very light sleep stages, or in the course of arousals, and least likely in deep SWS. This makes clear that sleep is not an all-or-none state, but that some voluntary and purposive behavior may persist into the lighter sleep stages.

Sleep Dysfunctions Associated with Diurnal Movement Disorders

A basic problem occurs when movement disorders prevent sleep or arouse patients from sleep. However, such direct effects of movement disorders are not the only effects on sleep. Additional problems arise because the movement disorder, or its treatment, may bring about disturbed sleep. Movement disorder patients may also be at risk for additional sleep disturbances, such as sleep apnea or parasomnias. Moreover, many movement disorder patients are elderly and even demented and may have the impaired sleep often seen with aging or dementing disease.

Sleep Fragmentation

In many disorders, a primary concomitant of a degenerative movement disorder is disrupted sleep—increased awakenings, more stage transitions, and partial and complete arousals. This disruption is called sleep fragmentation.[164] The result is usually a sleep characterized by more time awake, less SWS, and, perhaps, less REM sleep. This has been reported as a complication of many different movement abnormalities. It should be remembered, however, that many of these movement disorders occur primarily in older patients and that sleep quality declines even in the relatively healthy elderly.[165] Sleep may improve once effective therapy is found for the underlying condition.[166] Therapy for movement disorders may also interfere with sleep, and this must be considered in assessments of sleep problems. Because both the primary disease and its therapy may cause sleep disruption, completely successful management may not be possible. Instead, one must seek the optimal compromise between sleep dysfunction and treatment of the primary disorder.

Respiratory Disturbances

A major problem for movement disorder patients is the prevalence of respiratory disturbances during sleep. Respiratory disturbances are common in the motor disorders that include neuronal degeneration. Especially vulnerable are those patients with degenerative diseases that involve brain stem loci. In the more widespread degenerative diseases such as olivopontocerebellar atrophy or multiple system atrophy (MSA), there may be respiratory disturbances based on disturbed central regulation of breathing, problems with neuromuscular function leading to obstruction or laryngeal stridor, or impaired feedback control of respiration.

Dyssomnias and Parasomnias

There are a number of movement disorders in which parasomnias or other motor disturbances of sleep are more likely to occur than in the general population. Children with tics are reported to have an increased incidence of parasomnias such as somnambulism and somniloquy. Increased prevalence of PLMS or RLS has been reported with a variety of movement disorders, such as Huntington's disease[46] or PD.[167–169] A number of movement disorders, especially PD and related syndromes, may be associated with RBD.[170,171]

The degree to which such additional motor abnormalities are seen in patients with diurnal movement disorders is not yet clear. However, although good epidemiologic studies have not been done, it seems increasingly likely that these abnormalities may be common. Therefore, the frequency of associations reported does indicate that additional motor abnormalities during sleep must be considered in patients who present with a diurnal movement disorder.

Circadian Rhythm Disturbances

Circadian rhythm disturbances, especially changes in sleep phase or chaotic sleep rhythms,[172,173] are seen especially in the degenerative conditions. Many of these patients are elderly, severely incapacitated, or demented, all features that may weaken the circadian regulation of activity. Patients may have multiple factors that upset the circadian rhythm, including their medications. Nocturnal confusion or "sundowning" often occurs in this setting. Circadian rhythm disturbances are difficult to treat, especially in patients with cognitive compromise. Careful adjustment of medication, attempts to maintain wakefulness during the day, and good sleep hygiene may help. Sleep medications may be counterproductive, leading to additional difficulties such as confusion. Since these patients are often homebound or institutionalized, they may lack adequate bright light exposure to reset their circadian rhythms. A trial of bright light therapy should be considered in suitable patients. Patients with PD are prone to endogenous and reactive depressions.[174,175] They may show a classic pattern of sleep phase advance with increased and early-onset REM periods. In this situation, they may respond to judicious use of antidepressants.

Excessive Daytime Somnolence

Because of the varied difficulties associated with movement disorders—such as inadequate sleep, sleep fragmentation, sleep apnea, and circadian rhythm disturbances—excessive daytime somnolence (EDS) may be a major problem for patients.[176] This problem can be aggravated by medications such as L-dopa or the dopamine agonists, which can induce sleepiness at peak blood concentration or disrupt sleep at night. In recent years, this has become an important issue with reference to PD and its treatment, beginning with the recognition of "sleep attacks"[177] and then widening to understand the fundamental difficulties in sleep and daytime alertness in PD. (This is discussed at greater length later in the chapter.)

A Few Comments on Therapy

The first step in tailoring therapy is to determine whether the sleep problem is a direct consequence of the movement disorder itself or due to a coexisting sleep disorder, which may be primary (sleep apnea) or secondary (e.g., insomnia due to depression). Therapy should then be appropriately addressed to the movement disorder itself, or to the coexisting sleep disorder or its underlying cause. Most sleep disorders coexisting with movement disorders would be treated in the usual fashion—for example, with continuous positive airway pressure (CPAP) for obstructive sleep apnea (OSA) or antidepressants for insomnia due to depression.

A second consideration is whether behavioral measures, such as good sleep hygiene, can help with the sleep problem. Even demented patients with highly disrupted circadian rhythms may benefit from some imposed temporal order on their daily activity. Bright light therapy can regularize circadian rhythms[178] and improve sleep-maintenance insomnia.[179,180] Such therapy may then be applied even to those in whom degeneration has damaged the sleep and circadian regulatory circuits of the brain.[181] Exercise may also improve sleep and circadian cycling.[182]

Third is to begin pharmacologic therapy, especially in the elderly or those with degenerative neurologic disease, with low doses and only gradually build up to full dose schedules. This cautiousness may avoid many side effects. Of course, in some cases, slow buildup may be too discouraging to the patient, who may be looking for a more rapid effect; then the process of building up to a therapeutic dose may need to be modified.

Fourth is to avoid, if possible, regular, protracted use of sedative-hypnotic medications. In some cases, they may be used for a short time to regularize sleep or on an occasional basis to avoid particularly difficult nights. Antihistamines such as diphenhydramine or anticholinergic antidepressants such as amitriptyline may substitute for benzodiazepines. However, if appropriate for specific sleep disorders (e.g., RBD), benzodiazepines such as clonazepam may be beneficial on a protracted basis without dose escalation or tolerance[183]; one study found that clonazepam therapy in PD was associated with less EDS.[184] One new agent, eszopiclone,[185] has been tested for more long-term use and has maintained efficacy over a period of weeks.

Sleep-Associated Problems of the Hypokinetic Disorders

While most movement disorders have some associated sleep-related disturbances, more has been studied concerning the hypokinetic disorders.

Parkinson's Disease

While it long has been recognized that sleep is impaired in PD,[186–188] two specific findings have made the problems of sleep in PD particularly salient:

1. The discovery that a particular sleep problem, RBD (see later), is commonly associated with PD.[189] Furthermore, RBD could be the presenting feature of PD.[190]
2. The report that PD patients might be subject to sudden onset of sleep ("sleep attacks") that could cause automobile accidents.[177] Many studies have confirmed the fact that sleep is a major issue for PD patients and their quality of life.[191,192]

Sleep problems in PD can be due to a variety of causes,[193,194] and solving the sleep problems may require disentangling the different factors involved.[164,195–199] These factors, which are often similarly applicable to other movement disorders, include

1. PD itself (e.g., discomfort due to bradykinesia/akinesia and inability to change position[200] or reactivated symptoms such as tremor during arousal, which may be altered by treatment during the night[201] or benefit from longer acting medication[202,203])
2. Sleep disorders closely related to PD (e.g., RBD)
3. Consequences of PD, such as depression and related sleeping dysfunction[204,205]
4. Coincident sleep disorders common in adults, such as sleep-related breathing disorders
5. Side effects of medication, such as nightmares or insomnia

But sleep can also influence PD; in some patients sleep can reduce parkinsonian disability and alleviate symptoms,[206–208] perhaps due to the circadian peak of dopamine in the morning.[209] This may be particularly true of patients suffering from early-onset parkinsonism such as that due to the most common recessive *Parkin* (*PARK2*) mutation.[210] Sleep benefit is less consistent in those with the recessive *Pink1* (*PARK6*) mutation.[210,211] Sleep benefit in the group of early-onset patients is often associated with some degree of dystonia and the diurnal pattern associated with DRD. In others, disrupted sleep can lead to fatigue and increased symptoms, including daytime somnolence.

In recent years, several questionnaires have been developed and validated that can be used to assess sleep-related problems in PD.[212–216]

RBD in PD. Since its initial description, RBD has been linked to PD.[189,190,217] This association may be due to the parkinsonian degeneration affecting brain areas and systems responsible for sleep-wake regulation.[100,218] One scheme postulates that the synuclein pathology of PD (Lewy body pathology) ascends from the brain stem to the basal ganglia and finally to the cortex,[219,220] with early involvement of sleep regulatory nuclei before development of motor symptoms.[221] The combination of RBD with olfactory dysfunction may be a strong predictor for later development of PD.[222] In general, RBD patients show subtle motor, cognitive, autonomic, olfactory,[223] and visual changes that are associated with PD,[224,225] as well as brain perfusion changes determined by SPECT imaging.[226] One finding is that markedly reduced cardiac [123]I-*meta*-iodobenzylguanidine uptake, consistent with the loss of sympathetic terminals, in idiopathic RBD is consistent with a similar deficit in PD.[227]

One study suggests that RBD occurs primarily in PD patients who have the nontremor form of PD.[228] The authors also suggested that RBD will not precede early-onset PD, an observation supported in cases of *PARK6* (*PINK1*) early-onset familial PD.[229] RBD later in the course of PD may be associated with additional complications such as hallucinations[230,231] (which may represent REM intrusions[194]) and cognitive decline.[232]

A detailed analysis of movements in five patients with PD and RBD found that they had many more movements in sleep than controls, but that most movements were brief and restricted in scope[233]; 3.6% of all movements were violent, while 10.5% involved vocalizations. It has also been proposed that RBD-related movements may show "normalization" of motor production with reduction in bradykinesia and vocal hypomimia.[234]

EDS and Sleep Attacks in PD. Fatigue, somnolence, and EDS are common symptoms in PD.[198] Tandberg and colleagues,[235] for example, found that daytime somnolence was significantly more frequent in PD patients compared to healthy controls (26.8% vs. 10%), and appearance of EDS was even more frequent (15.5% vs. 1%). Compared to patients not reporting daytime somnolence, patients with EDS had significantly higher staging of PD, were more disabled, and showed a higher frequency of cognitive decline and of depressive symptoms.[205] They also had significantly more hallucinations and had taken levodopa for a longer time. Snoring may be associated with greater daytime somnolence.[198] EDS was also somewhat more frequent in patients taking dopamine agonists.[235]

The significance of this sleepiness was underscored by the reports in PD of sleep attacks—sudden episodes of sleep that appear without warning on a background of normal alertness.[177] Since the original report in 1999, numerous studies have examined the basis for and associations of somnolence and sleep attacks in PD.[198,236–247] While different studies have emphasized different variables as having greater impact on daytime sleepiness and sleep attacks, the following factors have emerged from the studies[248]:

1. Daytime somnolence is intrinsic to PD.
2. Sleep attacks do occur,[249] but are relatively rare compared to more ordinary sleepiness of which the patient is aware.[250]
3. Markers of PD—such as duration of illness or severity of illness—are associated with greater daytime somnolence.
4. Any dopaminergic medication can cause somnolence or sleep attacks.
5. The amount of medication is more important than the class of medication, although dopamine agonists generally, and nonergot agonists specifically, may be more likely to cause somnolence.
6. Daytime somnolence can exist without evidence for severely disrupted sleep.
7. Ordinary measures of sleepiness, such as the Epworth Sleepiness Scale (see Chapter 19), can predict many cases of excess somnolence and potential for sleep attacks, but not all patients with sleep attacks have sleepiness evident on a Multiple Sleep Latency Test (MSLT).[251]
8. Genetic variants of the pre-prohypocretin receptor[252] and dopamine D_2 receptor[253] genes have been associated with predisposition to sleep attacks.

Sometimes the somnolence seen in PD patients can mimic narcolepsy (see later), including a finding of sleep-onset REM periods.[254,255] This can be seen as 2 or more episodes of REM-onset sleep on an MSLT (four or five naps scheduled during the day at 2-hour intervals). The picture in PD, however, is often more complex, while cataplexy, a key finding in narcolepsy, is rare.[256] Consistent with narcolepsy, hypocretin neurons are progressively lost with more severe PD.[257]

Treatment of daytime sleepiness may include the use of stimulants. Some studies have supported the use of modafinil as a relatively well-tolerated stimulant,[258–260] but one double-blind, placebo-controlled study failed to support efficacy.[261]

Insomnia in PD. Insomnia is very common in PD.[262] Patients with PD may have difficulty getting to sleep and even more difficulty maintaining sleep; they may have increased arousals, awakenings, and periods awake during the night.[167,263] A key summary term for this is *sleep fragmentation*, the loss of sleep continuity with multiple intrusions of light sleep and wake.[264–266] Sleep can be improved in many cases by appropriate therapy, including dopaminergic medications to cover the night[267,268] and, in some cases, deep brain stimulation.[201,269–271] But

recommendations are complicated by the finding that, in some cases, dopaminergic treatment itself can increase fragmentation.[193]

Sleep-Related Respiratory Disturbances in PD. Respiratory disturbances are common in PD and other neurodegenerative disorders due to changes in upper airway function or disturbed central regulation of breathing. Altered upper airway function may be based on weakness of respiratory and upper airway muscles or on altered muscle tone and coordination. Patients with PD may have stridor or laryngeal spasm associated with off-times or dystonic episodes.[272,273] Abnormal vocal cord function with regular rhythmic movements or irregular jerky movements in the glottic area may also produce changes of airflow and contribute to intermittent airway closure.[274] Similar activity persisting during sleep can lead to OSA or upper airway resistance syndrome.[275] It has not been definitely established that the incidence of respiratory dysfunction during sleep in patients with PD as a whole is any higher than in healthy elderly persons.[276,277] However, in some studies sleep-disordered breathing was more frequent and occurred in up to 50% of patients with PD.[278] Snoring has occurred in the majority of subjects in some series.[198] Patients with parkinsonism and autonomic impairment more often develop sleep apnea and related respiratory abnormalities, including central and obstructive apneas and nocturnal hypoventilation. In the presence of sleep apnea, patients with autonomic impairment are probably more likely than other patients to have nocturnal cardiac arrhythmias.

Other Sleep Disorders in PD. Another association of PD has been to RLS and periodic limb movements (PLM). Studies have suggested that RLS is increased in PD,[198,279–281] including association in one family with a parkin mutation.[282] However, this association is only poorly understood.[283–285] Some studies report that most RLS develops after onset of PD,[279] suggesting that RLS may be provoked by dopaminergic treatment, which can induce RLS through a process of "augmentation," even in those who do not have RLS[286] (see later). In one report, subthalamic stimulation may have induced RLS,[287] but this may have been due to decreased medication doses. PLM (see later) are closely connected to RLS: at least 80% of patients have a significant number of the movements. Some studies have found increased PLM in PD patients,[288,289] but one small study of de novo patients found no such elevation.[290] Therefore, at this point, we cannot be sure that there is a strong link between PD and RLS or PLM, independent of PD therapy.

Postencephalitic Parkinsonism

While not studied extensively, respiratory problems appear to be more common in patients with postencephalitic parkinsonism than in patients with PD, perhaps due to the more widespread brain stem pathology found in these patients.[291] They have been found to have poor voluntary respiratory control[292] as well as hypoventilation,[293] even while awake, which has been linked to a decreased sensitivity of central chemoreceptors regulating breathing.[293,294] These patients may also have greater sleep problems than idiopathic PD patients, including greater respiratory compromise in sleep.[275] While most cases of postencephalitic parkinsonism followed the flu epidemic of 1918–1920, occasional cases still occur.[295,296]

Progressive Supranuclear Palsy

A number of studies have been made of sleep in patients with progressive supranuclear palsy (PSP). These patients have been reported to have severe sleep disruption with reduced total sleep, marked diminution in sleep spindles, reduced REM sleep time with abnormal REMs, disordered sleep architecture, and frequent awakenings.[297–303] Patients may develop RBD,[304,305] which in one case was presaged by the development of somniloquy.[306] Sleep disruption was noted to increase with severity of the motor abnormalities in three studies,[299,301,307] but not to be related in a fourth.[300] The greater sleep abnormalities of PSP compared to PD[305] may be due to the greater brain stem pathology, especially that in the pedunculopontine tegmentum, a region linked to control of REM sleep.[303] One report found that cerebrospinal fluid hypocretin levels were lower in PSP than in PD patients.[308] Little is known about treatment of the sleep dysfunctions in this condition.

Multiple System Atrophy

In MSA (for reviews, see Wenning et al.,[309] Dickson et al.,[310] and Gilman et al.[311,312]; see also Chapter 29), patients have more severe sleep problems than do those with other movement disorders[312–316] and may even lack normal circadian regulation of sleep.[317] They may be especially sensitive to the sleep-inducing properties of levodopa.[318] It has been suggested that sleep dysregulation be considered one of the primary features of MSA.[316] MSA patients commonly have PLMS,[74,288,316] and also manifest two distinctive sleep problems. First, many, if not most, of these patients have been found to have RBD[74,313,316,319,320] (see Chapters 29 and 35). This presumably follows from the widespread brain stem pathology encountered in this disorder[321] and is an additional example of disordered motor control. RBD is unlikely to be seen in pure autonomic failure and provides one means of differentiating the two conditions.[319] Second, many MSA patients have an atrophic paralysis of the laryngeal abductor muscles,[322] or sleep-related hyperactivity of the adductors,[320] that has been described as dystonic,[320] leading to a coarse, snoring-like sound[323] referred to as laryngeal stridor.[316] In fact, stridor has been reported as the first sign of MSA[324] or may even be the only apparent sign.[325] It is a potentially life-threatening

condition, which varies in severity.[326] Higher grades of paralysis, observed during the day as well as at night, likely predispose to sudden respiratory death. Milder cases may be managed with CPAP[327]; more severe cases require tracheostomy. These interventions reduce, but do not eliminate, the possibility of sudden respiratory arrest and death.[328,329]

Sleep-Associated Problems of the Hyperkinetic Disorders

The hyperkinetic disorders are a diverse group characterized by excessive involuntary movement, often coupled with a deficiency of voluntary movement such as bradykinesia. In some cases, the conditions are known to have a very specific etiology, as in Huntington's disease (HD), which is presumed to be due always to a single genetic defect. As a general rule, these conditions are associated with fragmented sleep, some instances of which will be associated with persistent motor activities in sleep. Patients with more severe disease are more likely to have significant sleep problems.

Chorea

Chorea consists of movements that occur in a flowing or irregular pattern and appear to migrate from one part of the body to another.[330] They may be increased with action and typically are seen in the face and distal limbs.

The best known cause of chorea is HD, a dominant disease with a known mutation of the *IT15* gene located on the short arm of chromosome 4.[331] The mutation in HD is the expansion of a CAG repeat in the DNA that leads to increased length of a polyglutamine tract in the protein product, now called *huntingtin*. Currently, research is directed at finding the function of huntingtin in the normal brain and the elucidation of the toxic effect of the mutated protein. Although huntingtin is widely distributed in the brain,[332] the pathology of HD is more restricted. Patients also have prominent psychological symptoms, including depression, psychosis, and character disorders. Onset is typically between the ages of 25 and 50, although it may occur even in the first decade or in late adult life. Progression is slow but relentless, with eventual debility, dementia, and inanition occurring in those with onset before old age.

Sleep has been studied by a number of investigators in HD. These investigators have shown a variable persistence of chorea during sleep, with most chorea present in the lighter stages of NREM sleep (stages 1 and 2).[333–335] Fish and colleagues[26] found that most choreiform movements occurred during awakening, during lightening of sleep stages, or in stage 1 sleep, similar to other dyskinesias. One study reported an increase in overall sleep movements in HD.[336] Alterations in sleep spindles in HD have been inconsistent: whereas one study found sleep spindles to be largely absent,[192] other studies have found that their frequency increased.[337,338]

Sleep has been found to be variably impaired in HD, although only some studies have used matched control groups. In HD, excessive motor activity during the sleep period has been shown by actigraphy,[339] perhaps associated with altered circadian rhythms.[340] The general finding has been that sleep is disturbed, and especially fragmented, particularly in those patients with more advanced disease. Deficits include prolonged sleep latency, excessive waking, decreased SWS and REM sleep, and decreased sleep efficiency.[335,338,341,342] In one study, these sleep abnormalities were specifically correlated with caudate atrophy.[343] Some studies have reported that many patients have essentially normal sleep architecture and stages.[344] Unlike patients with parkinsonism, HD patients have not been found to have a significant number of sleep apneas contributing to impaired sleep.[341,342,345]

Sleep has not been well studied in other conditions with predominant chorea. Broughton et al.[346] reported that four patients with Sydenham's chorea, which follows a streptococcal infection, had reactivation of their movements during REM sleep. Because sleep complaints are not prominent in HD, little is known about the response to therapy or the effects of treatment for the motor manifestations of HD on sleep features.

Dystonia

Dystonia[347] is a condition characterized by sustained distorting or twisting postures, often mixed with a variety of more jerklike or oscillatory movements (see Fahn et al.[348] for a general discussion). Dystonia can be primary or secondary and can be of variable extent, either focal, segmental, or generalized, depending on the area of involvement. Dystonia includes a number of different conditions, some of which, like early-onset torsion dystonia, have a single-gene basis. The protein for early-onset torsion dystonia, torsin A, has been found to bind adenosine triphosphate, but how it causes dystonia itself remains unresolved.[349–353] Not all idiopathic dystonia patients have been shown to have a genetic mutation, however, and there are many cases of secondary dystonia that do not appear to depend on common dystonia genes.[354] One problem in evaluating sleep studies in dystonia is that the studies have often examined a fairly heterogeneous collection of patients with different distributions of dystonia and different etiologies. This will change, however, because patients can now be selected for studies on a genetic basis.

Although they usually subside significantly, dystonic movements may persist during sleep at a reduced frequency and amplitude. They are maximally reduced during SWS and may be partially reactivated during REM sleep episodes.[334,355] In the study by Fish et al.[26] of dyskinetic movements, both primary and secondary dystonic patients followed the general pattern of more frequent dyskinetic movements during awakening or lightening epochs; fewer movements in stage 1 sleep; only infrequent movements

in stage 2, REM, and SWS; and no movements during epochs of deepening sleep. In a study including focal and segmental dystonias, Silvestri and colleagues[356] found that Meige's syndrome (oromandibular dystonia), blepharospasm, and tonic foot syndrome all showed persistent abnormal activity during sleep, with reduced amplitude, duration, and frequency of EMG bursts. The greatest suppression was in SWS and REM sleep.

A number of studies have reported the presence of exaggerated sleep spindles in dystonia.[334,355,357] One study, however, found that this was, at best, a variable finding in a carefully studied group of patients with primary and secondary dystonia.[358]

It has been suggested that inhibitory mechanisms are defective in dystonia.[359] This prompted Fish and colleagues[360] to study whether REM inhibition is intact in both primary and secondary dystonics. They found that both types of dystonics had normal chin EMG atonia. No patients had complex abnormal activity during REM sleep. In an attempt to analyze motor excitability, the authors successfully stimulated three normal subjects and four dystonics with a magnetic coil over the vertex to evoke a motor response in the fifth finger abductor (abductor digiti minimi). Whereas response amplitudes were highly variable, dystonics, like controls, showed a decrease in the mean response relative to responses obtained before and after the sleep study in relaxed wakefulness. Latencies were prolonged on average in all groups. The findings of decreased amplitude and prolonged latency were consistent with REM motor inhibition. Occasional high-amplitude responses may have corresponded to periods of phasic excitation. These results indicate that, whatever the decreased inhibitory processes in dystonia, they do not involve the descending inhibitory pathways of REM sleep.

Studies of sleep in dystonia have not been systematic; they have involved small numbers of patients on diverse medications, some of whom had prior thalamic surgery. In these studies, sleep has been found to be inconsistently disrupted,[334,357] with more severe fragmentation seen in more advanced cases.[361] The major therapeutic effort in these patients is the attempt to reduce the dystonic movements (for review of therapy, see Fahn[347] and Fahn et al.[348]). Successful therapy of the movements should also improve sleep.[362]

It is not known to what degree different forms of dystonia—early- versus late-onset, focal versus generalized—have different relationships to sleep, although one striking form of dystonia, variably called *hereditary progressive dystonia with marked diurnal fluctuations*, DRD, and the *Segawa variant*, often shows distinct circadian variability.[363,364] These patients typically present at a young age (often in the middle of the first decade) with postural dystonia, usually affecting one leg and sparing the trunk and neck. Thereafter, the dystonia spreads and parkinsonian signs, which are present at onset in a minority of patients, become more prominent. The condition is usually inherited in an autosomal dominant mode with a mutation in the gene for GTP cyclohydrolase I (*GCHI*).[365] A number of different mutations in *GCHI* have been described,[366,367] but, less commonly, it seems that the condition can be inherited recessively with a mutation in the gene for tyrosine hydroxylase.[368] Some studies have found that even patients thought to have more typical idiopathic torsion dystonia may harbor a mutation in the *GCHI* gene.[369] These patients may obtain significant symptomatic relief from sleep and therefore are minimally impaired early in the day,[363] although this is not true of all patients (57 of 86, in one review[370]), and some dystonic patients unresponsive to L-dopa may have similar benefit from sleep.[371,372] Patients with PD may also show sleep benefit.[206–209] Whether only REM sleep[363] or NREM sleep or even rest can improve symptoms remains controversial.[371]

Patients do show abnormal sleep motility. Segawa and colleagues[363,373] obtained movement counts from PSG with multiple EMG channels (8–12 surface recordings on trunk and limbs) and found that, in DRD, there is a decrease in gross body movements in stage 1 sleep, an increase in stage 2 sleep, and a decrease in REM sleep. In contrast, localized twitch movements were depressed in all sleep stages, but followed the normal relative distribution between stages.[363,373]

Patients with diurnal dystonia or the nocturnal sleep abnormalities of DRD are responsive to low doses of L-dopa,[363] often as little as 50–200 mg/day with decarboxylase inhibitor. Some patients can maintain a stable therapeutic effect with doses every other day. Patients with long-standing disease (24–45 years before treatment) may benefit as well as those with recent onset.[370,374,375] DRD patients can use L-dopa without the development of the dyskinetic side effects that are so prominent in juvenile parkinsonism.[371,375,376] A few patients may develop "wearing off" phenomena, the re-emergence of symptoms several hours after an oral dose of L-dopa.[375] Older family members may present with a "parkinsonian picture," but still show the same persistent, positive response to L-dopa.[371,376,377] This finding is consistent with the idea that a single underlying disease has different manifestations that vary with age, dystonia being prominent early and parkinsonism late.[377]

With fluorodopa PET scanning, it has been shown in a number of families that patients with DRD have normal to modestly reduced striatal uptake of fluorodopa,[378] including those who present with parkinsonian features later in life.[377] Because of this finding, it can be concluded that these patients have relatively intact dopamine uptake, decarboxylation, and storage systems in the striatum. The genetic abnormalities so far uncovered are involved with the dopamine synthetic system. Gordon[379] reviewed the genetics of Segawa's disease, including the dominant and recessive forms, as well as mutations in *GCHI* and the tyrosine hydroxylase gene. Some authors have speculated

that the diurnal fluctuations that characterize DRD may be due to the circadian variation in dopamine production, with greater synthetic activity possible at night.[374]

One study found that acute dystonia secondary to neuroleptic medication also shows a circadian pattern,[380] with maximal dystonia present between 12:00 noon and 11:00 PM. This could not be accounted for by sleep, fatigue, or time since the last dose of medication (in this case, injections twice daily). Some of this circadian variability may be accounted for by circadian variations in the dopamine system, which seem to show the least activity in the evening hours with maximal activity in the morning.[381]

Myoclonus

The myoclonias (for a general discussion, see Fahn et al.[382]) are a diverse group of conditions with abnormal movements generated at various levels of the neuraxis, from cortex (cortical reflex or epileptic myoclonus) to spinal cord (spinal or segmental myoclonus). The basic abnormal movement is a single, repeated, or periodic jerk, most typically abrupt and "lightning-like." The categorization of these disorders is in a state of flux, and some conditions (e.g., nocturnal myoclonus, now known as *periodic limb movement disorder* [PLMD]), are likely to be removed from the overall myoclonus category, primarily because they lack the lightning-like quality of the movements in "true" myoclonus. The most typical myoclonus arises from higher motor centers, whereas more rhythmical movements, less truly myoclonic, appear to arise from segmental motor centers.

Most of the studies of myoclonus and sleep have focused on the persistence of myoclonic movements during sleep. Some of these dyskinesias are highly persistent. Lugaresi and colleagues[383] studied a range of patients with myoclonus and found that persistence of the movements during sleep depended on the source of the abnormal discharge: myoclonus with a cortical source showed suppressed movements during sleep while (as in epilepsy) cortical discharges persisted, myoclonus of presumed subcortical origin was rapidly suppressed during sleep, and myoclonus of lower level origins (spinal cord or secondary to peripheral damage) persisted during sleep. Myoclonic jerks associated with startle disease also persist during sleep, although with diminished intensity.[384]

Among persistent myoclonic conditions, palatal myoclonus, now called *palatal tremor*, has been found to persist in sleep and even during anesthesia.[385] Electrophysiologic studies in a small number of patients with palatal and associated eye and sometimes limb movements[386,387] have demonstrated that palatal contractions persist during sleep, albeit with shifts in amplitude and frequency or even altered rhythmicity. The eye or limb movements show a greater decrease during sleep. One study found that patients with symptomatic palatal myoclonus (caused by a recognized disorder) were more likely to show sleep persistence than patients with essential palatal myoclonus.[388] The range of such cyclic motor dyskinesias may be broader than currently known: A similar tongue movement was reported to persist largely unchanged in sleep.[389] The finding of persistent rhythmicity suggests a relatively autonomous oscillator, consistent with the idea that these segmental myoclonias may represent release of a primitive rhythmic center.[385] In contrast to other forms of myoclonus, these dyskinesias appear to arise at a segmental level and to be associated with decreased motor control from higher centers. This dissociation may explain their resistance to modulation by descending inhibitory influences during sleep.

The dyskinesias are not completely removed from higher motor centers or the periphery, however, because they may disappear in sleep, change with state, and be influenced by attention.[390,391] In one interesting case, palatal myoclonus was associated with time-locked respiration, suggesting a coupling of these two rhythms.[392] Spinal myoclonus, another segmental myoclonus, although more likely to disappear in sleep,[393,394] can also persist (see Walters et al.[395]). A similar observation was one of auricular myoclonus that persisted in sleep.[396] One patient was also reported with generalized, repetitive disabling myoclonus throughout the ocular and branchial musculature (including the eyes, face, pharynx, larynx, and diaphragm) associated with inhibition of limb muscles (negative myoclonus).[397] This apparently brain stem–mediated myoclonus persisted during sleep. The variable persistence of different segmental myoclonias is consistent with the suggestion of Lugaresi et al.[383] that these myoclonias should persist during sleep.

A conclusion to be drawn from these findings is that, when the sleep system is intact, dyskinesias arising from dysfunction of the higher motor centers are blocked from expression by the normal inhibitory controls of sleep. Dyskinesias from lower centers—segmental and effector levels (e.g., fasciculations)—may be associated with damage to descending control systems and, therefore, be less regulated by the sleep-wake cycle.

Little is known about sleep in the myoclonic conditions. When movements persist, they are likely to disrupt sleep to some extent, although the movements of palatal myoclonus are usually too modest and continuous to be a source of arousals. Standard therapy for myoclonus may improve any sleep disruption related to the movements themselves.[398]

Three other myoclonic conditions—propriospinal myoclonus (PSM) at sleep onset, sleep-related faciomandibular masticatory myoclonus (FMM), and opsoclonus-myoclonus syndrome (OMS)—may cause sleep disturbance. PSM was first described in 1997[399] and is characterized by muscle jerks in axial muscles occurring in the relaxation period preceding sleep, causing severe insomnia. A PSG study using multiple muscle montage documented rostral and caudal propagation at a very slow speed, which is typical of propriospinal pathways. PSM has also been observed in patients with RLS during relaxed wakefulness preceding sleep onset, which is different from PLMS noted during sleep.[400] In the ICSD-2, PSM is listed among the "isolated symptoms, apparently normal variants and unresolved issues." FMM[401,402] is characterized by myoclonic jerks involving facial and masticatory muscles during NREM sleep (especially stage 1 [N1], which may cause sleep-onset insomnia), is different from bruxism, and may sometimes be familial.[403] OMS in children may cause sleep disruption (e.g., fragmented sleep, prolonged sleep latency, nonrestorative sleep) and rage attacks, which may respond to trazodone treatment.[404]

Tics

Tics are typically brisk, stereotyped, complex, often repetitive movements.[405,406] Usually, any given patient has a somewhat limited repertoire of movements that may change over a period of months to years. Tic disorders include Tourette's syndrome, athetoid cerebral palsy, neuroacanthocytosis, hemiballism and hemifacial spasm, and paroxysmal dystonic choreoathetosis.

Tourette's Syndrome. The prototypical tic disorder is Gilles de la Tourette's syndrome, a condition involving multiple motor tics with vocalizations that usually begins in childhood or adolescence, and may subside in later adult life. Tics may be associated with a sensory penumbra and an urge to move.[407] Tourette's syndrome patients also have a number of commonly associated behavioral abnormalities, especially obsessive-compulsive disorder. Most sleep studies have been done in Tourette's syndrome patients.

Typically, younger Tourette's syndrome patients, who are the more severely affected in most cases, have been studied with PSG or sleep monitoring.[408–410] Tics in Tourette's syndrome have been found to persist during sleep in most cases, mostly in stages 1 and 2 of NREM sleep, with fewer during SWS or REM sleep.[411,412] In addition, bodily movements in general may be increased in tics. Hashimoto and colleagues[409] found that both twitchlike and gross body movements were increased over controls during all stages of sleep, with total movements in tic patients markedly increased during REM sleep. Those authors did not attempt to analyze such movements in detail, so it is not clear what fraction of them were actual tics.

Sleep has been reported to be impaired in patients with tics.[411,413–416] Various investigators have reported increased sleep disruption, an elevated prevalence of parasomnias, and respiratory disturbances during sleep in Tourette's syndrome patients.[410] In one study, 22 of 50 patients (44%) were reported to have disturbed sleep based on patient and family report.[408] One large study ($N = 57$ in each group) that found increased parasomnias used two control groups, one of children with learning disorders and another of children with seizures.[412] Somnambulism occurred in 17.5% of tic patients, significantly more than either of the two control groups. Sleepwalking is a frequently noted problem of younger Tourette's syndrome patients.[417]

In one study, patients were monitored after successful treatment of their movements with tetrabenazine and it was found that sleep was also improved.[418]

Athetoid Cerebral Palsy. In athetoid cerebral palsy, abnormalities of REM sleep have been noted. Hayashi and colleagues[419] reported on a group of adolescent and young adult patients with severe disease. The significant motor abnormalities were associated with REM sleep: three patients had decreased numbers of REM, two had increased chin muscle tone, and seven had reduced numbers of muscular twitches. The authors suggested this may be related to brain stem pathology in these birth-injured patients. It has also been noted that this patient group is commonly affected by childhood OSA and may benefit from surgical management[420] or, as reported in one case, intrathecal baclofen.[421]

Neuroacanthocytosis. Neuroacanthocytosis, or chorea-acanthocytosis, is the most common form of hereditary chorea after HD, presenting with tics, chorea, vocalizations, and self-mutilation together with frequent seizures, associated with elevated acanthocytes (spiked red cells) in blood smears.[422–424] Silvestri and colleagues[425,426] reported that abnormal movements persisted during sleep, but with decreased amplitude, duration, and frequency. Patients frequently vocalized during REM sleep. Sleep was fragmented and of poor quality. Two siblings with neuroacanthocytosis showed EEG slowing (predominantly delta) both while awake and during REM sleep,[427] indicating abnormal cerebral function. RLS has been reported to occur in this condition.[428]

Hemiballism. In hemiballism, there are proximal flinging movements of one side of the body, which may be of a violent nature, associated with damage to the contralateral subthalamic nucleus.[429] It was initially thought that the movements totally subsided in sleep. Askenasy,[334] however, reported a patient whose movements persisted in sleep, and Silvestri and colleagues[425] found that the movements were present during stages 1 and 2 NREM sleep as well as during REM sleep, although diminished in intensity and frequency. Puca and colleagues[430] reported one case in which spindle density and amplitude were greater ipsilateral to the damaged subthalamic nucleus. There was also disrupted sleep, with prolonged latency and an absence of both SWS and REM sleep. Successful treatment with haloperidol improved the sleep and decreased the spindling. In most cases, hemiballism is a transient phenomenon

after local injury to the subthalamus (usually ischemic), although it may be transformed into a chronic choreiform disorder.

Hemifacial Spasm. Hemifacial spasm is a synchronous contraction of one side of the face that is usually repetitive and jerklike, but may sometimes be sustained.[162,431] It is thought to arise from damage to the facial nerve or nucleus. EMG recording shows highly synchronous discharges in upper and lower facial muscles. Montagna and colleagues[161] studied 16 patients, recording from upper and lower facial muscles during sleep studies. In most patients, the dyskinesias decreased during sleep, being approximately 80% less frequent in SWS and REM sleep. One patient showed almost no change in the prevalence of spasms. Current therapy for hemifacial spasm includes medications such as carbamazepine, botulinum toxin injection[432–434] into the affected muscles, or varied surgical treatments, such as vascular decompression of the facial nerve.[435,436] Combined treatment with pregabalin and botulinum toxin injections has been reported.[437] We are aware of no reports of sleep studies after successful therapy, but it seems likely that the dyskinesias are relieved.

Paroxysmal Dystonic Choreoathetosis. One family with five generations affected by paroxysmal dystonic choreoathetosis with dominant transmission was found to show substantial benefit from even brief periods of sleep.[438] In a Serbian family with mutations in the myofibrillogenesis regulator 1 gene, sleep was reported to be the most effective means of terminating attacks.[439]

Sleep-Associated Problems of the Ataxic Disorders

Relatively little study has been given to the ataxic disorders. Today, a large number of different genetically based variants of spinocerebellar ataxia have been described, and some of these have been examined with respect to sleep. Patients with Machado-Joseph disease (spinocerebellar ataxia type 3 [SCA3]) may have both RLS and RBD[440,441] as common sleep-related problems. Patients with SCA2 can have REM sleep without atonia.[442,443] One report suggested increased PLMS and RLS in SCA6.[444] SCA6 patients also have impaired subjective sleep quality and tend to greater daytime sleepiness.[445] It seems likely that the paucity of associations reported to date is more due to the lack of studies than the absence of sleep problems in these disorders.

MOVEMENT DISORDERS EVOKED BY SLEEP

Movement disorders evoked by sleep are now generally categorized as a separate diagnostic group in the ICSD-2.[2] However, some conditions are only classified as temporary disorders (excessive fragmentary myoclonus) or as PSG findings. The scoring of these movements has been summarized.[3]

Periodic Limb Movements

PLM are repetitive, often stereotyped involuntary movements that typically recur at intervals of 15–40 seconds during NREM sleep. They usually involve the legs, where they may consist of extension of the great toe associated with flexion at the ankle, knee, and hip. These movements were first called nocturnal myoclonus,[446] although they are not usually myoclonic in speed.[447] The term *periodic limb movements in sleep* (PLMS) is preferable compared to periodic leg movements in sleep because, although less common, the arms may also be involved.[448] In the classification of sleep disorders, the disorder associated with PLMS is known as *periodic limb movement disorder* (PLMD).[449]

The individual leg movement of PLMS has been described as resembling Babinski's reflex (extension of the great toe with fanning of the other toes)[450] or a triple flexion reflex.[451] Most movements are too slow to be called myoclonus, and they typically last a few seconds (see Fig. 12–9). However, the movements may begin with one or more brief, myoclonic jerks that then blend into a more tonic phase; alternatively, a more sustained movement may terminate in a jerk.[46,451,452] Movements are often bilateral, involving both legs, but may be predominant in one leg or alternate between legs. They are quite varied in their manifestations, and attempts to find a modal pattern have led to contradictory results.[453–455] Their most characteristic feature is their repetitive, often strikingly periodic nature. In the typical moderate to severe patient, PLMS occur in bouts of dozens to a hundred or more movements that last for many minutes. While most movements occur in the lighter stages of NREM sleep (stages 1 and 2), some movements may occur in SWS and REM sleep as well as during the wake state.[49] Because PLMS may occur when awake, a broader term, *periodic limb movements*, has been used to designate these movements independent of the state in which they occur.

PLMS are generally diagnosed by PSG recording or ambulatory sleep monitoring (for PSG standards, see Kushida et al.[456]). The ICSD-2[2] and the current AASM manual[28] will count movements if they occur in series of four or more movements during any sleep stage (wake excluded) at intervals of 5–90 seconds (in some publications, intervals as short as 4 seconds or as long as 120 seconds have been accepted). EMG bursts must last 0.5–5 seconds. A proposal to increase the duration limit to 10 seconds[457] has been adopted in the current AASM scoring manual.[28] The number of movements associated with arousals may also be counted.[458] Table 28–2 lists the diagnostic features of PLMS. Although PLMD patients may also have movements during wakefulness, only movements that occur during sleep are typically counted. A new measure, the periodicity index, is a measure of how frequently leg movements fall into typical trains by

TABLE 28–2 Diagnostic Features of Periodic Limb Movements in Sleep

- Repetitive, often stereotyped movements during NREM sleep.
- Usually noted in the legs and consisting of extension of the great toe, dorsiflexion of the ankle, and flexion of the knees and hips; sometimes seen in the arms.
- Periodic or quasiperiodic at an average interval of 20–40 seconds (range 5–90 seconds from onset to onset of EMG activity) with a duration of 0.5–10 seconds, and as part of at least 4 consecutive movements.
- The onset of leg movement is defined as the beginning of an 8-μV increase in EMG amplitude above the baseline.
- The ending of leg movement is defined as the point when EMG amplitude falls below 2 μV above baseline resting EMG for at least 0.5 second.
- Movement in one leg separated by less than 0.5 second from a movement in the other leg should be counted as a single leg movement.
- May occur as an isolated condition or may be associated with a large number of other medical, neurologic, or sleep disorders and medications.
- Seen in at least 80% of patients with restless legs syndrome.
- If associated with clinical sleep disturbance (e.g., insomnia or excessive daytime sleepiness) not otherwise explained and a PLMS index (number of PLMS/hr of sleep) exceeding 5 in children and 15 in most adult cases, a diagnosis of periodic limb movement disorder can be made.

EMG, electromyogram; NREM, non–rapid eye movement; PLMS, periodic limb movements in sleep.

examining the interval before and after each leg movement.[459] This measure recognizes that true periodicity, rather than simple frequent recurrence (which the operational definition provides for) is the key element of PLMS.

Individuals with elevated frequency of PLMS are often asymptomatic, but severely affected patients may complain of difficulty maintaining sleep or EDS. Bed partners may complain more about the movements than the patients and are often an excellent source of information about the condition and its severity. The importance of PLMS has been questioned by several authors and in certain contexts,[447,460] but some sleep specialists believe that severe cases do cause significant sleep disturbance and warrant therapy. This is particularly true in patients with RLS, whose PLMS can be quite severe.[461] As noted, the ICSD-2 requires that the PLMS impact on either sleep continuity (insomnia) or daytime functioning (sleepiness) for a diagnosis of PLMD.[2]

PLMS may begin at any age, but prevalence increases markedly in healthy elderly people, with as many as 58% having a PLMS index greater than 5.[462,463] Some studies have found no association between PLMS and either objective measures of sleep or symptomatic reports in the elderly, or only very weak associations.[462] Because of these findings, elderly patients with PLMS should only be treated when the PLMS can be linked to their sleep complaints, which usually means excluding other sources of sleep dysfunction. Rather than the sheer number of

PLM, the number (or index per hour) of those associated with arousal may be a better predictor of disturbed sleep and clinical significance.[464]

PLMS may occur as an isolated condition or may be associated with a large number of sleep, neurologic, or other medical disorders, and with medications such as neuroleptics and antidepressants (Table 28–3). Among sleep disorders, the more striking associations are with narcolepsy[465–467] and RLS, because PLMS are common in these patients even at a relatively young age. PLMS are also common in patients with OSA[468] and RBD,[47] but these patients are elderly. Patients with OSA may have a significant degree of PLMS, sometimes resulting in significant sleep fragmentation, after successful treatment of their apnea. The PLMS may then cause residual sleep difficulty.[468] The presence of PLMS in basal ganglia disorders, including PD,[167,168,469] dopa-responsive dystonia,[470] and MSA,[169,288,316] is also noteworthy and may contribute to sleep problems in these disorders. Among medical conditions, the association of PLMS with uremia is likely to be an important one.[471] It has been reported that intrinsic and extrinsic lesions of the spinal cord may be associated with PLMS. This has been noted for multiple sclerosis,[451,472,473] radiculopathy,[474] transection,[451,475] and extrinsic lesions causing cord compression.[473]

A number of studies have examined the relationship between PLM and other measures of central nervous system (CNS)/autonomic activity such as EEG, heart rate, and blood pressure. A general summary is that PLM are linked to periodic changes in activity level in different neural and neuroresponsive systems; furthermore, these modulations do not appear to be caused by the movement of the PLM, but are likely to be parallel phenomena that can be independent of PLMS.[476] One suggestion is that the sympathetic nervous system may actually have a role in generating PLMS.[477]

A specific feature of NREM sleep, the cyclic alternating pattern (CAP), mentioned earlier, is a recurrent alternation between "baseline" and more activated EEG patterns.[30,478,479] PLM almost always occur during the activated, A phase of CAP.[34] A phases can be further subcategorized depending on the EEG frequencies most common in them: A1 activations consist primarily of slow waves while A3 activations are dominated by faster rhythms. The A3 phases are very strongly related to AASM-defined arousals. It has been proposed that a hierarchy of activations may be correlated to PLMS, with milder activations consisting solely of autonomic changes, slow waves, or K complexes while more intense ones are associated with EEG desynchronization and arousals.[480,481]

Because PLMS are associated with heart rate increases[476] and rises in blood pressure,[482,483] it has been suggested that, untreated, they may lead to persistent diurnal hypertension. This connection remains to be established, but provides a potential rationale for treating PLMS that occur without a related sleep complaint. Treating PLMS in RLS patients might be less effective than in those without RLS, because arousals may persist in RLS patients even when movements are effectively suppressed.[484] In RLS patients, there may be a different relationship between movements and arousals than in those without RLS[485]: in RLS, the PLMS may be more closely connected to an underlying abnormality. These suggestions need to be confirmed and their implications for treatment better understood.

Restless Legs Syndrome

RLS is a sensorimotor disorder predominantly characterized by an urge to move or restlessness that is provoked by rest, relieved by movement or CNS arousal, and increased with a circadian pattern during the evening and night.[486–488] RLS is a common disorder in the North American population,[489,490] perhaps due to its European origins.[491–494] Five genetic linkages have been described,[495] and associations to specific allelic variants have been found by genome-wide association studies.[496,497] However, the degree of familiality is low.[498] In an ongoing, methodologically rigorous study, the relative risk (Risch's lambda[499]) in first-degree relatives is in the range of 3 to 5.[500] This is due to the relatively modest risk seemingly conveyed by genetic factors and the likelihood that there are many contributing genetic factors as well as strong environmental influences. Therefore, like other common disorders, RLS is a genetically complex disease.

RLS occurs with elevated frequency in several discrete conditions, including iron deficiency[501] and pregnancy,[502] rheumatoid arthritis,[503] and uremia,[504–506] all of which have been associated with iron deficiency. As a result of

---

TABLE 28–3 Periodic Limb Movements in Sleep (PLMS): Comorbid Conditions

- Primary sleep disorders
  - Restless legs syndrome
  - Rapid eye movement sleep behavior disorder
  - Narcolepsy
  - Obstructive sleep apnea syndrome
- Neurologic disorders
  - Parkinson's disease
  - Multiple system atrophy
  - Dopa-responsive dystonia
  - Intrinsic and extrinsic lesions of the spinal cord
  - Multiple sclerosis
  - Radiculopathies
  - Myelopathies
  - Amyotrophic lateral sclerosis
- Medical disorders
  - Uremia
  - Heart failure
  - Chronic obstructive pulmonary disease
- Pregnancy (especially multiple pregnancies)
- Antidepressants
  - Selective serotonin reuptake inhibitors
  - Tricyclic antidepressants
  - Lithium

these findings, it seems likely that RLS is a complex disorder with multiple genetic and environmental determinants. A unifying theme may be a local deficiency of iron in critical brain neurons.[507–511] Table 28–4 lists risk factors for RLS.

The cause of RLS remains unknown, though the functional abnormality is almost certainly neural in origin.[512,513] A striking finding has been the almost universal response of RLS patients to medications that enhance dopamine system function.[514] Measures of dopamine dysfunction, however, have been equivocal or mixed,[512,515] and the reason that dopaminergic agents relieve the condition remains unclear.[516] Drugs that antagonize the dopamine system may also unmask RLS symptoms, especially in treated patients.[517,518] Studies have supported a deficiency of brain iron in RLS[508,509,519] that might influence dopamine function,[507] perhaps through decreased synaptic strength.[511] Autopsy studies have suggested that the iron deficiency is associated with abnormal levels of cellular iron regulatory proteins.[510] In this model of RLS causation,[507] iron deficiency is expected to act through a dysregulation of brain dopamine function, perhaps related to altered amplitude of circadian dopamine variation. There is no evidence of neurodegeneration in RLS.[509,520] Thus, RLS may be a functional abnormality in which all brain systems are intact, but interacting abnormally.

TABLE 28–4 Restless Legs Syndrome Risk Factors

Demographic and Lifestyle Factors

- Increasing age
- Female sex
- Family history (early onset)
- Living at high altitude
- Smoking
- Sedentary lifestyle
- Caffeine
- Alcohol consumption

Medical, Surgical, Neurologic, or Other Conditions

- Medical
  - Renal failure
  - Diabetes mellitus
  - Iron deficiency and anemia
  - Rheumatoid arthritis
  - Magnesium or vitamin B_{12} deficiency
  - Hypothyroidism
  - Heart failure
- Surgical
  - Gastric resection
  - Lung transplantation
- Neurologic
  - Polyneuropathies and radiculopathies
  - Parkinson's disease
  - Multiple sclerosis
  - Spinocerebellar ataxia (SCA3 or Machado-Joseph disease)
- Others
  - Pregancy
  - Blood donations
  - Medications

RLS significantly impacts patient health and quality of life.[493,521,522] Cross-sectional surveys have found RLS occurrence to be associated with general poor health, both physical and mental,[490,491,494,523–525] as well as specific disorders such as diabetes[490] and heart disease.[494,526,527] RLS, in turn, relates to a diminished quality of life[493,528] and may be responsible for varied forms of psychological distress[529,530] and impaired daily functioning.[531] In vulnerable populations, such as dialysis patients, RLS occurs with increased mortality.[504,532] Thus, there is evidence that RLS is provoked by a number of different disorders and also contributes to both morbidity and mortality. Much of this effect may occur through the impairment of sleep (Fig. 28–1) caused by RLS.[492,533] Almost all studies have found RLS to be a

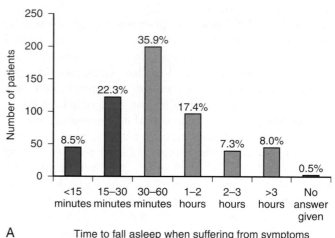

A   Time to fall asleep when suffering from symptoms

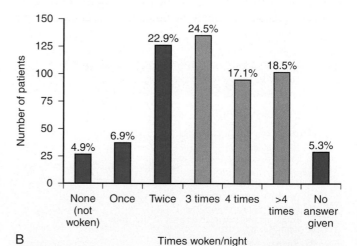

B   Times woken/night

FIGURE 28–1 Time to fall asleep **(A)** and number of reported awakenings **(B)** for RLS patients on nights when bothered by symptoms. *Unshaded bars* indicate those in the range considered abnormal and consistent with insomnia. Data are derived from RLS, Epidemiology, Symptoms and Treatment (REST) general population study in the United States, France, Germany, Italy, Spain, and the United Kingdom. *(Reproduced with permission from Hening W, Walters AS, Allen RP, et al. Impact, diagnosis and treatment of restless legs syndrome [RLS] in a primary care population: the REST [RLS Epidemiology, Symptoms, and Treatment] primary care study. Sleep Med 2004;5:237.)*

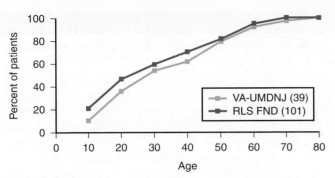

FIGURE 28–2 Cumulative prevalence of restless legs syndrome before a given age (*x* axis) gauged from date of onset of symptoms in two case series: 39 patients studied by Dr. Walters and colleagues at the UMDNJ–Robert Wood Johnson Medical School and at the Lyons, New Jersey, Department of Veterans Affairs Medical Center, and 101 patients interviewed by a team directed by Dr. Walters who were initially contacted through the RLS Foundation by Virginia Walker, secretary. *(Modified from Walters AS, Hickey K, Maltzman J, et al. A questionnaire study of 138 patients with restless legs syndrome: the 'Night-Walkers' survey. Neurology 1996;46:92.)*

chronic disease with both increasing prevalence[489,490,492] (Fig. 28–2) and generally increasing severity with age.[534] Thus, RLS presents a cumulative burden substantially contributing to loss of quality of life and decreased health status in old age. Subjects with RLS have as poor a general sense of health-related quality of life on the Medical Outcomes Short Form-36 as do those with other chronic diseases such as hypertension, congestive heart failure, and angina.[528]

Clinical Features and Diagnosis of RLS

RLS was first extensively described by Karl Ekbom, a Swedish neurologist who named the condition and elucidated its clinical features.[535,536] Over the last decade, the key clinical features required for diagnosis have been determined through a consensus process[488,537] and include the following symptoms:

1. An urge to move, usually caused by or associated with unpleasant sensations in the legs
2. Provocation of symptoms by rest
3. Relief of symptoms by activity
4. A circadian pattern of symptoms whereby, in patients with a normal day-night activity pattern, symptoms are worse in the evening and night[486,487]

While other body parts, especially the arms,[538] can be involved in RLS, the legs are generally involved first and more prominently. RLS without leg symptoms at onset is at least rare.[539]

Supportive and associated clinical features have also been noted (Table 28–5). Supportive features, which are not required for diagnosis,[488] include familial aggregation,[498,540] significant numbers of PLM,[541,542] and prominent response to dopaminergic agents.[514] There have been attempts, however, to use these supportive clinical features to improve diagnostic accuracy in uncertain cases. There are also diagnostic criteria suggested for

special populations (e.g., children under 12 years, cognitively impaired elderly). Tables 28–6 and 28–7 list such criteria (see Allen et al.[488]).

Because frequent PLM are associated with RLS, the measurement of PLM has been proposed as a diagnostic test. The Montreal group has taken the lead in validating such a test, finding that the number of PLMW during a sleep study best discriminates RLS patients from normal subjects.[542] They also use the Suggested Immobilization Test, a provocative test in which the subject is required to remain without activity sitting reclined in a bed for a sustained period (usually an hour) for diagnosis. Both sensory and motor features (PLMW) are measured. An increase in sensory discomfort combined with PLMW from the PSG was found to yield a fairly reliable diagnostic test: in a comparison of RLS patients and those with no sleep complaint, sensitivity for RLS was 82% and specificity was 100% (no false-positive diagnosis of RLS among the normal subjects).

To study responsiveness to dopaminergics, a test dose of L-dopa was used. A greater than 50% improvement of symptoms was strongly associated with a true RLS diagnosis, and a positive response to this test was a reliable indicator that a patient would subsequently benefit from dopaminergic treatment.[543]

Because there is, as of yet, no adequate laboratory marker for RLS, the standard for diagnosis remains a clinical one and is derived from the patient's history.[544] Laboratory evaluation is useful mainly to confirm the diagnosis of RLS and to identify any possible underlying medical condition (e.g., uremia).[544] To determine RLS, in the clinic or the community, it is necessary to first establish the presence of the four diagnostic features noted previously. While earlier epidemiologic studies used ad hoc questions to ascertain the presence of RLS,[489,490] more recent ones have generated probes based on the four diagnostic features.[492–494,524,531,545,546] However, a study at Johns Hopkins University has demonstrated that up to 16% of individuals without RLS may meet all four diagnostic criteria.[547] Definitive diagnosis, therefore, requires discriminating RLS from its mimics. The differential diagnosis of RLS includes conditions of restlessness and conditions of leg discomfort (Table 28–8).

Questionnaires for RLS can be used to screen patients in clinical practice or to ascertain cases of RLS in epidemiologic studies of large populations. A single question has proven highly sensitive in detecting RLS patients and has reasonable specificity in many populations.[548,549] Available in several languages (for many European languages, see Ferri et al.[550]), the English version runs: "When you try to relax in the evening or sleep at night, do you ever have unpleasant, restless feelings in your legs that can be relieved by walking or movement?"

Several multiquestion instruments have been developed for epidemiologic studies. Two have been validated. One three-question instrument developed by Klaus Berger and

TABLE 28–5 Clinical Diagnostic Criteria for Idiopathic Restless Legs Syndrome (RLS)

Essential Diagnostic Criteria for RLS

- An urge to move the legs, usually accompanied or caused by uncomfortable and unpleasant sensations in the legs. (Sometimes the urge to move is present without the uncomfortable sensations, and sometimes the arms or other body parts are involved in addition to the legs.)
- The urge to move or unpleasant sensations begin or worsen during periods of rest or inactivity such as lying or sitting.
- The urge to move or unpleasant sensations are partially or totally relieved by movement, such as walking or stretching, at least as long as the activity continues.
- The urge to move or unpleasant sensations are worse in the evening or night than during the day or only occur in the evening or night. (When symptoms are very severe, the worsening at night may not be noticeable but must have been previously present.)

Supportive Clinical Features

- **Family History**
  - The prevalence of RLS among first-degree relatives of people with RLS is 3–5 times greater than in people without RLS.
- **Response to Dopaminergic Therapy**
  - Nearly all people with RLS show at least an initial positive therapeutic response to either L-dopa or a dopamine receptor agonist at doses considered to be very low in relation to the traditional doses of these medications used for the treatment of Parkinson's disease. This initial response is not, however, universally maintained.
- **Periodic Limb Movements** (during wakefulness or sleep)

- Periodic limb movements in sleep (PLMS) occur in at least 85% of people with RLS; however, PLMS also commonly occur in other disorders and in the elderly.
- In children, PLMS are much less common than in adults.

Associated Features of RLS

- **Natural Clinical Course**
  - The clinical course of the disorder varies considerably, but certain patterns have been identified that may be helpful to the experienced clinician.
  - When the age of onset of RLS symptoms is less than 50 years, the onset is often more insidious; when the age of onset is greater than 50 years, the symptoms often occur more abruptly and more severely.
  - In some patients, RLS can be intermittent and may spontaneously remit for many years.
- **Sleep Disturbance**
  - Disturbed sleep is a common major morbidity for RLS and deserves special consideration in planning treatment. This morbidity is often the primary reason the patient seeks medical attention.
- **Medical Evaluation/Physical Examination**
  - The physical examination is generally normal and does not contribute to the diagnosis except for those conditions that may be comorbid or secondary causes of RLS.
  - Iron status, in particular, should be evaluated because decreased iron stores are a significant potential risk factor that can be treated.
  - The presence of peripheral neuropathy and radiculopathy should also be determined because these conditions have a possible, although uncertain, association and may require different treatment.

Adapted from Allen RP, Picchietti D, Hening WA, et al. Restless legs syndrome: diagnostic criteria, special considerations, and epidemiology. A report from the Restless Legs Syndrome Diagnosis and Epidemiology Workshop at the National Institutes of Health. Sleep Med 2003;4:101.

endorsed at the National Institutes of Health (NIH) diagnostic consensus conference[488] had an interrater kappa of 0.67 between two experts who, however, had access to the questionnaire results.[551] Another questionnaire developed at Johns Hopkins University was validated by independent clinician interview and had a sensitivity of 89% and specificity of 80% in an American primary care practice.[552] A slightly revised version of the questionnaire validated by telephone diagnostic interview[553] had a sensitivity of 87% and a specificity of 94% in a population of blood donors.[554]

Two different approaches have been taken to make more definitive diagnoses for clinical or research purposes. First is a telephone interview, the Hopkins Telephone Diagnostic Interview for RLS (HTDI).[553] This includes questions that address the diagnostic features, but also questions to assist with differential diagnosis and uncover mimics. Finally, there are questions concerning key aspects of the disorder. Agreement with expert interviews was found to be 92%, approaching the interrater reliability of two-expert face-to-face interviews of 96%.[553] A second approach is a protocol that begins with questions about diagnostic features but then includes tests related to the supportive and associated features (see Table 28–5). This diagnostic interview includes questions on family history,

a sleep study to look for PLM, a physical examination to exclude other causes for symptoms, and a dopaminergic challenge test.[555] Because it gives higher scores to patients with more frequent symptoms, it may not correctly identify those with sporadic symptoms. Its diagnosis is basically one of clinically significant RLS.

Epidemiology, Pathophysiology, and Genetics of RLS

Prevalence of RLS in Different Ethnic Groups. It is not clear whether substantial and true differences exist between different ethnic groups in the prevalence of RLS. Because RLS must be defined clinically from history, different groups with different languages (some of which still have no consensus term for RLS) may respond differently when asked apparently equivalent questions about their medical history. It is also an issue that population studies, even using several questions to diagnose RLS, may vary in how many individuals detected have true RLS and how many of those with RLS are missed.[551] A rough guide is that the positive predictive value—how many of those identified with RLS actually have the disorder—is on the order of 40–60% in studies using

---

TABLE 28–6 Criteria for Diagnosis of Probable Restless Legs Syndrome (RLS) in Cognitively Impaired Elderly

Essential Criteria (all five are necessary for diagnosis)

1. Signs of leg discomfort (e.g., rubbing or kneading the legs and groaning while holding the lower extremities) are present.
2. Excessive motor activity in the lower extremities (e.g., pacing, fidgeting, repetitive kicking, tossing and turning in bed, cycling movements of the lower limbs, repetitive foot tapping, rubbing the feet together, and the inability to remain seated) are present.
3. Signs of leg discomfort are exclusively present or worsen during periods of rest or inactivity.
4. Signs of leg discomfort are diminished with activity.
5. Criteria 1 and 2 occur only in the evening or at night or are worse at those times than during the day.

Suggestive Criteria

- Dopaminergic responsiveness
- Patient's past history—as reported by a family member, caregiver, or friend—is suggestive of RLS
- A first-degree, biological relative (sibling, child, or parent) has RLS
- Observed periodic limb movements while awake or during sleep
- Periodic limb movements of sleep recorded by polysomnography or actigraphy
- Significant sleep-onset problems
- Better quality sleep in the day than at night
- The use of restraints at night (for institutionalized patients)
- Low serum ferritin level
- End-stage renal disease
- Diabetes
- Clinical, electromyographic, or nerve conduction evidence of peripheral neuropathy or radiculopathy

Adapted from Allen RP, Picchietti D, Hening WA, et al. Restless legs syndrome: diagnostic criteria, special considerations, and epidemiology. A report from the Restless Legs Syndrome Diagnosis and Epidemiology Workshop at the National Institutes of Health. Sleep Med 2003;4:101.

TABLE 28–7 Diagnostic Criteria for Restless Legs Syndrome (RLS) in Children Under 12 Years

Criteria for the Diagnosis of *Definite* RLS

1. The child meets all four essential adult criteria for RLS
   AND
2. The child relates a description in his or her own words that is consistent with leg discomfort (the child may use terms such as *owies, tickle, spiders, boo-boos, want to run*, and *a lot of energy in my legs* to describe symptoms. Age-appropriate descriptors are encouraged.)
   OR
1. The child meets all four essential adult criteria for RLS *and*
2. Two of three of the following supportive criteria are present

Supportive Criteria for the Diagnosis of Definite RLS
a. Sleep disturbance for age
b. A biological parent or sibling has definite RLS
c. The child has a polysomnographically documented periodic limb movement index of 5 or more per hour of sleep

Criteria for the Diagnosis of *Probable* RLS

1. The child meets all essential adult criteria for RLS, except criterion 4 (the urge to move or sensations are worse in the evening or at night than during the day) *and*
2. The child has a biological parent or sibling with definite RLS
   *OR**
1. The child is observed to have behavior manifestations of lower extremity discomfort when sitting or lying, accompanied by motor movement of the affected limbs. The discomfort has characteristics of adult criteria 2, 3, and 4 (i.e., is worse during rest and inactivity, relieved by movement, and worse during the evening and at night) *and*
2. The child has a biological parent or sibling with definite RLS

Criteria for the Diagnosis of *Possible* RLS

1. The child has periodic limb movement disorder *and*
2. The child has a biological parent or sibling with definite RLS, but the child does not meet definite or probable childhood RLS definitions

*This last probable category is intended for young children or cognitively impaired children, who do not have sufficient language to describe the sensory component of RLS.
Adapted from Allen RP, Picchietti D, Hening WA, et al. Restless legs syndrome: diagnostic criteria, special considerations, and epidemiology. A report from the Restless Legs Syndrome Diagnosis and Epidemiology Workshop at the National Institutes of Health. Sleep Med 2003;4:101.

---

well-established diagnostic criteria (based on the consensus diagnostic criteria). This means that less than half may actually have RLS. It is generally considered that false positives in such studies are more likely than false negatives.

Despite methodologic limitations, repeated studies have shown that there is a high prevalence of RLS in Western (European and European-derived) populations.[489,490,492–494,524,526,531,545,546,556,557] It seems reasonable that the true rate in Western adults is on the order of 4–10% for RLS at any frequency. One large-scale study, the REST population study conducted in the United States and Europe, found an overall prevalence of 7.2% in adults.[493] That study used a questionnaire later found to have a positive predictive value of 59%.[554a] The study also looked at a measure of clinically significant RLS, a frequency of twice a week or more and moderate or greater distress when symptoms occurred, and found a frequency of 2.7%. A later study that confirmed questionnaire diagnoses with the HTDI[553] found that RLS frequency was approximately 4.4% and clinically significant RLS frequency was 2.7% as judged by diagnosing clinicians[554a]; those cases with a high impact of symptoms on patient life made up 0.8% of the total.

While a substantial number of studies have suggested a lower prevalence in non-Western countries,[281,558–560] other studies have found a higher prevalence in the general population.[561,562] In two methodologically rigorous studies, which used personal interviews to verify diagnosis, the frequency in Japanese elderly was around 1%[563] and among Korean adults, 7.5%.[564] The information on African Americans is scant. Very few African Americans seek treatment for RLS in clinics, and the previous published epidemiologic studies have not addressed the prevalence of RLS among African Americans. One preliminary study in Baltimore did not find a lower frequency in African Americans.[565] Given these uncertainties, it is not completely established that RLS is much more common in whites than in other ethnic populations.

TABLE 28–8 Disorders and Conditions That Can Be Confused with Restless Legs Syndrome

Presenting with Excess Restlessness

- Akathisia
  - Neuroleptic induced
  - Antidepressant induced
  - Related to central nervous system degenerative disease
- Disorders of abnormal muscular activity
  - Myokymia
  - Hypnic jerks
  - Essential myoclonus
  - Orthostatic tremor
- Anxiety/depression
- Periodic limb movement disorder
- Restlessness due to orthostatic hypotension
- Attention-deficit/hyperactivity disorder

Presenting with Nocturnal Leg Discomfort

- "Growing pains"
- Small fiber neuropathies
- Claudication
- Venous stasis–varicose veins
- Myalgias
- Arthritis
- Radiculopathies
- Delusional parasitosis

Presenting with Unusual Motor Activity, Combined with Leg Discomfort

- Painful muscle cramps, including nocturnal leg cramps
- Syndrome of painful legs and moving toes
- Variant of painless legs and moving toes
- Causalgia-dystonia syndrome
- Muscular pain–fasciculation syndrome

Reproduced with permission from Chokroverty S. Differential diagnosis of restless legs syndrome. *In* WA Hening, RP Allen, S Chokroverty, CJ Earley (eds), Restless Legs Syndrome. Philadelphia: Elsevier/Saunders, 2009:111.

TABLE 28–9 Important Associations with Restless Legs Syndrome and Potential Causes

Polyneuropathies and lumbar radiculopathies, including:
- Diabetic neuropathy
- Familial amyloid neuropathy
- Cryoglobulinemic neuropathy
- Charcot-Marie-Tooth disease, type 2
- Saphenous nerve entrapment
- Meralgia paresthetica

Iron deficiency
- With anemia; may be:
  - Due to blood donation
  - Due to internal bleeding
- Without anemia

End-stage renal disease
- With ongoing dialysis
- Without ongoing dialysis

Pregnancy
Parkinson's disease
Multiple sclerosis
Pulmonary disease, including:
- Chronic obstructive pulmonary disease
- Sleep apnea

Miscellaneous disorders
- Hyperthyroidism and hypothyroidism
- Hyperparathyroidism
- Myelopathy
- Stiff-man syndrome
- Isaac's syndrome
- Hyperekplexia
- After gastric resection

Medications
- Dopamine-blocking agents
  - Neuroleptics
  - Sedative blockers
  - Antinausea agents
  - Gastrointestinal medications (metoclopramide)
- Antidepressants
  - Tricyclic antidepressants
  - Serotonin and norepinephrine reuptake blockers
  - Lithium
- Centrally acting antihistamines
- Calcium channel blockers
- Lipid-lowering agents
- Nonsteroidal anti-inflammatory drugs

Reproduced with permission from Chokroverty S. Differential diagnosis of restless legs syndrome. *In* WA Hening, RP Allen, S Chokroverty, CJ Earley (eds), Restless Legs Syndrome. Philadelphia: Elsevier/Saunders, 2009:111.

Besides ethnicity, age and gender reportedly are strongly associated with RLS (see Table 28–4). Almost all studies[489–494,524,531,545,546] have reported positive correlations of RLS with age (but see Sevim et al.[560]) and somewhat to markedly increased frequency in women. The first systematic study of RLS frequency in children[566] found that 1.9% of those 8–11 years of age and 2.0% of those 12–17 years of age reported symptoms of RLS; 0.5% of the younger group and 1% of the older group had clinically significant RLS (twice a week and bothersome when occurring).

Secondary or Comorbid RLS. Elevated prevalences (>20%) of RLS have been reported in studies based on clinical samples of persons with a number of medical conditions such as iron deficiency,[502,567–569] anemia,[570] pregnancy,[571,572] rheumatoid arthritis,[503] and uremia[504] (Table 28–9). Their causative role is supported by the reversibility of symptoms of RLS after treatment or resolution of iron deficiency or anemia,[569,571,573] pregnancy,[572] and uremia.[505] Also, considerably higher prevalence among those with these comorbid conditions (pregnancy,[574] uremia[558,575]) has been reported even in Asian countries with

low prevalence of RLS in the general population. One constant factor noted in these conditions is that they typically predispose to low iron stores.[507] Decreased iron stores may also explain the finding that RLS may be aggravated by blood donation[576] and may be more common among blood donors[577] (but see the results of Burchell et al.[578] contradicting these findings) or among those who have been regular users of nonsteroidal anti-inflammatory medications that can cause gastrointestinal bleeding.[579] Such conditions may not only provoke RLS, but increase liability later in life. It has been also hypothesized that pregnancy may cause lasting changes that predispose to increased RLS in later life.[546,580]

In some neurologic conditions, the association with RLS is not so clearly related to iron metabolism. It has long been suggested that neuropathy might predispose to RLS. Neuropathic findings have been reported in RLS patients.[581,582] However, one earlier study did not find an unusual prevalence in a neuropathy clinic[583]; a more recent study reported that 30% of neuropathy patients had RLS.[584] Radiculopathies[474] and myelopathies may also cause RLS. There has also been an association between RLS and certain neurodegenerative conditions, including Machado-Joseph disease (SCA3),[585,586] multiple sclerosis,[587] and PD.[279] In PD, RLS often starts after beginning dopaminergic therapy, suggesting some analogue of the augmentation seen with dopaminergic therapy of RLS (see later).

RLS Pathophysiology. The functional abnormality in RLS is almost certainly neural in origin.[512,513] A striking finding has been the almost universal response of RLS patients to medications that enhance dopamine system function,[514] but the reason that dopaminergic agents relieve the condition remains unclear.[516] One attractive possibility is that the A11 dopamine system, which descends to the spinal cord, could be involved in RLS, acting through D_3 dopamine receptors[588]; D_3 knock-out mice show increased activity, as do mice with A11 lesions.[589] Studies have supported a deficiency of brain iron in RLS[508,509,519] that might influence dopamine function,[507,590] perhaps through decreased synaptic strength.[511] Animal models of iron-deficient mice demonstrate increased activity[591] that can occur in the period before the sleep period, similar to RLS.[592] In this model of RLS causation,[507] iron deficiency is expected to act through a dysregulation of brain dopamine function, perhaps related to altered amplitude of circadian dopamine variation.[593]

Familial Aggregation and Genetics in RLS. A striking finding in series of RLS cases is the high proportion of patients with family members who also have RLS.[540,594–596] One obvious explanation would be that the disorder is under a large degree of genetic control. The existence of numerous large families with affected members of both genders and presumed inheritance routes through both males and females led to an early idea that there might be a major dominant gene causing much of idiopathic RLS.[597] Two segregation analyses have supported this conclusion, although in one a major gene model worked only in families with younger onset RLS.[598] The second study fit a major gene model to all RLS families and noted that age of onset was itself under both genetic and environmental control.[599] Two studies suggested that RLS might show progression (earlier onset in succeeding generations), a finding typical of trinucleotide repeats disorders such as HD.[597,600,601] However, no repeat abnormalities were found in RLS,[602,603] and CAG repeats in disorders characterized by them do not influence RLS.[603] Three twin studies have suggested an elevated risk to monozygotic co-twins of affected individuals.[601,604,605] The first two studies suffered from major methodologic limitations.[601,604] The first study[604]

was restricted to monozygotic twins; the probands consisted of twins (10 female, 2 male) who were in treatment or volunteered from a patient organization; co-twins were interviewed by an RLS expert to determine status. A very high case concordance was noted (83%; 10 of 12 pairs), but there was considerable variability in the clinical presentations of co-twins. This study was suitably criticized for its biased sampling[606] and lack of a comparison sample of dizygotic twins. A second study was done on a preexisting twin registry of female twin pairs but used rather general questions for postulating RLS.[601] Because of the nonspecificity of these questions, it is unclear that these results give any clear information about the true heritability of RLS. The third study used another preexisting twin sample, used accurate diagnoses, and found modest evidence for a greater concordance in monozygotic twins.

The search for genetic determinants of RLS has been limited by two factors. First, the risk to first-degree relatives of patients has only been modest, on the order of three- to sevenfold.[498,500] Second, the frequency of RLS (4–10% of adults) is quite high for a genetic disorder. One initial approach to finding genetic deterimants, searching for candidate genes active in the dopamine and iron pathways presumed to be involved in RLS,[607,608] did not reveal specific mutations contributing to RLS (one exception was the association of a fast metabolizer allele of monoamine oxidase A with RLS in women[609]). A second approach to finding genetic determinants for RLS relied largely on linkage analyses conducted on large families. This approach did find suspect regions of the genome. As of now, five loci have been reported as linked to RLS susceptibility (but two additional loci have been presented in abstract form or as personal communications). One linkage was found in a French-Canadian population, using a recessive model (locus on 12q[610]); another in Italian families, using a dominant model (locus on 14q[611]); and the third in American families, using nonparametric linkage (locus on 9p[612]), confirmed in 2 of 15 families using a dominant model. Two other linkages have been reported on 20p (in a large French Canadian family using a dominant model)[613] and 2q (in an isolated Tirolean population).[614] However, it is clear that these linkages are only prominent in selected families and may be restricted to particular populations.[615] There have been some confirmations in different populations than those in which the loci were originally reported (12q,[616] 14q,[616,617] and 9p[618]). However, there remains an active question of how many loci contribute to idiopathic/familial RLS and how general is their effect. Intensive searches within the linkage regions were initially negative; a candidate gene in the 12q region coding for neurotensin, an endogenous opioid neurotransmitter, could not be linked to RLS risk.[619] More recently, a genetic variant has been found in 12q through a case-control association study that may play a role in RLS causation. Different variants in the neuronal nitric oxide synthase 1 gene (*NOS1*) in the linked region of chromosome 12q are associated with RLS.[620] This gene is active in the nitric oxide/arginine pathway that is involved in sensory processing and affects both dopamine and endogenous opioid transmission.

The more recent approach to finding genetic determinants has relied upon genome-wide association studies in case-control populations. Two groups have now reported significant associations in three genes[496,497]: *BTBD9* (6p), *MEIS1* (2p), and *MAP2K5/LBXCOR1* (15q). These genes do not have clearly known functions in adults, but are active during development, especially in formation of the limbs. These genes are expressed within the nervous system.[621] One group found that *BTBD9* was better linked to the presence of increased PLM than to the purely subjective symptoms of RLS,[497] underscoring the important connection between RLS and PLM. The group also found that serum ferritin, the best marker of body iron stores, was decreased in a dose-response fashion in patients with the RLS-PLM predisposing variant. Interestingly, all the variants are in intronic (noncoding) portions of the genes. It has been estimated that variants in these three genes can account for up to 80% of individuals with RLS. Differences within different populations in the frequency of the variants may explain ethnic or regional differences in RLS frequency.

Treatment of RLS and PLMD

A spectrum of treatment options, both nonpharmacologic (Table 28–10) and pharmacologic (Table 28–11), are available to adequately address the wide range in severity and frequency of RLS symptoms. Before embarking on a decision to treat RLS some general comments about treatment guidelines are warranted (Table 28–12). For the purpose of treatment guidelines, RLS patients can be classified (Table 28–13)[622,623] into mild (or intermittent), moderate, severe, and refractory (or intractable) depending on the intensity and frequency of symptoms, impairment of quality of life, and International Restless Legs Syndrome Study Group (IRLSSG)[624–626] or Johns

---

TABLE 28–10 Nonpharmacologic Treatment of Restless Legs Syndrome (RLS)

- Follow sleep hygiene measures (see Table 19–17 in Chapter 19).
- Consider discontinuing or reducing medications that can worsen RLS (see Table 28–9).
- Avoid substances that may trigger RLS (e.g., alcohol, smoking, caffeine-containing drinks).
- Exercise regularly at moderate intensity (avoid vigorous exercise, which may exacerbate RLS symptoms).
- Participate in mentally alerting activities (activities promoting alertness benefit RLS symptoms).
- Use counterstimulation measures (e.g., hot or cold showers, massage, getting up and walking).
- Participate in patient support groups.

TABLE 28–11 Pharmacologic Agents used in Restless Legs Syndrome

- Dopaminergic medications
  - Dopamine agonists: pramipexole (approved), ropinirole (approved), rotigotine patch, cabergoline
  - Levodopa combined with a decarboxylase inhibitor
- Anticonvulsants
  - Gabapentine and related drugs (most commonly used)
  - Others (e.g., valproic acid, lamotrigine, levetiracetam, topiramate, carbamazepine, oxcarbazepine)
- Opioids (mild, moderate, strong)
- Benzodiazepines (particularly clonazepam)
- Iron supplements (in those with low serum iron or ferritin below 50 ng/ml)

TABLE 28–12 General Treatment Guidelines for Restless Legs Syndrome (RLS)

- Does the patient have RLS?
  (This must be established first.)
- Does the patient have primary RLS or comorbid (secondary) RLS?
  (This distinction is important as the comorbid conditions must be identified and treated.)
- Whom to treat and when to treat?
  (It is important to determine if mild or intermittent symptoms without significant disability require drug treatment or nonpharmacologic measures are sufficient.)
- How to define severity?
  (This can be determined based on the IRLSSG or JHRLSS rating scale score [see Tables 28–14 and 28–15], effectiveness of daytime function, and overall clinical impression.)
- How to define end points in therapy?
  (Some examples are: elimination of RLS symptoms, reduction or elimination of leg jerks during sleep as obtained by history from bed partner or polysomnography study, a significant reduction of IRLSSG scale score, and quality-of-life improvement.)

TABLE 28–13 Classification of RLS for Treatment Purpose

Categories	Key Features
Mild (Intermittent) RLS	• Intermittent mild symptoms • Sometimes bothersome • Often predictable and situational • IRLSSG score of 1–10 (see Table 28–14)
Moderate RLS	• Symptoms (significantly bothersome) occurring at least twice a week interfering with quality of life • IRLSSG score of 11–20
Moderately Severe RLS	• Same as moderate RLS symptoms • IRLSSG score of 21–30
Severe RLS	• Significant and intense symptoms occurring daily interfering with daytime function and quality of life • IRLSSG score of 31–40
Refractory or Intractable RLS	• Severe daily symptoms despite adequate doses of dopaminergic medication • Severe sleep disturbance • Impairment of quality of life and severely impaired daytime function • IRLSSG score of 40

IRLSSG, International Restless Legs Syndrome Study Group; RLS, restless legs syndrome.
Modified and adapted from Hening et al.[622] and Silber et al.[623]

TABLE 28–14 International Restless Legs Syndrome Study Group (IRLSSG) Rating Scale

The subject is asked, "*In the past week...*"

1. Overall, how would you rate the RLS discomfort in your legs and arms?
   4—Very severe
   3—Severe
   2—Moderate
   1—Mild
   0—None
2. Overall, how would you rate the need to move around because of your RLS symptoms?
   4—Very severe
   3—Severe
   2—Moderate
   1—Mild
   0—None
3. Overall, how much relief of your RLS arm or leg discomfort did you get from moving around?
   4—No relief
   3—Mild relief
   2—Moderate relief
   1—Either complete or almost complete relief
   0—No RLS symptoms to be relieved
4. How severe was your sleep disturbance due to your RLS symptoms?
   4—Very severe
   3—Severe
   2—Moderate
   1—Mild
   0—None
5. How severe was your tiredness or sleepiness during the day due to your RLS symptoms?
   4—Very severe
   3—Severe
   2—Moderate
   1—Mild
   0—None
6. How severe was your RLS as a whole?
   4—Very severe
   3—Severe

   2—Moderate
   1—Mild
   0—None
7. How often did you experience RLS symptoms?
   4—Very often (6–7 days in 1 week)
   3—Often (4–5 days in 1 week)
   2—Sometimes (2–3 days in 1 week)
   1—Occasionally (1 day in 1 week)
   0—Never
8. When you had RLS symptoms, how severe were they on average?
   4—Very severe (8 hours or more per 24 hours)
   3—Severe (3–8 hours per 24 hours)
   2—Moderate (1–3 hours per 24 hours)
   1—Mild (less than 1 hour per 24 hours)
   0—None
9. Overall, how severe was the impact of your RLS symptoms on your ability to carry out your daily affairs—for example, carrying out a satisfactory family, home, social, school, or work life?
   4—Very severe
   3—Severe
   2—Moderate
   1—Mild
   0—None
10. How severe was your mood disturbance due to your RLS symptoms—for example, angry, depressed, sad, anxious, or irritable?
    4—Very severe
    3—Severe
    2—Moderate
    1—Mild
    0—None

Each question is scored from 0 for no problem or RLS symptoms to 4 for very severe. As a rough guide, the overall score can be divided into different levels of severity:

0	No RLS
1–10	Mild RLS
11–20	Moderate RLS
21–30	Severe RLS
31–40	Very severe RLS

Adapted from Walters et al.,[624] Allen et al.,[625] and Abetz et al.[626]

Hopkins Restless Legs Severity Scale[627] rating scale score (Tables 28–14 and 28–15).

Important pharmacologic treatment options for RLS (see Table 28–11) include the dopaminergic agents, the anticonvulsants (particularly gabapentin), the opioids, and the sedative-hypnotics. Table 28–16 lists some

TABLE 28–15 Johns Hopkins Restless Legs Syndrome Rating Scale (JHRLSS)*

No restless legs syndrome (RLS)	0
Less than almost daily	0.5
Symptoms at bedtime or during sleep	1
Symptoms begin after 6:00 PM but before bedtime	2
Symptoms begin before 6:00 PM	3
Symptoms begin before noon	4

*Before applying, a diagnosis of RLS must be made and the rating applied strictly to RLS symptoms.
Reproduced with permission from Allen RP, Earley CJ. Validation of the Johns Hopkins restless legs severity scale. Sleep Med 2001;2:239.

general principles of pharmacotherapy for RLS. The first review and standards for RLS treatment were published in 1999 by the AASM.[628,629] They established that clinicians managing RLS should be able to make an accurate diagnosis, understand primary and secondary RLS and the comorbidities of RLS, and follow patients at appropriate intervals to adjust treatment as needed. Subsequent published evidentiary reviews include an update of the AASM standards restricted to dopaminergics[630] and a review by the European Federation of Neurological Societies.[631] An evidentiary review sponsored by the Movement Disorder Society with participation by the World Association of Sleep Medicine and the IRLSSG has been published, covering articles at least electronically published by the end of 2006.[632] A management paradigm was published in 2004 by the Medical Advisory Board of the RLS Foundation.[623] While somewhat out of date, it provides a workable scheme for approaching the diagnosis of different classes of RLS patients (intermittent, daily,

TABLE 28–16 Principles of Pharmacotherapy for Restless Legs Syndrome

- Individualize the therapy.
- Start with monotherapy rather than polytherapy.
- Begin with a very small dose, and gradually increase every 3–5 days to an optimal or maximal tolerable dose.
- Try monotherapy even in an apparently severe case using small to medium dose (a surprising number of such patients will respond satisfactorily).
- Try to convert patients on polytherapy (placed on treatment before referral to you) to monotherapy if possible (it is possible to do so in many such patients).
- Try to reduce the dose or eliminate some medications if patients complain of undesirable side effects from multidrug treatment.
- Perform regular follow-up to monitor for side effects, progression of the disease, augmentation, tolerance, and rebound.

TABLE 28–17 NIH Workshop Diagnostic Criteria for RLS Augmentation

RLS augmentation can be diagnosed if either of the following two criteria are met:
- Criterion 1: RLS symptoms occur at least 2 hours earlier than was typical during the initial course of beneficial stable treatment.
- Criterion 2: Two or more of the following key features of RLS augmentation are present:
  - An increased overall intensity of the urge to move or sensations is temporally related to an increase in the daily medication dosage, or a decreased overall intensity of the urge to move or sensations is temporally related to a decrease in the daily medication dosage.
  - The latency to RLS symptoms at rest is shorter than the latency either during initial therapeutic response or before treatment was instituted.
  - The urge to move or sensations are extended to previously unaffected limbs or body parts.
  - The duration of treatment effect is shorter than the duration during initial therapeutic response.
  - Periodic limb movements while awake occur for the first time or are worse than either during initial therapeutic response or before treatment was instituted.

In addition to meeting one of these two criteria, the diagnosis requires both of the following:
- Augmented symptoms meeting these criteria are present for at least 1 week for a minimum of 5 days.
- No other medical, psychiatric, behavioral, or pharmacologic factors explain the exacerbation of the patient's RLS and the augmented symptoms meeting these criteria.

NIH, National Institutes of Health; RLS, restless legs syndrome.
Adapted from Allen RP, Picchietti D, Hening WA, et al. Restless legs syndrome: diagnostic criteria, special considerations, and epidemiology. A report from the Restless Legs Syndrome Diagnosis and Epidemiology Workshop at the National Institutes of Health. Sleep Med 2003;4:101.

refractory). The basic scheme includes as-needed medication for infrequent RLS, dopamine agonists as first choice for daily RLS, and an array of strategies (switching agents, trying nondopaminergics, combination treatment, strong opioid agents) for refractory patients who fail first-line treatments. These reviews and the algorithm provide an easy route into the RLS therapeutic literature.

Pharmacologic Treatment of RLS.

Levodopa. Akpinar[633] and Montplaisir et al.[634] first reported a profound response of RLS symptoms to small doses of levodopa. Subsequent studies have consistently found that levodopa and the dopamine agonists have high response rates. They quite reliably ameliorate RLS symptoms, decrease PLM, and improve sleep.[628,635] Unfortunately, after the initial success, a prominent side effect was noted with levodopa therapy in many RLS patients, termed *augmentation.*[286] Augmentation is an iatrogenic increase in the severity of RLS[488]; its primary manifestation is the progression of symptoms earlier in the day. Initially defined at the NIH RLS consensus conference,[488] it has subsequently been redefined according to new standards (Tables 28–17 and 28–18).[636] Based on a study of levodopa patients in which 60% developed augmentation, a validated severity questionnaire has been developed.[637] A diagnostic interview for augmentation has been devised and is under development (Diego Garcia-Borreguero, personal communication, *dgb@iis.es*).

Although many patients used levodopa successfully for years, levodopa augmentation rates have been reported to occur in as high as 80% of RLS patients, with 50% of them requiring a change in medication.[286] Augmentation appears to occur more often at higher doses of levodopa (>200 mg on a daily basis). Dopamine agonists have lower rates of augmentation (20–30%)[638,639] and may provide sustained relief throughout the night, and for this reason they are now usually the first line of therapy for RLS patients with daily symptoms.[623,630] Augmentation is more common with levodopa and less commonly occurs with dopaminergic agonists, probably due to their longer half-life. Augmentation should be differentiated from natural progression of RLS, tolerance, rebound, and comorbid conditions exacerbating RLS (e.g., medications, sleep deprivation, iron deficiency, alcohol use). Augmentation has characteristic symptoms (see Tables 28–17 and 28–18) and generally manifests within 2 years of drug treatment, whereas natural progression of RLS generally is manifested by worsening of symptoms 2.5 years after onset of significant symptoms. An increasing dose requirement for relief of increasingly intense symptoms may suggest tolerance, but tolerance does not cause an earlier onset of symptoms. Rebound is an end-of-dose effect and is easy to differentiate from augmentation based on diagnostic criteria (see Tables 28–17 and 28–18). The cause of augmentation remains undetermined, but suggested theories include down-regulation of dopamine receptors (similar to that suggested for tolerance; in fact, some investigators[639] think augmentation goes through a stage of tolerance), with hyperstimulation of D_1 more than D_2 receptors.[640] Iron deficiency may be a predisposing factor for augmentation by reducing dopamine transporter function.[640] Another factor predisposing to augmentation is a positive family history.

The treatment of augmentation could be challenging and depends on the intensity and timing of symptoms. The following are some suggested strategies (therapy should be individualized):

TABLE 28–18 WASM–IRLSSG–Max Planck Institute Diagnostic Criteria for Augmentation

In addition to A, either B or C (or both) need to be satisfied (i.e., A+B, A+C, or A+B+C)

A. Basic features (all of which need to be met)
- The increase in symptom severity is experienced on 5 of 7 days during the previous week.
- The increase in symptom severity is not accounted for by other factors, such as a change in medical status, lifestyle, or the natural progression of the disorder.
- It is assumed that there has been a prior positive response to treatment.

B. Persisting (although not immediate) paradoxical response to treatment
- RLS symptom severity increases some time after a dose increase and improves some time after a dose decrease.

C. Earlier onset of symptoms
- An earlier onset by at least 4 hours *or*
- An earlier onset (between 2 and 4 hours) occurs with one of the following compared with symptom status before treatment:
  - Shorter latency to symptoms when at rest
  - Extension of symptoms to other body parts
  - Greater intensity of symptoms or increase in periodic limb movements if measure by polysomnography or the suggested immobilization test
  - Shorter duration of relief from treatment

Reproduced with permission from Garcia-Borreguero D, Allen RP, Kohnen R, et al. Diagnostic standards for dopaminergic augmentation of restless legs syndrome: report from a World Association of Sleep Medicine–International Restless Legs Syndrome Study Group consensus conference at the Max Planck Institute. Sleep Med 2007;8:520.

- If augmentation occurs after levodopa, slowly taper off levodopa and add a dopamine agonist in gradually increasing doses.
- Abruptly discontinue levodopa and add a medium- to high-potency opioid for a few weeks and use a dopamine agonist, gradually increasing the doses.
- Switch to a different class of medication (e.g., from dopaminergics to opioids, anticonvulsants, or a combination) or rotation of drugs as suggested for refractory RLS (see Table 28–19 later).

Expert centers report that augmentation after dopamine agonists can often be managed without withdrawing the medication,[638,639] but the full extent of augmentation with agonists, the time course of development, and the degree of clinical significance remain to be determined in suitably monitored long-term studies.[636]

Dopaminergic Agents. Dosing of dopaminergic agents for RLS differs from the typical dosing schedule in PD. Many RLS patients can be successfully managed with low doses given 2 hours before symptom onset. Generally, a single dose taken at night can benefit those with late evening and bedtime symptoms, while more severe patients with significant evening symptoms can take one dose in the early evening and a second before bedtime. For the patient who develops a rapid escalation in RLS severity, with increasing medication requirements in the first 2 years of therapy, augmentation should be considered; if

TABLE 28–19 Treatment Strategies for Mild, Moderate, Severe, and Refractory or Intractable Restless Legs Syndrome (RLS)

Categories	Treatment Strategies
Mild or Intermittent RLS	- Nonpharmacologic measures (NP) plus gabapentin initially if needed - If failed, pramipexole or ropinirole
Moderate to Moderately Severe RLS	- NP plus pramipexole or ropinirole - If needed, add clonazepam or mild- to moderate-potency opioids
Severe RLS	- NP plus pramipexole or ropinirole with increasing dose - If needed, add gabapentin or medium- to high-potency opioids or clonazepam - Multiple doses, including daytime medication, may be needed
Refractory or Intractable RLS	- Multiple doses (e.g., evening, bedtime, middle of night, and if needed during daytime) - Polytherapy with combination of 2, 3, or 4 drugs from different classes - High-potency opioids - Drug holidays or rotation among 2 or 3 drugs - Consider augmentation, tolerance, comorbid conditions (including iron deficiency or low serum ferritin)

suspected, the patient should be changed to another dopaminergic agent or another class of agents. Because of reports of fibrosis and valvulopathy with ergot-derived agonists (pergolide, bromocriptine, cabergoline),[641,642] non–ergot-derived agonists are currently more recommended. Ropinirole and pramipexole have been approved for treatment of RLS after several large multicenter studies[643 647]; they have also been shown to markedly decrease PLMS in RLS.[645,648] Rotigotine, another non–ergot-derived agonist that is delivered through a patch, has been approved for PD and is being studied for use in RLS.[649,650] Unlike oral agents, the transdermal route allows for continuous delivery over 24 hours and sustains a near-constant blood level. However, rotigotine patches have been recalled because of a problem with local crystallization. It is considered likely that longer half-life agents such as cabergoline,[651] which do not have more rapid changes in blood level, may result in less augmentation. Other agonists and formulations are likely to follow in the near future.

Anticonvulsants. Among the anticonvulsants, gabapentin has been demonstrated effective in a double-blind, placebo-controlled trial that used the IRLSSG criteria for RLS and reported both PLMS reduction as well as reduced severity in RLS symptoms.[652] Carbamezapine had earlier studies demonstrating successful use in RLS. However, clinical experience has not demonstrated as good a response as that seen with gabapentin. Gabapentin can also be taken as a single nighttime dose, but for evening symptoms, twice-daily dosing (noon or afternoon and night) results in better coverage. The dosage of gabapentin varies, but in the double-blind trial the mean dose for the study was 1855 mg/day divided in two doses.[652] There are only limited case reports or small series with other anticonvulsants, such as lamotrigine, pregabalin, and topirimate; thus these are usually tried only in patients who are unable to tolerate other agents. A gabapentin prodrug[653] has also been evaluated in one large multicenter clinical trial for RLS with favorable results.[653a]

Opiates. Because of the success of dopaminergic agents and gabapentin, opiates are generally reserved for treatment of refractory RLS. Opiates have been documented to be effective in RLS.[654,655] Because of individual variation in response to the different classes of opiates, it is often worthwhile trying more than one agent. Longer acting medications such as methadone often provide relief for some of the most severely affected patients, including those who have failed dopaminergic therapy. One opioid agent, tramadol, which also has serotoninergic properties, has been reported to cause augmentation.[656,657]

Sedative-Hypnotics. Despite the early use of benzodiazepines for treating RLS and PLMD, the sedative-hypnotic agents do not have reliable effectiveness in eliminating RLS sensations or eliminating PLMS. They are best reserved for mild cases with primary sleep disruptions or as adjunctive therapy.

Pharmacologic Treatment of Mild Intermittent RLS.
For those patients with mild intermittent symptoms, a hypnotic agent may help induce sleep; alternative treatments for these patients include as-needed levodopa or an opioid. For aggravating situations such as long car rides, regular-strength levodopa has the benefit of having a more rapid onset of action, making it suitable for as-needed dosing. Occasional use at low doses will probably avoid the problem of augmentation. Dopamine agonists may also have a role in treating intermittent RLS.[658–660] Table 28–19 outlines treatment strategies for mild, moderate, severe, and refractory RLS.

Pharmacologic Treatment of PLMD.
Treatment of PLMD starts with dopamine agents to gauge if the PLMS are dopamine-responsive as in RLS. Low-dose L-dopa may be useful, or low doses of dopamine agonists. Otherwise a variety of medications are tried, especially gabapentin and clonazepam. Opioids are probably not helpful. Clonazepam was demonstrated to improve sleep in earlier studies,[628] but because recent studies have not been done, it cannot be known whether these patients had RLS or some other undetected sleep disorder. In cases of daytime somnolence, it is sometimes advisable to target the somnolence itself with such stimulant medications as modafinil.[661]

Summary

RLS is the most common neurologic movement disorder and is often misdiagnosed, underdiagnosed, under-recognized, and mistreated or undertreated. RLS should be strongly considered in any subject complaining of leg discomfort or excessive restlessness of the legs while lying in bed in the evening and of having difficulty falling asleep or maintaining sleep or of nonrestorative sleep. The vast majority of patients get relief from treatment with dopamine agonists.

Sleep-Related Bruxism

Bruxism or teeth grinding can interrupt sleep and cause significant dental wear; this nocturnal bruxism is clearly differentiated from daytime bruxism. Tooth grinding itself is not abnormal; what characterizes abnormal sleep bruxism is the frequency and intensity of grinding.[662] While bruxism declines in prevalence with age,[489] it does cause dental problems for many adults. Bruxers may also have increased movements during sleep in general, which could suggest an underlying motor hyperactivity.[663] Bruxism is associated with arousals and autonomic activation during sleep,[664,665] which may serve as precipitating events[666]; bruxism also occurs with swallowing during sleep, which may be more common in the supine position.[667]

Bruxism may need to be distinguished from other dyskinetic movements that involve the jaws, including oromandibular dystonia and idiopathic myoclonus in the oromandibular region during sleep.[668–670] Idiopathic myoclonus in the oromandibular region during sleep is an apparently isolated, nonepileptic condition that occurs predominantly in stages 1 and 2 NREM sleep.[668] It consists of isolated or short runs of shocklike jaw movements with brief EMG bursts.

Bruxism has been treated with various modalities: dopaminergic agents,[671] anticonvulsants,[672] and botulinum toxin injections.[673] Dental devices may also help,[667,674] but some studies suggest caution in their use.[675,676] However, a paradigm for treatment is not yet clear. SPECT studies show an asymmetry in D_2 dopamine receptor binding in bruxism patients at the level of the basal ganglia compared to controls, suggesting that dopaminergic cell dysfunction may play a role in the pathogenesis of bruxism.[677]

According to the new AASM manual for the scoring of sleep and associated events,[3,28] bruxism can be divided into brief (phasic) EMG elevations of 0.25–2 seconds and sustained (tonic) EMG elevations of >2 seconds. (An alternate term for the phasic type of bruxism is *rhythmic masticatory muscle activity.*[28]) These EMG elevations must be at least twice the amplitude of the background EMG. Phasic bruxism events must occur in a sequence of 3 or more, and this sequence can be said to comprise a bruxism episode. At least 3 seconds of stable EMG must be present before a new episode of bruxism can be scored. Bruxism can be reliably scored by audiotape in combination with PSG by a minimum of 2 audible tooth-grinding episodes/night of PSG in the absence of epilepsy. In addition to chin EMG, additional masseter electrodes may be placed at the discretion of the investigator or clinician for optimal detection of bruxism.

Sleep-Related Rhythmic Movement Disorder

Rhythmic movement disorder (also known variably as jactatio capitis nocturna, head banging, or body rocking) may need to be distinguished from tremor or segmental myoclonias, as well as RBD or nocturnal seizures. While rhythmic movement disorder is most common in prepubertal children, there are older children[678] and also adults[82,679-684] who will show persistent or emergent rhythmic movement. Rhythmic movement disorder can also cause significant injury.[685] Most movements occur at sleep onset or in NREM sleep, but a rare case may show a REM predominance.[686,687] Bouts of movements may be related to a CAP.[688] Most older children with persistent disorder are usually suffering from organic brain dysfunction.

Few studies have looked into treatment of rhythmic movement disorder. Since most childhood cases are self-limited, there may be no need. Clonazepam has been reported to be effective.[680] Treatment with sleep restriction and initial sedative-hypnotics was suggested to be beneficial in a small series.[689]

According to the ICSD-2,[2] the term *sleep-related rhythmic movement disorder* is reserved for patients in whom the movements have some biological consequence such as interference with normal sleep, significant impairment in daytime function, or self-inflicted bodily injury that requires medical treatment (or would result in injury if preventable measures were not used). In the absence of any of these biological consequences, the term *sleep-related rhythmic movements* is used but the word "disorder" is not appended.[2] According to the AASM manual,[3,28] the minimal frequency for scoring rhythmic movements is 0.5 Hz and the maximum frequency for scoring rhythmic movements is 2.0 Hz. The minimum number of individual movements to make a cluster of rhythmic movements is 4 movements, and the minimum amplitude of an individual rhythmic burst must be at least two times the background EMG activity.[28]

Isolated Symptoms, Apparently Normal Variants, and Unresolved Issues

These conditions include a variety of nocturnal phenomena whose morbidity is unclear or that, though unusual, might best be considered normal variants, such as small sharp spikes on an EEG. Until their status becomes clearer, they are consigned to this general wastebasket category.

Benign Sleep Myoclonus of Infancy

Formerly known as benign neonatal sleep myoclonus, this condition is a transient, sometimes familial condition that begins soon after birth and resolves within months.[690-692] The reason for the change in terminology is that it is now appreciated that the disorder may extend beyond the neonatal period up to 6 months of age. Although not well known, this condition may not be rare.[693] The myoclonic jerks are brief, asynchronous, and repetitive, involving primarily the distal limbs (especially the arms but also the trunk); the jerks are often generalized. The jerks occur during all stages of sleep, with most occurring in NREM sleep, and typically do not arouse or wake the infant[694,695]; waking the child will cause them to cease promptly. The movements do not occur continually in sleep and, when not present in sleep, they may be precipitated by rocking the infant.[696] The movements can also be evoked by gentle restraint during sleep.[695] The pathophysiology of this disorder is unknown. It is not typically associated with other nervous system disease and the EEG is not epileptogenic, distinguishing this condition from a seizure disorder,[697,698] although it can sometimes suggest status epilepticus.[699] The lack of other features can distinguish it from the sleep myoclonus seen in hyperekplexia.[700,701] It may be an exaggeration of the normally greater sleep-related movements in infants.[702]

Hypnagogic Foot Tremor and Alternating Leg Muscle Activation During Sleep

These movements were incidental discoveries in the course of serial investigation of unusual phenomena found in sleep studies. Hypnagogic foot tremor was first described by Broughton[56] and found in 7.5% of PSGs in a later study.[703] Alternating leg muscle activation (ALMA) was first described by Chervin's group, found in just over 1% of reviewed PSGs[704]; most of those showing the phenomenon were taking antidepressants. Both types of movements occur in series that last for a few up to many seconds, with movements at a frequency between 0.3 and 4 Hz. The duration of an individual movement varies between 100 and 1000 msec.[28] At least 4 movements must be present in a row to make the diagnosis. Both occur during lighter sleep and in transitional states into and out of sleep. ALMA requires the presence of alternating activity and has been suggested to be an equivalent of a locomotor rhythm.[38] Diagnosis of either requires a PSG recording. Because variant patterns are reported in each, there is at least some plausible degree of overlap, and further investigation may be required to ascertain whether they are distinct or merely variant conditions. It has also been suggested that both may be variants of rhythmic movement disorder. Convincing evidence of any definite clinical consequence of these movements is yet to be presented.

In one patient, pramipexole reduced ALMA and improved sleep,[38] together with a reduction of an associated CAP.

Propriospinal Myoclonus at Sleep Onset

Propriospinal myoclonus is a form of suprasegmental myoclonus in which the excitatory impulses are believed to travel through relatively slow-conducting intersegmental propriospinal pathways.[705–707] The myoclonic movements typically involve the trunk with possible extension into the limbs. In a newly described form of this myoclonus, the myoclonic jerks are only evident during relaxation or recumbency,[54,707–710] especially when the patient is drowsy. Unlike PLM, the movements are relatively easily abolished by even light sleep. They may, however, produce a substantial difficulty with sleep induction and can therefore be a cause of significant insomnia. Some cases have been associated with RLS.[710]

One case of propriospinal myoclonus that occurred during sleep was reported after a thoracic spine fracture that progressed to "myoclonic status" and respiratory failure.[711] An important consideration in the differential diagnosis of propriospinal myoclonus at sleep onset are the more myoclonic forms of PLMW seen while sitting or lying in patients with RLS.[712]

Excessive Fragmentary Myoclonus in NREM Sleep

Excessive fragmentary myoclonus (EFM) in NREM sleep is also considered a variant PSG finding that may not generally cause any sleep problems.[2,28] If movements are present at all, they are small movements involving the corners of the mouth or small movements of the fingers or toes. In some cases no movement across a joint space occurs and the movements may resemble fasciculations, mere dimplings seen over the muscle associated with very brief EMG potentials (<50 msec). If movements across large joint spaces occur, such as at the hips or knees, EFM should not be considered. The movements occur primarily during the light stages of NREM sleep,[66] although they may occur in REM.[713] In EFM, the EMG pattern resembles the normal phasic twitches seen in REM sleep except they are more evenly spread throughout an individual epoch and not clustered as are phasic REM twitches. They are least common in SWS.[713] The associated EMG shows brief bursts (typically <150 msec) of variable amplitude.

EFM may be associated with a variety of sleep disorders or occur in isolation.[66,714] This condition may be another in which inadequate inhibitory drive fails to block descending activation from higher centers, or it may represent a condition of excessive activation of higher centers during sleep. The condition has been found in degenerative developmental diseases (Niemann-Pick disease[715]) and as a consequence of brain stem lesions.[44] Convincing evidence is yet to be presented that EFM has any biological consequence. The disorder is usually detected as an incidental finding on PSG. EFM may sometimes be seen in wakefulness. To be diagnosed as having EFM, a patient must have at least 20 minutes of NREM sleep recorded with the characteristic EMG pattern present, and at least 5 EMG potentials per minute must be recorded.[28]

Sleep Disorders Associated with Conditions Classifiable Elsewhere

Fatal Familial Insomnia (see also Chapter 29)

Fatal familial insomnia (FFI)[716,717] is a prion disorder that involves progressive insomnia with derangement of sleep states,[718] loss of circadian rhythm and associated endocrine cycles,[719,720] autonomic abnormalities,[721] and abnormal motor signs, especially ataxia (loss of coordination) and myoclonus.[722] The prominence of different features and the order of their appearance may vary,[723] even within the same family.[724,725] While onset in middle age (fifth, sixth, or seventh decade) is common, some younger onset cases have been described.[726]

FFI is not classified as a specific sleep disorder in the current classification.[2] In some patients, the motor symptoms are the first to be noted.[716] The condition appears to be inherited in an autosomal dominant pattern (with parent-to–children of both sexes transmission).[725] Genetic linkage studies have established that the disease is related to a mutation in the prion protein that also causes Creutzfeldt-Jakob disease (CJD), a rapidly progressive dementia often accompanied by myoclonus. Indeed, the mutation in FFI is identical to that of one familial form of CJD (asparagine substituted for aspartic acid at locus 178 of the prion protein).[727] Familial manifestation as either FFI or CJD apparently depends on which common polymorphism occurs in the mutant allele at locus 129: methionine results in FFI while valine yields CJD,[725] although more recent studies suggest this distinction may not be as clear cut as first proposed.[728]

One study indicates that, compared to other prion diseases, the degeneration seen with FFI is more selective.[729] The primary pathology is a degeneration of the thalamic nuclei.[730] In the presymptomatic state, thalamic hypometabolism associated with loss of sleep spindles (sigma rhythm)—signs of FFI—may occur, anticipating symptoms by 12 or more months,[731] although these changes are not generally discovered until disease onset. The clinical picture of FFI—inability to sleep consistently associated with motor and sympathetic overactivation due to dysfunction of the sleep generation mechanisms—has been called "agrypnia excitata,"[732] This picture is also found in Morvan's chorea[733] and delirium tremens.[734]

While the disorder appears to be inexorably fatal, one report has suggested some relief from insomnia may be obtained with γ-hydroxybutyrate.[735]

Nocturnal Paroxysmal Dystonia and Related Conditions

Nocturnal paroxysmal dystonia (NPD) was first described by Lugaresi's group as a condition that might be considered analogous to diurnal paroxysmal movement disorders.[736,737] Attacks of NPD with short duration (seconds to minutes) together with two other conditions, paroxysmal arousals[738,739] and episodic nocturnal wanderings,[740–742] were later found to represent variant forms of frontal lobe epilepsy[743] (see Chapter 30). They share the main features of sudden arousals or awakenings from NREM sleep and dyskinetic or semipurposeful movements and vocalizations.

It is now clear that most of the patients who fit the diagnosis of NPD have a form of sleep-activated focal epilepsy.[739,741,743–747] Most may be considered to have nocturnal frontal lobe epilepsy (NFLE),[743] which in many cases is inherited as an autosomal dominant trait.[748] Others may have a temporal focus.[749] Consistent with an epileptic etiology, there is an increased prevalence of clinical seizures in patients, there are interictal EEG abnormalities, and many patients respond to anticonvulsants (especially carbamazepine). Meierkord and colleagues demonstrated that the episodes of NPD overlap substantially in character with nocturnal attacks of patients with an established diagnosis of epilepsy.[745] It is also possible that there is some overlap in the pathophysiology of epileptic motor attacks and nonepileptic dystonia. Both are largely dependent on motor tracts descending from the cortex to cause abnormal muscle activation and, in certain conditions, there may be a common basis (e.g., deSaint-Martin et al.[750]).

The characteristically brief attacks associated with epileptic NPD begin with arousal, including an abrupt autonomic activation that can include substantial tachycardia, followed by dystonic choreoathetoid or ballismic movements and large-scale semipurposeful movements of all limbs. Vocalizations are common. The attacks are quite diverse if considered between patients, but appear to be stereotyped in a single patient. Attacks last about a minute (range 15 seconds to 2 minutes for typical attacks) and may be vaguely remembered. Neither tongue biting nor urinary incontinence is common. In addition, it is not uncommon for there to be little or no postictal confusion, which is one of the reasons that it was not appreciated early on that at least the brief attacks are a form of epilepsy. In some patients, the attacks are decidedly unilateral.[751] Other patients have been described with paroxysmal dystonic movements both during the day and night, with both types of attacks thought to be epileptic.[750] Paroxysmal arousals[739] are brief attacks lasting several seconds in which patients awaken abruptly from NREM sleep, perhaps with a start or cry, and have fleeting dyskinetic movements, then fall back to sleep. Episodic nocturnal wanderings[741,752] are attacks of sudden motor activity, including violent ambulation, loud vocalizations, and a variety of forceful gestures that can cause significant injury. The attacks commonly occur in stage 2 NREM sleep. Recent studies have suggested that the attacks may be associated with unstable sleep in a CAP.[753] Patients may also have disturbed sleep and daytime sequelae.

However, there may still remain a residual group of disorders that may not be of epileptic origin. In the original description, two cases had longer duration (2 to 50 minutes) attacks, with no epileptic associations.[736] In one case, a patient afflicted with such attacks for 20 years developed HD. There are a number of more recently described disorders of at least uncertain etiology. Lugaresi's group described a periodic form of NPD[754] that recurs every 30 seconds to 2 minutes with usually quite brief attacks (2–13 seconds in duration) and associated arousals that they called "atypical periodic movements in sleep." While showing overlap with the short-lasting NPD, this condition was unresponsive to seizure medications, even though one patient in the original series had a vascular orbital frontal tumor on computed tomography and spikes on depth recording. Other such disorders include dystonic attacks provoked both by sleep and by exercise,[755] apnea-associated paroxysmal dyskinetic movements,[756] and post-traumatic paroxysmal nocturnal hemidystonia.[757]

NPD events must be studied (best with video-PSG and multichannel EEG) to determine whether they are consistent with epilepsy.[758] They also must be distinguished from other eruptive motor events of sleep such as PLMS, RBD, nightmares, sleep terrors, and other parasomnias. A recently developed scale may help in the differentiation.[759] In the absence of clear-cut evidence for an epileptic focus, the main distinction between NPD and RBD often hinges on the clear association of the latter with REM and the response of NPD to anticonvulsants.

While treatment of the epilepsy-like attacks with anticonvulsants, especially carbamazepine, is usually successful, treatment of the various nonepileptic attacks of NPD remains uncertain. A report indicates that one of the newer anticonvulsants, topiramate, may also benefit most patients with NFLE.[760] Some patients with NFLE will remain refractory to medical treatment, and surgery may be needed to reduce seizures and improve sleep.[761]

METHODS FOR STUDYING SLEEP-RELATED MOVEMENTS

Standard sleep studies have been held to be of established worth in evaluating motor disturbances of sleep.[762] A standard PSG, with at least one EMG lead for the legs, provides a fair amount of information about motor disturbances. This should be supplemented by technician observations, wherever feasible, to explain motor events on the record. Where motor disturbances are the primary concern and seizures are in the differential diagnosis, it is helpful to perform video-PSG.[233,763] In an optimal setup, this may include multiple EEG channels, as for a regular EEG study (8–12 channels in a montage that can span the head and provide information about frontal and temporal activity), split-screen recording, and a facility for playing back the EEG record at the conventional daytime paper speed of 30 mm/sec.

The following sections make a number of suggestions about the use of different modalities for studying motor phenomena in sleep, then comment upon alternate schemes from the regular PSG for assessing sleep-related motor disturbances. Polysomnography, together with the MSLT, has been accepted as having established value for studies of PLMD as well as movements that can provoke violence in sleep (which includes RBD, seizures, somnambulism, and related conditions).[456,762,764,765] However, in sleep problems associated with diurnal movement disorders, a broad range of sleep problems may be under consideration and attention directed to them.[766]

Polysomnography

In deciding how to proceed with PSG, it is important to think about what conditions are being studied. Since the differential diagnosis of unknown motor disorders of sleep is relatively broad, it is usually important to monitor breathing as well as to make extensive EEG and EMG recordings. Accurate technician observation and videotaping may be extremely helpful in conducting studies that yield accurate diagnoses. Polysomnography also offers the chance to do close analysis of a wide variety of sleep events, including arousals that can disrupt sleep and reduce its quality.[767] Respiratory monitoring is a regular component of PSG and may be important to detect sleep-related breathing disorders associated with diurnal movement disorders.[766] Current standards for respiratory monitoring include abdominal and chest belts to measure effort together with airflow or nasal pressure measures to establish air movement and resistance.

EEG Montages

The standard sleep study may use only two EEG leads: a central lead (C3-A2 or C4-A1) together with an occipital lead (O1, O2, or Oz linked to an ear electrode). The AASM manual[28] recommends three EEG leads. However, in cases in which seizures may be in the differential, as in unknown motor disorders of sleep, more elaborate montages may be necessary to adequately rule out seizure activity (see Chapter 11). Special electrodes may be required.

EMG Recording

Standard sleep recording uses the chin EMG and leads on one or both legs for evaluation of possible PLMS. Where a specific motor complaint is noted that involves movement of other body parts (arms, trunk, abdomen, neck, or face), additional leads can be applied. Most laboratories perform EMGs with a standard EEG filter setting (bandpass of 5–70 Hz), but more artifact-free recordings can be obtained if a higher bandpass (e.g., 50–1500 Hz) is employed. These frequencies better match the frequency of actual muscle potentials. It is also useful to set the amplitude before the study so that a maximal voluntary contraction is near or slightly above the full pen excursion for a polygraphic recorder.

Videotaping

Videotape studies, especially video-PSG, can be extremely helpful in sorting out various abnormal movements or gaining some insight into their severity.[758,768] This can permit correlation of records of movement or EMG potentials with actual movements and allow the clinician, in some cases, to further distinguish the character of the movements. Split-screen studies, with polygraphic montages correlated directly with videotaping of the associated behavior, are especially helpful in this regard. Patients may also have different categories of movements that may be distinguished by the videotape record, but not the PSG.

In one study of the utility of video-PSG, Aldrich and Jahnke[763] found that, in 86 patients without known epilepsy who had reported abnormal motor activity in sleep, these studies provided useful diagnostic information for 52 patients. Fully 69% of those with prominent motor activity received such information. In 36 patients with known epilepsy, the studies provided useful diagnostic information about unclear motor phenomena in 28 (78%). The authors emphasized that ability to play back the record at slower speed, afforded by some digital EEG systems, improves the ability to discriminate seizure activity from other motor phenomena. Even without PSG monitoring, videotaping can give some insight into both normal and abnormal movements.[769] In recent years, video-PSG has become a standard technique for studying diverse movement abnormalities in sleep.[74,770–776]

Home-Based Polysomnography

A variety of systems are available for home or ambulatory monitoring of sleep, with capacity that can now include 16 or more channels. Most of the customary sleep monitors can be used in the ambulatory setting. Generally, technicians prepare the patient for study either in the laboratory or at home. The various channels are recorded on tape for later display and analysis with computer systems. The advantage of these systems is that they reduce the personnel required and can reduce cost. This may permit analysis of less frequent phenomena than those profitably studied in the laboratory or permit repeated studies to guide therapeutic options. In addition, the patient is studied under his or her normal conditions in the more relevant home environment. However, because these systems lack supervision, clear identification of abnormal events may not be feasible. Therefore, for diagnostic purposes, they may best be used as screening procedures, rather than a full substitute for laboratory-based PSG. Once a clear question is available—How well is the patient sleeping? How many typical events occur?—they may provide more exact answers.

Activity Monitoring

Activity monitoring or actigraphy is the technique of quantifying and recording movements. A value for movement is determined and assigned to a sample period that can range from a few milliseconds up to many hours. Actigraphy can be used for various purposes: to measure the degree of movement, to demonstrate circadian or other cyclical patterns of movement, and to discriminate wakefulness from sleep.[1,777]

Advantages and Limitations of Actigraphy

Activity monitoring has a number of *advantages* over sleep laboratory PSG or even ambulatory PSG monitoring. First, it can be efficiently and inexpensively used for extended periods of time. Depending on the equipment and technique used, recordings can be made for many days or even months. In assessing sleep disorders, this extended recording can allow for the capture of rare events, overcoming the problem of variability that can limit the accuracy of more abbreviated studies, and for repeated measurement of sleep in different conditions (disease progression or remission, therapeutic responses). One of the major problems with the movement disorders in sleep is the large night-to-night variation in expression of the disorder. Sleepwalking may occur only once a week or even less often. PLMS correlate across 3 consecutive nights at significant but relatively low levels (r^2 = .36–.64),[778] and the average absolute difference between consecutive nights in one study was slightly over 50% of the average rate of PLMS per hour[779] and about 30% in a similar study.[780] The amount of wake time during a night has even greater variability over nights, and the wake times between consecuting nights are often not even significantly correlated. (r^2 = .30–.62).[778] Thus, although a 1-night PSG may suffice for diagnosis of severe cases of movement dysfunction in sleep, it is less satisfactory for determining severity. Even for diagnostic purposes, the 1-night PSG is likely to miss some significant movement features. Indeed, a 3-night study of 46 healthy seniors (28 with PLM) included one who had no PLM on one night and 37/hr on another night.[781] Another study noted that the diagnosis from 2 consecutive nights for elevated PLMS per hour disagreed for 19% of the cases.[782] Moreover, the night-to-night variation in PLM rate for the elderly is estimated to be four times larger than that for sleep-related breathing disorders.[783]

Although adequate for evaluating sleep-related breathing disorders, the 1-night PSG is probably not satisfactory for evaluating the rate of occurrence of PLMS and other motor dysfunctions in sleep. This instability seriously hampers both clinical treatments and research studies. For example, the degree of morbidity due to PLMD remains controversial. Clinical studies in the elderly indicate that PLMD is a major cause of insomnia in the elderly,[784] but surveys have been inconsistent in finding relations between PLMs and subjective symptoms.[463,757,785] Data, also indicate that PLM events occur with autonomic arousal, including significant transitory elevations in blood pressure.[482,527,786] The marked lack of stability for rates of occurrence across nights for these events significantly complicates evaluating the clinical significance of PLM. The clinical presentation of RLS syndrome similarly shows marked night-to-night variation that may be reflected in marked differences in PLM rates across nights shown by these patients.[782] A reasonably stable metric for PLM of RLS patients requires recording over about 4–5 nights. Thus, given the large variability between individuals and across nights, and in some cases the unpredictable nature of a significant but rare event, the study of many movement disorders of sleep needs to involve fairly large sample sizes and multiple-night recordings. The inconvenience and expense of PSG currently makes this technique impractical for such extended or repeated studies.

The second major advantage for activity monitors occurs because PSG, and even the usual ambulatory PSG alternatives (such as the Vitalog or Oxford Medilog systems), are both expensive and inconvenient, and all require staff intervention (e.g., for applying EMG electrodes). The activity monitors, in contrast, are usually small, lightweight, and self-contained. They can be used in multiple settings, including the home or even a spacecraft,[787] and in varied activity states. The activity monitors can be taken out of the laboratory, self-applied, and even transmitted by mail. They may be particularly useful in uncooperative patient groups with degenerative disease who would not tolerate a laboratory sleep study,[788,789] and may simplify large studies of therapeutic interventions in insomnia or other sleep disturbances.

Third, some PSG channels, such as EMG, may indicate muscle activity that is not, in fact, significant for the patient. Activity monitoring can discriminate actual movement from EMG potentials, which may occur without any discernable displacement of a limb. Moreover, the uncalibrated surface EMG used for PSG cannot provide a quantitative measure of the amplitude of the leg movement.

The *limitations* on activity monitoring result from the relatively nonspecific results and the limited information monitored. The results are generally nonspecific because all movement, even transmitted movement, is recorded. The information obtained by activity monitoring is limited because there may be no information about cerebral state (EEG), eye movements (too small to be reflected in a limb monitor), or breathing. Therefore, they do not provide much useful information about physiologic state or crucial information about exact sleep stages.

Device Specifications

Typically, activity monitoring devices use accelerometry to quantify movement. Several small self-contained devices currently available on the market provide a direct assessment of the amount of activity or body movement at the point of the body where they are attached. These are all derived from the work of Colburn and Smith, who produced the first of these meters and documented the methods for others to use.[790] Virtually all of these devices use a piezoelectric sensor (usually a ceramic bender unit). The ceramic bender generates its own electric current that is directly proportional to the amount of acceleration. The activity devices usually include a volatile memory chip and a small computer or microcontroller chip. They are programmed to determine the amount of activity in a unit time and record that amount at a determined storage rate. The activity accepted by these devices is usually filtered so that they cover the dominant frequency ranges for human movement of about 0.5–15 Hz.[791] Later the data are downloaded to a computer, typically a desktop or laptop PC, usually through a special interface device. Various manipulations can then be performed on the downloaded data for further quantification or illustration. The activity data are maintained with a time-date code so that the activity can be analyzed by the time of each day recorded.

The self-contained units are battery powered; current models provide batteries capable of actively recording for from 14 days to 4 years. Although shorter battery life does limit the maximum duration of the recording, battery life may increase as this technology develops. Another limitation on the duration of monitoring is the amount of computer memory available to retain the stored values. Currently, the memory size available for these monitors is 4 megabytes to 1 gigabyte. Duration of monitoring is inversely proportional to the rate at which values are stored. For low storage frequencies (e.g., once every minute), these capacities translate into a total monitoring period of 3–720 days. However, at the high storage rates useful for examining individual movements (e.g., 10/sec), total monitoring would only be from about 7 minutes up to 29 hours. These devices all use internal circuitry to sample the output voltage at a certain frequency (sample frequency or rate). The amount of activity can be determined by checking the number of times the voltage reaches or exceeds a minimum criterion (threshold crossing) or by some integration or summation of the total voltage from the individual samples. Integration provides the more sensitive approach, especially for examining individual movements as opposed to total activity. After a certain number of samples, the result either in total threshold crosses or integrated voltage is stored. The storage frequency or rate limits the time resolution of this technique. For assessing total activity occurring in spans of a few seconds to minutes, the digital sampling can be at relatively low rates (e.g., 4–8 Hz) and still provide an adequate measurement. But for higher storage frequencies designed to examine individual movements, a sampling frequency of 10–40 Hz is probably necessary. Storage rates of 10 Hz or more would be ideal, although slower movements can be analyzed with storage rates perhaps as low as 1 Hz.

Uses of Actigraphy

One main use of activity monitoring has been in the multiday assessment of sleep and wakefulness. The determination of circadian activity patterns through activity monitoring is well worked out,[792] and is accepted as a standard of practice.[777] The assessment of sleep for total sleep time or sleep onset times has not been accepted as adequate. Sleep as determined by activity monitoring, with monitors typically placed on the nondominant wrist, has been compared to that indicated on PSG and shows both random and systematic errors.[793] In one study, three-fourths of 36 patients with insomnia assessed for 3 days with both actigraphy and PSG showed a mean discrepancy of less than 1 hr/night, but one-fourth showed a larger discrepancy.[794] Thus the standards of practice do not include use of activity meters for determining sleep times except in special situations (e.g., insmonia or sleep apnea in elderly patients) and evaluation of some special treatment responses.[668] Some efforts have been made to increase the accuracy of sleep detection by further processing the activity measures.[795] One of the authors (R.A.) and colleagues have shown that activity during the night's sleep has a small hysteresis effect for state changes between sleep and waking, so that the duration of inactivity preceding sleep onset after a period of wakefulness depends on the prior state as defined by length of the preceding awakening.[796] This further limits the use of activity measures for evaluating sleep times and waking during sleep.

For movement disorders, the activity monitor is placed at the site of the abnormal movement. In general, the goal of such recording is to count and quantify such movements, not merely to indicate when movement occurs. Various earlier studies showed that abnormal movements associated with hyperkinetic disorders could be quantified using actigraphy,[797,798] if appropriate filtering was used to select for frequencies associated with the movements. Early studies attempted such a quantitation in PLMS. The total movement activity during sleep for patients was determined from activity monitors worn on the ankle of the affected leg, but the correlations between overall activity and the number of PLM were not high (r values of about .6).[799]

More recently, sophisticated systems for counting movements have been developed and validated,[800–803] making these systems useful for therapeutic monitoring or assistance in diagnosis of PLMD and RLS.[804,805] A much better correlation between total activity and specific abnormal movements may be obtained with finer grained analyses.[806] Recognizing the distinctive profile of individual movements requires matching the descriptive powers of an EMG record. To detect the onset and end of a specific movement requires sensitivity to higher frequency components of the movement, necessitating sampling rates in the range of 10–40 Hz. Moreover, there are major data-storage problems for this condition. PLM are, by definition, greater than 0.5 seconds in duration.[457] Activity measurements to detect PLM should have storage frequencies of at least 4 Hz and preferably 8–10 Hz to enhance measurement accuracy. A fine-grained analysis with 40-Hz sampling and storage at 10 Hz available from one of these monitors (the PAM-RL; Respironics, Pittsburgh, PA) provides a description closely matching the EMG recordings for these movements. The recording at 10 Hz can then be saved for up to 7 days depending on the memory size in the units.

In the more advanced activity meters, such as the PAM-RL designed to be worn on the ankle to measure leg movements (Fig. 28–3), detections are based on sampling at 40 Hz with data stored for the activity summed over four samples (10-Hz data storage). The descriptive information about the movement, along with total activity per 0.1 second, permits a review of machine scoring to determine if criteria are met for periodic movements of sleep. The data provide an excellent agreement with EMG recordings from the legs (Fig. 28–4) and thus with

the nocturnal PSG for number of leg movements (with a correlation of $r = .997$ and an average error for rates per hour of less than 1.0) when done in the laboratory setting with calibrated meters.[807] The monitors when used off the shelf in a standard clinical setting also have very good agreement with results from the PSG and are considered validated for this use.[802] The PAM-RL has an advantage for home recordings since it records

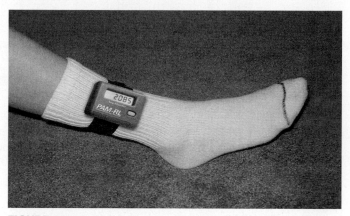

FIGURE 28–3 Example of a high-precision activity monitor worn on the ankle to detect leg movements.

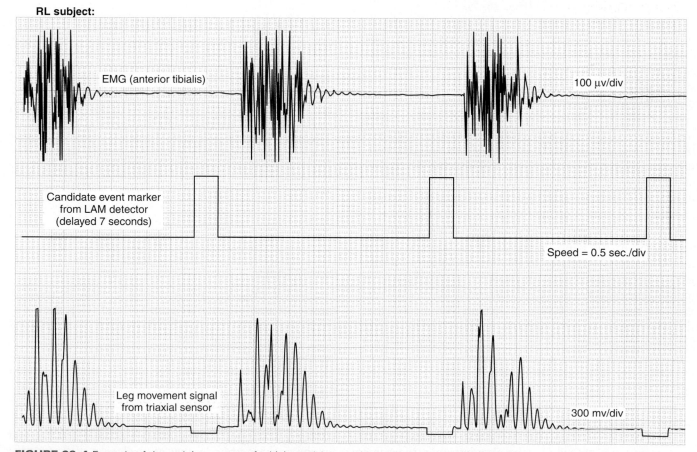

FIGURE 28–4 Example of the real-time output of a high-precision activity monitor worn on the ankle (*bottom line*) compared to anterior tibialis EMG activity (*top line*). The *middle line* shows the real-time automatic detection of a significant leg movement made by the activity meter. The decision rules for the real-time leg movement detector create a 7-second delay in the detection.

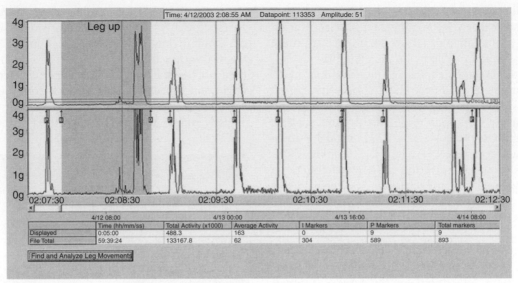

FIGURE 28–5 Example of computer display of stored leg activity and leg position data from a high-precision activity monitor worn on the ankle. The lighter areas on the graph (*white background*) indicate the leg is in a mostly horizontal position.

separately the PLM rates when the legs are stretched out versus when they are upright (subject sitting or standing). Thus they give the PLM rates for the sleep position (although not sleep, per se) (Fig. 28–5).

The use of the new ambulatory monitors that provide this fine-grained analysis of movements might be further extended to assess other movement disorders in sleep, such as RBD or rhythmic movement disorder. But even such a development would fail to provide relevant information about the patient's sleep-wake state. This can be approached by adding illumination[788,808] or position information. To detect body position, a system developed by one of the authors (R.A.) and colleagues requires wearing small monitors on the trunk and also on the leg just above the knee. Each monitor records position in three-dimensional space for each epoch (30 seconds to 1 minute), and the combination of the two provides a description of the overall body position as standing, sitting, reclining, supine, prone, or lying on the right or left side. These monitors, when compared to direct observation of a subject's body position, show an excellent overall agreement (contingency coefficients [C] = 0.85–0.91, maximum value of C for these data = 0.913).[809] Activity data collected at the same time as position data permits differentiating abnormal movements that occur while the patient is lying down from those while standing or sitting. It also permits the detection of events during the sleep time when the patient sits or stands up, such as occurs for sleepwalking.

For examination of overall movement, a meter on the dominant wrist is best for assessing daytime activity while a meter on the nondominant wrist can best track trunk movement at night.[810] A related movement recording device is the static charge–sensitive bed, which can record respiration,[811,812] heartbeats, and movements such as

periodic leg movements.[813] This technology is used primarily in Finland and has not had much spread to other countries.

Daytime and Evening Evaluation

Patients with sleep motor disturbances can be evaluated with the MSLT for EDS, as can sleep patients generally (see Chapter 16). The American Academy of Neurology[762] and the American Academy of Sleep Medicine[764,814] accept those studies as useful for patients with a variety of sleep disorders who complain of EDS.

Daytime sleep studies, sometimes done with sleep deprivation the night before, can occasionally be useful in disclosing sleep motor disturbances such as RLS or PLMS, or may assist in the evaluation of a patient with possible epilepsy. However, negative studies under these conditions are not helpful, and the limited yield of daytime studies makes full nighttime monitoring far more desirable.

SUMMARY

The past 3 decades have witnessed a great increase in knowledge about the motor disorders and sleep. New disorders such as RBD and NPD have been described, and other disorders, such as RLS, have been clarified. The importance of sleep dysfunction in the diurnal movement disorders, especially PD and related conditions, has been established. From the viewpoint of treatment, new therapies, both for long-known and recently described disorders, have been developed.

Newly developed techniques such as brain imaging and genetic analysis promise that an explosion of knowledge about brain function will also lead to much better answers about why sleep is needed and how it is regulated. We may also gain a much better understanding of how motor disturbances of sleep intrude on normal function. These answers should help provide guides for more specific therapy. Advances in understanding the genetics of a number of conditions, both diurnal movement disorders and sleep disorders such as RLS, may provide specific clues as to how the sleep-regulating system is disordered.

Currently, we are beginning to develop a sharper picture of how both normal and abnormal movements are controlled during sleep. In the normal or "ideal" case, there are three discrete states: wake, NREM sleep, and REM sleep.[43] Both sleep states act to provide two key functions: a relative dissociation of higher sleep centers from the external world and from lower levels of the nervous system and a partial suppression of overt motor activity. The wake state, in contrast, attempts to optimize association between higher centers, lower centers, and the world, and to facilitate motor expression. The two sleep states differ in the autonomous activity of higher centers, which appears to be much greater in REM sleep. Both normal movements and most abnormal movements due to diurnal movement disorders show a characteristic pattern in sleep. They are most likely to occur during the lightest stage of sleep (stage 1 NREM), often in association with lightenings or arousals. They are less likely to occur in stage 2 NREM or REM sleep and least likely to occur in SWS or during deepening sleep. This pattern seems to be followed by those movement disorders whose presumed generator is in a higher motor center, either cortical or subcortical. In contrast, movements generated at the segmental level or at the level of the motor neuron are relatively resistant to modulation by sleep, perhaps because their mere presence is evidence for a reduced degree of higher control.

NREM and REM sleep disorders involve separate but interrelated sensorimotor dysfunctions. NREM disorders, such as many parasomnias, RLS, and PLMD, are activated by repose and sleep. In the case of RLS, the activation may begin in the predormital phase, as relaxation and drowsiness overshadow awake alertness. Presumably, these conditions arise, especially RLS and PLMD, because of some changing control from higher centers that allows the expression of a more primitive motor rhythmicity. In the case of parasomnias that are similar to normal motor behavior, such as somnambulism or somniloquy, the major defect may be an excessive activity of higher centers or a relative failure of the NREM motor inhibitory system. NREM disorders probably would occur during REM sleep as well, as seen with PLMD in RBD[47] and narcolepsy,[465,466] but the additional inhibition that occurs during REM sleep suppresses them. REM disorders, by contrast, involve some shift in the critical REM sleep balance between excitation and inhibition. Although the exact changes are not clear, it seems most likely that this is a change in higher influence and most likely a deficiency in inhibitory systems in the brain stem, analogous to the animal lesion models of REM sleep without atonia.[37] A unifying thesis for both NREM and REM disorders is that they can involve a failure of descending inhibition. The different conditions are likely to involve partially distinct, but related inhibitory processes.

NREM and REM disorders, then, are likely to be activated by processes that impinge on the inhibitory systems of the brain stem. Because the balance between excitation and inhibition is fairly exacting, a variety of different influences, such as neurodegenerative disorders or even normal aging, may result in the emergence of disorders. Conditions that are associated with poor state regulation, such as narcolepsy, are very likely to be associated with additional NREM and REM disorders—hence the report that narcoleptics at a young age may have both PLMD and RBD.[50] The overall interrelatedness of failures of sleep inhibitory control can be seen in two further facts. First, REM and NREM disorders often overlap. For example, there is a high incidence of PLMD and fragmentary myoclonus in RBD. Second, certain medications, such as the benzodiazepines and dopaminergic agents, may be useful in a number of the NREM and REM motor disturbances, as well as in state dyscontrol conditions such as narcolepsy.

The further resolution of the pathophysiology of motor disturbances of sleep will now await a more exact understanding of the sleep regulatory systems of the brain, especially those responsible for the descending inhibition of the segmental and effector levels of the motor system.

REFERENCES

A full list of references are available at www.expertconsult.com

CHAPTER 29

Sleep, Breathing, and Neurologic Disorders

Sudhansu Chokroverty and **Pasquale Montagna**

INTRODUCTION

To understand the effects of neurologic lesions on sleep-wake cycles and sleep states, and to understand the normal interactions of sleep and breathing, it is important to have a clear understanding of the functional anatomy of sleep and breathing. In the first section of the chapter, therefore, a brief overview of the anatomy and physiology of sleep is presented. The section on the functional anatomy of sleep is followed by a short discussion of the control of breathing during sleep. For details, readers are referred to some excellent reviews and monographs,[1–10] and to Chapters 4, 5 and 7 in this volume.

Most of the anatomic structures that control sleep and breathing are located in the central nervous systems (CNS). These regions are influenced not only by other CNS structures but also by inputs from the peripheral neuromuscular system and other body systems. It is very common to encounter in practice a variety of neurologic disorders that affect sleep and breathing. It is important to understand not only that the neurologic illnesses may affect sleep and breathing but also that alterations of sleep and breathing may adversely affect the natural history of a neurologic disorder. A number of excellent sources provide systematic descriptions of the effects of neurologic lesions on the pattern and control of breathing.[11–21] The effect of acute and chronic neurologic disorders on the state of sleep and the resulting interaction on breathing has received scant attention. An understanding of such an interaction is essential for treatment and prognostic purposes in various neurologic disorders. In neurologic illnesses, breathing disorders may manifest as hypopnea, apnea, irregular or periodic breathing, or cessation of breathing. Similarly, sleep disturbances may manifest as hypersomnia, hyposomnia (insomnia), parasomnia, or circadian rhythm sleep disorders. The sections after those on functional anatomy and physiology of sleep and breathing deal with the clinical manifestations, laboratory assessment, and treatment of sleep and breathing disorders that accompany neurologic illnesses. The discussion is grouped into two major sections: (1) sleep and breathing disorders secondary to somatic neurologic illness and (2) sleep and breathing disorders secondary to autonomic failure. The somatic neurologic disorders are subdivided into CNS disorders and peripheral neuromuscular disorders.

FUNCTIONAL ANATOMY OF SLEEP AND WAKEFULNESS

The neuroanatomic substrate of wakefulness, rapid eye movement (REM) sleep, and non–rapid eye movement (NREM) sleep are located in separate parts of the CNS.[1,22] There are no discreet sleep/wake-promoting centers; rather, these states are produced by changes in the interconnecting neuronal systems modulated by neurotransmitters and neuromodulators.

Neuroanatomic Substrates of Wakefulness

The ascending reticular activating system (ARAS), containing glutamatergic, cholinergic, aminergic, and hypocretinergic neurons, determines the state of wakefulness.[1,23]

Cerebral cortical activation during wakefulness is maintained by projections from the ARAS terminating in the thalamus and by thalamocortical projections to widespread areas of the cerebral cortex. In addition, there are extrathalamic projections from the brain stem reticular neurons ending in the posterior hypothalamus and the basal forebrain regions; the latter in turn project to the cerebral cortex to help maintain wakefulness. All these pathways regulating the wakefulness system utilize cholinergic, noradrenergic, dopaminergic, and histaminergic neurons. The cholinergic neurons fire at the highest rate during wakefulness and REM sleep but decrease their rates of firing at the onset of NREM sleep. The wake-promoting aminergic neurons include noradrenergic neurons in the locus ceruleus (LC), serotoninergic neurons in the dorsal raphe of the brain stem, histaminergic neurons in the tuberomammillary nucleus of the hypothalamus, and possibly also dopaminergic neurons in the ventral tagmental area, substantia nigra, and ventral periaqueductal area. Although the role of dopamine is uncertain, pharmacologic, biochemical, and physiologic studies suggest that dopamine—probably through D_1 and possibly through D_2 receptors—along with noradrenergic system promotes wakefulness. Noradrenergic neurons in the LC show the highest firing rates during wakefulness, the lowest during REM sleep, and an intermediate rate during NREM sleep. Pharmacologic studies suggest that posterior hypothalamic histaminergic neurons are also important in maintaining wakefulness.

The excitatory amino acids glutamic and aspartic acids, intermingled within the ARAS and present in many neurons projecting into the cerebral cortex, forebrain, and brain stem, are released maximally during wakefulness. The discovery of hypothalamic hypocretin neurons with their widespread CNS projections directs our attention to the role of the hypocretinergic system in controlling sleep-wake regulation. De Lecea and coauthors[24] described two neuropeptides in the lateral hypothalamus and perifornical region that were termed hypocretin-1 and hypocretin-2. In the same year, independently, Sakuri et al.[25] described two neuropeptides in the same region that they named orexin A (corresponding to hypocretin-1) and orexin B (corresponding to hypocretin-2). It was shown thereafter that these hypocretin systems have widespread ascending and descending projections to the LC, dorsal raphe nucleus (DRN), ventral tagmental area, tuberomammillary nuclei of the posterior hypothalamus, laterodorsal tagmental (LDT) and pedunculopontine tagmental (PPT) nuclei, ventrolateral preoptic (VLPO) nucleus in the hypothalamus, basal forebrain, limbic system (hippocampus and amygdala), cerebral cortex, thalamus (intralaminar and midline nuclei), and autonomic neurons (nucleus tractus solitarius, dorsal vagal nuclei, and intermediolateral neurons of the spinal cord).[26–28] Hypocretin systems promote wakefulness mainly through excitation of tuberomammillary histaminergic, LC

noradrenergic, and midline raphe serotoninergic and dopaminergic neurons. Sleepiness may partly be induced by a reduction of activity of the hypocretin systems. These systems also participate in REM sleep regulation through activation of the aminergic neurons (REM-off), which in turn inhibit REM-generating neurons in the LDT/PPT (REM-on).[22]

Neuroanatomic Substrates of REM Sleep

Transection experiments in cats through different regions of the midbrain, pons, and medulla[22,29,30] established the existence of REM sleep–generating neurons in the pons (Fig. 29–1). A transection at the junction of the pons and midbrain (level A) produced all the physiologic findings compatible with REM sleep caudal to this transection, whereas rostral to the section, in the forebrain region, the recording showed no signs of REM sleep. The structures rostral to a section between the pons and medulla (level B) showed signs of REM sleep but structures caudal to the section showed no signs of REM sleep. Following transection at the junction of the spinal cord and medulla (level C), REM sleep signs were noted in the rostral brain areas. Finally, transections at the pontomesencephalic (A) and pontomedullary (B) junctions produced an isolated pons that showed all the signs of REM sleep. The pons is, therefore, sufficient and necessary to generate all the signs of REM sleep.

To explain the mechanism of REM sleep, three animal models are available. The earliest and most generally well known is the McCarley-Hobson reciprocal interaction model (Fig. 29–2) based on reciprocal interaction of REM-on and REM-off neurons[1,22] (see also Chapter 4). The cholinergic neurons in the PPT and LDT nuclei in the pontomesencephalic region are REM-on cells responsible for REM sleep, showing highest firing rates at this stage. The aminergic neurons located in the LC and DRN are REM-off cells and are inactive during REM sleep.

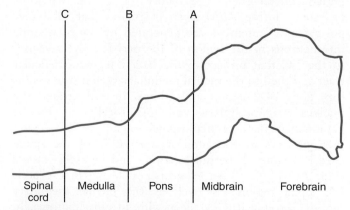

FIGURE 29–1 Schematic sagittal section of the brain stem of the cat. **(A)** Junction of midbrain and pons. **(B)** Junction of pons and medulla. **(C)** Junction of medulla and spinal cord. *(Modified from Jouvet[29] and Siegel.[30])*

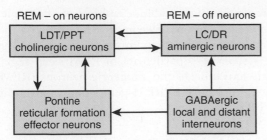

FIGURE 29–2 Schematic diagram of McCarley-Hobson model of REM sleep mechanism. (GABA, γ-aminobutyric acid; LC/DR, locus ceruleus/dorsal raphe; LDT/PPT, laterodorsal tegmental/pedunculopontine tegmental nuclei.)*(Modified from McCarley RW. Neurobiology of REM and NREM sleep. Sleed Med 2007;8:302.)*

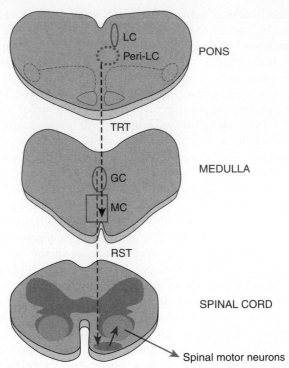

FIGURE 29–3 Schematic diagram to explain the mechanism of muscle atonia in REM sleep. (GC, gigantocellularis; LC, locus ceruleus; MC, magnocellularis; Peri-LC: peri–locus ceruleus alpha; RST, reticulospinal tract; TRT, tegmentoreticular tract.)

Histaminergic neurons in the tuberomammillary region of the posterior hypothalamus can also be considered as REM-off cells. Thus, the cholinergic REM-on and aminergic REM-off cells are all located within the transections of the pons as described previously. LDT-PPT cholinergic neurons promote REM sleep through pontine reticular formation (PRF) effector neurons, which in turn send feedback loops to the LDT-PPT. Cholinergic neurons of the PPT and LDT project into the thalamus and basal forebrain regions as well as to the PRF and are responsible for activation and generation of REM sleep. Aminergic cells play a permissive role in maintenance of the REM sleep state. In the latest modification of the reciprocal interaction model, McCarley[22] suggested that γ-aminobutyric acid (GABA) also plays a role in the REM sleep generation. At the onset of REM sleep, there is activation of GABA neurons in the pons that causes inhibition of the LC/DRN (REM-off neurons) as well as activation of (or disinhibition of) cholinergic neurons in the pons.[31] The reason for GABA activation is not known, and the source of GABAergic neurons is probably both local (e.g., a subgroup of PRF GABA neurons) and distant (e.g., GABAergic neurons in the ventrolateral periaqueductal gray). The theory for muscle hypotonia or atonia during REM sleep postulates that inhibitory postsynaptic potentials are generated by dorsal pontine interneurons in the region of the peri-LC alpha ventral to the LC that project to the lateral tegmentoreticular tract and then to the medial medullary region (the inhibitory zone of Magoun and Rhines in and around the nucleus magnocellularis and gigantocellularis in the paramedianus); the reticulospinal tract from this region then projects to the anterior horn cells of the spinal cord, causing hyperpolarization and muscle atonia (Fig. 29–3).[1,2,32–36] An experimental lesion in the peri-LC alpha region[37] as well as the medial medullary region[38] produced REM sleep without muscle atonia. In human REM sleep behavior disorder, causing dream-enacting behavior associated with REM sleep without muscle atonia, a structural or functional alteration of the

pathway maintaining muscle atonia during REM sleep is most likely responsible.[39]

In the model proposed by Luppi's group[40,41] (Fig. 29–4), neurons active during REM sleep are identified in a small area in the dorsolateral pontine tegmentum called the sublaterodorsal (SLD) nucleus in rats (corresponding to the dorsal subceruleus or peri-LC alpha region in cats). The onset of REM sleep is thought to be due to activation of REM-on glutamatergic neurons from the SLD. During NREM sleep and wakefulness, these neurons in the SLD would be inhibited (hyperpolarized) by tonic GABAergic input from GABAergic REM-off neurons located in the SLD, deep mesencephalic and pontine reticular nuclei, and ventrolateral periaqueductal gray (vlPAG) as well as by monoaminergic REM-off neurons. Ascending SLD REM-on glutamatergic neurons can cause cortical activation through projections to thalamocortical neurons along with REM-on cholinergic and glutamatergic neurons from the LDT/PPT mesencephalic and pontine reticular nuclei and basal forebrain regions. Descending REM-on glutamatergic SLD neurons would cause muscle atonia through excitatory projections to glycinergic premotor neurons in the magnocellularis and parvocellularis reticular nuclei in the medulla, causing hyperpolarization of the motor neurons. In the Luppi model, therefore, GABAergic and glutamatergic neurons play a crucial role in REM

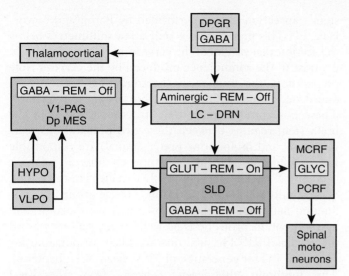

FIGURE 29–4 Schematic diagram of Boissard-Luppi model to explain REM sleep mechanism. (DPGR, dorsal paragigantocellular reticular nucleus; Dp-MES, deep mesencephalic; GABA, γ-aminobutyric acid; GLUT, glutamatergic; GLYC, glycinergic neurons; HYPO, hypothalamus [hypocretinergic neurons in lateral hypothalamus]; LC-DRN, locus ceruleus–dorsal raphe nuclei; MCRF, magnocellular reticular formation; PCRF, parvocellular reticular formation; SLD, sublaterodorsal nucleus; Vl-PAG, ventrolateral periaqueductal gray; VLPO, ventrolateral preoptic region.)*(Modified from Luppi and Fort[40] and Boissard et al.[41])*

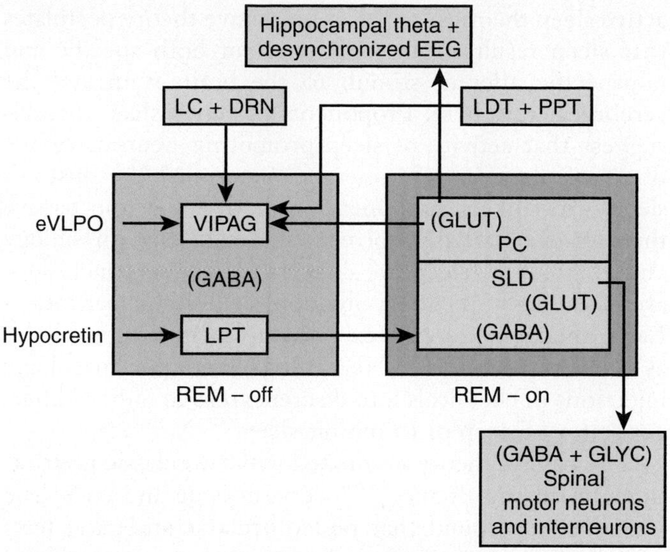

FIGURE 29–5 Lu-Saper "flip-flop" model shown schematically to explain REM sleep mechanism. (eVLPO, extended region of ventrolateral preoptic nucleus; GABA, γ-aminobutyric acid; GLUT, glutamatergic neurons; GLYC, glycinergic neurons; LC + DRN, locus ceruleus + dorsal raphe nuclei; LDT + PPT, laterodorsal tegmental + pedunculopontine tegmental nuclei; LPT, lateral pontine tegmentum; PC, preceruleus; SLD, sublaterodorsal nucleus; VlPAG, ventrolateral periaqueductal gray.)*(Modified from Lu J, Sherman D, Devor M, Saper CB. A putative flip-flop switch for control of REM sleep. Nature 2006;441:589.)*

generation. GABAergic neurons are also responsible for inactivation of monoaminergic neurons during REM sleep, and cholinergic neurons do not play a crucial role in activating REM executive neurons in this model.

In the third model, proposed by Lu and coworkers[42] (Fig. 29–5), there is a "flip-flop" switch interaction between GABAergic REM-off neurons in the deep mesencephalon, vlPAG, and lateral pontine tegmentum (LPT) and GABAergic REM-on neurons in the SLD, and a dorsal extension of the SLD named the preceruleus. These mutually inhibitory neuronal populations (SLD GABA-ergic REM-on and GABA-ergic REM-off neurons in the deep mesencephalon–lateral pontine tegmentum) serve as a flip-flop switch. Ascending glutamatergic projections from preceruleus neurons to the medial septum are responsible for the hippocampal electroencephalographic (EEG) theta rhythm during REM sleep. Descending glutamatergic projections from the ventral SLD directly to the spinal interneurons, apparently without a relay in the medial medulla, inhibit spinal ventral horn cells by both glycerinergic and GABAergic mechanisms. Cholinergic and aminergic neurons play a modulatory role and are not part of the flip-flop switch. McCarley[22] suggested that this model is based on c-*fos* labeling only without electrophysiologic recordings. Furthermore, this model does not address how REM periodicity occurs in this flip-flop switch utilizing two mutually inhibitory neuronal populations. Finally, this model also does not

explain the gradually increasing duration of REM sleep throughout the night and generally absent REM sleep during daytime naps. It should be noted that Brooks and Peever[43] challenged the glycinergic and GABAergic neurochemical mechanism of REM motor atonia based on experimental evidence in rats that REM atonia persists even when glycine and GABA receptors are blocked and after simultaneous application of glutamatergic agonists to the trigeminal motor pool. Multiple biochemical pathways are responsible for controlling muscle tone in REM sleep.

Neuroanatomic Substrates of NREM Sleep

Neurophysiologic studies of sleep really began after astute clinicopathologic observations by von Economo, who examined patients with encephalitis lethargica at the beginning of the 20th century.[44] It was noted that lesions of encephalitis lethargica, which severely affected the posterior hypothalamic area, were associated with the clinical manifestation of extreme somnolence, whereas morphologic alterations in the anterior hypothalamic region were associated with sleeplessness. These observations led scientists to believe in the existence of the so-called sleep-wake centers.[44–47]

Before the middle of the last century, the emphasis of sleep physiologists was on the passive[47–49] theories of sleep. Beginning in the late 1950s, thought shifted toward active sleep theories.[3,5,50–59] The passive theory postulates that sleep results from withdrawal of both specific and nonspecific afferent stimuli to the brain stem and the cerebral hemisphere. Proponents of active sleep theories suggest that activity of sleep-promoting neurons or the fibers of these so-called centers determine the onset of sleep. Most likely, proponents of both active and passive theories are partially correct, as far as the physiology and anatomy of sleep are concerned. These conclusions are based on stimulation, ablation, or lesion experiments. Later, these studies were extended to include extracellular as well as intracellular recordings, and pharmacologic injections of chemicals into discrete areas to induce different states of sleep or to inhibit sleep.[60]

The passive theory originated with two classic preparations in cats by Bremer[48,61]: cerveau isolé and encephale isolé. Bremer found that midcollicular transection (cerveau isolé) produced somnolence in the acute stage and that transection at the C1 vertebral level, to disconnect the entire brain from the spinal cord (encephale isolé), caused EEG recordings to fluctuate between wakefulness and sleep. From these experiments, Bremer concluded that in cerveau isolé preparations all the specific sensory afferent stimuli were withdrawn and thus sleep was facilitated, whereas such stimuli maintained the activation of the brain in encephale isolé preparations. These conclusions, however, have been modified since the discovery by Moruzzi and Magoun[49] in 1949 of the existence of nonspecific groups of neurons and fibers in the center of the brain stem called the reticular formation. Moruzzi and Magoun[49] stated that the brain stem ARAS energized the forebrain and that withdrawal of this influence in cerveau isolé preparation resulted in somnolence or coma. The observations of Moruzzi and Magoun[49] that EEG desynchronization results from activation of the midbrain reticular neurons, which directly excite the thalamocortical projections, have been confirmed by more recent intracellular studies.[62,63] It was thought that wakefulness resulted from activation of the ARAS and diffuse thalamocortical projections.[1] After stimulation of these structures, the EEG shows diffuse desynchronization, whereas lesions in these structures produce EEG synchronization or the EEG NREM sleep pattern. This also supports the suggestion of Steriade et al.[64] that, at the onset of NREM sleep, there is deafferentation of the brain due to blockage of afferent information first at the thalamic level, causing the waking open brain to be converted into a closed brain resulting from thalamocortical inhibition (see also Chapter 5). It has been demonstrated that the origin of the sleep spindles are related to the reticular nucleus of the thalamus.[1] Stimulation of this nucleus produces spindle-like activity, whereas destruction of it abolishes the spindles unilaterally and bilateral destruction abolishes the spindles on both sides.

The passive sleep theories were challenged by findings that came in the wake of midpontine pretrigeminal brain stem transection in cats performed by Batini and coworkers.[51,52] This preparation is only a few millimeters below the section that produces the cerveau isolé preparation. In contrast to the somnolence produced by the cerveau isolé preparation, the midpontine pretrigeminal section produced persistent EEG and behavioral signs of alertness. These observations imply that structures located in the brain stem regions between these two preparations (cerveau isolé and midpontine pretrigeminal) are responsible for wakefulness. Data demonstrate cholinergic neurons in the PPT nucleus and in the LDT nucleus in the region of the midbrain-pontine junction.[1] These groups of cholinergic neurons have been shown to have thalamic and basal forebrain projections as well as projections toward the medial PRF. The neurons are likely responsible for activation and for generation of REM sleep (see Chapter 4). The forebrain cholinergic neurons from the basal nucleus of Meynert project to the cerebral hemisphere, particularly to the sensorimotor cortex, and lesions in these neurons disrupt the EEG waves and elicit diffuse slow waves.[1] The finding of cholinergic neurons at the mesopontine junction confirms the conclusions drawn by Batini and colleagues[51,52] after midpontine pretrigeminal transections.

The active hypnogenic neurons for NREM sleep are thought to be located in two regions[1]: (1) the region of the nucleus tractus solitarius (NTS) in the medulla and (2) the preoptic area of the hypothalamus and the basal forebrain area (see Chapter 4). The evidence is based on stimulation, lesion, and ablation studies, as well as extracellular and intercellular recordings.[1] The active inhibitory role of the lower brain stem hypnogenic neurons on the upper brain stem ARAS has been clearly demonstrated by Batini et al.'s[51,52] experiment of midpontine pretrigeminal sectioning. Similarly, electrical[56] stimulation of the preoptic area, which produced EEG synchronization and a behavioral state of sleep, supported the idea of the existence of active hypnogenic neurons in the preoptic area.[1] Nauta's[47] experiments in 1946 that showed insomnia after lesions of the preoptic region also supported the hypothesis of active hypnogenic neurons in the forebrain preoptic area. Experiments by McGinty and Sterman[58] in 1968 confirmed Nauta's observations. More recently, ibotenic lesions in the preoptic region have been found to produce insomnia, and these results support the active hypnogenic role of the preoptic area.[1,65] In the same experiments, however, injections of muscimol (a GABA agonist) in the posterior hypothalamus transiently recovered sleep, suggesting that the sleep-promoting role of the anterior hypothalamus is dependent on inhibition of posterior hypothalamic histaminergic awakening neurons. It should also be emphasized that in 1934 Dikshit[66] induced sleep by intrahypothalamic injection of acetylcholine, suggesting the presence of a sleep center in the hypothalamus. Contemporary theory suggests that NREM sleep-promoting neurons are found in the VLPO area of the anterior hypothalamus as well as in the region of the NTS in the medulla. VLPO neurons consist of two subgroups—"clustered" and "diffuse" or extended—depending on the distribution pattern.[67,68] The tightly clustered neurons project to the tuberomammillary nuclei, inhibiting them and promoting NREM sleep, whereas diffusely distributed neurons project to and inhibit the aminergic nuclei in the LC and the dorsal raphe region of the brain stem participating in REM sleep. The VLPO neurons fire actively during NREM sleep, and their lesion induces insomnia. The GABA- and galanin-containing VLPO neurons project to and inhibit the LC, dorsal raphe, and tuberomammillary aminergic nuclei, which in turn inhibit VLPO neurons.

The contemporary theory for the mechanism of NREM sleep thus suggests a reciprocal interaction between two antagonistic neuron types in the VLPO of the anterior hypothalamus and wake-promoting neurons in the tuberomammillary nuclei of the posterior hypothalamus, as well as the LC, dorsal raphe, basal forebrain, and mesopontine tagmentum.[1,22,67–69] Reciprocal interaction between sleep-promoting neurons in the region of the NTS and wake-promoting neurons within the ARAS of the brain stem independent of the reciprocal interaction of the neurons of the forebrain also plays a role in the generation of NREM sleep, as stated earlier. In summary, the active and passive theories of sleep may be viewed as complementary rather than mutually exclusive mechanisms.[1] The role of postulated humoral sleep factors (e.g., prostaglandin D_2, growth hormone–releasing factor, muramyl peptides) remains undetermined in the absence of experiments to test their role at the cellular level in critical brain areas. It has been suggested that adenosine, a neuromodulator, may act as a physiologic sleep factor modulating the somnogenic effects of prolonged wakefulness.[70] This has been postulated after experiments in cats have shown that adenosine extracellular concentration in the basal forebrain cholinergic region increased progressively during prolonged spontaneous wakefulness.

Many important unanswered questions remain regarding the mechanism of sleep. Why do VLPO neurons fire at sleep onset? What initiates the cascade of dysfacilitation in the brain stem wake-promoting neurons? What initiates activation of LDT-PPT neurons at REM onset? What causes activation of GABAergic pontine neurons at the onset of REM sleep? What causes activation of wake-promoting neurons at sleep offset? And, finally, what maintains NREM-REM cycling? We here provide a speculative summary to answer some of these questions. VLPO excitation at NREM sleep onset is initiated by progressive accumulation of adenosine (a sleep-promoting factor in the forebrain region accumulated during prolonged wakefulness) and probably also an excitatory drive from the suprachiasmatic nucleus (SCN) as well as reciprocal inhibition of aminergic and orexin wake-promoting

neurons; progressive inhibition of aminergic REM-off neurons causes disinhibition of REM-on neurons and initiates REM sleep; and a simultaneous cascade of dysfacilitation of the brain stem arousal system with decreased environmental afferent stimuli culminates in blockade at thalamic levels. Physiologically, facilitation (or disinhibition) after a certain period (perhaps determined in the case of sleep-wake regulation by the SCN regulatory neurons connected anatomically to sleep-wake neurons) will be followed by inhibition (or dysfacilitation), and thus the cycle will begin again. For additional discussion on the functional anatomy of sleep, the reader is referred to Chapters 4 and 5.

Marked impairment of the arousal and cognition systems may result in coma or severe sleepiness. The reversibility of this state of awareness differentiates sleep from coma. There are also physiologic and metabolic differences between sleep and coma. Coma is a passive process (loss of function), whereas sleep is an active state resulting from physiologic interactions of various systems in the brain stem and cerebral cortex. Metabolic depression of the cerebral cortex and brain stem characterizes coma and stupor, whereas in sleep oxygen use and metabolic rhythm remain intact. By disrupting the arousal system and stimulating the sleep-promoting neurons, focal neurologic lesions may also cause excessive sleepiness. For example, lesions of the brain stem, thalamus, hypothalamus, and PAG regions may produce excessive sleepiness, stupor, and coma. These lesions may also affect REM-generating neurons in the pons and cause various REM sleep alterations. Thus, these lesions may also cause symptomatic narcolepsy.

FUNCTIONAL ANATOMY OF RESPIRATION IN SLEEP AND WAKEFULNESS

The neuroanatomy of respiration, its control, and physiologic changes during sleep in healthy individuals are described in detail in Chapter 7. Briefly, respiration is controlled by the automatic or metabolic and behavioral systems.[11–14,71–74] The two systems are complemented by a third system known as the *arousal system*, which may also be called the *system for wakefulness stimulus*.[74,75] These respiratory systems work in concert with the various peripheral and central inputs to maintain acid-base regulation and respiratory homeostasis.[9] The location of the respiratory neurons makes them easily vulnerable to a variety of central and peripheral neurologic disorders, particularly central neurologic disorders involving the brain stem. Many acute and chronic neurologic illnesses may affect central or peripheral respiratory pathways, giving rise to acute respiratory failure in wakefulness and sleep. Some conditions may affect control of breathing only during sleep. Such a condition may cause undesirable, often catastrophic, results, including cardiorespiratory failure and even sudden death.

SLEEP-RELATED RESPIRATORY DYSRHYTHMIA IN NEUROLOGIC DISORDERS

Many types of sleep-related respiratory dysrhythmia have been noted in association with neurologic illnesses[73,76,77] (Fig. 29–6). The most common types are sleep apnea and sleep hypopnea.

Sleep Apnea

Three types of sleep apnea have been noted[78]: central, upper airway obstructive, and mixed. Normal individuals may experience a few episodes of sleep apnea, particularly central apnea, at the onset of NREM sleep and during REM sleep. To be of pathologic significance, the sleep apnea should last at least 10 seconds and the apnea index

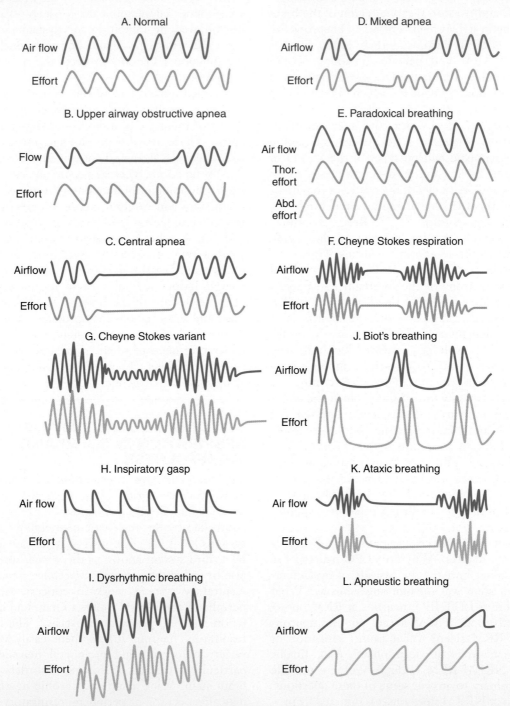

FIGURE 29–6 Schematic diagram to show different types of breathing patterns in neurologic illnesses. **(A)** Normal breathing pattern. **(B)** Upper airway obstructive apnea. **(C)** Central apnea. **(D)** Mixed apnea (initial central followed by obstructive apnea). **(E)** Paradoxical breathing. **(F)** Cheyne-Stokes breathing. **(G)** Cheyne-Stokes variant pattern. **(H)** Inspiratory gasp. **(I)** Dysrhythmic breathing. **(J)** Biot's breathing (a special type of ataxic breathing characterized by 2–3 breaths of nearly equal volume followed by long period of apnea). **(K)** Ataxic breathing. **(L)** Apneustic breathing.

(number of apneas per hour of sleep) should be at least 5. In the American Academy of Sleep Medicine (AASM) scoring criteria,[79] in addition to a duration of 10 seconds, apnea is scored when the peak amplitude drops by 90% or more of the baseline, and this amplitude reduction must last for at least 90% of the event's duration.

Cessation of airflow with no respiratory effort constitutes central apnea. During this period there is no diaphragmatic and intercostal muscle activity or air exchange through the nose or mouth. Upper airway obstructive sleep apnea (OSA) is manifested by absence of air exchange through the nose or mouth but persistence of diaphragmatic and intercostal muscle activity.

During mixed apnea, initially airflow ceases, as does respiratory effort (central apnea); this is followed by a period of upper airway OSA. On rare occasions this pattern may be reversed, resulting in an initial period of OSA followed by central apnea (Fig. 29–7).

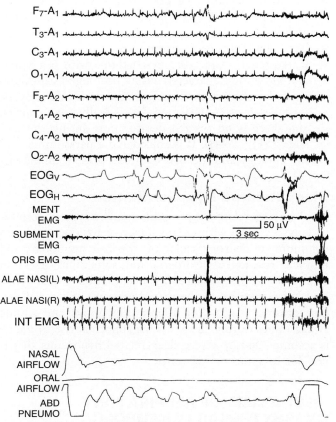

FIGURE 29–7 Polysomnographic recording in a patient with narcolepsy and sleep apnea showing the electroencephalogram (EEG; top eight channels); vertical (EOG$_V$) and horizontal (EOG$_H$) electro-oculograms; mentalis (MENT), submental (SUBMENT), orbicularis oris (ORIS), left (L) and right (R) alae nasi, and intercostal (INT) electromyogram (EMG); nasal and oral airflow; and abdominal pneumogram (ABD PNEUMO). Note unusual type of mixed apnea (initial obstructive apnea for a period of 14 seconds followed by central apnea for a period of 8 seconds) during REM sleep.

Sleep-Related Hypopnea

Sleep-related hypopnea is manifested by decreasing airflow at the mouth and nose and decreased thoracoabdominal movement causing a reduction in tidal volume. Until recently, there was no standard definition of hypopnea and investigators used one of two definitions: that proposed by the 1999 consensus report of the AASM Task Force and the AASM Clinical Practice Review Committee definition.[80] However, in the AASM scoring criteria[79] the recommended definition for hypopnea is a reduction of nasal pressure signal excursion (or that of the alternative airflow sensor) by 30% or more of the baseline amplitude lasting for a period of at least 10 seconds and accompanied by a 4% or more desaturation from the pre-event baseline. Furthermore, at least 90% of the event's duration must meet the amplitude reduction criteria for hypopnea. An alternative suggestion in the same manual is a reduction of the amplitude excursion in the nasal pressure signal (or that of the alternative airflow sensor) by 50% or more of the baseline lasting for at least 10 seconds and accompanied by oxygen desaturation of 3% or more from the pre-event baseline, or the event is associated with an arousal. This amplitude reduction must be present for at least 90% of the event's duration. An apnea-hypopnea index (AHI; defined as the number of apneas plus hypopneas per hour of sleep) of 5 or less is considered normal. The respiratory disturbance index (RDI), a term often incorrectly used interchangeably with AHI, includes respiratory effort–related arousals in addition to apneas and hypopneas per hour of sleep. Most investigators consider an AHI or RDI of 10 or more to be clinically significant.

Sleep-related apneas and hypopneas in neurologic diseases are secondary sleep apnea syndromes, in contrast to primary OSA syndrome, in which in many cases no cause except for minor deviations of the upper airway anatomic configuration is found to account for the appearance of apnea. The neurologic illness may be aggravated by the secondary sleep apnea because of the adverse effects of sleep-induced hypoxemia and hypercapnia, and repeated arousals with sleep fragmentation. In long-standing cases there may be pulmonary hypertension, congestive cardiac failure, and other manifestations of chronic sleep deprivation.

Paradoxical Breathing

The thorax and abdomen move in opposite directions during paradoxical breathing, indicating increased upper airway resistance. In upper airway resistance syndrome, this may be noted without any change in oronasal airflow; in OSA, however, paradoxical breathing is accompanied by reduction or absence of oronasal airflow.

Cheyne-Stokes and Cheyne-Stokes Variant Patterns of Breathing

Cheyne-Stokes breathing (CSB) is a special type of central apnea manifested as cyclic changes in breathing with a crescendo-decrescendo sequence separated by central apneas (see Fig. 19–2).[81–83] The Cheyne-Stokes *variant pattern* of breathing is distinguished by the substitution of hypopneas for apneas.[19,21] In neurologic disorders, the Cheyne-Stokes type of breathing is mostly noted in bilateral cerebral hemispheric lesions[12,13] and it worsens during sleep, whereas Cheyne-Stokes variant patterns of breathing may also be noted in brain stem lesions, in addition to bilateral cerebral hemispheric disease. In the AASM scoring manual,[79] CSB is scored if there are at least 3 consecutive cycles of cyclical crescendo-decrescendo change in breathing amplitude accompanied by at least one of the following: five or more central apneas and hypopneas per hour of sleep; and a cyclic crescendo-decrescendo change in breathing amplitude and duration of at least 10 consecutive minutes. The cycle length is most commonly in the range of 60 seconds but must be at least 45 seconds in duration. The arousals typically occur in the middle of the hyperventilation cycle. This breathing pattern is most prominently seen in NREM sleep, particularly stages 1 and 2, and attenuates or disappears during REM sleep. Besides neurologic lesions, this pattern of breathing is noted in patients with severe congestive cardiac failure.

Dysrhythmic Breathing

Dysrhythmic breathing[81,84] is characterized by nonrhythmic respiration of irregular rate, rhythm, and amplitude during wakefulness with or without O_2 desaturation that becomes worse during sleep. Dysrhythmic breathing may result from an abnormality in the automatic respiratory pattern generator in the brain stem.

Apneustic Breathing

Apneustic breathing is characterized by prolonged inspiration with an increase in the ratio of inspiratory to expiratory time.[82] This type of breathing may result from a neurologic lesion in the caudal pons that disconnects the so-called apneustic center in the lower pons from the pneumotaxic center (parabrachial and Kölliker-Fuse nuclei) in the upper pons in association with vagotomy.[85,86]

Inspiratory Gasp

Inspiratory gasp is characterized by a short inspiration time and a relatively prolonged expiration (reduced inspiratory-expiratory time ratio).[87] Gasping or irregular breathing has been noted after lesion in the medulla.[16,82]

Ataxic Breathing

This type of breathing is characterized by clusters of cyclic irregular breathing followed by recurrent periods of apnea. The apnea length is greater than the ventilatory phase. Ataxic breathing is often noted in medullary lesions.[88]

Biot's Breathing

Biot's breathing is a special type of cluster breathing (ataxic breathing) characterized by breaths of nearly equal volume separated by long periods of apnea.[88] This is really a variant of ataxic or cluster breathing and may be found in patients with medullary lesions.

Other Abnormal Breathing Patterns

The following abnormal breathing patterns have also been noted in neurologic disorders, particularly in patients with Shy-Drager syndrome (multiple system atrophy [MSA])[74,76]:

- Nocturnal stridor causing severe inspiratory breathing difficulty
- Periodic central apnea in the erect position accompanied by postural fall of blood pressure in Shy-Drager syndrome[89]
- Prolonged periods of central apnea accompanied by mild O_2 desaturation in relaxed wakefulness, as if the respiratory centers "forgot" to breathe[81,84]
- Transient occlusion of the upper airway or transient uncoupling of intercostal and diaphragmatic muscle activity[84]
- Transient sudden respiratory arrest
- Catathrenia (respiratory dysrhythmia with bradypnea and groaning), characterized by prolonged expiration with the characteristic groaning noise. This may be mistaken for a central apnea but is really not an apnea, and there is no oxygen desaturation during the episode[90] (Fig. 29–8). It is considered a parasomnia, and the etiology and mechanism are at present unknown.

Sleep-Related Hypoventilation

Finally, sleep-related hypoventilation,[91] a type of respiratory dysrhythmia without any apnea or hypopnea, is seen commonly in neuromuscular and intrinsic pulmonary and thoracic restrictive disorders, and sometimes in brain stem lesions. Sleep-related hypoventilation is characterized by an increase in the partial pressure of arterial carbon dioxide (Pa_{CO_2}) of 10 mm Hg above the supine awake values during sleep.[79] This abnormal rise in Pa_{CO_2} is accompanied by severe sleep-related hypoxemia that is not due to apnea or hypopnea.

MECHANISM OF RESPIRATORY DYSRHYTHMIAS IN NEUROLOGIC DISEASE

Several mechanisms may be responsible for the respiratory abnormalities in sleep associated with neurologic disorders[74,81]:

1. Direct involvement causing structural alterations of the medullary respiratory neurons (automatic or metabolic respiratory controlling system) may result

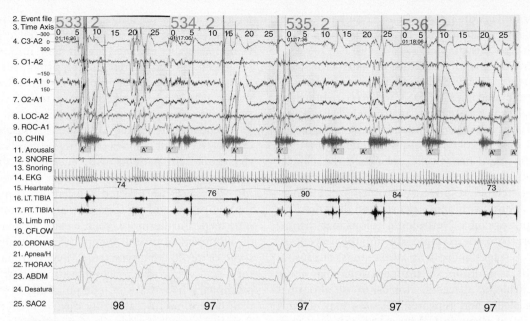

FIGURE 29–8 Catathrenia (expiratory groan). A polysomnographic segment of a 120-sec epoch showing the electroencephalogram (EEG: C3-A2, O1-A2, C4-A1, O2-A1); left and right eye movements (LOC-A2; ROC-A1); chin, left tibialis (LT.TIBI), and right tibialis (RT. TIBI) electromyograms (EMGs); snoring (SNORE); electrocardiogram (EKG); oronasal airflow (ORONAS); thoracic (THORAX) and abdominal (ABDM) effort channels; and oxygen saturation (Sao₂). Note prolonged expiration in the flow and effort channels followed by arousals without oxygen desaturation in stage 2 NREM sleep. *(Reproduced with permission from Siddiqui F, Walters AS, Chokroverty S. Catathrenia: a rare parasomnia which may mimic central sleep apnea on polysomnogram. Sleep Med 2008;9:460.)*

in apnea or hypopnea during NREM and REM sleep. During REM sleep, this problem may be aggravated because of the additional complicating factor of oropharyngeal or other upper airway muscle hypotonia contributing to upper airway OSA.

2. Involvement of the voluntary respiratory control system causes respiratory dysfunction during wakefulness and may give rise to respiratory apraxia.

3. Functional or neurochemical alteration of the respiratory neurons may cause respiratory dysrhythmia.

4. Interference with the afferent inputs to the medullary respiratory neurons (e.g., compromise of the peripheral chemoreceptors located in the vagal and glossopharyngeal nerve endings), supramedullary pathways, and central chemoreceptors in the ventrolateral medulla may cause abnormal breathing.

5. Direct involvement of the efferent mechanism through respiratory muscle weakness may result from either direct involvement of the muscles, as in myopathies, or involvement of the lower motor neurons to the respiratory muscles. In patients with weakness of the principal respiratory and the accessory respiratory muscles, the central respiratory neurons may increase their rate of firing or recruit additional respiratory neurons during wakefulness to maintain ventilation at a level adequate to drive the weak respiratory muscles. Because of the normal vulnerability of the respiratory neurons during sleep, the central respiratory neurons may not be able to participate in such

compensatory mechanisms during sleep in patients with respiratory muscle weakness. Ventilatory problems may thus be aggravated, causing more severe hypoventilation and even apnea during sleep. In addition, weakness of the upper airway muscles, which in fact are respiratory muscles and receive phasic inspiratory drive from the respiratory neurons in the brain stem, may cause obstructive apnea.

SLEEP AND BREATHING DISORDERS SECONDARY TO SOMATIC NEUROLOGIC ILLNESS

Neurologic disorders may affect sleep/wake-generating neurons, causing profound sleep disturbances that may include insomnia, hypersomnia, parasomnia, circadian rhythm disorders, and abnormal movements in sleep at night. An adverse interaction between neurologic illness and sleep dysfunction exists. The sleep disturbances may adversely affect the natural course of the neurologic illness. Sleep dysfunction may result from central or peripheral somatic or autonomic neurologic disorders.

A complaint of insomnia may be related to sleep onset or maintenance difficulties. Insufficient or fragmented night sleep may result in nonrestorative sleep, fatigue, muscle aches and pains, and poor attention and concentration as well as irritability, anxiety, depression, and impairment of daytime function with daytime somnolence. Most of the neurologic disorders cause hypersomnia, but sometimes insomnia is the predominant complaint[92,93]; an important but rare example, fatal familial insomnia (FFI), is described later in this chapter.

Hypersomnia is generally noted in patients with sleep-related respiratory dysrhythmias. Hypersomnia includes excessive daytime sleepiness (EDS) and irresistible sleep attacks. Associated complaints may include daytime fatigue, lack of concentration, impaired motor skills, morning headaches, and absence of symptom relief from additional sleep. In acute neurologic disorders, the clinical features of neurologic dysfunction may overshadow the sleep and sleep-related respiratory problems.[81] Furthermore, many patients with acute neurologic disorders are actually in stupor or coma. Neurologic lesions may disrupt the sleep architecture, for example, altering the percentage of different sleep stages, increasing awakenings, or causing sleep stage shifts. In addition, sleep apnea (which may occur in various neurologic diseases), intrusion of abnormal movements in sleep, and repeated seizures may disrupt the morphology of sleep and sleep stages. Sleep disturbances may impair memory, cognition, or behavior, or cause cardiopulmonary changes secondary to repeated hypoxemia. These effects, secondary to sleep disturbance, can aggravate the primary neurologic condition. Neurologic causes of hypersomnia have been described in Chapter 3.

The parasomnia (excessive motor activity and abnormal behavior intruding during sleep) most commonly noted in neurologic illnesses is REM sleep behavior disorder (RBD). This is characterized by intense motor activity related to dream-enacting behavior and absence of muscle atonia during REM sleep (see Chapter 35). It has been suggested that, in the setting of degenerative dementia or parkinsonism, RBD is a manifestation of evolving synucleinopathies (e.g., Parkinson's disease [PD], MSA, diffuse Lewy body disease [DLBD] with dementia) but is rare in tauopathies (e.g., Alzheimer's disease [AD]). Patients with RBD generally do not complain of EDS, and the Multiple Sleep Latency Test (MSLT) rarely documents increased somnolence. There is potential for injury to self and others in patients with RBD and, therefore, early recognition and treatment are very important. Circadian sleep-wake rhythm disturbances are noted in some neurologic disorders; most prominently, AD may present as a cyclic agitation syndrome. An excessive amount of nocturnal motor activity may be related to the primary neurologic disease (e.g., dystonia in patients with torsion dystonia and nocturnal frontal lobe epilepsy).

Clinical Manifestations

The clinical manifestations of sleep and breathing disorders in chronic neurologic illnesses may be divided into specific and general features.[74,81] The specific manifestations depend on the nature of the neurologic deficit. The general features that are relevant to the diagnosis of sleep-related hypoventilation and apnea include EDS,

fatigue, early morning headache, unexplained pedal edema, disturbed nocturnal sleep, intellectual deterioration, personality changes, and in men, impotence. Breathlessness is generally not an important feature of CNS disorders except those illnesses that affect the lower motor neurons to the respiratory muscles. The general symptoms of daytime fatigue, somnolence, and morning headache may be related to frequent arousals at night secondary to repeated apnea or hypopnea and carbon dioxide retention.[94] In patients with neurologic disorders, it is very important to recognize alveolar hypoventilation during sleep because assisted ventilation at night improves the symptoms and protects patients from fatal apnea during sleep. Furthermore, such treatment may prevent the development of serious complications resulting from episodic or prolonged hypoxemia, hypercapnia, and respiratory acidosis in sleep, complications that may include pulmonary hypertension, cor pulmonale, congestive cardiac failure, and occasionally cardiac arrhythmias. Occasionally, neurologic disorders may cause an inversion of the sleep-wake rhythm that is manifested by excessive somnolence during the day and insomnia with agitation during the night.[95]

To make a clinical diagnosis of sleep disorders or sleep-related breathing disorders (SRBDs), a careful history—from the patient and the caregiver—and a physical examination are essential.

Mechanisms of Sleep Disturbances

Neurologic disorders can be metabolic or structural (e.g., head injury, tumor, infection, toxic-metabolic brain dysfunction, vascular and degenerative CNS disease, headache from any cause, painful peripheral neuropathy, or other neuromuscular disorder). The following are the suggested mechanisms of the sleep disturbances associated with neurologic disorders[74,81,96]:

1. Direct involvement of the hypnogenic neurons. Hypofunction of the hypothalamic VLPO neurons or the lower brain stem hypnogenic neurons in the region of the NTS and dysfunction of the thalamus may alter the balance between the waking and the sleeping brain, causing wakefulness or sleeplessness. Similarly, a disorder of the posterior hypothalamic, ARAS, or other brain regions responsible for waking and alertness causes hypersomnolence.
2. Indirect mechanisms associated with the disorder, such as pain, confusional episodes, changes in the sensorimotor system, and movement disorders, can interfere with sleep.
3. Medications used to treat neurologic illnesses (e.g., anticonvulsants, antidepressants, dopamine agonists, anticholinergics, hypnotics, sedatives) may have a direct effect on sleep and breathing.
4. Neurologic diseases (e.g., hyperkinetic movement disorders, Rett syndrome) may change the

neurochemical environment of the sleep-generating and sleep-promoting neurons.[97]

5. Comorbid depression or anxiety in neurologic illnesses may disrupt sleep.

6. Certain neurologic disorders may alter circadian rhythm in the suprachiasmatic nuclei (e.g., dementia, PD, traumatic brain injury), causing insomnia.

7. Finally, neurologic disorders may cause sleep-disordered breathing (e.g., MSA, DLBD, and other neurodegenerative and neuromuscular disorders), resulting in sleep fragmentation and insomnia, and sleep apnea syndrome.

Sleep and Breathing Disturbances in Central Nervous System Disorders

Alzheimer's Disease and Related Dementias

Dementia is characterized by progressive deterioration of memory and cognition (as assessed by mental status and neuropsychological testing), followed by language dysfunction, hallucinations, other psychotic features, depression, and sleep disturbances. In the advanced stage of the illness, the patient becomes bedridden, mute, and incontinent. Sleep dysfunction with or without abnormal motor activity during sleep is increasingly recognized in patients with irreversible chronic dementing illness. It has been estimated that approximately 10% of the adult population over the age of 65 years suffer from some kind of dementing illness. AD is the most common cause of chronic dementia, accounting for at least 60% of all cases. Other conditions include DLBD, accounting for at least 15–20% of the cases; PD with dementia and frontotemporal dementia (FTD) in about 10%; and corticobasal degeneration (CBD), progressive supranuclear palsy (PSP), multi-infarct or vascular dementia, Huntington's disease (HD), Creutzfeldt-Jacob disease (CJD), and FFI (described later in the chapter), accounting for the rest of the cases.

Dementia can be classified according to location or according to molecular neurobiologic abnormalities (Table 29–1). In terms of location, dementia is classified into cortical dementia, consisting of AD, FTD, and vascular dementia; subcortical dementia, consisting of PD with dementia, PSP, and HD; and mixed cortical-subcortical dementia, including DLBD, CBD, CJD, and FFI. Most of the degenerative dementing illnesses are proteinopathies due to excessive protein misfolding and intracellular protein aggregation.[98] They are mainly classified into tauopathies, synucleinopathies, prion diseases and polyglutamine disease. Tau proteins belong to the family of microtubule-associated proteins involved in maintaining the cell shape and serve as tracts for axon transport. The main tauopathies include AD, PSP, CBD, argyrophilic grain disease, Pick's disease, and FTD with parkinsonism associated with chromosome 17. α-Synuclein is a presynaptic protein that helps transportation of dopamine-laden vessels from the cell body to the

TABLE 29–1 Classification of Dementia

According to Location

- Cortical dementia
  - Alzheimer's disease
  - Frontotemporal dementia
  - Vascular dementia
- Subcortical dementia
  - Parkinson's disease
  - Progressive supranuclear palsy
  - Huntington's disease
- Mixed cortical-subcortical dementia
  - Diffuse Lewy body disease
  - Corticobasal degeneration
  - Creutzfeldt-Jacob disease
  - Fatal familial insomnia

According To Molecular Neurobiology

- Taupathies
  - Alzheimer's disease
  - Frontotemporal dementia
  - Progressive supranuclear palsy
  - Corticobasal degeneration
- Synucleinopathies
  - Diffuse Lewy body disease
  - Parkinson's disease
  - Multiple system atrophy (Shy-Drager syndrome)
- Prion diseases
  - Fatal familial insomnia
  - Creutzfeldt-Jacob disease
- Polyglutamine disorder
  - Huntington's disease

synaptic cleft. Synucleinopathies are a group of disorders with abnormal deposition of α-synuclein in the cytoplasm of neurons or glial cells as well as in extracellular deposits of amyloid. The main synucleinopathies include PD, DLBD, and MSA, including Shy-Drager syndrome, striatonigral degeneration, and sporadic olivopontocerebellar atrophy.

Types of Sleep Disturbances in Dementia. The major sleep disturbances in dementing illness include insomnia, hypersomnia, circadian sleep-wake rhythm disorders, excessive nocturnal motor activity, "sundowning," and respiratory dysrhythmias. Circadian sleep-wake rhythm disturbances are noted, most prominently in AD, and may present as a cyclic agitation syndrome that is popularly known as sundown syndrome. Commonly encountered excessive nocturnal motor activity that may occasionally cause sleep disturbance to the patient but very often causes sleep disturbance to the bed partner includes periodic limb movements in sleep (PLMS), which may be noted in many of these dementing illnesses. Sleep-related respiratory dysrhythmias and loud snoring (see later) during sleep occur in some of these conditions, particularly in patients with AD, PD, and DLBD. Sleep dysfunction in AD may occur even in the early stage but is more common and severe in advanced stages. In addition to sundowning, these patients often sleep early in

TABLE 29–2 Criteria for the Clinical Diagnosis of Alzheimer's Disease

I. The criteria for the clinical diagnosis of probable Alzheimer's disease include

Dementia established by clinical examination and documented by the Mini-Mental Status Examination, Blessed Dementia Scale, or some similar examination, and confirmed by neuropsychologic tests;

Deficits in two or more areas of cognition;

Progressive worsening of memory and other cognitive functions;

No disturbance of consciousness;

Onset between ages of 40 and 90 years, most often older than age 65; and

Absence of systemic disorders or other brain diseases that could account for the progressive deficits in memory and cognition.

II. The diagnosis of probable Alzheimer's disease is supported by

Progressive deterioration of specific cognitive functions such as language (aphasia), motor skills (apraxia), and perception (agnosia);

Impaired activities of daily living and altered patterns of behavior;

Family history of similar disorders, particularly if confirmed neuropathologically; and

Laboratory results as follows:

Normal lumbar puncture as evaluated by standard techniques;

Normal pattern or nonspecific changes in EEG, such as increased slow-wave activity; and

Evidence of cerebral atrophy on computed tomography with progression documented by serial observations.

III. Other clinical features consistent with the diagnosis of probable Alzheimer's disease, after exclusion of causes of dementia other than Alzheimer's disease, include

Plateaus in the course of progression of the illness;

Associated symptoms of depression; insomnia; incontinence; delusions; illusions; hallucinations; catastrophic verbal, emotional, or physical outbursts; sexual disorders; and weight loss. Other neurologic abnormalities seen in some patients, especially those with more advanced disease, include motor signs such as increased muscle tone, myoclonus, and gait disorder;

Seizures in advanced disease; and

Computed tomography normal for age.

IV. Features that make the diagnosis of probable Alzheimer's disease uncertain or unlikely include

Sudden, apoplectic onset;

Focal neurologic findings such as hemiparesis, sensory loss, visual field deficits, and lack of coordination early in the course of the illness; and

Seizures or gait disturbances at the onset or very early in the course of the illness.

V. Clinical diagnosis of possible Alzheimer's disease

May be made on the basis of the dementia syndrome in the absence of other neurologic, psychiatric, or systemic disorders sufficient to cause dementia, and in the presence of variations in the onset, presentation, or clinical course;

May be made in the presence of a second systemic or brain disorder sufficient to produce dementia but not considered to be the cause of the dementia; and

Should be used in research studies when a single, gradually progressive, severe cognitive deficit is identified in the absence of other identifiable cause.

VI. Criteria for the diagnosis of definite Alzheimer's disease include the clinical criteria for probable Alzheimer's disease and histopathologic evidence obtained from a biopsy or autopsy.

VII. Classification of Alzheimer's disease for research purposes should specify features that may differentiate subtypes of the disorder, such as

Familial occurrence;

Onset before age 65 years;

Presence of trisomy 21; and

Coexistence of other relevant conditions, such as Parkinson's disease.

Reprinted with permission from McKhann G, Drachman D, Folstein M, et al. Clinical diagnosis of Alzheimer's disease: report of the NINCDS-ADRDA work group under the auspices of Department of Health and Human Services Task Force on Alzheimer's Disease. Neurology 1984;34:939.

the evening, waking up frequently, and staying awake most of the night. Their sleep is fragmented and fractionated throughout a 24-hour period. The patients remain somnolent most of the time and bedridden in the advanced stages of the illness.

Sleep Dysfunction in Alzheimer's Disease. AD, or senile dementia of the Alzheimer's type, is characterized by progressive intellectual deterioration occurring in middle or later life associated with characteristic neuropathologic findings, including cerebral cortical atrophy and neuronal loss in the nucleus basalis of Meynert. There is also evidence of alterations in the forebrain cholinergic, and in many cases also in the noradrenergic system.[99] Sleep disturbances in AD may be related partly to the severity of the loss of the cholinergic neurons in the basal forebrain regions, as well as to changes in the brain stem aminergic systems. For the diagnosis of probable, possible, and definite AD, readers are referred to the clinical criteria developed by the National Institute of Neurological and Communicative Disorders and Stroke–Alzheimer's Disease and Related Diseases Association

(NINCDS-ADRDA) work group (Table 29–2).[100] Since the introduction of the work group criteria in 1984, there have been significant advances in the development of reliable biomarkers for AD based on structural magnetic resonance imaging (MRI), molecular neuroimaging with positron emission tomography, and cerebrospinal fluid (CSF) analysis. Based on these advances, in addition, diagnostic criteria have been established for non-AD dementias (e.g., FTD, DLBD with dementia, CBD, and vascular dementia). Many of these entities may fulfill the original NINCDS-ADRDA criteria, but the diagnostic accuracy of the original criteria ranges from 65% to 96% and the specificity ranges from 23% to 88%. It is therefore now time to revise the diagnostic criteria, taking into consideration recent advances given the rapid growth of knowledge about the potential pathogenic mechanisms of AD. Dubois et al.[101] have offered a new approach to the definition of AD (Table 29–3). The purpose of these new diagnostic criteria is to identify patients in the early stages with significant episodic memory impairment so that the newly developed drugs aimed at changing the pathogenesis of the tauopathies can be introduced early

TABLE 29–3 Newly Proposed Diagnostic Criteria for Alzheimer's Disease (AD)

Probable AD Criteria

Category A and one or more supportive features in B, C, D, or E

Core Diagnostic Criteria
A. Presence of an early and significant episodic memory impairment with gradual and progressive alteration in memory function over the previous 6 months or more associated with objective evidence of impaired episodic memory

Supportive Features
B. Presence of medial temporal lobe atrophy on MRI
C. Abnormal cerebrospinal fluid biomarker with low amyloid β concentrations with increased tau concentrations
D. Specific pattern on functional neuroimaging with PET showing reduced glucose metabolism in temporal parietal regions bilaterally
E. Proven AD autosomal dominant mutation within the immediate family

Exclusion Criteria

- History of sudden onset and early occurrence of vague disturbance, seizures and behavioral changes.
- Clinical features of focal neurological findings or early extrapyramidal signs
- Other medical disorders accounting for memory and related symptoms

Definite AD Criteria

- Both clinical and histopathological evidence of AD as well as both clinical and genetic evidence (mutation in chromosome 1, 14, or 21) of AD

MRI, magnetic resonance imaging; PET, positron emission tomography.
Reprinted with permission from Dubois B, Feldman HH, Jacova C, et al. Research criteria for the diagnosis of Alzheimer's disease: revising the NINCDS-ADRDA criteria. Lancet Neurol 2007;6:734.

to slow down the progress of the disease. The new diagnostic criteria, however, need validation studies to optimize their sensitivity and specificity.

Sleep disorders in AD may increase cognitive and behavioral dysfunction. Such sleep disorders may arise directly from the disease itself, as a consequence of the degeneration of the brain stem and other centers that regulate sleep,[102] or indirectly from changes in sleep associated with aging (see Chapter 36). Sleep disorders can have a number of undesirable consequences, including increasing cardiovascular and even cerebrovascular morbidity as well as impairing daytime alertness and functioning.[78,103]

A number of studies have examined the differences between demented patients and normal elderly individuals and have demonstrated higher prevalence of sleep apnea and poorer sleep quality when patients are compared to age-matched controls.[103,104] Although the results vary somewhat from study to study, these investigations have shown deterioration of sleep parameters, including reduced total length of sleep, decreased REM and stage 4 NREM sleep, loss of phasic components (spindles and

K complexes) of NREM sleep, and sleep-wake rhythm disturbances, in demented patients.[104–109] Montplaisir et al.[109] documented EEG slowing during both wakefulness and REM sleep in AD patients. The authors suggested that degeneration of the nucleus basalis of Meynert, which is the main source of cholinergic input to the cerebral cortex, may be responsible for EEG slowing and REM sleep changes. This pattern of disorder is different from that of depressed elderly patients, who most clearly show poor sleep maintenance, often with increased REM sleep.[105] Most of the studies, however, have not used current diagnostic criteria for dementia and have lumped together patients with different forms of it. When more accurate diagnostic groupings were made, similar results were found for AD patients, usually defined by clinical course. Some studies have shown a clear association between greater sleep disturbance and impaired mental functioning or severity of dementia.[102,110–112]

Some of the inconsistencies noted in the sleep architecture in AD patients[113,114] may be related to the fact that, in many studies, mild, moderate, and severe AD patients were grouped together and not necessarily analyzed separately. Another point to remember is that it is often difficult to separate the effects of the disease on sleep from the effects of medication and of PLMS or sleep apneas, both of which are common in elderly patients. Additionally, sleep architectural alterations noted during overnight sleep studies in the laboratory may be partly environmentally determined, as AD patients may become confused, displaying features of sundowning, in the artificial and foreign environment of the laboratory.

Vitiello and coworkers[115,116] and others[104,105,108,117–120] reported sleep disturbances in AD associated with a decrease in slow-wave sleep and an increase in nighttime awakenings. In a study of 45 control subjects and 44 mild AD patients, Vitiello's group[121] confirmed their previous findings of disturbed sleep-wake patterns in AD patients, but the phenomenon of sleep disturbances was not diagnostically useful for discriminating between those with a mild stage of AD and control subjects.

A meta-analysis by Benca et al.[113] clearly showed significant sleep disturbances in dementia. Reduced sleep efficiency, increased stage 1 NREM sleep, and increased number of awakenings are some of the prominent findings noted in the various studies.[104,105,108,115–127] In some studies, there is a relationship between the severity of sleep disturbance and the severity of dementia.[121] Contradictory findings have been noted regarding decrement of slow-wave sleep. Reduction of sleep spindles is noted by Prinz et al.[108] as well as by Montplaisir et al.[128] REM sleep abnormalities have given inconsistent results (decreased in some studies[108,121] but not in others[124,127]), and this discrepancy may have been related to the degree of severity of dementia. It should be kept in mind that more severe sleep disturbances have been noted in depression than in dementia, and sometimes differentiating these two conditions, particularly in the early stage of AD, may be difficult. Other sleep architectural changes in AD include sleep-wake cycle[129] and sleep rhythm[130] disturbances and alterations in physiologic delta waves.[131] These sleep quality changes may cause EDS.[132,133]

Sleep is disturbed early in the disease process, and sleep disturbances are noted even in the presence of mild cognitive impairment.[134,135] It has been suggested that sleep disturbances and cognitive dysfunction are positively correlated in AD—that is, sleep disturbances increase with severity of disease process.[136] Disruption in sleep-wake patterns, circadian rhythmicity, increased amount and frequency of nighttime wakefulness, and reduction of slow-wave sleep occur at the early stages of AD and worsen with disease progression. In later stages of AD, there is a reduction of REM sleep, increased REM latency, and alteration of the circadian rhythm resulting in daytime sleepiness. The daytime sleep, however, consists essentially of NREM stages 1 and 2 and does not compensate effectively for the loss of slow-wave sleep and REM sleep. Thus daytime napping and somnolence increase as the disease progresses.

The phenomenon of sundowning is noted in many AD patients, contributing to sleep disturbance. Sundowning can be described as cyclic nocturnal agitation syndrome with inversion of sleep schedule (wakefulness at night and somnolence in the daytime). It is most likely related to the severity of dementia and remains a common cause of institutionalization in AD patients. Factors such as going to bed early, increased use of sedatives, advanced cognitive impairment, associated medical conditions, and circadian rhythm disturbances may all contribute to sundowning. Sleep-wake rhythm disturbances are common in AD.[116] Circadian rhythm disturbances are frequently seen and pronounced in AD.[137] It has been suggested that an alteration in the biological clock in the SCN and the pineal gland are considered to be the biological basis for the circadian rhythm disturbances in AD. Wu and Swaab[137] found disruption of pineal melatonin secretion and pineal clock gene oscillations in AD patients. They noted even in the earliest AD stage a functional disruption of the SCN as manifested by decreased vasopressin RNA, a clock-controlled major output of the SCN. The functional disconnection between the SCN and the pineal gland noted in the earliest stage of AD seems to account for the pineal clock gene and melatonin changes accounting for the circadian rhythm disturbances in AD. They also noted decreased melatonin MT_1 receptor in the SCN in late-stage AD patients and therefore suggested that, in the advanced stages of AD, supplementary treatment with melatonin may not improve the circadian rhythm disturbances. Wu and Swaab[138] previously suggested that circadian disorders, such as sleep-wake cycle disturbances, associated with aging and advanced stages of AD causing disruptive melatonin production and rhythms may result from presumed degeneration of the retina-SCN-pineal axis. They further suggested that reactivation of the circadian system (retina-SCN-pineal pathway) by use of light therapy and melatonin supplementation to restore the circadian rhythm and relieve clinical circadian disturbances has shown promising results.

However, there are contradictory reports.[139,140] Dowling et al.[139] tested the effectiveness of time to bright-light therapy given in the morning and early afternoon in 70 institutionalized patients with AD and controls. They did not find any significant differences in actigraphy-based measures of nighttime sleep or daytime wakefulness between the groups. They therefore concluded that 1 hour of bright-light treatment in patients with AD in the morning or early afternoon did not improve nighttime sleep or daytime wakefulness compared to the control group. In another study, Dowling et al.[140] tested the effect of morning bright-light therapy in 46 AD subjects fulfilling the NINCDS-ADRDA criteria in two nursing home facilities in California. They gave 1 hour of bright-light exposure (≥ 2500 lux) to the experimental group and gave usual indoor light (150–200 lux) to the control group. By means of actigraphy, they assessed nighttime sleep efficiency, total sleep time, and number of awakenings. They also determined circadian rhythm parameters from the actigraphy data using core cosinor analysis and nonparametric techniques. They concluded that morning bright-light exposure did not induce an overall improvement in measures of sleep or rest activity in all treated patients compared to control subjects. However, they found that only subjects with the most impaired rest activity rhythm responded significantly and positively to a brief (1 hour) light therapy. Singer et al.[141] conducted a multicenter, placebo-controlled trial of melatonin for sleep disturbance in 157 individuals with AD recruited by 36 AD centers. They measured nocturnal total sleep time, sleep efficiency, wake time after sleep onset, and day-night sleep ratio during a 2- to 3-week baseline and 2 months of treatment with melatonin. The sleep measures were obtained from the actigraphic data. They did not find any statistically significant differences in objective sleep measures between baseline and treatment for any of the group. Therefore, they concluded that melatonin is not an effective agent for treating sleep disturbances in patients with AD. The results of these studies, therefore, contradict the earlier findings of Mishima et al.[142] of altered melatonin secretion rhythms in patients with AD having disturbed sleep-wake patterns.

Sleep apnea has been observed in approximately 33–53% of demented patients with probable AD[102,111,112,143] (Fig. 29–9). Although sleep apnea may be associated with disease severity, no longitudinal studies have been conducted to determine whether sleep apnea increases the severity of disease in individual patients and whether sleep apnea may be associated with more rapid progression of the disease. Such a deleterious effect of sleep apnea is to be expected, as it is thought to increase the intellectual

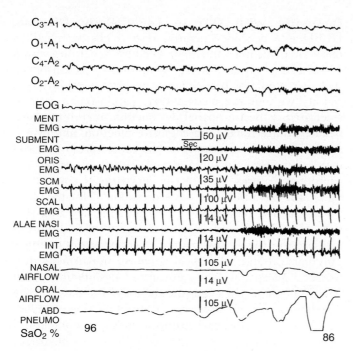

FIGURE 29–9 Polysomnographic recording of a patient in an advanced stage of Alzheimer's disease shows a portion of mixed apnea during stage 2 NREM sleep accompanied by oxygen desaturation. Top four channels represent the electroencephalogram (EEG) (Key: international electrode placement system). Electromyograms (EMG) of mentalis (MENT), submental (SUBMENT), orbicularis (ORIS), sternocleidomastoid (SCM), scalenus anticus (SCAL), alae nasi, and intercostal (INT) muscles are shown. Also shown are nasal and oral airflow, abdominal pneumogram (ABD PNEUMO), and oxygen saturation (Sao_2%). (EOG = electro-oculogram.) *(Reproduced with permission from Chokroverty S. Sleep and breathing in neurological disorders. In NH Edelman, TV Santiago [eds], Breathing Disorders of Sleep. New York: Churchill Livingstone, 1986;225.)*

deficit of demented patients.[110,111] Because sleep apnea may be treated by a number of modalities, it is possible that therapy may improve behavior and cognitive function, although as yet there are no reports of the effects of treatment of sleep apnea in AD or dementia. According to Smallwood and colleagues,[112] the incidence of sleep apnea in male AD patients is similar to that in healthy elderly subjects. Reynolds and coworkers[144] reported a higher prevalence of sleep apnea in female AD patients during the later stage of the illness than in controls. These findings have been confirmed by Vitiello et al.[115] and Mant et al.[145] A key genotypic marker of AD is the apolipoprotein E4 (*APOE4*) allele. In recent years the demonstration of an association between *APOE4*-genotype AD and sleep apnea has kindled interest in the possible association between sleep apnea and AD.[146–148] Gehrman et al.[149] suggested sleep apnea or sleep-disordered breathing (SDB) may be related to agitation in AD. These authors recorded sleep for 1 night and measured agitation with behavioral observations and ratings by nursing staff in 38 patients (29 women, 9 men) in a nursing home population. They found that SDB was very prevalent in this sample and was related to some types of agitation during the day but not in the

evening and night. They further suggested that treatment of SDB may decrease agitation in these patients. In a later study by this group[150] utilizing 66 patients with mild to moderate AD in a home polysomnographic (PSG) study, the authors observed that the patients with SDB spent less time in REM sleep than those with no SDB, but they did not find any differences in other sleep stages. They concluded that decreased REM sleep may be due to the presence of SDB in AD. They further speculated that treating these patients' SDB may increase their amount of REM sleep, which may result in improved daytime functioning. Chong et al.[151] randomly assigned 39 community-dwelling elderly patients with mild to moderate probable AD with SDB to receive 6 weeks of therapy with continuous positive airway pressure (CPAP) titration or 3 weeks of sham CPAP followed by 3 weeks of therapeutic CPAP. They measured Epworth Sleepiness Scale (ESS) scores at baseline, 3 weeks, and 6 weeks to measure the changes in daytime sleepiness. Their results of reduction of ESS scores after therapeutic but not sham CPAP treatment supported the effectiveness of CPAP in reducing subjective daytime sleepiness in AD patients with SDB.

Pseudodementia in elderly depressed patients presents a frequent diagnostic dilemma in differentiating depression from dementia of the Alzheimer's type. It has been noted that depressed elderly patients have shortened REM latency and increased REM density; in contrast, AD patients tend to have greater reduction in the amount of REM sleep and lower REM density.[152,153] These findings, however, are not useful as a predictive indicator on a case-to-case basis.

Hallucinations may occur in AD patients but are noted much less frequently than in DLBD (see later). Sinforiania et al.[154] administered a sleep questionnaire in the presence of a caregiver to 280 patients in order to evaluate the relationship between hallucinations and sleep-wake cycle in patients with early to moderate AD. They noted hallucinations, mainly visual, in 12% of the sample, and 69% of the hallucinations occurred when the patient was awake. Vivid dreams were reported in 11% and violent sleep-related and dream-related behaviors (probable RBD episodes) were noted in 10% of the subjects. The authors concluded that the higher occurrence of vivid dreams and RBD in AD patients with hallucinations compared with those without hallucinations indicates a potential role of disordered REM sleep in the occurrence of hallucinations in AD. It should be noted that, in most of the reports, RBD has not been seen frequently in tauopathies such as AD. Although RBD is rare, REM sleep without atonia may be noted relatively frequently in patients with probable AD.[155] EDS is very common in AD, and in order to assess daytime sleep propensity in a cohort of patients with mild to moderate AD, Bonanni et al.[156] studied 20 drug-free AD patients meeting the NINCDS-ADRDA criteria for probable AD and a group of 12 healthy subjects free of dementia as controls.

They used Multiple Sleep Latency Tests and overnight PSG recordings to evaluate daytime sleepiness. Their findings of significantly reduced daytime sleep latencies indicated an increased sleep propensity during the daytime in patients with mild to moderate AD. Park et al.[133] observed that AD patients with excessive daytime napping had more parkinsonian motor signs, suggesting that this subgroup may have an increased propensity for sleepiness resembling PD. The authors cautioned that longitudinal studies with objective measures are needed to determine whether a causal relationship exists between sleepiness and parkinsonism in AD.

The pathogenesis of sleep disturbances in AD is multifactorial, resulting from possible degeneration of neurons regulating sleep-wake cycles, SDB, and disruptive chronobiology. However, no longitudinal studies are currently available correlating sleep apnea with the severity or progression of the disease. Suprachiasmatic nuclei regulating circadian rhythm show degenerative loss of neurons in AD, which may explain inversion of rhythm in many patients. Other factors include normal age-related physiologic changes in sleep, medication effects, increased prevalence of PLMS causing arousal and sleep fragmentation in the elderly AD patients, environmental factors (e.g., artificial environment of the institution, laboratory, and nursing homes), and comorbid medical disorders or depression. Finally, there may be a genetically increased risk of sleep disruption in AD. Craig et al.[157] surveyed 426 AD patients diagnosed according to standard criteria and performed genotyping of APOE. They found that increased susceptibility to sleep disturbance is associated with genetic variation at the enzyme monoamine oxidase A.

In summary, it is known that sleep dysfunction is common in AD. It is unclear, however, whether a specific set of sleep abnormalities will be found to be associated with AD that are different from those observed in other dementias. Reynolds and coworkers[105] suggested that sleep dysfunction in AD may be related to the progression of the disease and may cause ongoing deterioration of the alertness, orientation, and cognitive function. Table 29–4 summarizes the sleep dysfunction in AD.

TABLE 29–4 Summary of Sleep Dysfunction in Alzheimer's Disease

- May occur in the early stage
- More common and severe in advanced stages
- Sleep onset in the early evening; waking up frequently or staying awake most of the night
- Sleep architectural changes, including decreased sleep efficiency, reduced slow-wave sleep with eventual disappearance as the disease advances, increased awakenings after sleep onset, and reduced REM sleep in later stages
- "Sundowning"
- Fragmented and fractionated sleep throughout the 24-hour period with increased daytime napping
- Sleep apnea: 33–53%; more with APOE4 allele
- Visual hallucinations with nocturnal agitations
- In advanced stage, somnolent most of the time

Dementia with Diffuse Lewy Body Disease. DLBD is a neurodegenerative disease characterized by onset of dementia (impaired executive function) within 12 months of onset of motor symptoms of parkinsonism such as akinesia or bradykinesia, postural instability, and rigidity without the characteristic parkinsonian tremor, associated with visuospatial dysfunction, recurrent visual hallucinations, fluctuating cognitive function, and hypersensitivity to neuroleptics. The clinical features of DLBD may be divided into three groups: core, suggestive, and additional features.[158] A recent international consortium on DLBD has resulted in revised criteria[159] for the clinical and pathologic diagnosis, incorporating new information about the core clinical features and improved measures for their assessment. The core features are typically cortical and subcortical cognitive impairment with worse visuospatial and executive dysfunction than AD.[158] In the early stage, the memory dysfunction may be relatively spared. Other core features include recurrent visual hallucinations, parkinsonism, and fluctuating attention. Suggestive features consist of RBD, severe neuroleptic sensitivity, and low dopamine transporter uptake in the basal ganglia on functional neuroimaging. Additional features supporting the diagnosis but occurring less commonly include repeated falls and syncope, transient loss of consciousness, severe autonomic dysfunction, systematized delusions, olfactory and tactile hallucinations, depression, neuroimaging finding of relative preservation of medial temporal lobe structures, reduced occipital activity in functional neuroimaging, EEG slowing, and myocardial scintigraphy showing low uptake.[158] The pathologic criteria include the presence of Lewy bodies in limbic, paralimbic, and neocortical regions in addition to the midbrain substantia nigra, LC, and raphe nuclei. Senile plaques are present in the majority of individuals with DLBD, although neurofibrillary tangles are typically absent.

Studies inquiring about sleep disturbance in DLBD are few given its recent recognition and its clinical overlap with AD and PD. Sleep disturbances in DLBD are very common and more prominent in DLBD than in AD patients. The significant sleep disturbances in DLBD consist of insomnia, daytime hypersomnolence, RBD, sleep apnea, and nocturnal visual hallucinations. Grace and colleagues[160] made a comparative study of sleep profiles in patients with DLBD and AD. They reported more overall sleep disturbances, more movement disorders in sleep, and more abnormal daytime sleepiness in DLBD patients in comparison with AD patients. RBD is very common in DLBD (present in 50–80% of DLBD patients), and sometimes may be the initial presentation without other core diagnostic features.[161,162] Boeve and colleagues in a series of studies[39,163–167] suggested that RBD is a manifestation of an underlying α-synucleinopathy (e.g., PD, DLBD, and MSA) and may be a forerunner or precursor of the disease. Neuropathologic studies by

Uchiyama et al.[168] and Boeve et al.[163–167] supported the conclusion that idiopathic RBD may be a preclinical sign of DLBD. Disturbance of the circadian rhythm has been noted and is a potential factor underlying the nocturnal sleep fragmentation and daytime sleepiness in many AD and DLBD patients. Harper et al.[169] studied circadian variation of core body temperature and motor activity in a total of 32 institutionalized patients with probable AD by NINCDS-ADRDA criteria, 9 of whom also met pathologic criteria for DLBD, and in 8 elderly male controls. They noted that patients with a postmortem diagnosis of DLBD manifested greater disturbances of locomotor activity circadian rhythms than patients with AD, which may reflect the greater sleep disturbances seen in this population. Bauman et al.[170] reported EDS with normal CSF hypocretin in 10 DLBD patients.

Sleep Disturbances in Frontotemporal Dementia. FTD is a type of cortical dementia and a tauopathy resembling AD, but there are many features differentiating these two entities. Sleep disturbances are noted in many FTD patients but have not been adequately characterized. The clinical features of FTD include core and supportive features.[171] Core features include insidious onset and progression, and early loss of insight, social decline, personal conduct, and emotional blunting with relative preservation of perception, praxis, and memory. Supportive features include perseveration, hyperorality, impersistence, mental inflexibility, decline in personal hygiene, and altered speech and language dysfunction such as echolalia, mutism, reduced speech output, and lack of spontaneity in speech. Physical findings may include akinesia, rigidity, and appearance of primitive reflexes. Laboratory tests may include normal EEG, and neuropsychological tests show frontal lobe impairment. Computed tomography (CT) and MRI of the brain may show frontal or temporal lobe atrophy.

In a retrospective review of the clinical records, Seeley et al.[172] studied the natural history of the temporal variant of FTD and divided FTD into three stages according to the progression of symptoms. Stage 1 is characterized by either semantic loss characterized by anomia with word-finding difficulties and repetitive speech or an early behavioral syndrome characterized by emotional distance, irritability, and disruption of sleep, appetite, and libido. In stage 2, appearing on an average after 3 years, patients have both semantic and behavioral syndromes. In stage 3, generally 5–7 years after onset, in addition to the above features patients now have disinhibition, compulsions, impaired face recognition, altered food preference, and weight gain. The authors concluded that the temporal variant of FTD follows a characteristic cognitive and behavioral progression, suggesting early spread from one anterior temporal lobe to the other, and the latest symptoms implicate ventromedial frontal, insular, and infero-posterior temporal regions. However, they caution that

precise anatomic correlates need to be confirmed. Liu et al.[173] compared the behavioral features in the frontal and temporal variants of FTD and performed volumetric measurements of the frontal, anterior temporal, and ventromedial frontal cortex and the amygdala in 51 patients with FTD and 20 normal controls as well as 22 patients with AD serving as dementia controls. They found that the group with the frontal variant of FTD showed more anxiety, apathy, and eating disorders, and the group with the temporal variant of FTD showed a higher prevalence of sleep disturbances, than patients with AD. The behavior between the two variants may be differentiated: there is greater apathy in the frontal variant and more sleep disturbances in the temporal variant of FTD.

Hemispheric/Diencephalic Stroke

Stroke is an acute neurologic deficit resulting from vascular injury to the brain and is the third leading cause of death and disability. Vascular injury could be ischemic (thrombotic or embolic) or hemorrhagic. In this section, sleep and breathing disorders in cerebral hemispheric and thalamic strokes are described. Those resulting from brain stem stroke are discussed in a later section.

There are a few scattered reports of sleep complaints after stroke and several reports of SRBDs after cerebral infarction, but there is a dearth of well-controlled studies of the relationship between sleep disorders and cerebral vascular disease. Such studies are important from prognostic and therapeutic points of view.

Hemispheric Stroke. Sleep disruption and sleep complaints resulting from sleep-related breathing dysrhythmias have been reported in many patients with cerebral hemispheric stroke. Sleep apnea, snoring, and stroke are intimately related. Sleep apnea may predispose to stroke and stroke may predispose to sleep apnea. There is increasing evidence based on case-control, epidemiologic, and laboratory studies that snoring and sleep apnea are risk factors for stroke. Confounding variables that are common risk factors for snoring, sleep apnea, and stroke (e.g., hypertension, cardiac disease, age, body mass index (BMI), smoking, and alcohol consumption) should be considered when attempting to establish relationships among snoring, sleep apnea, and stroke. A history of habitual snoring (established through questionnaire studies and interviews with a bed partner or other family members) is a clear risk factor for stroke. There is an increased frequency of sleep apnea in both infratentorial and supratentorial strokes. Sleep apnea may adversely affect the short-term and long-term outcomes in patients with stroke in terms of both morbidity and mortality. It is important to make the diagnosis of sleep apnea in stroke patients, as there is effective treatment for sleep apnea that can decrease the risk of future stroke.

Case-control and epidemiologic studies have established an association between hypertension and habitual snoring[174–177] and between habitual snoring and stroke.[177–182] The prospective study by Koskenvuo et al.,[177] adjusting for other risk factors, found that habitual snorers have a significantly increased risk of new stroke or ischemic heart disease. Neau et al.[183] also found a significantly increased adjusted risk of stroke in habitual snorers. Spriggs et al.[184] found that, in addition to increasing the risk for stroke, snoring adversely affected the prognosis after a stroke. In a prospective study, Bassetti et al.[185] used PSG to determine the frequency of habitual snoring and sleep apnea in 36 of 59 subjects within 12 days of acute hemispheric stroke or transient ischemic attack (TIA) and in 19 age- and sex-matched controls. Habitual snoring was reported in 58% of patients with TIA or stroke, in addition to an increased frequency of sleep apnea in patients with TIA and acute stroke.

There is considerable evidence based on several recent large epidemiologic and many case-control studies showing an independent association between obstructive sleep apnea syndrome (OSAS) and stroke. Sleep apnea has been found in more than 50% of patients with acute stroke. The pathogenesis is not clearly known and most likely is multifactorial, involving sympathetic nervous system hyperactivity, activation of inflammatory molecular pathways, endothelial dysfunction, metabolic dysregulation, abnormal coagulation, dyslipidemia, and insulin resistance.[186] There are several well-established risk factors for the development of stroke, including arterial hypertension, cardiac disease, diabetes mellitus, smoking, and dyslipidemia. Although the evidence of association between OSAS and stroke is strong based on mainly cross-sectional, case-control, and some limited longitudinal studies, large-scale collaborative studies including patients with OSA controlled adequately for potential confounders are needed to evaluate the relationship between OSAS and stroke and the potential interactions between different basic mechanisms. The Sleep Heart Health Study[187] is a cross-sectional study including a sample of 6424 individuals who underwent unattended overnight PSG at home. Sleep apnea was significantly associated with development of stroke, coronary artery disease, and congestive cardiac failure independent of known cardiovascular risk factors. A higher prevalence of OSA has also been shown in patients with TIAs compared with controls by Bassetti and Aldrich.[188] Cross-sectional studies, however, cannot make a definite conclusion about the cause-and-effect relationship, and therefore prospective longitudinal studies are needed. A prospective cohort study of patients admitted for stroke or TIA by Parra et al.[189] demonstrated a higher prevalence of OSAS than in the general population. However, this was contradicted in a small case-control study involving 86 patients with TIA matched for age and sex with controls that showed no significant difference in the severity of prevalence of OSAS between the two groups.[190] A study by Wierzbicka et al.[191] involving 43 patients found a high

prevalence of sleep apnea in patients with acute stroke and TIA. The authors suggested that overnight screening for SDB should be routinely performed in every patient admitted with stroke or ischemic attack. Grigg-Damberger,[192] in a review article, made a similar suggestion, and noted that such screening and treatment for OSAS should be incorporated into stroke prevention programs.

In an important observational cohort study, Yaggi et al.[193] performed PSG in 1022 consecutive patients enrolled in the study and verified subsequent events such as strokes and deaths. Proportional-hazards analysis was used to determine the independent effect of OSAS on the composite outcome of stroke or death. At baseline, 697 patients (68%) had a mean AHI of 35 as compared with 2 in controls. After a median follow-up period of 3.4 years, the OSAS syndrome was associated with stroke or death from any cause with a hazard ratio of 2.24. After adjusting for age, sex, smoking habits, alcohol consumption, BMI, and the presence or absence of diabetes mellitus, hyperlipidemia, atrial fibrillation, and hypertension, OSAS retained its statistically significant association with stroke or death with a hazard ratio of 1.97. The authors concluded that OSAS significantly increases the risk of stroke or death from any cause and the increase is independent of other risk factors. Several other studies confirmed an independent association between OSAS and stroke.[194–202] Harbison et al.[194] performed a prospective, uncontrolled observational study at week 2 and weeks 6–9 following stroke utilizing paired respiratory sleep studies, modified ranking score, Barthel score, Scandinavian Neurological Stroke score, and ESS score. They concluded that SDB improved in the first 6–9 weeks following stroke but remained highly prevalent. They made a surprising observation of the presence of SDB in patients with lacunar stroke. Marin et al.[195] did an observational study to compare the incidence of fatal and nonfatal cardiovascular events, including stroke, in simple snorers. They included patients with untreated OSAS, patients treated with CPAP titration, and healthy men recruited from the general population. The subjects were followed up at least once a year for a minimum of 10.1 years, and CPAP adherence was checked with a built-in meter. The study included 264 healthy men, 377 simple snorers, 403 patients with untreated mild to moderate OSAS, 235 with untreated severe disease, and 372 with the disease who were treated with CPAP. They found that patients with untreated severe disease had a higher incidence of both fatal cardiovascular events (deaths from myocardial infarction or stroke) and nonfatal cardiovascular events than did untreated patients with mild to moderate disease, simple snorers, patients treated with CPAP, and healthy participants. The authors concluded that, in men, severe OSAS significantly increased the risk of fatal and nonfatal cardiovascular events and CPAP treatment reduced this risk. Munoz et al.[196] performed a prospective 6-year longitudinal population-based study in subjects ages

70–100 years. After adjustment for confounding factors, the authors confirmed that patients with severe OSAS at baseline had an increased risk of developing stroke independent of known confounding factors. Artz et al.[197] also demonstrated after a cross-sectional longitudinal analysis of subjects from the general population that there was a strong association between moderate to severe SDB and prevalence of stroke independent of the confounding factors. These authors also provided the first prospective evidence that SDB preceded stroke and may contribute to the development of stroke. In a prospective 10-year follow-up study, Sahlin et al.[203] obtained overnight sleep recordings at a mean of 23 days after the onset of stroke in 132 patients. They found that the risk of death was higher among the 23 patients with obstructive apnea (AHI $\geq$15) than controls (AHI <15), with an adjusted hazard ratio of 1.76 independent of all the confounding factors. There was no difference in mortality between central sleep apnea (CSA) patients and controls.[203]

Several studies[204–206] evaluated the role of CPAP in treatment of patients with OSAS and found significant protection against new vascular events after ischemic stroke. Bassetti et al.[206] found a beneficial effect of CPAP in a small percentage of patients. In contrast, after a randomized control trial of CPAP in patients with stroke with an AHI of 30 or more, Hsu et al.[207] found no benefit from CPAP treatment. These authors advocated that CPAP treatment should be used for patients with stroke only if there are symptoms of SDB. Similar to the findings of Bassetti et al.,[206] Palombani and Guilleminault[208] found that the majority of stroke patients with OSAS rejected CPAP treatment, and they suggested that better education and support of patients and families, and special training sessions, will be needed to improve adherence in such patients.

OSA is the most common form of SDB in stroke victims, and the prevalence in stroke patients exceeds the figure quoted for the general population.[190,201,209–217] Bassetti et al.[212] suggested that the presence of OSA should be suspected in men and elderly patients with diabetes mellitus and nighttime onset of TIA or stroke. The increased prevalence of OSAS in patients with TIA and stroke suggests that OSAS does not commonly precede but rather follows the onset of cerebrovascular events.[188,189] It is notable that acute stroke may aggravate preexisting SDB or even may cause it de novo.[188] Improvement of SDB often occurs in the recovery phase after stroke.[189,212] In addition to OSA, patients with stroke may have central apnea, including central periodic breathing and CSB.[218–220] Nopmaneejumrusler et al.[220] suggested that, in patients with stroke, CSA and Cheyne-Stokes respirations are associated with hypocapnia and occult left ventricular systolic dysfunction but are not related to the location or type of stroke. Hermann et al.[219] found central periodic breathing during sleep in 3 of 31 patients with first-ever stroke in absence of cardiopulmonary dysfunction. They assessed the patients using PSG, MRI of the brain, and echocardiography. They concluded that central periodic breathing during sleep may be present in strokes involving the autonomic (insular) and volitional (cingulate and thalamus) respiratory networks, and that breathing improved in all patients during stroke recovery.

Some studies have addressed circadian variations of stroke onset. In a study of 53 stroke patients, Kapen et al.[221] confirmed their previous reports of prevalence for the onset of stroke in the morning during a 6-hour period after awakening from sleep. This is similar to the peak incidence in the morning hours for myocardial infarction and sudden cardiac death. All of these conditions may be aggravated by a combination of circadian increase of corticosteroids and catecholamines, increased blood pressure and heart rate in the morning, and increased platelet "aggregability." (Normal subjects exhibit increased platelet aggregability in the early morning.[222]) In several other studies, the incidence of stroke was highest during sleep at night[223] or during early morning hours after awakening from nocturnal sleep.[178,224–226] In order to investigate circadian variations in situations at stroke onset, Omama et al.[227] analyzed 12,957 cases of first-ever stroke onset diagnosed from the Iowa Stroke Registry between 1991 and 1996 by CT or MRI of the brain. They noted that patients who had cerebral infarctions showed a bimodal pattern with a higher peak in the morning and a lower peak in the afternoon, whereas intracerebral hemorrhage and subarachnoid hemorrhage patients had the same bimodal pattern but with a lower peak in the morning and a higher peak in the afternoon. The authors concluded that sleep tends to promote ischemic stroke and suppresses hemorrhagic stroke. Another study from Japan[228] found that intracerebral hemorrhage during the sleep period may be more detrimental compared with the intracerebral hemorrhage during awake periods, causing larger hematoma and higher mortality rates. In a 10-year follow-up study of 1986 men ages 59–69 years, completing a questionnaire on sleep patterns, Ellwood et al.[198] found that the risk of an ischemic stroke is increased in men with a history of sleep disturbance, including EDS and sleep apnea.

Stroke may predispose to a number of sleep disorders. Kleine-Levin syndrome can occur after multiple cerebral infarction.[229] Narcolepsy-cataplexy has been reported to follow cerebral hypoxia-ischemia.[230] Insomnia is commonly noted after cerebral infarction, but this may be partly due to the depression that typically follows stroke.[231] Hermann and Bassetti[232] reported an increased prevalence of sleep-wake disturbances in at least 20–40% of stroke patients, mainly in the form of increased sleep need (hypersomnia), EDS, or insomnia. They listed several factors contributing to sleep-wake disorders in such patients, including depression, anxiety, SDB, complications resulting from stroke (e.g. nocturia, dysphagia, and urinary or respiratory infections), and medications. In another study by Palomaki et al.,[233] the authors concluded that insomnia is a common complaint after ischemic stroke. Total dream loss (Charcot-Wilbrand syndrome) after acute bilateral infarction of the deep occipital lobe as well as after parietal and deep frontal infarcts has been described by Bischof and Bassetti[234] and Solms.[235] Sleep architectural changes involving NREM and REM sleep have also been noted after cerebral hemispheric stroke.[236–239]

Diencephalic Stroke. Freund[240] should probably be credited with the first report of patients with hypersomnolence following paramedian thalamic strokes. Thalamic stroke may cause ipsilateral loss of sleep spindles,[241] and bilateral paramedian thalamic infarcts may be associated with hypersomnia.[242,243] Bassetti et al.[243] evaluated 12 patients with MRI-proven isolated paramedian thalamic stroke and hypersomnia. The patients were evenly divided between groups of severe and mild hypersomnia. Nocturnal PSG findings included increased stage 1 NREM sleep, reduced stage 2 NREM sleep, and a reduced number of sleep spindles. Bassetti et al.[243] found intact REM sleep as well as circadian, ultradian, and homeostatic sleep regulation in their patients, however. The authors concluded that hypersomnia after paramedian thalamic stroke is accompanied by deficient arousal during the day and insufficient spindling and slow-wave sleep production at night. Their observation supported the hypothesis of a dual role of the paramedian thalamus for the maintenance of sleep-wake regulation.

In contrast, Guilleminault et al.[244] reported three patients with pseudo-hypersomnia and presleep behavior with bilateral paramedian thalamic lesions. These authors used long-term monitoring with an infrared video camera and polygraphic study to document that their patients did not develop the normal NREM cycling during the day; rather, the EEG indicated a mixture of low-amplitude theta and alpha frequency waves during the day, with "sleep-like behavior." The patients exhibited the behavioral aspects of sleep during the day, suggesting to Guilleminault et al.[244] that these subjects did not present hypersomnia but a "de-arousal" and were left in the transition between wakefulness and sleep. These authors[244] cited a report by Catsman-Berrevoets and von Harskamp[245] of a similar patient with compulsive presleep behavior and apathy due to bilateral thalamic stroke who responded to bromocriptine. There are a few other scattered cases reported of hypersomnolence following bilateral paramedian thalamic infarct.[246–251]

Basal Ganglia Disorders

Sleep disturbances and sleep-related respiratory dysrhythmias are noted in many patients with basal ganglia disorders, but a systematic study to evaluate such dysfunction has not been undertaken in a large number of patients. A review of sleep and movement disorders is provided in Chapter 28.

Disorders of the Cerebellum and Brain Stem

Olivopontocerebellar atrophy (OPCA) defines chronic progressive hereditary (usually dominant, occasionally recessive, rarely sporadic) cerebellar degeneration manifested by cerebellar-parkinsonian or parkinsonian-cerebellar syndrome and associated with atrophy of the pontine nuclei and cerebellar cortex, and degenerative lesions of the olivopontocerebellar regions.[252–254] There have been a few reports on sleep disturbances and sleep-related respiratory dysrhythmias in OPCA.

Cerebellar influence on the sleep-wakefulness mechanism has been clearly demonstrated in experimental animal studies.[255] The role of the cerebellum in the respiratory control mechanism in sleep, however, is not known. Brain stem neurons, which are known to be degenerated in OPCA,[253,254] lie close to the hypnogenic[61] and respiratory neurons.[72] Thus, dysfunction of respiratory control, in parallel with the somatic structural dysfunction in OPCA, may be expected. The known morphologic changes of OPCA[253,254] are adequate to explain the sleep disturbances and sleep apnea in this condition. Several authors[256–259] described EEG sleep alterations in degenerative cerebellar atrophy. Reduced or absent REM sleep, reduced slow-wave sleep, and increased awakenings are the essential PSG findings. In several cases of OPCA, REM sleep without muscle atonia accompanied by the typical features of RBD has been described.[260–262] Jouvet and Delorme[37] produced REM sleep without atonia in cats by bilateral pontine tegmental lesions. A similar lesion in OPCA may be also responsible for RBD in this condition. OPCA has also been associated with hyposomnia.[263]

Sleep apnea has been described in several cases of OPCA.[259,263–266] It should be noted that patients with sporadic OPCA associated with prominent autonomic failure are now classified as having MSA or Shy-Drager syndrome (see *Sleep and Breathing Disorders in Autonomic Failure* later in this chapter). Chokroverty and colleagues[264] described five patients with OPCA and sleep apnea. PSG study showed repeated episodes of central, upper airway obstructive, and mixed apneas during sleep; the apneic episodes lasted from 10 to 62 seconds and the apnea index was 30–55. Pure central apnea was noted in three patients, but all three types of apnea were seen in two, and most of the apneic episodes occurred during NREM sleep stage 2. Thus, these findings suggested central neuronal dysfunction in an area where respiratory and sleep-waking systems are closely interrelated, such as the NTS and the pontomedullary reticular formation. Salazar-Grueso and associates[259] described a 37-year-old man with a 19-year history of autosomal dominant OPCA and EDS whose PSG demonstrated episodes of mixed and central (predominantly central) sleep apnea and no sleep spindles or REM sleep. Trazodone treatment normalized the sleep architecture and reduced the apneic episodes.

Occasionally, sleep disturbances are associated with other types of cerebellar lesions, although systematic studies are lacking. Bergamasco and colleagues[267] made a polygraphic study of a 13-year-old girl with a diagnosis of dyssynergia cerebellaris myoclonica (Ramsay Hunt syndrome). An all-night sleep study showed no REM sleep and increased slow-wave sleep. The EEG showed multiple spike-and-wave discharges accompanied by myoclonic generalized seizures, and on other occasions a desynchronized EEG was noted during tonic seizure.

Brain Stem Lesions

The metabolic and autonomic respiratory neurons and the lower brain stem hypnogenic neurons are located in the medulla. These neurons are influenced by the supramedullary respiration-controlling inputs and hypothalamic preoptic nuclei, as well as by the peripheral afferent inputs to the respiratory centers (see Chapter 7). Therefore, sleep and respiratory disturbances should be common manifestations of lesions in the brain stem, and many such cases have been described. Such disorders have included brain stem vascular lesions, tumors, traumatic lesions, multiple sclerosis (MS), bulbar poliomyelitis and postpolio syndrome, brain stem encephalitis, motor neuron disease affecting the bulbar nuclei, syringobulbia-syringomyelia, and Arnold-Chiari malformation.[81] In addition, several cases in which brain stem and diencephalic lesions caused symptomatic or secondary narcolepsy have been described.[160–165,251,268] Generally, all the characteristic features of narcolepsy are not seen in the secondary syndrome. The causes have included infarction,[251] trauma, tumors[268] (including third ventricle tumor[269]), and arteriovenous malformation invading the third ventricle and affecting the hypothalamus,[270] and some cases have been associated with MS.[271–273] Scammell et al.[274] described a narcolepsy-like syndrome with low CSF hypocretin-1 in a 23-year-old man after diencephalic stroke following removal of a craniopharyngioma.

Brain Stem Vascular Lesions. Brain stem vascular lesions include infarction, hemorrhage, arterial compression, and localized brain stem ischemia. Sleep disturbances have been described in brain stem infarction by Markand and Dyken[275] and several other authors.[19,21,276,277] Polysomnographic findings generally consisted of increased wakefulness after sleep onset and decreased REM and slow-wave sleep. Several reports of EEG or PSG studies to document sleep disturbances have been described in patients with locked-in syndrome, which is characterized by quadriplegia associated with de-efferentation and results from ventral pontine infarction. Patients are generally aware of their surroundings and are conscious. They cannot speak because of facial muscle paralysis but can respond by moving the eyes, whose control is spared. Sleep EEG recordings of locked-in syndrome patients have been reported by Feldman,[278] Freemon and coworkers,[279]

Markand and Dyken,[275] Cummings and Greenberg,[280] Oxenberg and colleagues,[281] and Nordgren et al.[282] The EEG findings in these reports generally showed reduced or absent REM sleep and variable changes in NREM sleep, including reduction of slow-wave sleep and total sleep time. Oxenberg's group,[281] however, described only minor alterations in the initial recording in contrast to the more marked alterations noted in the other reports. The authors thought that the difference could be related to the extent of the lesion. Feldman[278] found in his patient reduced REM, stage 4 NREM, and total sleep time. Markand and Dyken[275] noted in five of seven locked-in syndrome patients total absence of REM sleep and variable changes in NREM sleep. Cummings and Greenberg[280] described one patient who had reduced slow-wave sleep and another with reduced NREM sleep and no REM sleep. Autret and coworkers[283] also found a reduction of REM and NREM sleep in four patients after medial pontine tegmental stroke.

Kushida and associates[284] described marked asymmetry in the EEG of REM sleep in a 24-year-old woman with a left pontine hematoma, suggesting to the authors that a unilateral pontine lesion may cause disruption of the normal REM sleep EEG in the ipsilateral hemisphere. The lesion did not affect the other characteristics of REM sleep, such as REMs and muscle atonia.

The term *Ondine's curse*, or the *syndrome of primary failure of automatic respiration*, was coined by Severinghaus and Mitchell[285] to describe three patients who experienced long periods of apnea even when awake but could breathe on command. They became apneic after surgery involving the brain stem and high cervical spinal cord and required artificial ventilation while asleep. When their consciousness was altered by nitrous oxide or thiopental, they became apneic. Carbon dioxide response to breathing showed low sensitivity. One patient died in apnea and the two others improved in 1 week. The authors suggested that Ondine's curse resulted from damage to the medullary carbon dioxide chemoreceptors. It is notable that the term *Ondine's curse* was derived from the sea nymph in German mythology, whose curse rendered her unfaithful lover incapable of automatic respiratory function and caused his death. This eponymic syndrome generated considerable controversy and confusion.[286] The syndrome of Ondine's curse is usually caused by bilateral lesions anywhere caudal to the fifth cranial nerve in the pons down to the upper cervical spinal cord in the ventrolateral region. Levin and Margolis[277] described a 52-year-old man with unilateral medullary infarction, however, who lost automatic respiratory control. At autopsy, the lesion was found to extend from the left lower pons through the left lateral medullary tegmentum to the upper cervical spinal cord and to involve the left paramedian PRF. Thus, in some patients, automatic respiratory control can reside unilaterally in the pontomedullary tegmentum.

A case of inverse Ondine's curse syndrome in a patient with selective paralysis of voluntary respiration but preservation of automatic respiration was described by Munschauer et al.[287] This was a 36-year-old man with sudden onset of quadriparesis and bulbar dysfunction in whom MRI demonstrated a well-demarcated lesion restricted to the ventral basilaris pontis. His hypercapnic ventilatory response and breathing during sleep were normal. Emotional stimuli producing laughter, crying, or anxiety appropriately modulated automatic respiration, but the patient could not voluntarily modify any respiratory parameters. The findings in this case suggested that descending limbic influences on automatic respiration are anatomically and functionally independent of the voluntary respiratory systems.

Bogousslavsky et al.[288] reported a clinical pathologic correlation in two patients who had central hypoventilation and unilateral infarct in the caudal brain stem. The authors suggested that unilateral involvement of the pontomedullary reticular formation and nucleus ambiguus is sufficient for generating a loss of automatic respiration, whereas associated lesion of the NTS may lead to more severe respiratory failure involving both automatic and voluntary responses.[288]

Respiratory rate and pattern were studied by Lee and colleagues[19] by impedance pneumography in 14 patients with acute brain stem or cerebral infarction, and in a subsequent study they reported on another 23 patients with acute brain stem infarction.[21] They found frequent abnormalities of respiratory pattern and rate in such patients, and these abnormalities became worse during sleep. The abnormal pattern included CSB and Cheyne-Stokes variant types of breathing, in addition to tachypnea and cluster breathing in some patients. In contrast to the observations of Plum and coworkers[11–13,289] that such breathing patterns are associated with bilateral cerebral hemispheric and diencephalic lesions but rarely with lesions in the upper pons, Lee's group[21] observed Cheyne-Stokes respirations in patients with extensive bilateral pontine lesions. They suggested that the size and the bilaterality of the lesions determined the types of respiratory pattern abnormalities.

Devereaux and coworkers[276] reported sleep apnea that required ventilatory support in two women who breathed normally while awake. Ages 36 and 59 years, they had bilateral infarctions limited to the lateral medullary tegmentum. In one of these patients the carbon dioxide response was markedly depressed. Although the authors stated that acute automatic respiratory failure did not generally evolve into a chronic alveolar hypoventilation syndrome, their second patient continued to have sleep-induced apnea after many months.

Sleep apnea after bulbar stroke was also described by Askenasy and Goldhammer.[290] Their patient had a left-sided Wallenberg syndrome (lateral medullary syndrome), and 2 nights' PSG recordings documented mostly obstructive or mixed apneas and hypopneas. This was a clinical diagnosis, and neuroimaging did not define the exact anatomy of the lesion. Their report, however, should direct attention to the possibility that unilateral brain stem lesions can cause sleep apnea syndrome. In such patients, it is important to diagnose and promptly treat ventilatory dysfunction during sleep.

Miyazaki and associates[291] described a 5-year-old boy with CSA (documented by PSG recording) associated with compression of the ventral medulla by abnormal looping of the vertebral artery as documented by MRI. The authors suggested that the aberrant vertebral artery might have compressed the respiratory center, although the hypercapnic ventilatory response, which reflects central chemoreceptor function, was normal during sleep in this case.

Periodic breathing, apnea, and cyanosis were described in a 57-year-old woman after carotid endarterectomy.[292] The authors suggested that respiratory depression resulted from midbrain hypoxia and edema.

Brain stem ischemic damage may also cause respiratory dysfunction. Beal and colleagues[293] described a 19-year-old man who had failure of automatic respiration and other signs of brain stem dysfunction after nearly drowning. He had sleep apneas, and PSG study confirmed the presence of CSAs. During wakefulness, his breathing was normal. Hypercapnic ventilatory response was markedly impaired, but hypoxic ventilatory response appeared to be normal. Autopsy findings 8 months later, after sudden death, documented marked bilateral neuron loss in the tractus solitarius, ambiguus, and retroambigualis nuclei. This most likely resulted from anoxia or ischemia.

Parenti et al.[294] described two patients ages 38 and 53 years with CSA who died during sleep. At autopsy, the authors described acute bilateral hypoxic lesions at the level of the solitary tract nuclei.

Lassman and Mayer[295] described a 70-year-old woman with right lateral medullary infarction who developed recurrent episodes of life-threatening central hypoventilation requiring diaphragm pacing with a phrenic nerve pacemaker and nocturnal mechanical ventilation via a tracheostomy.

Brain Stem Tumor. Brain stem glioma with automatic respiratory failure was mentioned by Plum.[13] Ito et al.[296] described two children with brain stem gliomas and sleep apnea. Brain stem tumor may cause disorganization of the tonic and phasic events of REM sleep, as described in a patient whose pontine tumor caused a marked decrease in the atonia of REM sleep.[297] Lee et al.[298] reported a 74-year-old woman with recurrent acoustic neuroma at the cerebellopontine angle presenting as central alveolar hypoventilation. The patient had shallow breathing during sleep and had hypersomnolence during the daytime. Arterial blood gases showed increased $PaCO_2$ and decreased partial pressure of arterial oxygen (PaO_2). Tumor resection eliminated hypersomnolence and respiratory failure. A patient seen by the senior author with a medullary tumor that caused severe hypoventilation during sleep required tracheostomy (unpublished observation). The central apneic episodes in the same patient became prolonged when the tracheostomy tube was occluded.

Brain Stem Trauma. Traumatic brain injuries (TBIs) include concussion, contusion, laceration, hemorrhage, and cerebral edema. After a severe TBI, brain stem function is severely compromised and the patient becomes comatose. There have been many EEG studies in patients with coma, and some patients may demonstrate sleep patterns such as spindles and K complexes. Such patterns are designated as *spindle coma*.[299] It is often stated that the presence of EEG sleep patterns indicates a favorable prognosis,[300] but this may not be necessarily true. On recovering from the coma during this stage of rehabilitation, many patients may have sleep-wake disturbances. However, there have been no adequate studies addressing the sleep-wake abnormalities in such patients. This is surprising, considering that one editorial labeled TBI a silent epidemic.[301] There is a dearth of studies addressing sleep-wake abnormalities after minor brain injuries that did not result in coma but caused a transient loss of consciousness. Many of these patients experience so-called postconcussion syndrome, characterized by a variety of behavioral disturbances, headache, and sleep-wake abnormalities.[302] A few reports[302–305] list subjective complaints of sleep disturbances but do not include formal sleep studies. In one report by Prigatano et al.,[306] PSG studies in patients with post-traumatic insomnia documented sleep maintenance insomnia with an increased number of awakenings and decreased night sleep in closed-head injury patients. The mechanism of these sleep abnormalities is unknown. All-night studies of 105 patients with brain damage after TBI were performed by Harada et al.,[307] showing a normalization of sleep organization and a parallel improvement of REM sleep recovery and cognition.

Insomnia, hypersomnia, and circadian sleep disturbances may occur after TBI, but objective sleep studies rather than anecdotal reports or single-case reports are necessary to determine this.[302] Post-traumatic hypersomnolence has been listed in the second edition of the International Classification of Sleep Disorders (ICSD-2).[308] Guilleminault et al.[308a] evaluated 20 patients with post-traumatic hypersomnia using PSG and the MSLT. The causes were multiple, including cases secondary to sleep apnea syndrome. TBI may cause central and upper airway obstructive sleep apnea by inflicting functional or structural alterations of the brain stem respiratory control system. It is important to remember, however, that many patients may have sleep apnea syndrome before sustaining TBI.

North and Jennett[18] recorded irregular breathing patterns in patients with traumatic lesions of the medulla

and pons. However, they did not discuss the changes in the breathing patterns during sleep in these patients. In contrast to the findings of Posner and colleagues,[289] they did not find that long- or short-cycle Cheyne-Stokes respirations helped localize the site of brain damage.

Okawa et al.[309] described disturbance of circadian rhythms in severely brain-damaged patients. Patten and Lauderdale[310] reported a case of delayed sleep phase syndrome in a 13-year-old boy after a minor head injury sustained in a motorcycle accident (5 minutes' loss of consciousness followed by headache and drowsiness without other objective neurologic findings). Billiard et al.[311] reported a reversal of the normal circadian rhythmicity in seven of nine severely head-injured patients. Quinto et al.[312] reported a case of a delayed sleep phase syndrome in a 48-year-old man after TBI.

There are several recent studies investigating the frequency of sleep disorders in TBI patients with hypersomnia and insomnia. Baumann et al.[313] prospectively assessed CSF hypocretin-1 levels in 44 consecutive patients with acute TBI. They found abnormally lower hypocretin-1 levels in 95% of patients with moderate to severe TBI compared with controls. Later on, this group of authors[314] enrolled 96 consecutive patients within the first 4 days after TBI, attempting to delineate the frequency and clinical characteristics of post-traumatic sleep-wake disorders. Six months later, they studied 65 of these patients using questionnaire, CT scan of the brain, CSF hypocretin-1 levels, overnight PSG, and MSLT and actigraphy. They found new-onset sleep-wake disorders following TBI in 72% of these patients, objective EDS in the MSLT test in 25%, post-traumatic hypersomnia (increased sleep need of 2 or more hours within 24 hours compared to the pre-TBI period) in 22%, and insomnia in 5%. They found low CSF hypocretin-1 levels in 4 of 21 patients 6 months after TBI compared to 25 of 27 patients in the first few days after TBI. The patients with post-traumatic sleep-wake disorders also had impaired quality of life. The authors suggested that sleep-wake disturbances are common and involvement of the hypocretin system is possible in the pathophysiology of post-traumatic hypersomnia.

Castriotta et al.[315] evaluated 87 adult patients at least 3 months after TBI using overnight PSG, MSLT, ESS, and neuropsychological testing. They found a high prevalence of sleep disorders (46%) and of EDS (25%) in subjects with TBI. Sleep dysfunction in these patients included a high prevalence of OSA (23%), post-traumatic hypersomnia (11%), and post-traumatic narcolepsy (7%). Ouellet and co-investigators[316] evaluated 452 subjects ages 16 years and older with minor to severe TBI utilizing a questionnaire related to quality of sleep. They found overall insomnia symptoms in 50.2% and diagnostic criteria for an insomnia syndrome in 29.4%. Risk factors for insomnia included mild TBI and high levels of fatigue, depression, and pain. Ouellete and Morin[317] studied

14 patients with mild to severe TBI compared to 14 healthy good sleepers using a sleep diary and 2 nights of overnight PSG. The authors found a higher proportion of stage 1 sleep in the TBI participants than in controls, but the percentages of stage 2, slow-wave, and REM sleep did not differ between the two groups. TBI patients, however, had more awakenings lasting longer than 5 minutes and a shorter REM sleep latency. The authors concluded that these results were similar to those found in patients with either primary insomnia or insomnia comorbid with depression.

Schreiber et al.[318] observed alterations in both timing and sleep architecture in 26 adult patients with a past history of minor head trauma (no structural brain imaging findings). In contrast, Gosselin and investigators[319] observed only subjective complaints but no objective sleep architectural abnormalities in 10 athletes with a history of sport-related concussion within the past year compared with 11 non-concussed athletes. EDS in adults with TBI was also reported prospectively in case series of subjects by Masel et al.[320] and Castriotta and Lai.[321] These investigators found a high prevalence of sleep apnea-hypopnea syndrome, PLMS, and post-traumatic hypersomnia as well as post-traumatic narcolepsy. Post-traumatic narcolepsy in mild to moderate head injury in nine patients was also reported by Lankford et al.[322] utilizing overnight PSG and MSLT.

Demyelinating Lesion in the Brain Stem. Sleep disturbances are very common in MS, and may be seen in over 50% of patients.[323–342] Surprisingly, there is a lack of adequate evaluation and characterization of such dysfunction in a systematic manner using subjective and objective measures in MS patients. Most MS patients suffer from an unexplained fatigue. An important reason for such fatigue may be an unsuspected sleep disorder, such as SDB or insufficient nocturnal sleep. Sleep disturbances in MS may include insomnia, hypersomnia, SDB, narcolepsy, restless legs syndrome (RLS)–PLMS, and RBD.[323–341] We do not know if such sleep disturbances have an adverse impact on the natural history of MS. Also, we have inadequate knowledge about the effects of treatment of MS with immunomodulating therapies on sleep-wake disturbances. It is not known if sleep-wake disorder is related to the severity of the illness as there have not been adequate studies in a large number of MS patients complaining of sleep-wake disorder correlating with Kurtzke's expanded disability scale score.

Sleep-Disordered Breathing in MS. In individuals with MS, a demyelinating plaque may involve the hypnogenic and respiratory neurons in the brain stem, giving rise to sleep disturbance and SRBDs. A few such cases have been described in MS patients. An interesting patient, a 38-year-old man who had a clinical diagnosis of acute demyelinating lesion in the cervicomedullary junction, was described by Newsom Davis.[323] The patient had an autonomous breathing pattern, but he could neither take a voluntary breath nor stop breathing, thus illustrating the apparent independence of the mechanisms controlling metabolic and behavioral respiratory control systems. A patient reported by Rizvi and coworkers,[324] whose brain stem dysfunction was consistent with MS, became apneic when asleep but was able to breathe when awake. His hypercapnic and hypoxic ventilatory responses were normal. Boor and associates[325] described a 40-year-old patient with paralysis of automatic respiration. During relaxation, the patient had recurrent apnea, but the breathing was stable when the patient was alert. The discovery at postmortem examination of a large, demyelinating lesion in the central medulla involving the medullary respiratory neurons explained the respiratory failure.

There are other reports of SDB in MS, including failure of automatic respiration (Ondine's curse) with sudden respiratory arrest and nocturnal death, CSA, hypoventilation, and paroxysmal hyperventilation. It is important to consider such a possibility when patients complain of EDS, fatigue, and nonrestorative sleep associated with snoring.[342,343] Most of the cases of SDB consisted of CSA rather than OSA.[327,343] Figure 29–10 and Figure 29–11 show a sample of the hypnogram and overnight PSG recording from a 51-year-old woman with a history of MS showing frequent obstructive, mixed, and central apneas and hypopneas during both NREM and REM sleep associated with mild to moderate oxygen desaturation and frequent arousals, as well as REM sleep dysregulation with longer REM sleep in the early part of the night.

Insomnia in MS. In addition to sleep-related breathing abnormalities, other sleep difficulties have been commonly reported in MS patients, including insomnia, EDS, and depression.[326–330] Sleep disturbances in MS may result from immobility, spasticity, urinary bladder sphincter disturbances, and sleep-related respiratory dysrhythmias due to respiratory muscle effects or impaired central control of breathing. Tachibana et al.[329] evaluated 28 consecutive patients with MS, 15 of whom had sleep problems that included difficulty initiating sleep, frequent awakenings, difficulty maintaining sleep, habitual snoring, and nocturia. All-night oximetric study showed sleep-related O_2 desaturation in three patients, two of whom had sleep apnea on PSG investigations. The authors concluded that sleep disturbance in MS is common but poorly recognized and is usually due to leg spasms, pain, immobility, nocturia, or medication but not commonly associated with nocturnal respiratory dysfunction. Ferini-Strambi et al.[330] performed PSG studies in 25 MS patients and compared the results with 25 age- and sex-matched controls. They found reduced sleep efficiency with increased awakenings during sleep and an excess of PLMS in patients as compared with the controls. An important cause of insomnia in MS is depression, which

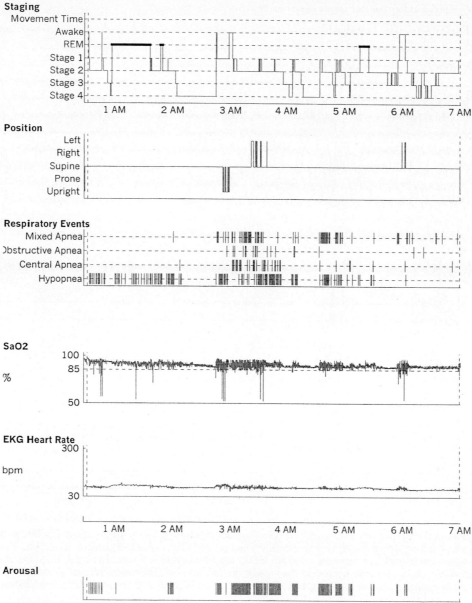

FIGURE 29–10 A case of SDB in a 51-year-old woman with a history of multiple sclerosis diagnosed 7 years ago. Her sleep difficulties started approximately 3 years ago and are described as frequent night awakenings, sleepwalking, and brief episodes consisting of sudden sleepiness or impairment of consciousness resulting in falls and multiple fractures but never accompanied by jerky movements of the limbs, tongue biting, or incontinence, with spontaneous recovery in 5–10 minutes without residual confusion. These episodes occur during the early morning hours as well as during the day. Her neurologic examination is significant for the presence of decreased visual acuity and impaired saccades bilaterally, horizontal nystagmus on looking to the left, intention tremor (left more than right) on finger-to-nose testing, mild ataxia in the lower extremities on heel-to-shin testing, tandem ataxia, and impaired joint and position sense in the toes bilaterally. She was clinically evaluated with a differential diagnosis of SDB related to multiple sclerosis, narcolepsy-cataplexy secondary to multiple sclerosis, and sleepwalking. Unusual nocturnal seizures remained unlikely given the clinical features, the several negative electroencephalograms, and the negative long-term epilepsy monitoring. This hypnogram is significant for REM sleep distribution abnormality (longest REM in the early part of the night); frequent obstructive, mixed, and central apneas and hypopneas both during NREM and REM sleep; mild-moderate O_2 desaturation; and frequent arousals. Sleep-related respiratory dysrhythmias due to brain stem involvement are a common finding in multiple sclerosis patients.*(Reproduced with permission from Chokroverty S, Thomas RJ, Bhatt M [eds]: Atlas of Sleep Medicine. Philadelphia: Elsevier, 2005.)*

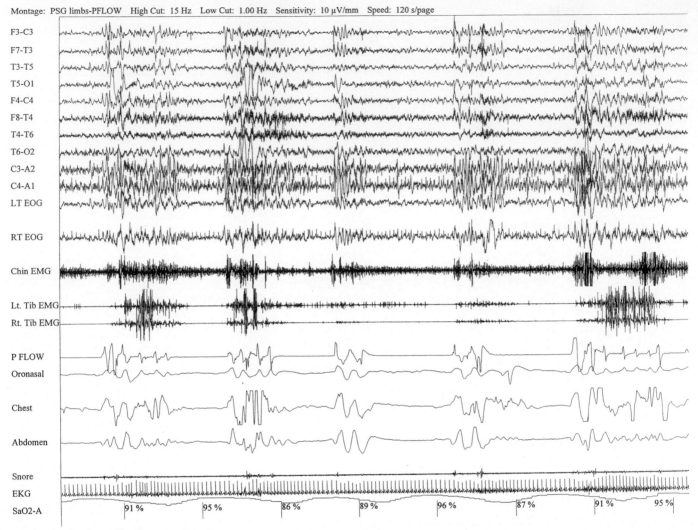

Montage: PSG limbs-PFLOW   High Cut: 15 Hz   Low Cut: 1.00 Hz   Sensitivity: 10 µV/mm   Speed: 120 s/page

FIGURE 29–11 A 120-second excerpt from an overnight polysomnographic recording (same patient as in Fig. 29–10) showing repeated central apneas with O₂ desaturation. An increase in muscle tone is noted on chin (Chin EMG) and tibialis anterior (Tib.) electromyography (EMG) channels following some central events. Electroencephalogram (EEG): top 10 channels. (Lt., left; Rt., right; EOG, electro-oculograms; P Flow, peak flow; oronasal thermistor; chest and abdomen effort channels; snore monitor; EKG, electrocardiography; Sao₂, oxygen saturation by finger oxymetry.)*(Reproduced with permission from Chokroverty S, Thomas RJ, Bhatt M [eds]: Atlas of Sleep Medicine. Philadelphia: Elsevier, 2005.)*

has a high prevalence (up to 50%); it is important to recognize depression as treatment may improve sleep dysfunction and quality of life.[344–346]

RLS-PLMS has a high prevalence in MS patients and in the general population.[330,346,347] RLS-PLMS is an important cause of insomnia in these patients. Manconi et al.[347] studied 156 MS patients using a structured questionnaire and assessing the ESS; about one-third of their subjects satisfied the criteria for RLS. These authors noted that the primary progressive form of MS was more representative of the RLS group, which showed a higher ESS score than those without RLS. In a later multicenter Italian REMS study, Manconi and colleagues[348] reported that the prevalence of RLS was 19% in MS and 4.2% in controls. They identified the following risk factors: older age, longer duration, primary progressive MS form,

higher disability and the presence of leg jerks at sleep onset.

Fatigue, Sleep Dysfunction, and MS. Most patients with MS suffer from an unexplained fatigue. In the studies by Attarian et al.[336,349] and Kaynak et al.,[335] there is a significant correlation between fatigue and disrupted sleep with sleep fragmentation, alteration of sleep macrostructure and microstructure, poor quality of life, and depression.

Other Sleep Disturbances in MS. Hypersomnolence with low CSF hypocretin-1 levels in primary and secondary narcolepsy[350–354] and RBD have also been observed in some MS patients.[339] Plazzi et al.[339] described a 25-year-old woman with MS who presented with RBD as an initial presentation of MS, and this subsequently resolved after treatment with adrenocorticotrophic hormone.

Medications Causing Sleep Disturbance in MS. Treatment of MS with immunomodulating therapies such as interferon and methylprednisolone may cause sleep disturbances in the form of hypersomnolence, increasing fatigue, insomnia, and depression.[355,356] The newer medications such as glatiramer acetate (Copaxone) or mitoxantrone (Novantrone) have not been found to cause sleep disturbance in MS, but adequate studies have not been undertaken. There is a report[357] showing that, compared with oral baclofen, intrathecal infusion to treat severe spasticity in MS patients improved sleep continuity without affecting respiratory function.

Quality of Life and Sleep Dysfunction in MS Patients. Merlino et al.[340] studied 120 MS patients to assess the prevalence of sleep dysfunction in MS and to evaluate various factors affecting sleep quality and quality-of-life indicators. These authors found poor sleep in 47.5% of the patients and concluded that poor sleep is an independent predictor of impaired quality of life, directing our attention to assessment and treatment of sleep dysfunction in MS patients to improve the quality of life. They also confirmed significantly higher mean Kurtzke MS disability scores among poor sleepers than among good sleepers, supporting an earlier report by Lobentanz et al.[358] but contradicting other reports[329,331,339] showing no correlation with these scores.

Bulbar Poliomyelitis and Postpolio Syndrome. In the acute and convalescent stages of poliomyelitis, respiratory disturbances commonly get worse during sleep. Some patients are left with the sequelae of respiratory dysrhythmia, particularly sleep-related apnea or hypoventilation requiring ventilatory support, especially at night. Another group of patients decades later develop symptoms that constitute *postpolio syndrome*. Sleep disturbances and sleep apnea or hypoventilation are also noted in postpolio syndrome. Medullary respiratory and hypnogenic neurons are involved directly by the poliovirus infection, and this explains the patients' symptoms.

Bulbar Poliomyelitis. Hypoventilation syndrome in bulbar poliomyelitis was first documented quantitatively by Sarnoff and colleagues.[359] They described four patients who could breathe voluntarily on command but hypoventilated during periods of sleep and quiescence. The authors described irregular rate and rhythm of respiration, incoordination of the muscles of respiration, and hypoventilation resulting from decreased sensitivity of the respiratory center to $Paco_2$ as a result of direct involvement of the respiratory center by the poliomyelitis virus. Two of their patients benefited from electrophrenic respiration.

An extensive report on the clinical and physiologic findings in 20 of 250 poliomyelitis patients with central respiratory disturbances was given by Plum and Swanson.[16] These patients' respiratory disturbances could not be explained by involvement of the spinal motor neurons or airway obstruction. In acute bulbar poliomyelitis, the disordered breathing progressed through three successive stages. Stage I was characterized by disorder of respiratory rhythm during sleep, when breathing became irregular in rate and depth with periods of apnea ranging from 4 to 12 seconds. During stage II, normal breathing required increasing effort and concentration, and strong auditory or painful stimuli were necessary to maintain respiratory rhythmicity. At this stage the patients had impaired chemosensitivity of the central respiratory centers as evidenced by a reduction in ventilation and carbon dioxide retention after O_2 inhalation. Sleep exacerbated the breathing difficulty, and there were longer periods of apnea. The respiratory homeostasis was lost entirely in stage III, and there was no ventilatory responsiveness to reflex, chemical, or other neuronal stimuli. The respiratory pattern was chaotic, with varying periods of apnea. The patients required ventilatory support to maintain respiratory homeostasis. Severe inflammatory changes and small areas of necrosis in the ventrolateral reticular formation of the medulla were noted in two patients on neuropathologic examination.

The breathing abnormalities in this series rarely lasted more than 2 weeks, but two patients had sleep-related irregular respiration that persisted many months after acute poliomyelitis. These two patients also demonstrated impaired hypercapnic ventilatory response and hypoventilation during administration of 100% O_2. The physiologic abnormalities suggested severe and permanent dysfunction of the medullary respiratory neurons. In several convalescent spinal poliomyelitis patients, the authors also observed subnormal ventilatory response to carbon dioxide with reduction of maximum breathing capacity or vital capacity to less than 50% of predicted normal values. These findings implied that peripheral mechanisms that cause restriction of chest movements may also contribute to impaired ventilatory response to carbon dioxide.

Postpolio Syndrome. Postpolio syndrome is manifested clinically by increasing weakness or wasting of the previously affected muscles and by involvement of previously unaffected regions of the body, fatigue, aches and pains, and sometimes symptoms secondary to sleep-related hypoventilation, such as EDS and tiredness.[360,361] The exact mechanism of postpolio syndrome is not known.[362] Some of the symptoms (e.g., EDS, fatigue) could result from sleep-related hypoventilation or apnea and sleep disturbances.[363] Thus, it is important to be aware of sleep apnea in such patients. This syndrome has been described in patients who had poliomyelitis decades earlier. Guilleminault and Motta[364] reported on five such men who had a history of bulbar poliomyelitis 16 years earlier. All had EDS, and PSG study documented numerous episodes of apneas, which were predominantly central but also mixed and upper airway obstructive types associated with O_2 desaturation. Their longest apneas were seen during REM sleep. It is important to know that these patients resemble those with primary sleep apnea syndrome. Presumably, the lesions in these cases involved the medullary respiratory neurons, and thus central lesions were responsible for all three types of apneas. The patients' symptoms improved and daytime somnolence decreased after ventilatory assistance at night. A 41-year-old woman with a history of bulbar poliomyelitis 20 years earlier was reported by Solliday and associates.[365] This patient had chronic hypoventilation with marked hypoxemia and hypercapnia during sleep. Hypercapnic ventilatory response was impaired, but the hypoxic ventilatory response was normal, suggesting that the patient had impaired central chemoreceptors but functioning peripheral chemoreceptors.

Steljes and coworkers[363] performed PSG examinations on 13 postpolio patients, 5 of whom used rocking beds for ventilatory assistance and 8 of whom had no ventilatory assistance. Patients who required ventilatory assistance demonstrated severe sleep disturbances with decreased total sleep time, reduced sleep efficiency, and decreased percentages of stage 2 NREM sleep, slow-wave sleep, and REM sleep, but increased awakenings and percentage of stage 1 NREM sleep. Respiratory abnormalities in these patients consisted of hypoventilation, apneas, and hypopneas associated with significant O_2 desaturation. These patients did not respond to CPAP treatment with the rocking bed, but they showed improvement in sleep structure and respiratory function after mechanical ventilation via nasal mask. Five of the eight patients who required no ventilatory assistance also showed impairment of sleep architecture similar to the other group, but the findings were less severe. All but one patient from the second group had obstructive or mixed apneas, which were treated successfully with nasal CPAP. One patient with mixed apnea and marked hypoventilation improved after treatment with nasal ventilation by mask.

Polysomnographic and pulmonary function studies by Bye et al.[366] and Ellis et al.[367] documented respiratory failure and sleep hypoxemia, particularly during REM sleep, in patients with postpolio respiratory muscle weakness. Sleep studies by Ellis' group[367] under controlled conditions without respiratory support showed repeated arousals with disruption and fragmentation of the REM-NREM cycle. Bye's group[366] and Howard's group[368] found a direct relationship between forced vital capacity, sleep hypoxemia, and nocturnal hypoventilation in such patients.

In a retrospective review of medical records from 108 consecutive patients with postpolio syndrome and sleep disturbances encountered during an 11-year period at the Mayo Clinic, Hsu and Staats[369] reported PSG findings from 35 patients fulfilling the inclusion criteria. All patients had hypersomnolence as the most common

presenting symptom, and the authors identified three patterns of sleep disturbances: OSA, hypoventilation, and a combination of both. They concluded that SDB is a late sequela of poliomyelitis. Dean et al.[370] from the National Institutes of Health reported the PSG findings in 10 patients with clinical signs of postpolio syndrome. They noted disruption of sleep architecture due to sleep apnea (both central and obstructive), which was more frequent in patients with bulbar involvement who had more central than obstructive apneas. Bruno[371] reported abnormal movements during sleep studies (e.g., random myoclonus, brief ballistic and slow grasping movements, PLMS) in seven poliomyelitis survivors. A physiologic study to understand the sequence of events during REM sleep in 13 patients with postpolio syndrome by Siegel et al.[372] from the National Institutes of Health measured latencies to the onset of the first occurrence of muscle tone reduction, the first sawtooth waves, and the first REMs in 13 patients with postpolio syndrome. The latencies for the entire group were longer than those of the normal volunteers, and the latencies for the bulbar group were significantly longer than for the nonbulbar group of postpolio patients. The authors concluded that prolongation of these latencies may be due to prolonged recruitment time for neurons in the pontine tegmentum as a result of damage from the poliomyelitis virus in the past. In questionnaire studies, Cosgrove et al.[373] found sleep disturbances in 31% of postpolio patients. Van Kralingen et al.[374] reported sleep complaints (i.e., daytime sleepiness and fatigue, morning headache, restless legs) in almost 50% of 43 postpolio patients.

Syringobulbia-Syringomyelia. Some patients with syringobulbia-myelia may have alveolar hypoventilation and sleep-related apneas or irregular breathing and stridor. Haponik and colleagues[375] described such a case. The patient was a 35-year-old woman whose polygraphic examination showed 370 upper airway obstructive apneas lasting 10–170 seconds associated with hypoxemia during 7 hours of NREM stages 1 and 2 sleep. The patient died 9 months after the onset of the illness, and neuropathologic examination disclosed a syrinx that extended from the lower third of the medulla to the upper thoracic spinal cord. Nogues et al.[376] studied 30 patients with syringomyelia, including 17 with syringobulbia, using overnight PSG and pulmonary function tests that also included hypercapnic ventilatory response; they found SDB (central, mixed, and obstructive apneas) in 1 of 13 patients with syringomyelia and 13 of 17 patients with syringobulbia. Impaired hypercapnic ventilatory response was noted in patients with syringobulbia. They found that symptoms of dysphagia and dysphonia rather than the size of the cavity on MRI or muscle weakness were predictive of SDB. These authors[377] also reported PLMS during NREM stages 1 and 2 in 16 of 26 patients with syringomyelia, and periodic limb movements in wakefulness in

3 of these patients. The EMG latency delay between the upper and lower limb muscles suggested conduction along slowly conducting propriospinal pathways, indicating hyperexcitability of the spinal cord in these patients. An occasional report[378] of postural tachycardia syndrome (see later) in syringomyelia suggests intermediolateral column dysfunction in this condition.

Western Equine Encephalitis and Limbic Encephalitis. Cohn and Kuida[379] and White and coworkers[380] described alveolar hypoventilation, CSA, EDS, and subnormal hypercapnic ventilatory response after western equine encephalitis. The respiratory center was thought to have been damaged by the virus. Iranzo et al.[381] reported six patients with non-paraneoplastic limbic encephalitis associated with antibodies to voltage-gated potassium channels. Five of these patients had RBD associated with the onset of limbic encephalitis, and in three of these patients immunosuppression resulted in resolution of RBD in parallel with remission of the limbic syndrome. The authors suggested that RBD may be seen in the setting of voltage-gated potassium channel antibody-associated limbic encephalitis, which may be related to an autoimmune-mediated mechanism.

Arnold-Chiari Malformation. Arnold-Chiari malformation, particularly types I and II, may cause SDB, predominately CSA but also upper airway OSA, and central hypoventilation, including sudden respiratory arrest during sleep or postoperatively.[382–391] A repeat PSG in 6 of 12 patients out of 16 consecutive patients with Arnold Chiari malformation type I showed a decrease in the central apnea index following decompression surgery. In a study by Sergio et al.[391] reporting a large sample of patients affected with Arnold-Chiari malformation (36 with type I and 67 with type II), a video-PSG study showed RBD in 23 and SDB in 65, predominantly with CSA syndrome in 61 of the 65 patients. Bokinsky and colleagues[392] described an 18-year-old patient with Arnold-Chiari malformation and syringomyelia accompanied by dysfunction of the IXth, Xth, and XIIth cranial nerves. They noted absent hypoxic ventilatory response but normal hypercapnic ventilatory response in their patient. These findings are consistent with bilateral ninth cranial nerve dysfunction. Figures 29–12 and 29–13 show a hypnogram and a 120-second excerpt from a PSG recording from a 52-year-old man with Arnold-Chiari malformation type I. The hypnogram findings suggest REM sleep-related hypoventilation, and the PSG tracing shows obstructive apneas and hypopneas.

Diseases of the Spinal Cord

In spinal cord disorders, sleep disturbances occur as a result of sleep-related respiratory dysrhythmias causing sleep apneas, hypopneas, or hypoventilation associated with hypoxemia and repeated arousals. The voluntary or behavioral respiratory control system descends via the corticospinal tracts, and the metabolic or automatic respiratory control system descends via the reticulospinal tracts; the two systems are integrated in the spinal cord (see also Chapter 7). The behavioral system is located in the dorsolateral quadrant of the cervical spinal cord[13,14] and the automatic respiratory system in the ventrolateral quadrant. These two systems control the final common respiratory pathways of the spinal respiratory motor neurons, which send impulses along the phrenic and intercostal nerves to the main respiratory muscles. The anterior horn cells in the third, fourth, and fifth cervical spinal cord segments give rise to phrenic nerves, and the intercostal nerves originate from the ventral rami from the anterior horn cells in the thoracic spinal cord. It is known that transection of either the dorsolateral or the ventrolateral quadrant of the spinal cord may independently affect the voluntary and the automatic respiratory control systems.[73] Most reports, however, refer to transection of the ventrolateral tracts giving rise to dysfunction of the metabolic respiratory control system. Direct involvement of the lower motor respiratory pathways, either in the anterior horn or in the phrenic and intercostal nerves, may also give rise to respiratory dysfunction. Three patterns of respiratory dysfunction have been summarized by Krieger and Rosomoff[393]: (1) efferent motor impairment (e.g., phrenic nerve paralysis causing diaphragmatic weakness) associated with reduced vital capacity, (2) impaired hypercapnic ventilatory response without significant chest wall or diaphragmatic weakness and with normal vital capacity, and (3) a mixture of these two abnormalities. The lesions that cause such dysfunction in the spinal cord may include spinal surgery, spinal trauma, amyotrophic lateral sclerosis (ALS), syringomyelia, cervical spinal cord tumor, and cervical myelitis (demyelinating or nonspecific myelitis).

Spinal Surgery. Several cases of sleep apnea have been described after spinal surgery.[393–396] Belmusto and colleagues[394] noted ineffective breathing during sleep that required assisted ventilation in a patient treated with bilateral high cervical cordotomy for intractable pain. Damage to the reticulospinal tracts was thought to be responsible for the breathing difficulty. Tenicela's group[395] and Krieger and Rosomoff[393] also described sleep apnea after high cervical cordotomy. Krieger and Rosomoff[393] observed respiratory dysfunction within 24–48 hours of bilateral percutaneous cervical cordotomy in 10 patients. Although the authors concluded that the ascending reticular fibers in the ventrolateral segment of the spinal cord that relay afferent impulses to the medullary respiratory center had been damaged in their patients, it is most likely that selective damage to the descending automatic respiratory control fibers in the ventrolateral quadrant of the spinal cord was the lesion responsible. In two other patients, Krieger and Rosomoff[396] described sleep apnea that required assisted ventilation at night for several days

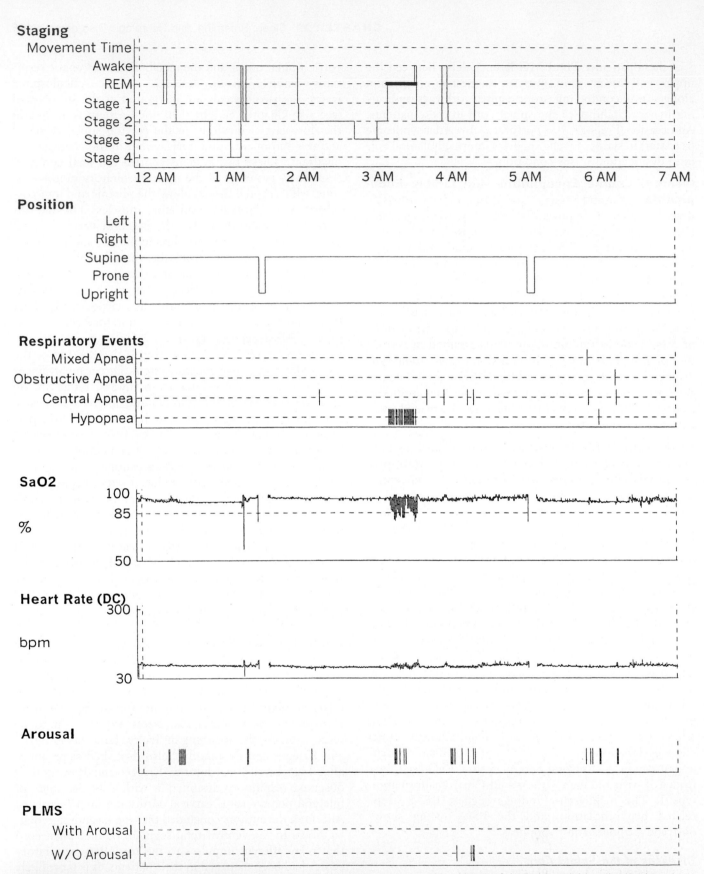

FIGURE 29–12 A case of Arnold-Chiari malformation and SDB in a 52-year-old man with a history of tiredness and excessive daytime sleepiness for many years but no cataplexy, sleep paralysis, or hypnagogic hallucinations. At the age of 27 years, he complained of gait problems, and magnetic resonance imaging examination revealed Arnold-Chiari malformation type 1. His neurologic examination is significant for the presence of a coarse horizontal nystagmus, minimal right lower facial weakness, minimal right wrist extensor muscle weakness, minimal to mild ataxia in upper and lower extremities on coordination testing, and presence of ataxia on tandem gait. This hypnogram shows a few periods of apneas and hypopneas accompanied by mild-moderate oxygen desaturation and arousals limited exclusively to a single REM sleep period recording during the night. A supine posture is maintained throughout the polysomnographic recording. These findings are suggestive of REM sleep–related hypoventilation. Central sleep apnea, obstructive sleep apnea, and hypoventilation have all been described in patients with Arnold-Chiari malformation, likely from brain stem involvement. *(Reproduced with permission from Chokroverty S, Thomas RJ, Bhatt M [eds]: Atlas of Sleep Medicine. Philadelphia: Elsevier, 2005.)*

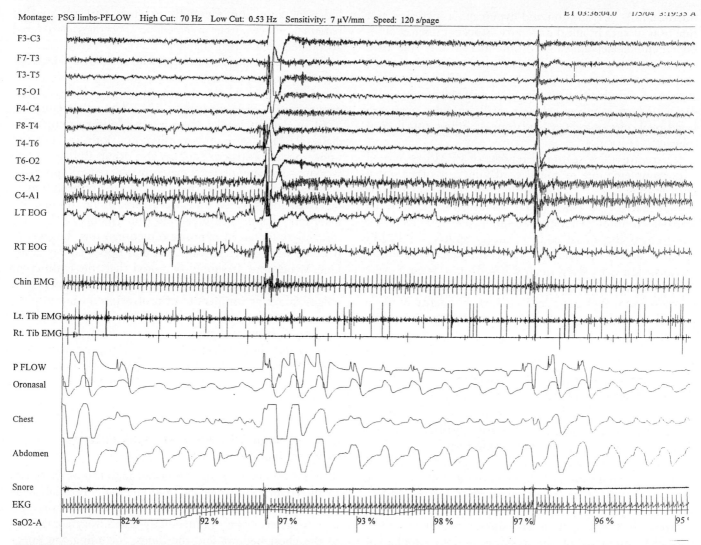

FIGURE 29–13 A 120-second polysomnographic excerpt from REM sleep (same patient as in Fig. 29–12) showing one obstructive apnea followed by two sequential hypopneas. Oxygen desaturation of 82%, likely from a prior respiratory event, is recorded at the onset of the epoch. The first two events are followed by an arousal response, and the epoch does not include the complete recovery phase of the third event. Phasic eye movements of REM sleep are noted on the electro-oculogram (EOG) channels in the early part of the epoch. Phasic muscle twitches of REM sleep are noted on both tibialis anterior electromyography (Tib. EMG) channels. Chin EMG channel shows electrocardiography artifact. Electroencephalogram (EEG): top 10 channels. (Lt., left; Rt., right; P Flow, peak flow; oronasal thermistor; chest and abdomen effort channels; snore monitor; EKG, electrocardiography; Sao$_2$, oxygen saturation by finger oxymetry.)*(Reproduced with permission from Chokroverty S, Thomas RJ, Bhatt M [eds]: Atlas of Sleep Medicine. Philadelphia: Elsevier, 2005.)*

after anterior spinal surgery at C3-4 interspace. Lahuerta et al.[397] performed high cervical cord percutaneous cordotomy for pain management in 12 patients, all of whom died during sleep postoperatively, presumably from respiratory dysrhythmia. These patients had lesions involving the anterolateral funiculus in the C2 segment, where respiratory fibers are intermingled with ascending pain fibers. Thus, these reports clearly document Ondine's curse as a sequela of high cervical spinal cord lesions.

Spinal Trauma. OSA has been described in patients with cervical spine fractures[398] or high spinal cord injury.[399,400] Additionally, alterations of EEG sleep patterns after high cervical lesions have been noted.[401]

Guilleminault[402] described eight victims of neck trauma who showed sleep apnea, hypoxemia, and EDS. The long-term prognosis of these patients is variable, and some may require tracheostomy. Guilleminault[402] suggested that mild compression of the lower medulla and upper cervical spinal cord might cause respiratory disturbances during sleep after severe whiplash injury or odontoid fractures. Bach and Wang[403] evaluated 10 C4-7 trauma tetraplegic individuals at least 6 months postinjury and again 5 years later. Five patients had an increased number of transient nocturnal O$_2$ desaturations, and eight of nine patients restudied by capnography were hypercapnic. However, the daytime blood gases were normal. The authors concluded that, in tetraplegic patients, this nocturnal O_2 desaturation and hypercapnia increased as a function of age. In another report, Stockhammer et al.[404] documented sleep apnea syndrome in 55% men and 20% of women in a series of 50 randomly selected patients with tetraplegia resulting from spinal cord injuries. The authors concluded that the incidence of sleep apnea syndrome is high in tetraplegia, especially in older men with large neck circumference and long-standing spinal cord injuries.

There are a few scattered reports of PLMS associated with paraplegia due to spinal cord injury or other spinal cord lesions.[403,405–408] The authors of these papers concluded that the PLMS resulted from disinhibition of the spinal locomotor generator. It should be noted that the question of the spinal cord as the generator for PLMS remains highly speculative and controversial. A cross-sectional study of sleep quality based on a basic Nordic sleep questionnaire in 230 patients with a spinal cord injury documented poor subjective sleep quality in those with higher ratings of pain intensity, anxiety, and depression.[409]

Sleep and Breathing Disturbances in Peripheral Neuromuscular Disorders

Sleep disturbances in peripheral neuromuscular disorders are most commonly due to respiratory dysrhythmias secondary to involvement of the respiratory pump, which includes the upper airway muscles (genioglossus, palatal, pharyngeal, laryngeal, hyoid, and masseter muscles), the intercostal and other accessory muscles of respiration, and the diaphragm, as a result of effects on the motor neurons, the phrenic and intercostal nerves, or the neuromuscular junctions of the respiratory and oropharyngeal muscles, and primary muscle disorders affecting these muscles.[69,410] The most common complaint is EDS resulting from repeated arousals and sleep fragmentation due to transient nocturnal hypoxemia and hypoventilation in addition to sleep-related respiratory dysrhythmias. Some patients, particularly those with painful polyneuropathies, muscle pain, muscle cramps, and immobility due to muscle weakness, may complain of insomnia. The most common neuromuscular disorders causing SDB and sleep dysfunction include motor neuron disease (amyotrophic lateral sclerosis [ALS]); myasthenia gravis, including myasthenic syndrome; acute inflammatory demyelinating polyradiculoneuropathies (Landry/Guillian-Barré/Strohl syndrome); muscular dystrophies, including myotonic dystrophy; and congenital myopathies. Many of these conditions are treatable; others show relentless progression but, even in these conditions, quality of life may be improved with prolongation of the natural course of the illness by timely and adequate treatment of SDB. It is therefore important for physicians taking care of patients with neuromuscular disorders to have a basic understanding of these disorders and a high

index of suspicion for SDB in such patients so that patients can be either referred to specialists or treated adequately in a timely manner.

SDB is commonly associated with insidiously developing chronic respiratory failure in neuromuscular disorders, especially in the advanced stages, but is often unrecognized and untreated.[411–413] The most common SDB in neuromuscular disorders is sleep related, especially REM-related, hypoventilation. Both central and upper airway obstructive apneas also occur. Bulbar muscle weakness in many patients may cause increased upper airway resistance, but adequate studies have not been undertaken to identify its true prevalence in neuromuscular disorders. Paradoxical breathing (movements of the thorax and abdomen in opposite directions) may be seen in patients with upper airway OSA and upper airway resistance syndrome. It should be noted that this is different from paradoxical inward movement of the abdomen with epigastric retraction instead of protrusion during inspiration as seen in patients with diaphragmatic paralysis. Nocturnal hypoventilation giving rise to hypoxemia and hypercapnia during sleep in the initial stage of neuromuscular disorders causes chronic respiratory failure; the abnormal blood gases may later present even during the daytime.

Mechanism of SDB and Respiratory Failure in Neuromuscular Diseases

Respiratory failure is defined as an inability of the lungs to effectively exchange gas and maintain normal acid-based balance as a result of failure of the respiratory system anywhere from the medullary respiratory controllers to the chest bellows and the lungs, including the upper airways. As a result of this failure, there is reduction in Pa_{O_2} and increased Pa_{CO_2}. A Pa_{O_2} of less than 60 mm Hg and a Pa_{CO_2} of more than 45 mm Hg at sea levels are commonly considered criteria for respiratory failure. Most neuromuscular disorders cause ventilatory failure, which is defined as an inadequate aveolar ventilation with reduced tidal volume causing low Pa_{O_2} and high Pa_{CO_2}.

Respiratory failure in neuromuscular disorders begins during sleep, followed by gradual or relentless progression unless interrupted by ventilatory support at night. A variety of physiologic changes occur in the central control of breathing and in the respiratory muscles during sleep (see Chapter 7) that are responsible for initiating respiratory failure in sleep in patients with neuromuscular disorders. Additionally, there may be a comorbid upper airway obstruction not related to neuromuscular disorders. However, in many of these patients the upper airway muscles are also affected, causing upper airway OSA. The accessory muscles of respiration maintain breathing during NREM sleep in patients with weakness of the diaphragm, the main muscle of ventilation; however, during REM sleep there is hypotonia or atonia of these accessory muscles, and ventilation then depends exclusively on the diaphragm. Therefore, in patients with diaphragmatic weakness, ventilation is severely affected during REM sleep, causing REM hypoventilation. This is the first stage of respiratory failure in neuromuscular disorders. As the disease advances to the second stage, the accessory muscles of respiration are affected severely, thus causing ventilatory disturbance during NREM sleep.[414] In the final stage of neuromuscular disorders, ventilation is affected even during the daytime, causing altered blood gases (e.g., hypoxemia, hypercapnia) during wakefulness. Stage two of respiratory failure may be related to either progression of the neuromuscular disorder or superimposed intercurrent infection (e.g., pneumonia), or both.

Several authors aimed at identifying daytime predictors of SDB and nocturnal hypoventilation and its onset.[415–417] These authors concluded that progressive ventilatory restriction in neuromuscular diseases correlates with respiratory muscle weakness and can be predicted from daytime lung and respiratory muscle function. Inspiratory vital capacity (IVC) and maximum inspiratory muscle pressure (PI_{max}) are the two important predictors of the onset of respiratory failure.[415,416] IVC of less than 60% and PI_{max} of less than 4.5 kPa predicted onset of REM hypoventilation, IVC of less than 40% and PI_{max} of less than 4.0 kPa predicted both REM and NREM hypoventilation, and IVC of less than 25% and PI_{max} of less than 3.5 kPa predicted daytime respiratory failure. However, Lyall et al.[417] and Morgan et al.[418] suggested that the noninvasive maximal sniff pressure measurement is more sensitive than vital capacity and static maximal inspiratory muscle pressure in patients with ALS and in assessing the risk of ventilatory failure. It has also been suggested that a significant (70% of the predicted value) fall of vital capacity from the erect to the supine position indicates the presence of diaphragmatic weakness.[419–421] A fluoroscopy will confirm the weak movement of the dome of the diaphragm during inspiration. A serial blood gas determination is important in detecting impending respiratory failure. It should be remembered that a normal daytime PaO_2 and $PaCO_2$ does not exclude REM-related hypoventilation.

In patients with weak respiratory muscles, regardless of cause, the waking breathing difficulties may worsen during sleep. While patients are awake, both voluntary and metabolic respiratory controls are intact and central respiratory neurons increase the rate of firing or recruit additional respiratory neurons to maintain ventilation adequately to drive weak respiratory muscles.[81] During sleep, however, voluntary control is absent and respiration is dependent entirely on the metabolic control system. Respiratory neurons are thus vulnerable during sleep, aggravating the ventilatory problems and causing more severe hypoventilation and even apneas and hypopneas. Functional impairment of the sensitivity of the central respiratory neurons, causing decreased metabolic respiratory control, may also give rise to apnea-hypopnea during both REM and NREM sleep. Oropharyngeal (upper airway) muscle weakness coupled with REM-related hypotonia or atonia of the muscles may contribute to possible upper airway OSA.

In summary, breathing disorders causing sleep-related hypoventilation in neuromuscular disorders may be related to the following factors:

1. Weakness of the respiratory and chest wall muscles causing impaired chest bellows
2. Increased work of breathing due to altered chest mechanics and reduced forced vital capacity caused by weakness of the chest wall muscles and diaphragm so that breathing is less efficient
3. Hyporesponsive chemoreceptors, which may be secondarily acquired or related to altered afferent inputs from skeletal muscle spindles, causing functional alteration of the medullary respiratory neurons
4. Weakness of upper airway muscles that increases upper airway resistance, adding respiratory muscle load or even upper airway OSA from complete closure of the upper airway
5. Decreased minute and alveolar ventilation during sleep
6. REM-related marked hypotonia or atonia of all the respiratory muscles except the diaphragm, causing increased diaphragmatic work load
7. Respiratory muscle fatigue due to increased demand on the respiratory muscles during sleep, particularly REM sleep
8. Kyphoscoliosis secondary to neuromuscular disorders, causing extrapulmonary restriction of the lungs with impairment of pulmonary functions, breathlessness, sleep apnea, and hypoventilation
9. Failure of central control of ventilation
10. Alteration of respiratory reflexes in upper airway and lung receptors and arousal responses

All these factors may lead to respiratory failure in neuromuscular disorders. As a result of alveolar hypoventilation and ventilation-perfusion mismatching, hypoxemia and hypercapnia occur, giving rise to chronic respiratory failure even during the daytime at an advanced stage of the illness.

Clinical Approach

The initial approach to clinical diagnosis of acute respiratory failure, as may occur in patients with acute inflammatory demyelinating polyradiculoneuropathies (e.g., Guillian-Barré syndrome) or myasthenic crisis is quite obvious. Patients may have irregular, rapid, shallow, or periodic breathing, intermittent cessation of breathing, and cyanosis. However, recurrent hypoventilation in neuromuscular disorders may present insidiously and may initially remain asymptomatic.[411,412,422–425] A high index of clinical suspicion is needed. Clinical clues include presence of EDS, nocturnal restlessness, frequent unexplained arousals, daytime fatigue, shortness of breath, orthopnea (breathlessness in supine position), morning headache, intellectual deterioration, and failure to thrive and declining school performance in children. Signs of impending cor pulmonale include insomnia, morning lethargy, headache, and unexplained leg edema. Patients with neuromuscular disorders manifesting these clinical features should be investigated to uncover nocturnal hypoventilation in order to prevent adverse consequences of chronic respiratory failure, such as congestive cardiac failure and cardiac arrhythmia. Special attention during physical examination should be paid to uncover bulbar and respiratory muscle weakness, use of accessory muscles of respiration, and paradoxical breathing. Neuromuscular disorders causing SDB, respiratory failure, and sleep disturbance include ALS or motor neuron disease, primary muscle diseases, acute and chronic inflammatory demyelinating polyneuropathies, hereditary sensory-motor neuropathy, phrenic neuropathy, and neuromuscular junctional disorders.

Amyotrophic Lateral Sclerosis

ALS is the most common degenerative disease of the motor neurons in adults, affecting the spinal cord, brain stem, motor cortex, and corticospinal tracts. It is characterized by a progressive degeneration of both upper and lower motor neurons manifesting as a varying combination of lower motor neuron (e.g., muscle weakness, wasting, fasciculation, dysarthria, dysphagia) and upper motor neuron (e.g., spasticity, hyperreflexia, extensor plantar response) signs. ALS can cause EDS as a result of repeated arousals and sleep fragmentation due to nocturnal hypoventilation, recurrent episodes of sleep apnea, hypopnea, hypoxemia, and hypercapnia. Insomnia related to other factors, such as decreased mobility, muscle cramps, anxiety, and difficulty in swallowing, may be present in some patients. In 18 ALS patients in the early stage without respiratory or sleep complaints, Kimura and colleagues[426] found no significant difference in the RDI between those with (11 patients) and those without (7 patients) bulbar dysfunction; however, three in the bulbar group had SDB, and the authors recommended respiratory monitoring at night even at an early stage to predict respiratory failure. SDB in ALS may result from weakness of the upper airway, diaphragmatic, and intercostal muscles due to involvement of the bulbar, phrenic, and intercostal motor neurons. In addition, degeneration of central respiratory neurons may occur, causing central and upper airway OSAs. Generally, respiratory failure in ALS occurs late, but occasionally this may be a presenting feature requiring mechanical ventilation.[427,428] Diaphragmatic weakness resulting from degeneration of phrenic neurons is noted frequently in ALS and is mainly responsible for nocturnal hypoventilation, initially during REM sleep. SDB causing sleep disturbance and daytime symptoms has also been noted in other types of motor neuron

diseases, such as Kugleberg-Welander syndrome, a variant of juvenile-type motor neuron disease, as well as spinal muscular atrophy types 1 and 2 in children and adolescents.[429–432]

Newsom Davis' group[433] described eight patients with diaphragmatic paralysis resulting from a variety of motor disorders. One of their patients had Kugelberg-Welander syndrome. The following features may be helpful in the diagnosis of diaphragmatic paralysis[81,433]:

1. Breathlessness and EDS, suggesting alveolar hypoventilation
2. Paradoxical inward movement of the abdomen with epigastric retraction instead of protrusion during inspiration
3. An elevated diaphragm on chest radiography and paradoxical movement or decreased excursion of the diaphragm on fluoroscopy
4. Documentation of a very sensitive measurement showing a lack of change in the transdiaphragmatic pressure during a maximum inspiration
5. Diaphragmatic electromyographic (EMG) findings
6. Respiratory function tests with evidence of a restrictive pattern
7. Blood gases showing hypoxemia and hypercapnia, suggesting alveolar hypoventilation
8. Documentation of sleep-related breathing abnormalities on PSG

Sleep-related respiratory dysrhythmia in two patients with ALS was described by the senior author,[434] who since has seen several other cases of central and obstructive sleep apneas, sleep hypoventilation, and respiratory failure associated with motor neuron disease (unpublished observations). Overnight polygraphic recording from one of these patients documented both central (Fig. 29–14) and upper airway obstructive apneas associated with severe oxygen desaturation.

Ferguson and colleagues[435] studied 18 ALS patients with mild to severe bulbar muscle involvement and 10 age-matched control subjects. Most patients complained of difficulty initiating and maintaining sleep. All patients and controls had overnight PSG study, and 13 ALS patients had a second night of PSG study. ALS patients had more arousals and stage changes per hour, more stage 1 NREM sleep, and shorter total sleep time than controls. ALS patients had mild SDB with greater AHI than controls. It is notable that SDB was similar in ALS patients with or without respiratory muscle weakness. The SDB consisted of REM-related nonobstructive and central apneas, and none had significant sleep apnea. In an early study, Minz and colleagues[436] described PSG findings in 12 ALS patients, six men and six women. Four patients had both central and obstructive apneas. Sleep structure was normal in eight, but the others had frequent awakenings.

Howard and colleagues[437] described 14 patients with motor neuron disease associated with respiratory

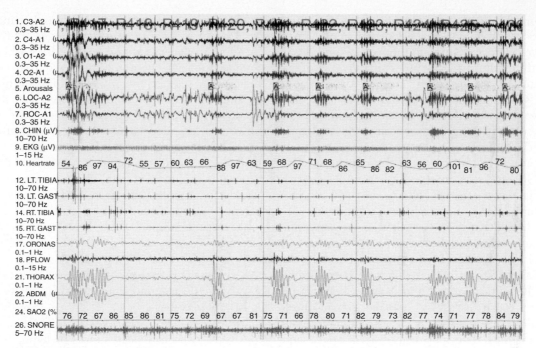

FIGURE 29–14 Overnight polysomnographic recording from a patient with amyotrophic lateral sclerosis presenting with upper and lower motor neuron signs, including bulbar palsy, showing recurrent periods of central apneas many of which are prolonged, followed by irregular ventilatory cycles (resembling ataxic breathing; see Fig. 29–6) accompanied by severe oxygen desaturation and sleep hypoxemia during REM sleep. Top four channels represent the electroencephalogram (EEG; international electrode placement system). (ABDM, abdominal breathing effort; CHIN, submental electromyogram (EMG); EKG, electrocardiogram; LOC, left electro-oculogram; LT.GAST, left gastronemius EMG; LT.TIBIA, left tibialis EMG; ORONAS, oronasal air flow; PFLOW, nasal pressure recording for air flow; ROC, right electro-oculogram; RT.GAST, right gastronemius EMG; RT.TIBIA, right tibialis EMG; SAO$_2$ %, oxygen saturation [%] by finger oximetry; SNORE, snoring recording; THORAX, thoracic breathing effort.)

dysfunction. Eleven received respiratory support, including CPAP and intermittent positive pressure ventilation (IPPV) at night with considerable benefit. The authors concluded that sleep-related respiratory dysrhythmia is a significant complication of motor neuron disease and contributes to daytime hypersomnolence.

Hetta and Jansson[438] reported that sleep disturbances in ALS patients can result from factors such as reduced mobility, muscle cramps, swallowing problems, anxiety, and respiratory problems. Based on interviews only, the authors reported insomnia in 25% of 24 patients with ALS. They mentioned sleep-onset and maintenance insomnia. They also stated that patients in the terminal stage of the disease had a higher frequency of sleep disturbance.

There have been some recent reports focusing on the role of noninvasive IPPV at night on the quality of life and the prognosis (see later in the section on *Treatment of Sleep and Respiratory Dysfunction Secondary to Neurologic Disorders*).[439–442] Atalaia et al.[443] studied 92 ALS patients with normal respiratory function tests and preserved diaphragmatic function. They concluded that the most common SDB in these patients was periodic mild oxygen desaturation independent of the sleep stage that might represent a dysfunction of central drive or respiratory muscle fatigue.

Polyneuropathies

The cardinal manifestations of polyneuropathies are bilaterally symmetric, distal sensory symptoms and signs, and muscle weakness and wasting (affecting the legs more often than the arms). Peripheral neuropathies may be caused by a variety of heredofamilial and acquired lesions. Disorders of the phrenic, intercostal, and other nerves supplying the accessory muscles of respiration can cause weakness of the diaphragm, intercostal, and accessory respiratory muscles, giving rise to breathlessness on exertion, hypoxia, and hypercapnia. These respiratory dysrhythmias become worse during sleep. Sleep disturbances in polyneuropathies may result from painful neuropathies, partial immobility owing to a paralysis of the muscles, or SRBDs.

Trauma, inflammatory polyneuropathy, and infiltrative lesions (e.g., neoplasms) may cause phrenic neuropathy. The most common cause of respiratory dysfunction in polyneuropathy is acute inflammatory demyelinating polyradiculoneuropathy (Landry/Guillain-Barré/Strohl syndrome). The characteristic clinical manifestations consist of predominantly motor deficits associated with rapidly progressive ascending paralysis beginning in the legs and manifesting maximally in 2–3 weeks. In approximately 20–25% of cases, severe respiratory involvement has been reported, and the critical period is usually the first 3–4 weeks of the illness. It is important to recognize and treat the ventilatory dysfunction. Even the mild respiratory dysrhythmia during wakefulness may worsen during sleep, causing sleep apnea and hypoventilation. Patients with Guillain-Barré syndrome (GBS) may also have vivid dreams and hallucinations with abnormalities of sleep structure in the form of sleep-onset REM, REM sleep without atonia, RBD, and autonomic dysfunction, which have been described in approximately one-third of the GBS patients admitted to an intensive care unit.[444] Phrenic neuropathy may also be secondary to varicella-zoster virus infection or diphtheritic neuropathy.[445] Goldstein and colleagues[446] described a patient with peripheral neuropathy and severe involvement of the phrenic nerves who presented with hypoventilation.

Diaphragmatic dysfunction has also been described in siblings with hereditary motor and sensory neuropathy (Charcot-Marie-Tooth disease).[447] Charcot-Marie-Tooth disease includes several inherited peripheral motor-sensory neuropathies that may cause sleep apnea and vocal cord dysfunction, possibly due to laryngeal nerve involvement.[448] Charcot-Marie-Tooth disease type 2, associated with predominant axonal atrophy, has been frequently associated with RLS-PLMS, which may cause sleep-initiation and maintenance insomnia.[449] Bilateral glossopharyngeal and vagal neuropathy can also cause respiratory and sleep dysfunction.[392]

Primary Muscle Diseases (Myopathies)

Myopathies are primary muscle disorders characterized by weakness and wasting of the muscles resulting from a defect in the muscle membrane or the contractile elements that is not secondary to a structural or functional derangement of the lower or upper motor neurons.[81] The characteristic clinical presentation consists of symmetric, proximal muscle weakness and wasting in the upper or lower limbs without sensory impairment or fasciculations. The causes include hereditary muscular dystrophies with or without myotonia; glycogen storage diseases; myoglobinuric myopathies; congenital nonprogressive myopathies with distinct morphologic characteristics; and various acquired metabolic, inflammatory, and noninflammatory myopathies. Some of these patients may report breathing disorders during sleep or worsening of the respiratory dysfunction during sleep. Generally, respiratory disorders show manifestations in the advanced stage, but a small number of patients may present with respiratory failure at an early stage. In many such patients, the true incidence of the sleep disturbances and sleep-related respiratory dysrhythmias cannot be determined without a systematic PSG study. Factors responsible for breathing disorders associated with hypoventilation and sleep apnea in these patients may be summarized as follows[81]: impairment of chest bellows owing to weakness

of the respiratory and chest wall muscles, increased work of breathing, and functional changes in the medullary respiratory neurons that could be due to hyporesponsive or unresponsive chemoreceptors acquired secondarily.[450] The other suggestion for carbon dioxide hyposensitivity is altered afferent input from the skeletal muscle receptors.[451] Sleep disturbances generally occur in muscle disorders secondary to sleep-related respiratory dysrhythmias. Alveolar hypoventilation, both during wakefulness and sleep, should be diagnosed early in these patients to prevent dangerous or fatal hypoventilation during sleep or during administration of drugs, general anesthetic agents, and respiratory infections.[81] Complaints of daytime hypersomnolence and breathlessness should direct attention to the possibility of SDB in these patients.

Muscular Dystrophy. A few cases of muscular dystrophy with sleep complaints and sleep-related respiratory dysrhythmias have been described. Smith and associates[452] described 14 patients with Duchenne's muscular dystrophy who had sleep apneas or hypopneas associated with marked O_2 desaturation. These authors stated that the severity of SDB in Duchenne's muscular dystrophy could not reliably be ascertained from daytime pulmonary function studies and asserted that sleep studies are essential.

Bye et al.[366] and Ellis et al.[367] also included patients with muscular dystrophy in their reports of patients with neuromuscular disorders who also had SRBDs. The REM sleep showed significant O_2 desaturation. Sleep study showed repeated arousals and sleep fragmentation.[367]

Gross and coworkers[453] described a 22-year-old patient with Duchenne's muscular dystrophy who was wheelchair bound and experienced breathlessness after meals. The blood gas studies showed hypercapnia and hypoxemia during wakefulness. A PSG study revealed nonapneic and hypopneic O_2 desaturation, which was more marked during REM than NREM sleep. After progressive inspiratory muscle training and administration of O_2 at a rate of 2 L/min via nasal prongs, the patient's subjective daytime symptoms of fatigue and breathlessness subsided.

Howard et al.[454] described nocturnal hypoventilation and respiratory failure in 84 patients with primary muscle disorders that included Duchenne's, Becker's, limb-girdle, and facioscapulohumeral muscular dystrophies; adult-onset acid maltase deficiency; myotonic dystrophy; polymyositis; congenital myopathies; and rigid spine syndrome. All patients needed ventilatory support in the form of negative or positive pressure ventilation or tracheostomy.

Sleep-related respiratory dysrhythmias (both obstructive and central apneas) accompanied by O_2 desaturation and daytime hypersomnolence have been described in many patients with Duchenne's muscular dystrophy.[411,455-464] Although respiratory failure is most commonly noted in

Duchenne's muscular dystrophy, sometimes it also occurs in the more advanced stages of Becker's, limb-girdle, and facioscapulohumeral muscular dystrophies.[464] In a pilot study, Kerr and Kohrman[455] described sleep apnea (obstructive and central) in 5 of 11 patients with Duchenne's muscular dystrophy. Khan and Heckmatt[457] studied 21 patients ages 13–23 years with Duchenne's muscular dystrophy and 12 age-matched controls using 2 consecutive nights of PSG. They noted apneas, 60% of which were obstructive in nature, with hypoxemia in 12 patients. Takasugi et al.[461] studied 42 patients with Duchenne's muscular dystrophy. PSG study documented three patterns of sleep-related respiratory disorders: obstructive apnea, central apnea, and paradoxical breathing without upper airway obstruction (nonobstructive paradoxical breathing). Obstructive apnea was the most common type. They concluded that sleep disorders are common in patients with Duchenne's muscular dystrophy. Obstructive apnea was the most common type of sleep disorder found, often accompanied by hypercapnia and central apnea in advanced cases, resulting from both respiratory muscle weakness and respiratory center abnormalities. It is important to make the correct diagnosis, which can be established by performing EMG, biochemical, histochemical, or morphologic examination of muscle biopsy samples and respiratory function testing. It should be noted that sleep architecture in Duchenne's muscular dystrophy appears better preserved as compared to the architecture in ALS. The respiratory care of patients with Duchenne's muscular dystrophy has been summarized in a consensus statement developed by the American Thoracic Society.[465]

Khan et al.[466] described eight children 6–13 years old with congenital myopathy, congenital muscular dystrophy, and rigid spine syndromes with respiratory failure. PSG documented nocturnal hypoxemia and severe hypoventilation. Sleep disturbances included repeated awakenings. Sleep complaints and sleep-related periodic respiratory dysrhythmias are also common in other congenital myopathies such as nemaline rod myopathy, centrotubular and central core disease, and merosin-deficiency myopathy.

Myotonic Dystrophy. *Dystrophica myotonica*, or myotonic dystrophy, is an adult-onset, dominantly inherited muscular dystrophy associated with myotonia. Benaim and Worster-Drought[467] were most probably the first to describe alveolar hypoventilation in myotonic dystrophy. Alveolar hypoventilation associated with hypoxemia, as well as impaired hypercapnic and hypoxic ventilatory responses, may be present in both the early and late stages of the illness. A few authors[411,463,468–470] performed polygraphic studies that showed central, mixed, and upper airway obstructive sleep apneas, and sleep-onset REM was noted in some patients. The latter finding may have been due to sleep deprivation secondary to sleep-related respiratory disturbances. Two fundamental mechanisms account for the SRBDs in this illness: (1) weakness and myotonia of the respiratory and upper airway muscles, and (2) an inherited abnormality of the central control of ventilation, most likely related to a common generalized membrane abnormality of the muscles and other tissues, including brain stem neurons that regulate breathing and sleep.[469–472]

Sleep studies by Bye and colleagues[366] in four patients with myotonic dystrophy showed REM sleep–related O_2 desaturation and sleep disorganization. Several other authors have described alveolar hypoventilation, daytime somnolence, and periodic breathing in patients with myotonic dystrophy in single case reports and small and large series.[411,473–487]

Begin et al.[482] found a high prevalence of chronic alveolar hypoventilation in a series of 134 patients with myotonic dystrophy. The authors suggested that the central ventilatory control mechanism is abnormal in myotonic dystrophy patients, contributing to chronic alveolar hypoventilation. These authors concluded that the chronic alveolar hypoventilation resulted from a combination of inspiratory muscle weakness and loading. In addition, the presence of EDS suggested reduced central ventilatory drive or sleep apnea in these patients. The clinicopathologic study by Ono et al.[486,487] of one patient with myotonic dystrophy, alveolar hypoventilation, and hypersomnia supported the hypothesis postulated by Begin et al.[482] On postmortem examination of this patient, Ono et al.[486,487] observed significant neuronal loss and gliosis in the midbrain and pontine raphe, as well as the pontomedullary reticular formation.

Park and Radtke[485] reviewed seven patients with myotonic dystrophy referred to their sleep disorders center. All patients had PSG. Five patients were subsequently given an MSLT. Each of the five who had an MSLT showed evidence of moderate hypersomnia. Three of these five patients had two sleep-onset REM episodes, only one of whom showed evidence of sleep apnea in the overnight PSG study. Human leukocyte antigen (HLA) typing was negative for DQW2 but DQW1 was present in two patients. The authors reviewed the literature available (they published their own paper in 1995) and found 86 patients, including their seven patients, with myotonic dystrophy who also had hypersomnolence. Ten percent of the reported patients with hypersomnolence had documented alveolar hypoventilation. Respiratory center hypoexcitability or myotonic muscle weakness is thought to be responsible for alveolar hypoventilation. Correction of hypoventilation does not always lead to improvement of EDS.[478] SDB events were noted in 57% of the reported patients with EDS, and both central and obstructive sleep apneas were observed. The presence of sleep-onset REMs in these patients supported the hypothesis of a primary CNS abnormality as the cause of EDS.[485] EDS in myotonic dystrophy patients often occurs in the absence of sleep apnea.[485] EDS in their patients[485] responded to methylphenidate treatment. Martinez-Rodriguez et al.[488] measured CSF hypocretin-1 levels in six patients with myotonic dystrophy type 1 complaining of excessive daytime sleepiness who were HLA-DQB1*0602 negative and found to have significantly lower hypocretin-1 levels compared to the control values. The authors concluded that the dysfunction of the hypothalamic hypocretin system may be responsible for hypersomnia in myotonic dystrophy type 1.

The danger of administering anesthetic agents to these patients was demonstrated by Kaufman[476]: 5 of 25 myotonic patients in this series had marked respiratory depression during operation, and another 4 died in the postoperative period. In some more recent studies, evidence of EDS and SRBDs have been noted in many patients with myotonic dystrophy.[489–491] Kumar et al.[489] evaluated 25 patients with type 1 myotonic dystrophy using PSG/overnight oximetry and pulmonary function tests. EDS and excessive tiredness were the most common presenting symptoms in their patients. Prevalence of SRBDs was found to be 36%. They noted that, of all the daytime pulmonary function measurements, forced vital capacity correlated best with $Paco_2$.

Quera-Salva et al.[490] prospectively studied 21 patients with childhood-onset myotonic dystrophy type 1 to assess sleep dysfunction using questionnaires, genetic testing, overnight PSG, and MSLT. In their patients, EDS was present in 52% of patients, and 76% were found to have sleep dysfunction as a result of microarousals caused by abnormal respiratory events (6 of 21 patients) or PLMS (8 of 21 patients).

Laberge et al.[491] surveyed 157 myotonic dystrophy type 1 patients using a modified version of the sleep questionnaire and assessment of wakefulness, measurement of muscular impairment rating, and the size of the trinucleotide repeat. They included 38 healthy family members as control subjects. They found EDS in 33.1% of their patients that was weakly related to the extent of muscular impairment but not to trinucleotide repeat size.

Striano and coworkers[472] described predominantly OSA associated with daytime hypersomnolence in a patient with dominantly inherited myotonia congenita. Because the patient was obese and also had obstructive pulmonary disease, the relationship between sleep apnea and myotonia congenita remains inconclusive.

Sleep disturbances have also been reported in proximal myotonic myopathy (PROMM), also known as myotonic dystrophy type 2. PROMM is an autosomal dominant multisystem disorder caused by a CCTG repeat expansion in intron 1 of the zinc finger protein 9 gene (ZNF9), which is differentiated from myotonic dystrophy type 1 by the absence of a chromosome 19 CTG trinucleotide repeat that is associated with type 1.[492–496] In a brief report, we described sleep disturbances in two sisters, ages 51 and 53, with PROMM.[495] The patients had difficulty initiating sleep, EDS, snoring, and frequent awakenings and movements during sleep. Overnight PSG study in these two patients showed decreased sleep efficiency, increased number of arousals, and sleep architecture abnormalities. One patient had absent REM sleep and the other patient had dissociated REM sleep characterized by phasic REM bursts associated with EEG patterns showing sleep spindles and alpha intrusions. These sleep abnormalities in PROMM suggested involvement of the REM-NREM generating neurons as part of a multisystem membrane disorder. In some patients (unpublished observations), upper airway OSA and REM-related hypoventilation have also been observed. The MRI findings of white matter hyperintensity in T_2-weighted images in six patients from three families with PROMM described by Hund et al.[494] suggested brain involvement in PROMM, but the relationship between the sleep disturbances and the MRI abnormalities remains to be determined.

Acid Maltase Deficiency and Other Glycogen Storage Disorders. Alveolar hypoventilation has been described in several cases of mild to moderate myopathy associated with adult-onset acid maltase deficiency, a variant of glycogen storage disease.[433,450,454,497–499] In this condition, correct diagnosis can be established by performing respiratory function testing; EMG; and biochemical, histochemical, or morphologic examination of muscle biopsy samples. Hypoxemia, hypercapnia, and impaired hypercapnic ventilatory response may be seen in these patients. Diaphragmatic dysfunction may account for the alveolar hypoventilation. Rosenow and Engel[497] suggested that the hypoxemia in their patients was secondary to a combination of hypoventilation due to muscle weakness and an impairment of the ventilation-perfusion ratio resulting from compression atelectasis due to an elevated diaphragm. The patient of Martin's group,[499] on polygraphic study, showed prolonged periods of hypopnea accompanied by O_2 desaturation. The patient improved considerably after inspiratory muscle training.

Bye and coworkers[366] described REM sleep–related hypoxemia and sleep disorganization in acid maltase deficiency, also known as Pompe's disease. An adult patient with acid maltase deficiency with severe OSA and respiratory failure was reported by Margolis et al.[500] The patient had mild daytime hypersomnolence, and the sleep study documented severe upper airway obstructive apnea with O_2 desaturation. Despite ventilatory support, the patient died. At postmortem examination, profound muscle replacement by fibrofatty tissue was noted in the tongue and diaphragm. The authors suggested that severe tongue weakness due to fatty metamorphosis associated with macroglossia contributed to the upper airway obstruction in this patient. The brain was not examined at the autopsy.

Other Varieties of Congenital Myopathies. Riley and coworkers[451] described alveolar hypoventilation in two patients with congenital myopathies (one with nemaline myopathy and the other with a myopathy of uncertain type). The patients' ventilatory response to carbon dioxide was absent, and the authors suggested that the alveolar hypoventilation may have been due to a primary defect in the central chemoreceptor control of breathing. Their other suggestion was that the sensory stimuli from skeletal muscle receptors (e.g., muscle spindles) may have played a role in the blunted hypercapnic ventilatory response by altering afferent input to the CNS.

Bye and colleagues[366] also studied a patient with central core myopathy who had sleep disruption and sleep hypoxemia. Kryger and colleagues[501] described two sisters with congenital muscular dystrophy, with CSA and blunted chemical drive to breathing in the index case. These abnormalities were thought to be out of proportion to the somatic and respiratory muscle weakness. The authors suggested that this patient's central control of breathing was defective. There are other reports of sleep hypoventilation in congenital myopathy.[466,502,503]

Miscellaneous Myopathies. Sleep-related hypoxemia and sleep disturbances have also been described in patients with polymyositis[366,411,454] and mitochondrial encephalomyopathy.[504,505] Sanaker et al.[506] described a patient with Kearns-Sayre syndrome, a mitochondrial encephalomyopathy presenting with polyendocrinopathy and acute respiratory failure. This patient required initially invasive ventilatory support and later noninvasive nocturnal bilevel positive airway pressure (BIPAP) treatment, demonstrating that respiratory failure is a treatable event in this disease.

Neuromuscular Junction Disorders

Myasthenia gravis, myasthenic syndrome, botulism, and tic paralysis are several neuromuscular junction disorders characterized by easy fatigability of the muscles, including the bulbar and other respiratory muscles, owing to failure of neuromuscular junctional transmission of the nerve impulses. The most important of these conditions is myasthenia gravis, an autoimmune disease characterized by a reduction in the number of functional acetylcholine receptors in the postjunctional region. Acute respiratory failure is often a dreaded complication of myasthenia gravis, and patients need immediate assisted ventilation for life support.[81,507] The respiratory failure, moreover, may be mild during wakefulness but may deteriorate considerably during sleep.

An important study by Quera-Salva and colleagues[508] reported the pulmonary function and PSG studies of 16 women and 4 men whose mean age was 40 years and who were diagnosed and treated for myasthenia gravis. Polysomnographic findings included moderately disturbed nocturnal sleep with an increase in stage 1 NREM and decreased slow-wave and REM sleep. Eleven patients had an RDI of 5 or higher. They had central, obstructive, and mixed apneas and hypopneas accompanied by decreased O_2 saturation. All patients with REM sleep–related apneas or hypopneas had disturbed nocturnal sleep with a sensation of breathlessness. Twelve patients had insufficient sleep owing to awakening in the middle of the night and early morning hours with a sensation of breathlessness. Four of the 12 patients also had daytime hypersomnolence. The authors suggested that those patients of advancing age, moderately increased BMI, abnormal pulmonary function results, and daytime blood gas concentrations are at particular risk for SDB. Before this report, brief reports of sleep disruptions and sleep apnea[509–511] appeared in the literature. Since this report, there have been a few other reports of SDB in patients with myasthenia gravis.[512–517]

Shintani et al.[511] studied 10 patients with myasthenia gravis using PSG and observed obstructive and central apneas in six of these 10 patients. Manni et al.[512] studied breathing patterns during sleep in 14 patients with mild generalized myasthenia gravis. Polysomnographic study documented infrequent central apneas, mainly during REM sleep, in five patients associated with O_2 desaturation. Putman and Wise[513] described a 54-year-old woman with myasthenia gravis and episodes of shortness of breath, which were more severe at night. The flow-volume loops suggested extrathoracic airway obstruction. They also surveyed a total of 61 myasthenia gravis patients referred to their pulmonary function laboratory during 42 months. They found a pattern of extrathoracic upper airway obstruction in 7 of the 12 patients who had flow-volume loops. Stepansky et al.[514] performed overnight PSG study in 19 middle-aged myasthenia gravis patients and 10 age-matched controls. In 60% of the myasthenics, they observed mild CSAs with O_2 desaturation without any impairment of the sleep profile. Nicolle et al.[516] randomly selected 100 patients with myasthenia gravis out of 400 patients from their database. Based on the Multivariate Apnea Prediction Index,[518] they performed PSG studies in those scoring more than 0.5 (50 patients). They found a prevalence of OSA of 36% compared to an expected prevalence of 15–20% of the general population. The prevalence of OSAS (those with daytime sleepiness) was 11% compared to 3% in the general population. The authors suggested that it is important to inquire about OSA symptoms in myasthenia gravis patients for adequate management of fatigue in these patients. Prudlo et al.[517] investigated sleep and breathing in 19 myasthenia gravis patients utilizing two consecutive overnight PSG studies. These authors found clinically relevant SDB in terms of OSA (defined as an RDI of >10/hr) in only four patients, who had also a few central apneas. The authors failed to confirm the high occurrence of central respiratory events during sleep and also failed to find a causal relationship between medically stable myasthenia gravis and OSA.

Myasthenic syndrome, or Lambert-Eaton syndrome, is a disorder of the neuromuscular junction in the presynaptic region and is often a paraneoplastic manifestation, mostly of oat cell carcinoma of the lungs. Patients complain of muscle weakness and fatigue involving the limbs accompanied by decreased or absent muscle stretch reflexes and characteristic electrodiagnostic findings that differentiate this from myasthenia gravis.

Botulism caused by *Clostridium botulinum* and tic paralysis caused by the female wood tic *Dermacentor andersoni* may also cause neuromuscular junctional transmission defects, which are due to released toxin.

SLEEP AND BREATHING DISORDERS IN AUTONOMIC FAILURE

Anatomically and functionally, sleep, breathing, and the autonomic nervous system (ANS) are closely interrelated.[81,519–524] To understand sleep and breathing disorders in autonomic failure, it is important to understand the functional anatomy of sleep, control of breathing, and the central autonomic network. A brief review of the functional anatomy of sleep is given in the beginning of this chapter, and the neurophysiology of sleep is also described extensively in Chapters 4 and 5. Functional neuroanatomy of respiration, control of breathing during sleep and wakefulness, and the central autonomic network with its integration of sleep and breathing are reviewed briefly in Chapter 7.

In all of these conditions, respiratory muscles may be affected and patients may require assisted ventilation. They can exhibit sleep hypoventilation and sleep apnea. Profound functional changes occur during sleep in circulation, respiration, thermoregulation, and the gastrointestinal and urogenital systems due to alterations in autonomic outflow[521,522] (see also Chapter 7). Thus sleep has an important effect on the functions of the ANS, and dysfunction of the ANS may have significant impact on human sleep. Sleep and breathing disorders have in fact been described in many patients with autonomic failure. It is also important to remember that the peripheral respiratory receptors, the central respiratory neurons, and the hypnogenic neurons in the preoptic-hypothalamic area and the region of the NTS in the medulla are intimately linked by the ANS, making it easy to comprehend why sleep and breathing disorders should be associated with autonomic failure.

Autonomic failure may be classified into primary and secondary types. Primary autonomic failure (without known cause) includes pure autonomic failure without any somatic neurologic deficits (Bradbury-Eggleston syndrome), MSA (Shy-Drager syndrome), postural tachycardia syndrome (POTS), familiar dysautonomia, and autoimmune autonomic neuropathy or acute pandysautonomia. The most well-known condition with autonomic failure in which sleep and respiratory disturbances have been reported and well described is MSA with progressive autonomic failure, or Shy-Drager

syndrome. In a consensus statement[525] sponsored by the American Autonomic Society and the American Academy of Neurology, *multiple system atrophy* is the favored term, replacing *Shy-Drager syndrome*. MSA defines a sporadic, adult-onset progressive disorder characterized by autonomic dysfunction, parkinsonism, and ataxia in any combination. *Striatonigral degeneration* is the term used when the predominant feature is parkinsonism. The term *sporadic olivopontocerebellar atrophy* is used when cerebellar features are present. Finally, when autonomic failure is the predominant feature, the term *Shy-Drager syndrome* is often used. Familial dysautonomia, a recessively inherited primarily autonomic failure, is also known to be associated with disturbances of breathing and sleep. A large number of neurologic and general medical disorders are associated with prominent secondary autonomic failure. In many patients with diabetic autonomic neuropathies, amyloid neuropathy, and GBS, sleep and sleep-related respiratory disturbances have been noted. In many neurologic conditions, sleep and respiratory disturbances are secondary to the structural lesions involving the central hypnogenic or respiratory neurons. Some examples of neurodegenerative diseases with autonomic failure are PD (see Chapter 28) and DLBD with dementia (see earlier section) and fatal familial insomnia (FFI), a rare prion disease with severe sleep disturbances and dysautonomia (see later in this chapter). Finally, upper airway OSAS, a very common primary sleep disorder, may be associated with autonomic deficits including cardiac arrhythmias.

Multiple System Atrophy with Progressive Autonomic Failure (Shy-Drager Syndrome)

In 1960, Shy and Drager[526] described a neurodegenerative disorder characterized by autonomic failure and MSA. Since their description, there have been many reports[76,77,84,89,252,521,527–537] of the condition, which has generally come to be known as *Shy-Drager syndrome* or *multiple system atrophy with progressive autonomic failure*. MSA defines a sporadic adult-onset progressive disorder of multiple systems characterized by autonomic dysfunction, parkinsonism, and cerebellar ataxia in various combinations (Table 29–5). A second consensus conference held in 2007 published new diagnostic criteria for definite, probable, and possible MSA (Table 29–6).[538]

Patients frequently manifest sleep and respiratory disturbances. Initially, they present with autonomic failure of both the sympathetic and parasympathetic systems. They may present with symptoms related to orthostatic hypotension (e.g., postural dizziness and faintness or even frank loss of consciousness in the erect posture), urinary sphincter dysfunction (e.g., frequency, urgency, hesitancy, dribbling, overflow incontinence), hypohidrosis or anhidrosis, and impotence in men. After 2–6 years, patients lapse into the second stage, showing some combination

TABLE 29–5 Salient Clinical Manifestations of Multiple System Atrophy[69]

Autonomic Features

Cardiovascular
- Orthostatic hypotension
- Postprandial hypotension
- Postural syncope
- Postural dizziness, faintness, or blurring of vision
- Orthostatic intolerance

Genitourinary
- Urinary bladder dysfunction (incontinence, hesitancy, frequency, nocturia)
- Impotence in men

Sudomotor
- Hypohidrosis or anhidrosis

Gastrointestinal
- Gastroparesis
- Intermittent diarrhea or constipation (intestinal or colonic dysmotility)
- Abnormal swallowing (esophageal dysmotility)

Ocular
- Horner's syndrome
- Unequal pupils

Nonautonomic Manifestations

Parkinsonism
- Rigidity
- Bradykinesis or akinesis
- Postural instability

Cerebellar dysfunction
- Ataxic gait
- Scanning speech
- Dysmetria
- Dysdiadochokinesia
- Intention tremor

Upper motor neuron signs
- Extensor plantar responses
- Hyperreflexia
- Spasticity

Lower motor neuron signs
- Muscle wasting
- Fasciculations

Respiratory
- Sleep apnea-hypopnea
- Other respiratory dysrhythmias

REM sleep behavior disorder
Normal sensation

TABLE 29–6 Criteria for the Diagnosis of Multiple System Atrophy (MSA) Based on Second Consensus Statement[538]

Definite MSA

A sporadic, progressive adult-onset (>30 years old) disease with neuropathologic demonstration of
- α-Synuclein–positive glial cytoplasmic inclusions in the CNS
- Evidence of neurodiagnostic changes in striatonigral or olivopontocerebellar structures

Probable MSA

A sporadic, progressive adult-onset (>30 years old) disease with
- Evidence of autonomic dysfunction (e.g., orthostatic fall of blood pressure by at least 30 mm Hg systolic or 15 mm Hg diastolic within 3 minutes of standing, urinary incontinence or erectile dysfunction in men)
- Parkinsonian features (e.g., bradykinesia, rigidity, tremor, postural instability) that are poorly levodopa-responsive or
- Cerebellar features (e.g., gait and limb ataxia, scanning dysarthria, cerebellar type of oculomotor dysfunction)

Possible MSA

A sporadic, progressive adult-onset (>30 years old) disease with
- Parkinsonian features or
- Cerebellar features or
- Evidence of at least one autonomic dysfunction (orthostatic fall of blood pressure should be significant, which may not meet the level required for probable MSA)
- Presence of at least one of the following additional features (either a clinical or a neuroimaging abnormality):
  - Stridor and hyperreflexia with Babinski sign
  - Possible MSA—parkinsonian or cerebellar features; dysphagia within 5 years of motor onset; olivopontocerebellar or putaminal atrophy on brain MRI; FDG-PET hypometabolism in putamen, brain stem, or cerebellum
  - Possible MSA—cerebellar features; presynaptic nigrostriatal dopaminergic denervation on SPECT or PET scan; olivopontocerebellar or putaminal atrophy on MRI; FDG-PET hypometabolism in putamen, brain stem, or cerebellum

CNS, central nervous system; FDG-PET, fluorodeoxyglucose positron emission tomography; MRI, magnetic resonance imaging; PET, positron emission tomography; SPECT, single-photon emission computed tomography.

of cerebellar, extrapyramidal, upper motor neuron, and lower motor neuron dysfunction, including bulbar deficits. Most patients manifest a parkinsonian-cerebellar syndrome. In some, atypical parkinsonian features (e.g., bradykinesia, rigidity, postural instability) predominate; in others, pancerebellar dysfunction predominates. In the later stages of the illness, a variety of respiratory and sleep disturbances add to the progressive disability. Occasionally, respiratory dysfunction, particularly dysrhythmic breathing in wakefulness that becomes worse during sleep, manifests in the initial stage of the illness. In the final stage, progressive autonomic and somatic dysfunction are compounded by respiratory failure. Ventilatory disturbances now may be present in both wakefulness and sleep. Pathologically, there are various combinations

of striatonigral degeneration, OPCA, and degeneration of the autonomic neurons. A distinctive neuropathologic alteration in MSA is thought to be the presence of argyrophilic oligodendroglial cytoplasmic inclusions in the cortical motor, premotor, and supplementary motor areas; extrapyramidal and corticocerebellar systems; brain stem reticular formation; and supraspinal autonomic systems and their targets.[535] This inclusion-bearing oligodendroglial degeneration may cause or contribute to the manifestations of clinical symptoms in MSA. In fact, Wenning et al.[536] recently hypothesized that MSA is a primary oligodendrogliopathy.

Sleep Disturbances

Sleep dysfunction is very common in MSA and includes insomnia with sleep fragmentation; RBD, which may occasionally be the presenting feature[539–541]; and sleep-related respiratory dysrhythmias. RBD is very common, being present in 80–95% of MSA patients.[39,542,543] The characteristic clinical features of RBD include intermittent loss of REM-related muscle atonia and appearance of a variety of abnormal motor activities during sleep. The patient presents a violent dream-enacting behavior during REM sleep, often causing self-injury or injury to the bed partner. RBD may precede the illness or may present concomitantly or after the onset of MSA.[543,544] Positron emission tomography (PET) and single-photon emission computed tomography (SPECT) studies by Gilman et al.[545] suggested that RBD in MSA is related to nigrostriatal dopaminergic deficit. In other cases, RBD in MSA may be due to the neuropathologic changes in the brain stem REM-generating neurons.

The most common sleep disorders in MSA result from a variety of sleep-related respiratory dysrhythmias similar to those described in other neurologic conditions (see Fig. 29–6). The most common types of respiratory dysrhythmias consist of sleep apnea and hypopnea associated with repeated arousals and hypoxemia,[67,74,546–558] dysrhythmic breathing,[74,546] and laryngeal stridor due to laryngeal abductor paralysis.[345–347,527,528,549,554,559–561] Less commonly, apneustic breathing[548] and inspiratory gasping[74,528,554] may occur. Hypersomnia often results from nocturnal sleep disruption. Sudden nocturnal death in patients with MSA in some cases probably is due to respiratory arrest and other cardiorespiratory abnormalities. Sleep-related respiratory dysrhythmias in MSA are present in almost 100% of the cases in the advanced stages of the illness. Polysomnographic studies may show the following: a reduction of total sleep time, decreased sleep efficiency, increased number of awakenings during sleep, a reduction of slow-wave and REM sleep, absence of muscle atonia in REM sleep in those with RBD, and a variety of respiratory dysrhythmias. Laryngeal stridor and excessive snoring resulting from laryngeal abductor paralysis have been described in cases of MSA by several groups.[527,529,549–554,559–562] The nocturnal stridor can be inspiratory, expiratory, or both and can cause upper airway obstruction during sleep. The stridor may result in a striking noise likened to a donkey's braying.[531] Williams's group[552] noted this abnormality in 8 of 12 cases. The stridor can be relieved by tracheostomy. The group led by Guilleminault[555–557] described eight patients with predominantly upper airway OSA associated with O$_2$ desaturation.

In our early study of four patients with MSA,[89] we observed periodic central apnea in the erect position and CSB in one patient during the last stage of the illness. Impaired hypercapnic ventilatory response and mouth occlusion pressure response in the supine position in one patient suggested impairment of the metabolic respiratory system, whereas normal hypercapnic and hypoxic ventilatory responses in another patient (in the presence of an abnormal respiratory pattern resembling that noted by Lockwood[547]) suggested that the chemoreceptor control and respiratory pattern generator were probably subserved by different populations of neurons rendered selectively vulnerable in MSA. The neuropathologic findings in the same patient with impaired chemoreceptor response—neuronal loss and astrocytosis in the pontine tegmentum—suggested involvement of the respiratory neurons in the brain stem. In a later study,[74] we described 10 other patients with MSA who showed central apnea, including CSB or Cheyne-Stokes variant type breathing and upper airway obstructive and mixed apneas accompanied by O$_2$ desaturation, predominantly during NREM sleep stages 1 and 2 and REM sleep (Fig. 29–15). During sleep, seven patients had central apnea, two had upper airway OSA, and three had mixed apneas. The RDI varied from 20 to 80; the duration of apneas ranged from 10 to 65 seconds. The variation in the heart rate during apneic and eupneic cycles was not seen in these patients with evidence of cardiac autonomic denervation. This finding was in contrast to the bradyarrhythmias and tachyarrhythmias noted during apnea and immediately after resumption of normal breathing in patients with primary sleep apnea syndrome.[81] Four patients had several episodes of central apneas during relaxed wakefulness; it was as if the

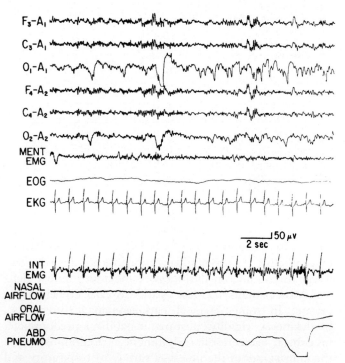

FIGURE 29–15 A portion of an episode of mixed apnea during stage 2 NREM sleep associated with oxygen desaturation in a patient with multiple system atrophy. The electroencephalogram (EEG) is shown in the top six channels. Also shown are electromyography (EMG) of the mentalis (MENT) and intercostal (INT) muscles, electrocardiogram (EKG), nasal and oral airflow, and abdominal pneumogram (ABD PNEUMO). *(Reproduced with permission from Chokroverty S. Sleep and breathing in neurological disorders. In NH Edelman, TV Santiago [eds], Breathing Disorders of Sleep. New York: Churchill Livingstone, 1986;225.)*

respiratory center "forgot" to breathe. Two patients had inspiratory gasps and two required tracheostomy for respiratory dysrhythmia. All-night PSG studies in two patients revealed the following sleep abnormalities in addition to recurrent episodes of sleep apneas accompanied by O_2 desaturation: marked reduction of NREM sleep stages 3 and 4 and REM sleep, increased awakenings after sleep onset, snoring, and excessive body movements and frequent arousal responses in the EEG. In 8 of 10 patients, dysrhythmic breathing occurred mostly during sleep, although in 4 of these 8 it was also present during wakefulness; this finding suggests that this type of respiratory dysrhythmia is very common in MSA. These observations are in agreement with the suggestion of McNicholas and colleagues[84] that such findings imply an impaired respiratory pattern generator in these patients.

Mechanisms of Ventilatory Dysrhythmia

There is ample evidence in the literature[252,526] of pathologic involvement of the pontine tegmentum, reticular formation, NTS, nucleus ambiguus, hypoglossal nucleus, and, in some patients, anterior horn cells of the cervical and thoracic spinal cord. Lockwood[547] and Chokroverty and colleagues[89] correlated the physiologic and clinical findings of respiratory dysrhythmias with direct involvement of the regions of the brain stem that contain the respiratory neurons. In addition, physiologic studies of respiratory control[84,89] showing impairment of hypercapnic and hypoxic ventilatory and mouth occlusion pressure responses indirectly suggested an impairment of the metabolic respiratory control system. Vagal and sympathetic denervation in these patients is firmly established.[252,526] The pathogenic mechanisms for the respiratory dysrhythmia include all that had been postulated in the beginning of this chapter for the respiratory dysrhythmias in neurologic disorders. Additional mechanisms for the respiratory dysrhythmia have been suggested[74]: interference with the forebrain, midbrain, and pontine inputs to the medullary respiratory neurons causing dysrhythmic and apneustic breathing; involvement of the direct projections from the hypothalamus and central nucleus of the amygdala to the respiratory neurons in the NTS and nucleus ambiguus; involvement of the vagal afferents from the lower and upper airway receptors, which would reduce the input to the central respiratory neurons, causing respiratory dysrhythmia; sympathetic denervation of the nasal mucosa causing increased nasal resistance, thus promoting upper airway obstructive apnea; and discrete neurochemical alterations that may interfere with normal regulation of breathing.

There is experimental evidence that noradrenaline, serotonin, and dopamine play distinct roles in the control of breathing.[563] Patients with MSA have been found to have low levels of dopamine and noradrenaline in the basal ganglia, the limbic-hypothalamic regions including the septal nuclei, and the LC.[564] Furthermore, these patients may also have specific catecholamine enzyme deficits in the brain and sympathetic ganglia.[565] SPECT findings by Gilman et al.[566] suggested decreased pontine cholinergic projections to the thalamus contributing to OSA in MSA. Finally, in a series of postmortem studies of brains obtained from patients with MSA, Benarroch and colleagues reported depletion of catecholaminergic neurons in the ventrolateral medulla,[567] A5 noradrenergic neurons,[568] cholinergic neurons in the medullary arcuate nucleus,[569] corticotrophin-releasing factor neurons[570] in the putative pontine micturition center, mesopontine cholinergic neurons in the PPT and LDT nucleus,[571,572] ventrolateral medullary neurokinin 1 receptor–like immunoreactive neurons,[573] chemosensitive glutamatergic and serotoninergic neurons in the arcuate nucleus in the ventral medullary surface as well as serotoninergic neurons in the medullary raphe,[574] serotoninergic neurons in the pontomedullary raphe,[575] and neurons in the ventrolateral nucleus ambiguus innervating the heart and dorsal vagal nucleus–innervating enteric neurons,[576] as well as loss of hypocretin (orexin) hypothalamic neurons.[577] Loss of these cell groups may contribute to the respiratory disturbances, including loss of automatic respiration and other autonomic dysfunction involving various systems in MSA.[578]

Vetrugno et al.[579] performed video-PSG study in 19 consecutive MSA patients and documented RBD in 100% of the patients, stridor in 42%, OSA in 37%, and PLMS in 88%. Plazzi et al.[542] documented RBD in 90% of 39 consecutive MSA patients. RBD preceded in 44%, appeared concomitantly in 26%, and followed the onset of MSA symptoms in 30% of the patients. They also noted OSA, stridor, and PLMS in some patients. Ghorayeb et al.,[580] based on a standard sleep questionnaire, reported a variety of sleep disorders in 70% of 57 unselected patients with MSA: sleep fragmentation (52.5%), vocalization (60%), RBD (47.5%), and nocturnal stridor (19%). They noted that severity of motor symptoms, disease duration, comorbid depression, and the duration of levodopa treatment correlated with sleep problems. Silber and Levine,[581] after reviewing 42 patients with MSA (17 with nocturnal stridor and 25 without stridor), concluded that survival is shorter in those with stridor than in those without stridor. There are several other reports of stridor, particularly nocturnal stridor and sudden nocturnal death resulting presumably from laryngeal obstruction, in some MSA patients. Iranzo et al.[582] reported sleep disturbances in all 20 patients with MSA and vocal cord abduction dysfunction in 14 (70%) of their 20 patients in a prospective study. Following CPAP treatment, laryngeal stridor and obstructive apneas were eliminated in three patients. Iranzo et al.[583] followed 13 MSA patients with stridor for months and reported beneficial effects of long-term CPAP therapy. In addition to improvement in the quality of sleep, these authors found similar median survival in patients with and without stridor. In a study of 22 MSA patients, Ghorayeb et al.[584] found 3 with OSA without stridor and 15 with stridor alone or accompanied by apnea. They administered CPAP treatment in 12 of these patients. Two, however, died shortly after CPAP titration and one died 17 months later. Five patients discontinued use of CPAP because of discomfort, and four continued CPAP with improvement of sleep and daytime alertness. The authors concluded that the severity of motor impairment at the time of initial CPAP is the most significant factor for long-term CPAP acceptance.

Postural Tachycardia Syndrome

POTS, also known as orthostatic intolerance syndrome, is an entity still in search of an identity, and the clinical manifestations are still evolving. Sleep dysfunction, which is often an important component of the clinical manifestations of POTS, has largely been neglected in the literature.[585] The clinical diagnostic criteria for POTS include symptoms of orthostatic intolerance accompanied by heart rate of 120 beats/min or more, or a heart rate increment of 30 beats/min or more on changing from supine to upright position within 5 minutes of standing or head-up tilt.[586] The symptoms of orthostatic intolerance include faint feelings, dizziness, palpitations, nausea, tremulousness, anxiety, and visual blurring on standing without significant orthostatic hypotension. The other symptoms of these patients include extreme fatigue, diffuse muscle aches and pains, and upper and lower gastrointestinal symptoms, as well as sleep dysfunction.[587] Some patients may complain of sleep-onset or maintenance insomnia, whereas others may have daytime hypersomnolence or circadian rhythm disorders. Some patients may complain of fatigue, which is a very common manifestation and may be difficult to differentiate from EDS. Sleep-onset and maintenance insomnia in patients with POTS may be related to PLMS, inadequate sleep hygiene, diffuse muscle aches and pains, and anxiety. Daytime hypersomnolence may be secondary to OSA or to sleep deprivation at night, as well as to depression in some patients. Circadian rhythm disorders suggest a dysfunction of the circadian clock in the SCN. It is important to pay attention to sleep dysfunction in these patients as treatment combining pharmacologic therapy (short-term hypnotic or selective serotonin reuptake inhibitor) and nonpharmacologic treatment (sleep hygiene, stimulus control therapy, relaxation techniques, appropriately timed bright-light exposure) may be beneficial in such patients. An adequate number of patients with POTS have not been studied to understand the pathophysiology of sleep dysfunction in this syndrome.

Familial Dysautonomia (Riley-Day Syndrome)

Riley-Day syndrome is a recessively inherited disorder associated with autonomic failure. The condition usually presents in childhood and is peculiar to the Jewish population. The clinical features consist of a variety of autonomic and somatic manifestations[588]: autonomic, neuromuscular, cardiovascular, gastroesophageal, skeletal, renal, and respiratory abnormalities; absence of the fungiform papillae of the tongue; defective lacrimation and sweating; vasomotor instability and fluctuation of blood pressure (postural hypotension and paroxysmal hypertension); relative insensitivity to pain; and absent muscle stretch reflexes. Sleep dysfunction, associated with both CSAs and OSAs, has been described in most of these patients.[589] Sleep abnormalities consist of increased awakenings; delayed sleep onset, including prolonged REM-sleep onset (but reduced REM sleep time); and sleep apneas. Patients with familial dysautonomia often have prolonged breath-holding spells, owing to defective responses of central respiratory neurons to changes in Pa_{CO_2}.

Gadoth and colleagues[589] performed PSG recordings in 13 patients (7 women and 6 men ages 5–31 years) with familial dysautonomia to investigate the role of ANS in sleep and breathing disorders in this condition. All had sleep apneas (an average of 73.5/night), 11 had central apnea, and 2 had OSA. REM latency was prolonged, with decreased amount of REM in some patients, and adults also had increased sleep latency. All had orthostatic hypotension, and cardiac responses during apnea were absent, indicating cardiac autonomic denervation.

Guilleminault and colleagues[557] described two adolescent girls with familial dysautonomia who had respiratory irregularities. One also had esophageal reflux during sleep that gave rise to sleep disturbances due to frequent awakenings. McNicholas and coworkers[84] described dysrhythmic breathing in a patient with familial dysautonomia similar to the irregular breathing noted in patients with MSA. Maayan and associates[590] described a 42-year-old woman with familial dysautonomia who had several episodes of apnea during both wakefulness and sleep. The patient had megaesophagus associated with constriction in the lower esophageal region, which caused recurrent aspiration and apnea. After gastrostomy, no apneas were noted. An infant with familial dysautonomia with episodic somnolence lasting for 4–15 hours during the neonatal period has also been reported.[591]

Secondary Autonomic Failure

Many medical and neurologic conditions have associated autonomic neuropathies with peripheral neuropathies, but in most of these conditions, sleep and respiratory dysfunctions have not been adequately studied.[76,592,593] However, there are many reports of such studies in diabetic polyneuropathies associated with autonomic neuropathy. This combination of somatic and autonomic neuropathies has been observed in some patients with acute inflammatory polyradiculoneuropathy (GBS), amyloidosis, and paraneoplastic autonomic neuropathy.

Rees and coworkers[594] observed 30 or more apneic episodes (in two patients mainly central and in one predominantly obstructive) during sleep at night in three of eight patients with diabetic autonomic neuropathy. In contrast, eight diabetes patients without autonomic neuropathy exhibited no sleep-related respiratory dysrhythmias. The authors speculated that sudden cardiorespiratory arrests that have been noted in some patients with diabetes may be related to autonomic failure and sleep apneas.

Guilleminault and coworkers[557] reported OSAs in two of four patients with juvenile diabetic autonomic neuropathy. One had central apnea and the other had irregular breathing associated with sleep-related esophageal reflux. Of the patients with primary sleep apnea syndrome described by Chokroverty and Sharp,[595] four had diabetes mellitus.

Mondini and Guilleminault[596] obtained PSG recordings for 12 type 1 and seven type 2 diabetics. They found obstructive and central apneas and an irregular pattern of breathing in five of 12 type 1 patients. They noted OSA in only one of seven type 2 diabetics. Autonomic neuropathy was present in all three type 1 patients with diabetes.

The findings of Catterall and coworkers[597] do not support the findings reported here of patients with diabetic autonomic neuropathy. They studied eight patients who had autonomic neuropathy and eight who did not and found no significant difference in frequency of apnea between the two groups.

Bottini et al.[598] described obstructive sleep apnea/hypopnea with a frequency of more than 30% in adult, nonobese diabetes with autonomic neuropathy independent of the severity of their dysautonomia.

Neurodegenerative Disease with Autonomic Failure and Sleep Dysfunction

Two neurodegenerative diseases, PD and DLBD, are associated with autonomic failure and sleep disturbances. They are considered synucleinopathies, which are a group of disorders with abnormal deposition of α-synuclein in the cytoplasm of neurons or glial cells. In PD, sleep dysfunction is present in 70–90% of cases, with progressive impairment with the progression of the disease (see Chapter 28). Sleep disturbances and sleep-related respiratory dysrhythmias are common in patients with PD, especially those with evidence of autonomic failure.[98] Distinguishing dopa-responsive idiopathic PD with autonomic failure from dopa-nonresponsive MSA with predominant parkinsonism and dysautonomia may be difficult but important for prognosis and treatment.

Symptomatic orthostatic hypotension, including syncope, occurs in up to 30% of patients with DLBD,[599-601] sometimes as the presenting feature. Other dysautonomic features in DLBD may include urogenital disturbance.

Fatal familial insomnia (see later) is also associated with significant dysautonomia, particularly sympathetic hyperactivity.

Cardiac Arrhythmias and Autonomic Deficits in Obstructive Sleep Apnea Syndrome

Several varieties of cardiac dysrhythmias are noted in patients with OSAS as a result of changes in the ANS. These are described in Chapter 33.

MISCELLANEOUS NEUROLOGIC DISORDERS

Sleep Apnea in Narcolepsy Syndrome

The narcolepsy syndrome is manifested by an irresistible desire to fall asleep at inappropriate times. Such attacks last a few seconds to as long as 20–30 minutes. They are often accompanied by cataplexy or other characteristic ancillary manifestations of narcolepsy (see Chapter 27). Narcolepsy may be associated with other comorbid sleep disorders such as RBD, OSA, PLMS, sleep-related eating disorder, sleepwalking, and nightmares. It is often associated with an increased BMI, which predisposes to the development of OSA. Narcoleptics have on average a BMI 10–20% higher than the normal population.[602,603] A reduced metabolic rate, decreased motor activity, and abnormal eating behavior[604] have been suggested as possible explanations. SDB is found in 10–20% of patients.[605,606]

Guilleminault's group[607] first reported CSA that lasted 20–90 seconds (during REM and NREM sleep) accompanied by O_2 desaturation in two patients with pure narcolepsy. In a later report, Guilleminault and colleagues[608] described 20 additional cases of narcolepsy with sleep apnea, which was predominantly central, although 5 also had mixed and obstructive apneas. The authors speculated that a dysfunction of the CNS structures that control sleep and respiratory centers was responsible for the combined syndrome of sleep apnea and narcolepsy. Laffont and colleagues[609] also described central, obstructive, and mixed apneas in 5 of 18 narcolepsy patients. Chokroverty[606] made polygraphic observations in 16 patients with narcolepsy syndrome, 11 of whom showed central apneas and 5 upper airway OSAs during both REM and NREM sleep stages associated with O_2 desaturation (Figs. 29–16 and 29–17).

The possibility of coexisting sleep apnea should be considered in a patient with narcolepsy, particularly when the patient is again complaining of EDS after initial improvement on stimulant therapy. OSA should be suspected in such a patient, particularly with increasing age

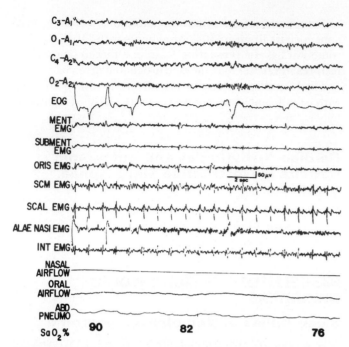

FIGURE 29–16 Polysomnographic recording of a patient with narcolepsy showing four channels of the electroencephalogram (EEG); vertical electro-oculogram (EOG); electromyograms (EMG) of mentalis (MENT), submental (SUBMENT), orbicularis oris (ORIS), sternocleidomastoid (SCM), scalenus anticus (SCAL), alae nasi, and intercostal (INT) muscles; nasal and oral airflow; abdominal pneumogram (ABD PNEUMO); and oxygen saturation ($Sao_2\%$; ear oximeter). The patient has central apnea during REM sleep (only 18–30 seconds are shown). Note decrease of Sao_2 from 90% to 76% during apnea.

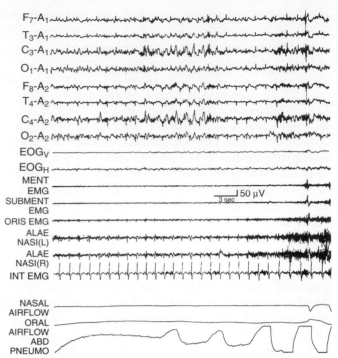

FIGURE 29–17 Polysomnographic recording in a patient with narcolepsy and sleep apnea showing the electroencephalogram (EEG: top eight channels); vertical (EOG_V) and horizontal (EOG_H) electro-oculograms; electromyography (EMG) of mentalis (MENT), submental (SUBMENT), orbicularis oris (ORIS), left (L) and right (R) alae nasi, and intercostal (INT) muscles; nasal and oral airflow, and abdominal pneumogram (ABD PNEUMO). Note mixed apnea (initial central apnea for a period of 13 seconds followed by obstructive apnea for a period of 19 seconds) during NREM sleep stage 2.

as prevalence of OSA increases in the elderly. Patients with comorbid narcolepsy and sleep apnea should receive treatment for both conditions.

Kleine-Levin Syndrome

An episodic disorder characterized by periodic hypersomnolence and bulimia was described first by Kleine[610] and later by Levin[611] occurring mostly in adolescent boys (but also described in girls[612]). Critchley[613,614] gave a comprehensive description after analysis of 15 cases from the literature and 11 personal cases. The episodes usually occur three to four times per year, and each episode lasts days to weeks. During the sleep "attacks," patients sleep 16–18 hours a day or more, and on awakening they eat voraciously. Other behavior disturbances during the episode may include dull appearance, withdrawal, confusion, hallucinations, inattentiveness, memory impairment, and hypersexuality. In a later report, Billiard and Cadilhac[615] reviewed 123 cases collected from the literature. The condition is generally sporadic and self-limited (although not always) and disappears by adulthood. Occasional familial cases have been described.[616,617] Polysomnographic studies show normal sleep cycling or nonspecific findings and

MSLTs show evidence of pathologic sleepiness without sleep-onset REM.[618–620] In a report on 10 patients, Huang et al.[621] observed a reduction of slow-wave sleep in the initial half of the symptomatic period and mild sleepiness in the MSLT, with two or more sleep-onset REM periods (SOREMPs) in 7 of 17 patients. Occasional atypical presentations with episodic alteration in sleep (hypersomnia and insomnia) and appetite (hyperphagia and anorexia) responding to carbamazine treatment have been reported.[622]

The cause of the condition remains undetermined, although a limbic-hypothalamic dysfunction has long been suspected but not proven. Reports of thalamic and hypothalamic hypoperfusion in SPECT study supports this hypothesis.[623,624] Previous reports by Gadoth et al.[625] describing episodic hormone secretion during sleep in Kleine-Levin syndrome, as well as the neuroendocrinologic assays by Chesson et al.[626] in a patient with Kleine-Levin syndrome during symptomatic and asymptomatic 24-hour periods, also supported a possible hypothalamic dysfunction. The earlier report by Gau et al.[627] of a 9-year-old Taiwanese boy with Prader-Willi syndrome associated with Kleine-Levin syndrome showing MRI evidence of a small hypothalamus further supports the hypothesis of a possible hypothalamic dysfunction in Kleine-Levin syndrome. Brief reports of decreased CSF hypocretin-1 levels in occasional patients also speak in favor of a recurrent dysfunction at the hypothalamic level.[628,629] Finally, there is a suggestion of an autoimmune hypothesis based on HLA study showing increased DQB1*0201 allele frequency in some patients with Kleine-Levin syndrome.[630]

Traditional treatment for this condition has been unsatisfactory, but lithium treatment has been found to be effective.[627,631–633] Some other reports also show beneficial effect of treatment with valproic acid,[622,634–637] carbamazepine,[622,636] and lamotrigine.[638] Readers are referred to Arnulf et al.,[639,640] Huang and Arnulf,[636] and Orlosky[641] for review of the Kleine-Levin syndrome.

Idiopathic Recurrent Stupor

Idiopathic recurrent stupor (IRS) is a condition of episodic loss of consciousness. In 1990, Cirignotta et al.[642] reported a patient with recurring coma and abnormal behavior in the absence of toxic, metabolic, or vascular factors. In 1992, Tinuper et al.[643] described a similar patient, and they described three more patients in 1994[644] in more detail. The clinical features are characterized by recurrent episodes of stupor in all of these patients, in whom no metabolic, toxic, or structural brain dysfunction was noted. Tinuper et al.[643] coined the term *idiopathic recurrent stupor* for this condition, describing a characteristic EEG during an episode of stupor in these patients. The EEG showed nonreactive, diffusely distributed fast rhythms (14–16 Hz). The frequency of the episodes of stupor varied between 1–2 and 26 per week, and the duration varied between 2 and 48 hours. A characteristic feature is that the patients were all briefly arousable from the stupor. In all three patients, the AHI or RDI was higher than normal, somewhat complicating the issue. However, the characteristics of this disorder, including EEG and pharmacologic response, have not been described in patients with sleep apnea syndrome. Benzodiazepine-like activity identified as endozepine-4 in plasma and CSF was markedly elevated in all patients. The clinical manifestations and the EEG abnormalities rapidly reversed to the normal state after administration of flumazenil (0.5–1.0 mg intravenously), a benzodiazepine-receptor antagonist. Lemesle et al.,[645] in a letter to the editor, confirmed the efficacy of flumazenil in IRS. Several other cases have subsequently been reported worldwide.[646–649] Lotz et al.[650] described a somewhat similar patient with recurrent attacks of unconsciousness but with several differences from the patients described by Tinuper et al.[644] The patient described by Lotz et al.[650] had a characteristic EEG showing diffuse alpha-like activity with frontal predominance, and this patient was unarousable. The duration of each attack varied from 2 to 24 hours and the frequency of attacks was two to three per week. In addition, this patient had a family history with a similar illness in the father and two siblings. The patient responded to flumazenil treatment. Additional differences in the patient described by Lotz et al.[650] included prolonged I-IV latency in brain stem auditory evoked response, a nocturnal peak of melatonin secretion, and distal sensory-motor polyneuropathy. No consistent treatment for the prevention of the attacks exists in IRS but, in the patient reported by Scott and Ahmed,[649] modafinil proved effective in preventing recurrent episodes of stupor and coma at a dose of 200 mg/day for a period of 6 months. Upon withdrawal of the drug, the patient experienced recurrent episodes that abated following reinstitution of modafinil.

The description of these cases points to the role of benzodiazepine-like receptors in stupor and coma. Endozepines, benzodiazepine-like $GABA_A$ receptor modulators, are present in physiologically significant amounts in the brain.[651] Endozepines do not seem to play a role in sleep disorders with EDS,[652] but it is notable that they accumulate in hepatic coma, in which flumazenil injection also causes transient arousal.[653] It was therefore suggested that IRS results from accumulation of endozepine substances, and the term *endozepine stupor* was suggested for this condition.[654] In 1998, however, the original authors who described IRS[655] reported a case of covert lorazepam intoxication misdiagnosed as endozepine stupor and called attention to the need to perform refined toxicologic analyses (mass spectroscopy with high-performance liquid chromatography) in order to exclude with certainty the presence of exogenous benzodiazepines, in particular lorazepam, that may mimic the action of endozepines. Subsequent reports also highlighted the need to exclude fraudulent exogenous benzodiazepines, in particular lorazepam administration, in cases of comas associated with fast EEG activities and response to flumazenil,[656–658] and have cast doubts on the true existence of a syndrome of recurrent comas due to endozepine accumulation.[658] However, endozepines do exist and accumulate in hepatic encephalopathy.[656] A review of endozepine stupor and a proposed algorithm for differentiating stupor related to endozepines from exogenous benzodiazepine accumulation has been published by Cortelli et al.[660]

Idiopathic Hypersomnia

Idiopathic hypersomnia (IH), a condition of excessive somnolence, has no known cause. A disorder of the CNS has been suspected but not proved.[661,662] The syndrome has been described under a variety of labels, including non–rapid eye movement narcolepsy; idiopathic central nervous system hypersomnia, and mono- or polysymptomatic idiopathic hypersomnia; *idiopathic hypersomnia* is the preferred term. IH closely resembles narcolepsy syndrome. The ICSD-2[91] defines the disorder as a condition characterized by EDS lasting for at least

3 months that is associated with either normal (6–10 hours) or prolonged (>10 hours) nocturnal sleep documented by history, actigraphy, sleep logs, or PSG. It is interesting to note that this division of IH into two forms in the ICSD-2 is reminiscent of the two forms of the disease described by Bedrich Roth,[663] who actually coined the term *idiopathic hypersomnia;* he described a monosymptomatic form manifested only by EDS and a polysymptomatic form characterized by EDS, nocturnal sleep of abnormally long duration, and signs of "sleep drunkenness" upon awakening. The onset of the disease is generally around the same age as narcolepsy (15–30 years). The sleep pattern, however, is different from that of narcolepsy. The patient generally sleeps for hours and the sleep is not refreshing. Because of EDS, the condition may be mistaken for sleep apnea or narcolepsy. However, the patient does not give a history of cataplexy, snoring, or repeated awakenings throughout the night. Sleep drunkenness is often seen in these patients and may manifest as automatic behavior with amnesia for the events. Physical examination uncovers no abnormal neurologic findings. The condition is disabling and generally lifelong, although spontaneous remissions have been noted in a few patients.[91,664] In a retrospective review of 77 patients with IH, Anderson et al.[664] stated that clinical features were heterogeneous and of variable severity, similar to the suggestion made by Aldrich.[665] Aldrich also suggested that clinical heterogeneity may reflect differences in etiology, such as the reports of preceding Epstein-Barr virus infection, infectious mononucleosis[666] or GBS, or human immunodeficiency virus infection.[667] Finally, Aldrich[665] argued for a re-evaluation of the diagnostic criteria for idiopathic disorders of sleepiness not associated with cataplexy. It has been suggested[668] that occasional patients with IH may be misdiagnosed as having adult-onset attention-deficit/hyperactivity disorder (ADHD) based on a self-reported ADHD questionnaire. The condition may be familial, and an autosomal dominant mode of inheritance has been suggested.[91,663,669]

The differential diagnosis of the condition should include other causes of EDS (see Chapter 3). Polysomnographic monitoring shows generally normal sleep structure and sleep cycling with either normal sleep duration (>6 but <10 hours) or prolonged nocturnal sleep duration (>10 hours). An increase of slow-wave sleep may be observed in some patients[91]; however, Sforza et al.[670] based on spectral analysis of the EEG found reduced power of slow-wave activity due to reduced amount of slow-wave sleep, suggesting that the homeostatic sleep regulatory mechanism is preserved but the sleep pressure indicated by slow-wave activity is reduced. The MSLT shows a mean sleep latency of less than 8 minutes but typically longer than in narcolepsy, and less than 2 SOREMPs. CSF hypocretin-1 levels are normal, in contrast to reduced levels in the majority of patients with narcolepsy-cataplexy syndrome.[628,671,672]

Montplaisir and Poirier[673] found an association with HLA-Cw2 and HLA-DR11 (a subtype of DR5) in a group of 18 subjects with IH. In contrast, Billiard[662] did not find this association in his population of 32 probands, but he found a significant increase of DQ3. Harada et al.[674] found no significant difference in the distribution of HLAs in patients with essential hypersomnia and control subjects. The treatment of IH is unsatisfactory and is somewhat similar to the stimulant treatment for narcolepsy. The behavioral approach of sleep hygiene techniques have been advised, but these do not have a significant impact on the disease. Compared with patients with classic narcolepsy with cataplexy, stimulants are less effective in those with IH. There are still unresolved and pending issues as raised by Billiard,[675] who questioned whether the two forms of IH are the same condition or two different conditions, and the pathophysiologic relationship between IH with a long sleep time and narcolepsy without cataplexy. Finally, the pathophysiologic mechanism of IH remains unknown.

Central Sleep Apnea and Sleep Hypoventilation Syndromes

Central Sleep Apnea

CSA is defined as an apnea of at least 10 seconds' duration due to an absence of central neural drive to the respiratory muscles associated with an absence of respiratory effort and airflow during sleep. Central hypopnea indicates a reduction in respiratory effort and airflow causing decreased tidal volume. In central hypopnea, there is no paradoxical thoracoabdominal motion nor flow limitation of the nasal pressure signal, which distinguish central hypopnea from obstructive hypopnea, wherein airflow decreases but respiratory effort continues. Sometimes it is very difficult to differentiate central hypopnea from obstructive hypopnea without intraesophageal or diaphragmatic EMG activity monitoring; these techniques are invasive and require specialized equipment, and therefore are not available in most sleep laboratories. Most sleep laboratories do not differentiate between obstructive and central hypopnea. Another caveat is that there is a lack of generally accepted standardized PSG diagnostic criteria for the CSA syndrome. The diagnostic criteria proposed by the Toronto group[676] consist of an AHI of 5–30 or more when at least 50% of events are central. CSA is a heterogeneous syndrome that includes primary or idiopathic CSA; CSA due to CSB pattern; high-altitude CSA with periodic breathing; CSA due to a variety of neurologic disorders, particularly brain stem dysfunction and other medical disorders; and CSA due to drug or substance abuse (e.g., use of opiates).[91] CSA can also be classified into two broad categories: hypercapnic CSA and hypocapnic (normocapnic) CSA.[677,678] Hypercapnic CSA includes a variety of neurologic disorders and sleep hypoventilation syndromes (see later). Neurologic causes of CSA include brain stem lesions, encephalitis, encephalopathy, neuromuscular and spinal cord disorders, and autonomic failure and have been described in an earlier section. Hypocapnic (normocapnic) CSA includes three major subtypes: idiopathic or primary CSA, high-altitude CSA with periodic breathing, and CSB-CSA.

Idiopathic CSA. Idiopathic or primary CSA is not a common condition.[91,678,679] A common complaint in patients with CSA is insomnia[680] with frequent awakenings during sleep at night, often accompanied by gasping for air or breathlessness. These patients may complain of EDS,[681] but EDS is less common in CSA than in upper airway OSA patients. These patients are not generally obese, and depression is noted in many of them. They have recurrent episodes of CSA accompanied by O_2 desaturation, cardiac arrhythmias, and sleep fragmentation. The patients may develop pulmonary or systemic hypertension.[682] A study by Podszus et al.,[683] however, found no change in pulmonary artery pressure during central apnea. Their awake $Paco_2$ is lower than normal (around 35 mm Hg), and they have an increased ventilatory response to CO_2 inhalation, but the reason for this is undetermined. Gas modulation, by adding CO_2 to the breath and increasing effective dead space, will eliminate apneas in these patients, supporting the role of hypocapnia in the pathogenesis, but this treatment is not used routinely because of practical difficulties.

High-Altitude Periodic Breathing and CSA. There is a decrease in the barometric pressure at high altitude associated with a decrease in O_2 tension, causing reduced arterial Pao_2 and tissue oxygenation. Hypoxia stimulates ventilation, which in turn causes hypocapnia and reduced $Paco_2$, thus lowering the $Paco_2$ apnea threshold. (The level of arterial CO_2 tension at which an apnea occurs is called the *apneic* or *apnea threshold*.[684]) The lowering of the apnea threshold results in central apnea and periodic breathing (Cheyne-Stokes respiration) causing repeated awakenings and sleep fragmentation. Acetazolamide, a carbonic anhydrase inhibitor, will produce metabolic acidosis causing a shift in the $Paco_2$ apnea threshold, and this has been used with success to treat central apnea at high altitude. This treatment may, however, cause OSA in some patients.[685]

Cheyne-Stokes Breathing–CSA. CSB (see also Chapter 33) is seen most commonly in congestive heart failure, particularly systolic heart failure[677,686,687]; in many cases of stroke; and sometimes in renal failure. CSB-CSA is characterized by repeated episodes of a crescendo-decrescendo pattern of breathing interspersed with central apneas or hypopneas. The cycle length (apnic-hypopneic phase) is more than 45 seconds in CSB-CSA and less than 45 seconds in CSA. Typically the cycle length of CSB in heart failure is around 60 seconds mainly due to prolonged hyperventilation. Arousals

are seen generally at the middle of the hyperventilatory phase and not immediately after termination of apnea-hypopnea, in contrast to OSAS, in which arousals are noted immediately on resumption of breathing at the end of apnea-hypopnea. The AASM Task Force[688] defined the following criteria for CSB-CSA:

1. A minimum of three consecutive cycles of crescendo-decrescendo pattern of breathing
2. Five or more central apneas-hypopneas per hour of sleep
3. The cycling crescendo-decrescendo pattern of ventilation lasting for 10 consecutive minutes or more

Sleep Hypoventilation/Hypoxemic Syndromes

Sleep hypoventilation/hypoxemic syndromes[91] include idiopathic or primary alveolar hypoventilation (PAH), congenital central hypoventilation syndrome (CCHS), sleep-related hypoventilation associated with neuromuscular and chest wall disorders, and sleep-related hypoventilation associated with pulmonary parenchymal diseases such as interstitial lung disease, cystic fibrosis, vascular pathology (e.g., pulmonary hypertension, sickle cell anemia and other hemoglobinopathies) and lower airway obstructive diseases (chronic obstructive pulmonary disease, bronchial asthma).

Primary Alveolar Hypoventilation. PAH is a syndrome of failure of automatic respiration without any recognizable disorder of the CNS or peripheral nervous system.[689] Central alveolar hypoventilation and central apnea syndrome associated with an organic neurologic disease should be differentiated from PAH.[405] The hallmark of PAH is a combination of arterial hypercapnia and hypoxemia during wakefulness that becomes worse during sleep.[690,691] Other manifestations include sleep apnea, congestive heart failure, pulmonary hypertension, and polycythemia. Central apnea is the usual type, but another feature in some cases is upper airway OSA. Impairment of hypercapnic ventilatory response is characteristic of this condition. The cause of the syndrome is unknown, and none of the reported cases of PAH showed evidence of CNS disease. Occasional postmortem reports showed no CNS structural lesions or produced nonspecific findings such as gliosis or mild loss of neurons in the medulla. A dysfunction of the medullary chemoreceptors is suspected, but no definite proof is available. Thus, the pathologic basis for PAH giving rise to the clinical manifestations of Ondine's curse remains undetermined. An important distinction from primary sleep apnea syndrome is that hypercapnic and hypoxic ventilatory responses during wakefulness are usually normal in primary sleep apnea syndrome.

Congenital Central Hypoventilation Syndrome. CCHS causes alveolar hypoventilation with CO_2 retention and repetitive central apneas during sleep, and the condition manifests within the first few days of life.[692–695]

These patients can ventilate normally during wakefulness but have marked hypoventilation, including episodes of CSA, during sleep. Ventilatory response to CO_2 is absent. In addition, they have symptoms of ANS dysregulation and, in a subset of cases, Hirschsprung's disease and later tumors of neural crest origin.[696-698] Patients with this rare disorder of failure of the automatic control of breathing lack arousal responses and sensation of dyspnea to the endogenous challenges of hypercapnia and hypoxemia, and require lifelong ventilatory support during sleep, but some will be able to maintain ventilation without assistance while awake once past infancy.[699] In the majority of patients with CCHS there is a typical mutation in the *PHOX2B* gene.[700] The characteristic mutation is a polyalanine repeat with 25–33 repeats in exon 3 arising usually de novo.[697,698,700,701] Late-onset central hypoventilation syndrome (LO-CHS) has been described in a few cases as late as adulthood.[702,703] Both CCHS and LO-CHS can result from heterozygous *PHOX2B* mutations. The adult cases have fewer polyalanine repeats in the gene than those presenting in the earlier years.[703] The condition seems to be due to a congenital defect of the central chemoreceptors in the medulla based on the frequent association of CCHS with ganglioblastoma and Hirschsprung's disease. Guilleminault and Challamel[704] hypothesized that CCHS is a disorder of autonomic cell integration. Conventional and diffusion tensor brain MRI studies in some CCHS patients suggested some neuroanatomic deficits in limbic and brain stem structures classically associated with autonomic and respiratory control.[705-707]

Complex Sleep Apnea

A new type of ventilatory pattern called complex sleep apnea has been described.[708-717] This is defined as an emergence of CSA and a breathing pattern somewhat similar to CSB following CPAP titration of OSAs patients. There is considerable current controversy about this entity, and its pathogenesis is unknown.[708-712] It has, however, been shown that low concentrations of CO_2 inhalation,[713] added dead space,[716] or adaptive servoventilation may eliminate complex sleep apnea.[714-717]

Sleep and Increased Intracranial Pressure

Increased intracranial pressure (ICP) may result from a variety of neurologic disorders (e.g., tumor, large infarction, intracranial hemorrhage, head trauma, focal abscess, diffuse encephalitis). Cooper and Hulme[718,719] found that the ICP of patients with intracranial lesions rose during REM and stage 2 NREM sleep. This was probably due to a combination of factors[720] (e.g., variations in cerebral blood flow, neurogenic reflex, cerebral vasoconstriction, enhanced brain metabolism). These observations have been confirmed by the findings of Munari and Calbucci[721] in 16 head trauma patients. In a study of children with craniosynostosis, Gonzalez et al.[722] observed both increased ICP and upper airway obstruction. They performed PSG studies along with continuous monitoring of ICP during sleep in 13 children with the syndrome of craniosynostosis and 7 control patients with isolated unicoronal synostosis only. In 11 of 13 patients with this syndrome, they found upper airway obstruction, and 8 of those 11 had frank OSAs. The other group of children showed no signs of upper airway obstruction during sleep. The causal relationship between upper airway obstruction and raised ICP in these children, however, remains undetermined. In a more recent report, Stephensen et al.[723] measured ICP levels during wakefulness and sleep in 29 adults with noncommunicating and 26 adults with communicating hydrocephalus. They found that ICP is normal in most adults with hydrocephalus; however, ICP is higher during sleep than during periods of wakefulness in the supine position and is not correlated with either symptoms or the rate of improvement after surgery. In idiopathic intracranial hypertension in adults, SDB may be noted in many patients.[724,725]

Headache Syndromes

Headaches and sleep complaints are common in day-to-day practice. Sleep disturbance (e.g., OSAS) may cause headache, and headache itself may cause sleep disturbances. The relationship between headache and sleep disorders is somewhat complex and remains ill understood. Sleep-related headaches include most daytime headache conditions, which also occur during sleep or on awakening in the morning. The ICSD-2[91] includes migraine, cluster headache, chronic paroxysmal hemicrania (CPH), and hypnic headache syndrome (HHS). Other causes of sleep-related headaches include medical (e.g., hypertension), neurologic (e.g., tumor, head trauma), and psychiatric (e.g., depression) disorders and primary sleep disorders (e.g., OSAS). Migraine headache can, of course, occur during both the day and night. There are several reports on headache and sleep disorders in the literature, but many of them are retrospective analyses and do not clearly eliminate other confounding factors. Despite these limitations, there are clear indications from the various reports that there is a reciprocal relationship between headache and sleep disorders.

Migraine headaches are common episodic headaches characterized by nausea, vomiting, photophobia, and phonophobia; they are generally unilateral and associated with throbbing pain. Dexter and Weitzman[726] made the first PSG recording in patients with chronic migraine and cluster headaches and found a clear relationship between REM sleep and attacks of headache. Attacks occurred during REM or within 9 minutes after it terminated. In later studies, Dexter[727] also found a relationship between NREM stages 3 and 4 and REM sleep, and arousals with migraine headaches. Kelman and Rains[728] evaluated 1283 migraineurs from 1480 consecutive headache patients attending a tertiary headache clinic. They reported that over half of migraineurs reported difficulty in initiating and maintaining sleep, and the migraine headaches were triggered by sleep disturbance in 50% of patients. "Awakening headaches," or headaches awakening them from sleep, were reported by 71% of patients. The authors concluded that there is a substantial sleep-migraine relationship, those patients who slept 6 hours per night exhibited more severe headache, and sleep complaints were more frequent during chronic episodic attacks. Gori et al.[729] after evaluating 100 patients suffering from migraine without aura, noted a preferential timing for occurrence of migraine attacks during the night and early morning hours.

Cluster headaches are unilateral severe headache in the periorbital or temporal region lasting for 15 minutes to 3 hours. As the name suggests, the headaches occur in clusters of one to three per day over a period of 1–2 months. Most of the patients have one cluster period each year, and the headache tends to occur at the same hour each day. A characteristic feature of cluster headache is the presence of autonomic features such as lacrimation, conjunctival injection, nasal congestion, rhinorrhea, and evidence of Horner's syndrome (e.g., absence of forehead and facial sweating, ptosis, small pupils). Cluster headaches are thought to be REM related,[727,730–732] but they may sometimes be triggered by NREM sleep.[733]

CPH[734] is probably a variant of cluster headache. The attacks of CPH occur unilaterally and are briefer and more frequent than cluster headaches. CPH is most commonly associated with REM sleep,[734] and it responds to indomethacin but in some cases may respond to calcium channel blockers.[735] Significant disruption of sleep architecture (decreased total and REM sleep time accompanied by increased number of awakenings during REM sleep) has been described in patients with CPH.[734] After a nocturnal polygraphic study, Conelli et al.[736] reported that CPH headache episodes were preceded by a sustained increase in blood pressure. There are occasional reports of the co-existence of OSAS and cluster headache with improvement of headache after CPAP titration.[737,738] An earlier report by Kudrow and colleagues[731] also found a high prevalence of CSA or OSAS in patients suffering from cluster headaches, especially episodic headaches.

The relationship between chronic headache and early morning headache has remained somewhat controversial. Patients with upper airway OSAS are thought to have an increasing incidence of morning headache as compared with controls,[739–741] and improvement in morning headache has been reported after treatment of OSAS.[742] Dexter[739] reported PSG-documented sleep apnea in 11 patients with chronic recurring headache syndrome. After surgical reconstruction in six patients with obstructive apneas, PSG demonstrated marked improvement in sleep apnea and considerable improvement in headache symptoms. In contrast, Aldrich and Chauncey[743] as well as Poceta and Dalessio,[744] after a survey, found that the complaint of morning headache was no different in patients with OSAS than in those with other sleep disorders. The Copenhagen Male Study,[745] however, found that heavy snoring was an independent risk factor for headache. This study evaluated 3323 men ages 54–74 years. Ulfberg et al.[746] confirmed the association between heavy snoring, OSA, and headache in both men and women based on a questionnaire survey as well as sleep apnea screening that included 4 hours of sleep on the back of a static charge–sensitive bed and finger oximetry. In a later report of 432 patients with a variety of sleep disorders studied with two nights of PSG comparing with 30 controls, Goder et al.[747] noted an increased frequency of morning headaches not only in OSAS but also in other sleep disorders. The authors concluded that morning headache might be associated with decreased total sleep time, sleep efficiency, and amount of REM sleep and an increase in the wake time during the preceding night.

Paiva et al.[748] evaluated 49 subjects successively seen in a headache clinic during a 6-month period with the predominant complaints of nocturnal or early morning headache. Based on the questionnaire and overnight sleep recordings, the authors found that headache was related to a specific sleep disorder (e.g., OSAS, PLMS, sleepwalking, sleep paralysis) in 55% of these subjects. They also found that treatment of these sleep disorders ameliorated the headaches. These findings confirmed the earlier observations of Paiva et al.[749] that morning or nocturnal headaches were frequent indicators of a sleep disturbance.

HHS is a rare benign headache syndrome of the elderly that usually occurs after the age of 60 years and awakens the patient from sleep at a consistent time each night.[91,750–752] HHS is differentiated from chronic cluster headache by its generalized distribution, age of onset, and the lack of autonomic manifestations. The disorder often responds to lithium, indomethacin, or caffeine treatment.

Another variety of unusual headache syndrome is "exploding head syndrome," which usually occurs in the transition from wake to sleep, abruptly arousing the patient with a feeling of an explosion or a sensation of bursting of the head.[753–755] The condition is benign and most likely represents a type of "sleep starts." Polysomnographic recordings[756,757] showed that the syndrome occurred during both wakefulness and REM sleep. In occasional cases, treatment with clomipramine may be effective.[756]

The exact pathophysiologic mechanism for association of headache and sleep is not known, but Dodick et al.[758] suggested a role for the hypothalamus, serotonin, and perhaps melatonin. The PET scan finding of hypothalamic activation in cluster headache[759] and the therapeutic response of melatonin[760] in migraine and other headache types lend some support to the suggested mechanism of Dodick et al.[758] The principles of treatment of sleep-related headaches include first the correct diagnosis of the type of the headache, investigations (including PSG recordings) to exclude other causes of headaches, practice of commonsense measures for sleep hygiene, treatment of underlying sleep disorders, and symptomatic treatment for specific headache using standard medications.

Familial and Sporadic Fatal Insomnia

Lugaresi and associates[761] originally described FFI in a family (14 affected members in three generations) as an autosomal dominant, rapidly progressive neurologic illness characterized by insomnia and dysautonomia that terminated in death. Later they found that two families with FFI harbored a mutation (associated with substitution of aspartic acid with asparagine) at codon 178 of the prion protein (PrP) gene *PRNP*, located on chromosome 20.[762,763] FFI therefore belongs to the so-called prion diseases, characterized by the accumulation of a pathologic isoform of the PrP that becomes resistant to the action of the proteases and called PrPres or PrPsc (sc for scrapie). It should be noted that the same mutation at codon 178 of *PRNP* is present in both FFI and familial CJD (178fCJD). These two conditions, however, are separated by the methionine-valine polymorphism at codon 129 on the mutated allele of *PRNP*, a common polymorphism that codes either for methionine or valine: FFI is invariably associated with methionine, while 178fCJD is associated with valine.[764–767] This genetic difference is expressed in a different type of PrPres being accumulated in the brain of affected individuals, whereby FFI brains accumulate a 19-kDa (type 2) PrPres while 178fCJD brains accumulate a 21-kDa (type 1) PrPres.[764]

Prion diseases can occur as infectious, sporadic, and hereditary forms, and are transmissible. Accordingly, FFI has been transmitted to experimental animals,[768,769] in particular to transgenic mice expressing a chimeric human-mouse *PRNP*.[770] A sporadic form of fatal insomnia (called sporadic fatal insomnia [SFI]) has also been described, characterized by the same clinicopathologic features of FFI and by type 2 PrPres and also transmissible, but in the absence of the defining *PRNP* 178 codon mutation.[771,772] Upon transmission of either FFI- or SFI-derived brain inoculates, the experimental animal accumulates the same type of PrPres and displays pathologic features comparable to those found in the donor brain, thus demonstrating that prion strains encipher and propagate the diversity of prion diseases.[770] FFI represents the third most frequent hereditary prion disease, and has been reported worldwide.[773,774] Age of onset of FFI is at about 51 years, but cases with young age of onset (23 and 24 years) are described. The clinical course runs from 7 to 72 months, with a mean of 18 months. A prolonged disease course (together with some differing clinical features) has been related to the presence of a valine 129 *PRNP* codon polymorphism on the *non*-mutated allele (heterozygote methionine/valine 129 *PRNP* codon FFI patients),[775] but this is controversial.

Clinical manifestations of FFI and SFI include impaired control of the sleep-wake cycle, including circadian rhythms; autonomic and neuroendocrine dysfunction; and somatic neurologic, cognitive, and behavioral manifestations.[761,775–779] Profound sleep disturbances and, in particular, severe insomnia are noted from the very beginning of the illness. Patients may remain in a state of subwakefulness, appearing drowsy, but are unable to sleep deeply and refreshingly. Polysomnographic study[761,776,779] showed almost total absence of deep sleep patterns and only short episodes of REM sleep lasting for a few seconds or minutes only, without muscle atonia associated with dream-enacting behavior in the form of complex gestures and motions, and myoclonus. As it progresses, there is progressive reduction of the total sleep time and reduced sleep cycles. The sleep cycle organization and stage shifts are altered from the very beginning. Sleep spindles and K complexes are markedly and progressively reduced and are absent in the later stage of the illness, and slow-wave sleep is never recorded. The terminal stage of the illness is characterized by progressive slowing of the EEG, and the patients remain in a coma. It is remarkable that the quasi-periodic sharp-wave EEG activities typical of CJD are not recorded in FFI, except in some patients with long evolution just before death.

Insomnia is associated with sympathetic activation in the form of hypertension, tachypnea and tachycardia, hyperhidrosis, and slight pyrexia. Autonomic function tests show evidence of sympathetic hyperactivity with preserved parasympathetic activity,[761,777,780,781] resulting in persistent elevation of plasma catecholamines with further increase after upright tilt of the table.[780] There is consistent elevation of blood pressure, heart rate, and core body temperature, and the nocturnal fall in blood pressure that occurs in normal individuals is lost from the early stages of the illness.[780,781]

Neuroendocrine functions[777,781–783] in FFI show a dysfunction of the pituitary-adrenal axis as manifested by striking elevation of serum cortisol but normal adrenocorticotrophic hormone and persistently elevated serum norepinephrine levels, associated with abnormal secretory patterns of growth hormone, prolactin, and melatonin: growth hormone showed no nocturnal secretory peaks, while the circadian rhythm of prolactin persisted. Circadian fluctuations of prolactin, however, tended to disappear with disease progression, and likewise the nocturnal rise in melatonin was progressively lost.[782] Fifty-two days of actigraphic monitoring in one patient showed up to 80% increased motor activity with a loss of circadian rhythmicity, and indirect calorimetry revealed a remarkably 60% metabolic increase in 24-hour energy expenditure.[784]

The somatic neurologic manifestations are present in all cases, particularly in the later stage of the illness, and consist of dysarthria and dysphagia, ataxia, evidence of pyramidal tract dysfunction, and myoclonus. Neuropsychological studies reveal impairment of attention and vigilance; memory deficits involving data manipulation but leaving semantic, retrograde, and procedural memory intact; and relatively intact intellectual skills so long as consciousness is preserved.[778] The disease progresses rapidly and, in the final stage of the illness, the patients may also have breathing disturbances and mutism, and then end in coma and death. CSF analysis for the 14-3-3 protein, a good marker of prion diseases, detects increased levels in only half of FFI patients. CSF hypocretin-1 levels are normal in FFI.[785]

Neuropathologically, the hallmark of FFI is severe atrophy of the thalamus, particularly the anterior ventral and dorsomedial thalamic nuclei, and of the inferior olives, associated with variable involvement of the cerebral cortex, striatum, and cerebellum.[761,786,787] In the thalamus, the loss of neurons is particularly striking, averaging 80% of neurons and associated with reactive astrogliosis.[786,787] There are no prominent spongiform changes, which are usually found in prion diseases, but a mild to moderate spongiform degeneration in the cerebral cortex has been noted in subjects with the longest duration of symptoms. These pathologic features in FFI are at variance with those found in 178fCJD, where spongiosis and cortical involvement predominate.[767] Moreover, deposition of PrPres in FFI brains is also characteristic, occurring to a much lesser degree than in sporadic CJD, especially in the neo- and limbic cortex and in those patients with prolonged disease course.[788] The amounts of PrPres indeed correlate with disease duration, though not in the thalamus, where deposition of PrPres is only moderate and unrelated to disease duration. This could probably reflect a selective thalamic vulnerability in FFI.[789] Severe hypometabolism of the thalamus along with a mild hypometabolism of the cingulate cortex was shown also by means of an in vivo fluorodeoxyglucose PET study in seven FFI patients by Cortelli et al.[790] Hypometabolism of other brain regions depended on the duration of symptoms, being more widespread in the methionine-valine heterozygotes at *PRNP* codon 129, who also had a more prolonged course. Comparison with the neuropathologic changes showed that the metabolic changes were more widespread than the pathologic alterations, correlating with the amount of abnormal PrPres deposited in the different brain areas.[790] In a fluorodeoxyglucose PET study[791] of 9 asymptomatic carriers of the FFI mutation, 10 noncarriers belonging to the same family, and 19 age-matched controls studied over several years, together with spectral EEG and PSG, the PET and all other examinations were normal at the beginning of the study. Four of the mutation carriers developed typical FFI during the study, but PET and the other examinations remained normal for 63, 56, 32, and 21 months before disease onset. Selective thalamic hypometabolism was found in the thalamus 13 months before the onset of symptoms, while spectral EEG analysis disclosed changes indicative of impaired thalamic sleep spindle formation. Following clinical disease onset, hypometabolism was found in the thalamus in all three patients examined. These findings were considered to demonstrate that the neurodegenerative process associated with FFI begins in the thalamus at close to 1 year before the clinical presentation of the disease.[791]

The study of FFI has opened a new era in the molecular biology of the prion proteins and their genes, being instrumental in the discovery of different prion strains in humans[764] and in establishing that prion strains alone encode prion disease diversity.[770,792] FFI has also been proposed as a model disease for sleep pathophysiology,[793] rekindling the role of the thalamus in sleep-wake regulating mechanisms[776,779,789,794] by demonstrating that the thalamus is essential for the generation of slow-wave sleep, and also suggesting a role for prions in sleep regulation. The consideration that FFI has clinical features in common with diseases such as delirium tremens and Morvan's chorea, an autoimmune limbic encephalitis, has finally led to the concept of "agrypnia excitata,"[795] a clinical condition characterized by loss of deep sleep and autonomic and motor hyperactivity and related to changes in the thalamolimbic circuitry. In agrypnia excitata, loss of slow-wave sleep occurs in the face of preserved light stage 1 NREM sleep, a fact that has been taken as evidence that NREM sleep is not a continuous process starting from stage 1 and progressing to stage 4, but that light sleep probably represents an independent state of sleep and should not be combined with deep sleep into a unique NREM sleep process.[795,796]

LABORATORY INVESTIGATIONS

The laboratory tests should be directed at a diagnosis of the primary neurologic disorder and an assessment of sleep disturbances resulting from the neurologic illness.

Laboratory Tests for the Primary Neurologic Disorders

It is beyond the scope of this chapter to delve into details of neurodiagnostic tests to assess the neurologic condition that gives rise to sleep and SRBDs, so readers are referred to some excellent neurologic texts available.[797–800] Laboratory tests must subserve the findings of the history and physical examination, as discussed in Chapter 19. Laboratory tests are essential for diagnosis, prognosis, and treatment of the primary neurologic disorders. These investigations can be broadly divided into neurophysiologic tests, neuroimaging studies, examination of the cerebrospinal fluid, and general laboratory tests, including blood work and urinalysis. Special procedures such as tests to uncover autonomic deficits; neuroimmunologic, neurovirologic, or neurourologic investigations; and brain biopsy are required to detect some neurologic disorders.

Neurophysiologic Tests

Neurophysiologic tests include EEG, evoked potential and nerve conduction velocity studies, and EMG. Electroencephalography, including 24-hour ambulatory and video-EEG examinations, is necessary to detect seizure disorder, metabolic-toxic-nutritional encephalopathies, and dementing illnesses (e.g., AD, CJD). Evoked potential studies include sensory (somatosensory, brain stem auditory, and visual evoked responses) and motor evoked potentials, and may be indicated in certain neurologic disorders, particularly demyelinating diseases such as MS. Nerve conduction measurements and EMG studies are necessary for diagnosis of various neuromuscular disorders, including neuromuscular junction diseases.

Neuroimaging Studies

Cerebral angiography, including digital subtraction arteriography, may be necessary to investigate for strokes. CT and MRI are important studies for structural lesions of the CNS (e.g., tumors, infarctions, vascular malformations). CT and MRI are also helpful in patients with demyelinating and degenerative neurologic disorders that can be responsible for sleep and SRBDs.

PET dynamically measures cerebral blood flow, O_2 uptake, and glucose utilization, and is helpful in diagnosis of dementing, degenerative (e.g., PD), and seizure disorders. It is very expensive, however, and is not available in most centers. SPECT, which dynamically measures regional cerebral blood flow, may be useful for patients with cerebral vascular disease, AD, or seizure disorders. PET and SPECT studies can also be performed to investigate D_2-receptor alterations in RLS-PLMS and narcolepsy.[801–807] Functional MRI can be useful to study the generators and the areas of activation in RLS-PLMS.[808] Doppler ultrasonography is an important test for investigation of stroke due to extracranial vascular disease. Myelography other than CT and MRI is important for diagnosis of diseases of the spinal cord.

In selected patients, fiberoptic endoscopy may be performed to locate the site of collapse of the upper airway, and cephalometric radiographs of the cranial base and facial bones may be obtained to assess posterior airway space or maxillomandibular deficiency (see Chapter 24). These are important when surgical treatment is planned. For research investigations, cross-sectional areas of the upper airway during wakefulness may be measured by CT and MRI.[809–814]

Cerebrospinal Fluid Examination and Other Laboratory Tests

CSF examination is important for the diagnosis of meningoencephalitis, Lyme disease, and MS, all of which may give rise to sleep disturbances. Hematologic tests and biochemical studies of blood and urine, as well as tests to assess endocrine, pulmonary, and cardiac disorders, are essential to uncover general medical disorders that may result in metabolic or toxic encephalopathies.

Laboratory Tests to Investigate Sleep and Sleep-Related Breathing Disorders

Polysomnography

The importance of PSG in the diagnosis of sleep and SRBDs is discussed in Chapters 11 and 19. Sleep can adversely affect breathing, and, conversely, respiratory dysrhythmias can have deleterious effects on sleep (see Chapter 7). Both alterations can affect the severity and course of a neurologic illness, causing such sleep disturbances, and so the sleep architecture should be studied. The technique of PSG is described in detail in Chapter 11.

Video-PSG is important for monitoring patients suspected of having epilepsy or parasomnias that may be associated with certain neurologic disorders (see Chapters 19 and 30).

Electroencephalography, Including 24-Hour Ambulatory EEG

Multiple channels of EEG recordings are essential to document focal and diffuse neurologic lesions and to accurately localize epileptiform discharges in patients with seizure disorders (see Chapter 12). Multiple orofacial muscle EMGs, in addition to the standard chin EMG, may help assess upper airway muscle hypotonia (see Chapter 12). Multiple muscle EMGs, including tibialis anterior EMG, are essential for diagnosis of RLS, PLMS, some parasomnias (e.g., RBD), and paroxysmal nocturnal dystonia (nocturnal frontal lobe epilepsy). Electroencephalography, including 24-hour ambulatory EEG, is essential if epilepsy is suspected, as it can cause sleep disturbances that may sometimes be mistaken for parasomnias or sleep apneic episodes. For further details see Chapters 12 and 30.

Multiple Sleep Latency Test

The MSLT is an important test to effectively document EDS. Narcolepsy is the single most important indication for performing MSLT. The presence of two sleep-onset REMs on four or five nap studies and sleep-onset latency of less than 8 minutes strongly suggest a diagnosis of narcolepsy[815] (see Fig. 19–3). Abnormalities of REM sleep regulatory mechanisms (e.g., OSAS, behaviorally induced insufficient sleep syndrome, use of REM-suppressant medications) or circadian rhythm sleep disturbance may also lead to REM sleep abnormalities during MSLT. Further details about the recording technique and the indications of MSLT are described in Chapter 16.

Maintenance of Wakefulness Test

The Maintenance of Wakefulness Test (MWT) is a variant of the MSLT measuring the subject's ability to stay awake. It also consists of four to five trials of remaining awake recording every 2 hours. Each trial is terminated if no sleep occurs after 40 minutes or immediately after the first 3 consecutive epochs of stage 1 NREM sleep or the first epoch of any other stage of sleep.[815] If the mean sleep latency is less than 8 minutes, it is then considered an abnormal test; values greater than this but less than 40 minutes are of uncertain significance. The MWT is less sensitive than the MSLT as a diagnostic test for narcolepsy but is more sensitive in assessing the effect of treatment (e.g., CPAP titration in OSAS and stimulant therapy in narcolepsy). For further details, see Chapter 17.

Actigraphy

Actigraphy is an activity monitor[816] or motion detector, designed to record acceleration or deceleration of body movements, that indirectly indicates the stage of sleep or wakefulness (see Fig. 19–4). This complements the sleep diary or sleep log data. It is a small watch-like device generally worn on the wrist, but that can also be worn at the ankle, for 1–2 weeks. The actigraph stores the activity data in epoch-by-epoch samples in its internal memory until the end of the recording period, when it is downloaded to a computer to pool the data graphically and generate a report of the sleep-wake pattern. It is assumed that sleep is represented by long periods with very little to no movement. Actigraphy is a cost-effective method for assessment of sleep-wake pattern. It can assess sleep-wake schedules in normal and sleep-disordered patients. Actigraphy is very useful in the diagnosis of circadian rhythm sleep disorders (see Fig. 19–5), paradoxical insomnia (sleep state misperception; see Fig. 19–6), and other types of insomnia. It also can be used to detect and quantify PLMS and other sleep-related movements. However, it is not suitable for assessment of SDB events. Sometimes it is difficult to assess sleep-wake schedule in subjects who may feign a sleep problem. Several models are commercially available. Actigraphy and overnight PSG sleep measures are highly correlated in clinical studies. For additional information about actigraphy, see Chapter 28.

Pulmonary Function Tests

Pulmonary function tests (PFTs) assess respiratory and ventilatory muscle function. PFTs include measurement of lung volumes (quantities of air within the lungs) and lung capacities (derived from lung volumes), arterial blood gases, PaO_2 and $PaCO_2$ obtained by arterial (radial or femoral) puncture, arterial oxygen saturation by finger oximetry and end-tidal CO_2 or transcutaneous CO_2. Spirometry is the most important pulmonary function test, measuring most of the lung volumes and capacities except residual volume, functional residual capacity, and total lung capacity, which require nonspirometry techniques (e.g., gas dilution technique). The important spirometric measurements[418–422,817] are forced vital capacity (FVC), forced expiratory volume in 1 second (FEV_1), and the ratio of FEV_1 to FVC. In order to obtain valid spirometric measurements, it is important to have patient cooperation and good patient-technician interaction. Values are expressed as percentage of predicted. Values of FVC, FEV_1, and peak expiratory flow of less than 80% predicted are considered abnormal. A value of less than 70% predicted for the ratio of FEV_1 to FVC is abnormal. The characteristic abnormalities in neuromuscular disorders include decreased FVC, FEV_1, and total lung capacity but increased residual volume. The airway obstruction shows less than predicted values of the ratio of FEV_1 to FVC, whereas restricted lung disease will show an increase in the ratio of FEV_1 to FVC combined with an absolute reduction in FVC and FEV_1. Table 29–7 lists the lung volumes and lung capacities, which are schematically shown in Figure 29–18.

Before a significant reduction in lung volume is appreciated, respiratory muscle strength must be severely reduced because pressure/volume characteristics of the respiratory system are not linear. Thus, static respiratory pressure measurements are often used to assess respiratory muscle strength: for example, maximal inspiratory pressure (PI_{max}) and maximal expiratory pressure (PE_{max}).[818] However, these measurements require the cooperation of patients, and the normal values have large ranges and variability that may be related to factors such as lung volume, type of mouthpiece, variable effort, and learning. In patients with bulbar muscle weakness, it may not be possible to measure PI_{max} and PE_{max}. In order to reduce the effects of these variables in the measurements of PI_{max}, investigators have used respiratory

TABLE 29–7 Lung Volumes and Capacities

Lung Volumes

- Tidal volume (TV): volume (ml) of air per normal inspiration or expiration
- Inspiratory reserve volume (IRV): volume of air during maximal inhalation following a normal breath
- Expiratory reserve volume (ERV): volume of air during maximal exhalation following a normal breath
- Residual volume (RV): volume of air remaining after maximal exhalation

Lung Capacities (derived from lung volumes)

- Vital capacity (VC): volume of air that can be exhaled maximally after maximal inspiration (IRV + TV + ERV)
- Inspiratory capacity (IC): inspiratory reserve volume plus tidal volume (IRV + TV)
- Functional residual capacity (FRC): volume of air remaining after a normal expiration (ERV + RV)
- Total lung capacity (TLC): vital capacity plus residual volume (VC + RV)

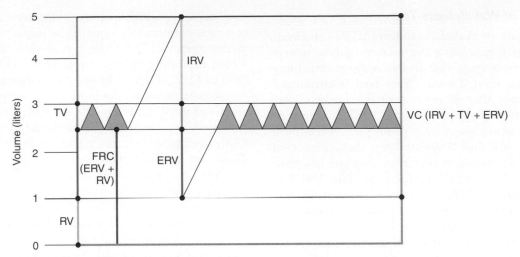

FIGURE 29–18 Schematic diagram to show lung volumes and capacities. (ERV, expiratory reserve volume; FRC, functional residual capacity; IRV, inspiratory reserve volume; RV, residual volume; TV, tidal volume; VC, vital capacity.)

pressures during the maximal sniff maneuver.[417,418] The maximal sniff pressure may be measured using transdiaphragmatic, esophageal, or nasal methods. Nasal pressure is often measured rather than esophageal pressure because it is much less invasive.

The definitive test for alveolar hypoventilation is an analysis of arterial blood gases showing hypercapnia and hypoxemia.[412,425] In the early stage of neuromuscular disorder, awake arterial blood gas values remain normal; only in advanced stages with chronic respiratory failure will these values be abnormal. To detect abnormal nocturnal arterial blood gases and hypoventilation, an indwelling arterial catheter needs to be placed throughout the night, which is invasive and rather impractical. Therefore, some investigators advocate noninvasive monitoring of arterial oxygen saturation and $PaCO_2$ only to detect hypoventilation; however, there are pitfalls to this line of investigation.[425] There is limitation to the usefulness of finger oximetry alone because of the hyperbolic shape of the oxyhemoglobin dissociation curves, which may show minor oxygen desaturation in the presence of significant hypoventilation and reduced PaO_2. The noninvasive end-tidal and transcutaneous carbon dioxide tension measurements are also unreliable and correlate poorly with actual $PaCO_2$.

Chemical control of breathing may be impaired if neurologic disease causes dysfunction of the metabolic respiratory controllers.[9] Such impairment may be detected by hypercapnic ventilatory response ($VE/PaCO_2$), hypoxic ventilatory response (VE/PaO_2), and mouth occlusion pressure ($P_{0.1}$) response, with or without loading.[9] Central respiratory drive and the inspiratory muscle strength independent of pulmonary mechanical factors are reflected in the $P_{0.1}$ response.

PFTs can exclude intrinsic bronchopulmonary disease, which may affect SRBDs.[817] For additional detail on PFTs, see Chapter 14.

Electrodiagnosis of the Respiratory Muscles

Electromyography of the upper airway, diaphragmatic, and intercostal muscles (see Chapters 7 and 12) may detect effects on these muscles in neurologic diseases.[819–825] In patients with MSA with laryngeal stridor, it is important to perform laryngeal EMG to detect laryngeal paresis.[826]

Phrenic nerve[827] and intercostal nerve conduction study[828] may detect phrenic and intercostal neuropathy, which may cause diaphragmatic and intercostal muscle weakness in some patients with neurologic disorders. Needle EMG of the diaphragm may reveal diaphragmatic denervation, which would suggest neurogenic dysfunction of the diaphragm.[829–831]

Chest Fluoroscopy

In patients suspected to have diaphragmatic paralysis, chest fluoroscopy in addition to measurement of transdiaphragmatic pressure using esophageal and gastric balloons inserted through the nasogastric route may be necessary.[832–834] The chest radiography is noninvasive and permits visualization of the diaphragm dome but provides little information regarding diaphragm function. Chest fluoroscopy of the diaphragm provides real-time examination of the start of diaphragm dome motion but carries the disadvantage of exposure to ionizing radiation and poor sensitivity and specificity.

TREATMENT OF SLEEP AND RESPIRATORY DYSFUNCTION SECONDARY TO NEUROLOGIC DISORDERS

Treatment is discussed under two broad categories: (1) therapy for the primary neurologic illness and (2) therapy for the secondary sleep disturbance.

Treatment of Primary Neurologic Illness

First and foremost is accurate diagnosis of the primary neurologic disorder. This is followed by vigorous treatment and monitoring of the neurologic illness. Such treatment may improve the sleep disturbances. It is beyond the scope of this volume to discuss the treatment of primary neurologic disorders, and readers are referred to some excellent texts.[797–800]

Treatment of Sleep-Related Breathing Disorders

Sleep disturbances in neurologic disorders include hypersomnia, insomnia, circadian rhythm sleep disturbances, and parasomnias. Treatment of these complaints is discussed in several chapters in this volume (see Chapters 24–28, 30, and 34–36). In this section, treatment of hypersomnia that results mainly from sleep-related respiratory dysrhythmias in neurologic disorders is discussed. In the following sections, general principles of treatment for sleep disturbances not related to the respiratory dysrhythmias in dementias and in PD are briefly reviewed.

The objective of treatment of SRBDs is twofold: (1) to improve the quality of life by improving the quality of sleep and (2) to prevent life-threatening cardiac arrhythmias, pulmonary hypertension, and congestive cardiac failure related to SDB. The quality of sleep may be improved by eliminating repeated apneas during sleep and thus preventing repeated arousals, sleep fragmentation, nocturnal hypoxemia, and daytime hypersomnolence. The treatment modalities for sleep-related respiratory dysrhythmias resulting from neurologic illness may be divided into five categories: (1) general measures, (2) pharmacologic agents, (3) mechanical devices, (4) supplemental O_2 administration, and (5) surgical treatment (Table 29–8).

General Measures

General measures of treatment include reduction or elimination of risk factors that can aggravate sleep-related respiratory dysrhythmias. Avoidance of alcohol and sedative-hypnotic drugs[835] (e.g., benzodiazepines, barbiturates, narcotics) that can depress breathing during sleep is an important step in eliminating the risk factors. Alcohol is known to increase the frequency and duration of apneas, probably by two mechanisms[836–838]: (1) selective depression of the genioglossus and other upper airway muscles, and (2) impairment of the arousal response by raising its threshold. For obese patients, weight loss is another important step in eliminating risk factors for sleep-related respiratory dysrhythmia. Other general measures include avoidance of sleep deprivation, avoidance of supine sleep position, and maintenance of a regular exercise program as much as possible from a practical point of view in the neurologically afflicted patient.

TABLE 29–8 Treatment of Sleep-Related Breathing Disorders in Neurologic Illness

General Measures

- Avoid alcohol and sedative-hypnotics, especially in the evening.
- Reduce body weight if overweight.
- Avoid sleep deprivation.
- Avoid supine sleeping position.
- Participate in regular exercise program if possible.

Pharmacologic Agents

- Protriptyline, medroxyprogesterone acetate, or SSRIs in mild cases (mostly ineffective)
- Nasal corticosteroids for OSAS in children (minimal benefit)
- Acetazolamide in central apnea at high altitude
- Modafinil as an adjunct treatment in a subset of OSAS patients with residual sleepiness and in some patients with myotonic dystrophy

Mechanical Devices

- Continuous positive airway pressure (CPAP) titration
- Bilevel positive airway pressure titration
- Auto-CPAP
- Assisted servoventilation
- Intermittent positive pressure ventilation
- Dental appliances, including mandibular advancement device
- Tongue retaining device

Supplemental O_2 Administration

Surgical Treatment

- Diaphragm pacing or electrophrenic respiration
- Tracheostomy (rarely performed nowadays)

OSAS, obstructive sleep apnea syndrome; SSRIs, selective serotonin reuptake inhibitors.

Pharmacologic Treatment

This therapy remains unsatisfactory.[839] The three most important agents that have been tried with partial success for mild to moderate sleep apnea are protriptyline, medroxyprogesterone acetate, and acetazolamide. Protriptyline may be used in a dose of 5–20 mg at bedtime. Suppression of REM sleep; a specific alerting property; increased upper airway muscle tone; and conversion of apnea to hypopnea are cited as mechanisms of action of this drug.[835,840] Anticholinergic effects and cardiac arrhythmias are the limiting side effects of this drug.

Medroxyprogesterone acetate has been tried in many patients with sleep apnea, but the results have been disappointing.[841–846] It is thought to act by increasing ventilatory drive. Impotence in men is a limiting side effect, and there are other side effects.[847]

Acetazolamide has been used with some success in central apnea, but development of obstructive apnea or aggravation of orthostatic hypotension owing to its diuretic and natriuretic effects should be kept in mind during treatment. Acetazolamide is a carbonic anhydrase inhibitor and will produce metabolic acidosis, causing a shift in the Pa_{CO_2} apnea threshold, and it has been used with some success to treat central apnea at high altitude.[679,848-851]

There have been isolated reports of the use of selective serotonin reuptake inhibitors in mild cases and topical nasal corticosteroids for OSAS in children with minimal benefit. In a subset of OSAS patients on CPAP titration (see later), complaining of residual daytime sleepiness, modafinil, a novel wake-promoting agent, has been used with success as an adjunct treatment.[852-858] Modafinil has also been used successfully for myotonic dystrophy patients with hypersomnia unrelated to alveolar hypoventilation or sleep apnea.[857,859-863] Modafinil may be initiated at 100 mg/day, increasing to a maximum of 400 mg/day to be taken in two divided doses. Methylphenidate and amphetamines may also be used if modafinil is not effective.

CSA, including CSB, associated with heart failure requires aggressive pharmacologic treatment for heart failure (e.g., beta blockers, digoxin, and diuretics) and, if needed, heart transplantation (see Chapter 33).

Mechanical Devices

Nasal Continuous Positive Airway Pressure. An important therapeutic advance in the treatment of OSAS, CPAP is described in detail in Chapter 25. It should be given a trial in neurologic disease patients with upper airway OSAs associated with intermittent CSAs or with mixed apneas. Such treatment often improves the quality of sleep and reduces daytime symptoms by eliminating or reducing sleep-related obstructive or mixed apneas and O_2 desaturation. The role of nasal CPAP for CSA is highly controversial. The Stanford University group[864] found CPAP helpful for central apnea patients who had associated OSA or who showed sleep fragmentation and repeated sleep-wake changes. In a subgroup of patients with CSA with insomnia who may show narrowing or occlusion of the upper airway via fiberoptic scope, nasal CPAP reversed the CSA.[865-867] Instead of CPAP, some patients require BIPAP (see Chapter 25 for further details).

Treatment of Cheyne-Stokes Breathing and Central Sleep Apnea. Patients with CSB-CSA should be given a trial with CPAP or BIPAP titration to improve ventilation in addition to pharmacologic treatment with acetazolamide or theophylline. Some patients may require oxygen inhalation and gas modulation with inert carbon dioxide through the nasal mask.[868] Another treatment besides CPAP-BIPAP that has been found to be useful in patients with CSB-CSA and complex sleep apnea includes adaptive servoventilation.[716,869-881] The role of adaptive servoventilation in terms of long-term prognosis, however, remains to be determined.

Other Ventilatory Supports. In the past, the mainstay of treatment for patients with neuromuscular disorders associated with SDB including hypoventilation was invasive ventilation through a tracheostomy (see later in this section), but this has now been largely replaced by noninvasive measures of ventilatory support consisting of negative and positive pressure ventilators.[425,882-884] These ventilators were developed during the early polio epidemics in the 1950s and the 1960s. Negative pressure ventilators include "iron lung" or tank respirators, the "rain coat" or "pneumo-wrap ventilator," and the cuirass or "tortoise shell."[882,885-889] Although the tank respirator is the most effective negative pressure ventilator, applying negative pressure to the entire body below the neck, it is bulky and limits the patient's acceptance.[882,887] Furthermore, negative pressure ventilators may cause upper airway OSA with oxygen desaturation both in normal subjects[890] and in patients with neuromuscular diseases.[891] The contemporary standard of care for chronic ventilatory failure in neuromuscular disorders is noninvasive IPPV using a nasal mask or prongs. Positive pressure ventilation includes CPAP, BiPAP, and IPPV. For upper airway OSAS, nasal CPAP is the ideal treatment. Following such treatment, sleep quality and daytime hypersomnolence often improve due to the reduction or elimination of sleep-related obstructive or mixed apneas and oxygen desaturation. However, such treatment has not been very useful in patients with relentlessly progressive disease; therefore, the role of CPAP in such diseases requires additional study. Some patients may not be able to tolerate the same high pressure during both inspiration and expiration and feel comfortable using BIPAP, which uses higher inspiratory than expiratory positive airway pressure.

The beneficial effect of nocturnal IPPV may be summarized as follows: improved nocturnal gas exchange as reflected in SaO_2 and transcutaneous CO_2 as well as improved daytime arterial blood gases; mild improvement of total sleep duration without significant improvement of quality of sleep; improved FVC and PI_{max}; reduced number of days of hospitalization; and improved quality-of-life measures and long-term survival.

The benefits of noninvasive ventilation through a nasal mask for 6–8 hours during sleep in neuromuscular disorders have been clearly shown in many studies.[413,423,439-442,892-919] IPPV generally uses no expiratory positive pressure, but in some patients, positive end-expiratory pressure up to 5 cm may be required. In some patients during initial nights of IPPV, there may be upper airway closure for the first time[414,463] during the expiratory phase. The mechanism for such closure may include driving up CO_2 below the inspiratory threshold and marked reduction of muscle tone as a result of REM rebound. Treatment of these patients is by the addition of a positive end-expiratory pressure valve by maintaining a positive pressure (up to 5 cm) during expiration. Noninvasive IPPV can be used even in those patients with bulbar muscle weakness utilizing the full-face mask. Either pressure-cycled ventilators delivering air at a fixed pressure or volume-cycled ventilators delivering a fixed volume of air may be used. Many clinicians prefer pressure-cycled ventilators to deliver IPPV, but there is variation in individual patient response.[919] There does not seem to be a difference between these two types of ventilators in terms of long-term survival[920] and short-term studies showing correction of hypoventilation.[921] The volume-cycled ventilators deliver tidal volume and pressure-cycled ventilators deliver fixed pressure (usually 10–20 cm H_2O) set by the clinician. One of the following three ventilator modes may be used: control mode, wherein the ventilator starts and ends inspiration according to prescribed settings; assist-control mode, wherein either the patient's effort or a programmed setting initiates inspiration; and spontaneous assist, wherein the patient's effort starts and ends inspiration.

Following such treatment, patients show improvement in daytime somnolence, arterial blood gases, sleep efficiency, and sleep architecture as well as reduction in the need for prolonged hospitalizations and increased longevity. Long-term follow-up and prospective randomized controlled trials in neuromuscular disorders such as ALS are limited. In one of the largest prospective, although not randomized, blinded studies, Mustafa et al.[901] proved the efficacy of noninvasive ventilation in ALS patients. There were striking improvements in blood gases and a variety of quality-of-life measures following noninvasive ventilation within 1 month that were maintained for up to 12 months in 26 patients with ALS showing respiratory muscle weakness. These authors also studied in parallel 15 age-matched patients without respiratory muscle weakness but with similar severity of ALS. These ALS patients showed improvement in quality-of-life measures despite progression of the disease. It was also shown that noninvasive ventilation in patients had no impact on most quality-of-life measures for caregivers and did not increase caregiver burden or stress. In another study,[904] 26 patients with congenital neuromuscular or chest wall diseases having daytime normocapnea and nocturnal hypercapnia were randomized either to nocturnal noninvasive ventilation or to a control group without ventilatory support. These authors found increased mean SaO_2 and decreased mean percentage of the night with peak transcutaneous CO_2 tension in the group using noninvasive ventilation as compared with controls. The authors suggested that such patients may benefit from nocturnal IPPV before daytime hypercapnia ensues. In the only randomized controlled trial, Bourke et al.[442] assigned 22 patients to noninvasive ventilation and 19 patients to standard care when these ALS patients developed orthopnea with PI_{max} less than 60% of predicted value or symptomatic hypercapnia. They found a median survival benefit of 205 days with improvement in quality-of-life measures in patients receiving noninvasive ventilation. In patients with severe bulbar involvement, however, survival benefit was not noted but there was improvement in sleep-related

symptoms. A survival benefit was also observed by Pinto et al.[892] and Kleopa and coworkers.[898] In a small study including 9 patients with ALS and sleep disturbance caused by nocturnal hypoventilation and 10 similar patients without ventilation problems (control group), Newsom-Davis et al.[440] showed that the cognitive dysfunction that may be noted in ALS patients having nocturnal hypoventilation and sleep disturbance may be partially improved by IPPV over a 6-week period. Improvement in nocturnal ventilation and sleep quality following IPPV has been noted by several authors in patients with nocturnal respiratory failure as a result of restrictive or neuromuscular disorders.[439,463,922,923]

Indications for Intermittent Positive Pressure Ventilation. A European consensus conference in 1993 listed the following criteria for long-term noninvasive nasal ventilation for patients with neuromuscular disorders[924]: presence of clinical symptoms associated with $PaCO_2$ level $\geq$45 mm Hg, PaO_2 <60 mm Hg in the daytime arterial blood gas analysis, or pronounced nocturnal oxygen desaturation. The patient's obstructive symptoms and arterial blood gases should be monitored. A later U.S. consensus conference in a 1999 report listed the criteria for IPPV for patients with neuromuscular disorders.[925] First the diagnosis must be established via history and physical examination followed by appropriate laboratory tests. The patients should have received treatment for associated (e.g., OSAS diagnosed by performing PSG studies) or underlying conditions. The suggested indications for use of noninvasive ventilation include clinical symptoms and one of the following physiologic criteria:

1. $PaCO_2$ $\geq$45 mm Hg
2. Nocturnal oxygen desaturation (by finger oximetry) of $\leq$88% for 5 consecutive minutes
3. PI_{max} of < 60 cm H_2O or FVC <50% of predicted value in cases of progressive neuromuscular diseases

A follow-up in 1–3 months for assessment of compliance and monitoring awake arterial blood gases is also suggested. Overnight oximetry may be helpful for monitoring such patients. It should be remembered that different neuromuscular disorders evolve and progress at different and varying speeds depending on the etiology of the disease process and other associated variables and, therefore, the setup guidelines may need further modifications depending upon the disease process involved.

There have been some attempts to document daytime predictors that will indicate nocturnal hypoventilation and hence the need for IPPV, and these have been discussed previously in this chapter. There is no controlled study implementing these predictors to evaluate the progression of disease and efficacy of treatment, but finger oximetry is the most widely used. In addition, transcutaneous or end-tidal CO_2 concentration can also be used. Electromyography of the accessory respiratory muscles may help in indicating evidence of ventilatory failure;

however, repeat PSG study remains the best test for evaluating quality of sleep and effectiveness of IPPV. Guilleminault and Shergill[410] suggested that even if there is no change in clinical symptoms, a PSG is recommended at least once a year as respiratory changes can occur without accompanying clinical symptoms. There are, however, no standard guidelines for this recommendation.

The complications of IPPV are similar to those noted with CPAP or BIPAP (see Chapter 25). One particularly annoying complication is nasal stuffiness or rhinorrhea, which may be relieved by using a warm humidifier or nasal corticosteroids. Some patients complain of claustrophobia when using a nasal mask, particularly those with breathing problems. In such patients, a nasal pillow instead of a nasal mask may be useful. Leaks around the mask causing arousals, sleep fragmentation, and subsequent decrease in efficacy of IPPV are also common, and correction of these leaks is important to improve sleep quality and architecture. Long-term use of a nasal mask can lead to a maxillary hypoplasia in young subjects. Children using nasal ventilation should be seen monthly to adjust mask size, particularly in the first 2 years of life, as a child's face grows quickly during infancy and childhood. Furthermore, airways develop and remodel during this time, and repetition of nocturnal PSG has been suggested approximately every 3 months.[410]

Mechanism of Improvement Following IPPV. Several mechanisms have been suggested but not proven for improving SDB and related symptoms in patients with neuromuscular disorders following noninvasive IPPV.[412,413,423,425,926,927] Improvement of respiratory muscle fatigue and restoration of the sensitivity of the respiratory center to carbon dioxide are the two important mechanisms cited. Changes in pulmonary mechanics (e.g., increasing lung volumes, improvement of lung compliance, reduction of dead space) may also contribute to improvement in symptoms and gas exchanges.

Oxygen Supplementation

The role of supplemental oxygen therapy using low-flow oxygen (1–2 L/min) in the treatment of SDB in neuromuscular diseases remains controversial. According to most investigators, oxygen therapy in restrictive thoracic disorders caused by neuromuscular diseases is ineffective and may be dangerous, leading to marked CO_2 retention.[928]

Supplemental O_2 therapy may decrease the severity of OSA in certain patients.[929] The recommended treatment of nocturnal hypoxemia is administration of O_2 at a low flow rate (1–2 L/min) via a nasal cannula (see Chapter 33). Oxygen administration may not be safe for all patients with sleep apnea syndrome. Motta and Guilleminault[930] and Chokroverty and coworkers[931] observed prolongation of apneas after O_2 administration during sleep in patients with OSAS. Gay and Edmonds[932] directed our attention to the possible exacerbation of hypercapnia after administration of low-flow O_2 in patients with neuromuscular disorders. In eight patients with neuromuscular disease and diaphragmatic dysfunction (patients with poliomyositis, ALS, or inflammatory motor neuropathy), mean $PaCO_2$ increased considerably after administration of low-flow supplemental O_2 (0.5–2.0 L/min). Four patients needed subsequent nocturnal assisted ventilation. The authors suggested that nocturnal assisted ventilation can be considered for patients with O_2-sensitive hypoventilation. In such patients, it may be possible to safely administer O_2 during the daytime.

Surgical Treatment

Diaphragmatic Pacing or Electrophrenic Respiration. Sarnoff and coworkers[933] first used electrophrenic stimulation in patients with poliomyelitis in 1951, but the technical difficulties at that time prevented its regular use for such treatment. Glenn and associates[934] improved the technique and extensively studied electrophrenic respiration by diaphragm pacing (DP). This form of treatment is used successfully in patients with respiratory center involvement with CSA syndrome. Superimposed OSA may complicate the procedure, which may then require both electrophrenic respiration and tracheostomy for treating such patients. Glenn's group[934] used such treatment successfully in three groups of neurologic disease patients: those with respiratory center involvement, either direct or through interruption of the afferent or efferent neurons to the respiratory center; those with high cervical spinal cord lesions; and those with PAH. Chervin and Guilleminault[935] reviewed the topic of DP. The authors stated that the "gold standard" of treatment of hypoventilation due to neurologic (including neuromuscular) disorders is BIPAP or IPPV. For those patients who require ventilatory assistance during both the day and night, however, DP is advantageous. The indications for DP include those patients with partial or total ventilatory failure, either during sleep or continuously. The causes for hypoventilation include neurologic disorders proximal to the phrenic motor neurons. The causes include both idiopathic CSA syndrome and CCHS in infants. Most of the patients on long-term DP require minimal or no additional ventilatory support, and most show improvement in the quality of life.

Complications of DP include precipitation of upper airway OSA requiring CPAP or tracheostomy in many patients, damage to the phrenic nerve, diaphragmatic damage due to fatigue, equipment malfunction, surgical complications, neuromuscular junction failure, local infection, and interference with cardiac pacemakers. Finally, DP is an invasive procedure. Despite the complications and disadvantages, DP is the preferred procedure for those requiring ventilatory assistance during both the day and night. In June 2008, the U.S. Food and Drug Administration (FDA) approved the $NeuR_x$ Diaphragm

Pacing System (DPS) only for spinal cord injury patients who depend on ventilators because of a paralyzed diaphragm. This approval was based on data obtained from a multicenter clinical trial.[936] Whether this device can be used in patients with neuromuscular disorders will depend on future clinical trials in such patients.

Tracheostomy. Tracheostomy remains the only effective measure for emergency treatment of patients with marked respiratory dysfunction with severe hypoxemia, patients with sudden respiratory arrest after resuscitation by intubation, and patients with severe laryngeal stridor due to laryngeal abductor paralysis. This used to be the definitive treatment for patients with severe OSAS, but it has been largely replaced by CPAP or BIPAP since they became available. On improvement after emergency tracheostomy, patients may later be weaned from the tracheostomy. Permanent tracheostomy may still be needed for patients with neuromuscular diseases: those with central respiratory drive abnormalities showing persistently elevated $PaCO_2$ despite using noninvasive IPPV; those who are unable to handle oropharyngeal secretions and show continued deterioration of neuromuscular disorders with very brief periods of spontaneous ventilation; and those patients with sleep apnea who fail to improve after nasal CPAP and nasal ventilation.[425,882] In such patients, ventilatory assistance is provided at night with plugging of the tracheostomy tube during the daytime, or the patient may use a commercially available portable ventilator continuously if needed, using the assist control mode.[882] Potential complications of tracheostomy and the care needed for maintenance of the tracheostomy should be discussed in detail with the patients and their families. Besides its invasiveness, the complications of tracheostomy include disfigurement, difficulty with speaking, tracheal stenosis, and tracheomalacia.[425,937]

Treatment of Sleep Disturbances in Alzheimer's Disease and Related Dementias

Treatment of acute confusional states associated with dementia is described in Chapter 36. In this section, general principles of treatment of sleep disturbance in patients with dementia are outlined.[938] Table 29–9 lists some certain general principles of treatment. Medications that could have an adverse effect on sleep and breathing should be reduced in dose or changed. Associated conditions that could interfere with sleep (e.g., pain due to arthritis and other causes) should be treated with analgesics. Depression is often an important feature in patients with AD, and a sedative antidepressant may be helpful. Frequency of urination in such patients may result from infection or enlarged prostate and may disturb sleep at night. Appropriate treatment should be directed toward such conditions. Patients should be encouraged to develop good sleep habits. They should be discouraged

TABLE 29–9 Treatment of Sleep Disturbance in Alzheimer's Disease and Related Dementias: General Measures

- Reduce or eliminate medications that may contribute to sleep disturbance or sleep apnea.
- Treat associated depression or anxiety and other comorbid conditions (e.g., pain causing sleep disturbances).
- Eliminate alcohol and caffeine in the evening.
- Institute regular sleep-wake schedule and sleep hygiene as much as possible.
- Avoid daytime naps.
- Encourage regular exercise (e.g., walking).
- Attend to environmental factors.
- For insomnia, try a nonbenzodiazepine agonist (e.g., zolpidem, eszopiclone) or melatonin receptor agonist (e.g., ramelteon)
- For extreme agitation or nocturnal confusional episodes, try small doses of antipsychotics, such as haloperidol (0.5–1.0 mg/day), risperdone (1–1.5 mg/day), or quetiapine (12.5–100 mg/day).
- Timed exposure to bright light in the evening and in the morning may be helpful.

from taking daytime naps and should be encouraged to exercise (e.g., walking during the day). They should not drink caffeine before bedtime or in the evening. For sleeplessness, a trial with a nonbenzodiazepine agonist such as zolpidem (including zolpidem-CR) and eszopiclone as well as a melatonin receptor agonist (e.g., ramelteon) should be tried for a short period (see Chapter 26). For nocturnal agitation and sundowning, the patient should be treated with antipsychotics, including the newer agents (haloperidol, 0.5–1.5 mg; thioridazine, 10–100 mg; risperdone, 1–1.5 mg; olanzapine, 5–10 mg; quetiapine, 12.5–100 mg) (see Chapter 32).

In some patients, timed exposure to bright light may be helpful.[939–942] In limited studies, Satlin et al.[939] and Okawa et al.[940,941] reported improvement in nighttime sleep and a decrease in daytime sleepiness after bright-light exposure in the evening. These findings were confirmed in some later reports.[137,943–945] In contrast, Dowling et al.[139] did not find any improvement in nighttime sleep or daytime wakefulness (actigraphically documented) following morning exposure to bright light (2500 lux) for 1 hour in a group of institutionalized AD patients compared to controls. However, in a later study Dowling and coworkers[946] observed that a combination of nighttime melatonin (5 mg) and bright light (2500 lux) exposure for 1 hour the next morning improved daytime activity levels and wake time in a group of institutionalized AD patients but not those receiving placebo and bright light only. Further studies are needed to confirm these observations.

Treatment of Sleep Disturbances in Patients with Parkinson's Disease

Sleep has not been consistently improved in patients with PD following antiparkinsonian medications. In those patients with reactivation of parkinsonian symptoms during sleep at night, adjustment in the timing and choice of medication may be helpful. Dopamine agonists or longer acting preparations of levodopa at bedtime may benefit sleep in some patients. Antihistamines such as diphenhydramine may promote sleep in addition to their modest antiparkinsonian effect. A small dose of carbidopa-levodopa at bedtime with a second dose later at night when the patient awakens may sometimes help those with insomnia. Nocturnal dyskinesias related to levodopa causing insomnia may respond to a reduction in the dopamine agonists or the addition of a small dose of a benzodiazepine or nonbenzodiazepine agonist as mentioned previously. In patients with psychosis and severe nocturnal hallucinations, clozapine or newer drugs such as olanzapine may be used with considerable benefit. During clozapine treatment, the usual precautions of monitoring blood counts and testing liver functions should be taken. Patients with PD associated with RBD should be treated with a small dose of clonazepam. Patients with PD with OSAS associated with oxygen desaturation and repeated arousals should be treated with CPAP titration. In some patients with insomnia, judicious short-term use of hypnotics may be recommended. Some patients with PD showing the phenotype of narcolepsy with EDS not associated with OSAS may be treated with a small dose (100 mg in the morning) of modafinil (not approved by the FDA), although the results have been inconsistent.[947–950]

CONCLUSION

The science of sleep is beginning to advance and probe even deeper into the significance and pathogenesis of sleep and its disorders. Dement[951] stated aptly that sleep medicine focuses on the sleeping brain and on all phenomena and pathologic effects that derive therefrom. This chapter has summarized how sleep, sleep disorders, and breathing interact in the brain and other neural structures, and how dysfunctions result in sleep and SRBDs. Progress in research involving molecular neurobiology and neurophysiology of sleep, chronophysiology, chronobiology, and functional imaging of the brain (e.g., functional MRI, PET, and SPECT scanning) holds great promise to unravel the mysteries of sleep even further and to direct our attention to finding more promising therapies for the unfortunate millions suffering from chronic disorders of sleep and wakefulness.

⊙ REFERENCES

A full list of references are available at www.expertconsult.com

CHAPTER 30

Sleep and Epilepsy

Sudhansu Chokroverty and **Pasquale Montagna**

INTRODUCTION

The relationship between sleep and epilepsy has intrigued researchers and thinkers since antiquity. Passouant[1] mentioned Hippocrates' description of "fears, rages, deliria, leaps out of bed, and seizures during the night." Aristotle observed that in many cases epilepsy began during sleep. Despite these early observations, the intriguing relationship between seizure and sleep was neglected by the medical profession until the end of the 19th century. Echeverria,[2] Fere,[3] and Gowers[4] gave clear descriptions of the relationship of epilepsy to the sleep-wake cycle. In a study of hospitalized epileptics, Fere[3] noted that in more than two-thirds of 1985 patients the attacks occurred between 8:00 PM and 8:00 AM. It is interesting to note that, even in those days, Fere mentioned the effect of epilepsy on sleep—he noted apparently associated difficulties with falling asleep and impairment of sleep efficiency, suggesting the facilitation of seizures by sleep deprivation. In the beginning of the 20th century, Turner,[5] Gallus,[6] and Amann[7] emphasized that many seizures were nocturnal and occurred at certain times of the night. These reports were followed by those of Langdon-Down and Brain,[8] Patry,[9] Busciano,[10] and Magnussen.[11]

All of these early observations were made on the basis of clinical features alone and without the benefit of electroencephalography (EEG), which was not described until 1929. The observation of Gibbs and Gibbs[12] in 1947 of the occurrence of paroxysmal discharges in the EEG twice as often during sleep as during the waking state marks the beginning of the modern era in the study of the relationship between epilepsy and sleep. Combining clinical and EEG observations showed that indeed a distinct relationship between epilepsy and sleep exists. This report was followed by many original observations, notably those of Janz,[13] Passouant,[14] Gastaut and coworkers,[15] Cadilhac,[16] Niedermeyer,[17] Montplaisir,[18] Broughton,[19] Billiard,[20] Kellaway,[21] and other researchers.

This chapter provides an overview of the effect of sleep on epilepsy as well as the effect of epilepsy on sleep. The usefulness of sleep in the diagnosis of epilepsy and the practical relevance to understanding the relationship between sleep and epilepsy are also discussed.

INTERRELATIONSHIP BETWEEN SLEEP AND EPILEPSY: PHYSIOLOGIC MECHANISMS

There is a reciprocal relationship between sleep and epilepsy: Sleep affects epilepsy, and epilepsy in turn affects sleep. To understand this relationship, it is important to review briefly the mechanism that generates paroxysmal EEG discharges and clinical seizures as well as the mechanism of initiation of sleep.

Basic Mechanism of Epilepsy

An understanding of the basic mechanism of epilepsy is derived primarily from studies of animal models and human clinical epilepsy.[22] Experimental animal models of epilepsy are produced by topical application of agents or focal electrical stimulation to the neocortex and limbic cortex to provoke partial seizures, whereas electric shock or systemic injection of convulsants and penicillin have been used for generalized epilepsy models.[22] Neuronal synchronization and neuronal hyperexcitability are fundamental physiologic factors that may transform an interictal to an ictal state.[22] Factors enhancing synchronization are conducive to active ictal precipitation in susceptible individuals. These factors include nonspecific influences, such as sleep, sleep deprivation, and so on. In addition, seizure itself may produce sleep disturbance. Neuronal mechanisms of focal and primary generalized epilepsies differ. A fundamental mechanism in generating focal epileptiform discharges (spikes or sharp waves) is a paroxysmal depolarization shift (PDS) in the epileptic neurons,[23] originally described by Matsumoto and Ajmone-Marsan,[24] followed by after-hyperpolarization.[25] PDS can be considered a giant excitatory postsynaptic potential (EPSP) caused by an abnormally prolonged depolarization of millions of neurons with positivity inside and negativity on the surface (spikes or sharp waves). The oscillation of a PDS involving a large area of cerebral cortex causes an alteration of behavior, manifesting as focal or secondarily generalized jerking movements. An understanding of the basic mechanism of human focal epilepsy is derived mainly from studying patients with mesial temporal lobe epilepsy (MTLE), and the fundamental pathologic substrate most often associated with temporal lobe epilepsy is hippocampal sclerosis.[22,26]

Nonspecific thalamic reticular nuclei are responsible for recruiting, and specific thalamic nuclei are responsible for augmenting, responses; both are also responsible for triggering generalized seizures by synchronizing afferent inputs to the cortex from these nuclei.[27,28] This thalamocortical interaction is responsible for changing the name of centrencephalic epilepsy to corticoreticular epilepsy for petit mal absence seizure.[29] A synchronous burst-pause firing pattern of the thalamocortical volleys of alternating EPSPs and inhibitory postsynaptic potentials (IPSPs) generates sleep spindles.[30,31] Similar mechanism takes place during generalized epileptic discharges, with enhancement of the discharges from the potentially epileptic neurons in the cerebral cortex generating spikes or multiple spikes followed by a prolonged γ-aminobutyric acid (GABA)–mediated inhibitory mechanism causing slow waves. These primary generalized epileptiform discharges begin simultaneously from the cerebral cortex bilaterally as a result of a diffuse cortical hyperexcitability.[32,33] This abnormal thalamocortical oscillation in primary generalized epilepsy is determined mainly by genetic factors.[32]

Epileptogenesis of the neurons is dependent on factors, both genetic and acquired, that maintain increased neuronal hyperexcitability and increased neuronal synchronization as well as factors encouraging failure of inhibitory mechanisms.[22] Examples of some of these factors are decreased dendritic spines and branches, cortical sprouting of surviving axons to cause increased synchronization, altered ionic microenvironment in and around the epileptic neurons,

attenuation of inhibitory influences causing enhanced synchronization, and alteration of calcium and chloride ion channel distribution.[22]

It is important to understand the interictal and ictal states as well as the mechanism of ictal termination and postictal state. The hallmark of an interictal state from the physiologic point of view is the focal or diffuse interictal EEG spike-and-wave discharge.[22] The epileptic neuronal aggregates show increased synchronization but with a decrease in firing rates, which may explain hypometabolism of the interictal focus as noted on positron emission tomography using ^{18}F-fluorodeoxyglucose scans.[22] Prevention of ictal spread and maintenance of the interictal state are determined by strong inhibitory influences that also keep the neurons in an excessively synchronous state.[22]

The ictal onset is determined by a combination of a failure of inhibitory interictal mechanisms and enhancement of excitatory synaptic activities, which may be initiated by an excess of subcortical synchronizing afferent input, as in generalized seizures or focal hypersynchronous discharge.[22] The true ictus in a generalized seizure is initiated in the cortex and may depend on a failure of inhibitory mechanism coupled with synchronizing thalamocortical input, as well as the influence of the reticular formation of the brain stem, particularly in the pontine region for the tonic phase.[22] A combination of diminution of synaptic inhibition, nonspecific excitation, propagation along the efferent projection pathways, and trans-synaptic alteration in excitation determines the appearance of partial ictus.[22] Investigations into both human and animal studies have revealed the presence of abnormal high-frequency (200- to 600-Hz) oscillations, named "fast ripples," which are seen in interictal spikes and are capable of precipitating ictal onset.[34–36] For the ictal termination, the two most important mechanisms are active inhibition and the failure of synchronization.[22] If these mechanisms fail, the patient may develop status epilepticus. Postictal phenomena (neuronal depression, neuronal deficit, EEG slowing, etc.) are sequelae to events that cause termination of the ictus. In the postictal state, there is neuronal hyperpolarization and neuronal depression causing termination of seizure and postictal EEG slowing.

Mechanism of Sleep

In humans there are two sleep states: desynchronized or rapid eye movement (REM) sleep and synchronized or non-REM (NREM) sleep. These sleep states are determined by two different mechanisms.[37] NREM or synchronized sleep seems to act as a convulsant because this state is characterized physiologically by an excessive diffuse cortical synchronization mediated by the thalamocortical input.[38] This predisposes to activation of seizure in an already hyperexcitable cortex. In REM or desynchronized sleep there is inhibition of thalamocortical synchronizing influence as evidenced by depression of recruiting rhythms generated by low-frequency electrical stimulation of the nonspecific thalamic nuclei.[38] Thus, there is attenuation of bilaterally synchronous epileptiform discharges at this stage of sleep. During REM sleep there is also a tonic reduction in the interhemispheric impulse traffic through the corpus callosum.[39] This also contributes to the limitation of propagation of the generalized epileptiform discharges.

Cortical excitability for epileptogenesis is higher during sleep than during wakefulness.[38] This observation was based on the finding of a significant drop in the threshold for electroconvulsive shock in the sleep deprivation (specifically desynchronized sleep deprivation) experiments in rats, suggesting heightened neural excitability. Studies in human epilepsy[40,41] utilizing a paired-pulse technique during transcranial magnetic stimulation, showing an increased cortical excitability following sleep deprivation, support the previous observations in rats.[38] This factor of cortical excitability coupled with the fact that the inhibitory mechanism (e.g., postspike hyperpolarization and afferent inhibition) may be less effective during sleep favors activation of focal cortical epileptiform discharge.

Physiologic synchronization can be defined as a state during which there is appearance of the same frequency in two or more oscillators due to coactivation of a large number of neurons.[31] In NREM sleep, spindles and slow waves result from synchronization. As stated earlier, a synchronous burst-pause firing pattern of the thalamocortical volleys of alternating EPSPs and IPSPs generates sleep spindles.[30] Extensive study by Steriade and colleagues has shown the importance of thalamocortical participation in the genesis of sleep spindles, delta waves, and very slow (infra-slow) oscillations.[31,42–51] Sleep spindles are generated in the thalamic reticular nucleus, resulting from synaptic interactions in a network involving the GABAergic reticular thalamic nucleus, glutamatergic thalamocortical neurons, and cortical pyramidal neurons.[52] Cortical pyramidal neurons project to the thalamic reticular nucleus, which in turn has two-way connections with thalamocortical neurons of the dorsal thalamus, which in turn projects to the cerebral cortex. Sleep spindles are abolished after isolation of the reticular nucleus from the rest of the thalamus and cerebral cortex[53]; however, spindle oscillations persist in the reticular thalamic nucleus disconnected from dorsal thalamic and cortical inputs.[54] Delta waves are generated at both cortical and thalamic levels. Hyperpolarization of thalamocortical pathways causing functional deafferentation from the sensory input is responsible for generation of delta waves.[49] Very slow oscillations (<1 Hz) are generated in the cortex (see also Chapter 5). The very slow oscillations must be generated in cortical networks because these are present in athalamic preparations[46,47] and absent from the thalamus of decorticate animals.[45,55] It has been proposed

that the vast majority of K complexes appearing during sleep are generated by the very slow (<1 Hz) cortical oscillations.

Lesions and stimulation experiments have shown the existence of structures responsible for cortical synchrony in the forebrain as well as in the hindbrain.[31,56] More than 60 years ago, Morison and Dempsey[57] observed recruiting synchronizing cortical responses after low-frequency electrical stimulation of the midline thalamic nuclei, evidence of an intimate thalamocortical relationship. In 1944, Hess[58] even suggested the existence of a thalamic sleep center. Later studies, however, have shown that the thalamus is responsible for the genesis of spindles and not for sleep slow waves or the behavioral aspect of sleep.[31,56]

The theory about REM or desynchronized sleep suggests that there are anatomically distributed and neurochemically interpenetrated "REM-on" and "REM-off" cells in the brain stem[59] (see also Chapters 4 and 29). REM sleep is dependent on an interaction between REM-on cells and REM-off cells in the brain stem. Thus the interaction and oscillation between the REM-promoting and REM-inhibiting neurons generate the REM-NREM cycle. The various chemical mechanisms (e.g., cholinergic, aminergic, GABAergic, glutamatergic) participating in NREM and REM sleep may also be responsible for activation or inhibition of epileptiform discharges during sleep.

An understanding of the basic mechanism of epilepsy and sleep helps us understand the mechanism of activation and suppression of seizure discharges during sleep and in particular during different stages of sleep. Sleep-induced seizures result from an altered interaction among sleep-generating neuronal networks, arousal systems, and the generators for epileptogenesis. In other words, there is a complex interaction between cortical and subcortical mechanisms. The activation of ictal and interictal seizures during NREM sleep seems to be related to the existence of a thalamocortical synchronizing mechanism, whereas suppression during REM sleep is due to depression of the thalamic synchronizing mechanism and a tonic reduction of interhemispheric transmission during REM sleep.[38,39] The role played by the arousal mechanisms in facilitation of seizures remains somewhat controversial. According to some investigators,[60,61] arousal mechanisms are important in facilitating the seizures, whereas other investigators[62] postulate that arousal mechanisms, particularly the posterior hypothalamic histaminergic system, exert an antiepileptic effect. In support of the arousal mechanism facilitating seizures is the suggestion[60] that sudden bursts of excitatory inputs from the wake-promoting neurons in the histaminergic posterior hypothalamic neurons and basal forebrain cholinergic neurons to the already hyperexcitable neocortical neurons might exacerbate the cortical hyperexcitability precipitating seizures.[32] Frontal lobe epilepsy is predominantly nocturnal, and strong thalamocortical projections to frontal lobes might anatomically explain the preferential occurrences of nocturnal seizures in frontal lobe epilepsy. Seizures occurring shortly after awakening in juvenile myoclonic epilepsy (JME) and generalized tonic-clonic seizures on awakening may be cited as clinical examples in support of the role of the arousal mechanisms facilitating sleep-related seizures.[63]

Interrelationship Between Epilepsy and Sleep

The activation of 3-Hz spike-and-wave discharges during NREM sleep is supported by the hypothesis of corticoreticular epilepsy of Kostopoulos and Gloor[64] and Gloor.[29] Kostopoulos and Gloor[64] presented evidence that the 3-Hz spike-and-wave discharges of primary generalized corticoreticular or petit mal epilepsy resulted from an excessive response of cortical neurons to those thalamocortical volleys that are responsible for production of normal sleep spindles. These abnormal thalamocortical oscillations in primary generalized epilepsy are determined by genetic factors.[22] In 1942, Morison and Dempsey[57] produced recruiting responses after intralaminar thalamic stimulation. In 1947, Jasper and Droogleever-Fortuyn[65] succeeded in producing 3-Hz spike-and-wave discharges after similar stimulation in the presence of cortical hyperexcitability. Spencer and Brookhart[66] and Spencer and Kandel[67] showed similarities between recruiting responses and cortical sleep spindles in the cat. Both of these waves resulted from summated postsynaptic potentials of cortical neurons due to low-frequency thalamocortical volleys. Gloor[68] confirmed and extended these observations with the feline model of generalized epilepsy induced by intramuscular penicillin and concluded that spike-and-wave discharges resulted from summated postsynaptic potentials of the cortical neurons as a result of the thalamocortical volleys that would normally produce sleep spindles and recruiting responses. Penicillin obviously caused cortical hyperexcitability.

In this connection, it is important to note that Niedermeyer[69] was the first to suggest that generalized synchronous spike-and-wave discharges originated from the physiologic K complex. It was previously suggested that the delta waves are enhanced after deafferentation of the cortex, suggesting that subcortical white matter participates in the production of EEG slow waves.[70,71] The initial observation of Neidermeyer[17] in 1965 was followed by other reports from the same author and his collaborators, and subsequently other authors.[72,73] Elegant studies by Steriade and colleagues clearly showed the propensity of spike-and-wave discharges occurring during sleep as a result of transformation of the very slow sleep oscillations into paroxysmal discharges.[43,45,48,49] It has been suggested that the depolarizing phase of the very slow oscillations progressively increases in amplitude and

decreases in duration, resembling a PDS. The actual mechanism converting the very slow sleep oscillations into rhythmic spike-and-wave discharges is not clearly understood, however, but involves an interaction between neurons, glia, and ions.[45] A good neurophysiologic explanation has been given by Steriade and McCarley for seizures being triggered by K complexes.[74] A synchronous burst-pause firing pattern of the thalamocortical volleys will cause enhancement of the discharges from the potentially epileptogenic neurons, generating spikes or multiple spikes. The interictal spike-and-wave discharges may be triggered by arousal mechanism generating epileptic K complexes and terminating in ictal discharges accompanied by clinical seizures. Thus all these studies show a close interrelationship among spike-and-wave discharges, K complexes, and sleep spindles, confirming common mechanisms and circuits for transmission shared by the epileptic neurons and normal phasic events of sleep.[17,75,76] The spike-and-wave discharges are triggered by the very slow cortical oscillations, which disappear after decortication but survive after thalamectomy.[43]

Wyler[77] studied epileptic neurons during sleep and wakefulness in 14 normal and 17 abnormal neurons recorded from alumina gel–induced chronic neocortical epileptic foci in four male *Macaca mulatta* monkeys during transition between sleep and wakefulness. During sleep, the neurons that were mildly epileptic during wakefulness changed their firing pattern drastically and behaved like neurons that were grossly epileptic during wakefulness; normal neurons and those neurons that were grossly epileptic during wakefulness did not change the firing pattern significantly. The author concluded that the neurons may represent the "critical mass" for initiation of seizure activity during synchronized sleep, which is characterized by burst-synchronizing events such as sleep spindles.

Shouse et al.[78] studied the mechanism of seizure suppression during REM sleep in cats. They created two seizure models in 20 cats, systemic penicillin epilepsy and electroconvulsive shock, and produced two types of lesions: bilateral electrolytic lesions in the mediolateral pontine tegmentum producing a syndrome of REM sleep without atonia, and systemic atropine injection producing REM sleep without thalamocortical EEG desynchronization. These authors made the following conclusions based on these experiments:

1. REM sleep retarded the spread of epileptiform discharges in the EEG.
2. The descending brain stem pathways responsible for lower motor neuron inhibition during REM sleep also protected against generalized motor seizure during REM sleep.
3. The mechanism to prevent spread of seizure discharge used a separate pathway in the ascending brain stem structures that caused thalamocortical EEG desynchronization during REM sleep.

4. The data thus suggest a cholinergic mechanism for thalamocortical EEG desynchronization and for retardation of EEG discharges during wakefulness and REM sleep.

They further concluded that, for generalized epilepsy, REM sleep was the most potent antiepileptic state in the sleep-wake cycle. It is important to note that Cohen et al.[79] found a lowered convulsive threshold during REM deprivation in cats. REM deprivation thus may exacerbate epilepsy.

EFFECT OF SLEEP ON EPILEPSY

Because of the awareness of an intimate relationship between sleep and epilepsy, various authors have classified seizures according to the time of occurrence of the seizures (clinical and electrical) during certain times in the sleep-wake cycle. Thus, seizures have been classified as waking, sleep, diffuse (both diurnal and nocturnal), circadian, ultradian, and infradian epilepsies. Table 30–1 lists biorhythmic (according to timing) classification of seizures.[60] Diurnal (waking) seizures are mostly primary generalized epilepsies that are mainly genetically determined. Nocturnal (sleep-related) seizures are most often localization-related seizures. Diffuse epilepsies (those occurring randomly during the night and day) show both ictal and interictal discharges during sleep and waking states. These are often associated with diffuse central nervous system dysfunction and are symptomatic generalized seizures. They are often medically refractory.

As early as 1885, Gowers[4] analyzed 840 institutionalized patients with a variety of seizure disorders and observed that 21% of seizures occurred exclusively at night; 42% exclusively in the daytime; and 37% at random, both during the day and night. According to Gowers, the two most susceptible periods were the onset of sleep and the end of sleep. Langdon-Down and Brain[8] and Patry[9] made similar observations. In all three series, the analysis was based on institutionalized patients.

TABLE 30–1 Biorhythmic Classification of Seizures

Diurnal (Waking) Epilepsies

- Absence seizures
- Juvenile myclonic epilepsy
- Generalized tonic-clonic seizure on awakening

Nocturnal (Sleep-Related) Epilepsies

- Nocturnal frontal lobe epilepsy
- Autosomal dominant nocturnal frontal lobe epilepsy
- Benign epilepsy of childhood with centrotemporal spikes with or without occipital paroxysms
- Continuous spike-and-wave discharges during slow-wave sleep
- Landau-Kleffner syndrome

Diffuse Epilepsies (Randomly Occurring During Night and Day)

- Lennox-Gastaut syndrome
- West's syndrome (hypsarrhythmia)
- Progressive myoclonus epilepsies

Langdon-Down and Brain[8] observed that, in a series of 66 patients, 24% had sleep, 43% had diurnal, and 33% had diffuse epilepsies. In a sample size of 31, Patry[9] found 19% sleep, 45% diurnal, and 36% diffuse epilepsies. Using the average of these three groups of institutionalized epileptics, the incidence of each of these three types of seizures in relation to the sleep-wake cycle is 22% sleep, 44% diurnal, and 34% diffuse epilepsies. Thus, the incidence is similar in these three series. Langdon-Down and Brain[8] found the peak incidence of waking epilepsies to be 1–2 hours after awakening, approximately 7:00–8:00 AM; smaller peaks were found at approximately 3:00 PM and 6:00–8:00 PM. Sleep epilepsies had two peaks, 10:00–11:00 PM and 4:00–5:00 AM (i.e., early and late at night, similar to that noted by Gowers[4]).

Among the contemporary epileptologists, Janz[13,80] has contributed most toward classification of seizures based on the sleep-wake cycle. He analyzed two large series of outpatients with tonic-clonic generalized seizures. In the first series of 2110 patients,[13] Janz found 45% sleep, 34% diurnal, and 21% diffuse epilepsies. In the second series of 2825 similar patients,[80] the incidence was 44% sleep, 33% diurnal, and 23% diffuse epilepsies. Therefore, the two series were similar. Janz called diurnal seizures *awakening epilepsies* because of the high prevalence of seizure during awakening from sleep.[13] In a sample size of 314 outpatient seizure patients, Billiard[20] found 15% sleep, 53% diurnal, and 32% diffuse epilepsies. It should be noted that Billiard included a variety of types of epilepsies in his analysis. Earlier, Hopkins[81] analyzed a series of outpatient tonic-clonic generalized seizures and found 51% sleep, 30% diurnal, and 19% diffuse epilepsies. Janz[13,80] also noted increased frequency at the beginning and end of the night in sleep epilepsies, similar to that observed by Gowers.[4] It is important to note that the earlier classification was based only on clinical studies and no nighttime EEGs were obtained. The contemporary epileptologists and neurologists had the benefit of obtaining the EEG and all-night polysomnographic (PSG) studies using standard sleep scoring criteria. As regards stability of type, Janz[13] reported that 10% of awakening epilepsies later became sleep epilepsies, whereas only 6% became diffuse epilepsies. According to Janz[13,80] and Hopkins,[81] sleep and diffuse epilepsies lasting for 2 years rarely become awakening epilepsies.

The differences in the incidence of the three types of seizures may be due to the selection of patients (i.e., outpatient, institutionalized, generalized or partial seizures). The importance of classification based on sleep-wake cycle is that this classification may shed light on the prognosis and etiology. Patients with diffuse epilepsies often have intractable seizures and structural neurologic deficits, with poor prognosis as compared to patients with awakening or sleep epilepsies.[82] Analyzing the various data, Shouse[82] stated that idiopathic type is generally awakening type, those associated with organic structural lesions are of the diffuse type, and the sleep epilepsies are intermediate in terms of organicity. D'Alessandro et al.[83] analyzed 1200 patients visiting the epilepsy center during a 5-year period (1974–1979). They found that 90 of the 1200 (7.5%) had sleep epilepsy (i.e., had one or more seizures exclusively during sleep). This frequency is lower than that found by Janz[13] and Kajtor[84] but similar to that noted by Gibberd and Bateson.[85] The authors concluded that pure sleep epilepsies have a good prognosis. They rarely have waking seizures during the first few years after the onset of epilepsy.

A number of investigators have studied the question of whether epilepsy manifests biorhythmicity—specifically, whether there are circadian, ultradian, or infradian epilepsies. Kellaway et al.[21,86] cited the specific relationship of epileptic phenomena to the sleep-wake cycle as an example of a circadian rhythm. It should be noted, however, that Autret et al.[87] noted an increase in focal discharges during NREM stages 1 and 2 and in generalized discharges during NREM stages 3 and 4, and a reduction or disappearance of the discharges in REM sleep during any time of the day and night. This evidence argues against a circadian rhythmicity. Kellaway and coworkers[21,86,88] suggested that epileptiform activity is linked to two rhythms: circadian and ultradian, related to NREM-REM cycle at 90–100 minutes. Stevens et al.[89] suggested that focal EEG discharges in adults may at times show an ultradian 90- to 100-minute periodicity in phase with prior NREM-REM sleep cycles throughout the day and night. Binnie[90] and Martins da Silva and Binnie[91] also noted periodicities of interictal discharges, both during diurnal waking and nocturnal sleep EEG recordings. In most of their patients, periodicities were longer or shorter than the typical 90- to 100-minute REM-NREM cycle. However, Kellaway et al.[86] failed to document waking ultradian rhythmicity in petit mal spike-and-wave discharges. In one case of petit mal absence, Broughton et al.[92] provided strong evidence for ultradian daytime variations of spike-and-wave discharges, mainly at the REM cycle rate. However, these observations have been made based only on one case study.

There are clear methodologic problems in studying biorhythmicity in epilepsy.[90] The classic methods include temporal isolation to observe the free-running rhythms (entrainment) and shifting the time zone. Such studies in epilepsy, however, have not been performed in detail.[90] Circadian rhythm, sleep, and epilepsy have been studied by Quigg[93] and others.[94] These authors have reported transient dysfunction of normal circadian function during seizures. Transient disruption of hormones under circadian modulation (e.g., an increase in prolactin secretion within 15 minutes of onset of seizures, particularly generalized seizures) is well known. There is a suggestion that there may be possible damage to suprachiasmatic nuclei as a result of repeated seizures. Quigg[93] noted subtle functional defects in primary circadian regulation in

rats, but no gross abnormalities were noted. Quigg et al.[95] demonstrated that electrically induced seizures in rats isolated from time cues and light for 3-week trials induced advances and delays in circadian rhythm of temperature. Based on these findings, the authors suggested that circadian dysregulation may contribute to some of the altered endogenous cycles associated with epilepsy. Several studies show circadian influence on the occurrence and timing of seizures. MTLE appears to be particularly vulnerable to circadian effects, but there is no conclusive evidence for this, and further study is needed. Both animal studies[96,97] and human studies[98] have provided evidence for circadian influence in MTLE. Frontal lobe seizures most commonly arise from NREM sleep.[99–102] In an analysis of 613 seizures in 133 patients, Herman et al.[101] noted that 57% of frontal lobe seizures occurred during NREM sleep, particularly stage 2, compared with 40% of mesial temporal lobe, 24% of neocortical temporal lobe, and about 13% of occipitoparietal lobe seizures. Quigg[93] suggested that melatonin might have an anticonvulsant effect and may be responsible for limbic seizures not occurring predominantly during sleep. However, the relation between melatonin and seizures remains controversial.[103,104]

Finally, the question of infradian rhythmicity in epilepsy, as exemplified by catamenial epilepsy (i.e., menstrual-related epilepsy), remains controversial. Almqvist[105] found a periodicity in 47 of 146 long-stay patients with epilepsy. The author noted that in some of the patients the interval of the attacks was equal to the period of the menstrual cycle. As mentioned by Newmark and Penry,[106] however, the concept of catamenial epilepsy, although generally accepted, remains questionable as far as published evidence is concerned.

In conclusion, epilepsy in some patients may show a circadian temporal periodicity and an association with sleep periodicity, but it is not known if this periodicity is "state" linked (sleep vs. wakefulness) or "time" linked (nocturnal vs. diurnal).[107] Webb[107] considered epileptic events to be "state dependent," whereas Martins da Silva and Binnie[91] considered them to be "time dependent." Thus, little is known about why a seizure occurs at a particular time of the day or night. This understanding may be important for effective control of epilepsy by optimization of the drug regimen. It should also be recognized that there are circadian variations of drug absorption, interaction, and metabolism (e.g., valproate absorption is reduced at night because of gastrointestinal physiologic changes at night, and carbamazepine shows circadian variation in autoinduction) complicating management of seizures.[108] Binnie[90] raised the question without an answer: Can we improve patient care if we learn about biorhythms in epilepsy? Because of inconsistencies and contradictions in terms of classification related to biorhythms, modern epileptologists use the International Classification of Epilepsy[109] (Table 30–2).

TABLE 30–2 International Classification of Epilepsy

International Classification of Epileptic Seizures

- Primary generalized
- Partial with or without secondary generalization
- Unclassified epileptic seizures

International Classification of Epilepsies and Epileptic Syndromes

- Localization-related epilepsies and syndromes
  - Idiopathic
  - Symptomatic
- Generalized epilepsies and syndromes
  - Idiopathic
  - Symptomatic
- Epilepsies and syndromes: undetermined

EFFECT OF SLEEP ON SPECIFIC SEIZURE TYPES

In this section, we briefly describe the effect of sleep on clinical seizures as well as on the interictal EEG epileptiform discharges in both generalized and partial seizures.

Clinical Seizures

Generalized Epilepsies

Generalized epilepsies commonly include generalized tonic-clonic (grand mal) epilepsy, petit mal (absence epilepsy), juvenile myoclonic epilepsy, infantile spasms (West's syndrome), and Lennox-Gastaut syndrome. Diurnal or *awakening epilepsy*, a term introduced by Janz[110] to differentiate from sleep and diffuse epilepsies, also belongs to the category of generalized epilepsies, which include generalized tonic-clonic, absence, and benign juvenile myoclonic seizure. Some varieties of diffuse epilepsies (e.g., Lennox-Gastaut and West's syndromes, progressive myoclonic epilepsies) also belong to generalized seizures.

Primary Generalized Grand Mal Seizure. Primary generalized grand mal seizure occurs almost exclusively in NREM sleep[111] and is most frequently seen 1–2 hours after sleep onset and at 5:00–6:00 AM, as noted originally in 1885 by Gowers[4] and later by others.[8,9,13] Grand mal seizure may occur only during sleep or only during the daytime, or be randomly distributed. In a study of 171 patients, Billiard et al.[112] found exclusively nocturnal seizures in only 8%. This study also confirmed the observations of Passouant et al.[113] and Bessett[111] that primary generalized seizure occurs exclusively in NREM sleep. Passouant et al.[114] called the seizure occurring exclusively during sleep *l'epilepsie morpheique*; this is considered a benign form of epilepsy. These patients rarely go on to develop waking epilepsies, and when they do, it is after the first 2 years from onset.[83]

Petit Mal (Absence) Epilepsy. Absence seizures occurring during sleep are difficult to diagnose, and clinical absence seizures are observed in the waking state.

According to Niedermeyer,[17] there may be fluttering of the eyelids during the spike-and-wave discharges in sleep. Gastaut and colleagues,[115] Gastaut and Broughton,[116] and Patry et al.[117] described occasional cases of petit mal status in REM sleep.

Juvenile Myoclonic Epilepsy. Meier-Ewert and Broughton[118] noted increased myoclonic seizures shortly after awakening in the morning, and the duration of the attack is longer on awakening from NREM than from REM sleep. Occasionally, these attacks occur on awakening in the middle of the night or later in the afternoon.[9,13,119]

Lennox-Gastaut Syndrome. In Lennox-Gastaut syndrome, the clinical seizures consist of tonic, myoclonic, generalized tonic-clonic, atonic, and atypical absence.[120] Information regarding the effect of sleep on the clinical seizures in this syndrome is lacking in the literature.[121] Tonic seizures, however, are typically activated by sleep,[122] are much more frequent during NREM sleep than during wakefulness, and are never seen during REM sleep.[123]

West's Syndrome (Infantile Spasms). Maximum clinical seizures, often spasms in series, are seen on arousal from sleep or before going to sleep.[124] Less than 3% of spasms are obtained in sleep.

Partial Epilepsies

Clinical seizures in simple partial seizures and complex partial seizures (CPS) are more frequent during the day.[20,83] In Billiard's[20] study of 156 patients, 61.5% had daytime and 11.5% had nocturnal seizures only. According to Montplaisir and coworkers,[125–127] Laverdiere and Montplaisir,[128] and Rossi et al.,[129] REM sleep did not facilitate temporal lobe seizure. However, other authors[113,130–132] observed ictal phenomena during both stages of sleep. In fact, Epstein and Hill[132] described a case of temporal lobe seizure with unpleasant dreams during REM sleep associated with increased epileptiform activities in the EEG in the temporal region. Frontal lobe epilepsies occur more commonly during sleep than during the waking state.[101]

Pure sleep epilepsies mostly present as focal seizures with or without secondary generalization.[13,20] Benign epilepsy of childhood with centrotemporal spikes (BECTS) and continuous spike-and-wave discharges during slow-wave sleep (CSWS) are also typical examples of sleep epilepsies and are described in the next section.

Interictal Epileptiform Discharges

Primary Generalized Grand Mal Tonic-Clonic Seizures

Interictal EEG discharges (Fig. 30–1) generally increase in NREM sleep and disappear in REM sleep.[18,20,70,87,116,133–135] Mostly the discharges are prominent at sleep onset and during the first part of

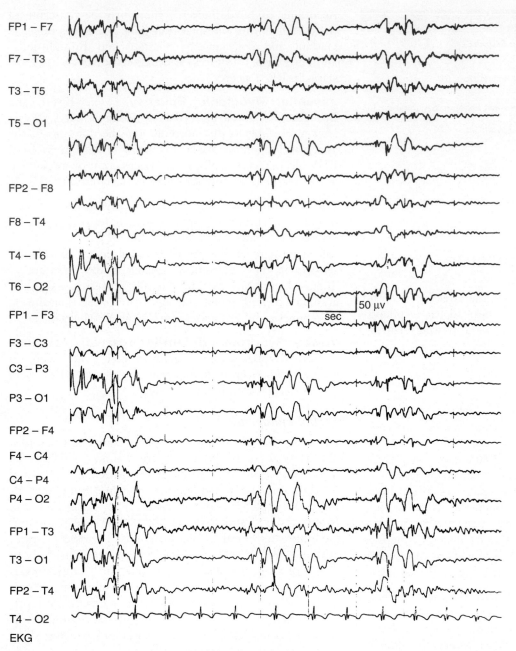

FP1 – F7

F7 – T3

T3 – T5

T5 – O1

FP2 – F8

F8 – T4

T4 – T6

T6 – O2

FP1 – F3

F3 – C3

C3 – P3

P3 – O1

FP2 – F4

F4 – C4

C4 – P4

P4 – O2

FP1 – T3

T3 – O1

FP2 – T4

T4 – O2

EKG

50 μv

sec

FIGURE 30–1 Interictal, primarily generalized epileptiform discharges (4- to 5-Hz spike-and-wave and multiple spike-and-wave discharges) seen synchronously and symmetrically with frontal dominance of amplitude in a patient with generalized tonic-clonic seizures. (EKG, electrocardiography.)

the night. Sometimes the discharges are activated during NREM sleep in the late part of the night, possibly resulting from reduced serum levels of antiepileptic medications.[18] Interictal discharges may be fragmented or may appear as polyspikes or focal spikes during NREM sleep. According to Billiard,[20] interictal discharges are more frequent during NREM than during REM sleep (41% vs. 9%) in pure sleep epilepsy, but in waking or random epilepsy, interictal discharges are seen throughout the day and night. With nocturnal epilepsies, the daytime EEG remains normal in a high percentage of patients.[136]

Petit Mal (Absence Epilepsy)

According to Sato et al.,[137] Tassinari et al.,[138] and Billiard et al.,[112] interictal EEG discharges (Fig. 30–2) in absence attacks are present during all stages of NREM sleep. These are more marked during the first sleep cycle[137] but generally absent in REM sleep. The pattern during REM sleep is similar to that during wakefulness with reduced duration.[137,138] Sato et al.[137] described alterations of spike-and-wave discharge morphology during different sleep stages: regular or irregular spike-and-wave discharges in NREM stages 1 and 2, and irregular polyspikes and slow waves during NREM stages 3 and 4.

FIGURE 30–2 Three-Hertz spike-and-wave discharges noted synchronously and symmetrically with dominance of the amplitude anteriorly in a patient with absence spells (petit mal). Note the paper speed on the panel to the left at 30 mm/sec (*sec*), and to the right at 10 mm/sec (*3 secs*; between the *arrows*).

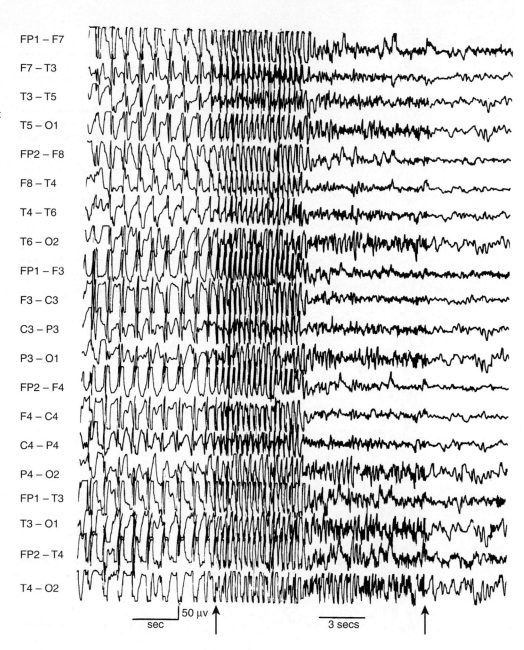

In addition, fragmentation or focalization of spikes can be seen over the frontal regions during NREM sleep.

Juvenile Myoclonic Epilepsy

Interictal discharges (Fig. 30–3) in these patients are prominent at sleep onset and on awakening but are virtually nonexistent during the rest of the sleep cycle.[18,139] According to Touchon,[119] induced awakening is a better facilitator than spontaneous awakening in these patients.

Lennox-Gastaut Syndrome

The typical EEG finding (Fig. 30–4) in Lennox-Gastaut syndrome is slow spike-and-wave discharges (1.5–2.5 Hz).

In sleep, these may be intermixed with trains of fast spikes of 10–25 Hz lasting 2–10 seconds (so-called grand mal discharges) as interictal abnormalities. The spike-and-wave discharges characteristically increase in NREM sleep.[121] Sometimes bursts of electrodecremental activity alternate with bursts of polyspikes, giving rise to a burst-suppression–like pattern.[121] According to Markand,[140] prognosis is better in those patients with significant increase of interictal EEG abnormalities during sleep.

West's Syndrome (Infantile Spasm)

The characteristic EEG finding of West's syndrome (Fig. 30–5) is hypsarrhythmia (high-amplitude slow waves

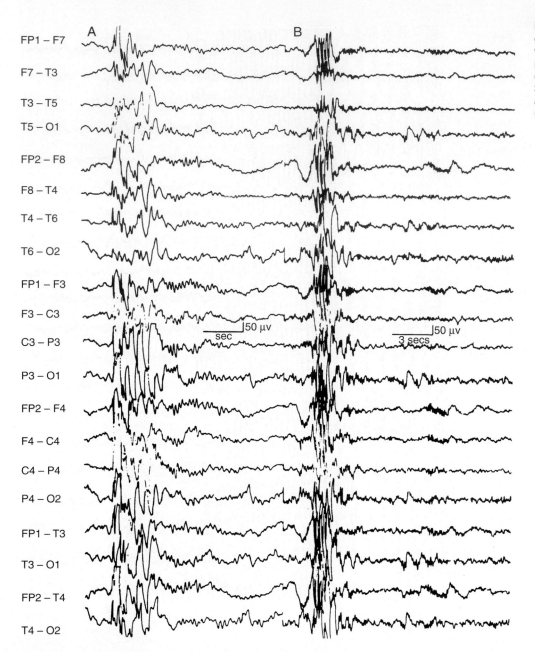

FIGURE 30–3 Interictal generalized multiple spike-and-wave discharges in the EEG of a patient with juvenile myoclonic epilepsy. Note the recording at 30 mm/sec (*sec*) on the left **(A)** and at 10 mm/sec (*3 secs*) on the right **(B)**.

and spikes or sharp waves occurring irregularly), which may show progressive changes during sleep. The characteristic pattern seen during wakefulness may increase in NREM sleep. The hypsarrhythmic EEG of wakefulness may change during NREM sleep into a periodic bilaterally synchronous diffuse pattern interspersed with flattening, resembling "burst suppression,"[113] and may even normalize during REM sleep. Occasionally the waking EEG may be normal, but the NREM sleep EEG may show the irregular high-voltage slow waves and spikes.[141]

Partial Epilepsies

An increase of interictal EEG discharges (Fig. 30–6) during NREM and diminution or disappearance during REM sleep have been found both in surface and depth electrode studies as well as in animal studies.[131,142–147] Interictal epileptiform spike discharges increase generally at sleep onset, peak in slow-wave sleep, but then decrease in REM sleep.[127,145,148,149] Malow et al.[149,150] studied the relationship of spikes to absolute log delta power, a continuous measure of sleep depth, and found that interictal discharge spiking was maximum during slow-wave sleep, particularly

FIGURE 30–4 Generalized slow spike-and-wave (2.0- to 2.5-Hz) bursts in a patient with Lennox-Gastaut syndrome.

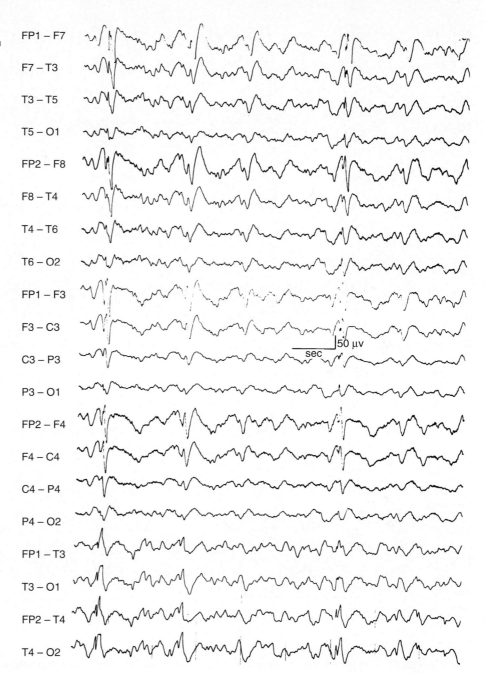

on the ascending slope of increasing log delta power. In another study, Malow et al.[151] concluded that temporal interictal epileptiform discharges observed during continuous overnight EEG studies provided important lateralizing information for the presurgical evaluation of temporal lobe epilepsy patients. However, Touchon,[119] Passouant et al.,[152] Mayersdorf and Wilder,[153] and Epstein and Hill[132] found an increase of focal temporal discharges during REM sleep. An important point to note is that during NREM sleep the discharges spread ipsilaterally and contralaterally from the primary focus, whereas during REM sleep the discharges seem to focalize maximally.[126,134,154] Localizing value of

REM sleep in temporal lobe epilepsy has also been shown in other studies.[147,155] Activation of discharges during REM sleep was also found by Frank and Pegram[156] in alumina cream monkey models of temporal lobe epilepsies. However, Mayanagi[157] did not confirm these findings in a similar monkey model.

Depth electrode studies in humans by Montplaisir et al.[127] and Lieb et al.[154] showed increased spike discharges during NREM sleep and a reduction of the discharges during REM sleep. Depth electrode studies also showed that during REM sleep the spike discharges became maximally focalized.[128,129,154]

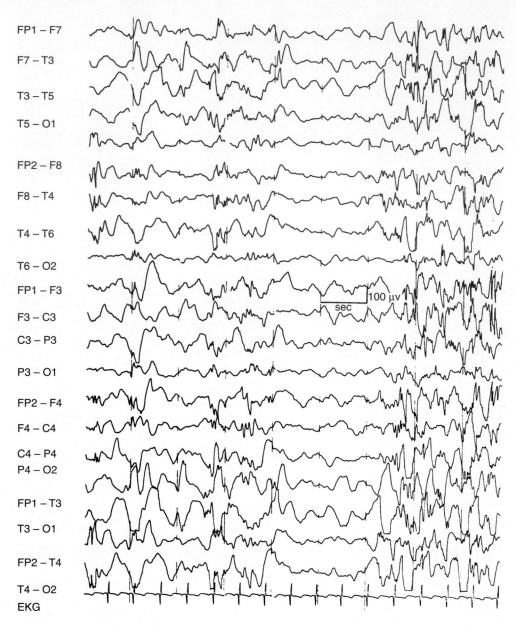

FP1 – F7
F7 – T3
T3 – T5
T5 – O1
FP2 – F8
F8 – T4
T4 – T6
T6 – O2
FP1 – F3
F3 – C3
C3 – P3
P3 – O1
FP2 – F4
F4 – C4
C4 – P4
P4 – O2
FP1 – T3
T3 – O1
FP2 – T4
T4 – O2
EKG

100 µv
sec

FIGURE 30–5
Electroencephalogram showing hypsarrhythmic pattern in a 9-month-old girl with infantile spasms.

Autret et al.[135] reviewed 236 adult epileptics attending outpatient clinics and classified the seizures in two ways: (1) according to the time of onset of seizures by history (e.g., diurnal, nocturnal, and diffuse epilepsies); and (2) according to the interictal activation during all-night PSG study. They found more frequent myoclonic attacks and increased seizure frequency in patients with diurnal epilepsy. Patients with increased incidence of interictal activities during sleep have less generalized motor seizure, more frequent CPS, a higher seizure frequency, and the appearance of new interictal activities during sleep. These authors did not find a significant relationship between the two classifications. It should be noted that these data are at variance with the results of Janz.[80]

Lieb et al.[154] performed all-night depth electrode recordings in 10 patients with medically refractory CPS

and used a computer spike recognition technique for depth spike activities arising from medial temporal lobe sites. They found the most frequent depth spike activity during deep sleep in six patients and during light sleep in three patients, and an equal number during deep and light sleep in one patient. They did not find a strong relationship between temporal lobe epilepsy and sleep pattern. Their findings that the discharge rates are greatest during NREM sleep and are suppressed during REM sleep are in agreement with the previous reports of temporal lobe epileptics. Similar depth electrode findings in temporal lobe epilepsies have been reported by Montplaisir and coworkers[125,128,158] and Passouant.[159] In some previous studies, however,[131,160] maximal spike activity was seen during light sleep. In the study by Lieb et al.,[154] the site showing maximal spike activity did not

FIGURE 30–6 Focal right anterior and midtemporal sharp and slow waves showing phase reversal at F8-T4 electrodes in a patient with complex partial seizure.

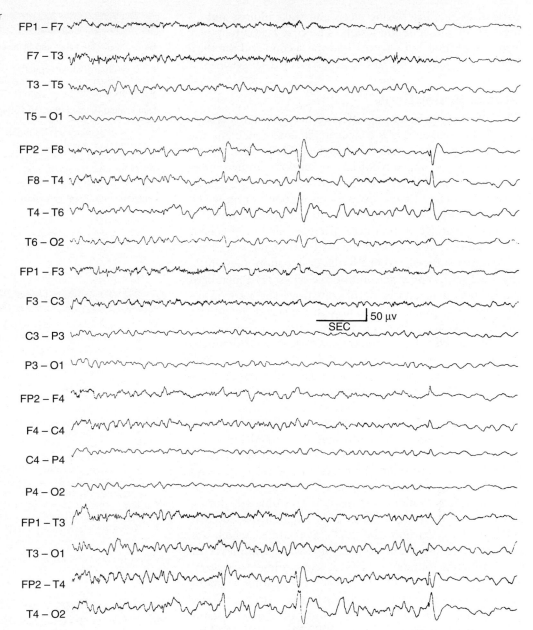

necessarily correspond to the site chosen for temporal lobectomy. This suggests that the interictal spikes and seizure-generating capacity may not bear a close relationship to underlying pathology.

Rossi et al.[129] obtained direct cerebral recordings (stereo-EEG) by stereotactic implantation of stainless steel electrodes on preselected brain sites in 19 patients with medically refractory partial epilepsy who were potential candidates for surgery. They found that interictal spiking increased at the onset of sleep, reaching a maximum level during deep NREM sleep and returning to a lower level during REM sleep. The level in REM sleep was slightly lower as compared with that during wakefulness. They further noted that the spike rate was not influenced by spike location but was affected by the local level of epileptogenicity (i.e., the higher the epileptogenicity, the lower the variation), and that the interictal spiking across sleep and wakefulness showed wide variation in different patients and in the different regions of the same patients.

In conclusion, NREM sleep is the stage of augmentation of interictal focal and generalized EEG discharges. In REM sleep, generalized discharges are usually suppressed but focal discharges may persist.

To explain the variation in spiking during sleep and wakefulness, three factors may be cited[129]: (1) subcortical-cortical interplay of the mechanisms for sleep and wakefulness as well as EEG synchronization, (2) alteration in the cortical excitability during sleep and wakefulness, and (3) location of the epileptic lesion. The first factor may play a role in generalized seizures, and the second and the third factors may play a role in the genesis of partial seizures.

Status Epilepticus

The information regarding effect of sleep on status epilepticus is limited, as this is a neurologic emergency and the first priority is treatment of the patient rather than spending time on prolonged recording. Therefore, limited information is available in certain types of status epilepticus. Gastaut[161] defined *status epilepticus* as a condition in which seizure persists for a sufficient length of time or is repeated frequently enough to produce a fixed and enduring epileptic condition. An arbitrary time of 30–60 minutes has been accepted as sufficient to justify the designation. Gastaut[161] classified status epilepticus into three types: (1) generalized status epilepticus consisting of convulsive and nonconvulsive types, (2) simple and complex partial status epilepticus, and (3) unilateral status epilepticus.

Generalized tonic-clonic (grand mal) status epilepticus occurs during the early part of the night.[162] Tonic status as may be seen in patients with Lennox-Gastaut syndrome, in whom it occurs almost exclusively during sleep and is seen mostly during NREM sleep.[108] Myoclonic status epilepticus can arise in two forms[161]: (1) as part of the primary generalized status epilepticus and (2) as the type associated with acute or subacute encephalopathies. In both these conditions, the myoclonic status epilepticus is markedly attenuated during sleep.[163] Petit mal status or absence status epilepticus may be terminated during sleep.[163] Gastaut and Tassinari[164] demonstrated that NREM sleep disrupts the EEG discharges, which are replaced by polyspikes or polyspike-wave complexes or even isolated bursts of spikes. According to several authors,[14,166] there may be recurrence of absence status on awakening during the night or in the morning. Occasionally the spike-and-wave discharges of petit mal status epilepticus may persist during NREM and REM sleep throughout the night.[14] In simple partial status epilepticus, both improvement and activation during sleep have been noted.[163] According to Froscher,[163] the role of nocturnal sleep in complex partial status epilepticus remains unknown. CSWS is discussed in the next section.

SPECIAL SEIZURE TYPES RELATED TO SLEEP-WAKE CYCLE

Certain epileptic syndromes occur predominantly or exclusively during sleep. These sleep-related epileptic syndromes (Table 30–3) may be classified similar to the suggestions by the International League Against Epilepsy (see Table 30–2) with some modifications.[63] The second edition of the International Classification of Sleep Disorders[167] listed certain diagnostic criteria for sleep-related epilepsy (Table 30–4).

TABLE 30–3 Sleep-Related Epilepsies

Generalized Epilepsies and Syndromes

- Juvenile myoclonic epilepsy
- Generalized tonic-clonic seizures on awakening
- Tonic seizures (as component of Lennox-Gastaut syndrome)

Localization-Related (Partial) Epileptic Syndromes

- Benign epilepsy of childhood with centrotemporal spikes with or without occipital paroxysms
- Nocturnal frontal lobe epilepsy
- Autosomal dominant nocturnal frontal lobe epilepsy
- Nocturnal temporal lobe epilepsy

Undetermined (Focal or Generalized) Epileptic Syndromes

- Epilepsy with continuous spike-and-wave discharges during slow-wave sleep, or electrical status epilepticus
- Landau-Kleffner syndrome or acquired epileptic aphasia

TABLE 30–4 Diagnostic Criteria for Sleep Seizures

- More than 70% of the episodes occur in sleep
- Patient complains of one or more of the following:
  - Sudden awakening
  - Abnormal sleep-related motor activities
  - Urinary incontinence
  - Tongue biting
- Patient has two of the following features:
  - Generalized tonic-clonic limb movements
  - Focal limb movement
  - Twitching of the face
  - Automatism
  - Postictal confusion and lethargy
  - PSG: ictal or interictal epileptiform discharge in any stage of sleep (an initial EEG may remain normal in many true cases of epilepsy)
- The symptoms do not meet the diagnostic criteria for another primary sleep disorder (e.g., RBD, partial arousal disorder, etc.)
- No medical, mental, or substance use disorder or medication use

PSG, polysomnography; RBD, rapid eye movement sleep behavior disorder.

Benign Epilepsy of Childhood with Centrotemporal Spikes

A clear description of BECTS, or benign focal epilepsy of childhood with rolandic spikes, was given by Nayrac and Beaussart in 1958.[168] Later, Beaussart[169] drew attention to the benign nature of the condition. This is a childhood seizure occurring between 3 and 13 years of age, at an average age of onset of 7, seen mostly during drowsiness and sleep. The clinical seizures are characterized by focal clonic facial seizures often preceded by perioral numbness. In many cases the patients have generalized tonic-clonic seizures that appear to be secondary generalization. On occasion, there is speech arrest. Consciousness is preserved. The EEG shows centrotemporal or rolandic spikes or sharp waves (Fig. 30–7) with a typical morphology of a triphasic sharp wave of high amplitude localized to the centrotemporal region but sometimes spreading to the contralateral hemisphere. Epileptiform discharges sometimes may occur outside the centrotemporal

FIGURE 30–7 Left centrotemporal spikes and sharp waves in patient with benign focal epilepsy of childhood with rolandic spikes.

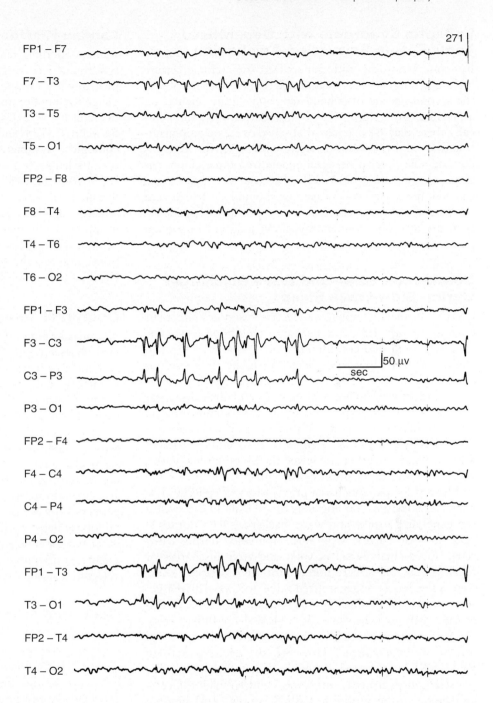

region and show occipital paroxysms in children exhibiting symptoms similar to those noted in BECTS.[170] These discharges are present throughout the night in all stages of sleep. The prognosis is excellent, with cessation of seizures by the age of approximately 16 years, without any neurologic sequelae. The patients respond to anticonvulsants satisfactorily.

Juvenile Myoclonic Epilepsy of Janz

JME, an electroclinical syndrome, was described by Janz and Mathes[171] and later published in detail by Janz and Christian.[172] The onset of the syndrome is usually between 13 and 19 years and is manifested by massive bilaterally synchronous myoclonic jerks, which are most commonly seen in the morning shortly after awakening.[172,173] The EEG is characterized by generalized spike-and-wave and typically multiple spike-and-wave discharges (see Fig. 30–3), seen in a synchronous and symmetric manner. Photosensitivity[174] and the phenomenon of perioral myoclonia[175] of the lips, tongue, jaw, or throat (precipitated predominantly by talking) may occur in a large number of patients with JME. The excellent response to anticonvulsants makes this condition benign and easily distinguishable from the malignant syndrome of progressive myoclonus epilepsies.

Epileptic Syndrome with Generalized Tonic-Clonic Seizure on Awakening

Epileptic syndrome with generalized tonic-clonic seizure on awakening[173,176] is manifested by the occurrence in the second decade of generalized tonic-clonic seizures on awakening from sleep. This is a rare syndrome, and clinically there may be occasional absence or myoclonic manifestations and photosensitivity resembling JME. There is considerable overlap between generalized tonic-clonic seizures on awakening and JME. Patients with generalized tonic-clonic seizures on awakening should have had at least six generalized tonic-clonic seizures, and in JME patients, there are relatively frequent myoclonic jerks and infrequent generalized tonic-clonic seizures.[63]

Continuous Spike-and-Wave Discharges During Slow-Wave Sleep

CSWS, formerly known as electrical status epilepticus during sleep (ESES), is a disease of childhood characterized by generalized continuous spike-and-wave EEG discharges during slow-wave sleep. All-night PSG study is necessary for diagnosis. The patients display progressive behavioral disturbances, although the seizures disappear within months or years. This entity is rare and found in children between 5 and 15 years old. ESES was first described by Patry et al.[117] in 1971 in six children. Later, Tassinari and coworkers reviewed the literature and gave a comprehensive description of the entity.[177–179]

Most of the patients had a prior history of epilepsy. The characteristic EEG finding consists of 2.0- to 2.5-cycles/sec generalized spike-and-wave discharges seen during at least 85% of NREM sleep and suppressed during REM sleep. Occasional bursts of spike-and-wave discharges or focal frontal spikes were noted during REM sleep. There were a few bursts of generalized spike-and-wave discharges seen in the EEG during wakefulness. These EEG discharges disrupted the stages of NREM sleep. In particular, the vertex sharp waves, K complexes, and spindles could not be well recognized. However, the cyclic pattern of REM-NREM persisted normally. Generally, there were no sleep disturbances but some children had difficulty awakening in the morning. CSWS is now considered an epileptic encephalopathy of childhood characterized by cognitive and motor impairment and epilepsy.[178,179] The etiologic heterogeneity of CSWS has been emphasized by Veggiotti and colleagues.[180] The EEG findings of continuous epileptic discharges generally disappear within 3 years of appearance.[177–179] Focal abnormalities, in the EEG may persist, however. It is not clear whether CSWS is a focal epilepsy or a generalized epilepsy with heterogeneous presentation, and hence it is classified under the category of undetermined epileptic syndromes. Seizures show a benign course and respond well to antiepileptic medications, with disappearance of seizures by the mid-teens. The psychological impairment, however, persists.

Landau-Kleffner Syndrome

Landau-Kleffner syndrome (LKS) is an acquired aphasic syndrome occurring in a previously normal child and probably is a variant of CSWS.[181] The characteristic language dysfunction in LKS is an apparent "word deafness" or auditory verbal agnosia. There are many similarities between CSWS and LKS, and the type of neuropsychological dysfunction may depend on the location of the discharge (e.g., frontal in CSWS and temporal in LKS). Most CSWS patients have no evidence of language dysfunction. Approximately 70–80% of children have seizures that are characterized by eye blinking, head dropping, or minor automatisms with secondary generalization. These patients respond to antiepileptic medications and remain seizure free by the mid-teens. The EEG pattern is similar to that noted in CSWS.

Nocturnal Temporal Lobe Epilepsy

Nocturnal temporal lobe epilepsy (NTLE) has not been well characterized. It has been described by Bernasconi and co-investigators[182] in a subgroup of 26 patients with refractory temporal lobe epilepsy without structural lesion, with more than 90% of seizures occurring during sleep. Focal seizures with transient impairment of consciousness, staring, automatism, and experiential or other sensory components occurring predominantly during sleep characterize the clinical syndrome. These simple partial staring seizures are frequently followed by secondary generalization. The following features differentiate patients with NTLE from the typical nonlesional temporal lobe epilepsy patients with diurnal seizures: a rare family history of epilepsy, low prevalence of childhood febrile seizures, infrequent and nonclustered seizures, and favorable surgical outcome.[63,182]

Nocturnal Frontal Lobe Epilepsy

In the early 1980s, Lugaresi and Cirignotta[183] and Lugaresi et al.[184] reported cases of paroxysmal attacks occurring during NREM sleep characterized by prominent motor behaviors in the form of dystonic posturing, tremors, and ballistic movements of the limbs, lasting 15 seconds to 2 minutes and not associated with epileptic abnormalities on the scalp EEG (Table 30–5). The attacks could respond to low doses of carbamazepine, posing the question of whether they represented epileptic seizures or sleep-related movement disorders. These attacks, termed *nocturnal paroxysmal dystonia*, were later demonstrated to represent a form of nocturnal frontal lobe epilepsy (NFLE).[185–187] Subsequently, the spectrum of frontal lobe epilepsy manifestations was enlarged to include the so-called paroxysmal arousals, characterized by abrupt arousals from NREM sleep with stereotyped motor activity of head movements, frightened expression, and dystonic posturing, lasting less than 20 seconds,[188–190] and

TABLE 30–5 Nocturnal Frontal Lobe Epilepsy: Salient Features

- Movements: tonic, clonic, bipedal, bimanual, bicycling, choreoathetoid, ballismic
- Retropelvic thrust
- Motor and sexual automatisms
- Contralateral dystonic posturing
- Contralateral arm abduction with or without eye deviation
- Oftentimes exclusively nocturnal
- Sudden onset and termination in NREM sleep
- Duration: usually less than a minute
- Short postictal confusion
- Often in clusters
- Mistaken for nonepileptic seizures
- Ictal EEG may be normal
- Interictal EEG may or may not show spikes

the so-called epileptic nocturnal wanderings,[191,192] more complex events lasting 2–4 minutes and associated with agitated ambulation and jumping about. Paroxysmal arousals, often recurring quasi-periodically every 20–40 seconds for long stretches during NREM sleep, are often associated with attacks of nocturnal paroxysmal dystonia and epileptic nocturnal wanderings in the same patient, and can represent the initial manifestations of the more prolonged attacks.[193] The orderly complexity of the attacks was taken to indicate progression of the ictal discharge to involve wider brain regions in a graded fashion.

The peculiar features of NFLE thus consist of its nocturnal recurrence, related to NREM sleep stages in over 80% of the seizures,[194] and of the characteristic motor pattern with truncal and bipedal gross and often violent movements with dyskinetic features; the latter have led to the definition of hypermotor or hyperkinetic seizures. Recently however, the application of deep brain electrodes (stereo-EEG) in presurgical cases has led to the recognition that "hypermotor seizures" may also be found in seizures originating from the temporal lobe and the insula.[195–198] In such cases, the hyperkinetic features appeared 8–15 seconds after the beginning of the discharge in the temporal lobe, when the discharge spreads to extratemporal (cingulate, frontal, parietal) structures.[195] Functional brain imaging in frontal lobe seizures (nocturnal paroxysmal dystonia and paroxysmal arousals) indeed confirms that the peculiar motor patterns are related to involvement of mesial, especially cingulate, motor areas.[199,200]

Autosomal Dominant Nocturnal Frontal Lobe Epilepsy

Scheffer et al.[201] described an autosomal dominant form of frontal lobe epilepsy in six families. Brief motor seizures usually occurred in clusters during sleep. The disorder usually started in childhood and persisted through adult life. Patients were of normal intellect and had normal neurologic examination and neuroimaging. Response to carbamazepine was excellent. In most cases, interictal EEGs were normal, although one family with daytime attacks had epileptiform discharges. Videotelemetry during the attacks confirmed

their epileptic nature. They called this condition autosomal dominant nocturnal frontal lobe epilepsy (ADNFLE). The clinical features of ADNFLE were later confirmed by Thomas et al.[202] in one family with very frequent seizures during infancy, in which carbamazepine therapy again was dramatically effective, and by Oldani et al.,[203] who studied 33 patients and found similar results. In 1995 Phillips et al.[204] mapped a gene responsible for ADNFLE in a large Australian kindred to chromosome 20q13.2, and Steinlein et al.[205] demonstrated that epileptic nocturnal frontal lobe (ENFL) type 1 was due to mutations in *CHRNA4*, the gene encoding the A4 subunit of the acetylcholine (ACh) neural receptor. Another linkage site was later reported to chromosome 15q24 accounting for ENFL type 2,[206] and mutations in *CHRNB2*, the gene encoding for the B2 subunit of the ACh neural receptor localized on chromosome 1 as accounting for ENFL type 3.[207] Another linkage locus to chromosome 8p12.3-8q12.3 and a missense mutation in the gene *CHRNA2* encoding for the neural ACh receptor A2 subunit have been reported in familial seizures characterized by complex and finalized ictal behavior resembling epileptic nocturnal wanderings,[208] as well as mutations in the corticotropin-releasing hormone gene.[209]

Genetic findings thus implicate the nicotinic ACh receptors in ADNFLE. Mutations responsible for ADNFLE work by increasing the receptor sensitivity to ACh,[210] indicating that a gain of function of the mutant receptors underlies the neuronal dysfunction responsible for the epileptic seizures. Mutated nicotinic receptors responsible for ADNFLE were also found to be more sensitive to carbamazepine, which works as a noncompetitive inhibitor of the nicotinic ACh receptors.[211] On the basis of the genetic findings and functional imaging data,[212] the pathogenesis of ADNFLE has been attributed to dysfunction in the dorsal cholinergic ascending arousal system, and a common background with the arousal parasomnias[213] has been hypothesized based on preliminary epidemiologic and clinical data.

EFFECT OF SLEEP DEPRIVATION ON EPILEPSY

The diagnostic value of sleep-deprived EEG has been well documented.[142,214–217] What is the mechanism of activation during sleep deprivation? This is probably not a sampling effect and not related to sleep alone.[214,215,217] In a study using paired-pulse transcranial magnetic stimulation in 30 patients with untreated newly diagnosed epilepsy (15 idiopathic generalized and 15 focal epilepsies) and 13 healthy control subjects before and after sleep deprivation, Badawy et al.[40] noted an increase in cortical excitability following sleep deprivation at a short interstimulus intervals. This change was most prominent in the patients with idiopathic generalized epilepsy. The authors' findings confirmed the hypothesis that sleep deprivation increases cortical excitability in epilepsy. Sleep deprivation increases the epileptiform discharges mostly in the transition period between waking and light sleep and also has a localizing value.[215,217] Although the original study by Rodin et al.[218] in 1962 found epileptiform discharges in healthy subjects after sleep deprivation, later studies[217,219] failed to confirm these observations.

Rowan et al.[215] studied 43 consecutive patients using two types of activation: sleep deprivation (24 hours in adults and partial deprivation in children) and sedated sleep (after oral secobarbital). They obtained useful information in 44% of sleep-deprived as opposed to 14% of sedated sleep records. The patients were referred because of doubtful diagnosis of epilepsy or because seizure types could not be determined. They also found sleep deprivation superior to sedated sleep for differentiating those with a final diagnosis of seizure. It should be noted that sleep alone does not explain the activating effect of sleep deprivation. The mechanism remains largely unknown. Rowan et al.[215] suggested increased cerebral excitability after sleep deprivation in normal individuals.

Degen[216] studied 127 waking and sleep EEGs after sleep deprivation in 120 epileptic patients on anticonvulsant medication. He found seizure activity in 63% of the patients, although in the previous EEG records of these patients only 19% had shown seizure activity; thus, sleep deprivation increased the incidence of seizure activity. Approximately 48% of discharges occurred during slow-wave and 25% during REM sleep.

It is interesting to note that in 1896 Patrick and Gilbert[220] apparently performed sleep deprivation studies in human beings. The studies by Bennett[221] in 1963 and Mattson et al.[222] in 1965 established the value of sleep deprivation as a diagnostic tool in patients with seizure disorders. Rodin[223] computed the incidence of activation after sleep deprivation from an analysis of the literature and came up with a figure of approximately 45%. Later studies by Frucht et al.,[224] Ropakiotis et al.,[225] and Teraita-Adrados et al.[226] confirmed the value of sleep deprivation in activating EEG epileptiform discharges. There is, however, a contrasting observation by Malow et al.,[227] who failed to note increasing seizure frequency after partial sleep deprivation in inpatient video EEG monitoring in a group of 84 patients with medically refractory epilepsy.

PHENOMENA DURING SLEEP THAT CAN BE MISTAKEN FOR EPILEPSY (NONEPILEPTIFORM DISORDERS)

Certain paroxysmal arousal disorders in NREM sleep may be mistaken for seizures, particularly for CPS. Some examples of these disorders are night terrors (pavor nocturnus), somnambulism (sleepwalking), confusional arousals, tooth grinding (bruxism), rhythmic movement disorder, benign sleep myoclonus of infancy, hypnagogic foot tremor, and nonepileptic seizure (nocturnal pseudo-seizure). Two other parasomnias usually associated with REM sleep, REM sleep behavior disorder (RBD) and nightmares (dream-anxiety attacks), may be mistaken for seizures. These conditions are described in Chapter 35 and listed in Table 30–6. Table 30–7 lists some salient features of nonepileptic seizures that may help differentiate this condition from a true seizure.[228]

Arousal parasomnias, in particular pavor nocturnus and somnambulism, are nocturnal events arising during NREM sleep that may be mistaken for seizures, in particular for NFLE. The differential diagnosis is complicated by the fact that there are no obligate PSG markers for the parasomnias, and even ictal EEG recordings may sometimes remain inconclusive in frontal lobe seizures.[194] Moreover, small sharp spikes or benign epileptiform transients of sleep, as noted in the EEG (Fig. 30–8) in stages 1 and 2 NREM sleep, may resemble true epileptiform spikes even though the distribution, morphology, and occurrence during particular stages of sleep without any clinical accompaniments differentiate these from true epileptiform spikes.[229]

Thus these nocturnal events (clinical and electrographic) of nonepileptiform significance discussed earlier must be differentiated from true epileptic attacks; otherwise, unnecessary medications and tests will be used. Characteristic clinical features combined with EEG and PSG recordings are important to differentiate these conditions. It should be noted that presence of EEG epileptiform discharges independent of nocturnal attacks may not be proof sine qua non that the attacks are of an epileptic nature.[19] However, video-EEG recordings to correlate

---

TABLE 30–6   **Conditions That May Mimic Nocturnal Seizures**

- Confusional arousals
- Sleep walking
- Sleep terror
- REM sleep behavior disorder
- Rhythmic movement disorder
- Tooth grinding (bruxism)
- Benign sleep myoclonus of infancy
- Hypnagogic foot tremor
- Nonepileptic seizure (nocturnal pseudo-seizure)

TABLE 30–7   **Features of Nonepileptic Seizure (Pseudo-Seizure)**

- Predominantly diurnal; sometimes nocturnal
- Gradual onset and gradual termination
- Prominent pelvic thrusting, mainly forward
- Asynchronous (out-of-phase) clonic limb movements
- Eyes usually closed
- Prominent head movements (horizontal—"no-no"—or rotary)
- Lack of concern about symptoms (*la belle indifference*)
- Urinary incontinence and self-injury: extremely rare[231]
- Video-EEG: normal awake EEG

FIGURE 30–8 Small sharp spikes (benign epileptiform transients of sleep) seen in channels 5–8 and 13–16 from the top.

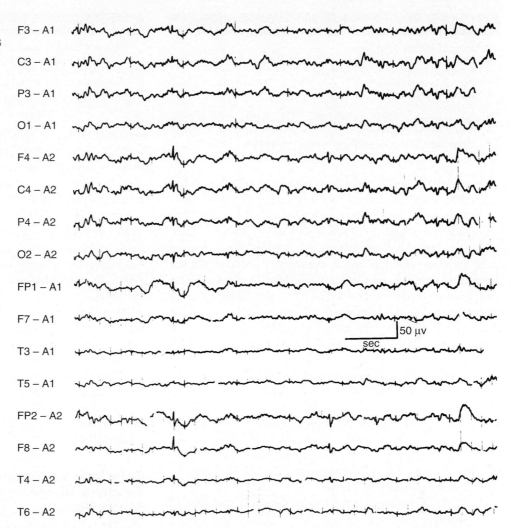

behavior with EEG manifestations may establish or exclude the diagnosis. Sometimes the two conditions (epileptic and nonepileptic attacks) may coexist. Finally, an improvement after empiric treatment with an anticonvulsant medication does not necessarily prove the epileptic nature of the condition.[19] Practical suggestions for differential diagnosis between the arousal parasomnias and NFLE seizures have been proposed[194,230]: NFLE should be suspected if attacks recur several times during the same night; if they occur in a stereotyped fashion; if tremor, dystonia, or ballism are noted during the attack; if the attacks arise in or persist into adulthood; and if there is a good response to low doses of carbamazepine.[231] Unfortunately, however, these suggestions rely on expert opinion and are not validated against any "gold standard."

EFFECT OF EPILEPSY ON SLEEP

An objective evaluation of the states of sleep in epileptic patients reveals that they are altered in a large percentage of patients studied. Although the utility of sleep in the diagnosis of epilepsy is well established, the altered sleep characteristics in epileptics are not well known. One of the difficulties has been that most of the studies have been conducted in patients who have been on anticonvulsants, thus adding the confounding factors of the effect of anticonvulsants on sleep architecture. Furthermore, there have not been good longitudinal studies to determine the effect of epilepsy on sleep in the early versus late stage of the illness. Despite these limitations, there have been several studies from which a general consensus has been reached regarding the effect of epilepsy on sleep and sleep structure. A variety of sleep disturbances have been observed in epileptics and can be summarized as follows[131,133,152,232]: a reduction in REM sleep; an increase in wake after sleep onset (WASO); increased instability of sleep states, such as unclassifiable sleep epochs; an increase in NREM stages 1 and 2; a decrease in NREM sleep stages 3 and 4; a reduction in the density of sleep spindles; and an increase of sleep-onset latency.

Table 30–8 lists effects of epilepsy on sleep architecture (macrostructure and microstructure). In patients with

TABLE 30–8 Effect of Epilepsy on Sleep Architecture
• Increased sleep-onset latency • Increased number and duration of awakenings after sleep onset • Increased cyclic alternating pattern • Reduced sleep efficiency • Reduced sleep spindles and K complexes • Reduced REM sleep • Increased stage shifts • Abnormal sleep cycling • Sleep state instability (unclassifiable sleep epochs)

TABLE 30–9 Causes of Excessive Daytime Sleepiness in Epileptics
• Clinical seizures, particularly nocturnal seizures • Frequent ictal and interictal epileptiform EEG discharges • Coexisting disorders (e.g., sleep apnea, polycystic ovary syndrome) • Depression

absence spells, sleep macrostructure may be normal but microstructural alterations showing increased cyclic alternating patterns may have relevance to the postulated physiologic mechanism of spike-and-wave generation utilizing the same thalamocorticothalamic pathways that are used for sleep spindles and K complexes. Sleep structural alterations are related to frequency of nocturnal seizures and increased interictal epileptiform discharges during sleep. Severe sleep disruption related to spike-and-wave discharges may be partly responsible for cognitive impairment in epileptics, including patients with CSWS and LKS.

Nocturnal seizures may alter sleep architecture by five mechanisms: (1) effects of seizures (ictal discharges); (2) effects of interictal discharges; (3) effects of antiepileptic medications; (4) associated organic brain disorders; and (5) comorbid primary sleep disorders (e.g., sleep apnea, insomnia, restless legs syndrome/periodic limb movements in sleep). Three questions may be asked regarding the effect of epilepsy on sleep:

1. Is sleep quality related to the duration and type of seizures?
2. Is sleep quality related to repeated episodes of seizures or poorly controlled seizures?
3. Can epilepsy lead to a sleep disorder?

These questions are discussed in the next sections.

Sleep Complaints in Patients with Epilepsy

Patients with epilepsy may complain of excessive daytime sleepiness (EDS), insomnia (inability to fall or maintain sleep and early morning awakening), and adverse daytime consequences related to insomnia and EDS, as well as unusual movements and behaviors intruding into sleep. EDS in epileptics may result from clinical seizures, particularly nocturnal seizures and ictal or interictal EEG epileptiform discharges; comorbid conditions such as obstructive sleep apnea syndrome (OSAS; see later) and polycystic ovary syndrome (PCOS); and effects of antiepileptic medications (see later). Table 30–9 lists causes of EDS in epileptic patients. Maganti et al.[233] reported that EDS and sleep complaints are common among adults with epilepsy, and in some patients these may be due to underlying sleep disorders such as sleep apnea. Khatami et al.[234] assessed sleep-wake habits and EDS using a standardized questionnaire in 100 consecutive outpatients with epilepsy and 90 controls. Sleep complaints were more common in epilepsy patients than in controls, and sleep maintenance insomnia as well as EDS were found frequently; they noted that loud snoring and restless legs symptoms are the only independent predictors of EDS in epilepsy patients. Jenssen et al.,[235] based on a questionnaire and chart review of a tertiary referral center, noted subjective somnolence to be related mainly to depression rather than to obstructive sleep apnea (OSA) and other variables.

Manni and Terzaghi[236] described two elderly men with late-onset sleep-related tonic-clonic seizures and RBD. The authors hypothesized that RBD may facilitate seizure occurrence. In a later study, Mani et al.[237] reported co-occurrence of epileptic seizures and RBD in six cases. The authors cautioned that further investigations of the occurrence of RBD episodes and epilepsy are needed to understand the neurobiological significance of this comorbidity.

Relationship Between Seizure Type, Severity of Seizure, and Extent of Sleep Deficits

The relationship between seizure type, severity of seizure, and extent of sleep deficits remains somewhat controversial, and the reports are contradictory. WASO, sleep stage shifts, and sleep fragmentation are found in all seizure types.[111,232,238–241] Reduction of REM sleep and an increase in NREM stages 1 and 2 are in part dependent on the type of epilepsy. Declerck et al.[232] found an increase of NREM stages 1 and 2 and a reduction of REM sleep in 258 patients with primary generalized or partial seizures with secondary generalization as compared with 223 nonepileptic subjects. Seizure occurrence during sleep accentuates sleep deficits, which are more marked in primary generalized and partial seizures with secondary generalization than in other types. In 25% of epileptics, Declerck et al.[232] could not evaluate PSG recordings because of severe encephalopathies associated with seizures. Similar findings were obtained by Bessett.[111] Baldy-Moulinier[238] noted a decrease of REM sleep in patients with CPS occurring during sleep. However, Baldy-Moulinier found markedly reduced REM sleep in patients having only one attack of secondary generalized seizure during the night. It is interesting to note that Bessett[111] in human epileptics and Baldy-Moulinier[238] in temporal lobe epilepsy models found no rebound REM sleep in subsequent recordings after REM sleep loss, which is contrary to the usual findings of REM rebound after REM deprivation. In summary, WASO and sleep fragmentation are found in all types of epilepsy, and generalized seizures are associated with an increase of NREM stages 1 and 2 and a reduction of REM sleep. In CPS there is often REM reduction only. Bessett[111] could not discriminate NREM stages or REM sleep in the EEG because of disrupted sleep architecture due to the seizures (ictal and interictal).

Hoeppner et al.[242] studied self-reported sleep disorder symptoms in epilepsy. They gave a questionnaire relating to six aspects of sleep: delayed sleep onset, night awakenings, dreams, night terrors, sleepwalking, and fatigue on awakening. They evaluated four groups of subjects: (1) 4 patients with simple partial seizures, (2) 18 patients with CPS, (3) 8 patients with generalized seizures, and (4) 23 controls (14 women and 9 men ages 16–53 years). They found significantly more sleep disorder symptoms (particularly frequent awakenings at night) in patients with simple partial seizures and CPS. The generalized group behaved like the control group. Patients with the most frequent seizures, irrespective of type, had the most sleep disturbances.

Roder-Wanner et al.[243] obtained polygraphic sleep recordings in 43 patients with different types of epilepsies. They found that patients with generalized epilepsy had a higher percentage of deeper stages of sleep (NREM 3 and 4) than patients with focal epilepsy. These observations are correlated with the factor of photosensitivity, which was noted in a subgroup of these patients. The authors concluded that there was no real relationship between sleep structure and the type of epilepsy. Thus, there is some controversy regarding the relationship between seizure type and sleep. It can be concluded, however, that the severity of sleep deficits is in part correlated with severity of the seizure disorder. Animal studies support such a conclusion.[244,245] In previous studies, sleep structure abnormalities may have been related to clinical or subclinical seizure activity preceding the PSG investigation or to the medication received during the study.

There are contradictory reports regarding REM sleep disturbance.[133] On seizure-free nights, REM sleep is usually normal, but REM decrement is noted when there are primary or secondary generalized seizures during the night. There is no REM suppression during partial seizure without secondary generalization.[111,238] Bowersox and Drucker-Colin[246] stated that increased cortical neuronal excitability and reduced seizure threshold may result from chronic REM sleep deprivation secondary to repeated and frequent nocturnal generalized seizures.

In a series of 15 patients with temporal lobe seizure disorders, Touchon et al.[247] found increased WASO, shifting of the sleep stages, and increases in NREM sleep stages 1 and 2. In a study of 23 patients with temporal lobe epilepsy, Kohsaka[248] found significantly decreased sleep efficiency and increased awakenings in both treated and untreated patients. He also noted increased NREM stage 4 in untreated patients compared to healthy controls. The site of the primary focus may determine the type of the sleep disturbances.[18] Foci in the amygdalohippocampal region may lead to increased WASO and decreased sleep efficiency. Frontal lobe epileptics, however, may show a specific reduction in stages 3 and 4 NREM sleep.

In a questionnaire-based study of 40 children with tuberous sclerosis, Hunt and Stores[249] found that concurrent epilepsy was significantly associated with sleep disturbances in these children. This observation was corroborated by Bruni and coworkers,[250] who found a more disrupted sleep architecture in patients with tuberous sclerosis and epilepsy compared with seizure-free children. In large series of children with epilepsy, there was a correlation among seizure frequency, incidence of interictal epileptiform discharges, duration of seizure disorders, behavior problems, poor quality of sleep, and disturbed breathing during sleep.[251,252] Becker et al.[253] noted that 80% of 30 children complaining of sleep disturbance had PSG documentation of OSA, abnormal sleep architecture, and fragmentation.

de Weerd et al.[254] reported poor quality of life and sleep disturbances that were more common in adults with focal seizures with or without secondary generalization compared with controls. A variety of PSG-documented sleep abnormalities have been described in patients with JME[103,255,256] and focal temporal lobe epilepsy. Bazil et al.[103] documented reduction of REM sleep by seizures in temporal lobe epilepsy. Sleep abnormalities in absence seizures gave conflicting results.[134] In BECTS, no sleep architectural abnormalities are noted.[30,257]

Several authors have noted that sleep abnormalities are more common in patients with primary or secondary generalized seizures than in those with partial focal epilepsies,[30,257,258] but other studies have shown that patients with severe or medically refractory temporal lobe seizures may have equally severe sleep structural abnormalities.[256,257] Several investigators have reported severe sleep abnormalities in symptomatic epilepsies associated with neurologic deficits.[120,259–264] In all of these patients, both sleep dysfunction and seizure disorders must be treated simultaneously to obtain best results.

In several reports, PSG findings and sleep abnormalities have been described in partial seizures, especially frontal lobe[265,266] and temporal lobe[103,266] seizures. Tachibana et al.[265] showed an improvement in sleep structure after treatment with appropriate antiepileptic drugs (AEDs) (Fig. 30–9).

Can Epilepsy Lead to a Sleep Disorder?

It is generally thought that sleep deficits in seizure disorders are secondary to the severity of the seizure disorder and are a direct result of seizures during sleep. However,

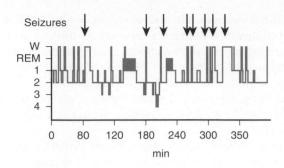

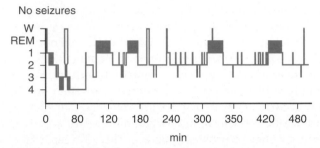

FIGURE 30–9 (Top) Polysomnogram showing increased slow-wave and REM sleep along with frequent awakenings during the night with eight nocturnal seizures. **(Bottom)** Sleep architecture showing remarkable improvement in the same patient following treatment with carbamazepine. *(Modified from Tachibana N, Shinde A, Ikeda A, et al. Supplementary motor area seizure resembling sleep disorder. Sleep 1996;19:811.)*

studies by Tanaka and Naquet[267] demonstrated progressive sleep deficits in amygdala kindling models. In addition, the sleep deficits persisted 1 month after discontinuation of kindling procedures.

Shouse and Sterman[244] produced amygdala kindling in 10 adult cats and studied their sleep and waking patterns chronically. They found a progressive sleep disturbance and retention of the deficit over a prolonged period after termination of amygdala stimulation. These findings suggest the "kindling" of a sleep disturbance in addition to a seizure disorder. The authors further stated that sleep abnormalities cannot be viewed as a simple or temporary side effect of epileptiform activity. It appears that a permanent change in sleep physiology occurs in epilepsy. These observations of Shouse and Sterman[244] partially answer the question posed by Passouant[1]: "Can epilepsy lead to a sleep disorder?" Effective treatment of epilepsy with anticonvulsant medications or surgical methods normalizes sleep disturbances in human epilepsy.[240]

Can a Sleep Disorder Lead to Epilepsy?

In 1995, Silvestri et al.[268] reported six patients who were diagnosed in childhood as having disorders of arousal and later developed epileptic seizures. The sleep disorders consisted of sleepwalking and night terrors, all confirmed by PSG studies. The seizures noted were complex partial in five and generalized tonic-clonic in one. Nocturnal monitoring confirmed the epileptic

nature of these events. The authors hypothesized that, because both disorders of arousal and epilepsy are related to sleep and share other common factors such as age of onset and precipitating factors, these disorders share common functional substrates, and it is possible that disorders of arousal may later turn into epileptic seizures. It should be noted, however, that sleepwalking and sleep terrors are frequently noted in children, and seizures may simply coexist with these NREM parasomnias. Most sleep specialists and epileptologists simply do not believe that such parasomnias can later turn into epileptic seizures. It should also be remembered that cases of typical disorders of arousal not associated with epileptic discharges in epileptic children have been described.[14,116,269]

EFFECT OF ANTICONVULSANTS ON SLEEP AND SLEEP ARCHITECTURE IN EPILEPTICS

Malow and coworkers[270] noted increased Epworth Sleepiness Scale scores in 28% of 158 adult epilepsy patients. Peled and Lavie[188] described bursts of generalized spike-and-wave complexes during stages 2 and 3 of NREM sleep, preceded by K complexes and associated with arousals causing sleep disruption, and daytime sleepiness. Some patients with epilepsy may have EDS as a result of sleep apnea (see later) and PCOS, which is more common in women with epilepsy, especially those patients taking valproic acid, than those without epilepsy.[271] Betts et al.[272] reported 30% of women treated with valproic acid, 6% with lamotrigine or carbamazepine, and 14% of age-matched controls with clinical biochemical evidence of PCOS. PCOS is associated with increased prevalence of OSAS.[148,273]

Some patients with epilepsy may complain of insomnia, which may be difficulty falling asleep or maintaining sleep, or early morning awakening associated with adverse daytime consequences of sleepiness, inability to concentrate and pay attention, and impairment of the quality of life. Insomnia in epileptics may be related to sleep fragmentation and repeated arousal as a result of nocturnal seizures and interictal EEG epileptiform discharges, some AEDs, depression and anxiety, or withdrawal or tapering of AEDs during video-EEG monitoring for presurgical evaluation of refractory seizures or may be due to an associated primary sleep disorder (Table 30–10). Some AEDs (lamotrigine and felbamate) may cause insomnia. Sadler[274] reported a 6.4% incidence of dose-dependent insomnia

TABLE 30–10 Causes of Insomnia in Epileptics

- Nocturnal seizures and interictal epileptiform discharges causing repeated arousals
- Some antiepileptic drugs (AEDs; e.g., lamotrigine, felbamate)
- Withdrawal or tapering of AEDs during video-EEG monitoring
- Depression and anxiety
- Associated primary sleep disorder

among patients taking lamotrigine. In contrast, Foldvary et al.[275] failed to observe any effect of lamotrigine in a PSG study in seven subjects with epilepsy on sleep efficiency, sleep latency, or total sleep time. The other antiepileptic medication that was found to have stimulant-like effects in patients with epilepsy is felbamate[276,277]; however, because of serious toxicity, felbamate has largely been withdrawn from the market and is rarely used nowadays to treat epilepsy.

There is a dearth of well-controlled, careful studies documenting the effects of anticonvulsant medications on sleep architecture that properly take into account the effects of seizures on sleep. Only limited data are available. It is somewhat daunting to study the effects of AEDs in epileptics taking into consideration all the confounding factors. Objectively, the sleep architecture should be studied by PSG recordings before starting the patient on medication—that is, in the drug-free state—and then restudied with the patient on chronic therapy with one rather than multiple drugs. From a practical point of view, this is somewhat difficult because, when the patient presents to the physician, he or she must be treated before performing these investigations. Furthermore, the pharmacokinetic and pharmacodynamic effects of AEDs show considerable variation depending on the age and genetic predisposition. There may be a circadian effect of the drugs, and comorbid conditions may also affect sleep. Furthermore, AEDs may have residual effect on sleep architecture even after withdrawal of the medication.[278] Johnson[240] reviewed the literature up to about 1981 showing the effects of acute and chronic exposure to anticonvulsant drugs in relation to the sleep pattern. Acute exposure to anticonvulsants may reduce REM and NREM stages 3 and 4 and increase stage 2 NREM sleep. Acute and chronic drug trials in epileptics suggest that the main effects of anticonvulsants consist of sleep stabilization, however, which includes a reduction in WASO and an increase in NREM stages 2, 3, and 4, along with sleep spindle density. These improvements are concomitant with the reduction of seizures. The bulk of the evidence in the literature points to the fact that effective anticonvulsant treatment and seizure control result in reduction of sleep disturbance. Thus, the effects may be due to the reduction of seizures and not to any specific effect of the anticonvulsants on sleep architecture.

In a survey of experimental epilepsy in animals, Wauquier et al.[279] observed that sleep fragmentation as obtained in epileptic animals as well as in humans may be the consequence of microarousals. Anticonvulsants may suppress microarousals because of their sedative properties and hence lead to stabilization of sleep fragmentation and normalization of sleep. Anticonvulsants may normalize sleep, however, because of a specific action on particular abnormal EEG patterns. Thus, despite the suggestion that anticonvulsants themselves may be responsible in part for the fragmentation and disruption of sleep architecture, the general consensus is that anticonvulsant medications normalize sleep architecture, most probably by reduction of the seizures.

AEDs have both detrimental and beneficial effects.[280] Most AEDs, however, normalize and stabilize sleep[80,240,256,281] due to the suppression of clinical seizures and interictal discharges or a direct consequence of AEDs. In addition, the AEDs may also have neuromodulatory effects causing sleep disruption.[282–284] Most of the first-generation AEDs may delay REM sleep onset or suppress REM sleep percentages.[30,281,285] Some AEDs cause weight gain[286] (e.g., valproic acid, vigabatrin, pregabalin, gabapentin, and probably also carbamazepine) and decrease upper airway muscle tone (e.g., benzodiazepines and phenobarbital), which may have deleterious effects on the upper airway muscles causing sleep apnea in some patients[30] (see later). The effects of AEDs in sleep can be divided into general effects consisting of reduction of REM and slow-wave sleep, reduction of sleep latency, increased percentage of NREM stages 1 and 2, and specific effects depending on the individual AEDs (Table 30–11). In the following paragraphs, effects of the traditional or first-generation and some of the newer AEDs are briefly discussed.

Older Antiepileptic Drugs

In most of the studies, phenobarbital is found to increase stage 2 NREM sleep and decrease sleep-onset latency, REM sleep, and WASO without any significant effect on slow-wave sleep.[259,287,288] Wolf et al.[287] reviewed the literature to assess the effect of barbiturates, phenytoin, carbamazepine, and valproic acid treatment on sleep. They noted significant reduction of REM sleep, a reduction in total awake time, and an increase in NREM stage 2 sleep as the short-term effects of barbiturates. The long-term effects of barbiturates are similar in general, but in some cases the sleep pattern returned to the premedication level. Wolf et al.[287] performed a prospective polygraphic study of sleep in epileptic patients before and after medications using a crossover design. They studied phenobarbital, phenytoin, ethosuximide, valproic acid, and carbamazepine. The authors included 40 unmedicated patients to study the effect of phenobarbital and phenytoin. The short-term effects of phenobarbital included reduction of WASO and REM sleep and increase of stage 2 NREM sleep. There was no relationship with the serum drug levels.

Manni et al.[289] performed an objective and subjective assessment of daytime sleepiness using the Multiple Sleep Latency Test (MSLT), clinical, and psychometric data on 10 patients with generalized epilepsy treated chronically with phenobarbital, 10 patients with cryptogenic partial epilepsy treated with carbamazepine, and 10 healthy

TABLE 30–11 Effects of Antiepileptic Drugs (AEDs) on Sleep Architecture*

AEDs	SE	Sleep LAT	Stage 1	Stage 2	SWS	REM	WASO
Phenobarbitol	D	D	I	I	—	D	D
Phenytoin	D	D	I	I	D	—	D
Primidone	?	D	?	?	I	D	?
Carbamazepine	I	D	—	—	I	D *(Tr)*	D
Valproic acid	—	—	?	—	I	?	I
Ethosuximide	D	I	I	—	D	I	I
Benzodiazepines	D	D	D	I	D	?	D
Felbamate	D	?	?	?	?	?	?
Gabapentin	I	D	D	—	I	I	D
Lamotrigine	—	—	—	—	D	I	—
Levetiracetam	—	—	—	I	D	—	—
Oxcarbazepine	?	?	?	?	?	?	?
Pregabalin	I	D	—	—	I	—	D
Tiagabine	I	—	—	—	I	—	—
Topiramate	—	—	—	—	—	—	—
Zonisamide	?	?	?	?	?	?	?
Vigabatrin	?	—	?	?	?	?	?

*D, decreased; D *(Tr)*, transiently decreased; I, increased; —, no change; ?, unknown.
SE, sleep efficiency; Sleep LAT, sleep latency; SWS, slow-wave sleep; WASO, wake after sleep onset.

controls. These authors found that patients on phenobarbital had a greater daytime sleep tendency and performed worse on the digit symbol substitution test compared to the other two groups. In a similarly designed study,[290] they noted a shorter mean sleep latency in patients on phenobarbital compared with patients on sodium valproate and controls. Psychomotor functioning was also poor in patients on phenobarbital compared to controls, whereas patients on valproate had some attentional impairment and a tendency toward longer motor movement time. However, they did not find a correlation between the assessed parameters and serum drug concentrations.

Phenytoin generally causes a reduction of sleep-onset latency, REM sleep, and slow-wave sleep as well as sleep efficiency, but causes increased stage 1 and 2 NREM sleep.[264,284] Phenytoin also increases daytime sleepiness. The short-term effects of phenytoin included no change in the percentage of WASO, a decrease in NREM sleep stages 1 and 2, and an increase in sleep stages 3 and 4; there was no change in REM sleep and no relationship with the serum drug levels. Wolf et al.[287] studied the long-term effects of phenytoin in 12 patients. The long-term effects were in general a reversal of the short-term effects and consisted of an increase of NREM sleep stages 1 and 2 with a decrease of slow-wave sleep. REM sleep, however, remained unaltered.

Carbamazepine has been studied fairly extensively in various studies. This AED is found to increase sleep efficiency and slow-wave sleep but decrease REM sleep in healthy subjects[288] and transiently decrease REM in epileptics. Baldy-Moulinier[238] reported normalization of disturbed sleep pattern in temporal lobe epileptics after carbamazepine treatment. After acute carbamazepine administration in cats, Gigli et al.[291] reported an increase of NREM stage 1 sleep and total sleep time, a decrease of REM sleep, and reduced duration of awakenings. Some

studies examined the effects of carbamazepine in treated versus untreated epileptic patients.[247,255,256] Studies in healthy normal subjects showed that carbamazepine can increase slow-wave sleep, decrease REM sleep, and consolidate sleep.[292–294] In some studies, the EEG effects in epileptics have been contradictory. For example, Legros and Bazil[284] failed to find any EEG effects during sleep in 10 epileptics treated with long-term carbamazepine, but Bell et al.[282] found increased slow-wave sleep and decreased stage 2 NREM sleep with carbamazepine monotherapy.

There have been very limited studies to describe effects of primidone on the sleep EEG. In one study using 30 healthy subjects, a single dose of primidone (250 mg) resulted in an increase of slow-wave sleep and a reduction in REM sleep.[295] Treating epileptic patients with 750 mg primidone daily for 3 months resulted in reduced sleep-onset latency and REM density but not percentage.[296]

The effects of ethosuximide included disrupted sleep, increased sleep latency, increased stage 1 sleep, decreased slow-wave sleep, and increased REM sleep and awakenings.[287,297]

Valproic acid in general has minimal effects on sleep architecture in patients with epilepsy.[281,287–289,298] Findji and Catani[298] reported an improvement of sleep organization and increase of slow-wave sleep in epileptic children after treatment with valproic acid. At higher doses, however, Harding et al.[299] observed a decrease of delta and REM sleep.

The benzodiazepine group of drugs is generally used for status epilepticus (e.g., lorazepam, diazepam, midazolam) but sometimes clonazepam is used in some drug-resistant seizures and certain types of seizures (e.g., myoclonic seizures and Lennox-Gastaut syndrome). These drugs generally cause decreased sleep efficiency, sleep-onset latency, stage 1 NREM and slow-wave sleep, and arousals.[240,281,300]

Newer Antiepileptic Drugs

Several newer AEDs have come onto the market to treat patients with seizure disorders; most of them have been indicated to use as add-on drugs, but some are being used as primary AEDs. These drugs have not been studied extensively to determine their effects on sleep architecture.

Felbamate is one of the earlier drugs in the newer generation but has largely been discontinued because of severe hepatotoxicity. This drug has been reported to cause insomnia in epileptic patients.[276,301]

Gabapentin was originally developed to treat seizure disorder but later was found to be useful in many other conditions, such as neuropathic pain and restless legs syndrome/periodic limb movements in sleep. In healthy subjects, gabapentin increases slow-wave sleep.[296,302,303] Placidi et al.[304] studied the effects of long-term gabapentin treatment on nocturnal sleep in drug-resistant epileptics and observed an increase in slow-wave and REM sleep, and a reduction of arousals and stage 1 NREM sleep.

Lamotrigine has minimal effects on sleep in general.[264,284] Lamotrigine may cause increased REM sleep and decreased slow-wave sleep.[288] Sadler[274] reported insomnia (difficulty initiating and maintaining sleep shortly after administration of the drug) requiring reduction in dosage or discontinuation of the drug in over 6% of 109 patients treated with lamotrigine. This finding, however, was contradicted by Foldvary et al.,[275] who did not find any insomnia in any of 10 adult patients with focal epilepsy on lamotrigine treatment.

Levetiracetam in general has minimal effect on sleep architecture in normal volunteers. Bell et al.[282] studied levetiracetam in normal volunteers and patients with epilepsy in a double-blind, placebo-controlled study. They found increased stage 2 NREM sleep in both epileptics and controls, and increased REM sleep latency only in the healthy subjects and diffuse slow-wave sleep in patients. In a double-blind, crossover, placebo-controlled study in 14 healthy volunteers using PSG and the MSLT after oral administration of levetiracetam up to 2000 mg/day or placebo for 3 weeks, Cicolin et al.[305] found increased total sleep time and sleep efficiency and decreased WASO. MSLT findings did not differ between the two groups. The authors concluded that levetiracetam in healthy volunteers consolidated sleep without causing any daytime sleepiness.

Oxcarbazepine has not been adequately studied but has been noted to cause excessive sleepiness.[259]

Pregabalin is a more recent AED and has been studied in a limited manner. Hindmarch et al.[306] studied 24 healthy volunteers and measured sleep objectively using PSG and subjectively using a questionnaire. Compared with the placebo, pregabalin significantly increased slow-wave sleep and reduced sleep-onset latency and REM sleep percentage. Subjective evaluation showed significant improvement in sleep quality, but ratings of behavior following awakening were impaired.

Tiagabine, a selective GABA reuptake inhibitor, has been used for partial and secondary generalized seizures. In healthy elderly subjects, tiagabine significantly increased slow-wave sleep and sleep efficiency.[307,308] In patients with primary insomnia, tiagabine increased slow-wave sleep and reduced WASO in a dose-dependent manner.[309,310]

Topiramate, tiagabine, zonisamide and vigabatrin, which are used in some partial secondary generalized seizures, especially in those not responding to other AEDs, have not been adequately tested to study the effects of these drugs on sleep architecture in epileptic patients. Bonanni et al.,[283] following topiramate monotherapy in an open-label trial with 14 epileptics, found no difference in sleep architecture and daytime sleepiness as measured objectively by multiple sleep latency testing. Bonanni et al.[311] studied the effects of carbamazepine and vigabatrin on daytime sleepiness in patients with partial epilepsy by measuring with MSLT and overnight PSG. The results suggested that vigabatrin did not significantly affect sleep architecture in their patients with epilepsy. Vigabatrin treatment in medically refractory epilepsy, however, causes weight gain, making these patients susceptible to developing OSAS.[312]

Nonpharmacologic Treatment

Vagus nerve stimulation has been used with some success in patients with refractory or intractable seizure disorder. However, in addition to improving the seizure state and daytime alertness, vagus nerve stimulation caused OSA in some patients.[313–315]

Summary

A survey of the literature thus reveals that we need more studies to understand the interactions among anticonvulsants, sleep, and epilepsy. Based on the literature and their own investigations, Declerck and Wauquier[281] emphasized the importance of the use and development of automatic methods to assess antiepileptic-induced sleep changes in patients with epilepsy. It may be that the anticonvulsants disrupt the circadian distribution of interictal discharges during the night, and this may have practical relevance in terms of treatment.

SLEEP, EPILEPSY, AND AUTONOMIC DYSFUNCTION

There are a number of autonomic nervous system (ANS) changes, particularly involving the respiratory and cardiovascular systems, during sleep[316] (see also Chapter 7). Furthermore, epilepsy itself may cause changes in the ANS, and thus there is a close interrelationship between sleep, epilepsy, and the ANS.

ANS changes involving the cardiovascular system during sleep consist of reduction of blood pressure and heart rate during NREM sleep and wide fluctuation of these during REM sleep.[316] Respiration shows considerable changes during NREM and in particular during REM sleep (see Chapter 7). Sleep adversely affects breathing, even in normal individuals, and often triggers seizures in epileptic patients. Knowledge of the central autonomic network makes it easy to understand why this relationship between ANS, sleep, circulation, and respiration exists.[317] The nucleus tractus solitarius, a structure in the region of the medulla important for sleep and for cardiovascular and respiratory regulation, is reciprocally connected with the limbic-hypothalamic and other forebrain structures[317] (see also Chapter 7). This connection explains why epileptic seizures triggered by the limbic-hypothalamic or other forebrain structures may interact with the cardiovascular and respiratory regulation during sleep. Respiratory dysrhythmia during generalized seizures, after seizure discharges in the limbic system, and after experimental stimulation of the limbic areas is documented.[318] The coexistence of sleep apnea and epilepsy, once thought to be rare, is increasingly recognized (see later).

It is well known that, in generalized tonic-clonic seizures and CPS, transient abnormalities of ANS functions may occur and may consist of alterations in cardiac rhythm, blood pressure, and respiration.[319] In addition, it is well known that epileptiform discharges without any clinical accompaniments may produce a variety of autonomic abnormalities. In patients after electroconvulsive[320] treatment and in animal models after pentylenetetrazol injection,[321] there are intense changes in blood pressure and cardiac rhythms. Similar changes have been observed in patients with focal temporal lobe discharges. Furthermore, the phenomenon of unexpected sudden death in patients with epilepsy[322,323] may account for up to 15% of deaths in epileptic patients and may be the result of some unexplained autonomic dysfunction affecting the cardiac rhythm.

EPILEPSY AND SLEEP APNEA

The association of epilepsy and sleep apnea was once thought to be a rare combination; however, in 1981 Wyler and Weymuller[324] described a 26-year-old man with medically intractable CPS and upper airway OSA, whose seizure control improved after treatment of sleep apnea with tracheostomy. Since then, sleep apnea has been increasingly recognized as a comorbid condition of patients with epilepsy. Sleep, epilepsy, and breathing are all interrelated. Both sleep and seizures may adversely affect breathing, and disordered breathing during sleep may in turn adversely affect seizures. Also, while the cause of sudden unexpected death in epilepsy is not definitely known, it has been suggested that the combination of postictal central apnea and neurogenic pulmonary edema may be responsible.[325] There is sufficient theoretical justification for why epilepsy and sleep apnea may coexist. Sleep adversely affects breathing even in normal individuals; for example, sleep is associated with increased upper airway resistance, mild alveolar hypoventilation, mild hypoxemia and hypercapnia, impaired central chemosensitivity with decreased hypoxic and hypercapnic ventilatory responses, and decreased number of functioning medullary respiratory neurons (see Chapter 7). These adverse effects may cause sleep apnea or sleep-disordered breathing (SDB) in susceptible individuals such as patients with seizures. It is well known that sleep and sleep deprivation may trigger seizures in patients at risk.

There is clinical and experimental evidence to suggest that generalized seizures as well as seizure discharges in the limbic-hypothalamic system may cause SDB.[317,318] Reciprocal connections between central respiratory neurons in the medulla (in the region of nucleus tractus solitarius) and the limbic-hypothalamic and other forebrain structures may explain why epileptic seizures triggered during sleep by the discharges in the limbic-hypothalamic and orbitofrontal regions may interfere with respiratory regulation, causing SDB.[317] Experimental stimulation in animals in the limbic area, including the orbitofrontal cortex, may cause respiratory dysrhythmia.[318] Stimulation of the limbic areas in humans, including that during depth recording, may cause SDB.[318] Furthermore, severe hypoxemia during prolonged seizure or status epilepticus may cause SDB. It should also be remembered that apnea causing severe hypoxemia may trigger seizures in susceptible individuals during prolonged apnea. Sleep apnea, in most cases, however, does not trigger seizures in those who do not have a propensity toward epilepsy. Recurrent apneas during the night in patients with sleep apnea syndrome cause sleep fragmentation and sleep deprivation, which may trigger seizures in susceptible individuals. Other factors that may trigger seizures associated with sleep apnea include decreased cerebral blood flow in epileptics due to cardiac arrhythmias and decreased cardiac output. Some other factors contributing to sleep apnea in seizure patients include weight gain related to AEDs (e.g., valproate, carbamazepine, grabapentine, pregabalin, vigabatrin),[286,312,326] alteration of upper airway muscle tone by AEDs, or endocrine disorders caused by AEDs.

The frequently quoted figure for the prevalence of sleep apnea from the Wisconsin Cohort study by Young et al.[327] is 4% in men and 2% in women. An estimated prevalence of epilepsy in the general population is approximately 1%.[328] Therefore, by chance association some patients may have both sleep apnea and epilepsy. A perusal of the literature reveals a few scattered case reports and letters to the editor to document the coexistence of sleep apnea and epilepsy. Wyler and Weymuller[324] were the first to document improvement of both sleep apnea and seizures after tracheostomy treatment for OSAS. Daytime PSG recordings by Chokroverty et al.[329] documented obstructive, mixed, and central apneas in eight patients with partial complex seizures with secondary generalization. In a retrospective survey from a tertiary care sleep medicine division, we reported a prevalence of approximately 6% of sleep apnea in epileptics.[330] This survey almost certainly underestimated the prevalence of seizure in sleep apnea patients, because the diagnosis was made on the basis of questionnaire only and not by direct interview. Many patients did not answer all relevant questions. Our survey, however, is somewhat similar to the retrospective survey by Sonka et al.[331] that included 480 adult patients with sleep apnea syndrome, 19 of whom (4%) had a history of seizures. Devinsky et al.[332] reported an improvement in seizure frequency and severity in six of seven patients with refractory partial epilepsy and sleep apnea after treatment. Vaughn et al.[333] identified 10 patients with recurrent seizures and OSA. Following continuous positive airway pressure (CPAP) and positional therapy, there was considerable reduction of seizure frequency. Koh et al.[334] reported improvement of seizure control after treatment of sleep apnea in children with neurodevelopmental disorders and intractable epilepsy. Malow and collaborators[335] documented OSA in one-third of 39 patients with medically refractory epilepsy undergoing PSG prior to epilepsy surgery. They concluded that sleep apnea is common among men, older subjects, and those with nocturnal seizures.

In a retrospective review of 63 adult epilepsy patients who had PSGs, Malow and colleagues[336] identified 45 (71%) with obstructive sleep apnea. Twenty-eight patients with OSA were treated with CPAP, and most reported improvement in seizure control. Subsequent studies by Malow and collaborators[326,337] confirmed this improvement of OSA in epileptics after CPAP therapy. Chihorek et al.[326] provided evidence that OSA is a risk factor for epilepsy in older adults and its treatment by CPAP may improve seizure control in this population. The limitation of this study is the small number of patients in each group (11 with late-onset or worsening seizures and 10 seizure-free individuals over the age of 50 years), but this is an important study that should encourage larger prospective studies in the future documenting increasing association of OSA with epilepsy and the effect of treating OSA. In a more recent study, Malow and colleagues[337] randomized 22 adult subjects with medically refractory epilepsy and coexisting OSA to therapeutic CPAP therapy and 13 similar subjects to sham CPAP. Based on their observations of a significant reduction of the apnea-hypopnea index in the therapeutic group as compared to the sham group, the authors concluded that this pilot study provided valuable information for designing a comprehensive trial to test the hypothesis that treating OSA in epileptics would improve seizure control. The literature survey thus gives a high prevalence of sleep apnea in epilepsy and documented improvement of seizure control following effective treatment of sleep apnea.[270,326,337–342]

UTILITY OF SLEEP IN THE DIAGNOSIS OF EPILEPSY

Utility of sleep in the diagnosis of epilepsy was well established after the landmark paper by Gibbs and Gibbs[12] in 1947 showing activation of epileptiform discharges in the sleep EEG. For the diagnosis of epilepsy, the following sleep recordings are recommended: (1) a standard sleep EEG recording, (2) an EEG recording after sleep deprivation, (3) an all-night PSG study, (4) a video-PSG study, (5) an MSLT, and (6) a 24-hour ambulatory EEG and sleep recording. Table 30–12 outlines a suggested protocol for EEG recording in patients suspected to have epilepsy.

Sleep EEG Recording and Sleep Deprivation Study

The usefulness of sleep EEG recording and sleep deprivation is discussed in detail in the previous paragraphs. For such recordings, a full complement of electrodes should be used and various montages have been suggested (see Chapter 11). Broughton[19] listed some of the main indications and objectives of the daytime sleep EEG recording as follows: (1) normal EEGs in patients suspected of epilepsy to establish the diagnosis of true epilepsy; (2) normal waking EEGs in patients with known epilepsy to clarify the type of epilepsy; (3) patients with febrile convulsions showing normal waking EEGs; (4) assessment of the familial predisposition to epilepsy in family members; and (5) assessment of the degree of drug control, for example, in patients with hypsarrhythmia.

Interictal EEG findings can help in the confirmation of the diagnosis of epilepsy, in the classification of seizures, and in identification of specific epileptic syndromes. Epilepsy is a clinical diagnosis, and a single

---

TABLE 30–12 Suggested Protocol for Electroencephalography Recording in Patients Suspected of Epilepsy

1. Routine EEG recording with hyperventilation and photic stimulation.
2. If negative for interictal epileptiform activity (IEA), EEG with sleep (natural or induced) recording.
3. If negative for IEA, EEG study with partial (at least 4 hr) or total (24 hr) sleep deprivation.
4. If negative for IEA after three to four EEGs, prolonged (4- to 6-hr) daytime EEG with sleep recording.
5. If negative for IEA, overnight polysomnographic (PSG) study, preferably video-PSG study for electroclinical correlation. Change the monitor speed to 30 mm/sec instead of the usual sleep recording speed of 10 mm/sec during interpretation of the recording. Use appropriately devised seizure montage with full complement of electrodes (see Chapter 11) or special electrode placements (e.g., T1 and T2 electrodes).
6. If still negative for IEA, cassette ambulatory 24-hour EEG recording.
7. If still negative for IEA, long-term video-EEG monitoring for 24–72 hr or longer if necessary.
8. Finally, in some patients, invasive intracranial EEG monitoring using subdural grids, strips, or depth electrodes may be necessary for localizing and lateralizing a focus.

normal EEG in a patient with suspected epilepsy does not exclude the diagnosis of true epilepsy. The reason for a normal EEG in such a patient may be a sampling problem or the fact that the epileptic foci are located in a deeper brain region (e.g., oribitofrontal and medial interhemispheric region). Surface electrodes may not pick up these discharges located in a deeper site. A third reason may be that the EEG recording was obtained without the benefit of sleep or sleep deprivation. In such patients, the protocol suggested in Table 30–12 should be followed. The EEG findings may help in the classification of seizures. Bilateral synchronous spikes or spike-and-wave complexes in the interictal EEGs suggest primary generalized epilepsy. Particular characteristics of generalized epileptiform discharges may help in diagnosing certain epileptic syndromes (e.g., slow spike-and-wave discharges seen synchronously and symmetrically in the Lennox-Gastaut syndrome; multiple transient spike-and-wave discharges in JME); focal spikes present consistently in one location may correlate with partial epilepsy.

All-Night Polysomnographic Recording

Broughton[19] listed the following important indications to perform all-night PSG study:

1. To differentiate between epileptic and nonepileptic nocturnal events (e.g., pseudoseizures, syncope due to cardiac arrhythmias, parasomnias)
2. To clarify the classification in patients with known sleep epilepsies
3. To diagnose CSWS
4. To diagnose benign epilepsy of childhood with rolandic spikes
5. To lateralize or localize the principal focus during REM sleep by use of stereo-EEG (this may be important before surgical treatment is considered)
6. To unmask the primary focus in a patient with secondary bilateral synchrony during REM sleep by causing suppression of the generalized discharges
7. To reveal abnormalities in patients with hypsarrhythmia, for whom waking EEGs rarely may be normal but sleep EEGs may, and to clarify focal abnormalities in such patients
8. To diagnose tonic seizures in patients with Lennox-Gastaut syndrome
9. To diagnose sleep apnea or other primary sleep disorders, which may be mistaken for or associated with epilepsy
10. To investigate patients complaining of excessive daytime somnolence that cannot be explained by their anticonvulsant medication

Two additional indications are (1) to document cardiac arrhythmias that may arise during sleep and may be confused with, or even give rise to, seizures; and (2) to document sleep disturbances and sleep architecture in epileptics so that these disturbances may be treated to prevent chronic sleep deprivation, which may in turn have deleterious effects on epilepsy itself. In suspected seizure disorders, all-night PSG recording should include multiple EEG leads and special montages (see Chapter 11). Figure 30–10 is a representative sample showing upper airway OSA in a patient with CPS and sleep apnea.

Video-Polysomnographic Study

The value of video-PSG for the diagnosis of parasomnias and seizure disorders has been well documented by Aldrich and Jahnke[343] (see also Chapter 19). Figure 30–11 is a PSG showing the onset of a partial seizure recorded at 10 mm/sec and 30 mm/sec paper speed.

Multiple Sleep Latency Test

The MSLT[344] is indicated in patients complaining of EDS that is not explained on the basis of anticonvulsant medication. Seizure during sleep may lead to repeated arousals, causing EDS with further increase of seizure frequency, thus creating a vicious cycle. Sometimes narcolepsy may be mistaken for epilepsy, and an important diagnostic test for narcolepsy is the MSLT. Finally, as discussed earlier, patients with epilepsy may have sleep apnea, which can be diagnosed by showing reduced sleep-onset latency on the MSLT that is causing EDS.

Ambulatory 24-Hour EEG Recording and Sleep Scoring

Ambulatory 24-hour EEG recording and sleep scoring allow for recording of the EEG discharges throughout the day to understand the circadian and ultradian rhythmicity and the effects of sleep on the interictal discharges. The question of whether epilepsy manifests biorhythmicity was discussed earlier. Technical problems associated with unattended recordings, however, are serious limitations. Ambulatory EEG recording permits 24 hours of continuous recording of the patient's normal day-to-day environment. This type of recording is very valuable in documenting interictal epileptiform discharges in the presence of normal routine EEGs. The presence of movement and muscle artifacts and lack of video documentation of the behavior are distinct disadvantages of ambulatory recording.

Long-Term Video-EEG Monitoring

In some patients, simultaneous video and EEG monitoring in the inpatient unit for several days is necessary to document an ictal epileptiform discharge and its characteristic behavioral correlate, thus providing indisputable evidence of a true seizure episode. Documentation of an ictal epileptiform discharge during long-term video-EEG monitoring

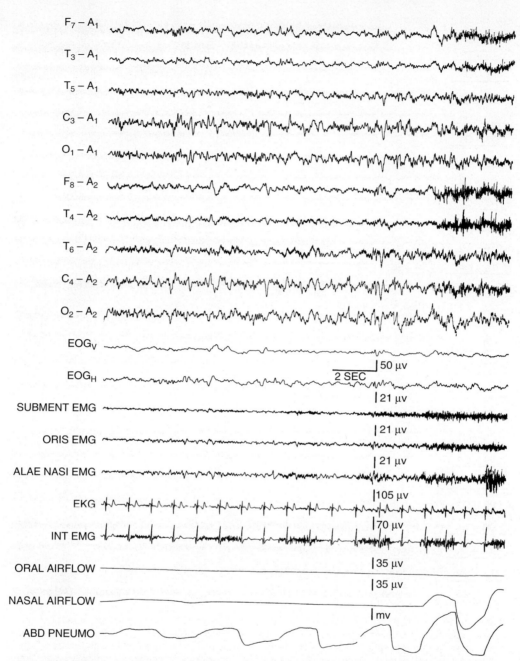

FIGURE 30–10 Polysomnographic recording in a patient with partial complex seizure and sleep apnea showing EEG (top 10 channels); vertical (EOG$_V$) and horizontal (EOG$_H$) electro-oculograms; submental (SUBMENT), orbicularis oris (ORIS), alae nasi, and intercostal (INT) electromyograms (EMG); electrocardiogram (EKG); oral and nasal airflow; and abdominal pneumogram (ABD PNEUMO). Note upper airway obstructive apnea during NREM stage 2 sleep. No epileptiform discharges are seen in the EEG during the episodes. Paper speed is 15 mm/sec.

permits unambiguous evidence of the presence of true seizure. Persistent normal background EEG activity (alpha rhythm in an adult) and absence of postictal slowing after an apparent seizure episode are inconsistent with a diagnosis of true seizure.

Intracranial Recordings

If the results of EEG, including long-term monitoring and neuroimaging (see later), are discordant in localizing the focus, patients should be referred to a specialized epilepsy center for intercranial recordings. Recommended procedures include stereotactically implanted depth electrodes and subdural strips or grids recording from the surface of the cerebral cortex. For a suspected neocortical focus (based on the patient's ictal spells), subdural electrodes are preferred, whereas for a suspected limbic focus, depth recording is the recommended procedure.

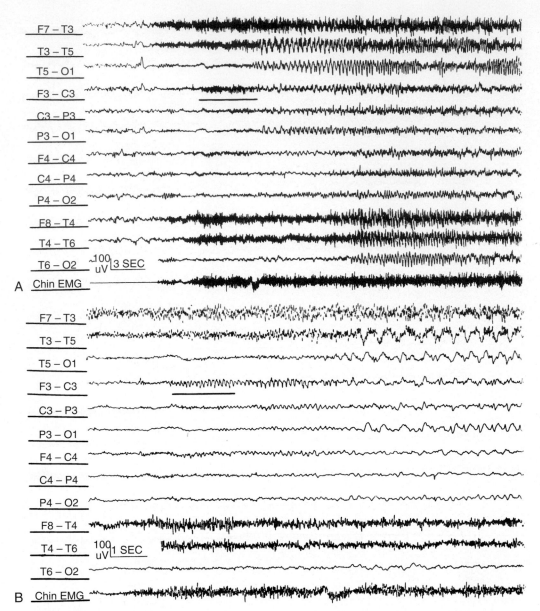

FIGURE 30-11 A portion of a PSG recording using 12 channels of EEG showing the onset of a partial seizure recorded at 10 mm/sec paper speed. The *underlined* activity represents rhythmic ictal discharges beginning over the left hemisphere (F3-C3) and spreading rapidly to the right hemisphere, and is accompanied by clinical seizure. Although at 10 mm/sec paper speed **(A)** the underlined activity superficially resembles muscle artifacts, at 30 mm/sec paper speed **(B)** it becomes obvious that this activity is the beginning of the rhythmic epileptiform discharges in the EEG. *(Reproduced with permission from Aldrich M, Jahnke B. Diagnostic value of video-EEG polysomnography. Neurology 1991;41:1060.)*

NEUROIMAGING

Neuroimaging studies are indispensable in investigating the presence of structural lesions that may serve as epileptogenic foci. Anatomic studies (computed tomography and magnetic resonance imaging) are usually performed in all adults with new-onset seizures and in children without any characteristic epileptic syndromes to identify any structural brain disorders. Specialty magnetic resonance imaging of the brain is more sensitive than computed tomography, and that is the preferred procedure.

Functional or physiologic studies (single-photon emission computed tomography and positron emission tomography) may be able to identify seizure foci by revealing areas of cerebral hypermetabolism or hyperperfusion during an ictal episode and areas of hypometabolism during the interictal period.

PRACTICAL RELEVANCE TO UNDERSTANDING THE RELATIONSHIP BETWEEN SLEEP AND EPILEPSY

An understanding of the relationship between sleep and epilepsy is important for three main purposes:

1. Such an understanding can aid in the diagnosis of seizure and in differential diagnosis between epileptic and nonepileptic events and among different types of seizures.
2. An understanding of this relationship can increase the understanding of the pathogenesis of triggering mechanisms of seizures during sleep and the mechanism and nature of sleep disturbances induced by epilepsy.
3. Therapeutic manipulation can be guided by the knowledge obtained through an understanding of the relationship between epilepsy and sleep. It may be possible to adjust the timing of the drug dose, but this really has not been useful from a practical point of view. An understanding of the biorhythmicity and the relationship between sleep and epilepsy may be important to choosing the type of anticonvulsant, so that one may avoid those with marked hypnotic effects in nocturnal seizure patients and use drugs with less sedative effects (e.g., carbamazepine, valproic acid, lamotrigine). Finally, one may manipulate sleep stages—that is, give anticonvulsants that may increase REM or NREM stages 3 and 4—to reduce the ictal or interictal discharges.

Finally, as Broughton[19] stated, it may be necessary to put some patients on a strict program of sleep hygiene (see Table 19–17 in Chapter 19) or to treat the sleep disorders with pharmacologic agents because of the deleterious effects the epilepsy has on sleep and sleep on epilepsy. Such patients may be advised to avoid sleep deprivation, alcohol in the evening, and late evening exercise, and to maintain regular sleep and waking hours. Broughton[19] suggested that the improvement of nocturnal sleep after such a regimen may be associated with definite reduction of seizure frequency and overall improvement in general well-being.

☯ REFERENCES

A full list of references are available at www.expertconsult.com

CHAPTER 31

Dreaming in Neurologic Disorders

Mark Solms and **Susan Malcolm-Smith**

BACKGROUND

Historically, there has been little systematic investigation of changes in dreaming due to neurologic damage, despite numerous clinical reports of marked abnormalities. Accordingly, the subject remains poorly understood. This reflects the lack of development in the field of dream research itself: an understanding of the brain mechanisms of dreaming has lagged behind that of other mental functions. There are two main reasons for this. First, unlike most mental functions that were the focus of 19th- and 20th-century behavioral neuroscience, dreaming is almost entirely subjective. The observable data are retrospective, single-witness qualitative descriptions, only indirectly related to the phenomenon of dreaming itself. This poses special methodologic problems.

The second reason for the undeveloped state of this field is closely related to the first. Researchers seeking an objective approach to dreaming eagerly alighted on a physiologic state that correlates closely with it: rapid eye movement (REM) sleep.[1–4] This physiologic state was then conflated with dreaming itself, resulting in the development of neuropsychological models of dreaming that were in fact models of REM sleep (e.g., Hobson and McCarley[5]). This conflation was confounded by the fact that the models were empirically grounded in animal studies (where dream reports are of course precluded) rather than human lesion studies of the kind that informed models of most other mental functions. When the conventional human lesion studies were belatedly performed, it became apparent that dreaming and REM sleep are in fact doubly dissociable states.[6]

A traditional neuropsychology or behavioral neurology grounded in the systematic application of clinico-anatomic correlation—which has been widely applied to other mental functions since the mid–19th century—is little more than 20 years old in the case of dreaming. Incidental reports of changes in dreaming associated with focal cerebral damage did neverthelsess accumulate in the literature over a long period, albeit without any attempt to synthesize the scattered observations into a coherent picture. Systematic clinico-anatomic group studies were first published in the 1980s,[7–9] but the available evidence was not comprehensively reviewed before the 1990s.[10–12] The clinico-anatomic studies have since been complemented by a slew of functional brain imaging studies, with strongly convergent findings.[13] Rigorous pharmacologic probes of the neurochemistry of dreaming (as opposed to REM sleep) have not yet been conducted.[14]

An understanding of the brain mechanisms of dreaming is now beginning to emerge. Systematic observation of abnormalities of dreaming in neurologic disease has contributed fundamentally to this emerging picture. The bewildering array of abnormalities may perhaps best be grouped under two headings: (1) deficits of dreaming and (2) excesses of dreaming.

DEFICITS OF DREAMING

The earliest clinical observations of changes in dreaming with neurologic disease concerned *cessation* of dreaming (or cessation of aspects of dreaming). The terms *Charcot-Wilbrand syndrome* and *anoneira* have been used to describe this abnormality, which is typically (but not exclusively) seen in the acute phase of focal neurologic pathology.

Charcot-Wilbrand Syndrome

The concept of this syndrome, based on two case reports by Charcot[15,16] and Wilbrand,[17,18] was first articulated by Pötzl,[19] who defined the syndrome as "mind-blindness with disturbance of optic imagination" (p. 306). Nielsen[20] defined it as "visual agnosia plus loss of the ability to revisualise" (p. 74). Critchley's widely cited definition[21] was: "a patient loses the power to conjure up visual images or memories, and furthermore, ceases to dream during his sleeping hours" (p. 311).

Critchley described prosopagnosia and topographic agnosia or amnesia as associated features. The localization of the lesion producing this syndrome was never precisely defined, but the occipital cortex (especially area 19) was implicated by most early authors—usually bilaterally. The Charcot-Wilbrand syndrome remained in late 20th century nosographic usage, although the condition was (until recently) considered rare. A modern definition of the syndrome reads: "the association of loss of the ability to conjure up visual images or memories and the loss of dreaming . . . [indicating] a lesion in an acute phase affecting the posterior regions" (Murri et al.,[8] p. 185).

Deficient revisualization (called "irreminiscence" in the nomenclature of Nielsen[20]) was the fundamental deficit in almost all definitions of the syndrome. Cessation of dreaming ("or at least, an alteration in the vivid visual component of the dreaming state" [Critchley,[21] p. 311]) was seen as a secondary consequence of the visual imagery deficit. The associated visual agnosias, too, were originally considered to be caused by defective revisualization, since visual agnosia was classically understood as a loss of "visual memory images."[22,23]

Subsequent advances in the agnosia concept, and a misreading of the original case reports, have resulted in considerable nosologic confusion regarding this syndrome.[12,24] It is widely assumed that Wilbrand's case—an elderly female patient with bilateral posterior cerebral artery thrombosis—could not *visualize* familiar places.[20,21,25,26] However, the original report stated only that she was unable to *recognize* familiar places. This symptom (which we would today call topographic *agnosia*) was conceptualized, in accordance with classical theory, as a disorder of "topographical *memory*" (Wilbrand,[17] p. 52 [emphasis added]). This conceptualization was then misconstrued by secondary authors as a disorder of topographic *revisualization*. The original report reveals that Wilbrand's case actually lacked the cardinal feature of the so-called Charcot-Wilbrand syndrome. As the patient herself clearly stated: "With my eyes shut I see my old Hamburg in front of me again" (Wilbrand,[17] p. 56). Charcot's case—also a probable posterior cerebral artery thrombosis (autopsy findings were lacking)—was quite different. He described a striking absence of visual mental imagery. The Charcot-Wilbrand syndrome is therefore misnamed.

It is also misconceived. Charcot's patient ceased to dream in visual images, but he continued to dream in words. Wilbrand's patient, in contrast, dreamed "almost not at all anymore" (Wilbrand,[17] p. 54). The original report is ambiguous as to whether Wilbrand's patient merely dreamed infrequently or actually lost the capacity to dream completely (and then gradually recovered it); either way, there is no question of an isolated loss of *visual* dream imagery, which is what Charcot's patient unequivocally described. The "Charcot-Wilbrand syndrome" therefore appears to be two different (but related) syndromes, one characterized by loss of *visual* dream imagery and the other by *global* cessation or suppression of dreaming. This distinction is supported by a review of the world literature.[12]

Charcot's Variant: Isolated Loss of Visual Dream Imagery

At least 10 case reports of isolated loss of visual dream imagery have been published, together with five further reports of patients who experienced deficits of specific *aspects* of visual dream imagery (e.g., color, movement, faces). Cessation of visual imagery or aspects thereof results from various pathologies, usually of acute onset (thrombosis, hemorrhage, trauma, carbon monoxide poisoning), but it has also been described in cases of neoplasm, probable Alzheimer's disease, callosal dysgenesis, and Turner's syndrome. The lesion is typically localized to the mesial occipitotemporal or lateral occipitoparietal regions, and is usually bilateral, but precise localizing information is often lacking.[12,15,26–41]

Defective revisualization (irreminiscence) is a constant feature in these cases, although it is typically restricted to the disordered aspect of vision (e.g., color, movement, faces) in cases in which the loss of visual dream imagery is partial. This strongly suggests a common underlying image-generation deficit causing the same disorder in both waking and dreaming cognition. Various forms of visual agnosia are commonly associated features, but agnosia is definitely absent in some cases and therefore cannot be considered integral to the syndrome.[12]

Most published reports of deficits in visual dream imagery derive from retrospective accounts in a clinical setting. However, the reports have been confirmed directly upon REM awakening in at least three cases.[32,33,35]

Negative Findings

Interestingly, modality-specific deficits of dream imagery outside the higher visual sphere have never been demonstrated. Thus although achromatopsic, akinetopsic, prosopagnosic, and hemineglect disorders are duplicated in dreams, cortically blind and hemianopic patients invariably report normal vision (full fields) in their dreams. Moreover, hemiplegic patients experience normal somatomotor and somatosensory functions in their dream imagery (as do acute-phase paraplegic and quadriplegic patients). The same applies to the extrapyramidal movement disorders. Similarly, nonfluent aphasics claim to speak normally in their dreams.[12]

Of related interest, perhaps, is the fact that the dreams of patients with substantial impairments of executive function due to dorsolateral prefrontal lesions are indistinguishable from the dreams of controls (Badenhorst and Solms, 2007, unpublished paper). These findings point to a differentiated network of forebrain structures involved in dream cognition.

Wilbrand's Variant: Global Loss or Suppression of Dreaming

At least 106 cases of global loss or suppression of dreaming have been reported, excluding leucotomy cases, which are discussed separately later (see Solms[12] for a full listing of these cases). A larger number of cases in group studies, for which individual case data were lacking and in which "not dreaming" was defined in variable ways,[7–9] have also been reported.

As with Charcot's variant, global anoneira is typically—but not invariably—associated with acute-onset, focal cerebral lesions (thrombosis, hemorrhage, and trauma are the most commonly reported pathologies). The first systematic attempt to identify the lesion site responsible for global cessation of dreaming pointed to the inferior parietal lobule.[12] Unilateral lesions of either hemisphere were shown to be commonplace, with no lateralizing bias. However, at least two cases have since been reported in which the parietal lobe was unequivocally spared,[42,43] as indeed it appears to have been in Wilbrand's original case.[18] A reanalysis of Solms' data by Yu[44] revealed that the lesions in his parietal cases almost always extended into adjacent occipitotemporal tissues (especially Brodmann areas 22, 19, and 37). It is therefore still not possible to make a more precise localizing statement than the one offered by Murri et al.[8]: "a lesion in an acute phase affecting the posterior regions" (p. 185). The reference to an *acute phase* is not superfluous. Solms[12] observed that almost all cases of global anoneira recover the capacity to dream within 12 months. This fact, which suggests diaschetic effects, may help explain the imprecise localization of the causal lesion.

Of particular clinical interest is Solms' observation that hydrocephalus is associated with cessation of dreaming, which recovers after successful VP shunting.[12] Cessation of dreaming might therefore be used as an indicator of shunt malfunction.

Defective revisualisation (irreminiscence) is a common but by no means essential feature of these cases. It was overrepresented in the earlier case reports for the probable reason that patients were only asked about their dreams once irreminiscence had been established. The more recent cases reported by Solms[12] were part of an unselected clinical series and are therefore more likely to be representative. Global cessation of dreaming (unlike visually deficient dreaming) therefore cannot be reduced to irreminiscence.

Not surprisingly, considering the lesion site, global anoneira is frequently associated with disorders of spatial cognition, including visuospatial short-term memory.[12] The lack of association between cessation of dreaming and *long-term* memory disorder of any kind excludes the possibility that cessation of dreaming is really a memory disorder—failure to remember dreams as opposed to cessation of dreaming per se.[45–47] This applies also to the various language disorders that were previously thought to explain loss of dreaming.[10,48–51] In his systematic survey, Solms found no relationship between language disorder of any kind and reported cessation of dreaming.[12]

Retrospective reports of absence of dreaming on morning awakening has repeatedly been confirmed by the REM sleep awakening method.[42,43,52,53] This further supports the assumption that this disorder concerns cessation of dreaming per se, as opposed to loss of memory for dreams. Even severe amnesies with bilateral hippocampal lesions report dreams on awakening from REM sleep and at sleep onset[54,55] (V.S. Ramachandran, personal communication, 2004).

Cessation or Suppression of Dreaming Following Prefrontal Leucotomy

In a survey of 200 cases of prefrontal leucotomy, Frank[56] observed that a common result of the procedure was "a poverty or entire lack of dreams" (p. 508). In a later report on the same series of cases, then comprising more than 300 patients, he confirmed this finding.[57] Replication of Frank's observations was forthcoming from other authors[26,58–61] (Slater, cited in Humphreys and Zangwill[62]). Moreover, Jus et al.[58] confirmed the absence of dream reports following prefrontal leucotomy by the REM sleep awakening method.

In apparent contradiction to these reports, however, Humphrey and Zangwill,[62] Cathala et al.,[7] Murri et al.,[8,9] and Doricchi and Violani[10] all observed a relatively *low* incidence of cessation of dreaming with anterior versus posterior cerebral lesions. The same applies to the observation noted previously to the effect that the dreams of frontal convexity patients are indistinguishable from those of controls (Badenhorst and Solms, 2007, unpublished paper). This apparent contradiction was resolved when Solms reviewed the lesions in the previously reported cases and described nine new cases with cessation of dreaming following naturally occurring bifrontal lesions.[12] His conclusion was that dreaming was entirely spared with *dorsolateral*

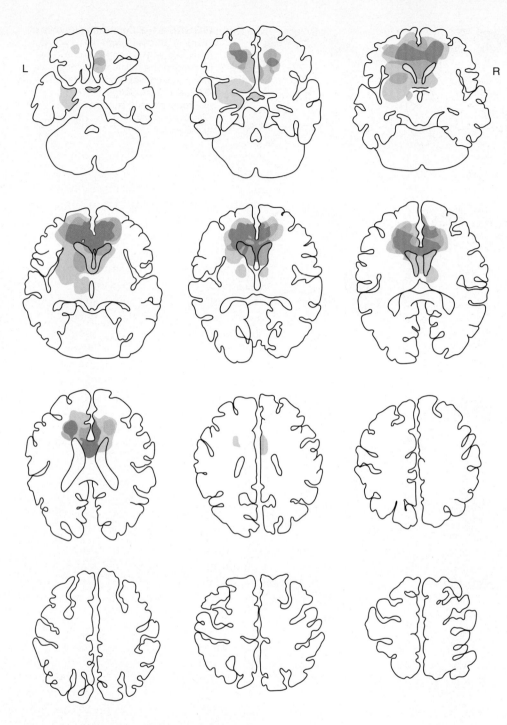

FIGURE 31–1 Combined facsimile of scans in nine cases with global cessation of dreaming caused by deep frontal lesion, illustrating the strong involvement of the white matter surrounding the frontal horns of the lateral ventricles. *(Modified from Solms M. The Neuropsychology of Dreams: A Clinico-anatomical Study. Hillsdale, NJ: Erlbaum, 1997.)*

prefrontal cortical lesions, and affected only with *deep* white-matter lesions in the ventromesial quadrant of the frontal lobes (Figs. 31–1 and 31–2). The lesion site in his nine cases coincided exactly with the area that was targeted by prefrontal leucotomy[63]: "a circumscribed lesion just anterior to the frontal horns of the ventricle, in the lower medial quadrant of the frontal lobes" (p. 177). A reanalysis of the original data in 35 cases from Solms' series with global cessation of dreaming associated with subcortical lesions revealed that the lesion was located in either the deep frontal white matter (areas F09 and F14 in the classification of Damasio and Damasio[64]) (Fig. 31–3), or the head of the caudate nucleus, or both.[65] The lesion is typically bilateral. Of theoretical importance is the fact that the region defined as the "head of the caudate nucleus" in this study included the nucleus accumbens (which is situated immediately beneath it).

It is noteworthy that the psychotropic medications that replaced prefrontal leucotomy as the treatment of choice for psychotic disorders block dopamine (DA) transmission in a mesial forebrain pathway that projects primarily to the nucleus accumbens. Probably related to this is the

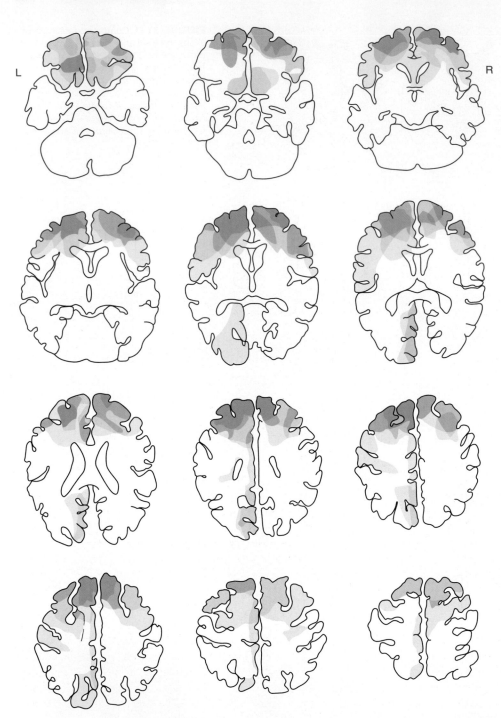

FIGURE 31–2 Combined facsimile of scans in 14 cases with preserved dreaming with bifrontal lesions, illustrating the relative preponderance of cortical convexity involvement. *(Modified from Solms M. The Neuropsychology of Dreams: A Clinico-anatomical Study. Hillsdale, NJ: Erlbaum, 1997.)*

observation that both prefrontal leucotomy in general and cessation of dreaming in particular, due to lesions in this general area, are associated with reduced motivational incentive,[12] as indeed are most antipsychotic medications.[66] Also of interest in this connection is the observation by Piehler[60] and Schindler[61] to the effect that early recovery of dreaming after prefrontal leucotomy typically coincided with psychiatric relapse, suggesting that absence of

dreaming could serve as an index of the clinical success of the operation. Dreaming is, after all, a psychotic state.

Effects of Pontine Brain Stem Lesions

Cessation of dreaming following circumscribed pontine lesions—with or without cessation of REM sleep—has never been demonstrated (see Solms[6,12] for reviews), despite the longstanding assumption that dreaming is

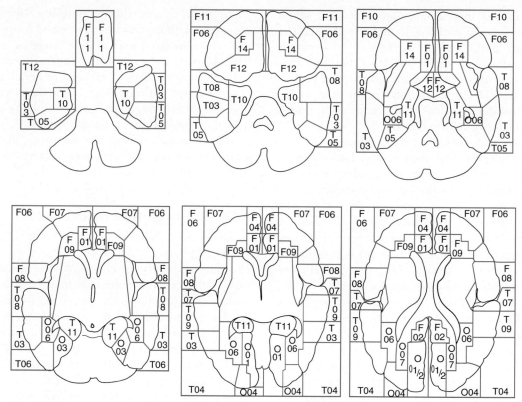

FIGURE 31–3 The subdivision of frontal subcortical areas (after Damasio and Damasio), showing areas F09 and F14. *(Modified from Damasio H, Damasio A. Lesion Analysis in Neuropsychology. New York: Oxford University Press, 1989.)*

caused by—if not identical with—the cyclical, spontaneous activation of acetylcholinergic (ACh) cells in the mesopontine tegmentum during the REM state, together with reciprocal inhibition of serotonergic (5-HT) and noradrenergic cells in the dorsal raphe and locus ceruleus complex.[67,68] Consciousness in general is of course frequently compromised by pontine lesions, but at least eight cases with cessation or near-cessation of REM sleep have been reported in which patients were capable of communicating meaningfully about their dreams.[69-72] Indeed, one such patient did actually report loss of dreaming,[69] but the lesion—caused by a ruptured traumatic aneurysm of the basilar artery—almost certainly extended beyond the pontine brain stem and included the visual-spatial cortical areas discussed earlier. Even this isolated case therefore does not support the old equation of pontine brain stem mechanisms with dream generation. (The relationship between dreaming and REM sleep is discussed further later.)

EXCESSES OF DREAMING

Dream/Reality Confusion

Solms loosely grouped together 12 case reports in the literature and 10 of his own cases under the heading of dream/reality confusion (or "anoneirognosis").[12] These patients reported excesses of dreaming, ranging from increased frequency and/or vivacity of dreams to intrusions of dreaming and dreamlike thinking into waking cognition. The principal justification for collecting these cases under a unitary nosologic heading was that the focal lesions (representing a wide variety of pathologies) that cause "anoneirognosis" were typically located in the transitional zone between the anterior diencephalon and the basal forebrain. Kindred phenomena are, however, also observed with visual deafferentation, peduncular hallucinosis, delirium, parkinsonian syndromes, Guillain-Barré syndrome, and a variety of toxic and metabolic conditions. The common denominator in these cases may therefore simply be degradation of constraints on consciousness. Certainly, any suggestion at this stage that dream/reality confusion may be considered a focal symptom is unjustified.

Dream/reality confusion in parkinsonian syndromes is difficult to interpret. Increased dreaming and hallucinations are frequently seen with Parkinson's disease (PD), but this may be iatrogenic. It is well established that hallucinations and excessive dreaming can be provoked by the administration of L-dopa, both in patients with PD[73] and in normal subjects, independently of any concomitant changes in REM sleep.[74] Accordingly, it has been shown that reduction of dopaminergic medication and administration of dopamine blockers reduces hallucinations and excessive dreaming in PD.[75] However, visual hallucinations in PD may also be an indication of the presence of Lewy body pathology, with involvement of parieto-occipital and limbic regions.[76,77] Excessive dreaming in parkinsonian syndromes may therefore have a different mechanism in cases with and without cortical Lewy bodies. In PD, hallucinations occur late in the course of the disorder, whereas they are an early feature of dementia with Lewy bodies (DLB).

Hallucinations and dream/reality confusion are also common in narcolepsy.[78] In these cases, hallucinations may accompany or follow attacks of cataplexy and sleep paralysis. Hallucinations of a presence of someone nearby ("sensed presence") or a pressure on the chest with breathing difficulties ("incubus/succubus"), and floating/flying and "out-of-body" experiences, are typical in these cases. Dreams can occur at sleep onset (at night or during daytime naps) as well as on awakening (Rosenthal's syndrome). The retention of elements of normal waking mentation, such as volitional control or environmental awareness, is characteristic of narcoleptic dreams.

Various other rare disorders are associated with dream/reality confusion. Idiopathic hypersomnia manifests in excessive daytime sleepiness, prolonged unrefreshing sleep, and "sleep drunkenness" on attempting to wake up. Habitual dreaming, hypnagogic hallucinations, and sleep paralysis are common in these cases.[78] Kleine-Levin syndrome is a rare disorder characterized by recurrent episodes of hypersomnia, compulsive eating behavior, and various psychopathologic changes such as hypersexuality, irritability, and apathy. Hallucinations, delusions, and "dreamy states" are reported in 14–24% of patients with Kleine-Levin syndrome.[79] In fatal familial insomnia, a variant of Creutzfeldt-Jakob disease, progressive insomnia is coupled with an oneiric stuporous state in which patients perform complex, jerky movements that correspond to dream content that patients are later able to report.[80] Dream/reality confusion with hallucinations also occurs in sporadic Creutzfeldt-Jakob disease.[81]

Nightmares

Nocturnal seizures (and complex partial seizures in particular) sometimes present as recurring nightmares.[82,83] Solms identified 24 cases of this type in the literature and 9 in his own series.[12] Of theoretical interest is the fact that such nightmares typically occur during non-REM sleep. The content of the nightmares frequently coincides with that of the patient's typical aura or "dreamy state" seizures.[12,84] Penfield was able to artificially generate a waking aura resembling the recurring nightmare in one case by stimulating exposed cortex in the region of the epileptogenic focus.[85–87] Successful pharmacologic or surgical treatment of the seizure disorder invariably results in disappearance of the recurring nightmares. These facts further support the interpretation of the nightmares in these cases as seizure equivalents (and indeed as non-REM phenomena).

As with dream/reality confusion (which frequently co-occurs with nightmares), increased frequency of nightmares is associated with a wide range of toxic and withdrawal states and metabolic abnormalities. The grounds for detaching these two "excesses of dreaming" from each other are not entirely clear. The common denominator here may therefore, once again, simply be general degradation of constraints on consciousness.

It is important to note that nocturnal panic attacks and sleep terrors are not instances of nightmares. Detailed dream recall is lacking in such attacks.[88,89]

REM Sleep Behavior Disorder

In REM sleep behavior disorder (RBD), dreamed behaviors are physically acted out. This is due to disruption of pontomedullary mechanisms that induce REM atonia.[90] The enacted behaviors may be dramatic or even violent, and usually relate to vivid, frightening dreams. A fair proportion of patients injure their bed partners.[91] The disorder is most common in males, and onset is often in the sixth or seventh decade. RBD manifests mainly in the second half of the sleep cycle (where REM is predominant). Increased slow-wave sleep and increased periodic limb movements across all sleep stages are also seen.[92–95]

Of special interest is the association of RBD with the parkinsonian syndromes discussed previously. The presence of RBD in PD patients is associated with cognitive deficits and appears to predict dementia.[96,97] Disorders with Lewy body pathology often involve RBD. The incidence of RBD in PD is 25–50%, and more than 50% in DLB and multiple system atrophy (MSA). In contrast, disorders without Lewy bodies rarely involve RBD. Notably, idiopathic RBD may present many years prior to the other symptoms of an incipient parkinsonian syndrome.[91,98–103] The prognostic significance of RBD as a precursor to PD, DLB, and MSA is now well established, resulting in the suggestion that the term *cryptogenic* RBD should replace "idiopathic" RBD.[104–106]

PHARMACOLOGIC FINDINGS

The chemical and pharmacologic evidence is extremely difficult to interpret. This is due partly to the dynamic interactions that characterize neurotransmitter systems, and the paucity of rigorous pharmacologic studies.[14] Mention is made here only of more recent findings that seem particularly relevant to understanding dream generation, and the distinction between dreaming and REM sleep.

The neurochemical signature of the REM state is well established: autochthonous activation of ascending pontine ACh cells (which is thought to produce characteristic ponto-geniculo-occipital waves), and reciprocal inhibition of pontine aminergic (5HT and noradrenergic) cells (which is thought to demodulate the dreaming forebrain).[107]

Equally well established is the fact that non-REM sleep has the opposite pattern. Less widely known is the fact that, unlike other aminergic brain stem cells, the source cells in the ventral tegmental area (VTA) of the mesocortical DA pathway described earlier in connection with prefrontal leucotomy continue to fire at equal rates during sleeping and waking.[108,109] These cells also fire with greater interspike variability during REM than non-REM sleep.[108] This has recently been shown to indicate prominent burst activity in the REM state,[110] resulting in greater terminal DA release. Dopamine delivery to the nucleus accumbens is in fact maximal during REM sleep when compared with non-REM sleep and waking.[111]

The REM state is also characterized by minimal prefrontal glutamate release,[111] which presumably coincides with the observation noted previously to the effect that dorsolateral prefrontal lesions have no obvious effect on dream content (and with the observation that this region is strongly deactivated in positron emission tomography [PET] imaging studies of REM sleep[112]). The chemical signature of the REM state, as regards the neurotransmitter interactions underlying the observed regional patterns of forebrain activation and deactivation, is certainly more complex than was previously assumed.[113]

This complexity is underscored by the impenetrable thicket of psychopharmacologic evidence. Of particular value is any evidence that could clarify the pathophysiology of dream cessation following deep ventromesial frontal lesions. Since the sleep cycle is unaffected by such lesions,[58] it is reasonable to assume that they impair a mechanism that is *specific* to dream generation (as opposed to REM generation). Two competing hypotheses have been advanced to account for dream cessation following deep ventromesial frontal lesions (and the commensurate hyperactivation of this region in functional magnetic resonance imaging and PET imaging of dreaming sleep and schizophrenic hallucinations[112,114]). The first hypothesis is that it reflects activation of ACh cells in the basal forebrain; the second is that it reflects activation of DA cells in the VTA.

Against the former hypothesis is the observation that ACh antagonists (e.g., scopolamine), rather than suppressing dreaming and dreamlike thinking, have the opposite effect: they produce dream/reality confusion.[115] In fact, in this respect anticholinergic drugs mirror the effects of lesions in cholinergic basal forebrain nuclei.[116] These

and other considerations led Braun[117] to observe that activation of these nuclei during REM sleep may actually reflect *inhibition* of forebrain ACh in dreaming sleep.

In favor of the latter hypothesis is the observation that DA agonists (e.g., L-dopa) increase dream bizarreness, vivacity, complexity, and emotionality without having any commensurate effects on REM sleep.[74] (Dopamine agonists, of course, also provoke other symptoms of psychotic cognition.) Systematic studies of the effects on dreaming of DA antagonists have not yet been performed. However a preliminary study by Yu of the effects on dreaming of antipsychotic medications recently found significant dream-suppressing effects.[118]

Particularly incompatible with the view that dreaming and REM sleep are generated by the same pontine mechanisms is the accumulating evidence to the effect that 5-HT agonists (selective serotonin reuptake inhibitors [SSRIs]), like anticholinergics, have the opposite effect to what the "REM = dreaming" hypothesis would have predicted. SSRIs suppress REM sleep but produce *excesses* of dreaming, of both types described earlier.[119–125]

The available pharmacologic evidence therefore supports the view that dreaming—like other forms of psychosis—is primarily generated by (demodulated) DA mechanisms rather than ACh ones.[126] However, the neurochemical basis of dreaming is likely to be far more complex than this, the only conclusion that the limited current evidence reasonably allows.

CONCLUSION

Despite the minimal attention that neurologists typically pay to dreams, their assessment can be of diagnostic interest, and have prognostic and management implications. Dreams can also be a major source of distress to patients. There is also every reason to expect that systematic studies of clinical dream phenomena will continue to provide valuable new insights into the functions and malfunctions of the human brain and mind.

⊙ REFERENCES

A full list of references are available at www.expertconsult. com

CHAPTER 32

Sleep in Psychiatric Disorders

Peter L. Franzen and **Daniel J. Buysse**

INTRODUCTION

Numerous studies support a bidirectional relationship between psychopathology and poor sleep. The incidence of psychiatric disorders is elevated among sleep-disordered patient populations, and sleep disorders are likewise overrepresented in psychiatric patients. This overlap can complicate both the diagnosis and treatment of sleep and psychiatric disorders.

Sleep disturbances have long been considered as a function of an underlying psychiatric condition; however, chronic pain[1] and other medical illnesses, including sleep disorders, can interfere with sleep and lead to insomnia complaints. As an example, Forsell and Winblad[2] investigated the prevalence of psychiatric symptoms in the oldest old. Sleep disturbances were named as the most common psychiatric symptom observed. There are many other plausible reasons, however, that sleep disturbances would be frequently observed in an over-90 population, including age-related neurologic changes and increases in apnea rates.

The attribution of insomnia or "sleep difficulties" as exclusively indicative of a psychiatric symptom is problematic for several reasons: (1) sleep is a physiologically driven process, not simply a state of mind, with mounting evidence that sleep is biologically linked to mood disorders; (2) sleep disturbances can exist independent of psychiatric symptoms, or remain after a psychiatric disorder remits; and (3) sleep disturbances have been identified as an important underlying factor in eliciting psychiatric symptoms, as well as in their severity and recurrence. While insomnia may be a frequent consequence of some medical and psychiatric disorders (secondary insomnia), such as chronic

pain or major depression, it is now clear that insomnia can be a primary problem that precedes or co-occurs with another condition (comorbid insomnia). Thus, it is important to consider other factors in addition to psychopathology that can affect sleep. Such distinctions are important for understanding the pathophysiology of sleep disturbances, and may impact treatment.

This chapter reviews the various relationships between sleep and psychiatric disorders, focusing on sleep disturbances and psychiatric symptoms in a broad sense; on psychopathology in individuals with sleep disorders; and on sleep findings in various psychiatric disorders. The chapter concludes with some considerations for approaching sleep disturbances in the treatment of patients with psychiatric disorders.

SLEEP DISTURBANCES, SLEEP LOSS, AND PSYCHIATRIC DISORDERS

Both sleep loss and sleep disturbances can significantly impact mood and psychopathology. Sleep disturbances are frequently observed in psychiatric disorders, with 50–80% of individuals with a primary psychiatric disorder reporting sleep disturbances at some point during the course of their disorder.[3] Epidemiologic evidence shows that self-reported habitual sleep duration is associated with increased risk for psychopathology. Based on interviews of 4075 adults from northern Germany, short sleepers (≤5 hours of sleep) had significantly greater risk of having a current nicotine dependence, alcohol dependence, depressive disorder, or anxiety disorder, using

Diagnostic and Statistical Manual of Mental Disorders, Fourth Edition (DSM-IV) criteria.[4] Shorter sleep duration (<8 hours) and frequent nightmares were significantly associated with increased risk for suicidal ideation and suicide attempts in an epidemiologic sample of 1362 adolescents ages 12–18 from China[5]; the risk for suicide attempts remained significant after controlling for depressive symptoms. Similar findings for increased suicide risk in adults experiencing frequent nightmares have also been reported.[6] Sleep problems in childhood increase the risk for psychiatric problems in adulthood. In a longitudinal sample, 943 children with parent-reported sleep and psychiatric symptoms at ages 5, 7, and 9 were assessed for current anxiety and depression using standardized structured interviews at ages 21 and 26.[7] Persistent sleep problems in early childhood predicted adulthood anxiety disorders but not adulthood depression in this sample.

Both insomnia and hypersomnia symptoms are associated with increased incidence and severity of psychiatric disorders. A survey of 7954 people in scattered major U.S. cities between 1981 and 1985 as part of the National Institute of Mental Health Epidemiological Catchment Area study[8] revealed that 40% of those with insomnia and 46.5% of those with hypersomnia met the criteria for mental illness using criteria from the American Psychiatric Association's *Diagnostic and Statistical Manual of Mental Disorders, Third Edition, Revised.* Ten percent of the sample complained of insomnia and 3.2% of hypersomnia.[9] Fourteen percent of the patients with insomnia met criteria for major depression, compared to 9.9% of those with hypersomnolence. The rate of new psychiatric disorders at 1-year follow-up was greater among respondents with persistent sleep complaints. The numbers in this study were thought to be low due to strict criteria for defining insomnia and the omission of generalized anxiety disorder and personality disorders from the survey. In a study by Mosko and colleagues,[10] 66.5% of 206 patients presenting to one sleep disorders center reported one episode of major depression in the previous 5 years, and 25.7% described themselves as depressed on presentation. Additional studies have established substantial risk of developing major depression and generalized anxiety in patients with sleep disorders.[11–13] Both insomnia and hypersomnia are associated with worsening course of depression[14] and increased suicidal behavior.[15]

Sleep loss/deprivation also leads to mood dysregulation. Experimental studies manipulating sleep duration consistently demonstrate a negative impact on self-reported mood,[16] although mood can become dysregulated in the opposite direction as well (e.g., mood elevation, giddy laughter). Negative consequences from sleep deprivation are in general more common, and can impact functioning. For example, sleep deprivation can impair interpersonal transactions. Average nightly sleep duration was assessed in a sample of medical residents.[17] Reports of treating others badly or feeling belittled/humiliated by

colleagues increased as average nightly sleep decreased. Although reported by a smaller percentage of respondents, the incidence of violent behavior (i.e., hitting, kicking, and punching) showed the same inverse relationship with sleep duration.

Among patients with major depressive disorder, symptoms can improve following total sleep or selective rapid eye movement (REM) sleep deprivation, although symptoms may worsen in some. The improvement is transient, and only occurs in 40–60% of patients with endogenous depression.[18–20] Sleep deprivation can lead to an antidepressant response in patients with bipolar disorder as well.[21] Sleep deprivation can also lead to drastic consequences on psychiatric symptomatology. Irregular social rhythms and sleep deprivation can elicit mania in some patients with bipolar disorder.[22–25] It has also been suggested that sleep deprivation may induce bipolar disorder in vulnerable individuals. Lack of sleep has also been associated with the *development* of bipolar disorder,[26] as well as pre- and postpartum psychosis,[27–29] and greater rates of depression in both new mothers and new fathers have been attributed in part to the sleep disruption that occurs with the arrival of a newborn.[30] A sleep deficit has also been found to prospectively predict the development of depressive symptoms in patients with bipolar disorder.[31]

ASSOCIATIONS BETWEEN SLEEP DISORDERS AND PSYCHIATRIC SYMPTOMS/DISORDERS

Insomnia

Insomnia can be a primary disorder or it may co-occur with other medical or psychiatric illnesses. Insomnia independently places an individual at risk for future medical and psychiatric complications.[32] Not only is psychopathology more severe in people who complain of sleep disturbances, insomnia itself specifically confers an increased risk for the *future* development of a mood or anxiety disorder, even when controlling for baseline mood symptoms.[9,33] Mellinger and coworkers[11] reported that 21% of insomniacs had symptoms of major depression, and another 13% symptoms of generalized anxiety. Breslau et al.,[12] in a 3-year longitudinal study of 979 young adults, found a lifetime prevalence of 16% for insomnia. Patients with insomnia had a fourfold increase in risk for developing major depression compared to patients without insomnia; notably, sleep disturbance was a stronger predictor of the subsequent development of depression than any other factor.

The timing of chronic insomnia and psychiatric illness were assessed by telephone interview in a population-based sample of 14,915 Western European participants.[34] Of the 19.1% of the sample with insomnia, about one quarter had a current psychiatric diagnosis and another quarter had a psychiatric history. For those with mood disorders, insomnia either preceded (40%) or appeared at the same time (22%) as mood symptoms. In contrast, insomnia tended to appear at the same time as (38%) or after (34%) the development of an anxiety disorder. The strongest predictors of having a psychiatric history were severe insomnia, primary insomnia, or insomnia related to a medical condition, and insomnia persisting more than 1 year. Studies have shown a relationship between suicide and insomnia in depression[22] and panic disorder,[35] as well as higher rates of insomnia[36] and poor sleep quality[15] among suicidal individuals, again illustrating the bidirectional relationship between sleep and psychopathology.

Circadian Rhythm Disorders

Circadian rhythm disorders, such as delayed or advanced sleep phase syndrome, are characterized by abnormal timing of sleep. These disorders lead to secondary insomnia due to the difficulty in sleeping at desired, typically socially appropriate times, and thus can significantly impact functioning. For example, a severely delayed sleep schedule can significantly impede academic or occupational functioning; such stresses can easily lead to depression, which may in turn hamper the behavioral self-control needed to try to "normalize" the individual's schedule (e.g., taking melatonin at the appropriate time, engaging in a consistent sleep-wake schedule, chronotherapy). As many as three-quarters of individuals with delayed sleep phase syndrome have a past or current history of depression.[37]

Sleep Apnea

Sleep fragmentation and chronic intermittent hypoxemia induced by sleep-disordered breathing (SDB) lead to impairments in cognitive and affective domains (see El Ad and Lavie[38] for review). Affective consequences of SDB include elevated rates of depression, anxiety, and hostility symptoms based on self-report questionnaires,[39] although inconsistencies have been reported.[40] In a large cohort of Veterans Administration health care beneficiaries, those with sleep apnea had significantly greater prevalence of mood disorders, anxiety, post-traumatic stress disorder, psychosis, and dementia compared to patients without sleep apnea.[41] Patients diagnosed with obstructive sleep apnea often present to sleep disorders centers with concomitant symptoms of depression and other psychopathology. Successful treatment of SDB, usually positive pressure therapy, leads to improvements in quality-of-life measures. Studies of post-treatment improvement in depression symptoms, however, have been inconclusive,[42-44] perhaps in part to the many methodologic differences and reliance on self-report measures of depressive symptoms, such as the Beck Depression Inventory, rather than clinical interview.

The association between SDB and depression has been consistently found, with reports ranging from 24% to 58% of SDB patients meeting diagnostic criteria for depression.[10,45-47] In a recent general population study consisting of nearly 19,000 Western Europeans responding to a telephone survey, 0.8% were found to have both SDB and depression.[48] They found that that 17.6% of individuals with SDB also were diagnosed with depression and 18% of depressed individuals were diagnosed with SDB. After controlling for obesity and hypertension, an individual with major depression is still at increased risk of also having SDB. Because depression and SDB are both prevalent conditions in the general population, these findings are of particular relevance to psychiatrists and sleep specialists alike. That nearly one-fifth of individuals with one of these disorders may have the other underscores the importance of screening for SDB in people diagnosed with depression, and vice versa. By accurately identifying both disorders when present, treatment outcomes for both disorders may be improved (see Schroder and O'Hara[49] for further discussion).

Studies in children have tended to not clearly differentiate primary snoring from obstructive sleep apnea; however, cross-sectional evidence suggests a strong increase in behavior problems and neurocognitive abnormalities in children with SDB (see Schechter[50]). Surgical interventions seem to help. Many children who received adenotonsillectomy to treat their SDB have improved academic and behavioral functioning (e.g., aggression, inattention, hyperactivity, alertness),[51-53] although positive results have not always been reported.[54]

Restless Legs Syndrome/Periodic Limb Movements

Restless legs syndrome (RLS) is another prevalent sleep disorder that is associated with depression and anxiety,[55-58] as well as attention-deficit/hyperactivity disorder (ADHD). An increased association between RLS and depression, and RLS and ADHD, has been reported (see Cortese et al.[59] and Picchietti and Winkelman[56] for reviews). One retrospective review of 100 consecutive idiopathic RLS patients failed to find an association between RLS severity and Beck Depression Inventory scores.[60] However, Winkelmann and colleagues[61] found an increased risk of having 12-month depressive and anxiety disorders based in 130 adult RLS patients who were compared to over 2000 community respondents with other types of physical disorders. Whether the increased incidence of psychiatric disorders in RLS patients is due to sleep disruption, or to some shared pathophysiologic process, or is spurious cannot be determined by the epidemiologic associations found to date. Such findings, however, do support assessing psychiatric symptomatology in the diagnosis and treatment of RLS patients.

Narcolepsy

Patients with narcolepsy are at increased risk for psychopathology.[62,63] Narcolepsy patients were found to exhibit greater psychosocial impairments than two matched comparison groups (epilepsy patients and normal controls).[64] Hypnagogic hallucinations, part of the symptom tetrad of narcolepsy, do not occur in all cases of narcolepsy, nor do they typically indicate psychotic symptomatology. However, there are reports of an increased association between narcolepsy and psychotic disorders, although this association has been disputed.[65]

SLEEP IN PSYCHIATRIC DISORDERS

Studies of REM sleep architecture in various psychopathologic states have been conducted since Dement first evaluated REM sleep in schizophrenic patients in 1955. More recently, REM sleep changes have most often been associated with affective disorders. Subsequently, numerous studies have attempted to use measures of REM sleep latency, REM density, and REM sleep distribution to link affective disorders to various other psychiatric disorders such as schizophrenia, eating disorders, personality disorders, and substance abuse disorders. Others have attempted to use these same measures to distinguish various psychopathologic states from major depression. Unfortunately, a great deal of confusion has resulted from various methodologic issues and diagnostic uncertainties in psychiatric patients. Examples of methodologic differences in studies include the number of consecutive nights patients are studied, determination of the time between sleep onset and REM sleep onset (REM sleep latency), the definition of increased REM density, concurrent use of psychotropic drugs, period of withdrawal from psychotropic medications, sleep schedule, and the severity of the illness. Just as important is the overlap of symptoms among various disorders found in the Research Diagnostic Criteria, the DSM-IV, and other classifications for mental disorders. Although in theory psychiatric diagnoses are categorically distinct from one another, in clinical practice such distinctions are more difficult to make, and comorbid psychiatric diagnoses are common.

Mood Disorders

Major Depression

Major depression is the psychiatric disorder most studied by sleep researchers, and several theories of the mechanisms involved have been published.[66] In approximately 90% of cases, major depression results in insomnia. A smaller percentage of patients with major depression complain of excessive sleepiness; most are adolescents and young adults.[67] Whereas depressed adolescents and young adults may be more prone to be "long sleepers," studies of older depressed patients with the complaint of hypersomnolence have failed to show evidence of pathologic sleepiness.[68] Sleep disturbances can interfere with treatment response in depression. In a sample of depressed women treated with interpersonal psychotherapy, those with higher pretreatment subjective

sleep quality ratings showed significant post-treatment improvement in mood symptoms compared to treatment nonresponders.[69] Similar findings of worse subjective sleep quality being associated with worse treatment response have also been reported in patients with depression receiving combined pharmacologic and psychological treatments.[70] Conversely, improvement in subjective sleep quality following depression treatment is associated with lower recurrence rates of depression.[71] Treating insomnia in addition to depression may speed recovery from depression. In a double-blind study, adults with comorbid depression and insomnia who were assigned to fluoxetine and eszopiclone coadministration had improved sleep and higher rates of responders and remitters compared to those assigned to fluoxetine and placebo.[72]

Efforts have been made to distinguish major depression from other psychopathologic states by use of sleep electroencephalography (EEG) and other biological markers. The primary well-documented changes in sleep architecture include shortened REM sleep–onset latency, increased REM density, reduced total sleep time, reduced sleep efficiency, increased awakenings, decreased slow-wave sleep (SWS), and a shift of SWS from the first non-REM (NREM) cycle to the second (Fig. 32-1). More recently, high-amplitude fast-frequency EEG activity has been suggested as a marker for depression.[73] Sleep architecture changes found in depression may serve as a marker for the development of depression in those individuals genetically predisposed to depression.[74,75] In comparison with major depressive disorder, dysthymia has not been extensively studied. Hypersomnolence,[76] reductions in K complexes, vertex sharp waves, increased stage 1 sleep, decreased SWS, increased awakenings, spindles in REM sleep, theta bursts, and positive occipital sharp transients[77,78] have been cited in isolated studies.

Changes in sleep architecture, particularly in REM sleep and deep NREM sleep, are more pronounced with age in major depression. Prepubertal depressed children are less likely to show changes in sleep architecture than postpubertal depressives.[79,80] There has been some conflict in the literature about whether REM sleep latency in depressed children is normal or shortened.[81] Changes in sleep architecture in adolescents appear to depend on the severity of the illness. Inpatient, psychotic, or suicidal adolescents may exhibit the typical adult changes of major depression, whereas the sleep of adolescents who are not as severely depressed may show no changes.[82–84]

Aging has a marked influence on sleep, such as REM sleep latency, in depression; elderly depressed patients often have a REM sleep onset of less than 10 minutes. Older patients with a history of suicide attempts have longer sleep-onset latency, reduced sleep efficiency, and increased REM density than "nonattempters."[85] Depressed men have less SWS than depressed women,[86] but women may have more and higher amplitude beta activity.[87] Women with past depressive episodes appear to experience more

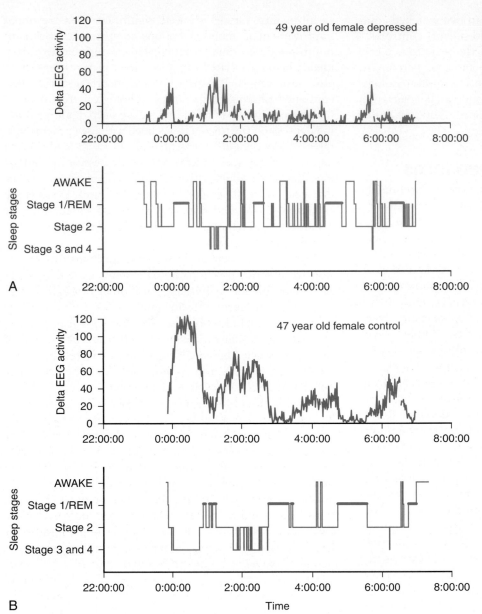

FIGURE 32–1 Representative sleep histograms for a patient with major depressive disorder **(A)** and an age- and sex-matched healthy subject **(B)**. In each figure, the *top panel* shows EEG delta activity during NREM sleep identified by computer algorithm, and the *bottom panel* shows the sleep histogram from visual sleep stage scoring. Relative to the control subject, the depressed patient has a longer sleep latency, more wakefulness during sleep, less visually scored stage 3/4 sleep and EEG delta activity, and shorter REM sleep latency.

sleep disruption and reduced REM sleep latency[88] in the immediate postpartum months.

Studies of the effects of antidepressant medication on REM sleep measures in patients with major depression have suggested that, when immediate and persistent anti-depressant-induced prolongation of the REM sleep latency, reduction of total REM sleep time, and REM density are observed, clinical response is better.[89,90] The occurrence of sleep-onset REM sleep episodes and shorter REM sleep duration during maintenance treatment with antidepressants has been associated with increased risk of relapse during treatment.[91] Studies of the effects of electroconvulsive therapy (ECT) on REM sleep architecture suggest that they are not as pronounced as those observed with most antidepressants.[92] As with

pharmacotherapy, patients with post-ECT EEG signs of depression are more likely to have recurrence of the illness.[93]

Bipolar Disorder

Patients in the manic phase of bipolar disorder have been shown to have much reduced total sleep time, which gradually extends as the manic phase passes.[94] There is also a reduction in stages 3 and 4 sleep. No consistent change in REM sleep has been found, probably due to excitability and subsequent reduction of total sleep in these patients, but most studies show the same changes as seen in major depression.[95,96] It has been suggested that the switch from euthymia or depression into the manic phase occurs during sleep.[97] Lithium, which is the primary drug used to treat the manic phase of bipolar disorder, has been found to increase SWS and reduce REM sleep.

Anxiety Disorders

Anxiety disorders are the most prevalent group of psychiatric disorders. As described earlier, anxiety symptoms and disorders co-occur with many sleep disorders. Anxiety has also long been associated with sleep disturbances, especially insomnia, as a quiet mind is a prerequisite to fall asleep. While less research has been done in this area compared to mood disorders, strong associations between sleep and anxiety have been reported.[98]

Generalized Anxiety Disorder

While anxiety symptoms are most often associated with sleep initiation difficulties, Belanger and colleagues[99] found a more varied pattern of sleep difficulties in generalized anxiety disorder (GAD). They examined self-reported insomnia symptoms both before and after a cognitive behavioral intervention targeting excessive worry in 44 primary GAD patients. Insomnia subtypes included difficulty initiating sleep (endorsed by 48%) or maintaining sleep (64%), and early morning awakenings (57%); 77% experienced at least one symptom, 41% two symptoms, and 26% all three. Comorbid depression, an important confounding variable, was not discussed and may have influenced study results. In polysomnographic studies, patients with GAD typically have prolonged sleep-onset latency, increased stages 1 and 2 sleep, less SWS, a smaller REM sleep percentage, and, with the exception of isolated reports, increased or normal REM sleep latency.[100,101] No difference has been found between patients with GAD alone and those with GAD and depression.[102]

Panic Disorder

Panic disorder has multiple somatic and emotional symptoms leading to diagnostic confusion. Similar presentations are seen in mitral valve prolapse syndrome, cardiovascular dysautonomia, and sleep choking syndrome. The diagnosis may depend on the presentation of psychiatric symptoms, as opposed to autonomic and respiratory symptoms. Controversy exists over the roles of increased brain stem carbon dioxide receptor sensitivity and dysautonomia in panic.[103–109] It has been suggested that a number of substances and situations provoke panic attacks, such as caffeine, nicotine, over-the-counter cold remedies, cannabis, cocaine, sleep deprivation, excessive sugar intake, exercise, relaxation, hyperventilation, stress, and even fluorescent lighting.[110]

As many as 70% of patients with panic disorder have difficulty with sleep-onset and maintenance insomnia,[111,112] and often report sleep paralysis[113] and hypnagogic hallucinations.[114] Overbeek and colleagues[112] compared 70 panic patients and 70 controls on six types of sleep complaints assessed with the Sleep-Wake

Experiences List (initiating sleep, sleep maintenance, early morning awakenings, tiredness upon awakening, difficulty waking up, and daytime sleepiness). Within the patient group, there were subsamples of patients with only panic disorder, patients with additional nocturnal panic, and patients with comorbid depression. The percentage of participants reporting sleep complaints was greater for the entire patient sample versus controls (67% vs. 20%), as well as for the panic-only subgroup (53%). Compared to the nondepressed panic group, the panic with comorbid depression subgroup were more likely to have sleep complaints (86% vs. 59%); specifically, there were significantly more sleep maintenance and daytime sleepiness complaints in the panic with comorbid depression subgroup. Patients with nocturnal panic were significantly more likely to report sleep maintenance problems, but the overall percentage of subgroup members reporting sleep complaints did not differ between these two subgroups, suggesting that neither the contribution of nocturnal panic attacks nor depression is the primary reason for sleep complaints in panic disorder, although a higher prevalence of sleep complaints was found in the panic with comorbid depression subgroup.

Panic attacks can occur in any stage of sleep, but most occur during NREM sleep just before the onset of SWS. Symptoms similar to those associated with nocturnal panic attacks may be observed in patients with arrhythmias, gastroesophageal reflux, sleep apnea,[115] sleep terrors, REM sleep behavior disorder, and paroxysmal hypnogenic dystonia.[116] More rarely, panic attacks can occur solely at night. It has been suggested that patients with sleep-only panic attacks experience depression more frequently than panic disorder patients who do not experience sleep-related panic attacks.[117] Of people diagnosed with panic disorder, 44–71% have a history of nocturnal panic,[118] and 30–45% experience episodes of recurrent episodes of nocturnal panic.[119] Nocturnal panic is typically experienced as more intense than daytime panic. Fear of sleep can develop and lead to restricted sleep, which in turn might facilitate nocturnal panic events.[119] Patients with nocturnal panic attacks tend to experience worse daytime panic attacks, more somatic symptoms,[120] and more comorbid psychiatric disorders[121] than daytime-only panic disorder patients.

Polysomnographic studies in nondepressed patients with panic disorder have reported normal sleep-onset latency and modestly reduced total sleep time and delta sleep.[122] However, studies in patients with panic and comorbid major depression have reported features typical of major depression, with substantially prolonged sleep-onset latency, reduced total sleep time, sleep disruption, reduced SWS, and early REM sleep onset.[123–126]

Post-traumatic Stress Disorder

Post-traumatic stress disorder (PTSD) is caused by exposure to an event or events in which a person witnesses or hears of a threat to the integrity (life) of themselves or a loved one, often in natural disasters, combat, torture, rape, or other situations involving physical and psychological abuse. Sleep complaints are nearly universal in individuals diagnosed with PTSD, and include nightmares,[127] difficulties initiating and/or maintaining sleep (in 70–90% of individuals with PTSD),[128–130] and sleep paralysis.[131] REM sleep behavior disorder has also been associated with PTSD,[132,133] as has sleep paralysis.[131] Sleep disturbances shortly after trauma exposure predict the development of PTSD at follow-up assessment.[134–136] PTSD patients who report more severe sleep symptoms also report more depression severity, suicidality, anxiety, and substance use.[137–139]

Current first-line interventions for PTSD do not directly target the nighttime symptoms in either pharmacotherapeutic (e.g., selective serotonin reuptake inhibitors [SSRIs]) or cognitive behavioral therapy (CBT) approaches; the former has minimal benefits on nightmares and insomnia,[140–142] and the latter had minimal benefits for 48% of PTSD patients who had a reduction in daytime symptoms in one study.[130] Fortunately, behavioral sleep interventions are effective in reducing nighttime symptoms in PTSD. For chronic nightmares, imagery rehearsal therapy has been found to reduce nightmare frequency and severity in both individuals with PTSD and those who have nightmares as a primary sleep disorder.[143] Nightmare reductions have lasted up to 30 months in follow-up studies,[144] and are associated with significant reductions in daytime PTSD symptoms, depression, anxiety, and quality of life.[145–148] Effective behavioral interventions for primary insomnia (i.e., stimulus control instructions, sleep restriction) can also effectively reduce PTSD-related insomnia.[147,149,150] More recently, prazosin, an α_1-adrenergic receptor antagonist, has emerged as promising treatment of PTSD-related sleep disturbance, including both nightmares and insomnia symptoms.[151]

Much like polysomnographic studies of insomnia, in which sleep variables do not significantly differ from those of controls, reports of polysomnographic abnormalities in PTSD have been inconsistent (see Kobayashi et al.,[152] for meta-analytic review). This disorder has been associated with increased sleep-onset latency, decreased sleep efficiency, increased wakefulness after sleep onset, decreased total sleep time, reduction in stage 2 sleep, and increased stage 1 sleep.[153] There is controversy over the effects on REM sleep: Some authors report normal REM sleep parameters,[153] whereas others report reduced REM sleep latency and increased REM density.[154–156] Nightmares have been found to occur during both NREM and REM sleep.[157,158] Authors have speculated that PTSD may be a disorder of REM sleep mechanisms.[159]

Obsessive-Compulsive and Social Phobia Disorders

Less work has been done in obsessive-compulsive disorder or social phobia, although these disorders too are common. Patients with social phobia show increased sleep-onset latency, awakening after sleep onset, and reduced total sleep time.[160] In obsessive-compulsive disorder, sleep can become restricted by repeatedly engaging in compulsive behaviors. Sleep studies in obsessive-compulsive disorder show decreased total sleep time, increased number of awakenings, shortened REM sleep latency, reduced stage 4 sleep, and reduced sleep efficiency.[161]

Eating Disorders

Most studies of patients with bulimia show very little change in REM sleep measures compared with controls. REM sleep architecture studies of patients with anorexia nervosa have been more contradictory: Some report no change in REM sleep parameters,[162] whereas others suggest that there are changes similar to those seen in major depression.[163] These findings may be due to high rates of comorbidity with affective disorders and frequent family history of affective disorders in anorexia patients. Patients with severe untreated anorexia nervosa often show reduced total sleep time, decreased sleep efficiency, increased wakefulness after sleep onset, increased stage 1 sleep, and decreased SWS. Sleep normalizes after weight is gained.[164,165] One study suggests that there is initial shortening of the REM sleep latency with severe weight loss but that, with recovery of weight, the REM sleep latency returns to normal.[166]

Schizophrenia

Patients with schizophrenia often sleep worse than healthy individuals, with sleep continuity disturbance, reduced SWS, decreased REM latency, and increased REM sleep, although there are contrasting studies showing relatively little change in sleep. Variability in documented sleep architecture changes and sleep quality are most likely due to differences in the age of patients, medications, study techniques, and other variables. Sleep efficiency, stage 2 sleep, sleep continuity, total sleep time, and total REM sleep decrease on withdrawal of neuroleptics.[167–169] In one study,[167] patients with tardive dyskinesia had an earlier onset of REM suppression after withdrawal of medication. Mean REM sleep latency was shorter, and total REM sleep time was greater, in patients with tardive dyskinesia than in those without tardive dyskinesia. NREM sleep parameters improved more on withdrawal of medication than REM sleep parameters. All patients had prolonged sleep-onset latencies. SWS was more abundant in patients without tardive dyskinesia. Studies have suggested an inverse relationship between SWS and sleep maintenance and brain ventricle size.[170–172] It has been suggested that reductions in SWS and increases in negative symptoms may be related to reduced anabolism and accelerated aging or atrophy of the brain.[173] SWS also does not rebound after sleep deprivation in patients with schizophrenia.[174]

Borderline Personality Disorder

Borderline personality disorder as defined by the DSM-IV encompasses a number of symptoms of other psychiatric disorders, including major depression. In numerous studies of borderline personality disorder, it has been shown repeatedly that the sleep architecture changes are very similar to those observed in patients with major depression.[175–178] Borderline personality disorder patients have less total sleep time, less sleep efficiency, reduced SWS, increased stage 2 sleep, reduced REM sleep latency, and increased REM density. Subjects with borderline personality disorder frequently have symptoms of depression and have been shown to have abnormalities of other biological markers associated with depression.[179]

Childhood Psychiatric Disorders

Sleep disturbances are associated with a variety of behavioral and emotional problems in childhood and adolescence: anxiety and depression,[180,181] attention/hyperactivity symptoms,[182,183] and behavioral problems such as acting out.[184] As reported in the adult literature, a number of studies have suggested a bidirectional association between sleep and behavioral/emotional problems in childhood.[185,186]

Sleep and behavioral/emotional problems were longitudinally assessed in 490 children between the ages of 4 and 15.[181] Sleep problems at age 4 were associated with an increase in behavioral/emotional symptoms in midadolescence, although evidence for a reciprocal relationship was inconsistent. Early childhood sleep problems (mother-reported overtiredness and trouble sleeping) were similarly found to predict the early-onset use of alcohol and other drugs during midadolescence in a longitudinal sample of 257 high-risk Caucasian Americans families[187]; sleep problems also predicted elevated attention and anxiety/depression symptoms during adolescence, although these problems did not mediate the relationship between early childhood sleep problems and substance use.

Childhood sleep problems are also associated with increased risk for adult psychopathology. Parent-reported sleep and psychiatric symptoms at ages 5, 7, and 9 were compared with current anxiety and depression using standardized structured interviews at age 21 and 26 in a longitudinal sample of 943 individuals.[7] Persistent sleep problems in early childhood predicted adulthood anxiety disorders (46%:33% ratio of adolescents with anxiety who did and did not have persistent childhood sleep problems, respectively), but not adulthood depression, in this sample. Although similar connections between sleep and depression are found in both pediatric and adult populations, polysomnographic differences in clinical populations with depression have been less consistent in the child and adolescent literature (see Ivanenko et al.[188]).

Tourette's syndrome often results in sleep disruption. Increased SWS and decreased REM percentages, and increased awakenings and motor tics, were observed in a sample of 14 Tourette's syndrome patients less than 23 years old compared to 11 matched controls.[189] Motor tics may disturb sleep, and patients with comorbid ADHD experience the most sleep disturbance.[190,191]

ADHD may be associated with childhood insomnia,[190] sleep deprivation, and snoring and obstructive sleep apnea,[50] and sleep problems are much more likely to be reported by adults with ADHD. Several polysomnographic studies in children with ADHD have reported relatively normal sleep parameters[192–194]; however, a more recent investigation of 38 school-age boys with ADHD and 64 control school-age boys using sleep diaries and actigraphy found increased instability in sleep onset and sleep duration in the patient group.[183] Objective and subjective sleep was measured in 20 adults with primary ADHD.[195] Compared to matched controls, patients had an increase in polysomnographically measured total sleep time and periodic limb movements in sleep; the latter were inversely related to subjectively perceived total sleep time. Subjective sleep quality was lower in patients than the controls. Sleep complaints were also more likely to be reported in a sample of 120 adults with ADHD compared to a control sample, including RLS symptoms and not feeling refreshed in the morning, although complaints of insomnia were related to comorbidity with depression.[196]

Alcohol and Substance Abuse Disorders

Dependence on alcohol or other drugs of abuse invariably leads to sleep problems both while on and when trying to get off the substance. Withdrawal effects can often lead to insomnia or hypersomnia symptoms. The impact on sleep can last for years into abstinence, as has been documented in alcohol abuse. Long-term chronic problem drinkers were found to have marked fragmented and shortened sleep that contains more light and less deep sleep, as well as elevated percentages of REM sleep, after 1–2 years of abstinence.[197–199] Sleep disturbances have been suggested as a pathway for the development of alcohol and substance abuse, and are associated with increased risk for relapse following substance abuse treatment. For example, the adolescent who finds she cannot fall asleep unless first smoking marijuana may shift from being an occasional to a habitual user. Alcohol is an oft-used self-medication for difficulty falling asleep; unfortunately, while alcohol is quite effective in hastening sleep onset, the effect wears off after a few hours, leading to sleep fragmentation.[200] Alcohol also has the unexpected effect of interacting with sleep loss, leading to marked daytime sleepiness.[201,202] Likewise, sleep disruption can be highly frustrating, and may be one of the motivating factors driving some back to substance use if disrupted sleep suddenly becomes very prominent during the initial withdrawal and subsequent abstinent period.

Both daytime sleepiness and insomnia symptoms can lead to self-medication with stimulants and to alcohol and marijuana use, which, given the negative effects these substances have on sleep, can lead to an escalating pattern of use and worsening sleep disturbance. Subjective sleep complaints consistently predict relapse in individuals with alcohol dependence, as do objective, polysomnographic markers of sleep disturbance. In the first few weeks of abstinence, elevated REM density was the best predictor of relapse 3 months post-discharge from a 1-month treatment program.[203,204] At 5 months, REM measures no longer predicted relapse at 1 year; however, objective sleep disturbances consistent with insomnia symptoms, including long sleep latency and poor sleep efficiency, were predictive. Sleep latency measured about 1 month into abstinence was the best predictor of patients who relapsed by the fifth month.[205]

Johnson and Breslau[206] reported a positive association between trouble sleeping and nicotine, alcohol, and other drugs of abuse in a large cross-sectional survey of 13,381 adolescents 12–17 years old, suggesting that sleep difficulty, psychiatric symptomatology, and substance use may co-occur within the same individuals. Thus, specific attention to sleep and psychiatric symptoms in people undergoing alcohol and other drug abuse treatment programs may well improve outcomes and decrease relapse rates in these populations.

Medication Effects and Substance Abuse

The reader is referred to Table 32-1 for a review of the acute, chronic, and withdrawal effects on sleep parameters of various medications and substances of abuse.

TABLE 32–1 Drugs That Affect Sleep

Drug	Effects on Sleep		Comments
Barbiturates	Acute:	↑ TST	Rapid development of tolerance
		↓ WASO	Withdrawal insomnia
		↓ REM	Daytime sedation
		↑ Stage 2, ↑ spindles	
		↑ or ↓ Delta	
	Withdrawal: ↓ TST		
Benzodiazepines	Acute:	↓ SL (most agents)	Agents vary in onset and duration of action
		↑ TST	Daytime sedation (with long-acting agents)
		↓ WASO	Tolerance develops (with short-acting agents)
		↓ REM	Withdrawal insomnia (with short-acting agents)
		↑ Stage 2, ↑ spindles	
		↓ Delta (most agents; some ↑ delta)	
	Withdrawal: ↓ TST		
Benzodiazepine receptor agonists (e.g., zolpidem)	Acute:	↓ SL	Sleep architecture not typically altered
		↑ TST	Withdrawal effects inconsistently seen
		→ REM	
		→ Delta	
	Withdrawal: → or ↑ WASO		
Chloral hydrate		↑ TST	Little information on tolerance or withdrawal
		→ REM	
		→ Stage 2	
		→ Delta	
L-Tryptophan		→ or ↑ TST	Effects are mild and inconsistent and may be delayed
		→ or ↑ REM	
		↑ Delta	
Alcohol	Acute:	↑ TST 1st half of night, ↓ 2nd half	Acute effects variable
		↑ WASO 2nd half of night	Degree of REM rebound may correlate with likelihood of withdrawal delirium
		↓ REM 1st half of night	
		↑ Delta	
	Chronic:	→ TST	
		→ REM	
		↓ Delta	
	Withdrawal: ↓ TST		
		↑ WASO	
		↑ REM	
		↓ Delta	
Narcotics	Acute:	↑ WASO	Effects vary with specific agents
		↓ REM	Hypersomnolence may occur during withdrawal
		↓ Delta (total), with ↑ delta "bursts"	
	Chronic:	→ WASO	
		→ Delta	
	Withdrawal: ↓ WASO		

Continued

TABLE 32–1 Drugs That Affect Sleep—Cont'd			
Drug	**Effects on Sleep**		**Comments**
Aspirin	Acute:	↓ Delta	May act via prostaglandin inhibition and temperature effects
Amphetamines	Acute:	↓ TST ↑ WASO, ↑ movements ↓ REM ↓ Delta	Sleep-wake cycle may be severely disrupted during acute use and withdrawal
	Withdrawal:	↑ TST ↑ REM	
Caffeine		↑ SL ↓ TST ↑ WASO ↓ REM ↓ Delta (1st half of night)	May have effects on sleep EEG even when no subjective disturbance occurs
Miscellaneous stimulants (e.g., nicotine, cocaine, pemoline, methylphenidate)		↑ SL ↓ TST ↓ REM	
Antidepressants (e.g., tricyclics and monoamine oxidase inhibitors, except trimipramine)	Acute:	↓ WASO ↓ REM ↑ Stage 2 ↑ Delta	Sleep effects vary with sedative potential of specific agent; MAOIs may cause ↑ WASO
	Withdrawal:	↑ WASO ↑ REM	
Selective serotonin reuptake inhibitors	Acute:	→ or ↑ WASO → TST ↓ REM → Delta	May cause insomnia or hypersomnia May produce eye movements in NREM sleep
Trazodone	Acute:	↓ WASO → or ↓ REM → or ↑ Delta	Less suppression of REM sleep than tricyclics and MAOIs
Lithium		↓ REM ↑ Delta	
Phenothiazine		↑ TST ↑ Delta	Effects mild and variable, according to specific agent REM effects inconsistent
Reserpine		↑ WASO ↑ REM ↑ Delta	Can cause insomnia, nightmares
Yohimbine		↑ REM ↓ Delta	
Clonidine		→ TST ↑ WASO ↑ Stage shifts ↓ REM	Can cause insomnia, daytime sedation
α-Methyldopa		↑ REM (1st half of night) ↓ Delta	Can cause nightmares
Diuretics		↑ WASO	Probably acts via nocturia, hemodynamic effects
Cimetidine		↑ Delta	Can cause daytime sedation
Baclofen		↑ TST	
L-Dopa		→ TST → or ↑ REM → Delta	In toxic doses, causes insomnia, delirium
Methysergide		→ TST → or ↑ REM ↑ Delta	
γ-Hydroxybutyrate		↑ TST	
Steroids		↑ WASO	

↑, increased; ↓, decreased; →, unchanged; EEG, electroencephalography; MAOIs, monoamine oxidase inhibitors; NREM, non–rapid eye movement; REM, rapid eye movement; SL, sleep latency; TST, total sleep time; WASO, wakefulness after sleep onset.

Adapted from Buysse DJ, Reynolds CF. Insomnia. *In* MJ Thorpy (ed), Handbook of Sleep Disorders. New York: Marcel Dekker, 1990:375.

TREATMENT OF SLEEP PROBLEMS IN PATIENTS WITH PSYCHIATRIC ILLNESS

Sleep disturbances and psychiatric symptoms frequently co-occur, and like the chicken and the egg question, it can be difficult to determine which came first, whether they are causally related, or even which to target first in treatment. Comorbidity and symptom overlap between sleep disorders and psychiatric disorders can complicate the assessment process for both the mental health specialist and the sleep generalist. For example, insomnia may be a symptom of depression, or it may be a precursor, a residual symptom, or a side effect of a depression treatment. Regardless of the classification, which can be difficult to determine, it is most important that the clinician assess for and try to resolve sleep symptoms, as there is clear risk for the onset of depression, exacerbating symptom severity, and insomnia is strongly related to depression relapse.[14]

Patients who present to sleep disorders centers frequently exhibit symptoms of psychopathology, which may or may not be due to psychiatric illness. Often, physicians who have exhausted all routine laboratory assessments and medical interventions in the effort to diagnose and treat a person with an undiscovered sleep problem refer the patient to a psychiatrist. Because many sleep practitioners do not have extensive psychiatric training, it is often necessary to engage the assistance of a psychiatrist or psychologist to evaluate a patient with suspected or known psychiatric illness. Psychological tests such as the Inventory of Depressive Symptoms, Beck Depression Inventory, and State Trait Anxiety Inventory are useful for screening patients with sleep disorders for psychopathology. These tests alone, however, are somewhat limited. Many patients with untreated organic sleep disorders such as sleep apnea show changes in psychological tests that are suggestive of psychopathology, but the changes may resolve following effective treatment of the disorder; continued assessment is warranted, however, as symptoms may not resolve.

Likewise, may patients with psychiatric illness often have sleep symptoms. The sleep disorders specialist may be called upon to help determine whether there is an underlying organic disorder such as sleep apnea, RLS, or periodic limb movements that may cause or contribute to the symptoms. In addition, the sleep specialist can be especially helpful in assessing and correcting behaviors that contribute to sleep impairment. The sleep disorders specialist may also be in a position to recommend sleep-specific pharmacotherapy, typically involving sedatives and stimulants (i.e., onset of action, duration of action, relative toxicity, drug interactions, drug withdrawal effects, and relative effects on alertness and sleep parameters).

There is mounting objective evidence to support the claim that behavioral/CBT interventions are useful in improving insomnia in patients with psychiatric illness (see Smith et al.[207] for a thorough review of relevant issues and outcome data for CBT interventions for secondary insomnia). Behavioral interventions include stimulus control instructions[208] and sleep restriction.[209] CBT interventions usually include an additional cognitive component, such as correcting dysfunctional beliefs about sleep (e.g., "If I don't get enough sleep tonight, I'll fall apart tomorrow"), although no evidence shows that CBT interventions are superior to straight behavioral interventions. In addition, there are data to support the argument that patients with chronic insomnia have sustained benefit with and without adjunctive sedative administration.[210,211] Most evidence comes from studies in depression and PTSD. Given the links between sleep and psychopathology described earlier, however, such behavioral interventions may prove quite valuable for individuals with other anxiety disorders, those with dementia, or within pediatric populations.

The severity of the insomnia of a psychiatric patient often parallels the severity of the illness. Therefore, the aggressiveness of medication and behavioral management of insomnia in psychiatric patients should parallel the severity of psychiatric symptoms. Patients with severe sleep disturbance due to schizophrenia or affective psychosis often require sedating neuroleptics as well as adjunctive sedative-hypnotics. Patients with schizophrenia and affective disorders with nocturnal hallucinations may need additional neuroleptic medication for better control of their illness to reduce nighttime hallucinations. Chronic psychiatric illnesses with associated insomnia are much more difficult to manage and may require long-term insomnia treatment with medications such as benzodiazepine receptor agonists. Psychiatric illnesses that are intermittent (e.g., major depression) may require hypnotics only during the active phase of the illness.

In some instances, medications used in psychiatric patients aggravate an existing organic sleep problem or insomnia. Antidepressants, antipsychotics, and antihistamines may aggravate RLS. Sometimes, nocturnal akathisia, which has symptoms very similar to RLS, is caused by neuroleptic compounds. Medications such as the monoamine oxidase inhibitors, fluoxetine, sertraline, bupropion, protriptyline, and buspirone, which have stimulant properties, may aggravate insomnia. Despite studies showing sleep disruption with stimulating antidepressants, however, patients placed on these compounds often report subjective improvement in their sleep, particularly with the SSRIs.

There is little evidence that treatment of insomnia due to depression without other interventions such as psychotherapy, antidepressant therapy, or ECT relieves depression.[212] Combinations of antidepressants and sedatives can improve insomnia without interfering with the antidepressant effectiveness or onset of action.[213,214] Pharmacotherapy for insomnia in patients with affective disorders can be addressed in one of several ways: The patient can be given an antidepressant alone, a combination of two antidepressants, a benzodiazepine sedative alone, or a combination of a sedative and an antidepressant. Some antidepressants, such as most of the tricyclic antidepressants and trazodone, have the advantage of causing sedation without the addition of another drug but are limited by side effects (e.g., dry mouth, constipation, myoclonus), toxicity, and daytime cognitive and alertness impairment. SSRIs are sometimes combined with other sedating antidepressants such as trazodone to improve sleep. The potential for drug interaction between some antidepressants[215] as well as development of the "serotonin syndrome" exists in this scenario. Additionally, there is little empirical evidence to support the use of trazodone in primary insomnia, despite recent surveys that suggest that trazodone is the most widely prescribed medication to treat insomnia in the United States. There are no studies of long-term use of trazodone for treating insomnia,[216] and unfortunately, little treatment outcomes research for secondary insomnia (due to psychiatric or other conditions) exists despite its widespread prevalence.

While there are case reports that tricyclic antidepressant and SSRIs can lead to or exacerbate RLS symptoms, this has not always been supported. Brown and colleagues[217] did not find an association between antidepressant use and RLS using a retrospective chart review sample of 200 consecutive patients presenting with sleep-onset insomnia. Leutgeb and Martus[218] compared RLS symptoms before and after 6 months of tricyclic or SSRI pharmacotherapy in a sample of 243 mood or anxiety disorders patients. Antidepressant pharmacotherapy was not found to be a significant risk factor for RLS symptoms, although nonopioid analgesics, usually with caffeine, were associated with increased risk of RLS.

The appropriate selection of a sedative-hypnotic for patients with psychiatric illness is often more difficult than for the general population. There is greater potential for adverse drug interactions with multiple psychotropic medications than between most sedatives prescribed along with medications used for other conditions. Particular attention must be paid to the duration of action of sedatives in patients with anxiety. There may be a tendency for increased daytime anxiety in patients taking short- and intermediate-acting sedative-hypnotics.[219] Alternative approaches include using multiple doses of intermediate-acting benzodiazepines (e.g., lorazepam, alprazolam, oxazepam) during the day, and using the same medication at bedtime as a hypnotic. Another approach is to use a long-acting antianxiety agent such as diazepam,

clonazepam, or chlordiazepoxide less frequently during the day and also as a hypnotic. As most of the intermediate- and long-acting benzodiazepine antianxiety agents have delayed onset, it is often best that they be given approximately an hour before bedtime for the sedative properties to have enough time to take effect. Patients with nocturnal panic attacks may benefit from benzodiazepines such as alprazolam, estazolam, or clonazepam. In addition, various antidepressants, β blockers, calcium channel blockers, and α agonists may be useful.

As with all patients, those with chronic psychiatric illness with associated chronic insomnia require careful follow-up to ensure that no long-term adverse effects result from psychotropic drugs and, in cases in which abusable medications are necessary, that the patients do not develop tolerance leading to excessive usage. When any patient presents to the sleep disorders center taking an excessive amount of a sedative with abuse potential, or taking a normal dose of a sedative for a prolonged period, it is very important to determine whether there is a psychiatric illness or any underlying tendency to abuse drugs. Some patients with sleep disorders such as persistent psychophysiologic insomnia and periodic limb movements may not have had the underlying causes of their insomnia identified, and therefore resort to long-term use of sleeping medication. These individuals may increase the dose of the sedative to quite large amounts to achieve sleep, yet do not experience the craving or euphoria often associated with substance abuse. For them, it is quite important to identify the underlying causes of the sleep problem. After long-term use of large doses of sedatives, it is very important that the patient be tapered gradually. After treatment of underlying organic sleep disorders and training in sleep hygiene and relaxation skills, these patients may be able to sleep without the help of habituating medication.

CONCLUSION

Although sleep quality and duration impact affective function, the pathophysiologic processes by which sleep is linked to daytime mood and functioning are poorly understood. Continued research efforts to expand our knowledge of sleep and its functions will improve our understanding of the pathophysiology of disordered sleep generally and its role in the development and maintenance of psychopathology, and pave the way for continued improvements in behavioral and pharmacologic interventions to improve outcome and functioning in individuals with sleep and/or psychiatric disorders.

⊗ REFERENCES

A full list of references are available at www.expertconsult.com

CHAPTER 33

Sleep Disturbances in General Medical Disorders

Sudhansu Chokroverty

INTRODUCTION

General medical disorders may cause a disruption of neuroanatomic substrates for sleep/wakefulness by indirectly affecting the sleep/wake-promoting neurons through metabolic, toxic, or anoxic disturbances. It is therefore incumbent upon the sleep specialist, general internist, and primary care physician to have a high index of suspicion for the presence of sleep disorders so that appropriate steps for assessment and management of these patients can be instituted. This chapter deals with medical disorders—excluding neurologic diseases—associated with sleep dysfunction, which may cause added distress to the existing complaints related to the medical disorders and which may need special attention. For example, if a patient suffering from bronchial asthma or coronary artery disease, complaining of difficulty initiating or maintaining sleep, not having restorative sleep, and excessive daytime sleepiness, seeks the attention of a physician, these complaints are obviously causing additional distress and need special attention. The second edition of the International Classification of Sleep Disorders (ICSD-2)[1] does not list a separate category of sleep disturbances associated with medical disorders, in contrast to the previous edition. These medical disorders are mentioned within the eight major categories of sleep disorders as well as in Appendix A of the ICSD-2.[1]

Gislason and Almqvist[2] did an epidemiologic study in a random sample of 3201 Swedish men ages 30–69 years. Difficulty initiating or maintaining sleep and too little sleep were the major complaints, followed by excessive daytime somnolence or too much sleep. Sleep maintenance problems became more frequent with increasing age. The following conditions were associated with the sleep complaints: systemic hypertension, bronchitis and bronchial asthma, musculoskeletal disorders, obesity, and diabetes mellitus. The authors suggested that the reported increased mortality among patients with sleep complaints might be related to the intercurrent somatic diseases.

In a questionnaire of 100 adult male medical and surgical patients in a teaching hospital in Melbourne, Australia, Johns and coworkers[3] found sleep duration to be the same as that in the general population. The sleep duration decreased from 20 to 50 years of age, then increased again after age 60. Daytime sleep duration increased with age. These authors found that increasing age and ischemic heart disease were mostly associated with long-term sleep disturbances. The aging process per se may not be the primary cause of sleep disturbances, particularly insomnia, among elderly people as noted from a 3-year longitudinal study comprising 6800 men and women age 65 and older.[4] Risk factors associated with insomnia in this study included several medical conditions such as heart disease, cancer, diabetes, and stroke as well as hip fractures and use of sedatives. Several other epidemiologic studies[5–7] attest to the frequent association of sleep disturbances with medical disorders.

When a patient presents to a sleep specialist with sleep disturbance, with the complaint of either insomnia or hypersomnia, the first important step is to obtain a detailed medical history and other histories, followed by physical examination to uncover a cause for the sleep disturbance. Often, the patient presents to an internist or a family practice physician, who may then refer for a consultation to a sleep specialist if there are sleep complaints. Therefore, a comprehensive knowledge of major medical disorders that may present with sleep disturbance is essential. In this chapter, a review of the salient clinical diagnostic points of some important medical disorders presenting with sleep disturbance is offered, along with information on key laboratory investigations.

MEDICAL DISORDERS THAT CAUSE SLEEP DISTURBANCES

Several medical disorders are associated with sleep disturbances, as listed here. The mechanisms and general features of sleep disturbances in medical disorders are also briefly described. For further details, readers should consult general textbooks of internal medicine.

- Cardiovascular diseases: cardiac arrhythmia, congestive cardiac failure, ischemic heart disease, nocturnal angina
- Intrinsic respiratory disorders: chronic obstructive pulmonary disease, asthma (including nocturnal asthma), restrictive lung disease
- Gastrointestinal diseases: peptic ulcer disease, reflux esophagitis
- Endocrine diseases: hyperthyroidism, hypothyroidism, diabetes mellitus, growth hormone deficiency and excess
- Renal disorders: chronic renal failure, sleep disturbances associated with renal dialysis
- Hematologic disorders
- Rheumatic disorders, including fibromyalgia syndrome
- Dermatologic disorders
- Acquired immunodeficiency syndrome
- Lyme disease
- Chronic fatigue syndrome
- Medical and surgical disorders of patients in medical and surgical intensive care units
- African sleeping sickness (trypanosomiasis)
- Cancer
- Medication-related sleep-wake disturbances

Mechanism of Sleep Disturbances in Medical Disorders

Sleep disturbance may have an adverse effect on the course of a medical illness. Thus, a vicious cycle may result from the effect of sleep disturbance on the medical disease and the effect of the medical illness on sleep architecture.

Sleep may be disturbed in medical disorders by a variety of mechanisms, including

- Indirect effects on the hypnogenic neurons in the diencephalon and brain stem, and respiratory neurons in the brain stem, by metabolic disturbances (e.g., renal, hepatic, or respiratory failure; electrolyte disturbances; hypoglycemia or hyperglycemia; ketosis; toxic states)
- Adverse effects on sleep organization and sleep structure by drugs used to treat medical illness
- Disturbances of circadian rhythm (i.e., sleep-wake schedule)
- Effects on the peripheral respiratory mechanism (including respiratory muscles) causing respiratory sleep disorder
- Esophageal reflux, which may be due to prolongation of acid clearance of the lower esophagus, aspiration, and reflex mechanism (see Chapter 7)
- Adverse effect on sleep structure after prolonged immobilization resulting from medical disorders
- Dysfunction of the autonomic nervous system caused by medical disorder (e.g., diabetes mellitus, amyloidosis)

General Features of Sleep Disturbances in Medical Illness

Sleep architecture, sleep continuity, and sleep organization may be affected in a variety of medical illnesses. Patients may present with either insomnia or hypersomnolence, but most medical disorders present with insomnia. Some patients may have a mixture of insomnia and hypersomnolence (e.g., those with chronic obstructive pulmonary disease or nocturnal asthma). Other sleep complaints include abnormal motor activity and behavior intruding into sleep (parasomnias), sleep-related breathing problems with sleep fragmentation and snoring during sleep, and disturbances of normal sleep-wake rhythm (circadian rhythm disorders). Table 33–1 lists the medical causes of insomnia. For medical causes of hypersomnolence, see Table 3–1 in Chapter 3.

Patients with insomnia may complain of lack of initiation of sleep, inability to maintain sleep, repeated arousals at night, and early morning awakening. Daytime symptoms of fatigue, inability to concentrate, irritability, anxiety, and sometimes depression may be related to the sleep deprivation. Polysomnographic (PSG) findings include prolonged sleep latency, reduction of rapid eye movement (REM) sleep and slow-wave sleep (SWS), more than

---

TABLE 33–1 Medical Causes of Insomnia

- Congestive heart failure
- Ischemic heart disease
- Nocturnal angina
- Chronic obstructive pulmonary disease
- Bronchial asthma, including nocturnal asthma
- Peptic ulcer disease
- Reflux esophagitis
- Rheumatic disorders, including fibromyalgia syndrome
- Lyme disease
- Acquired immunodeficiency syndrome
- Chronic fatigue syndrome

10 awakenings per night, frequent stage shifts, early morning awakening, increased waking after sleep onset (WASO), and increased percentage of wakefulness and stage 1 non-REM (NREM) sleep.

Patients with hypersomnolence may present with repeated daytime somnolence, fatigue, depression, headache, and intellectual deterioration related to repeated sleep-disordered breathing (SDB) and hypoxemia.[8] PSG findings consist of SDB, repeated arousals with oxygen desaturation at night, sleep fragmentation, sleep stage shifts, reduced SWS, shortened sleep-onset latency on the Multiple Sleep Latency Test, and sometimes REM sleep abnormalities.[8]

Systemic medical disorders may cause neurologic disturbances, which in turn may cause sleep disturbances either directly by affecting sleep-wake systems in the central nervous system (CNS) or indirectly by affecting breathing. Sleep-related breathing dysfunction and neurologic illness are described in Chapter 29.

SPECIFIC MEDICAL DISORDERS AND RELATED SLEEP DISTURBANCES

Cardiovascular Disease

It is generally well known that sleep disturbances may occur in cardiovascular diseases, particularly in patients with ischemic heart disease, myocardial infarction, or congestive cardiac failure (CCF). Cardiac arrhythmias and sudden cardiac death at night are also known to occur, although adequate objective tests, including PSG study to document such disturbances, are lacking.

Ischemic Heart Disease

A careful inquiry into history is most important in making the diagnosis. The patient complains of a sense of tightness in the middle of the chest and a bandlike feeling around the chest. The pain is often induced by exertion and relieved by rest. Generally, it lasts only a few minutes. When the patient complains of pain on lying supine, it is known as *angina decubitus*, whereas pain that awakens the patient at night is known as *nocturnal angina*. Infrequently, the pain results from coronary artery spasm accompanied by transient ST-segment elevation in the electrocardiogram (ECG), and the entity is then known as *Prinzmetal's* or *variant angina*. The condition is most common in middle-aged men but may affect postmenopausal women. Complications include cardiac arrhythmias; left ventricular failure; acute myocardial infarction; and sudden cardiac, often nocturnal, death.

Sleep disturbances are very common in patients with ischemic heart disease. Pain may awaken the patient, causing frequent awakenings and reduced sleep efficiency. Obstructive sleep apnea syndrome (OSAS) is associated with arterial hypoxemia causing cardiac ischemia. Simultaneous recording of an ECG may show ST-segment depression at least 1 mm below the horizontal, whereas ST-segment elevation occurs in Prinzmetal's or variant angina. Often, the patient complains of discomfort in the arms during the retrosternal pain. Pain may sometimes radiate to the epigastrium or to the neck and the jaw. It may be accompanied by shortness of breath. An ECG is essential for the diagnosis of ischemic heart disease or myocardial infarction. Coronary angiography provides information about the site of coronary artery occlusion.

Treatment consists of avoiding exertion for patients susceptible to angina attacks and administration of drugs such as nitrates, β blockers, and calcium channel antagonists. Patients with severe symptoms that persist despite medical treatment may need surgical treatment in the form of coronary artery bypass grafting or stenting.

Factors contributing to myocardial ischemia, infarction, or arrhythmia include increased sympathetic surge during REM sleep, increased platelet aggregability, hypotension associated with SWS and altered balance between fibrinolytic and thrombotic factors, oxygen desaturation, and increased ventricular diastolic pressure and volume associated with supine posture. There is also increased risk of CCF among patients with the onset of myocardial infarction at night.[9] Patients with diabetes, advancing age, and impaired ventricular function are at an increased risk for developing nocturnal myocardial infarction.[10–13]

"Non-dippers" (those hypertensive patients whose blood pressure during sleep does not decline or declines less than 10% from daytime to nighttime readings) have significant risk for developing cardiac arrhythmias, stroke, and death from cardiovascular disease.[14–16] Newman et al.[17,18] have shown that daytime sleepiness associated with sleep disturbances in elderly patients, especially women, is a predictor of cardiovascular morbidity and mortality and CCF.

Nocturnal Angina, Myocardial Infarction, and Sleep Disturbance. Nocturnal angina or myocardial infarction may cause frequent arousal, sleep maintenance insomnia, and impaired sleep efficiency. Nocturnal angina is known to occur during both REM and NREM sleep stages. Karacan and coworkers[19] found increased sleep-onset latency, reduced SWS, decreased sleep efficiency, and very little change in REM sleep on PSG study in 10 patients with a history of nocturnal angina. In a later study, Karacan and coworkers[20] followed four patients with myocardial infarction in the intensive care unit (ICU) continuously from the second to the sixth day and found increased wakefulness, reduced REM sleep, absent SWS, and a partial breakdown in the circadian cycling. It should be noted that circadian susceptibility to myocardial infarction (attacks are most likely between midnight and 6:00 AM) has been described.[21,22] Broughton and Baron[23] found decreased sleep efficiency, increased sleep stage shifts, increased awakenings, and decreased REM sleep in 12 patients with acute myocardial infarction studied in the ICU. Sleep patterns became normal by the ninth day of the illness.

In several epidemiologic studies there is a clear relationship between increased cardiovascular morbidity and mortality and sleep disturbances associated with SDB. Patients with coronary artery disease (CAD) and obstructive sleep apnea (OSA) may have an increased cardiac risk due to nocturnal myocardial ischemia triggered by apnea-associated oxygen desaturation. In many case-controlled studies in the past, an association between sleep apnea and increased risk of myocardial infarction was noted.[24–29] Epidemiologic data from the Sleep Heart Health Study demonstrated a linear relationship between the apnea-hypopnea index (AHI) and risk of CAD, including myocardial infarction.[30] In a population-based prospective study including a postal questionnaire regarding sleep complaints in a random sample of 1870 subjects, Mallon et al.[31] provided evidence at the 12-year follow-up that there was an association between difficulty falling asleep and CAD mortality in men.

A high prevalence of OSA in patients with CAD has been noted in several studies.[26,28,29,32–39] An important study was done by Marin et al.[39] This was an observational and not a randomized controlled study, recruiting men with OSA or simple snorers from a sleep clinic and a population-based sample of healthy men matched for age and body mass index with untreated severe OSA patients (total $N = 1651$). All had PSGs and were followed up at least once per year for a mean of 10.1 years; compliance with treatment of OSA with continuous positive airway pressure (CPAP) was checked with a built-in meter. Multivariate analysis adjusted for confounders showed that untreated severe OSA increased the risk of fatal and nonfatal myocardial infarction and stroke compared with healthy participants; CPAP treatments reduced this risk. The authors also noted that mild to moderate untreated OSA patients had an intermediate risk for these events, indicating a dose-effect relationship. A similar effect was also observed by Schaffer et al.[35] The survival benefit to CPAP therapy in these patients as shown by Marin et al.[39] is also supported by other studies.[36,40,41] Prior to the study by Marin et al.,[39] long-term beneficial effects of CPAP treatment in patients with OSA and CAD were shown by Milleron et al.[42] These authors treated 25 of 54 patients with OSA and CAD (29 declined treatment). At a mean follow-up of 87 months, the treatment significantly reduced the risk of occurrence of cardiovascular death, acute coronary syndrome, hospitalization for heart failure, or need for coronary revascularization. Similar results were observed by Doherty et al.,[43] who reported that deaths from cardiovascular disease were more common in an untreated group (61 patients who were intolerant to CPAP) than in a CPAP group (107 patients) after follow-up of 7.5 years.[43]

In an important study, Kripke and associates[44] noted increased mortality rates among patients with ischemic heart disease, stroke, and cancer who slept 4 hours or less, or more than 10 hours. Wingard and Berkman,[45] in their study of approximately 7000 adults over a period of 9 years, also found excessive mortality from ischemic heart disease in short sleepers (less than 7 hours) and long sleepers (more than 9 hours). Poor sleep was thus associated with increased risk of future cardiovascular morbidity or mortality. These results, however, were contradicted by a later study by Mallon et al.[31] observing that short or long sleep duration did not influence the risk of CAD mortality or total mortality for either gender. In a later study, Meisinger et al.[46] reported a modest association between short sleep duration and difficulty maintaining sleep, and risk of occurrence of myocardial infarction in middle-aged women, but not men, from a general population sample in Germany.

Heart Failure

Heart failure is the leading cause of disability in individuals older than 65 years. Prevalence increases with age. Heart failure may be systolic (with reduced ejection fraction) or diastolic (with preserved ejection fraction), and both obstructive and central apneas, including periodic breathing (Cheyne-Stokes breathing [CSB]), have been observed in such patients, although the incidence of sleep apnea in diastolic failure is not definitely known.[47] A large percentage of the OSA population has heart failure.[30] About 40–80% of patients with systolic heart failure (decreased ejection fraction accompanied by shortness of breath and pulmonary congestion) have sleep apnea. Thirty percent to 60% of patients with systolic heart failure have predominantly central apnea and 5–32% have predominantly obstructive apnea.[48–53] The prevalence of sleep apnea in isolated diastolic heart failure (heart failure with preserved ejection fraction) is not known but also appears to be high in limited studies.[54,55] Atrial fibrillation and hypertension are commonly associated with diastolic heart failure.[54,55] Diabetes mellitus, CAD, and hyperlipidemia are commonly associated with systolic heart failure.[54,55] Survival at 1–5 years in both groups is approximately equal. There is about 25% mortality at 1 year and 65% mortality at 5 years in patients with heart failure. Sleep apnea is more common in men with heart failure than in those without heart failure.

There is convincing evidence of an association of hypertension and sleep apnea,[56–63] and treatment of OSA with CPAP may improve such hypertension and prevent possible cerebrovascular disease and myocardial infarction.[64–76] A number of well-designed studies, however, have failed to show a significant improvement in blood pressure after CPAP treatment.[77–80] Systolic heart failure is also associated with OSA and central apneas, including CSB, which improve after treatment[81–86] (see later).

Mechanism of Central Apnea and Cheyne-Stokes Breathing in Heart Failure. CSB (see Fig. 29–6B in Chapter 29) is characteristic of systolic heart failure.

The following three factors may be responsible for CSB in heart failure[47,48,87–89]:

1. *Increased arterial circulation time* (due to cardiomegaly, decreased cardiac output, and increased pulmonary blood volume). This is very common in systolic heart failure, but in diastolic heart failure circulation time may be normal.

2. *Central and peripheral chemoreceptor gain;* for example, increased chemoreceptor gain will cause increased ventilation in response to increased partial pressure of arterial carbon dioxide ($PaCO_2$) and decreased partial pressure of arterial oxygen (PaO_2).

3. *Decreased functional residual capacity (FRC),* due to a combination of pleural effusion, enlarged heart, and pulmonary congestion causing decreased pulmonary compliance in patients with heart failure. FRC decreases further in the supine position, promoting CSB. Decreased FRC causes underdamping—that is, for a given change in ventilation (e.g., transient cessation of breathing), there is an increased response to changes in PaO_2 and $PaCO_2$.[48] CSB occurs during sleep and wakefulness, although it is pronounced during sleep. In many patients with heart failure, there is low $PaCO_2$ and a failure of rise of $PaCO_2$ during sleep, unlike that which occurs in normal individuals as a result of increased venous return in the supine position, increased respiratory rate, and increased ventilation. Heart failure patients with $PaCO_2$ less than 35 mm Hg have a high probability for developing central apnea because the low $PaCO_2$ is close to the apnea threshold (i.e., the level of $PaCO_2$ at which breathing ceases due to a lack of chemoreceptor stimulation).

Mechanism of Obstructive Apnea in Heart Failure. CSB itself may predispose to obstructive apnea by decreasing the tone of the upper airway dilator muscles at the end of the ventilatory cycle (the lowest point or nadir). Other factors for obstructive apnea in heart failure include venous congestion in the oropharyngeal region in right heart failure, especially in the supine position, and comorbid obesity. The presence of periodic breathing (e.g., CSB) in heart failure may increase the morbidity and mortality and so it is important to be aware of this. Treatment with CPAP/bilevel positive airway pressure (BIPAP) with or without low-flow (1–2 L/min) supplemental oxygen inhalation may improve the pattern of breathing.

Clinical-Pathologic Consequences of Heart Failure and Sleep Apnea. The common symptoms of heart failure in obstructive apnea patients include paroxysmal nocturnal dyspnea, orthopnea, daytime sleepiness and fatigue, and sleep-onset and maintenance insomnia. Recurrent episodes of apnea and hypopneas accompanied by repeated arousals, hypoxemia, hypercapnia, and sympathetic activation adversely affect cardiovascular function, particularly in patients with CAD and incipient cardiac

dysfunction. Indications for overnight PSG in these patients include witnessed apneas, habitual snoring, nocturnal angina, and unrefreshing restless sleep; overnight PSG is also indicated in patients requiring cardioverters or defibrillators, those requiring cardiac transplantation, and those with cardiac arrhythmias.

There is an increased mortality associated with sleep apnea and heart failure.[90–92] He et al.[91] reported for the first time that, among 385 men with OSA, those with an apnea index of more than 20 per hour had an increased mortality when compared to those who had been treated with either CPAP or tracheotomy. This was a retrospective study, but later studies confirmed these earlier observations.[36,38] In a more recent study, Gami et al.[93] reported occurrence of sudden death from cardiac causes in 46% of patients with OSA as compared with 21% without OSA from midnight to 6:00 AM. It should be noted that several factors have been associated with the development and progression of CCF and increased mortality in OSA. The following factors are thought to be responsible for vascular endothelial dysfunction causing CAD, hypertension, and stroke: increased sympathetic activity, repeated hypoxemias, re-oxygenation, hypercapnia, hypercoagulopathy, release of endothelin, abnormal endothelial-dependent vasodilation and vascular growth factor and apoptosis, increased levels of inflammatory mediators, increased concentration of adhesion molecules, and oxidative stress.[48,94–97] Randomized controlled trials with CPAP in patients with OSA have shown improved cardiac function, sympathetic nervous system activity, quality of life, reduction of blood pressure, and reversal of the various neural, hormonal, and biochemical abnormalities, suggesting a cause-and-effect relationship.[98,99,100]

Principles of Treatment of Heart Failure and Sleep Apnea. Adequate treatment with diuretics, angiotensin-converting enzyme (ACE) inhibitors, and β blockers is the first prerequisite. For obstructive apneas, weight loss, nocturnal CPAP/BIPAP, and supplemental oxygen if needed are the recommended treatment (Table 33–2).

The gold standard for treatment of OSA in heart failure is treatment with CPAP or BIPAP (see Chapter 25). Adequate treatment of OSA in heart failure utilizing the measures outlined in Table 33–2 eliminates excessive daytime somnolence (EDS) and improves sleep of these patients. Such treatment may also decrease blood pressure in hypertensive patients and may help reduce the dose of antihypertensive medications. The treatment of OSA with CPAP increases ventricular ejection fraction significantly even within 1 month after therapy. The data on diastolic heart failure are limited. Arias et al.[101] reported that 15 of 27 consecutive patients with OSA had impaired left ventricular relaxation. The authors performed a double-blind sham-controlled crossover trial of CPAP for 12 weeks and noted an improvement in diastolic function.

TABLE 33–2 Principles of Treatment of Obstructive Sleep Apnea and Heart Failure

- Adequate treatment of heart failure
- Weight reduction if needed
- Follow general sleep hygiene measures
- Avoid alcohol and sedative-hypnotics
- Cessation of smoking
- Avoid supine position in subset of patients with positional OSA
- Treat any nasal abnormalities (e.g., septal deviation)
- Nocturnal CPAP/BIPAP
- Supplemental oxygen through CPAP if needed
- Dental appliances
- Upper airway surgery
- Tracheostomy

BIPAP, bilevel positive airway pressure; CPAP, continuous positive airway pressure; OSA, obstructive sleep apnea.

Treatment of central sleep apnea in heart failure is more difficult than treating OSA. The general measures for treating central apnea/CSB are listed in Table 33–3. Adequate treatment of heart failure may improve or eliminate periodic breathing and decrease circulation time due to increased stroke volume, decreased pulmonary congestion, increased FRC, and decreased sympathetic activity. Javaheri and others[53,86-88] have clearly shown improvement after aggressive treatment of heart failure with diuretics, ACE inhibitors, β blockers, and positive airway patient devices. CPAP treatment for central apnea has not produced as dramatic results as in OSA. Javaheri has shown that, in mild to moderate central apnea patients, overnight use of CPAP improved central apnea in 43% of patients with systolic heart failure.[102,103] The number of premature ventricular contractions, bigemini, and episodes of ventricular tachycardia also decreased. However, severe central apnea patients with heart failure did not respond to short-term CPAP treatment. Treatment lasting from 1 to 3 months with nasal CPAP in patients with heart failure showed a reduction in the AHI with desaturation and decrease in plasma and urinary norephenephrine, in addition to an increase in ventricular ejection fraction. There are other reports of quality of life[104] improvement and reduction of mortality in such patients after CPAP treatment,[39,81-85,105] although a large Canadian CPAP trial for congestive heart failure (CANPAP) contradicted this.[86] However, a later study by Arzt et al.[106] showed

TABLE 33–3 Principles of Treatment of Central Apnea and Cheyne-Stokes Breathing in Heart Failure

- Aggressive treatment of heart failure
- CPAP/BIPAP
- Adaptive pressure support servoventilation
- Atrial overdrive pacing or biventricular pacing
- Supplemental oxygen
- Cardiac transplantation
- Pharmacologic treatment (e.g., acetazolamide, theophylline, diazepam) in selective cases

BIPAP, bilevel positive airway pressure; CPAP, continuous positive airway pressure.

suppression of central sleep apnea by CPAP and transplant-free survival in heart failure. Cardiac transplantation will virtually eliminate central apnea, but a large number of such patients develop OSA due to the weight gain.[107] Cardiac pacing and cardiac resynchronization therapy have been shown to improve some patients with central apnea in heart failure.[108-112] Atrial pacing was thought to improve patients with obstructive apnea,[108,112] but other studies[113-116] did not support such an improvement. Nocturnal nasal supplemental oxygen therapy improves central apnea in heart failure patients.[117-121] Such treatment decreases muscle sympathetic nerve activity and improves left ventricular ejection fraction. Additional studies, however, are needed to determine if such treatment decreases the morbidity and mortality in patients with systolic heart failure.[48] Adaptive servoventilation has also been found to be useful in treatment of central apnea, including CSB, in patients with heart failure.[122-127]

Hypertension

A high prevalence (22–48%) of sleep apnea and related symptoms (e.g., EDS) has been noted in patients with systemic hypertension.[128-131] In contrast, studies by Escourrour and colleagues[132] found no significant difference between 21 hypertensive and 29 normotensive patients in sleep stage distribution and disorganization, AHI and duration, and arterial oxygen saturation (SaO_2). These 50 patients did not have airway obstruction as evidenced by values of forced expiratory volume in 1 second (FEV_1) or daytime hypoxemia, and were selected from 65 patients referred to a sleep clinic complaining of daytime hypersomnolence and snoring. The prevalence of hypertension in sleep apnea patients is approximately 50–90%.[5,133-144] In the Wisconsin Sleep Cohort study, a dose-response relationship between hypertension and the AHI as well as snoring has been described.[145,146] Furthermore, studies have confirmed that treatment of sleep apnea by nasal CPAP reduces blood pressure.[6,147]

Previously Stradling and Davies[148] made a persuasive argument based on a critical analysis of the literature, and taking into consideration the confounding variables (e.g., age, sex, smoking, obesity, and alcohol consumption), that there is no convincing evidence yet supporting the contention that OSA is a significant independent risk factor for sustained hypertension in humans. They suggested that a large randomized, controlled trial by CPAP on blood pressure in patients with a range of OSA severity is needed before CPAP can be recommended for asymptomatic OSA patients. Several other older reports support this conclusion.[7,149-152] Silverberg and Oksenberg,[153,154] however, contended that, even when the confounding factors are taken into consideration, OSA is an independent risk factor for hypertension and that treatment of OSA reduces daytime as well as nighttime blood pressure.

There is now convincing evidence of an association between hypertension and sleep apnea. Epidemiologic studies suggest that approximately 50% of patients with OSA have hypertension and about 30% of patients with hypertension develop OSA. Compelling evidence on the association between OSA and hypertension in humans has been provided by epidemiologic studies.[59,61,140,155] In drug-resistant hypertension, the prevalence of OSA is even higher; one study quoted a figure of 83%.[156] The Sleep Heart Health Study, in a prospective cross-sectional analysis of more than 6000 subjects, showed an independent association between hypertension and OSA.[59] A subgroup analysis by Bixler et al.[60] failed to show this association in subjects older than 65 years. The Wisconsin Sleep Cohort Study[61] was able to show that OSA is an independent risk factor for high blood pressure during a 4-year follow-up study that also showed a dose-response relationship between OSA and blood pressure independent of confounding factors. A population-based case-control study failed to show an association between OSA and high blood pressure in postmenopausal woman.[157] OSA has been considered to be an important risk factor for hypertension.[158] Several randomized, placebo-controlled studies revealed very significant reduction in mean blood pressure during sleep in the CPAP-treated group (see Chapter 25 for a detailed discussion). Although the results have so far been promising, further studies are needed to find the effect of CPAP therapy on high blood pressure in OSA patients.

"Non-dippers," those hypertensive patients whose blood pressure during sleep does not decline or declines less than 10% from daytime to nighttime readings, have significant risk for developing cardiac arrhythmias, stroke, and death from cardiovascular disease.[14–16]

In addition to systemic hypertension, OSA may also cause severe pulmonary arterial hypertension, particularly in patients with preexisting cardiopulmonary diseases.[48,158] Factors for developing pulmonary hypertension include several mechanisms such as repeated hypoxemia causing pulmonary vasoconstriction, left ventricular diastolic dysfunction resulting in increased left ventricular end-diastolic pressure, and possible pulmonary vascular remodeling.[48] It is important to remember that several long-term studies have shown improvement of pulmonary arterial hypertension following treatment of OSA with CPAP.

The recognition of the association of metabolic syndrome with OSA should direct attention to an early diagnosis and treatment with a view to preventing serious consequences such as stroke or myocardial infarction. The metabolic syndrome is a serious risk factor for cardiovascular disease and includes hypertension, hypertriglyceridemia (dyslipidemia), central obesity, glucose intolerance and insulin resistance (syndrome X) or hyperinsulinemia, and low levels of high-density lipoprotein cholesterol.[46,47,159] Kaplan[159] spoke about a deadly quartet: upper body obesity, glucose intolerance, hypertriglyceridemia, and hypertension.

Cardiac Arrhythmias

An understanding of the interaction between the autonomic nervous system (ANS), cardiac innervation, and sleep is important to appreciate the effects of sleep on cardiac rhythms. Readers are referred to Chapters 7 and 29 for such review. It is known that there is an imbalance between sympathetic and parasympathetic tone during REM and NREM sleep. During REM sleep there is an intermittent increase in sympathetic nerve activity, reaching even higher levels than in wakefulness. This surge causes intermittent increase in the heart rate and blood pressure, although at the same time, vagal tone (parasympathetic activity) is suppressed, causing irregular breathing, oxygen desaturation, and a few periods of apneas. These alterations in the sympathetic and parasympathetic balance can be clinically measured by recording heart rate variability (see also Chapter 7). The high-frequency (HF: 0.15–0.4 Hz) heart rate spectrum reflects parasympathetic tone, the low-frequency (LF: 0.01–0.05 Hz) spectrum reflects sympathetic tone, and the intermediate frequency (0.06–0.14 Hz) spectrum reflects a mixture of both activities. The LF/HF ratio is used in clinical practice to indicate overall sympathetic tone. Sudden cardiac death after myocardial infarction is associated with a decrease of heart rate variability. Based on heart rate variability studies, Bonnet and Arand[160] have clearly shown an increase in HF heart rate spectrum with a decrease of LF in NREM and an increase in LF and a decrease in HF in REM sleep and wakefulness.

A relationship between sleep and atrioventricular arrhythmias has been noted, but reports in the literature are somewhat contradictory. Atrial arrhythmias, such as atrial flutter, atrial fibrillation, paroxysmal atrial tachycardia,[161] and first- and second-degree atrioventricular block,[162] have been described in normal subjects during REM sleep, but no clear relationship between different sleep stages and atrial arrhythmias has emerged. A prominent sinus arrhythmia has been noted in several studies in normal subjects using Holter monitoring.[163] Brodsky and colleagues[164] monitored 24-hour continuous ECGs in 50 male medical students with no apparent heart disease and observed sinus pauses of 1.8–2.0 seconds' duration in 30% of them, as well as episodes of second-degree heart block (Mobitz type I) in another 6%. Guilleminault and associates[165] noted 42 episodes of sinus arrest in four young, healthy adults that lasted 2–9 seconds during REM sleep. No associated apneas or significant oxygen desaturation was observed. Osuna and Patino[166] observed REM-related sinus arrest in a subject without any associated OSA or oxygen desaturation. The incidence of nocturnal bradyarrhythmias decreases with advancing age.[167]

Contradictory results have been noted in human studies of the effects of sleep on ventricular arrhythmia, but the majority show an antiarrhythmic effect of sleep on ventricular premature beats (VPBs).[168] This seems to be due to enhanced parasympathetic tone during sleep, confirming protection against ventricular arrhythmia and sudden cardiac death. Pitzalis et al.[169] evaluated 45 patients with frequent premature ventricular contractions to find out whether the phenomenon of sleep suppression may be a sensitive and specific parameter for predicting the antiarrhythmic effect of β blockers and premature ventricular contractions. Based on Holter recordings, these authors concluded that sleep suppression of the premature ventricular contractions was a sensitive characteristic for identifying those patients with premature ventricular contractions who are likely to benefit from administration of β blockers. Ventricular arrhythmias are also noted to occur during arousal from sleep.[168] A classic example was provided by Wellens and colleagues,[170] who described a 14-year-old girl awakened from sleep by a loud auditory stimulus who had ventricular tachyarrhythmia. The authors postulated that increased sympathetic activity triggered these episodes, because they could be prevented by the β blocker propranolol.

Lown's group[171] noted reduction of VPBs by at least 50% in 22 subjects and 25–35% in 13 others during sleep. De Silva[172] noted reduction in VPBs in all stages except REM sleep, with stages 3 and 4 NREM sleep showing the most effect. Pickering and colleagues[173] described 12 untreated patients with frequent ventricular extrasystoles who showed a significant decrease in both the heart rate and extrasystoles during sleep. Intravenous propranolol, and to a lesser extent intravenous phenylephrine, produced a similar decrease in the heart rate and ventricular arrhythmias during wakefulness. These changes appear to be mediated by the ANS, the sympathetic system dominating the parasympathetic system. They found that the frequency of ventricular arrhythmias was similar in both REM and NREM sleep. Their findings are similar to those of Lown and colleagues.[171]

The observations of Pickering's group[173] also contrast with those of Smith and coworkers,[174] who studied 18 patients in a coronary care unit to document frequency of cardiac arrhythmias in wakefulness and sleep. They found no significant difference in the occurrence of ventricular or atrial premature contractions during sleep and wakefulness. Similarly, Richards et al.,[175] in a pilot overnight sleep study on nine patients with cardiovascular disease in the medical ICU, did not find any increase in incidence of dysrhythmias during any sleep stages or during sleep state in these critical care unit patients. Disturbed sleep in coronary care patients[23] may explain the discrepancies in these data.

Cardiac Arrhythmias, Autonomic Deficits, and Obstructive Sleep Apnea Syndrome. Several investigators[163,176–180] reported a variety of cardiac arrhythmias

in patients with OSAS. These arrhythmias are determined by the changes in the ANS. The most common is bradytachyarrhythmia alternating during apnea and immediately after termination of apnea. The other dysrhythmias consist of the following: sinus bradycardia with less than 30 beats/min; sinus pauses lasting from 2 to 13 seconds; second-degree heart block; and ventricular ectopic beats, including complex and multifocal ectopic beats, and ventricular tachycardia. There is a clear relationship between the level of SaO_2 and premature ventricular contractions and sleep apnea syndrome. Patients with SaO_2 below 60% are the most vulnerable. Hoffstein and Mateik,[181] using nocturnal PSG, prospectively studied 458 patients with OSAS. They found a prevalence rate of 58% of cardiac arrhythmias in these patients, and those with arrhythmias had more severe apnea and nocturnal hypoxemia than those without arrhythmias. Earlier studies showed a higher prevalence than more recent epidemiologic studies suggested. Roche et al.[182] performed a prospective study in 147 consecutive patients referred for assessment of OSAS. The authors found OSAS in over 45% with AHI ≥ 10. They found significantly more nocturnal paroxysmal asystole in OSAS patients than in controls (10.6% vs. 1.2%). They further noted that the number of episodes of bradycardia and pauses increased with the severity of OSAS. CPAP treatment followed for 1 year showed amelioration of arrhythmic events in OSAS patients, indicating the usefulness of CPAP treatment. The Sleep Heart Health Study[180] investigated 228 patients with severe sleep apnea (AHI > 30/hr) and 338 individuals without sleep apnea, and found a significant relationship between nonsustained ventricular tachycardia, bigeminy, trigeminy, or quadrigeminy and severe OSA.

ANS dysfunction was implicated in cardiovascular morbidity and mortality in OSAS (e.g., hypertension, left ventricular failure, increased risk of coronary or cerebral events).[183] CPAP treatment can prevent the cardiovascular risks associated with ANS dysfunction.

Gami et al.,[93] after reviewing the PSGs and death certificates of 112 Minnesota residents who have died suddenly from cardiac causes during the period from July 1987 to July 2003, concluded that OSAS patients had a peak sudden death from cardiac causes during sleeping hours, contrasting with the nadir of sudden death in those without OSAS and in the general population. Peltier et al.[184] recruited 32 patients complaining of EDS and snoring and performed PSG studies and 2-hour oral glucose tolerance tests as well as autonomic testing consisting of heart rate response to deep breathing, Valsalva maneuver, head-up tilt, and quantitative sudomotor axon reflex testing (QSART). These authors found that 19 of 24 patients with OSAS had abnormal glucose tolerance, and cardiac autonomic dysfunction was more strongly associated with impaired glucose regulation than OSAS. They concluded that cardiovagal and adrenergic dysfunction are responsible for cardiovascular adverse affects in OSAS, but the question remains whether impaired glucose regulation in such patients may have been responsible for such ANS dysfunction. Further studies using larger numbers of patients are needed to resolve this complex relationship between OSAS, autonomic function, and glucose regulation.

Sudden Cardiac Death

An analysis of the time of sudden cardiac death in 2203 individuals by Muller and associates[185] revealed a low incidence during the night and a high incidence from 7:00 to 11:00 AM. Similarly, nonfatal myocardial infarction and myocardial ischemic episodes are more likely to occur in the morning. It is known that sympathetic activity increases in the morning, causing increased myocardial electrical instability; thus, sudden cardiac death may result from a primary fatal arrhythmia.

LaRovere and associates[186] correlated increased cardiovascular mortality among patients with a first myocardial infarction with reduced baroreflex sensitivity. *Reduced baroreflex sensitivity* is defined as less slowing in heart rate for a given rise in arterial blood pressure, which indicates reduced vagal tone.

McWilliams[187] first suggested that ventricular fibrillation is the cause of sudden death and that sympathetic discharges play an important role in causing this fatal arrhythmia. During sleep, cardiovascular hemodynamic activity is decreased, as are heart rate and blood pressure, owing to withdrawal of sympathetic tone and increased vagal tone (see Chapter 7).

Reduced vagal tone, as measured by decreased heart rate variability in 24-hour Holter monitoring, was found by Kleiger and colleagues[188] to be a powerful predictor of increased mortality and sudden cardiac death after myocardial infarction. Autonomic imbalance (either sympathetic overactivity or parasympathetic underactivity) may trigger ventricular arrhythmias.[189]

Besides myocardial infarction, another clinical entity known as *long QT syndrome* may cause syncope or sudden death.[190–195] In long QT syndrome, the ECG shows a prolonged QT interval with abnormal U waves and torsades de pointes (polymorphic ventricular tachycardia).

Another cause of sudden death in young adults in the Western literature is the Brugada syndrome, described in 1992.[196–199] Patients with this syndrome present with life-threatening ventricular tachyarrhythmias without any structural cardiac lesions, and the ECG shows characteristic abnormalities of atypical right bundle branch block and ST-segment elevation over the right precordial leads. An involvement of the ANS is suggested, and abnormal ^{123}I-MIBG single-photon emission computed tomography (SPECT) uptake in Brugada syndrome indicating presynaptic sympathetic dysfunction of the heart has been reported by Wichter et al.[200] The Brugada syndrome has a genetic basis and links to mutation in *SCN5A*, the gene encoding the alpha subunit of the sodium channel. The ideal treatment suggested for this syndrome is implantation of a cardioverter-defibrillator. Sudden unexpected nocturnal death syndrome (SUNDS) is another disorder found in Southeast Asia with abnormal ECG findings similar to those noted in Brugada syndrome.[201,202] It has been suggested that both SUNDS and Brugada syndrome may have a common genetic and biophysical basis.[203]

Intrinsic Respiratory Disorders

Chronic Obstructive Pulmonary Disease

Chronic obstructive pulmonary disease (COPD), the fourth leading cause of death in the United States, is caused largely by cigarette smoking and also by α_1-antitrypsin deficiency. Patil et al.[204] in a retrospective review reported a 2.5% in-hospital mortality following acute exacerbation of COPD in 70,000 patients. The COPD is defined by the Global Initiative for Chronic Obstructive Lung Disease (GOLD) as an irreversible progressive airflow limitation causing an inflammatory response in the lung parenchyma giving rise to the clinical features of chronic bronchitis and emphysema.[205]

The salient clinical features include chronic cough, exertional dyspnea, tightness in the chest, and sometimes wheeze. Physical examination reveals inspiratory and expiratory rhonchi and crepitations. Patients with resting hypoxemia and hypercapnia may exhibit cyanosis. Investigations should include radiographic examination of the chest and pulmonary function tests. Complications include polycythemia, pulmonary hypertension, cor pulmonale, and cardiac arrhythmias.

To understand sleep disturbances, it is important to have some knowledge of gas exchange during sleep.[206] In COPD patients, Sao_2 and Pao_2 fall and $Paco_2$ rises during sleep; these values worsen during REM sleep.[207–210] In some patients SDB (e.g., apnea, hypopnea, or periodic breathing) is associated with reduced Sao_2 saturation, which is generally short lived (less than 1 minute) and mild to moderate in intensity.[211–213] Episodes of Sao_2 desaturation during REM sleep last more than 5 minutes and are more severe than in NREM sleep.[211,214,215] Physiologic changes in respiration, respiratory muscles, and control of breathing (see Chapter 7) during sleep adversely affect breathing in these patients. In COPD patients, two basic mechanisms worsen hypoxemia during sleep: alveolar hypoventilation, which is worse during REM sleep, and ventilation-perfusion mismatch.[216–219]

Other groups at risk for hypoxemia include the middle-aged and elderly (particularly men), postmenopausal women, and obese individuals.[206] Diminished ventilatory response to hypoxia and hypercapnia in some COPD patients contributes to increasing nocturnal oxygen desaturation.[206] Nocturnal hypoxemia causes repeated disruption and fragmentation of sleep architecture.[206]

COPD patients are traditionally divided into two groups, "pink puffers" and "blue bloaters."[220,221] Pink puffers generally have normal blood gases, hyperinflated lungs, no hypoxemia or hypercapnia, and no cardiomegaly or cor pulmonale.[206] In contrast, blue bloaters are generally hypoxemic and hypercapnic and have cor pulmonale, polycythemia, an enlarged heart, and reduced ventilatory response to hypoxemia and hypercapnia.[206] In general, blue bloaters have more severe hypoxemia of longer duration than pink puffers.[222,223] It should be noted that oxygen saturation for both groups is somewhat similar during wakefulness and in the upright position but is markedly different during sleep. The worse value is noted in blue bloaters. There are no absolute criteria for determining which groups of COPD patients has more severe nocturnal hypoxemia. Patients must be monitored at night, which is impractical considering the large number of patients who should be monitored. In some patients, COPD may coexist with OSAS—a condition called *overlap syndrome*, a term introduced by Flenley.[224] In a study[225] of 265 consecutive unselected OSAS patients, COPD was found to be present in 30 (11%) of these patients. Coexistence of COPD and OSAS results in a higher risk of pulmonary hypertension and CCF than in those with only OSAS.[216,217] In addition, Bednarek et al.[226] noted that the course of SDB is more severe in subjects with overlap syndrome, but these authors found that COPD in subjects with OSAS was as frequent as in the general population. OSAS has a major impact on quality of life in patients with overlap syndrome.[227] COPD patients who are hypoxemic during wakefulness become more hypoxemic during sleep, which is most severe during REM sleep. Alveolar hypoventilation and ventilation-perfusion mismatching are the two most important factors (alveolar hypoventilation being the predominant factor) for worsening of nocturnal hypoxemia in these patients. Hypoxemia is worse in patients with overlap syndrome.[228,229] The consequences of sleep hypoxemia include pulmonary hypertension due to hypoxic pulmonary vasoconstriction and cardiac arrhythmias.[230]

Changes in Sleep Architecture. Disturbances in sleep architecture in COPD patients have been reported by several authors.[208,231–238] These disturbances may be summarized as follows: a reduction of sleep efficiency, delayed sleep onset, increased WASO, frequent stage shifts, and frequent arousals. Arand and coworkers[231] correlated these findings with EDS. These patients are more likely to have difficulty with falling and staying asleep as well as EDS.[238] Chronic coughing and nocturnal wheezing in addition to nocturnal oxygen desaturation are mostly responsible for arousals from sleep in these patients.[239]

A number of factors cause sleep disturbances in COPD patients, resulting in disturbed electroencephalographic (EEG) sleep patterns, including the use of drugs that have a sleep-reducing effect, such as methylxanthines;

increased nocturnal cough resulting from accumulated bronchial secretions; and associated hypoxemia and hypercapnia.[216,240] In a study by Calverley,[236] administration of supplemental oxygen at 2 L/min by nasal cannula during sleep improved both oxygen saturation at night and sleep architecture, in terms of decreasing sleep latency and increasing all stages of sleep, including REM and SWS. Other reports did not note improved sleep quality, but the nocturnal hypoxemia did improve after oxygen administration.[231,232]

Aoki et al.[241] noted four patterns of SDB in the desaturation group of COPD patients: hypoventilation, paradoxical movement, periodic breathing, and unclassified pattern. Urbano and Mohsenin[237] listed the following eight mechanisms to explain nonapneic oxygen desaturation during sleep in COPD patients: decreased functional residual capacity, diminished hypoxic and hypercapnic ventilatory responses, impaired respiratory mechanical effectiveness, diminished arousal responses, respiratory muscle fatigue, diminished nonchemical respiratory drive, increased upper airway resistance, and the position of baseline saturation values while awake on the oxyhemoglobin dissociation curve.

Diagnostic Considerations. The most important test to document airflow obstruction and determine severity of COPD is spirometry. An FEV_1/FVC ratio (FEV_1 divided by forced vital capacity [FVC]) of less than 0.70 defines an obstructive defect. The COPD severity is determined by observing FEV_1 percent, predicted as follows: mild, less than 80%; moderate, 50–80%; severe, 30–50%; and very severe, less than 30%.[242] The spirometric measurements are performed before and after bronchodilator therapy, and other pulmonary function tests may also be important. In addition, pulse oximetry and arterial blood gas determinations, chest radiograph and high-resolution computed tomography chest scan, ECG, and determinations of α_1-antitrypsin levels may be useful. In patients suspected to have an associated OSA (overlap syndrome), an overnight PSG is essential.

Treatment Considerations. The cornerstone of treatment for COPD includes smoking cessation, bronchodilators or inhaled steroids, and pulmonary rehabilitation.[243] The ultimate goal is improvement of sleep quality and quality of life as a result of improvement of lung mechanics and gas exchange. All patients must avoid risk factors by instituting smoking cessation, getting early pneumococcal and influenza vaccinations, and receiving patient education and exercise training. The mainstay of COPD treatment is bronchodilators, which include anticholinergics and β_2-agonists. Metered-dose inhalers and nebulizers both work well. In severe cases, in addition to short- and long-acting bronchodilators, inhaled corticosteroids may be needed. In very severe cases, oral corticosteroids (but only on alternate days, using the lowest effective dose) combined with inhaled corticosteroids may have to be used. The role of supplemental oxygen therapy is discussed below. For patients not able to use inhaled medication, oral therapy including sustained-release theophylline in addition to a β_2-agonist or anticholinergic may have to be used. Theophylline can also be useful to control nighttime symptoms; however, nighttime symptoms may cause insomnia that itself needs separate treatment consideration. Insomnia is prevalent in COPD patients and needs to be treated to improve quality of life, however, use of hypnotics in the hypercapnic patient with severe COPD might be dangerous.[238,244] Benzodiazepines may be dangerous for elderly COPD patients, particularly those with overlap syndrome. Nonbenzodiazepine receptor drugs may be used with some benefit, but even these drugs may promote apnea, thus exacerbating hypoxemia in COPD patients. Ramelteon has been shown to be safe and efficacious in mild to moderate COPD and OSA patients; however, further research is needed to determine the safety in this population.[238] In patients with overlap syndrome, treatment with CPAP or BIPAP therapy may have to be used, but such treatment in these patients may not necessarily lead to an improvement in the coexistent COPD.[245] In very severe cases not responding adequately to medical therapy, lung volume reduction surgery or lung transplantation should be considered.

Treatment of Nocturnal Oxygen Desaturation.

Investigators have become aware of severe nocturnal hypoxemia in many patients with COPD.[207–210] This nocturnal hypoxemia may or may not be accompanied by sleep-related apnea, hypopnea, or periodic breathing and impairment of gas exchange.[211–213] It is clear that repeated or prolonged oxygen desaturation at night may cause cardiac arrhythmias and may lead to pulmonary hypertension and cor pulmonale.[246] In addition, patients with COPD show changes in sleep architecture[208,231–236] that may be related to the poor quality of sleep or may be secondary to nocturnal hypoxemia causing disruption of nocturnal EEG sleep stages. Oxygen desaturation during sleep in COPD patients can be identified only if PSG, using sleep staging or continuous monitoring of oxygenation, is performed. Several studies show episodes of oxygen desaturation during sleep in COPD patients. An important study by Wynne's group[211] showed that oxygen desaturation could be associated with two types of patients: those with SDB (apnea and hypopnea) and those without SDB. In patients with SDB, the desaturation typically lasts less than 1 minute and is mild. In the other group, the desaturation lasts 1–30 minutes and is associated with a profound decrease in oxygen saturation. The maximum episodes, lasting longer than 5 minutes, occur during REM sleep. Similar episodes of nocturnal oxygen desaturation have been described in patients with kyphoscoliosis,[247,248] in young patients with cystic fibrosis,[215,249,250] and in patients with interstitial lung disease.[251,252]

Modern treatment of nocturnal hypoxemia is administration of oxygen by nasal cannula at a slow flow rate, usually less than 2 L/min. The multiple-center study by the Nocturnal Oxygen Therapy Trial Group[253] and the Medical Research Council Working Party study[254] showed increased longevity for patients who used continuous supplemental oxygen at home. The Thoracic Society of Australia and New Zealand has published a position statement for oxygen therapy in COPD patients.[255]

Particular indications for supplemental oxygen can be summarized as follows: daytime PaO_2 below 55 mm Hg (SaO_2 below 88%) and daytime PaO_2 between 56 and 60 mm Hg (or SaO_2 of 89%) accompanied by signs of right-sided heart failure, unexplained polycythemia, pulmonary hypertension, and cor pulmonale,[240,256,257] as well as significant nocturnal or exercise-induced oxygen desaturation. Oxygen administration may also improve sleep architecture.[236] O'Reilly and Bailey[258] reviewed the published evidence for and against the use of long-term oxygen treatment in COPD, summarized the problems with current guidelines, and suggested important areas for future research. Earlier, Croxton and Bailey[259] published recommendations for long-term oxygen treatment for COPD for future research based on a National Heart, Lung and Blood Institute Workshop report.

The question of safety of oxygen administration has to be determined.[206] Some patients become more hypercapnic after oxygen administration.[208] Furthermore, Motta and Guilleminault[260] showed the worsening effects of administration of oxygen at night in patients with OSAS. Chokroverty et al.[261] reported worsening of apnea and prolongation of apnea after administration of 100% of oxygen in four patients with obesity-hypoventilation syndrome. Many patients with COPD may have OSA (overlap syndrome),[208,224,225] so physicians must be careful during administration of oxygen. Kearley and colleagues[262] have shown that administration of oxygen at 2 L/min reduces the episodic desaturation. Fleetham and associates[263] confirmed this finding, but Guilleminault and coworkers[213] contradicted these findings in five patients with excessive sleepiness associated with chronic obstructive airflow disease. The multiple-institution studies by the Nocturnal Oxygen Therapy Trial Group[253] showed the relative safety of oxygen therapy, however, including home oxygen. In COPD patients undergoing long-term oxygen therapy, it may be useful to monitor breathing and oxygen saturation by finger pulse oximetry during sleep at night.[264] The role of noninvasive intermittent positive pressure ventilation (NIPPV) to improve hypoxemia in COPD patients remains undetermined[265,266] in the absence of adequate clinical trials using a large number of patients.

Bronchial Asthma, Including Nocturnal Asthma

The characteristic clinical triad of asthma is the paroxysm of dyspnea, wheezing, and cough. The paroxysmal attacks of wheezing and breathlessness may occur at any hour of the day or night, and the nocturnal attacks are distributed at random without any relationship to a particular sleep stage. Nocturnal symptoms of wheezing and coughing at least once per week are noted in as many as 75% of asthmatics.[267] Breathing is characterized by prolonged expiration accompanied by wheezing and unproductive cough. There may be tightness of the chest and palpitation. The attacks typically last for 1–2 hours. When the attacks last hours, the disorder is called *acute severe asthma* or *status asthmaticus;* this is a life-threatening condition because of extreme respiratory distress and arterial hypoxemia.

Pulmonary function tests and radiographic examination of the chest are important for confirming the diagnosis of bronchial asthma. Abnormalities of certain pulmonary function tests (i.e., FEV_1, vital capacity [VC], peak expiratory flow [PEF]) suggest airflow obstruction. An overnight fall in PEF of over 15% associated with characteristic history is diagnostic of nocturnal asthma.[268] Chest radiography may reveal hyperinflated lungs and emphysema.

Sleep Disturbances in Bronchial Asthma. A variety of sleep disturbances have been noted in patients with asthma.[269–278] Janson and associates,[273] using questionnaires and sleep diaries, studied the prevalence of sleep complaints and sleep disturbances prospectively in 98 consecutive adult asthma patients attending an outpatient clinic in Uppsala, Sweden. Compared with 226 age- and sex-matched controls, the authors found a high incidence of sleep disturbances in asthma patients, including early morning awakening, difficulty in maintaining sleep, and EDS. Sleep disturbances in general consist of a combination of insomnia and hypersomnia. Polysomnographic studies may reveal disruption of sleep architecture as well as sleep apnea in some patients. Nocturnal exacerbation of symptoms during sleep is a frequent finding in asthma patients.[217,267,279]

There is evidence of progressive bronchoconstriction and hypoxemia during sleep in patients with asthma.[268,270] In an important study by Turner-Warwick,[271] 94% of 7729 asthmatics surveyed woke up at least once a night with symptoms of asthma, 74% at least 1 night a week, 64% at least 3 nights a week, and 39% every night. Nocturnal asthma is a potentially serious problem, as there is a high incidence of respiratory arrest and sudden death in adult asthmatics between midnight and 8:00 AM.[272,273]

To understand the relationship between the attacks of asthma and sleep stage and time of night, Kales and colleagues[274] studied six men and six women ages 20–45 years with PSG, each for 2–3 consecutive nights. They observed a total of 93 asthma attacks in these patients, 73 during NREM sleep and 18 during REM. They did not find a relationship between asthma attacks and sleep stage or time of night. Sleep pattern showed less total sleep time, frequent WASOs, early final awakenings, and reduced stage 4 sleep. Kales' group[275] observed similar findings in a PSG study of 10 asthmatic children. Montplaisir and colleagues[276] studied 12 asthmatics, eight of whom showed nocturnal attacks on sleep studies (six women and two men ages 20–51 years).

Two questionnaire surveys from the European community[277,278] found that bronchial asthma was associated with increased daytime sleepiness and impaired subjective quality of sleep (difficulty initiating sleep and early morning awakenings). One survey also noted increased prevalence of snoring and sleep-related apneas during sleep.[277] In the same survey, associated allergic rhinitis may have been a confounding variable. Twenty-six attacks were documented. No attacks occurred in stage 3 or 4 NREM sleep, nor were attacks more frequent during REM than NREM sleep. Thus, stage 3 and 4 sleep was "protective." Sleep efficiency was decreased. The number and duration of apneas were not significantly greater in asthmatics than in controls. Episodes of oxygen desaturation occurred only in the asthmatics. Sleep efficiency and waking time after sleep onset were altered in asthmatics. When there were no attacks, no difference in sleep architecture was noted between the controls and the patients, which suggested that sleep disturbances are characteristic of unstable asthma with nocturnal attacks.

A number of pathogenic mechanisms for sleep disturbances and nocturnal exacerbations of asthma have been suggested[217,267–269,280–283]:

- Sleep deprivation[284]
- Impaired ventilatory function in the supine posture[285]
- A decrease in circulating epinephrine at night, with an increase in histamine[286]
- Gastroesophageal reflux[287,288]
- Marked fluctuation in airway tone during REM sleep[289]
- Theophylline, a commonly used asthma drug that may cause insomnia[290,291] and increased episodes of gastroesophageal reflux[292,293] (a study by Hubert's group[294] found no such increase in asthmatics taking theophylline)
- Prolonged administration of corticosteroids in some asthmatics, which may have adverse effects on sleep and daytime functioning because of increased incidence of OSA[295,2960]
- Increased cellular inflammatory response in the bronchopulmonary region at night[282,297]
- Miscellaneous factors, including allergens (e.g., house dust); increased bronchial secretions combined with suppression of cough, especially during REM sleep; airway cooling at night; increased pulmonary resistance; altered bronchial reactivity; normal propensity for worsening of lung function during sleep; normally increased vagal tone during sleep, which may be a major cause of nocturnal bronchoconstriction as evidenced by circadian desynchronization studies and cholinergic blockade studies[298,299]; and suppressed

arousal response to bronchoconstriction in severe nocturnal asthma[282]

- Certain circadian factors[280–283]

Three pieces of evidence support the claim that circadian factors contribute to nocturnal exacerbation of asthma:

1. PEF typically is highest at 4:00 PM and lowest at 4:00 AM.[282] The variation is ordinarily approximately 5–8%, but if it reaches 50%, as it can in some asthmatics, there is the danger of respiratory arrest.[282] This circadian variation in PEF is related to sleep and not to recumbency or the hour.[281–283]

2. Airway resistance as measured breath by breath is not increased in normal individuals at night, but asthmatics show a circadian rhythm of increased airway resistance at night that is related to the duration of sleep and not to sleep stages.[282,300]

3. As with OSAS and COPD, nocturnal asthma is associated with SDB.[279,296,301,302]

Treatment of Bronchial Asthma. Treatment of bronchial asthma, including nocturnal asthma,[268,282] consists of judicious use of bronchodilators and corticosteroids, preferably inhaled in a compressor; oral theophylline, maximizing the serum concentration at around 4:00 AM when most nocturnal attacks occur; and, for a small subset of patients who show the lowest plasma cortisol levels accompanied by the lowest PEF at night or in the early morning, nocturnal steroids.[303] Other measures include treating the reversible factors such as allergens, nasal congestion, or bronchopulmonary infections, and using a humidifier.[282]

In a double-blind, placebo-controlled, crossover study, Kraft et al.[304] and Wiegand et al.[305] reported that salmeterol, an inhaled β_2-agonist with a prolonged duration of action, improved the number of nocturnal awakenings with nocturnal asthma. Wiegand et al.[305] found that salmeterol was superior to theophylline in maintaining nocturnal FEV_1 levels and in improving morning and evening PEF, and in an improvement in patient perception of sleep but not in PSG measures of sleep architecture. Previously, several studies showed efficacy of salmeterol in nocturnal asthma, primarily in combination with inhaled corticosteroids.[306–310]

Sleep disturbances in asthma caused by nocturnal asthma attacks should not be treated with hypnotic medicines; rather, the best treatment is vigorous treatment of the asthmatic attacks by using oral and preferably inhaled steroids (e.g., prednisone, beclomethasone, triamcinolone, fluticasone).[268,282] Other agents that may be helpful are salmeterol and anticholinergic medications (e.g., inhaled ipratropium bromide[243,305,311,312]). Patients with PSG evidence of OSA should be treated with CPAP, which not only is effective for OSA but also helps nocturnal asthmatic symptoms. Ciftci et al.[302] reported moderate to severe OSA based on an AHI of 15 in 16 of 43

asthmatic patients with nocturnal symptoms. CPAP treatment improved nocturnal symptoms but did not correct pulmonary function test abnormalities. Patients with gastroesophageal reflux disease (GERD) often have worse symptoms of the disease at night, which may worsen the nocturnal asthmatic symptoms. Treatment of GERD with proton pump inhibitors (e.g., omeprazole) at bedtime may improve nocturnal asthmatic symptoms and sleep quality.[313,314] However, the evidence is conflicting; Coughlan et al.,[315] after a systematic review, concluded that clear evidence or improvement of nocturnal asthmatic symptoms after treating GERD is lacking.

Restrictive Lung Disease

Restrictive lung disease is characterized functionally by a reduction of total lung capacity, FRC, VC, expiratory reserve volume, and diffusion capacity but preservation of the normal ratio of FEV_1 to FVC.[252] This may be due to intrapulmonary restriction (e.g., interstitial lung disease) or extrapulmonary restriction resulting from diseases of the chest wall (e.g., kyphoscoliosis) or pleura; neuromuscular diseases; obesity; or pregnancy, which may abnormally elevate the diaphragm.

Interstitial Lung Disease.

Etiopathogenesis. Interstitial lung disease may result from a variety of causes, including idiopathic pulmonary fibrosis, fibrosing alveolitis associated with connective tissue disorders, pulmonary sarcoidosis, occupational dust exposure, pulmonary damage resulting from drugs, or radiotherapy to the thorax.[316–319] The common features of all these conditions include alveolar thickening due to fibrosis, cellular exudates, or edema; increased stiffening of the lungs causing reduced compliance; and ventilation-perfusion mismatch giving rise to hypoxemia, hyperventilation, and hypocapnia.

Clinical Features. Features of interstitial lung disease include progressive exertional dyspnea, a dry cough, clubbing of the fingers, and pulmonary crepitations on auscultation of the lungs. The diagnosis is based on a combination of characteristic clinical features, radiographic findings (e.g., diffuse pulmonary fibrosis), and pulmonary function test results.

Sleep Abnormalities. Bye et al.,[251] Perez-Padilla et al.,[320] Hira and Shama,[321] and Prado and coworkers[322] reported on sleep studies in interstitial lung disease. Sleep abnormalities consist of repeated arousals with sleep fragmentation and multiple sleep stage shifts, increased stage 1 and reduced REM sleep accompanied by oxygen desaturation during REM and NREM sleep owing to episodic hypoventilation and ventilation-perfusion mismatch, and occasionally OSA.[319] Mermigkis et al.,[323] in a retrospective study, reported OSA in 18 patients with interstitial lung disease. These authors concluded that an increased body mass index and a significant impairment in pulmonary function tests may predict the occurrence of OSA in these patients, and it is important to make the diagnosis and treat comorbid OSA to improve quality of life.

There is no effective treatment for interstitial lung disease except to treat the comorbid conditions such as OSA. Corticosteroids are found to be effective in some cases. George and Kryger[252] advocated symptomatic treatment with supplemental nocturnal oxygen therapy according to the guidelines developed by the Nocturnal Oxygen Therapy Trial Group.[253] In summary, supportive care, treatment of comorbid conditions and ultimately, lung transplantation are the only therapeutic options available for these conditions.

Kyphoscoliosis. Kyphoscoliosis is a thoracic cage deformity that causes extrapulmonary restriction of the lungs and gives rise to impairment of pulmonary functions, as described earlier for restrictive lung diseases. The condition may be primary (idiopathic) or secondary to neuromuscular disease, spondylitis, or Marfan syndrome.[252]

In severe cases of kyphoscoliosis, breathing disorders during sleep (e.g., central, obstructive, and mixed apneas associated with oxygen desaturation) and sleep disturbances (e.g., disrupted night sleep, reduced NREM stages 2 through 4 and REM sleep, and EDS) have been described.[247,248,252]

The best treatment for patients with chronic respiratory failure secondary to severe kyphoscoliosis is NIPPV. This has been described in detail in Chapter 29. Long-term NIPPV treatment improves nocturnal and daytime blood gases, respiratory muscle performance, pulmonary function, and hypoventilation-related symptoms in patients with severe kyphoscoliosis.[324–326]

Gastrointestinal Diseases

Peptic Ulcer Disease

A peptic ulcer is an ulcer in the lower esophagus, stomach, or duodenum.[327] The prevalence of peptic ulcer in the general population is fairly high—approximately 10% of the adult population—and men are most often affected. The most common presentation of peptic ulcer is episodic pain localized to the epigastrium that is relieved by food, antacids, or other acid suppressants. The pain has a characteristic periodicity and extends over many years. The patient generally can localize the pain to the epigastrium. Occasionally, however, it is referred to the interscapular region at the lower chest and is usually described as burning or gnawing. Duodenal pain is often described as "hunger pain" and is relieved by eating. An important feature is that the pain awakens patients 2–3 hours after retiring to bed, disturbing sleep. An important physical sign is the so-called pointing sign and localized epigastric tenderness.

The natural history of the disease is episodic occurrence over a course of days or weeks, after which the pain disappears, to recur weeks or months later. Between attacks the patient feels well. Presentation may be secondary to complications of ulcer, such as an acute episode of bleeding or perforation, or even an episode of gastric obstruction. The differential diagnosis of ulcer pain should include cholecystitis, angina, gastroesophageal reflux, esophagitis, and pancreatitis. Definitive diagnosis is established by barium examination of the gastroduodenal tract and, if necessary, by endoscopic examination and biopsy.

In the last decade, it has been clearly established that the most common cause of peptic ulcer disease is *Helicobacter pylori* infection.[327–332] The second most common cause is ingestion of aspirin and other nonsteroidal anti-inflammatory drugs (NSAIDs).[327,328,332] *Helicobacter pylori* infection is responsible for 90% of duodenal and more than 75% of gastric ulcers.[327,328,332]

Sleep, Nocturnal Acid Secretion, and Duodenal Ulcer (see also Chapter 7). To understand the role of nocturnal gastric acid secretion in duodenal ulcer, Dragstedt[333] studied hourly collections of nocturnal gastric acid from patients with duodenal ulcer and from normal subjects. The study found 3–20 times greater volumes of nocturnal acid secretion in patients than in normal controls (see also Fig. 7–13). Vagotomy abolished this increased secretion and improved healing of ulcers. Studies by Orr and colleagues[334] have shown that patients with duodenal ulcer exhibit failure of inhibition of gastric acid secretion during the first 2 hours after onset of sleep. A study by Watanabe et al.[335] confirmed the findings of Orr et al.[334] and found that the intragastric pH values increased during NREM and REM sleep in healthy controls and gastric ulcer patients, but the intragastric pH of duodenal ulcer patients did not change. Schubert and Peura[336] reviewed the physiology and pathophysiology of acid secretion and its inhibition in the management of acid-related clinical conditions.

Sleep disturbances in duodenal ulcer patients characteristically result from episodes of nocturnal epigastric pain. These symptoms cause arousals and repeated awakenings, thus fragmenting and disturbing sleep considerably in these patients.

Treatment. In light of the evidence about the role of *H. pylori* infection and NSAIDs in the pathogenesis of gastroduodenal ulcers, the theory of hypersecretion of acid in peptic ulcer patients has been relegated to a secondary role.[327,332] The first step is to find the causes of ulcer based on the history and laboratory tests such as serology, urea breath test, and endoscopic biopsy and histology, particularly in patients with gastric ulcer.[327,331,332] The purpose of treatment is to relieve symptoms; heal the ulcer; and either cure the disease, in the case of *H. pylori* ulcers, or prevent recurrences, in the case of NSAID ulcers.[327,332] To cure the ulcer, the best approach is a triple combination of antimicrobial therapy as recommended and approved by the Food and Drug Administration as follows[327]: esomeprazole, amoxicillin, clarithromycin; lansoprazole, amoxicillin, clarithromycin; omeprazole, amoxicillin, clarithromycin; or rabeprazole, amoxicillin, clarithromycin. Antimicrobial agents effective against *H. pylori* infection include amoxicillin, clarithromycin, tetracycline, and metronidazole. Most commonly a 10- to 14-day regimen may be effective. To accelerate healing, the antimicrobial agent is combined with antisecretory agents (histamine$_2$ [H$_2$]–receptor antagonists such as cimetidine [Tagamet], ranitidine [Zantac], nizatidine [Axcid] or famotidine [Pepcid]). The most potent antisecretory agents are the proton pump inhibitors (e.g., esomeprazole, lansoprazole, omeprazole, rabeprazole). Kwok et al.[337] reviewed recent consensus statements, recommendations, and evidence-based indications for *H. pylori* eradication. Because of emergence of resistant strains of *H. pylori* and failure of eradication in 20–25% of cases, sequential therapy has been suggested for eradication of *H. pylori* infection.[338–340] Sequential therapy includes an initial 5 days of therapy with a proton pump inhibitor and amoxicillin followed by 5 days of a proton pump inhibitor plus clarithromycin and tinidazole. For treatment of NSAID ulcers, NSAID therapy should be stopped and treated with traditional antisecretory agents. Patients who require continued NSAID therapy, however, may be treated with misoprostol, a synthetic prostaglandin E$_1$ analog (200 μg two to four times a day).[327] General measures of treatment of peptic ulcer disease should consist of avoidance of tobacco and alcohol. For detailed management of uncomplicated, complicated, and resistant ulcers, the reader is referred to Feldman.[327]

Gastroesophageal Reflux Disease

Clinical Features. *Gastroesophageal reflux disease* is preferable to the term *reflux esophagitis*.[341] GERD frequently occurs in middle-aged and elderly women, and sometimes in younger women during pregnancy. Hiatal hernia is often associated with reflux esophagitis. The characteristic symptom is heartburn, described as retrosternal burning pain exacerbated by lifting or straining or when the patient lies down at night.[341–345] The nocturnal burning pain causes difficulty in initiating sleep, frequent awakenings, and fragmentation of sleep.[346–350] The nocturnal pain is characteristically relieved by sitting up or ingesting food or by acid-suppressant agents. An important differential diagnosis would be angina, particularly when the pain radiates to the neck, jaws, and arms, but an important point to remember is that the esophageal pain is usually not related to exertion. Other symptoms include transient or persistent dysphagia if the patient has developed stricture and regurgitation of gastric contents associated with coughing, wheezing, and shortness of breath due to the aspiration of the gastric contents into the bronchopulmonary region.[341–345] A serious complication of repeated episodes of gastroesophageal reflux and esophagitis is Barrett's esophagus, which may be a precursor to esophageal adenocarcinoma.[341,343–345,351–353] Another potential complication is exacerbation of nocturnal asthma.

Differential Diagnosis, Pathogenesis, and Diagnostic Tests. Peptic ulcer disease, ischemic heart disease, sleep apnea, abnormal swallowing, and sleep choking syndromes may be mistaken for gastroesophageal reflux.[341,343–345,347] It has been shown that the fundamental mechanism of GERD is the inappropriate, transient, and frequent relaxation of the lower esophageal sphincter, causing episodes of acid reflux.[341,344,345,354] The esophagitis resulting from acid reflux in the esophagus reduces the sphincter pressure and impairs esophageal contractility.[354] An additional mechanism is the presence of a hiatal hernia. Other factors, such as the acid clearance time, frequency of swallowing, and secretion of saliva, play an important role in the pathogenesis. The diagnosis of gastroesophageal reflux and prolonged acid secretion can be made by continuous monitoring of lower esophageal pH.[355] When the pH falls below 4, gastroesophageal reflux occurs.[356] Repeated prolonged episodes of gastroesophageal reflux during sleep at night can cause esophagitis.[357] Physiologic changes during sleep consisting of suppression of saliva, decreased swallowing frequency, and prolonged mucosal contact with the gastric acid all contribute to the development of esophagitis.[347,358–360] After repeated prolonged episodes of gastroesophageal reflux at night for many years, patients may develop Barrett's esophagus, which results from replacement of the squamous epithelium of the lower esophagus by the columnar epithelium of the stomach.[341,343–345,351–353] Documentation of spontaneous gastroesophageal reflux and prolonged acid clearance is important for diagnosis and treatment of esophagitis and of extraesophageal reflux and upper aerodigestive tract diseases resulting from repeated episodes of gastroesophageal reflux.[345,358,359,361–364]

Role of Gastroesophageal Reflux in Bronchopulmonary Disease. In some patients with asthma and chronic bronchitis or COPD, spontaneous gastroesophageal reflux at night plays a role in the pathogenesis of symptoms such as nocturnal wheeze, cough, or shortness of breath.[341,344,345,365–368] In such patients, intraesophageal pH monitoring has shown prolonged acid clearance.[366] This is important from a therapeutic point of view, because administration of acid suppressants to such patients improves pulmonary symptoms.[341,344] A study by Tan and coworkers,[369] however, casts doubt on the relevance of gastroesophageal reflux to asthma.

The mechanisms of pulmonary symptoms in gastroesophageal reflux include aspiration of the gastric contents in the lungs causing pneumonitis and acid contact with the lower esophagus initiating reflex stimulation of the vagus nerve, causing bronchoconstriction.

Actual aspiration of gastric contents into the lungs can be documented with the scintigraphic technique used by Chernow and associates.[368] These authors instilled a radionuclide into the stomach before sleep. A lung scan the next morning showed the radioactive material in the lung, suggesting nocturnal pulmonary aspiration. Children with asthma and bronchopulmonary disease may have sleep apnea, in addition to the other complications of gastroesophageal reflux.[370] Gastroesophageal reflux has been implicated in some cases of sudden infant death syndrome, possibly causing apnea and sudden death, but this has been found in only a small percentage of cases.[371,372] The relationship between GERD and OSAS remains undetermined, although there is an increased prevalence of GERD in OSAS patients and CPAP treatment in such patients improves GERD symptoms.[372–375]

Diagnostic Tests. No single test is diagnostic for GERD, but a combination of tests to assess the potential for reflux damage to the esophagus and actual presence of reflux is necessary to make the diagnosis. The diagnosis is confirmed by barium examination, and, if necessary, by endoscopic examination and biopsy.[345] Measurement of lower esophageal sphincter pressure and a diagnosis of hiatal hernia may detect risk factors for reflux.[341,343] Damage to the esophagus may be assessed by Bernstein's test (acid perfusion test), esophagography, esophagoscopy, and mucosal biopsy.[343,345] The actual presence of reflux may be established with the following tests: esophagography, acid reflux test, prolonged esophageal pH monitoring, and gastroesophageal scintigraphy.[341,343,345] The importance of 24-hour ambulatory esophageal pH monitoring has been emphasized by Triadafilopoulos and Castillo.[376]

Treatment. Treatment[341,343–345,354] includes general measures such as avoidance of fatty foods and stooping, weight reduction, and elevation of the head of the bed to reduce reflux at night. Smoking should also be avoided. These simple measures decrease the frequency and length of reflux episodes as demonstrated by 24-hour pH monitoring.[341] If the patients fail to improve as a result of these simple measures, H_2-receptor antagonists (cimetidine, ranitidine, famotidine, and nizatidine) in the usual dose range as used for peptic ulcer patients (see earlier) will improve the symptoms of GERD.[206,341,344,345,354] For patients who are resistant to H_2-receptor antagonists, a proton pump inhibitor may be used.[341,344,345,354] Proton pump inhibitors decrease gastric acid secretion through inhibition of the proton pump (H^+,K^+-ATPase) of the parietal cells (this is the most potent inhibitor of gastric acid secretion) and are in fact the treatment of choice for nighttime symptoms causing sleep dysfunction.[345,377–384] Several studies have shown improvement of subjective measures of sleep without evidence of objective measurement after pharmacologic treatment for GERD.[381,383] Other measures found to be useful are prokinetic agents (e.g., metoclopramide, 10 mg qid;

cisapride, 10 mg qid; bethanechol, 10 mg qid).[341] For patients who fail to respond to medical treatment, antireflux surgery (e.g., fundoplication) is indicated.[345,385] Rarely, a Roux-en-Y near esophagojejunostomy is necessary for those intractable GERD patients who failed prior antireflux surgery.[386]

In conclusion, an awareness of the role of sleep in the pathogenesis and treatment of peptic ulcer disease, particularly duodenal ulcer and esophageal reflux, is important for diagnosis and treatment. Facilities for all-night PSG study and 24-hour esophageal pH monitoring have contributed to an understanding of the association between sleep and these diseases. These disorders are good examples of diseases that benefit from a multidisciplinary approach to patient management by a gastroenterologist, a pulmonologist, and a sleep specialist. This review also shows that sleep adversely affects patients with GERD by increasing the episodes of reflux and prolonging the acid clearance time. Furthermore, repeated spontaneous reflux episodes adversely affect sleep by causing arousals, frequent awakenings, and sleep fragmentation.

Sleep in Functional Bowel Disorders

Functional bowel disorders include functional or nonulcer dyspepsia (NUD) and irritable bowel syndrome (IBS). NUD includes functional disorders of the upper gut and presents with upper abdominal pain or discomfort, nausea, gaseous distention, and early satiety.[387–390] A number of patients with functional bowel disorders have symptoms originating from the lower gut consistent with IBS, which is a common medical disorder characterized by symptoms of bowel dysfunction and abdominal pain.[391] In the last 2 decades, our understanding of IBS has grown considerably,[392] beginning with change in the classification and definition, which are the symptom-based Rome III criteria.[393] The basis for IBS symptoms is thought to be dysregulation of the brain-gut (central nervous system–enteric nervous system) relationship. The concept of IBS as a functional bowel disorder with no structural alteration has been dispelled by the functional and structural magnetic resonance imaging (MRI) findings of significant cortical thinning of the anterior cingulate cortex (ACC) and insula.[394] These findings confirm the investigators' previous observation of absent rectal pain–related functional MRI responses in the anterior insula and ACC in IBS.[395] These findings support the earlier abnormal EEG findings in IBS.[396] Davis et al.[394] also noted reduced gray matter in the anterior/medial thalamus and ACC on voxel-based morphometry in the IBS group relative to healthy controls.

Many patients with NUD and IBS have history of sleep complaints (e.g., frequent awakenings with or without pain and nonrestorative sleep).[397,398] Such functional disorders may be associated with fibromyalgia syndrome (FMS).[399–401] Patients with FMS complain of a variety of sleep problems (see later). Jarrett et al.[402] and Eisenbruch and coworkers[403] reported that women with IBS associated with gastrointestinal symptoms complain of poor sleep and nonrestorative sleep more often than women without IBS. In a previous study, Eisenbruch and collaborators[404] reported poor sleep quality in the absence of objective sleep abnormalities (PSG findings), suggesting an altered sleep perception. In contrast to these findings, Fass et al.[405] prospectively evaluated 505 new patients with functional bowel disorders and 247 healthy controls using validated bowel symptom and sleep questionnaires. They concluded that functional dyspepsia patients, but not IBS patients, reported sleep disturbances more frequently than healthy control subjects. Another important observation is that IBS patients, compared with controls, had greater sympathetic dominance as indicated by increased LF/HF heart rate variability ratio during REM sleep because of vagal withdrawal, suggesting that autonomic functioning during REM sleep may be an useful biological marker to identify IBS patients.[406] Treatment of IBS patients includes an integrated pharmacologic and behavioral approach depending on the severity of symptoms and disability.

Miscellaneous Gastrointestinal Disorders and Sleep

There is circumstantial evidence that sleep deprivation or sleep disturbance may trigger flare-ups of two chronic autoimmune inflammatory bowel disorders: Crohn's disease or regional ileitis, and ulcerative colitis.[407–409] Demonstration of exacerbation of colonic inflammation and tissue damage following acute and chronic sleep deprivation in a mouse model of colitis[410] supports such contention. Future research and clinical trials focusing on an improvement in the quantity or quality of sleep in patients with inflammatory bowel disorders are needed to provide definitive evidence.

Hepatic encephalopathy may cause hypersomnia, inversion of the sleep-wake rhythm, and recurrent stupor, which are most likely related to neurotransmitter alterations in the brain. There is an excessive accumulation of endozepines (benzodiazepine-like γ-aminobutyric acid [GABA] type A receptor modulators) in hepatic encephalopathy, explaining the recurrent stupor that is noted in some cases.[411]

Sleep disturbances have not been adequately studied in celiac disease (nontropical sprue or gluten-sensitive enteropathy) and Whipple's disease (a chronic multisystem disease due to infection with *Tropheryma whipplei*). Patients with celiac disease may have restless legs syndrome (RLS)–periodic limb movements in sleep (PLMS), and Whipple's disease patients may present with insomnia or sleep-wake cycle changes.

Endocrine Diseases

Thyroid Disorders

It is important to be aware of the association between thyroid disorders, disordered breathing, and sleep disturbances.

History and physical examination may direct attention to a thyroid disorder, in which case thyroid function tests should be performed to confirm the clinical diagnosis.

Hypothyroidism. The salient diagnostic features suggestive of myxedema consist of presentation in a middle-aged or elderly individual of fatigue, weight gain, decrease of physical and mental faculties, dryness and coarsening of the skin, pretibial edema, hoarse voice, cold sensitivity (sometimes presenting with hypothermia), constipation, and bradycardia or evidence of ischemic heart disease in the ECG. Both upper airway obstructive[412] and central sleep apneas,[413] which disappeared after thyroxine treatment, have been described in patients with myxedema. Mechanisms include deposition of mucopolysaccharides in the upper airways as well as central respiratory dysfunction as evidenced by impaired hypercapnic and hypoxic ventilatory response.[414]

In an important study, Jha et al.[415] evaluated 50 newly diagnosed consecutive patients with primary hypothyroidism using PSG in all patients. Thyroxine replacement therapy was associated with improvement, including the findings in the repeat PSG study. This supports the previous findings of Rajagopal and coworkers.[416] Grunstein and Sullivan[417] recommended nasal CPAP treatment in patients with hypothyroidism and concomitant OSA while the patient is receiving thyroxine treatment. Routine screening for hypothyroidism in OSAS remains controversial.[418–421] Hashimoto's thyroiditis, an autoimmune disease diagnosed on the basis of high titers of antithyroid antibodies and histologic findings, is associated with higher prevalence of sleep-related breathing problems compared with controls.[422]

Hyperthyroidism. Clinical features suggestive of thyrotoxicosis are presentation in a woman (female-to-male ratio, 8:1) of apparent increased energy, weight loss despite increased appetite, staring or bulging of the eyes (exophthalmos), tachycardia or atrial fibrillation, heat intolerance with excessive sweating, feelings of warmth, and a fine tremor of the outstretched fingers.

Few sleep studies have been made in patients with thyrotoxicosis. Dunleavy and colleagues[423] observed an increased amount of SWS, which returned to normal after treatment. In contrast, Passouant and colleagues[424] did not find any change in SWS but described an increase in sleep-onset latency in hyperthyroid patients. Johns and Rinsler[425] found no relationship between stages of sleep and alteration of thyroid function.

Ajlouni and co-investigators[426] reported eight cases of patients with new-onset sleepwalking coinciding with the onset of thyrotoxicosis resulting from diffuse toxic goiter. Disappearance of sleepwalking with successful achievement of a euthyroid state supported a cause-and-effect relationship.

Diabetes Mellitus

For a discussion of sleep disturbance and sleep apnea in diabetes, see the section on autonomic neuropathy in Chapter 29.

Growth Hormone Disorders

Growth Hormone Deficiency and Sleep. In eight adults with isolated growth hormone (GH) deficiency (ages 18–28 years), Astrom and Lindholm[427] found a reduction of stage 4 sleep but increases in stage 1 and 2 NREM sleep, with a net result of an increase of total sleep time. In a later paper, Astrom and others[428] studied these patients after daily treatment with GH for 6 months and found a decrease in total sleep time that was due mainly to a reduction in stage 2 sleep, unchanged slow waves, and an increase in REM sleep time. In contrast to these findings, Pavel et al.[429] found no difference in sleep efficiency and daytime sleepiness in 16 GH-deficient adults (7 women and 9 men with a mean age of 36.8 years) after GH substitution. The subjective sleep parameters improved, however, and the authors suggested that this improvement might be caused by other indices of general well-being in this study with a small sample size.

Excessive Growth Hormone Release and Sleep. Sullivan and colleagues[430] reported sleep apnea in association with GH release from the pituitary in patients with acromegaly. The most common explanation for sleep apnea in these patients is enlargement of the tongue and pharyngeal wall, which causes narrowing of the upper airway. Sullivan's group[430] studied 40 patients with acromegaly and observed central sleep apnea in 30%. Increased respiratory drive with increased hypercapnic ventilatory response is present in these patients. Sandostatin, a somatostatin analog, cured central apnea and normalized the ventilatory response.

Grunstein and coworkers[431] studied 53 patients with acromegaly who were consecutively referred for consultation. Sleep apnea was a reason for referral of 33 patients, whereas 20 patients were referred without any suspicion of apnea. Thirty-one patients of the group of 33 referred for apnea had sleep apnea; 12 of the 20 patients referred without suspected apnea were found to have apnea. Central apnea was predominant in 33% of patients. The authors concluded that sleep apnea is common in individuals with acromegaly and central sleep apnea is associated with increased disease activity as reflected by biochemical measurement. They speculated that alteration of respiratory control may be a mechanism for sleep apnea in these patients. In a later study of 54 patients with acromegaly, Grunstein and collaborators[432] found increased hypercapnic ventilatory responses in those patients with central sleep apnea but not in those with OSA or those without sleep apnea. These authors also found that acromegalic patients with central sleep apnea

have increased GH and insulin-like growth factor-I levels compared with their counterparts with OSA. The authors concluded that increased ventilatory responsiveness and elevated hormonal parameters of disease activity contribute to the pathogenesis of central sleep apnea and acromegaly.

In contrast, later investigators found a high prevalence of sleep apnea, predominantly obstructive type and rarely central apnea.[433,434] Suggested mechanisms for the development of OSA in acromegaly include an anatomic abnormality, especially at the base of the tongue[435]; craniofacial changes (e.g., increased vertical dolichofacial growth) causing narrowing of the posterior airway space; and displacement of the hyoid caudally.[436]

Octreotide, a long-acting somatostatin analog, has been found to be an effective noninvasive treatment for sleep apnea in acromegaly.[437–440] Sze and coworkers[441] reported a high prevalence of sleep apnea syndrome in acromegaly patients with resolution of SDB symptoms after transsphenoidal adenoidectomy. The relationship between sleep apnea and the GH level in active acromegaly remains unresolved.[431,434,439]

Miscellaneous Endocrine Diseases and Sleep

In the only controlled study in patients with Cushing's syndrome (hyperpituitarism with corticosteroid excess), about one-third of the patients were diagnosed with sleep apnea.[442] There is one report of decreased delta sleep and increased stage 1 sleep and sleep fragmentation.[443]

Addison's disease (adrenal gland insufficiency) patients may have increased sleep fragmentation and decreased REM sleep.[444]

The male hormone testosterone is a risk factor for sleep apnea, as exogenous administration of testosterone induces sleep apnea in both normal and hypogonadal men[445] and worsens sleep apnea in older men.[446]

There is an increased prevalence of OSAS, insulin resistance, and type 2 diabetes mellitus in patients diagnosed with polycystic ovary syndrome, the most common endocrine disorder in reproductive-aged women, characterized by chronic anovulation and hyperandrogenism.[447–449]

Renal Disorders

Sleep Disturbances and Chronic Renal Failure

Sleep dysfunction has been well described in cross-sectional studies of patients with chronic renal failure (CRF) on hemodialysis[450–461] and those not on hemodialysis,[462–465] and even in patients with renal transplantation.[466,467] Sleep dysfunction has been noted in up to 80% of patients with CRF.[454] There is, however, no clear relationship noted between indices of renal failure and sleep disturbance in these studies.

Several studies have used PSG to objectively document the sleep disturbances, which consist of reduced sleep efficiency, increased sleep fragmentation, frequent awakenings with difficulty in maintenance of sleep, decreased SWS, and disorganization of the sleep cycle.[450–454] Various studies have demonstrated a variety of sleep complaints in CRF patients that include poor-quality and nonrestorative sleep, difficulty in initiating and maintaining sleep, EDS, SDB, and sleep apnea.

In a prospective longitudinal study of 154 consecutive patients with CRF (78 completed the follow-up), Sabbatini et al.[468] determined sleep quality based on the Pittsburgh Sleep Quality Index (PSQI), and the data suggested that the progression of renal disease is accompanied by a progressive worsening of sleep quality. The data showed no correlation with creatinine clearance or with other indices of renal failure, but showed a correlation with age, which served as a confounding variable. Four patients had high PSQI score at baseline and had further deteriorated at 3-year follow-up.

There are several factors which may contribute to the sleep problems in CRF patients[469]:

1. Disease-related factors (e.g., symptoms related to uremia, anemia, comorbid conditions, metabolic changes, alterations in neurotransmitters)
2. Treatment-related factors (e.g., rapid changes in fluid, electrolyte, and acid-based balance; alterations in melatonin and thermoregulatory functions; medications; types of dialysis; alterations of cytokine metabolism in patients treated with hemodialysis causing abnormal somnolence[470] and proinflammatory cytokines (interleukin-1β), which might be associated with sleep complaints in hemodialysis patients[471])
3. Demographic factors (e.g., increasing age, male gender, white race)
4. Psychological factors (e.g., anxiety, depression)
5. Lifestyle factors (e.g., increased intake of coffee, cigarette use, poor sleep hygiene)

Sleep Apnea in Patients Receiving Dialysis

Sleep apnea is noted in up to 50% of patients with renal failure.[472] Sleep apnea could be upper airway obstructive or central, but mainly an obstructive type of apnea is noted in most of the patients.[451,470,473–483] This sleep apnea improves after nocturnal hemodialysis,[484] which may be due to a decrease in chemosensitivity, suggesting also that, in some patients with kidney failure, increased chemoreflex responsiveness may contribute to the pathogenesis of sleep apnea. Beecroft et al.[484] studied 23 patients on hemodialysis and found decreased hypercapnic ventilatory response in sleep apnea patients who showed a significant reduction of the AHI after conversion from conventional to nocturnal hemodialysis. The authors suggested that increased chemosensitivity, by destabilizing respiratory control during sleep, may be responsible for both obstructive[485] and central sleep apnea.[87,486,487] An important study from the Sleep Heart Health Study identified an association between conventional hemodialysis and severe sleep apnea with nocturnal hypoxemia.[488] It should be noted that the prevalence of sleep apnea is similar in patients before and after receiving peritoneal dialysis or hemodialysis.[489–491] Although sleep problems may not be as common among transplantation patients as those on dialysis, the problems are still higher than in the general population.[466,467] There are case reports indicating resolution of sleep apnea after renal transplantation[492]; however, many patients do not improve.[479,481,493]

The following are the suggested mechanisms for the pathogenesis of sleep apnea in CRF:

- Upper airway edema causing partial airway obstruction coupled with decreased muscle tone during sleep.[478]
- CNS depression during sleep resulting from so-called uremic toxins causing excessive reduction of upper airway muscle tone[478] (persistence of sleep apnea after dialysis speaks against this suggestion).
- Disturbance of the ventilatory control of breathing in renal failure and hemodialysis[452,453,470,484,492,494–496] making the respiratory control unstable, causing an imbalance between diaphragmatic and upper airway muscles. Beecroft et al.[497] reported an increased ventilatory sensitivity to hypercapnia in CRF patients with sleep apnea, suggesting an increase in respiratory control system "loop gain," which destabilizes central respiratory control and contributes to upper airway occlusion. Beecroft and colleagues[484] suggested that decreased chemoreflex sensitivity after conversion from conventional hemodialysis to nocturnal hemodialysis corrected sleep apnea by decreasing respiratory control system "loop gain," thus stabilizing the control of ventilation.
- CCF, which may occur in association with CRF, itself causing sleep apnea.[498]
- Chronic metabolic acidosis, as noted in patients with CRF.[499] (Kimmel's group,[473] however, did not find any relationship between disordered breathing events and hydrogen ion concentrations or carbon dioxide tension in the symptomatic patients.)
- Alteration of the hydrogen ion set point for stimulation of respiration.[494]
- Anatomic narrowing of the upper airway.[473,500] The same investigators also noted that there was an increase in pharyngeal size following conversion from conventional hemodialysis to nocturnal hemodialysis in those patients who previously had decreased pharyngeal cross-sectional area.[501]
- Hypertension associated with CRF.
- Metabolic derangement associated with uremia. (Soreide et al.[502] reported that an infusion of branched-chain amino acids stimulated nocturnal respiration and resulted in a decreased number of obstructive apneas.)

Restless Legs Syndrome in Chronic Renal Failure Patients

RLS has been described as symptomatic or comorbid in many patients with CRF, and the prevalence in hemodialyzed patients varies from 15% to 40%.[503–509] Symptomatic RLS is associated with CRF and not with the hemodialysis itself.[505,510,511] It should be noted that uremic RLS and idiopathic RLS resemble each other and cannot be distinguished clinically.[511] RLS after successful kidney transplantation may disappear or may improve considerably. Winkelmann et al.[508] investigated clinically the long-term course of 11 of 64 hemodialysis patients who underwent kidney transplantation. In all patients, RLS symptoms disappeared within 1–21 days after transplantation, and at follow-up visits up to 9 years, four patients remained free of RLS symptoms. In three other patients, RLS symptoms gradually reappeared. In 3 of 11 patients, transplantation failed and RLS symptoms reoccurred within 10 days to 2 months. In one patient RLS symptoms reoccurred with transplant failure but disappeared after a second successful transplant. The authors concluded that kidney transplantation has a positive effect on RLS symptoms in hemodialysis patients. In an important cross-sectional study, Molnar et al.[507] assessed the prevalence of RLS in 992 kidney-transplanted patients using an RLS questionnaire. They found a prevalence rate of RLS of 4.8% and concluded that the prevalence is significantly lower in kidney-transplanted patients than in patients with maintenance dialysis. The increasing prevalence of RLS in their series is associated with declining renal function. The authors found a significant association between the glomerular filtration rate, higher prevalence of iron deficiency and increased number of self-reported comorbid conditions. In a preliminary study, Benz et al.[512] treated 10 hemodialysis patients having sleep complaints with recombinant human erythropoietin; in 9 of 10 patients this therapy corrected the anemia and improved sleep quality.

Fibromyalgia Syndrome, Rheumatoid Arthritis, and Other Rheumatologic Disorders

All of these conditions are associated with chronic pain, and hence some knowledge of human pain pathways is essential for understanding the pathophysiology of these disorders.[513] Pain pathways include afferent (ascending) fibers, central pain processing regions, and descending (efferent) fibers modulating these pathways. Impulses from peripheral pain-sensitive receptors are transmitted via thinly myelinated A delta and unmyelinated C fibers to the dorsal horn of the spinal cord in the region of zone of Lissauer, from where the fibers cross within one to three spinal segments to the contralateral spinothalamic tracts. The sensory afferent neurons in the spinothalamic tracts terminate in the ventral posterolateral nucleus of the thalamus. The third-order neurons from the thalamus terminate in the somesthetic cortex for pain perception, discrimination, and central processing, as well as in the anterior cingulate cortex and amygdala for affective and emotional pain processing.[514–518] Sensory descending pathways originating from the periaqueductal gray region, locus ceruleus, and hypothalamus[519–521] modulate pain perception.[522,523] These anatomic pathways are influenced by several neurotransmitters and neuromodulators[524–528] (e.g., noradrenalin, serotonin, dopamine) as well as neuropeptides and their receptors. Dysregulation of ascending and descending pathways, and alteration of central sensitization may be responsible for chronic pain in articular and nonarticular painful syndromes. Electrophysiologic[529–531] and functional neuroimaging,[532,533] as well as SPECT and positron emission tomography (PET),[534–537] studies have lent support to these hypothesis. This section briefly reviews sleep disturbances in FMS; rheumatoid arthritis (RA), including juvenile rheumatoid arthritis; osteoarthritis; and miscellaneous other painful conditions (e.g., ankylosing spondylitis, systemic lupus erythematosus, Sjögren's syndrome, and scleroderma) causing sleep disturbances.

Fibromyalgia Syndrome

FMS is a common but poorly understood syndrome characterized by chronic diffuse soft tissue pain and tenderness accompanied by a variety of somatic symptoms, including sleep dysfunction, in the absence of any structural lesion and without a single laboratory diagnostic test. The condition affects approximately 6–10 million people, with a female-to-male ratio of about 9:1, and onset typically occurs between 20 and 50 years of age.[538] In this survey, the most common symptoms included morning stiffness, fatigue, nonrestorative sleep, pain, low back pain, impaired concentration, and memory "fog." Yunus and colleagues[539] originally listed specific diagnostic criteria for FMS, and this was followed by a description by Goldenberg[540] of an emerging but controversial condition. The American College of Rheumatology in 1990 published the formal diagnostic criteria for FMS.[541] According to these criteria, the diagnosis is based on the presence of widespread diffuse pain affecting both upper and lower extremities lasting for at least 3 months and present in a symmetric fashion accompanied by 11 of 18 "tender points" when applying pressure of about 4 kg/cm² by digital palpation using the thumb or two fingers (Table 33–4).

The diagnostic criteria based on tender spots was challenged in terms of its validity as a diagnostic disorder by Croft and colleagues[542] and Bohr.[543] Kissel,[544] in an editorial, agreed with Croft and colleagues and Bohr that, currently, there are no "gold standards," but he suggested that physicians should be encouraged to expand their knowledge in order to understand the pathophysiology of this entity, which afflicts a large segment of the population. The pathophysiology of the condition remains undetermined. However, based on the evidence that

TABLE 33–4 Diagnostic Criteria for Fibromyalgia

- Widespread diffuse pain lasting for at least 3 months
- Tender points in at least 11 of 18 anatomically defined sites (9 pairs of tender spots as listed below) after applying digital pressure of approximately 4 kg of force:
  - Second rib at the costochondral junctions
  - Lateral epicondyle 2 cm distal to the epicondyle
  - Suboccipital region
  - Midpoint of the upper border of the trapezius
  - Low cervical region
  - Supraspinatus above the medial border of the scapular spine
  - Gluteal region
  - Greater trochanteric region posteriorly
  - Medial fat pad at the knee joint proximal to the joint line

patients with fibromyalgia have dysfunctional pain processing in the CNS and perceive pain differently from the general population (see electrophysiologic, functional neuroimaging, SPECT, and PET studies cited above), suggested mechanisms included central sensitization, alterations in neurotransmitters, blunting of inhibitory pain pathways, and associated psychiatric comorbid conditions.[513] A positive family history of fibromyalgia is found in some studies, and this is supported by the findings of a specific polymorphism in the 5-hydroxytryptamine$_{2A}$ receptor gene[545] and the serotonin transporter gene,[546] which may predispose these patients to have psychiatric symptoms.[547]

An important item in the differential diagnosis is polymyalgia rheumatica, which is also characterized by diffuse muscle aches and pains but is often associated with accelerated erythrocyte sedimentation rate and evidence of temporal arteritis. Other differential diagnostic considerations include chronic fatigue syndrome (see later) and other myofascial pain syndromes. The etiology and pathogenesis of FMS remain undetermined.[539,540,548–550]

Sleep disturbance is very common in FMS.[539,540,548–556] The characteristic PSG finding is intermittent alpha activity during NREM sleep giving rise to the characteristic alpha-delta or alpha-NREM sleep pattern in the recording (Fig. 33–1). Another important association is the presence of PLMS on PSG examination.[554,555] It should be noted that, although alpha-delta sleep is seen in this condition, this variant is not specific for the syndrome. Alpha-NREM sleep has also been reported in other rheumatic disorders,[557] febrile illness, postviral fatigue syndrome,[558] psychiatric patients,[559] and even normal individuals.[560,561] Nonrestorative sleep associated with nonspecific PSG abnormalities of sleep fragmentation, increased awakenings, decreased sleep efficiency, and alpha-NREM sleep is the most prominent complaint in these patients. In two retrospective reviews of PSG records and medical charts, there is a high prevalence of sleep apnea and RLS in addition to the other sleep complaints noted previously.[554,555] Gold and colleagues[562] reported that, following CPAP treatment in women with FMS and upper airway resistance syndrome, the patients obtained considerable relief from

fatigue, pain, and gastrointestinal symptoms. The most prominent feature in all of these studies is the subjective perception of poor sleep, which is out of proportion to objective measures of sleep.[563] Another objective measurement of sleep is actigraphy, which gave inconsistent results in FMS.[564–566] In summary, patients with FMS have a high prevalence of sleep difficulty, with up to 99% reporting poor sleep quality.[567] The most common sleep difficulties reported are EDS, fatigue, and insomnia.[568] The observation of disassociation of subjective sleep complaints with objective sleep measures is strengthened by a pilot study showing high levels of dysfunctional beliefs and attitudes about sleep and perceived stress associated with poor sleep quality in FMS patients.[569]

Treatment of FMS remains unsatisfactory. Treatment options should include both pharmacologic and nonpharmacologic therapies.[570–572] The nonpharmacologic treatment should include an exercise program,[573] good sleep hygiene measures, education and reassurance, and cognitive behavioral therapy.[574] Pharmacologic treatment[563] found to be useful includes tricyclic antidepressants (e.g., amitriptyline), nonbenzodiazepine hypnotic drugs, selective serotonin reuptake inhibitors (e.g., fluoxetine), serotonin/norepinephrine reuptake inhibitors (e.g., venlafaxine, duloxetine, milnacipran), gabapentin,[575] and pregabalin.[576] Pregabalin, a centrally acting drug used to treat neuropathic pain and adults with partial epilepsy, is the only drug approved by the Food and Drug Administration for treating and managing fibromyalgia. The recommended dose of pregabalin is 300–400 mg/day in two divided doses beginning with smaller doses of 75 mg twice a day and gradually increasing. Patients should also be treated for comorbid conditions (e.g., depression, sleep apnea).

Rheumatoid Arthritis and Other Rheumatologic Disorders

Arthritis, including rheumatoid and nonrheumatoid types, is the leading cause of disability in the United States, affecting approximately 70 million individuals. These conditions include RA (including juvenile RA), osteoarthritis, seronegative spondyloarthritis (e.g., ankylosing spondylitis, a reactive arthritis that was formerly known as Reiter's syndrome; psoriatic arthritis; arthritis associated with ulcerative colitis, Crohn's disease, and Whipple's disease), systemic lupus erythematosis, Sjögen's syndrome, scleroderma, gouty arthritis, and polymyalgia rheumatica. Osteoarthritis is the most common type of arthritis, followed by RA. A systematic approach encompassing history, physical examination, and appropriate laboratory tests will help differentiate these conditions.[577] For appropriate diagnosis and differential diagnosis of these conditions, readers are referred to a standard text in internal medicine. Many of these patients suffer from sleep dysfunction, and in particular insomnia, fatigue, and depression; however, adequate scientific data correlating subjective with objective measures in a large number of such patients are lacking.[568,578]

In limited studies, sleep disturbances in osteoarthritis are commonly noted, consisting of sleep-onset and maintenance insomnia (including early morning awakenings), correlating with the severity of joint pain, physical function, and depression.[579] Polysomnographic findings are not specific but correlate with sleep complaints, showing increased stage 1 sleep and repeated awakenings and arousals.[580] Sleep disturbances in adult RA patients consisting of difficulty in sleep onset and maintenance and fragmentation of sleep associated with EDS and fatigue are noted. In a large percentage of patients,[581] PSG studies show normal sleep architecture associated with alpha intrusions and increased PLMS.[582–585] Studies generally show a positive correlation between sleep complaints and severity of the disease activity.[585–588] There is an increased prevalence of RLS in patients with RA.[582,584,589,590] There is also an increased prevalence of sleep apnea in these patients.[582,591,592] Similar sleep disturbances are also noted in juvenile RA.[593,594] Similar sleep disturbances, particularly insomnia and daytime sleepiness, are also noted in systemic lupus erythematosis, Sjögren's syndrome, and seronegative spondylotic arthritis.[322,552,595–600] Comorbid upper airway OSA and PLMS are noted in systemic lupus erythematosis and ankylosing spondylitis. Gastroesophageal reflux, pulmonary fibrosis,

Montage: SLEEP   High Cut: 70 Hz   Low Cut: 1.00 Hz   Sensitivity: 7 µV/mm   Speed: 10 s/page

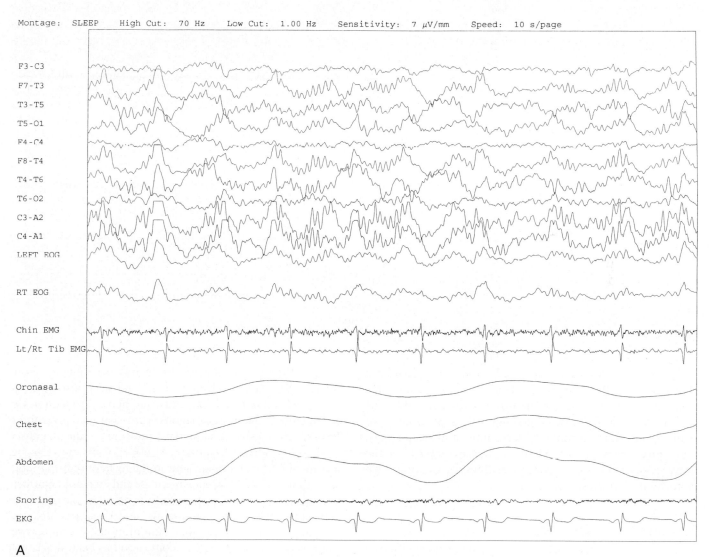

A

FIGURE 33–1 Ten- (A) and 30-second (B) excerpts from a nocturnal PSG showing alpha-delta sleep in a 30-year-old man with history of snoring for many years. He denied any history of joint or muscle aches and pains. The alpha frequency is intermixed with and superimposed on underlying delta activity. Alpha-delta sleep denotes a nonspecific sleep architectural change noted in many patients with complaints of muscle aches and fibromyalgia. It is also seen in other conditions and in many normal individuals. (EEG, top 10 channels; Lt. and Rt. EOG, left and right electrooculograms; chin EMG, EMG of chin; Lt./Rt. Tib. EMG, left/right tibialis anterior EMG; oronasal thermistor; chest and abdomen effort channels; snore monitor; EKG, electrocardiography.)(From Chokroverty S, Thomas RJ, Bhatt M [eds]: Atlas of Sleep Medicine. Philadelphia: Elsevier, 2005.)

Continued

Montage: SLEEP   High Cut: 70 Hz   Low Cut: 1.00 Hz   Sensitivity: 7 μV/mm   Speed: 30 s/page

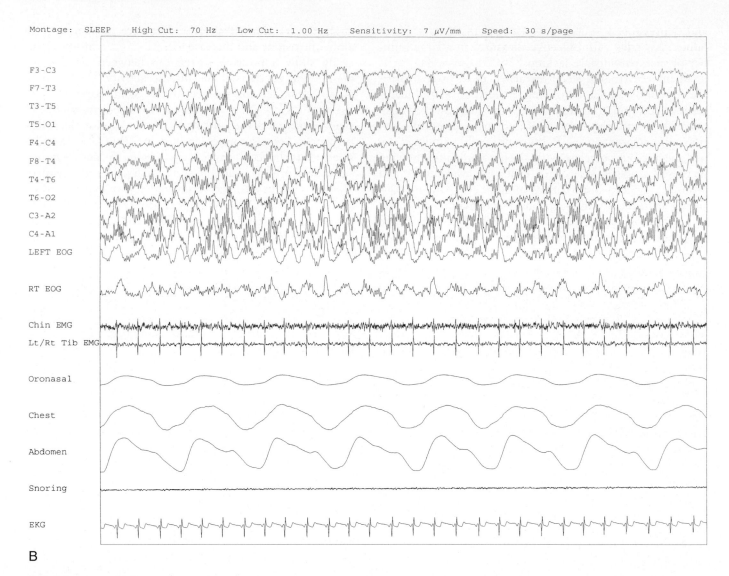

B

FIGURE 33–1—Cont'd.

and RLS are additional comorbid conditions disrupting sleep in scleroderma patients. Treatment of these conditions includes treatment of the primary diseases and associated sleep dysfunction following the general lines of management for insomnia, hypersomnia, and sleep apnea. Currently, there are no adequate studies describing the prevalence of and appropriate guidelines for treating sleep disturbances in these conditions.

Hematologic Disorders

The hematologic disorders that may be adversely affected by sleep include paroxysmal nocturnal hemoglobinuria (PNH), sickle cell anemia, and hereditary hemorrhagic telangiectasia. Hansen[601] noted increased levels of plasma hemoglobin in five of seven patients with PNH, and the maximum values were found at midnight or at 4:00 AM. However, the author did not record EEGs or electro-oculograms to document any relationship with different sleep stages. Patients with sickle cell anemia occasionally show reduced SaO_2 during sleep.[602] OSA and sleep disturbances resulting from reduced SaO_2 can occur in patients with sickle cell anemias; when these diagnoses are suspected, overnight PSG recording should be obtained to confirm the diagnosis so that appropriate treatment with CPAP titration can be instituted.[603] Sleep impairment in the form of reduced total sleep time and REM sleep percentage and increased number of awakenings and sleep stage shifts is noted in patients with clinically stable sickle cell anemia, and these findings are probably due to hemoglobin desaturation.[604] Progressive somnolence accompanied by confusion has been described in a patient with hereditary hemorrhagic telangiectasia.[605] Iron deficiency anemia in infancy is reported to be associated with altered temporal organization of sleep states and stages in childhood.[606] Zilberman et al.[607] reported an improvement of anemia in congestive heart failure following administration of erythropoietin and intravenous iron, along with an improvement of sleep-related breathing disorder and daytime sleepiness. Finally, sleep deprivation in healthy individuals may cause a hypercoagulable state as evidenced by increased levels of prothrombotic hemostasis factors, which are risk factors for cerebrovascular and cardiovascular diseases.[608,609]

Dermatologic Disorders

Dermatologic disorders may cause sleep disruption because of pruritus and painful skin diseases.[610,611] Patients may have sleep initiation and maintenance insomnia. In many dermatologic disorders, patients may have recurrent episodes of pruritus, which is most frequently noted during stages 1 and 2 NREM and least frequently noted in SWS; the intensity of symptoms is intermediate in REM sleep.[611] Patel et al.[610] reviewed the question of the high prevalence of nocturnal pruritus in many systemic and dermatologic diseases causing sleep disturbance and diminished quality of life. Singareddy et al.[612] reported skin picking or pathologic excoriation in nearly 2% of patients attending the dermatologic clinic in a mid-Western region of the United States. They found a significant correlation between skin picking and poor sleep as well as high anxiety. Mouzas et al.[613] reported a significantly higher occurrence of sleepwalking, sleep terrors, nightmares, and nocturnal enuresis in 116 patients suffering from vitiligo compared with 52 patients with other dermatologic diseases and 48 healthy controls.

Atopic dermatitis, a common skin disorder beginning in infancy, may also cause disturbance of sleep in children because of nocturnal itching and scratching.[614] This can be documented by questionnaire and actigraphic recording.[615] Lichen simplex chronicus is another common pruritic disorder in which nighttime pruritus is a common feature disturbing sleep. This was documented by overnight PSG study and the Epworth Sleepiness Scale in 15 patients with lichen simplex chronicus and 15 age-matched controls.[616] Polysomnographic findings in patients demonstrated increased arousals and awakenings associated with scratching bouts during sleep.

Miscellaneous Disorders

Acquired Immunodeficiency Syndrome

Acquired immunodeficiency syndrome (AIDS) is a multisystem disorder caused by infection with human immunodeficiency virus (HIV). Its manifestations are protean. Neurologic manifestations include both CNS and peripheral neuromuscular dysfunction. Encephalitis, due to either opportunistic infection or direct invasion by the virus, may cause a variety of disorders such as memory impairment, seizures, and pyramidal or extrapyramidal manifestations. Some patients have sleep disturbances, but adequate studies utilizing PSG recordings and validated sleep scales have not been performed in a large number of these patients.

Norman and colleagues[617–619] found alterations in sleep architecture in groups of asymptomatic HIV-positive men that progressed as the disease became symptomatic in 17 of the initial group of patients followed for 19–63 months. Several other authors[620–623] also reported sleep architectural abnormalities after PSG recordings in asymptomatic HIV-positive patients. Darko and co-investigators[622,623] also suggested that there is evidence to support a role for the somnogenic immune peptides tumor necrosis factor-α and interleukin-1β in the sleep changes and fatigue commonly seen in HIV infection. These authors[622] stated that these peptides were elevated in the blood of HIV-infected individuals, and are somnogenic in clinical use and animal models.

A more recent study utilizing the PSQI and the Medical Outcome Short-Form Health Survey in a sample of 144 HIV-infected African American women recruited from 12 health clinics and AIDS service organizations in three southern states in the United States showed a high prevalence of poor sleep quality associated with an impairment of health-related quality-of-life index in these patients.[624] Moyle et al.[625] also reported sleep disturbances and alterations of sleep architecture following initiation of efavirenz-containing triple antiretroviral therapy in HIV-positive individuals.

HIV infection can cause SDB. Epstein et al.[626] identified three HIV patients with OSA due to adenotonsillar hypertrophy. They also surveyed 134 patients with asymptomatic HIV disease with a self-administered questionnaire designed to detect OSA and EDS. Those patients whose responses suggested possible OSA were studied by overnight PSG recording. Twelve HIV-positive patients with OSA were identified. The consistent risk factor in this young and nonobese population was the presence of adenotonsillar hypertrophy, which was found in 11 of 12 patients with OSA. In a previous paper, these authors[627] reported the first cases of severe OSA in HIV-infected men. Garrigo et al.[628] obtained PSG recording in asymptomatic HIV-positive men and reported an elevated apnea index in 7 of 24 patients who did not have symptoms related to SDB. In a more recent retrospective review of the medical records of consecutively identified HIV-infected subjects, there was a high prevalence of SDB on PSG recordings. The authors suggested that clinicians caring for HIV patients should inquire about risk factors for OSA because overnight PSG study can aid the diagnosis of sleep disturbances in such patients.[629] This is important for treatment and improvement of quality of life.

Whether PSG can document significant and specific abnormalities in asymptomatic individuals or warn of the development of encephalopathy remains to be determined. A systematic study of a large number of cases needs to be done to answer these questions.

Lyme Disease

Lyme disease[630–638] is a multisystem disease caused by the spirochete *Borrelia burgdorferi* and transmitted to humans by tick bite. The clinical manifestations may be divided into three stages:

1. Initially there is a characteristic skin lesion, erythema migrans, which is followed in the course of time by a febrile illness (acute stage or stage I).
2. In the subacute stage or stage II, which occurs in several weeks to months after the onset of the illness, approximately 12–15% of patients may develop neurologic manifestations and approximately 4–10% may have cardiac involvement (conduction disturbance or cardiomyopathy).[638] Neurologic manifestations may present as axonal polyneuropathy, radiculoneuropathy, cranial neuropathy (particularly affecting the facial nerve), lymphocytic meningitis, encephalitis, or encephalopathy. Encephalitis is rare. Patients with CNS manifestations may have sleep disturbances.
3. In the chronic stage or stage III, which occurs weeks to as long as 2 years after the onset of illness, approximately 60% of patients develop arthritis.[638]

Sleep complaints are common in Lyme disease,[630] but no large-scale study using PSG is available to characterize the sleep disturbances in this condition. Greenberg et al.[639] obtained 2 nights of PSG in 11 patients meeting Centers for Disease Control and Prevention (CDC) criteria for late Lyme disease with serologic confirmation and 10 age-matched controls. In addition, the authors performed the Multiple Sleep Latency Test (MSLT) in the Lyme disease patients. All patients had complaints of difficulty initiating sleep, frequent nocturnal awakenings, and EDS; a small percentage had restless legs or nocturnal leg jerking. Polysomnographic findings included decreased sleep efficiency, increased arousal index with sleep fragmentation, and alpha intrusion into NREM sleep. These authors concluded that these sleep abnormalities may have contributed to the sleep complaints and fatigue that are commonly present in this disease.

Because Lyme disease is treatable, every attempt should be made to diagnose it accurately. Diagnosis depends on the serologic detection of antibodies against *B. burgdorferi* in the serum (or, in the case of CNS infection, in cerebrospinal fluid samples).[634] The usual method of testing is the enzyme-linked immunosorbent assay,[634] but antibodies usually are not detectable until 4–6 weeks after the initial infection. Diagnosis may be complicated by false-positive results and lack of a standardized technique to assay for antibodies. Polymerase chain reaction has been shown to be useful in demonstrating *B. burgdorferi* DNA in clinical material.[634,638] Recently developed serodiagnostic tools, such as the C6 assay, and appropriate use of Western blotting show considerable promise in improving the diagnostic accuracy.[640]

In most patients, oral antibiotics are efficient, but in severe cases, 2–4 weeks of parenteral therapy is needed. Practice parameters are available for treatment of nervous system Lyme disease developed by the American Academy of Neurology and Clinical Infectious Diseases Society of America.[637,641] The most effective oral antibiotics include amoxicillin 500 mg three times a day, doxycycline 100 mg twice a day, and cefuroxime 500 mg twice a day given for 2–3 weeks. Treatment of more than 4 weeks' duration is not needed and carries substantial risk but minimal benefit.[635,642,643]

Chronic Fatigue Syndrome

Chronic fatigue syndrome (CFS) is a complex, ill-defined heterogeneous debilitating condition. Patients complain of profound fatigue, functioning below their usual level of energy, that is not improved by bed rest. CFS affects more than 1 million in the United States and is more common in women than men. The diagnostic criteria for CFS are established from a consensus among international experts.[644,645] Diagnosis of CFS depends on the patient's history and the information obtained by physical examination as well as exclusion of other causes of the fatigue after extensive laboratory investigations. The patient must be suffering from severe chronic fatigue for 6 months or longer and must have at least four of the eight primary symptoms as outlined in Table 33–5.

There is controversy in this case definition as the condition overlaps with many other disorders and because it is based on a consensus of experts without availability of any laboratory diagnostic test.[563,646–648] The clinical course of CFS follows a randomly cyclical pattern, and studies conducted by the CDC[645] have found that 40–60% of the people with CFS report partial or total recovery, particularly those who have received early treatment. Certain comorbid conditions with CFS include IBS, fibromyalgia, depression, Gulf War syndrome, and interstitial cystitis. There is some suggestion of increased familial aggregation of CFS because of increased concordance rates in monozygotic compared with dizygotic twins.[647,649] The cause of CFS is undetermined. A variety of viruses, particularly herpes simplex, enterovirus, retroviruses, and Epstein-Barr virus, have been incriminated

TABLE 33–5 Diagnostic Criteria for Chronic Fatigue Syndrome

- Severe chronic fatigue for 6 months or longer
- Absence of other medical conditions explaining chronic fatigue
- Presence of 4 or more of the following features:
  - Impairment of short-term memory or concentration
  - Muscle pain
  - Sore throat
  - Tender lymph nodes
  - Multiple joint pain without swelling or tenderness
  - Headache different from any previous headache
  - Unrefreshing sleep
  - Postexertional malaise lasting longer than 24 hours

without any firm evidence. Several patients with CFS had orthostatic hypotension on tilt-table study, which was thought to be responsible for some of the symptoms.[650,651] However, further studies are needed to understand the significance and the prevalence of orthostatic hypotension in CFS.

Sleep disturbances (e.g., disturbed nighttime sleep, sleep disorganization, EDS) are important problems in some CFS patients, but in many cases these have not been adequately characterized by PSG studies. Sleep complaints and PSG abnormalities have been found in a few studies. Fischler et al.,[652] in a PSG study in 49 CFS patients and 20 healthy controls, found more sleep initiation and maintenance disturbances and a significantly lower percentage of stage 4 NREM sleep in the CFS patients than in the control group. However, they did not find any association between sleep disorders and the degree of functional impairment. In some studies,[653–655] PSG recordings in CFS patients have shown a high incidence of associated or coexistent primary sleep disorders such as sleep apnea, PLMS, or narcolepsy. Insomnia, hypersomnia, circadian rhythm sleep disorders, and sleep-related breathing disorders have been shown in various case reports of CFS.[656] However, in a population-based study of CFS patients and nonfatigued controls from Wichita, Kansas, utilizing overnight PSG and MSLT tests, Reeves et al.[657] did not provide evidence that altered sleep architecture is a critical factor in CFS. Guilleminault et al.[658] reported that complaints of unrefreshing sleep and chronic fatigue were associated with an abnormal EEG cyclic alternating pattern and an increase in respiratory effort and nasal flow limitation, suggesting subtle undiagnosed SDB. A PSG study by Fossey and colleagues[659] showed that more than 50% of patients with CFS had SDB or PLMS.

In conclusion, the entity of CFS remains ill-defined and the treatment, at present, should be symptomatic, using both pharmacologic and nonpharmacological treatment. Nonpharmacologic treatment includes sleep hygiene measures and cognitive behavioral therapy. Symptomatic treatment for depression using appropriate antidepressants and nonsteroidal medications for pain is suggested.

Sleep of Intensive Care Unit Patients (Medical and Surgical)

Generally patients are admitted to the medical ICU because of acute respiratory failure resulting from COPD, bronchial asthma, sleep apnea syndrome, restrictive lung disease, acute cardiovascular disorders (e.g., ischemic heart disease with or without myocardial infarction, cardiac arrhythmias, CCF), acute neurologic disorders causing respiratory disturbances (e.g., brain stem lesion, status epilepticus, high cervical cord lesions, neuromuscular disorders), renal failure, or gastroesophageal reflux causing acute respiratory

tract symptoms. All of these conditions can be associated with sleep disturbances (insomnia, hypersomnia, and sleep-related respiratory dysrhythmia), which become intense in severely ill patients admitted to the ICU who require life-saving cardiorespiratory support.[450,660–674]

Sleep disruption is very common in ICU patients; a figure of more than 50% incidence has been quoted.[670] The causes of the sleep disruption include a variety of factors, such as the ICU environment, the underlying medical or surgical illnesses, effects of many medications used to treat these critically ill patients, psychological stress, pain resulting from the surgical procedures, and therapeutic interventions (e.g., use of ventilators, noise generated by the monitors).[660–674] The ICU environment itself is deleterious to normal sleep and conducive to sleep deprivation with its attendant complications, such as ICU psychosis. In addition to sleep deprivation, physiologic and physical factors contribute to ICU psychosis. Noise, bright light, and constant activity on the part of the ICU personnel for monitoring and drug administration play significant roles in disturbing the sleep of ICU patients.

The ICU syndrome or ICU psychosis describes a cluster of psychiatric symptoms and is a characteristic mental state defined as a reversible confusional state developing 3–7 days after ICU admission secondary to sleep deprivation.[661,662,671–674] ICU psychosis is more common in surgical than in medical ICUs, and the prevalence has been estimated to be between 12.5% and 38.0% of patients admitted to the ICU.[661,662,671–674] Sleep deprivation has been cited as the major cause of the ICU syndrome.[661,662] In a study by Helton et al.,[672] 10% of patients with moderate sleep deprivation and 33% with severe sleep deprivation developed the ICU syndrome. There is evidence to suggest that the ICU syndrome is similar to delirium.[673] The question remains whether sleep deprivation is the cause of the delirium.[675] There is evidence that higher morbidity and mortality increases the length of stay and cognitive impairment associated with ICU delirium.[676,677]

An important cause of sleep disruption in the ICU is noise.[669,670,678–686] Technological advances in the ICU setting (e.g., monitors and meters, ventilator alarms, television, phones, beepers) have been cited as the major culprits for contributing to ICU noise and sleep disruption. The role of the noise in contributing to sleep disruption has been documented objectively by continuous sleep monitoring and recording of the environmental peak sound levels.[683,685,687]

In the surgical ICU, patients are usually admitted in the postoperative period because they are recovering from anesthesia, are beginning to suffer from pain, are experiencing metabolic disturbances, or have an infection related to surgical care. All these factors may cause severe disturbance of sleep and breathing.

Another condition noted in many patients admitted to the ICU is REM sleep behavior disorder. Schenck and Mahowald[688] evaluated over 200 adults with injurious, sleep-related behaviors during 8 years of clinical practice, and 20 of these had ICU admissions. Polysomnography with audio-video recordings documented REM sleep behavior disorder in 17 of these 20 patients.

Several authors have studied ICU patients using PSG to document disruption of sleep structure.[678,689–694] These disturbances consist of marked diminution of SWS and REM sleep, frequent awakenings, sleep fragmentation, and reduced total night sleep time. The total sleep over a 24-hour period appears to remain normal. Because of night sleep disturbances, ICU patients often have EDS.[689,692]

Some studies have suggested that an impairment of the melatonin rhythm may play a role in explaining sleep disturbances and delirium in ICU patients.[695–697] The questions of ultimate outcome and functional status of patients in the ICU and the impact of improving poor sleep in ICU patients are not clearly known, and further research is needed in this direction.[698] It is stated that, overall, physical recovery is more complete than psychosocial recovery.[699] There have been reports of posttraumatic stress disorder following ICU admission for critical illnesses.[700] Roberts et al.[701] reported experiencing vivid dreams, hallucinations, or delusions associated with a longer ICU stay among 41 participants in three ICUs 24 months postdischarge. The authors suggested that, because these dreams are disturbing, the patients should have information and counseling about delirium, particularly for those who remain in ICU for longer periods.

Treatment. The physicians and paramedical personnel who take care of ICU patients must be aware of the various ICU factors contributing to the problem of sleep disturbances, so that correct diagnosis and management of secondary complications (in addition to treatment of the primary disorders) can be effected promptly. The treatment for sleep disturbance in the ICU environment consists of nonpharmacologic and pharmacologic intervention. Nonpharmacologic treatment includes measures to decrease or eliminate many of the factors (noise, light, and others as described previously) causing sleep deprivation in ICU patients. Other nonpharmacologic measures include sleep hygiene rules, cognitive behavioral therapy, counseling the patients after discharge from the ICU, and adjusting ventilator settings to prevent dys-sychronous breathing and central apneas in those using mechanical ventilation.[663] Clinical practice guidelines to improve sleep in critically ill adults have been suggested.[702] These guidelines suggest an integrative approach to improve sleep in these patients, combining pharmacologic and nonpharmacologic measures. The suggested pharmacologic measures include hypnotics and benzodiazepine drugs (short and intermediate acting, such as alprazolam, lorazepam, and temazepam). These drugs should be used with caution because of adverse effects. Nonbenzodiazepine receptor agonists (e.g., zolpidem, eszopiclone, ramelteon) are preferable to benzodiazepine drugs because of the lesser side effect profiles. The newer antipsychotic drugs (e.g., olanzapine, risperidone, quetiapine) may be useful to treat delirium, but adequate studies have not been undertaken yet. Opiates and NSAIDs should be used for pain. In a report using a small sample size, significant improvement in postoperative delirium after surgery for esophageal cancer was noted following bright light therapy.[703]

In addition to treating the primary disorder, it is important to treat secondary sleep-related respiratory problems. If a sleep disturbance persists after the patient leaves the ICU, a primary sleep disorder may be suspected and appropriate investigations, such as PSG study and MSLT, should be performed.

African Sleeping Sickness (Trypanosomiasis)

African sleeping sickness is caused by *Trypanosoma gambiense* or *Trypanosoma rhodesiense* and is transmitted to humans by the bite of tsetse flies. The clinical features are characterized by lymphadenopathy, fever, and later (after several months or years) excessive sleepiness due to encephalopathy or encephalitis. In stage 1 of the disease, the parasites proliferate in the hemolymphatic system (hemolymphatic stage). In stage 2, the parasites invade the central nervous system, causing progressive neurologic dysfunction with disruption of sleep-wake patterns (meningoencephalitic stage).[704–706] The clinical manifestations in the type caused by *T. rhodesiense* (Rhodesian sleeping sickness) are more rapidly progressive, resulting in cardiac failure and acute neurologic manifestations.[707] Gambian sleeping sickness, caused by *T. gambiense*, is a more chronic illness with predominant neurologic manifestations.[704] Within 6 months to several years after the onset of the first symptoms, the Gambian type progresses into a late meningoencephalitic stage. CNS involvement is initially characterized by personality changes followed by delusions, hallucinations, and reversal of sleep-wake rhythm.[704] The patient remains somnolent in the daytime and progresses gradually into the stage of stupor and coma. The cerebrospinal fluid examination shows increased cells and protein.

Several PSG studies lasting for at least 24 hours and correlating with several plasma hormone levels have been conducted in patients with human African trypanosomiasis.[706–716] These studies documented disruption of the circadian sleep-wake rhythm, which is proportional to the severity of the illness. In less severely affected patients, the relationship between hormonal pulses (cortisol, prolactin, and plasma renin activity) and specific sleep stages persists. Circadian disruption of plasma cortisol, prolactin, and sleep-wake rhythms is noted in the most advanced patients, but not in patients with less severe illness.[712–715] These findings of circadian disruption suggest selective changes in the suprachiasmatic nucleus (SCN), resulting in circadian rhythm changes in the advanced stage of the illness. The association between SWS and GH secretion persisted in the patients, even in the presence of disrupted circadian rhythms.[710] In one study, circadian periodicity of the sleep-wake cycle was disturbed proportional to the severity of the illness, but the patients' melatonin rhythm was similar to that in normal individuals, suggesting additional control for melatonin besides the SCN.[711] In three advanced patients, the cytokine interferon-γ levels were increased 7- to 12-fold.[712] In an experimental study, rats infected with the parasite *Trypanosoma brucei brucei* showed selective changes in c-*fos* expression in the SCN, supporting the hypothesis that, in human trypanosomiasis, changes in the SCN are responsible for circadian rhythm dysregulation and changes in the sleep-wake pattern.[713] Lundkvist et al.[717] suggested that the parasites target circumventricular organs in the brain, causing inflammatory responses in hypothalamic structures that may lead to dysfunction of the circadian timing and sleep-regulatory systems in patients with African trypanosomisis.

The possible role of hypothalamic hypocretin was evaluated by measuring cerebrospinal fluid hypocretin 1 levels in 25 untreated patients with human African trypanosomisis.[718] The authors observed that the cerebrospinal fluid hypocretin 1 levels were significantly higher in these patients than in narcoleptic patients but lower than in neurologic controls. The authors observed undetectable hypocretin levels in only one stage 1 patient and intermediate levels in one stage 2 patient. These results do not suggest a unique implication of the hypocretin system in African sleeping sickness, but the authors proposed that a dysfunction of the hypothalamic hypocretin region may participate in sleeping disturbances observed in African trypanosomisis. The diagnosis of trypanosomiasis is based on history as well as confirmation that the organism is in the blood, bone marrow, cerebrospinal fluid, lymph node aspirates, or a scraping from the chancre.[704] The treatment of choice for patients in the meningoencephalitic stage is arsenical melarsoprol.[704,705,714]

Sleep and Cancer

Sleep disturbance, although very common in patients with cancer, has not been systematically studied adequately in such patients as this complaint has been overshadowed by other major problems related to cancer.[719] A prominent complaint in the patient is fatigue, which may be secondary to insomnia in many of these patients. It is important to differentiate primary fatigue from that secondary to insomnia. Given the opportunity for sleep (e.g., relaxing on a couch or lying in bed during the daytime), a patient whose primary complaint is fatigue will not be able to fall asleep and will not complain of heaviness or drooping of the eyelids or head nodding. These patients remain alert and do not doze off. In contrast, patients with secondary fatigue will doze off under these circumstances. The most common sleep complaints in cancer include sleep initiation or maintenance insomnia, nonrestorative sleep, and impaired daytime function as a result of nighttime sleep dysfunction. Savard and Morin[720] quoted a figure of 30–50% of patients with insomnia in newly diagnosed or recently treated cancer patients. This figure is much higher in patients with metastasis associated with pain.

The cause of sleep disturbance in cancer patients is multifactorial,[721] including severe anxiety and depression related to cancer, cancer chemotherapy (e.g., tamoxifen in breast cancer), corticosteroids given to such patients to alleviate the medication side effects, environmental factors (e.g., hospitalization for surgical intervention), severe pain in patients with bone metastasis or compression of nerves or nerve routes, and radiation therapy. In addition to insomnia,[719,722] which is the most common sleep complaint in cancer patients, some patients may have upper airway OSA after head and neck surgery as a result of edema in the pharyngeal space and reduction of upper airway dilator muscle tone.[723,724] Sleep dysfunction in cancer patients adds to the burden of impaired quality of life and may also cause EDS in many of these patients. Most of the studies have involved breast and lung cancer patients, but there are scattered reports in patients with cancers in other sites causing sleep disturbances.[722,725–728]

It is important to diagnose sleep dysfunction in both early and advances stages of cancer to improve the quality of life. The important first step is a history obtained from patients and the caregivers. Laboratory tests are not needed in most of the patients,[720] but if upper airway OSAS is suspected (e.g., if the patient complains of snoring and EDS and has witnessed apneas), an overnight PSG study is recommended so that this patient can be adequately treated to improve quality of life in advanced stages of cancer and to prevent long-term adverse consequences of OSAS in early stages of cancer with long-term good prognosis. Savard et al.[729] performed PSG recordings in breast cancer survivors and observed that nighttime hot flashes were associated with sleep disturbances in those complaining of insomnia. Actigraphy in conjunction with a sleep diary may be useful in patients with insomnia to diagnose and monitor treatment as well as to measure sleep-wake pattern and circadian rhythm activity, which may be disturbed in many cancer patients.[730]

Management of sleep disturbance in cancer patients will follow the same general principles of management of insomnia and sleep apnea as outlined in other chapters of this book. Adequate hypnotic therapy,[721] preferably with nonbenzodiazepine GABA agonists, should be tried first; for insomnia associated with pain in advanced stages of cancer, stronger hypnotics, including opiates, should be liberally used. Pharmacotherapy should always be combined with nonpharmacologic treatment (e.g., sleep hygiene and cognitive behavioral measures). It is important for physicians to be perceptive of sleep disturbance in cancer patients as treatment will largely improve the quality of life. Another important point to remember is that the patient's caregiver or spouse may also need treatment for insomnia as that individual's sleep is also disturbed as a result of a combination of psychological factors and sleep deprivation.[719,720,727]

MEDICATION-RELATED SLEEP-WAKE DISTURBANCES

Medications causing sleep-wake disturbances can be divided into five groups[611,731–733] (Table 33–6): (1) drugs used to treat general medical disorders; (2) drugs used to treat psychiatric disorders; (3) drugs used to treat neurologic disorders; (4) miscellaneous agents (drugs of abuse and alcohol); and (5) over-the-counter (OTC) medications. The importance of chronobiology, chronophysiology, and chronopharmacology should be kept in mind when discussing medication effects because biological responses to medications may depend on the circadian

---

TABLE 33–6 Medications Causing Sleep-Wake Disorders

Drugs Used to Treat General Medical Disorders

- Analgesics, including opioids
- Antiemetics
- Antihistamines
- Cardiovascular medications, including angiotensin-converting enzyme inhibitors and β blockers
- Bronchodilators
- Appetite suppressants
- Sleeping medications

Drugs Used to Treat Psychiatric Disorders

- Antidepressants (e.g., tri- and tetracyclics, MAO inhibitors, SSRIs, trazodone, nefazodone, bupropion, mirtazapine, venlafaxine, duloxetine, lithium)
- Antipsychotic drugs (e.g., haloperidol, phenothiazines, thioridazine, clozapine, olanzapine, quetiapine)

Drugs Used to Treat Neurologic Disorders

- Antiepileptic agents
- Antiparkinsonian medications

Miscellaneous Agents (Drugs of Abuse, Alcohol)

- Amphetamines
- Cocaine
- Marijuana
- Methylenedioxymethamphetamine (MDMA; ecstasy)
- Lysergic acid diethylamide (LSD)
- Phencyclidine (PCP or "angel dust")

Over-the-Counter (OTC) Medications

- Nasal decongestants
- Appetite suppressants
- Caffeine
- Sleeping medications

MAO, monoamine oxidase; SSRIs, selective serotonin reuptake inhibitors.

---

timing of administration of the drugs (see also Chapter 2). Responses of antibiotics to bacteria or cancer cells to chemotherapy may depend on the time of administration because pharmacokinetic or pharmacodynamic interactions vary depending on time of day.

Drugs for General Medical Disorders

Antihistamines (histamine₁ blockers), used to treat allergies, cause EDS as proven by the MSLT. These agents, however, are not recommended as hypnotics because of inadequate knowledge about their safety and efficacy as well as their daytime sedation and anticholinergic effects.

Narcotics (e.g., morphine, codeine, and other opioids), which are used to relieve severe pain and to induce sleep, can cause CNS sedation and respiratory depression. Other analgesic medications such as anti-inflammatory and antipyretic agents (e.g., acetaminophen, aspirin) have not been adequately studied to understand their effects on sleep, but they may have a mild hypnotic effect. It is shown in healthy individuals that the narcotics may increase wake time and reduce the amount of REM sleep and SWS. Antiemetics (e.g., metoclopramide, domperidone, phenothiazines, and the anticholinergic scopolamine) may produce drowsiness as a common side effect. Scopolamine may increase stage 2 NREM but decrease total REM sleep. Domperidone has the least side effects.

Cardiovascular drugs include ACE inhibitors, β blockers, and clonidine. ACE inhibitors, used to treat hypertension, may affect sleep adversely, causing impairment of performance and mood. The β blockers (e.g., propranolol, metoprolol, pindolol), which are used to treat hypertension, cardiac arrhythmias, and angina pectoris, may cause difficulty initiating and maintaining sleep with frequent nightmares. They may also cause insomnia by suppressing the production of melatonin. Clonidine, a centrally acting α-adrenergic receptor agonist used to treat hypertension, may disrupt the quality of sleep by inducing shift changes to stage 1 or wakefulness and by suppressing REM sleep. Clonidine, like the β blockers, may increase daytime sleep and sleepiness.

Bronchodilators used to treat COPD and bronchial asthma may cause insomnia. Theophylline may cause sleep fragmentation and increased awakenings during sleep.

Anorectics or appetite suppressants may act as CNS stimulants by increasing catecholaminergic activity, causing insomnia.

Sleeping medications such as benzodiazepine and non-benzodiazepine (e.g., zolpidem, eszopiclone) receptor agonists may have the opposite effect after prolonged use, and an abrupt withdrawal may disrupt sleep due to severe withdrawal effects. There is individual variation and susceptibility to the withdrawal effects. Transient disruption of sleep after cessation of hypnotic medication is common. All sleeping medications, particularly long-acting ones, may affect daytime functioning. The short-acting drugs may cause rebound insomnia, daytime anxiety, and amnesia. Although benzodiazepines affect cognition and memory, these drugs are relatively safe and have low risk of abuse, and the side effect profiles are predictable. All sleeping medications may have respiratory depressant effect, particularly in patients with COPD, bronchial asthma, and OSA. Sleeping medications should be used cautiously in the elderly as these may easily induce side effects because of alterations of metabolism and drug absorption in the elderly. All benzodiazepine agonists improve sleep quality by reducing latency to persistent sleep onset, reducing WASO, and increasing sleep efficiency and total sleep time. Benzodiazepine drugs may suppress SWS, but non-benzodiazepine agonists do not do so.

Drugs Used to Treat Psychiatric Disorders

Antidepressant medications such as tri- and tetracyclics, monoamine oxidase (MAO) inhibitors, selective serotonin reuptake inhibitors (SSRIs), and others (e.g., trazodone, bupropion, nefazodone, mirtazapine, venlafaxine, duloxetine, lithium) may disrupt sleep, alter sleep architecture, and suppress REM sleep. Some of the tricyclics and MAO inhibitors are sedating, whereas others are stimulating, but most of the SSRIs are stimulating drugs. These antidepressants suppress REM sleep, may increase latency to REM sleep, and reduce percentage of REM sleep. Sedative antidepressants (e.g., amitriptyline, doxepine, trazodone) may be used to treat insomnia, especially associated with depression. Most tricyclic antidepressants may cause daytime sedation. MAO inhibitors have alerting properties, so they are best used in the morning or early afternoon. Trazodone, a sedative antidepressant, increases SWS but is a weak REM suppressant. Fluoxetine has an alerting effect and can suppress REM sleep at high doses. Lithium increases SWS and has a mild REM suppressant effect. Sudden withdrawal of these REM suppressant medications may cause REM rebound. Anxiolytics (e.g., buspirone, alprazolam) may cause sedation.

Antipsychotic drugs such as haloperidol, the phenothiazines, thioridazine, and the newer antipsychotic agents (e.g., clozapine, olanzapine, risperidone, quetiapine) are used to treat psychotic conditions, including schizophrenia. Some of these drugs, particularly the phenothiazines, may cause drowsiness and impairment of performance. All neuroleptic drugs may produce serious side effects in combination with hypnotics, alcohol, or antihistamines. The newer antipsychotics have a better side effect profile.

Drugs Used to Treat Neurologic Disorders

Antiepileptic agents, especially benzodiazepines and barbiturates, cause sedation. However, well-controlled studies documenting the effects of antiepileptic agents and sleep architecture are lacking (see also Chapter 30). Effective control of seizures following treatment with antiepileptic agents results in reduction of sleep disturbance due to the reduction of seizures and not due to any specific effect of antiepileptic agents on sleep architecture. Antiparkinsonian medications such as L-dopa may cause nocturnal hallucinations and agitated confusion during sleep at night. Some of the dopaminergic agonists (e.g., pergolide, pramipexole, ropinirole, cabergoline) may cause nightmares.

Miscellaneous Agents

Drugs of abuse and alcohol (although not a drug, alcohol can be considered a social drug), have potentially deleterious effects on sleep. Stimulant drugs of abuse (e.g., amphetamines, cocaine) may cause insomnia. Amphetamines increases wakefulness, suppress REM sleep, and delay sleep onset. Cocaine reduces REM sleep and increases sleep latency and REM latency. On cessation, these may cause REM rebound. Hallucinogens such as lysergic acid diethylamide (LSD) and mescaline may cause a state resembling dreaming. Marijuana, through its active ingredient tetrahydrocannabinol (THC), may cause sedation at lower doses and hallucinations at higher doses. THC increases SWS and reduces REM sleep. Drugs of abuse mostly alter the amount and timing of REM sleep and produce REM rebound on discontinuation.

Alcohol has profound effects on sleep/wakefulness. Acute alcohol administration, by acting as a CNS sedative, will cause shortening of sleep onset, increase SWS, and reduce REM sleep. However, after the initial sedative effects lessen and as the blood alcohol level falls, the patient will have repeated awakenings causing sleep fragmentation and REM rebound. REM rebound is also noted on discontinuation after several nights of alcohol consumption. The sedative action of alcohol may be due to facilitation of GABA function and inhibition of glutamate. Alcohol, barbiturates, tricyclic antidepressants, and SSRIs may produce REM sleep behavior disorder and other complex phenomena such as status dissociatus.

Over-the-Counter Medications

OTC medications include nasal decongestants and anorectics, which are stimulants (e.g., pseudoephedrine, phenylpropranolamine) and will cause insomnia. Caffeine, which is present in coffee, tea, colas, and chocolates, also is a stimulant and may promote wakefulness by blocking adenosine A_{2a} receptors. As little as 150 mg of caffeine, which is the equivalent of 1–2 cups of coffee, may disturb sleep quality by increasing sleep latency and reducing total sleep time. During sleep deprivation, high doses of caffeine reduce total sleep time, increase stage 1 NREM sleep, and reduce SWS but do not affect neurocognitive functions.

OTC sleeping medications are widely used for the induction of sleep. The active ingredients in these agents are antihistamines (diphenhydramine and doxylamine), and these drugs represent the most common use of antihistamines in OTC preparations. These histamine$_1$ blockers have undesirable anticholinergic effects (e.g., dryness of the mouth, palpitations, dilation of pupils, tachycardia, difficulty in urination) and cause daytime sedation.

SUMMARY AND CONCLUSIONS

There has been explosive growth in sleep medicine and increasing awareness about the importance of sleep in everyday life. It is therefore important for sleep specialists, general internists, and family physicians to have adequate knowledge about sleep dysfunction in general medical disorders to practice their trade effectively. This chapter attempts to summarize in a comprehensive manner general medical disorders that may account for a variety of sleep complaints (e.g., insomnia, hypersomnia, parasomnias, sleep-related breathing disorders, and circadian rhythm sleep-wake dysfunction) or may be comorbid with sleep disorders. General medical disorders may affect sleep-wake neurons by indirect mechanisms through metabolic, toxic, or anoxic disturbances. The possibility of medically induced sleep disturbance should always be kept in mind because the natural history of medical illness may be altered by this comorbidity. It is unfortunate that the ICSD-2 eliminated medical disorders as a separate category of classification and introduced these conditions in a scattered manner throughout the eight major categories and appendices.

All major categories of general medical disorders were addressed in this chapter, and some conditions were addressed in greater details than others because of the importance of sleep complaints affecting quality of life and because of long-term adverse consequences of sleep-related breathing disorders in many of these medical conditions. In the final section, a brief description was also given of a variety of medications used to treat general medical, neurologic, and psychiatric illnesses that may affect sleep and breathing, causing acute and emergent events during the course of the practice of sleep medicine.

⊙ REFERENCES

A full list of references are available at www.expertconsult. com

CHAPTER 34

Circadian Rhythm Disorders

Mark W. Mahowald and Milton G. Ettinger

INTRODUCTION

Chronobiology—the study of biological rhythms, both normal and abnormal—is a field whose time has come. Although major advances have been made, much remains to be learned. The staggering medical, social, and economic consequences of chronobiologic dysfunction are imperatives for further advancement of this exciting field.

Disorders of these rhythms are of more than academic interest; they affect alertness, concentration, and performance that may be crucial for safety in certain occupations such as transportation and manufacturing. The *Report of the National Commission on Sleep Disorders Research* has underscored the startling socioeconomic consequences of sleepiness in our society—at personal, national, and global levels.[1] Wake/sleep scheduling conditions play a major role in these disastrous consequences. Job-related and social demands on the wake/sleep schedules of individuals may result in circadian rhythm disorders that can be life threatening. Studies have shown a circadian pattern of motor vehicle accidents, with severalfold higher incidence in early morning hours and a lesser peak in the afternoon.[2] Human death and birth show circadian patterns, with a tendency for both to occur in the late night or early morning.[3] Other circadian rhythm disorders may not have any obvious cause, but can nevertheless result in significant impairment if affected individuals are required to perform when sleepy or fatigued as they attempt to adjust to demands of the geophysical world.

Most living creatures follow a relentless and pervasive daily rhythm of activity and rest that is ultimately linked to the periodic energy flow from the sun to a spot on Earth as it rotates. Plants, animals, even unicellular organisms show daily variations in metabolic activity, locomotion, feeding, and many other functions.[4] When isolated from time cues such as sunlight, many creatures show intrinsic rhythms of nearly, but rarely exactly, 24 hours. Such a near–24-hour rhythm is called a *circadian rhythm*, a term coined by Franz Halberg[5] from the Latin *circa*, "about," and *dies*, "day."

In humans and other mammals, the suprachiasmatic nucleus of the hypothalamus controls most circadian rhythms, such as rest/activity rhythm[6] and drinking rhythm. There is good evidence that the circadian pacemaker promotes wakefulness.[7] The discovery of a retinohypothalamic tract in animals indicated that the biological clock is directly influenced by environmental light. This led to the application of bright light to reset rhythms of activity in animal studies and the wake-sleep cycle in humans.[8] The timing of exposure to bright light with respect to the animal's intrinsic rhythm controls the nature of the resetting. For example, in a diurnal or day-active animal, bright light administered just as activity is beginning, at 6:00 AM, will typically advance the onset of the next activity onset, which might occur at 5:00 AM the next day. Bright light administered in the middle of the day, at 1:00 PM, will usually have no effect on the timing of the next day's activity. This time interval of little effect is called the "dead zone." Bright light administered at the end of the day, a few hours before sleep onset, at 8:00 PM, will often delay the activity rhythms. The animal experiences a delay in activity onset, which in this example, might not occur until 7:30 AM instead of the usual 6:00 AM.

This has led to the concept of the phase-response curve (PRC), which indicates the various responses of advance, "dead zone," and delay of the cycle. The PRC is determined by exposing an individual or population to bright light or other stimulus at a variety of clock times in the free-running condition and noting the effects on subsequent activity onsets. The same stimulus will have dramatically different effects upon the underlying rhythm—depending upon the timing of administration within the rhythm. The effect is much greater during the subjective night, and may be negligible during the day. Light at the beginning of the "night" will delay the rhythm, and will advance it if administered toward the end of the "night."[8] The PRC may differ substantially among individuals, and will differ systematically with the intensity of the light stimulus.

The importance of the light-dark cycle upon the human biological clock is underscored by the fact that, in totally blind humans, only one-third will be entrained to the environment. Another third will have a cycle that is 24 hours but out of phase with the environment, with the remaining third experiencing a free-running pattern longer than 24 hours.[9] The fact that some blind individuals become entrained to the light-dark cycle is explained by the persistence of a retinohypothalamic tract that is independent of the tracts for vision.[10] This fact should be taken into account prior to bilateral enucleation in blind individuals with normal circadian entrainment.[11] Treatment of totally blind people with a variety of pharmacologic agents may be useful in demonstrating the effect of these agents upon biological rhythms.[12]

It is important to keep in mind that other influences such as changes in activity, posture, meals, timed caloric restriction, and the environment may also affect circadian rhythms.[13–15] There is some evidence that age may affect circadian rhythms, with a dampening and/or advancement of the rhythms in the elderly.[16,17]

In humans, many biological variables show circadian rhythms in isolation studies: temperature; sleep; serum potassium, sodium, and calcium levels; urine output; white blood cell count; attention; short-term memory; ability to perform calculations; and performance. Such isolation studies have been carried out for decades, and typically require a subject to live in a set of rooms sequestered from external time cues for weeks or longer. There are no windows, clocks, radios, televisions, or current newspapers or magazines. Instruments record activity, core temperature, and sleep electroencephalograms.[18]

The human biological clock has two "sleepy" periods—the primary one occurs during the conventional "night"

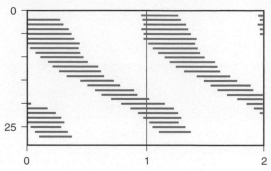

FIGURE 34–1 Schematic example of a free-run study. See text for details.

between midnight and 6:00 AM, with a secondary period in the early to mid-afternoon "siesta time." The magnitude of this post-lunch dip in performance and alertness is individually determined.[19]

Figure 34–1 displays a schematic example of the sleep-wake pattern typical of a free-run study. This is not from an actual recording, but is contrived to illustrate some conventions and terms that are used in the following discussion of circadian rhythm disorders. Black bars represent sleep, double plotted to highlight patterns. Two 24-hour intervals extend to the right of each number, which represents a day of the study. The left end of the first bar represents the first sleep onset, which occurs at about 11:00 PM on day 1. Just below that, on day 2, sleep begins also at 11:00 PM. The second sleep onset is represented to the right of the first and also below it. During the first 6 days of the study, the subject is "entrained," or synchronized with external time cues or *Zeitgebers*. The sleep onsets line up at 11:00 PM on virtually all days.

On day 7, isolation begins, after which the sleep onset delays to about 00:30 AM on day 8. From day 7 through day 17, there is a fairly constant delay of about 1 hour/day. Sleep onsets occur throughout the hours of the day. The average time between sleep onsets, which is one measure of the "period" of the cycle, is about 25 hours, typical for humans in free-running conditions. Such a free-running pattern is observed briefly in the transition from the chaotic wake-sleep pattern of the newborn infant to the well-developed wake-sleep/day-night pattern in normal adults.[20]

In addition to overall circadian wake/sleep schedule abnormalities, there may be ultradian (less than 24-hour) dysrhythmias of state (wake/rapid eye movement [REM]/ non-REM [NREM]). These are beyond the scope of this review.[21]

MEDICAL CHRONOBIOLOGY

Chronobiology is the study of the timing and mechanisms of biologic rhythms. Medical chronobiology is a developing field of medicine, and is concerned with two most important issues: (1) chronopathology—the effect of circadian rhythms and the manifestations of disease; and (2) chronopharmacology—the circadian variability of efficacy and toxicity of various treatments for a wide variety of medical conditions.[22]

Chronopathology

As more physiologic systems and disease states are studied, it has become apparent that many, if not all, have a predictable circadian variation in activity or severity. For instance, blood pressure is lowest at 3:00 AM; epidermal mitosis is maximal at midnight. The same holds true for disease states: asthma is worse at 4:00 AM, and cerebral hemorrhage peaks in the early evening.[23] Nocturnal asthma is probably one of the most studied medical conditions in which there are marked chronobiological aspects.[24,25] As more is learned about the peaks of occurrence of physiologic variables and disease states, more effective treatment approaches can be developed.

Chronopharmacology

Not only may pharmacologic agents influence biological rhythms, but, conversely, the timing of administration of a wide variety of (and perhaps all) medications and other therapies such as irradiation may have profound effects upon their efficacy and toxicity.[26–28] There is substantial work demonstrating that the therapeutic benefits may be maximized and the toxic side effects minimized by administration of the drug at the appropriate time of day. Circadian rhythms in rates of metabolism and inactivation have been demonstrated,[29] along with variations in blood volume and extracellular fluid volume, resulting in varying degrees of dilution of the drug, variations in the susceptibility of the target organ or organs to the circulating drug, and the like. All contribute to the net effect of circadian variation in response to a specific medication. There is compelling evidence of the importance of considering time of circadian cycle in drug administration from clinical areas such as cancer chemotherapy, use of anesthetics and antiepileptic drugs, and steroid administration.[30] Some specific examples of circadian variability include the following: evening medication with diltiazem is more effective than other dosage schedules,[31] and continuous intravenous infusion of heparin has a maximum anticoagulant effect between 4:00 and 8:00 AM, with a minimum effect at noon, indicating that laboratory control studies should be performed at fixed times.[32]

There has been very little work to date on the circadian considerations of drugs utilized in the treatment of sleep disorders. Narcolepsy is a good example of a sleep disorder requiring lifetime stimulant therapy. Data are not currently available to help plan timing of medication to maximize therapeutic effects and minimize toxic effects.

This concept presents a challenging new opportunity for investigation of drug therapy in sleep disorders.

CLINICAL EVALUATION

The wake/sleep schedule disorders fall into two categories: (1) primary (malfunction of the biological clock per se), and (2) secondary (due to environmental effects upon the underlying clock). The secondary disorders (such as jet lag and shift work) are usually immediately apparent upon simple questioning of the patient. The primary disorders may be much more difficult to diagnose, as they typically masquerade as other disorders such as hypersomnia, insomnia, substance (sedative-hypnotic or stimulant) abuse, or psychiatric conditions.

Clinical evaluation must include a thorough medical and psychiatric history, physical examination, and a detailed analysis of the wake-sleep pattern. Careful attention must be paid to medication (prescription and otherwise) use. One most important piece of historical information is that, once sleep has begun, it is uninterrupted and normal. It is not the sleep per se, but rather the *timing* of sleep, which is the abnormality. The patient's report of what his or her pattern would be (or has been) under free-running conditions may be invaluable. Even if there has been no opportunity to free-run, most individuals are amazingly accurate when asked to speculate what the pattern would likely be if they were to spend 2 weeks on a South Sea Island with absolutely no environmental time constraints (work, school, meals, family obligations, etc). When free-running, it is usually clear that the issue is the timing, not the duration or quality, of sleep.

A subjective log reflecting at least 2 weeks of the patient's wake-sleep pattern should be available at the time of the initial interview. Often, analysis of such sleep diaries is sufficient to suspect or establish a tentative diagnosis. If not, objective data may be invaluable. Such data may be obtained by actigraphy, a recently developed technique that provides an objective record of activity that supplements the log. An actigraph is a small wrist-mounted device worn for a week or two, during which the device records the activity per time epoch, which is often 1 minute for a 1-week study. When data collection has been completed, the results are transferred into a personal computer, where software permits display of activity versus time. Figure 34–2 shows an actigraphic report, and demonstrates how the pattern is apparent at a glance. There is high correlation between the rest/activity recorded by the actigraph and the wake-sleep pattern.[33]

TREATMENT MODALITIES

Until recently, the circadian rhythm disorders were only of academic interest, as no proven effective treatments existed. Fortunately, this has changed, and the majority of patients with these often incapacitating disorders will

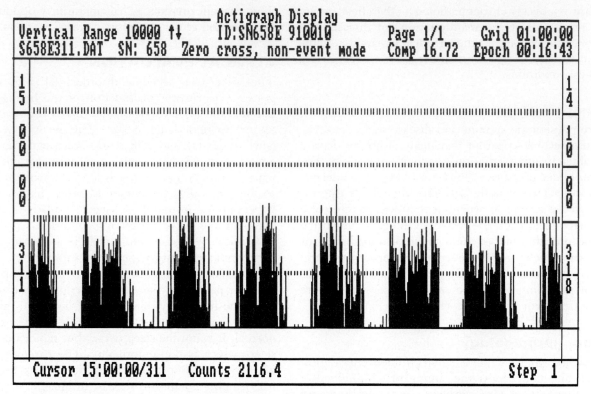

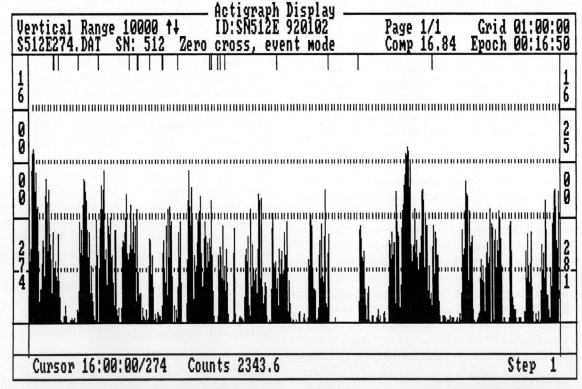

FIGURE 34–2 (A) Actigraphic report of rest/activity pattern in normal individual. **(B)** Actigraphic report of rest/activity pattern in an adult male with a chaotic rest/activity cycle.

benefit from accurate diagnosis and appropriate treatment. The mainstays of treatment are phototherapy and chronotherapy.[34] In addition, there are promising new pharmacologic treatments on the horizon. Unfortunately, some cases may be refractory to treatment.[35]

Chronotherapy

For chronotherapy, the desirable total sleep time is determined by sleep logs during a free-running period. The patient then delays or advances sleep onset by a few hours every day, sleeping only the predetermined number of hours until the sleep onset time is at the desired time, at which time the patient attempts to maintain that time. This method requires several days of free time, and can be derailed if sleeping quarters cannot be kept dark and quiet during the several day sleeps required.[36]

Phototherapy

Exposure to bright light at strategic times of the wake-sleep cycle results in a change in the underlying rhythm. This has afforded an opportunity to treat circadian dysrhythmias very effectively.[8,37,38] The timing of the phototherapy and the duration depend on diagnosis and individual response. The patient sits at a prescribed distance from a bright light, furnishing a luminance of more than 2500 lux at that distance. Fluorescent lights are commonly used. Commercially available light boxes for treatment of seasonal affective disorder typically provide 5000–10,000 lux, depending on the model. Distance from the light is critical in determining the luminance, according to the inverse square law: doubling the distance cuts the luminance to one fourth. The effect of light upon human rhythms varies with intensity, wavelength, timing, and duration of exposure. Much remains to be learned regarding these variables and the effectiveness of phototherapy in the clinical setting.[39]

The light should be angled with respect to the patient's eyes to diminish eyestrain. For a patient with a history of eye disorders, the patient's ophthalmologist should be consulted before beginning treatment. Light units should be safety-tested electrically, and should include measures to screen ultraviolet light.[39]

Adverse effects include headache, eyestrain, and excessive advance of sleep onset. Possible remedies for these problems include analgesics, change in light position, and decrease in exposure time, respectively. Bright light exposure has been reported to precipitate mania in bipolar individuals.[40,41] In such cases, light therapy should be discontinued immediately, and appropriate measures instituted to control the mania, such as neuroleptics, other mood-stabilizing medication, and hospitalization. Candidates for light therapy should be questioned about both personal and family histories of psychiatric disorders and should be warned about the possible precipitation of mania.

Little information exists regarding the interaction of light and a variety of commonly used medications. Caution is urged in the use of light with medication said to cause photosensitization.[39]

Pharmacologic Manipulations

Drugs that shift biological rhythms are called "chronobiotics." Numerous neurotransmitters and peptides that affect the circadian clock have been identified (see Chapter 6). There are a number of exciting therapeutic possibilities under development. Although promising, pharmacologic manipulation of biological rhythms is still in its developmental phase. None of these potential treatments is of proven efficacy for any given clinical application, and thorough review is beyond the scope of this chapter. There are compelling data to suggest that benzodiazepines are capable of affecting biological rhythms.[42] There have been scattered reports of the effect of vitamin B_{12} in some circadian rhythm abnormalities.[43] Tricyclic antidepressants, monoamine oxidase inhibitors, and lithium may also influence biological rhythms.[44,45]

One of the most promising pharmacologic treatment hopefuls is melatonin. Melatonin is secreted by the pineal gland. This secretion is suppressed by exposure to light, and is entrained by the light-dark cycle. It is coupled to the wake-sleep cycle and to the circadian cortisol rhythm and is a valuable marker of the underlying wake-sleep period. It is likely that melatonin plays an important role in biological rhythms, and there is evidence that administration of exogenous melatonin may alter the biological rhythm—with most important therapeutic clinical applications.[46] The discovery of melatonin receptors in the suprachiasmatic nucleus in humans suggests its importance in biological rhythms.[47] The timing of melatonin administration results in variable changes in the underlying rhythm, resulting in a PRC similar to that of light exposure but in the opposite direction (melatonin at the beginning of the "night" advances the sleep phase and vice versa). The effects of melatonin on sleep and performance are very complicated. Melatonin may affect the circadian rhythm, and also diminishes alertness (possibly by reducing body temperature) and impairs performance. The soporific effects of melatonin are minimal, and are likely independent from the circadian effects.[48,49] It should be remembered that melatonin is best thought of as a "dark" hormone, rather than a "sleep" hormone, as it is released during the dark phase in both light- and dark-active animals.

Other Possible Treatments

Exercise

There is preliminary evidence that appropriately timed exercise can phase-shift circadian rhythms, and therefore exercise might be used to promote circadian adaptation.[50]

More work needs to be done in this area to determine the true effect of exercise on human circadian timing. The timing and amount of exercise and its interaction with nonphotic and photic *Zeitgebers* are unknown.[51]

Light Exposure

There is evidence that bright-light exposure may improve alertness and performance during nighttime hours—possibly related to light-induced suppression of melatonin and the attendant nocturnal decrease in temperature.[52] The combination of bright light and caffeine has been shown to enhance alertness and performance during sleep loss.[53]

RELATIONSHIP WITH MAJOR PSYCHIATRIC DISORDERS

Although beyond the scope of this chapter, the striking relationship between circadian rhythms and psychiatric disorders—particularly seasonal affective disorder, primary depression, and bipolar affective disorder—must be mentioned.[54] These disorders are often associated with abnormalities of the wake-sleep cycle and of the cycling of REM and NREM sleep within the wake-sleep cycle.[55,56] Interestingly, many of the treatment modalities for these conditions (sleep deprivation, phototherapy, and many medications such as the tricyclic antidepressants, monoamine oxidase inhibitors, and lithium) affect the wake-sleep cycle and the REM-NREM cycle.[44,57–59] Conversely, psychotropic drugs such as selective serotonin reuptake inhibitors and haloperidol have been implicated as a cause for circadian dysrhythmias.[60]

PRIMARY CIRCADIAN DYSRHYTHMIAS

Delayed Sleep Phase Syndrome

In delayed sleep phase syndrome (DSPS), the patient falls asleep late and rises late. There is a striking inability to fall asleep at an earlier, more desirable time. For example, a college student is habitually unable to fall asleep until 2:00 AM, and has great difficulty getting up in time for her 8:00 AM classes Monday through Friday. She finds herself dozing off during morning classes. On Saturday and Sunday she sleeps in until about 10:00 AM, and feels rested upon arising, with no episodes of dozing during the day.

This disorder may represent 5–10% of cases with presenting complaints of insomnia at some sleep disorders centers.[61] Onset is often during adolescence, but some patients report onset in childhood. A history of DSPS in family members has been noted clinically, and specific gene markers have been identified.[62–64] DSPS may follow head trauma.[65,66]

Some individuals may suffer disruption of school and work. The complications depend partly on the tolerance of the patient's environment. A lenient employer and flexible schedule may allow a person to perform unimpaired if permitted to begin and end work a few hours later than others. More demanding or rigid work or school regimens may not allow this, and will require the patient to drop out if treatment is not possible. Disrupted family life may also result, if other family members do not have a similar schedule. The pervasive misperception that "sleeping in" is an undesirable personality characteristic such as laziness, slothfulness, or avoidance behavior often leads to interpersonal stress and hostility. Driving or operating machinery when sleepy can result in accidents. Victims of DSPS may use alcohol and sedative-hypnotics in an attempt to induce sleep earlier, sometimes developing alcohol or drug dependence.

Differential diagnosis includes irregular sleep-wake pattern and psychiatric disorders associated with disturbed sleep, such as major depression, mania, dysthymia, obsessive-compulsive disorder, and schizophrenia, as well as obstructive sleep apnea syndrome, narcolepsy (particularly during its development in adolescents),[67] and periodic limb movements disorder with or without restless legs syndrome. It may be very difficult to differentiate a true, physiologic DSPS from "sleep phase delay," which is a volitional wake/sleep schedule adopted by an individual to avoid family contact, school, or work.[68]

There appears to be an association between DSPS and depression; however, the cause-and-effect relationship is unclear.[69,70] Furthermore, there is some evidence that there is a correlation between DSPS and personality disorders, and that the DSPS may predispose to the development of personality disorders.[71,72]

Bright-light exposure upon awakening (toward the end of the PRC) has been shown to be effective in advancing sleep onset as well as in advancing temperature rhythm in a placebo-controlled study. The patient is asked to sit near a bright light, furnishing 5000–10,000 lux, for about 1 hour upon awakening every day. The response may not be evident for 2 weeks, and the treatment may have to be continuous.[38] There is some evidence that melatonin secretion may be suppressed by relatively low levels of illumination. Therefore, evening low-level light exposure could serve to maintain DSPS.[73] In support of this is a case report of a patient with non–24-hour sleep-wake syndrome who displayed intermittent changes in sleep onset attributed to exposure to light in the "delay" portion of the PRC.[74]

Other treatment for DSPS includes chronotherapy and schedule change. For example, the patient goes to sleep at 2:00 AM the first night, then at 5:00 AM, then at 8:00 AM, and so on, until reaching 10:00 PM. Patients are not always able to stop at the desired time, but keep delaying, sometimes ending up where they started. There are case reports of individuals who developed non–24-hour cycle disorder upon attempting chronotherapy for DSPS. Their sleep onsets never stopped changing once they were progressively delayed.[75]

Some individuals with DSPS report temporary resolution when in environments with strong time cues, for example, staying with friends or relatives who set limits on staying up late, and who assist the patients in arising at the desired time. There are isolated reports of response to vitamin B_{12},[43] benzodiazepines,[76] and melatonin.[77] The (often unconscious) secondary gain in the intentional "sleep phase delay" syndrome can make this condition very difficult to treat.

DSPS may be difficult to treat, and tends to relapse if the treatment is suspended. Combinations of approaches such as chronotherapy, phototherapy, and pharmacotherapy appear very promising.[78]

Case Example: DSPS

Ms. K is a 36-year-old female who referred herself to the sleep center to discuss treatment options for her nearly lifelong pattern of an inability to fall asleep before 4:00 AM, with a tendency to sleep until 2:00 PM. She has lost two jobs due to an inability to get to work on time, and her wake-sleep pattern played a role in her divorce. She currently works an afternoon shift, and has no wake-sleep complaints.

On her sleep center questionnaire, she stated:

"Over the past many years I have been unable to wake up in the morning by an alarm or naturally—my body's sleep cycle seems "stuck" in a schedule where I sleep all day and am awake during the night and early morning hours. It has *totally* baffled most physicians and I have and still am being treated for depression, since this is the "diagnosis"—which I feel is not the case. If I indeed do have delayed sleep phase syndrome, and it can't be cured by techniques or meds, I will then fully accept this condition after learning more about it. This condition has totally disrupted my life and has created financial hardship, and seeing friends and family is difficult with my schedule.

I would simply like to know if this condition is temporary or permanent. I would like to be awake during the day again! My life has changed drastically due to this condition, and I feel life is passing me by. Social activities and relationships are rare to non-existent."

There is no history of true psychiatric or neurologic disease. Her father has a similar wake-sleep pattern. She brought sleep diaries to the appointment, which exactly confirmed the report of her wake-sleep pattern (Fig. 34–3).

Treatment options discussed included:
1. Continuing to accommodate her wake-sleep pattern by working the afternoon-evening shift.
2. Combinations of chronotherapy, phototherapy, and possibly the use of sedative-hypnotic agents and melatonin.

Comment. This patient's response on her questionnaire emphasizes the devastating nature of this condition. This case also underscores the value of sleep diaries. The history and sleep diaries speak for themselves, and indicate that DSPS is a clinical diagnosis. (She had undergone a totally unnecessary formal sleep study at another sleep center.)

Advanced Sleep Phase Syndrome

Individuals suffering from advanced sleep phase syndrome (ASPS) fall asleep early and awaken early. They are unable to remain awake until the desired time, falling asleep in the early evening and awakening in the very early hours of the morning.

There are no studies of the prevalence and incidence of this disorder, but clinical experience suggests that it may be less common than DSPS. However, its prevalence may be underestimated, as the consequences are less bothersome than those associated with DSPS. The onset of the disorder occurs in later years, with most patients being over the age of 50. ASPS may be responsible for some of the deterioration in the wake-sleep pattern experienced by the elderly. In some cases, there is clearly a genetic component.[79–82]

Patients complain of interruption of evening activities by their sleepiness. They may avoid evening social activities, fearing the intrusive sleepiness. They are also distressed by the very early awakenings. Driving and operation of machinery while sleepy (particularly in the evening) may result in accidents.

Differential diagnosis includes psychiatric disorders with sleep disturbance. The early morning awakenings are often erroneously assumed to be a manifestation of depression. The early evening hypersomnia may be misinterpreted as a symptom of a primary sleep disorder such as obstructive sleep apnea syndrome or narcolepsy.

Bright light administered in the late afternoon or early evening (at the early portion of the PRC) has been reported effective in delaying both sleep onset and temperature rhythm.[4] The technique is the same as that for DSPS, except for the timing of exposure. Adverse effects are similar; however, there is no advance of sleep onset. Instead, there may be excessive delay of sleep onset, for example, until the early hours of the morning. Shorter light exposures may prevent this. Some flexibility may be needed in establishing the timing of the exposure, since the patient may have social activities in the early evening. Occasionally an exposure just before supper is convenient and effective. Chronotherapy, with a 3-hour advance every other day until the desired sleep-onset time has been reached, may also be effective.[83]

Contributing to the growing body of evidence suggesting that in many cases of insomnia there are underlying organic factors,[84,85] one study has suggested that early morning awakening insomnia may arise from phase-advanced circadian rhythms that result in early arousals from sleep.[86]

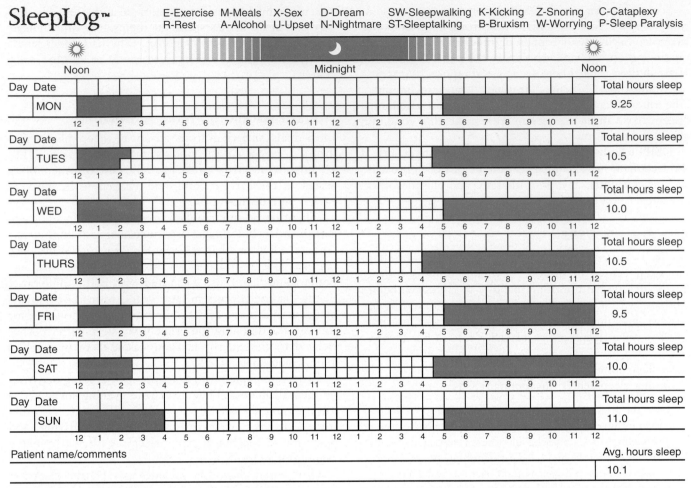

SleepLog™

| | E-Exercise | M-Meals | X-Sex | D-Dream | SW-Sleepwalking | K-Kicking | Z-Snoring | C-Cataplexy |
| | R-Rest | A-Alcohol | U-Upset | N-Nightmare | ST-Sleeptalking | B-Bruxism | W-Worrying | P-Sleep Paralysis |

Noon — Midnight — Noon

Day Date																										Total hours sleep
MON																										9.25
	12	1	2	3	4	5	6	7	8	9	10	11	12	1	2	3	4	5	6	7	8	9	10	11	12	

Day Date																										Total hours sleep
TUES																										10.5
	12	1	2	3	4	5	6	7	8	9	10	11	12	1	2	3	4	5	6	7	8	9	10	11	12	

Day Date																										Total hours sleep
WED																										10.0
	12	1	2	3	4	5	6	7	8	9	10	11	12	1	2	3	4	5	6	7	8	9	10	11	12	

Day Date																										Total hours sleep
THURS																										10.5
	12	1	2	3	4	5	6	7	8	9	10	11	12	1	2	3	4	5	6	7	8	9	10	11	12	

Day Date																										Total hours sleep
FRI																										9.5
	12	1	2	3	4	5	6	7	8	9	10	11	12	1	2	3	4	5	6	7	8	9	10	11	12	

Day Date																										Total hours sleep
SAT																										10.0
	12	1	2	3	4	5	6	7	8	9	10	11	12	1	2	3	4	5	6	7	8	9	10	11	12	

Day Date																										Total hours sleep
SUN																										11.0
	12	1	2	3	4	5	6	7	8	9	10	11	12	1	2	3	4	5	6	7	8	9	10	11	12	

| Patient name/comments | Avg. hours sleep |
| | 10.1 |

FIGURE 34–3 Sleep diary of a patient with the delayed sleep phase syndrome. It is clear that this patient's problem is the timing, rather than the duration or continuity, of sleep because she is unable to fall asleep earlier than approximately 5:00 AM and sleeps until 3:00 PM.

Non–24-Hour Sleep-Wake Disorder (Hypernyctohemeral Syndrome)

Individuals suffering from non–24-hour sleep-wake disorder, also known as hypernyctohemeral (or hypernychthemeral) syndrome, cannot maintain a regular bedtime, but find their sleep onsets wandering around the clock. Most patients will experience a gradually increasing delay in sleep onset, often about 1 hour per sleep-wake cycle. A typical pattern of sleep onsets might be 9:00 PM the first cycle, then 10:00 PM, then 11:30 PM, then 12 midnight, then 1:30 AM, then 3:00 AM, and so on, eventually progressing through daytime hours into the evening again. This likely reflects the fact that most humans have an intrinsic circadian rhythm of about 25 hours, slightly longer than the 24-hour geophysical day. Rarely, patients will experience a gradually increasing advance in sleep onset time. These individuals lack the ability to be entrained, or synchronized, by the usual time cues such as sunlight and social activity. In one large series, there was a male predominance, onset was during the teenage years, there was an increase in total sleep time, and psychiatric disorders more often followed, rather than preceded, the onset of symptoms.[87]

This disorder is apparently extremely uncommon. In our few cases, there have been major psychiatric diagnoses, including recurrent major depression, panic disorder with agoraphobia, and post-traumatic stress disorder. Two had a history consistent with DSPS before the onset of the non–24-hour sleep-wake disorder. In one, the onset of the non–24-hour sleep-wake disorder followed a period of shift work. The course is chronic, with many patients reporting years of this disturbance. There is some evidence that there is a relationship between the hypernyctohemeral syndrome and DSPS.[88]

Structural lesions of the central nervous system such as hypothalamic tumors or head injury have been associated with this disorder.[89] Magnetic resonance imaging studies of the head, with special attention to the hypothalamic and pituitary regions, are recommended in these patients.[61] Totally blind individuals, who have lost or suffered impairment of their retinohypothalamic pathway, frequently experience this disorder.[9]

Complications include severe disruption of work or studies, and accidents when attempting to drive or operate machinery while sleepy. As with DSPS, the tolerance of the patient's environment plays an important role in determining the degree of disruption. Some individuals with a flexible work schedule (such as freelance writers) may experience no disruption of work, which they accomplish when convenient. Others are disabled by this disorder, having been fired from work or expelled from school as a result of poor performance when sleepy or as a result of tardiness or absences associated with inopportune episodes of sleep.

The differential diagnosis includes the irregular sleep-wake pattern, DSPS, psychiatric disorders associated with changes in wake-sleep patterns, and primary sleep disorders such as narcolepsy and obstructive sleep apnea syndrome.

Treatment attempts have included strengthening time cues, with one individual reporting temporary resolution of symptoms when living with a relative who kept her to a strict schedule. Phototherapy,[90] benzodiazepine,[91] and vitamin B_{12} administration[43,92,93] have been successful in isolated cases, but controlled studies are not available. Melatonin was able to entrain a non–24-hour sleep-wake syndrome in a sighted man.[94]

Irregular Sleep-Wake Pattern

Individuals suffering from this disorder show a disorganized sleep-wake pattern with variable sleep and wake lengths. They complain of insomnia or excessive daytime sleepiness or both. Sleep onsets may occur at a variety of clock times. To meet the official criteria for this diagnosis, there must be at least 3 sleep episodes per 24-hour period.[61] The disturbance must be present for at least 3 months. The average total sleep time per 24 hours is normal for age. There must be objective evidence of disturbed rhythms by 24-hour polysomnographic monitoring or by 24-hour temperature monitoring. The patient must currently suffer no medical or psychiatric disorder that could explain the symptoms and not suffer from another sleep disorder that would account for insomnia or excessive daytime sleepiness. Patients may complain of insomnia or excessive sleepiness, cognitive disturbance, and fatigue.

The incidence and prevalence of this disorder are unknown. This uncontrollably irregular pattern of sleep may interfere with work and family activities. This disorder may occur in individuals with central nervous system disorders such as senile dementia of the Alzheimer type, head injury,[95] hypothalamic lesions,[96] or developmental disabilities.[97] In the demented or developmentally impaired patient, this disorder may have a high cost to society in forcing the institutionalization of a demented or developmentally impaired individual previously living at home. One major reason for institutionalization of demented elderly individuals is the inability of caregivers at home to monitor the irregular, round-the-clock activity of their impaired relative.[97]

Most nursing home residents and elderly individuals not in nursing homes receive very little exposure to natural light, spending nearly all day inside.[98] This relative lack of exposure to time cues may contribute to the development of this disorder. Stronger social time cues help some patients resume a regular 24-hour pattern. In uncontrolled reports, bright-light exposure[99] or vitamin B_{12} administration[100] have reportedly been effective.

Profound abnormalities of the wake-sleep cycle appear to be common (and disabling) for patients (and their caregivers) with static encephalopathies and some individuals following traumatic brain injury. No systematic studies are available in these groups.[101] Some associated diagnoses in patients at our center include alcohol abuse in remission and major depression.

Other sleep disorders such as obstructive sleep apnea syndrome, narcolepsy, periodic limb movements disorder, and restless legs syndrome could result in irregular patterns of sleep and wake, and should be ruled out. Medical disorders causing multiple awakening, such as those causing bladder or bowel dysfunction, could result in a similar pattern.

SECONDARY CIRCADIAN DYSRHYTHMIAS

In contrast to the primary circadian dysrhythmias that represent malfunctioning of the biological clock within the conventional geophysical environment, the secondary circadian dysrhythmias occur *because* the biological clock is working properly—but functioning out of phase due to an imposed shift in the geophysical environment. Technological advances such as electric lights and jet planes have allowed us to override or intentionally ignore our physiologic biological rhythms. The numbers of people involved in trans-meridian flight and shift work are startling (nearly one-fourth of all workers in industrialized countries work unconventional shifts). This coupled with the well-documented impairment of performance and judgment attendant to trying to buck the biological clock has staggering implications at the personal, national, and international levels.[1]

The changes associated with time-zone crossing are transient and self-limited; those associated with shift work persist as long as the shift work. The symptoms of these disorders have been experienced by most of us, and are well reviewed elsewhere.[102,103] Schedule-induced decrements in alertness and performance have enormous implications for shuttle diplomats, traveling athletic teams, and shift workers. Effective treatment to reduce or minimize the devastating consequences of the secondary circadian dysrhythmias is in the developmental stage and includes chronotherapy, phototherapy, and the administration of stimulant medications, sedative-hypnotics, or melatonin.[78,104-106] Such manipulations (particularly melatonin administration) are promising.[107,108]

The primary consequences of shift work are impaired performance, workplace accidents, family/social problems, and absenteeism.[109,110] In addition, there is some evidence linking shift work with increased cardiovascular morbidity and mortality, gastrointestinal disease, and breast cancer in women.[111-114] There is a high degree of variability in the short- and long-term adjustment to shift work.[115,116] This is in part due to the exposure to bright light on the drive home in the morning that can impair or prevent circadian adaptation.[117]

In the past, one approach to improving adjustment to shift work was to use sedative-hypnotic agents to promote sleep. Inasmuch as the human circadian pacemaker promotes alertness, it has been suggested that emulation of the biological function of the circadian pacemaker by administering wake-promoting agents may be more effective in combating the sleepiness experienced during working hours in shift workers.[118] Shift work schedules should be individualized to accommodate the goals of the employer, the desires of the employee, and ergonomic recommendations for the design of shift systems.[119] Night-shift workers rarely develop circadian adaptation to the night shift.

Symptoms due to jet lag may be alleviated by treatment with sedative agents, melatonin, and phototherapy.[78,120]

CONCLUSION AND FUTURE DIRECTIONS

The study of chronobiology has taught us much about circadian rhythms—both normal and abnormal. The dire consequences of all types of circadian dysrhythmias are just now becoming appreciated. The biological clock is a powerful physiologic force—and when out of synchrony with the environment may cause disabling and even dangerous symptoms. In the primary disorders, the clock is defective; in the secondary disorders, there is difficulty or delay in the clock's adjustment to a sudden shift in environmental time cues.

With the advent of effective treatments, the identification of these disorders is of the utmost importance. The primary circadian dysrhythmias are undoubtedly much more prevalent than previously thought, and are masquerading as psychiatric, substance abuse, or primary sleep disorders. Careful history taking, and the use of sleep diaries and actigraphy, will usually lead to a proper diagnosis with practical therapeutic implications. As with any field in its infancy, chronobiology is exploding with excitement as new treatments emerge. Few fields have such important implications for so many people.

⊘ REFERENCES

A full list of references are available at www.expertconsult.com

CHAPTER 35

Parasomnias

Jacques Montplaisir, Antonio Zadra, Tore Nielsen and Dominique Petit

INTRODUCTION

In the second edition of the International Classification of Sleep Disorders (ICSD-2), the American Academy of Sleep Medicine defines parasomnias as "undesirable physical events or experiences that occur during entry into sleep, within sleep or during arousals from sleep."[1] Parasomnias can sometimes be considered normal sleep phenomena, especially when occurring during childhood, and do not in general have serious impacts on sleep quality or quantity, or on daytime functioning. In some cases, however, injuries, psychological distress, and/or sleep disruption can ensue and seriously disturb the individual and his or her spouse or family.

True parasomnias are currently classified into (1) disorders of arousal, or non–rapid eye movement (NREM) parasomnias; (2) parasomnias associated with rapid eye movement (REM) sleep; and (3) other parasomnias. Disorders of arousal (from NREM sleep) comprise somnambulism (or sleepwalking), sleep terrors, and confusional arousals. Parasomnias associated with REM sleep consist of nightmare disorder, recurrent isolated sleep paralysis, and REM sleep behavior disorder (RBD). Other parasomnias include sleep enuresis and sleep-related groaning, among other conditions (see Chapter 20). Sleep-related bruxism, sleep-related rhythmic movement disorder, and somniloquy (or sleeptalking) were classified under parasomnias in the first edition of the International Classification of Sleep Disorders (ICSD) but not in the ICSD-2[1] (see Chapter 20). We have, however, included these topics in this chapter.

The clinical presentation, polysomnographic (PSG) characteristics, prevalence, associated factors, pathophysiology, and treatment of the diverse conditions forming this heterogeneous group are reviewed in this chapter. Secondary parasomnias (disorders of specific organ systems that manifest preferentially during sleep) are not discussed here.

DISORDERS OF AROUSAL (FROM NREM SLEEP)

The symptoms and manifestations of the disorders of arousal can be considered along a spectrum. The patient's emotional expression can range from calm to extremely agitated while the actual behavioral manifestations can range from simple and isolated actions (e.g., sitting up in bed, mumbling, fingering bedsheets) to complex organized behaviors (e.g., rearranging furniture, inappropriate sexual activity, playing a musical instrument, driving a vehicle). Moreover, an episode can be composed of two overlapping disorders such as a sleep terror followed by sleepwalking.

The three disorders of arousal share many characteristics. Generally episodes develop from sudden but incomplete arousals from slow-wave sleep (SWS: stages 3 and 4 NREM sleep)[2–4] and sometimes from stage 2 sleep.[4–6] As a consequence, these parasomnias tend to take place in the first third of the night when SWS is predominant. In all disorders of arousal, episodes are typically characterized by misperception and relative unresponsiveness to external stimuli, mental confusion, automatic behaviors,

591

and variable retrograde amnesia. Conditions that intensify sleep, such as sleep deprivation,[6-8] intense physical activity,[9] hyperthyroidism,[10] fever,[11-13] neuroleptics[14,15] or medications with depressive central nervous system effects,[16,17] can precipitate disorders of arousal in predisposed individuals. Finally, a common genetic component is suspected. People with an arousal disorder often have a positive family history for one of the three disorders.[18-20]

Somnambulism

Clinical Presentation

Somnambulism (or sleepwalking) is characterized by complex behaviors usually initiated during arousals from SWS; it may begin with simple movements (e.g., sitting up in bed) and culminate in walking, bolting from the room, or worse.[1] Table 35-1 presents the diagnostic criteria established by the American Academy of Sleep Medicine.[1] Although usually considered a benign condition in children, sleepwalking in adults is potentially injurious. Episodes of surprising complexity have been reported: cooking or eating,[21] driving a car,[22] even homicide.[23-27] Accordingly, the duration of episodes may vary from a few seconds to several minutes.[21] The number of legal cases of sleep-related violence is on the rise[28] and raises fundamental questions as to the medicoforensic implications of these acts.[22,23,29-34] Associated mental activity

includes instances of confusion, perceived threat, dreaming, and even pseudohallucination.

Experimental sleep deprivation can be used to trigger full-blown episodes of somnambulism in the sleep laboratory, since these rarely occur spontaneously in lab conditions. Indeed, a new method of total sleep deprivation for 38 hours has shown an increase of both the frequency and behavioral complexity of episodes during recovery sleep.[6,35] Diagnosis may be substantially aided by such techniques.

Analyses of sleep architecture reveal no significant differences between adult somnambulistic patients and control subjects,[36-41] except for a greater number of arousals selectively out of SWS in sleepwalkers, even for nights without sleepwalking episodes.[36,38] On quantitative analysis of their electroencephalograms (EEGs), sleepwalkers were found to have lower power in slow-wave activity (0.75–4.5 Hz) during the first NREM cycle.[38] They also had a higher number of awakenings during SWS than control subjects (Fig. 35–1).[38]

Several studies have documented the presence in the EEG of high-amplitude delta waves, termed *hypersynchronous delta* (HSD) activity, occurring during SWS or immediately prior to somnambulistic episodes.[3,36,39,42] The occurrence of HSD was assessed by our group,[35] and it was found that (1) HSD was present in 80% of controls during baseline recording but occurred more frequently in sleepwalkers' sleep EEGs, (2) sleep deprivation increased HSD during stage 4 sleep in both groups, and (3) there was no evidence that somnambulistic episodes are immediately preceded by a buildup in HSD. Therefore, although HSD seems to be related to the expression of sleep homeostatic process (HSD represents an

TABLE 35-1 ICSD-2 Diagnostic Criteria for Somnambulism and Sleep Terrors

Somnambulism

A. Ambulation occurs during sleep
B. Persistence of sleep, an altered state of consciousness, or impaired judgment during ambulation demonstrated by at least one of the following:
   i. Difficulty in arousing the person
   ii. Mental confusion when awakened from an episode
   iii. Amnesia (complete or partial) for the episode
   iv. Routine behaviors that occur at inappropriate times
   v. Inappropriate or nonsensical behaviors
   vi. Dangerous or potentially dangerous behaviors
C. The disturbance is not better explained by another sleep disorder, medical or neurologic disorder, mental disorder, medication use, or substance use disorder.

Sleep Terrors

A. A sudden episode of terror occurs during sleep, usually initiated by a cry or loud scream that is accompanied by autonomic nervous system and behavioral manifestations of intense fear.
B. At least one of the following associated features is present:
   i. Difficulty in arousing the person
   ii. Mental confusion when awakened from an episode
   iii. Amnesia (complete or partial) for the episode
   iv. Dangerous or potentially dangerous behaviors
C. The disturbance is not better explained by another sleep disorder, medical or neurologic disorder, mental disorder, medication use, or substance use disorder.

ICSD-2, International Classification of Sleep Disorders, second edition.

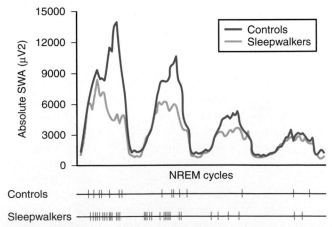

FIGURE 35-1 Slow-wave activity (SWA) over 4 consecutive NREM-REM cycles in 15 sleepwalkers and 15 healthy paired controls. Power is significantly reduced in the second half of the first NREM period. Awakenings from SWS are indicated on the two *horizontal lines* below the graph. (*Reproduced with permission from Gaudreau H, Joncas S, Zadra A, Montplaisir J. Dynamics of slow-wave activity during the NREM sleep of sleepwalkers and control subjects. Sleep 2000;23:755.*)

increased activity of the neural structures involved in the regulation of delta activity during NREM sleep), it has a low specificity for the diagnosis of somnambulism.

With regard to postarousal EEG, Schenck and coworkers[41] described three patterns that characterized the first 10 seconds of most SWS arousals in adults with sleepwalking/sleep terrors: pattern I, diffuse rhythmic and synchronous delta activity ($\leq 4\,Hz$), most prominent in bilateral anterior regions; pattern II, diffuse and irregular moderate- to high-voltage delta and theta activity intermixed with, or superimposed by, alpha and beta activity; and pattern III, prominent alpha and beta activity, at times intermixed with moderate-voltage theta activity. More recently, these patterns were assessed and it was found that the two more frequently observed forms of postarousal activity were patterns II and III.[43]

There is a strong genetic component to somnambulism.[18] About 80% of somnambulistic patients have at least one family member affected by this parasomnia, and the prevalence of somnambulism is higher in children of parents with a history of sleepwalking.[44–46] A population-based twin study[18] showed a considerable genetic effect in adulthood sleepwalking (proband-wise concordance five times higher in monozygotic than dizygotic pairs), although the effect in childhood sleepwalking was not as pronounced (1.5 times higher in monozygotic than dizygotic pairs). In fact, this parasomnia was recently found to be linked to excessive transmission of the human leukocyte antigen DQB1*05 and *04 alleles.[47]

Associated Factors and Pathophysiology

The exact pathophysiologic mechanisms of somnambulism remain unclear. Several factors have been proposed, including psychopathology, genetics, and deregulation of serotonergic systems.

Traditionally, the presence of somnambulism in adulthood has been viewed as a sign of major psychopathology.[42,48,49] However, several studies have shown that most adult patients do not have a *Diagnostic and Statistical Manual of Mental Disorders*–based[50] Axis I psychiatric disorder, nor do they necessarily present with highly disturbed personality traits.[40,51–53] However, anxiety may increase its occurrence in both children and adults.[54–56] Based on clinical and research experience, Rosen and colleagues[54] proposed that somnambulism and sleep terrors may be nocturnal expressions of repressed anger concerning major life events such as separation, divorce, marital conflict, or family relocation.

Serotonin has also been hypothesized to be involved in the pathophysiology of sleepwalking on the basis that certain factors implicating the serotoninergic system (e.g., certain drugs, fever) can precipitate sleepwalking.[57] In addition, sleepwalking episodes are four to nine times more common in conditions associated with abnormalities in the metabolism of serotonin, such as Tourette's syndrome or migraine headaches.[58–60]

Finally, one single-photon emission computed tomography study was performed during sleepwalking in a 16-year-old boy with a history of somnambulism.[61] It showed that sleepwalking arose from the selective activation of thalamocingulate circuits and the persisting inhibition of other thalamocortical arousal systems. During the episode, the EEG showed diffuse, high-voltage rhythmic delta activity. This supports the notion that sleepwalking is a dissociated state consisting of motor arousal and persisting mind sleep.

Prevalence

The peak incidence of somnambulism (approximately 17%) is around age 12 years.[62] For adults, a suggested prevalence of 2–2.5%[63,64] is probably an underestimate. Although many studies report no gender difference in older children, adolescents, or adults,[62,65] a study of two large cohorts of young children (2.5–6 and 4–9 years old) found it to be more common in boys than in girls.[66,67]

Treatment

Treatment is often unnecessary when the episodes are benign and not associated with potential injury.[68] In this case, reassuring the patient/family about the benign nature of the episodes and demystifying the events is often sufficient. However, identifying and avoiding the potential precipitating factors, such as sleep deprivation, stress, and environmental disturbances, is effective in preventing episodes. Precautions should also be taken to ensure a safe sleep environment.

In children, the preferred treatment for somnambulism consists of a behavioral technique called anticipatory or scheduled awakening.[69] The parents keep a diary of their child's episodes of confusional arousal and determine an average time at which the episodes take place. They then awaken their child about 15–20 minutes before the typical time of occurrence of the episode for a period of 1 month. It has been reported that the episodes cease as soon as this intervention is started, and the benefit is maintained on long-term follow-up.[70,71] Hypnosis (including self-hypnosis) has been found to be effective in both children and adults with sleepwalking or sleep terrors.[70,72–79]

Pharmacologic treatment should be considered only if the behaviors are hazardous or extremely disruptive to the bed partner or other household members.[80] Benzodiazepines (clonazepam or diazepam) and tricyclic antidepressants (imipramine) can be effective.[68,81–85] However, pharmacotherapy does not always result in adequate control of sleepwalking.[53] Treatment should always include instructions on sleep hygiene and stress management.

Sleep Terrors

Clinical Presentation

Sleep terrors (also known as night terrors or *pavor nocturnus*) are "arousals from SWS accompanied by a cry or piercing scream and autonomic nervous system and behavioral manifestations of intense fear."[1] The American Academy of Sleep Medicine[1] diagnostic criteria for sleep terrors are presented in Table 35–1. Historically, sleep terrors have been confused with nightmares, a distinct REM sleep parasomnia. In 1965, Gastaut and Broughton[86] first observed by PSG that sleep terrors were not associated with REM sleep but rather occurred suddenly during SWS. Typically, within 90 minutes after sleep onset, the individual will scream loudly and sit up in bed with a panic-stricken expression. There is usually intense autonomic activity (sweating, flushing of the skin, mydriasis, tachycardia, rapid breathing) and, less often, complex behavioral manifestations such as leaving the bed, fleeing the room, or thrashing around. Injuries may result in such cases. The distinction between sleep terrors and somnambulism is ambiguous, although the activity displayed during sleep terrors is usually more rapid and abrupt than it is during somnambulism.[87] Inconsolability is a key feature of sleep terrors; attempting to console or awaken an individual during an episode will only unduly prolong or intensify it. As is the case for somnambulism and confusional arousals (and contrary to a nightmare), the individual usually does not fully wake up and remains amnesic for the event the next day.

As for somnambulism, sudden awakenings from SWS (even without an actual episode starting) are typical of this condition, especially in the second half of the first two SWS sleep episodes. However, a normal PSG does not rule out a diagnosis of sleep terrors. Time spent in SWS preceding an episode appears to be positively correlated with severity of the episode.[87] Rarely, sleep terrors may arise from stage 2 sleep.

Associated Factors and Pathophysiology

Sleep terrors that occur in childhood are usually not associated with a neurologic condition, whereas onset in adulthood could indicate a neurologic disease. Sleep terrors in adulthood have been described in relation to various psychopathologies, but many studies have shown that such parasomnias can occur in otherwise mentally healthy individuals.[2,40,88] As is true for somnambulism and confusional arousals, genetic factors play a major role. Monozygotic twins are more concordant than dizygotic twins for sleep terrors,[89] and terrors are twice as frequent in children for whom one or both parents have a sleepwalking history than in children with nonaffected parents.[90] These data and the clinical similarities between these two parasomnias suggest a common genetic predisposition and similar pathophysiologic mechanisms.

As for somnambulism, the incidence of sleep terrors in the sleep laboratory is lower than in the patient's normal environment.[80,87,91] However, sleep terrors can be induced in predisposed individuals by auditory stimulation during SWS.[40,87] Indeed, in individuals with sleep terrors, the orienting response to auditory stimuli has been reported to be more intense and persistent than in normal subjects, suggesting a hyperexcitability of the nervous system in these individuals.[92] In the sleep lab, the severity of the sleep terror, as assessed by heart rate increase and maximum heart rate after arousal, has been found to be proportional to the duration of the preceding stage 3/4 sleep episode.[93] The prearousal delta power was also proportional to the sleep terror's intensity[94]; the EEG preceding sleep terrors contained significantly more delta power in central and frontal regions than control EEG (no event) sections. This was confirmed by Espa and colleagues,[2] who showed that sleep terrors were preceded by an increase of slow-wave activity with the main increase occurring immediately prior to the episode. During the sleep terror itself, the EEG activity demonstrated that the subject was neither fully asleep nor fully awake.[87]

Prevalence

Reported incidence estimates are wide ranging.[65,95–97] For childhood sleep terrors, the estimate is influenced by the age range studied, the sampling method and definition used. Further, some parents may fail to differentiate between nightmares and sleep terrors. When an operational definition was supplied to parents, a high overall prevalence (40%) was found for preschoolers.[67] As for somnambulism and confusional arousals, sleep terrors tend to resolve during adolescence and do not display a gender difference.[65,67] The prevalence in the general adult population is about 2.2% and declines gradually with age to attain about 1% at 65 years of age and older.[64] In adults, there is a high degree of overlap among the three principal disorders of arousal.

Treatment

The scheduled awakening technique was shown to be effective to treat sleep terrors in children.[98,99] Results of a randomized study in children with sleep terrors indicate satisfactory treatment with L-5-hydroxytryptophan.[100] In adults, when the episodes are not associated with injury potential, treatment is often unnecessary.[68] If a treatment is needed, the same pharmacologic and nonpharmacologic approaches as for somnambulism can be tried.

Confusional Arousals

Clinical Presentation

Confusional arousals (or sleep drunkenness) are defined as transitory states of confusional behavior or thought occurring during or following arousals from NREM sleep, typically from SWS early the night, but occasionally also upon awakening in the morning.[1] During an episode, the individual appears to be partially awake and partially asleep. The individual is confused and disoriented and may display automatic or inappropriate behaviors. Sleep-related abnormal sexual behaviors, such as prolonged or violent masturbation, sexual molestation, initiation of sexual intercourse, and loud sexual vocalizations during sleep, are now considered to be part of the spectrum of confusional arousals.[1] Most episodes last from a few to 15 minutes. Significant sleep mentation is usually not present.

Confusional arousals typically occur during the first two periods of SWS, but can also occur during other NREM sleep stages, later in the night, or during naps. Polysomnographic recordings usually show awakenings from SWS, even in the absence of confusional episodes.

Prevalence

The incidence is unknown, but episodes are frequent in early childhood and diminish in occurrence after the age of 5 years.[54] Children with persisting confusional arousals can become sleepwalkers in adolescence. The prevalence in adults is 3–4%,[101] and no gender difference has been reported. Confusional arousals should be considered benign in children, whereas, in adults, they are often associated with mental disorders or obstructive sleep apnea syndrome. As for the other disorders of arousal, they occur more frequently in conditions leading to sleep deprivation or to a change in sleep-wake schedules, such as in night-shift or rotating-shift work.[101] Drug or alcohol use can also trigger them. A family history of confusional arousals is a major risk factor.

Treatment

As for the other disorders of arousal (somnambulism and sleep terrors), confusional arousals in children can be alleviated by the technique of scheduled awakening. In adults, there is very little information on effective treatment for confusional arousals, which are usually not harmful.

PARASOMNIAS ASSOCIATED WITH REM SLEEP

Nightmare Disorder

Clinical Presentation

Nightmare disorder consists of persistent disturbing dreams that arise primarily from REM sleep (and more rarely from stage 2 NREM sleep) and that usually awaken the sleeper.[1,102] Nightmares are distinguished from bad dreams by the presence of an awakening from the dream. Awakenings are usually abrupt, not confused, and accompanied by recall of a detailed disturbing dream. However, there is typically a much lower level of autonomic activation in nightmares than in sleep terrors, as well as an absence of dream-enacting behaviors. Nightmares are associated with varying levels of heart rate and respiratory activation during REM sleep, but often the autonomic arousal appears much less than might be expected from the disturbing dream content.[103]

Associated Factors and Pathophysiology

Bad dreams among 29-month-old preschoolers are predicted by mother ratings of difficult temperament as early as 6 months of age and by parental ratings of child anxiety as early as 17 months.[104] Among adults, nightmares are also associated with psychopathologic traits[105–107] and personality variables such as physical and emotional reactivity,[105,108,109] fantasy proneness,[110,111] and thin boundaries.[112–119] Nightmares are more frequent and prevalent in psychiatric populations[120–124] and are associated with pathologic symptoms such as anxiety, neuroticism, posttraumatic stress disorder, schizophrenia spectrum symptoms, suicide risk, dissociative phenomena, problematic health behaviors, and sleep disorders (see review by Levin and Nielsen[102]).

Nightmares are also reactive to stressful life events.[105,109,125–129] This general pattern of comorbidity among nightmares, pathologic symptoms, and stress has been explained as due to an underlying distress-prone personality style.[102] Finally, genetic contribution to nightmares has also been suggested by one large population study. The estimated proportion of genetic effects to the phenotypic variance in childhood was 44% for males and 45% for females.[130]

A neurocognitive model has been proposed to explain nightmares.[131] The affect network dysfunction model of nightmare production is based on a combination of findings in brain imaging, sleep physiology, post-traumatic stress disorder, fear memory, and anxiety disorders. It goes together with a neurophysiologic description of nightmare formation referred to as the AMPHAC model (short for amygdala, medial prefrontal cortex, hippocampus, and anterior cingulate cortex).[102] According to these models, nightmares would result from dysfunction in a network of affective processes that, during normal dreaming, serves the function of fear memory extinction.

Prevalence

Prevalence of nightmare disorder is difficult to assess precisely because of different operational definitions, response scales, age ranges, and study samples used (see reviews by Levin and Nielsen[102] and Spoormaker et al.[132]). In addition, prevalence studies usually evaluate nightmares as an isolated symptom but rarely as a disorder per se. The prevalence of nightmare symptoms is estimated in tandem with their temporal frequency. Accordingly, nightmares as a symptom occur occasionally in over 85% of the general population, at least once a month in 8–29%, and at least once a week in 2–6%.[63,108,120,133,134] There is a consensus that a frequency of one nightmare per week reflects clinical pathology.

Surprisingly, bad dreams are not frequent among preschoolers (1.5–3.9% report them *often* or *always*). They can appear as early as 29 months, and the prevalence remains stable until age 6 years.[104] An Internet survey of

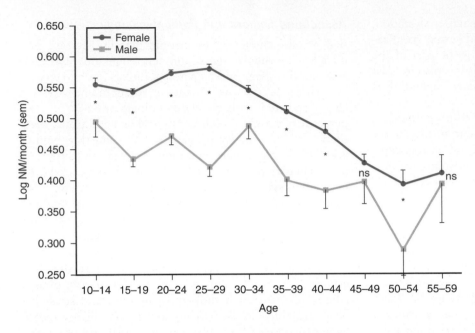

FIGURE 35–2 Retrospective estimates of monthly nightmare frequency by 5-year age strata in an Internet sample of 23,839 respondents. *Significant difference between female and male subjects at that stratum (p < 0.05). *(Reproduced from Nielsen TA, Petit D. Description of parasomnia. In CA Kushida (ed), Handbook of Sleep Disorders, 2nd ed. New York:Informa Health Care, 2008:459.)*

23,839 respondents found that the typical monthly recall of nightmares peaks between the ages of 20 and 29 and declines steadily. There is a gender difference in prevalence favoring girls that appears in adolescence[136,137] and continues throughout the lifespan (Fig. 35–2).[135]

Treatment

Treatments for nightmares include psychotherapy, systematic desensitization and relaxation techniques, imagery reversal, and hypnosis. Psychotherapy has been the treatment of choice for nightmares since Freud. However, it lacks empirical support. Systematic desensitization and relaxation techniques (including eye movement desensitization), in which a relaxation response to the nightmare content is learned, have proven effective to treat nightmares.[138–140] Imagery reversal, in which patients are asked to change and rehearse the scenario of their nightmare, has been successful in reducing nightmare frequency and associated distress.[141,142] Hypnosis has shown some success as well.[143]

Recurrent Isolated Sleep Paralysis

Clinical Presentation

Previously known as isolated sleep paralysis or simply sleep paralysis, recurrent isolated sleep paralysis is a common, generally benign, parasomnia characterized by brief episodes of motor or vocal paralysis combined with a waking state of consciousness.[1] During sleep paralysis episodes, fear-provoking dreamlike hallucinations often intrude and produce considerable distress. Episodes occur primarily at sleep onset (hypnagogic) and upon awakening (hypnopompic). Feelings of fear and terror are accompanying sleep paralysis experiences,[144] and they are often linked to a feeling of presence (i.e., a vivid impression that a sentient being is nearby, but without a clear visual image of it).[145,146]

Sleep paralysis episodes usually arise from sleep-onset REM periods,[147,148] suggesting that they are periods of state dissociation in which some REM sleep characteristics, muscle atonia and dreaming, intrude upon wakefulness.[149,150]

Associated Factors

Stress, shift work, and irregular sleep-wake schedules are factors associated with sleep paralysis episodes.[148,151–153] Several studies link sleep paralysis to various neurologic and psychiatric disorders. It is predicted by bipolar disorder, automatic behavior, and use of anxiolytic medications.[64] It is also comorbid with post-traumatic stress disorder,[154–156] depression symptoms,[157,158] anxiety disorder with agoraphobia,[159] panic disorder,[156,160–163] generalized anxiety disorder, and social anxiety.[164,165] This wide comorbidity has been attributed to mediation by an affect distress personality style ("sleep paralysis distress"[145]) in a manner analogous to that proposed for nightmare disorder ("nightmare distress"[102]).

Associations of sleep paralysis with psychiatric conditions vary among ethnic groups.[166] Some of these differences may stem from cultural interpretations of sleep paralysis hallucinations, sensed presence in particular, as a form of spiritual entity, such as "ghost oppression" in China,[153] "Old Hag" in Newfoundland,[167] and "the ghost that pushes you down" in Cambodia.[154] Finally, a genetic component has also been reported: 36% of respondents in a Japanese sample had family members who experienced sleep paralysis.[168]

Prevalence

Variations in prevalence estimates (5–40%) depend upon differences in operational definitions, age of subjects, and sociocultural factors.[64,151,152] Age of onset is typically 14–17 years. Accompanying sensed presence hallucinations occur in 60–69% of cases.[145,146,169,170]

Treatment

Snyder and Hams[171] report three cases of isolated sleep paralysis controlled by L-tryptophan.

REM Sleep Behavior Disorder

Clinical Presentation

RBD was first described as a clinical entity in 1986.[172] It is characterized by the loss of skeletal muscle atonia normally present during REM sleep and accompanied by complex dream-enacting motor activity. Behaviors can range from simple motor activities such as laughing, talking, shouting, or excessive body and limb jerking to complex, seemingly purposeful and goal-directed behavior, such as gesturing, punching, kicking, sitting up, leaping from bed, and running.[1] Sleep behaviors produce injuries to the patient or the bed partner such as ecchymoses, lacerations, fractures, and subdural hematomas. Injuries are a main reason for consultation, being reported by 79–96% of consulting cases.[112,113] RBD episodes may also cause severe sleep disruption for the bed partner and lead to major marital discord, mood changes, and even suicide attempts.[173] In addition, the dream process and its content appear altered. Most patients (87%) report that their dreams became more vivid, intense, action filled, and violent with the onset of RBD.[174] Dream themes associated with behaviors are largely stereotyped in structure and emotional content.[172,175] The most frequent pattern is that of vigorous defense against attacks by people (58.8%) and animals (23.5%) (see review by Nielsen[176]).

It has been observed that the aggressiveness displayed during nocturnal behaviors stands out against the good-natured daytime personality.[174] Indeed, a controlled study using content analyses of recently remembered dreams revealed an elevated proportion of aggressive content, yet normal levels of daytime aggressiveness.[177] The mechanism by which dream content is changed is unclear. However, it has been proposed that a hyperactivity (disinhibition through degeneration) at the brain stem level activating motor, perceptual, and affective pathways may be responsible for both REM sleep behaviors and altered dreams.[177] The fact that clonazepam reduces both behavioral manifestations and disturbed dreaming[174,178] supports the notion that the two phenomena share a common neurophysiologic substrate.

Clinical diagnostic criteria include (1) complaints of violent or injurious behaviors during sleep, (2) limb or body movements associated with dream mentation, and (3) one of the following: harmful or potentially harmful sleep behaviors, dreams that appear to be acted out, and sleep behaviors that disrupt sleep continuity. Polysomnographic recordings reveal an intermittent or complete loss of REM sleep muscle atonia and an excessive phasic electromyographic (EMG) activity during REM sleep.[179]

TABLE 35–2 ICSD-2 Diagnostic Criteria for RBD

1. Presence of REM sleep without atonia: electromyographic finding of excessive amounts of sustained or intermittent elevation of submental electromyographic tone or excessive phasic submental or (upper or lower) limb electromyographic twitching.
2. At least one of the following is present:
   - Sleep-related injurious, potentially injurious, or disruptive behaviors by history
   - Abnormal REM sleep behaviors documented during polysomnographic monitoring
3. Absence of electroencephalographic epileptiform activity during REM sleep unless RBD can be clearly distinguished from any concurrent REM-related seizure disorder.
4. The sleep disturbance is not better explained by another sleep disorder, medical or neurologic disorder, mental disorder, medication use, or substance use disorder.

RBD, REM sleep behavior disorder; REM, rapid eye movement; ICSD-2, International Classification of Sleep Disorders, second edition.

Diagnostic criteria are listed in Table 35–2. Early studies reported a substantial loss of REM sleep muscle atonia in patients with RBD. For example, three large series reported that 92–100% of patients had some loss of REM sleep muscle atonia.[180–182] Changes in REM sleep in patients with RBD seem to be restricted to the excessive tonic and phasic motor activity. All other features of REM sleep, including REM latency, REM percentage, REM density, number of REM periods, and REM/NREM cycling, are usually preserved.[40,183]

In contrast, Schenck and coworkers[180] originally reported an increase in the proportion of SWS in patients with RBD. In one series, 80% of patients over the age of 50 years had more than 15% of sleep time spent in SWS. This was not associated with prior sleep deprivation. In the Mayo Clinic series, 33% of patients over the age of 58 years had more than 15% SWS.[181] These observations were confirmed in a comparison with age-matched controls: RBD patients demonstrated a higher percentage of SWS and more delta power in NREM sleep.[184] Patients with RBD also showed lower occipital beta power during REM sleep,[185] as well as markedly higher theta power in frontal, temporal, and occipital regions, lower occipital beta power, and lower dominant occipital frequency during wakefulness.[185]

Another polygraphic characteristic of RBD is the presence of periodic leg movements in sleep (PLMS). In a study of RBD and restless legs syndrome (RLS) patients, RBD patients showed a mean PLMS index of 39.5 per hour of sleep, a value not significantly different from the mean PLMS index found in patients with RLS.[186] In this study, 70% of RBD patients had a PLMS index greater than 10. This percentage is similar to the prevalence of PLMS previously reported in RLS patients and significantly higher than the prevalence rate found in healthy subjects of the same age.[187] One difference between RLS and RBD patients is that, in RBD patients, a PLMS index occurred mainly during REM sleep. This is most likely due to the lack of motor inhibition during REM sleep in this condition, and this suggests that PLMS have a different pathophysiologic basis in RBD.

Also, PLMS were significantly less likely to be associated with microarousals in RBD compared to RLS patients,[187] and a markedly reduced amplitude of cardiac response was found in patients with RBD.[186] These findings suggest the presence of dysautonomia and/or reduced cortical reactivity in RBD.

Until recently, the diagnosis of RBD was based on clinical manifestations; PSG recordings of patients were not necessary for diagnosis. However, there are some limitations in using clinical criteria only. RBD-like features can occur with other sleep conditions, such as obstructive sleep apnea syndrome, sleepwalking, night terrors, and sleep-related seizures. Therefore, it is important to ensure that behavioral manifestations occur exclusively during REM sleep. In addition, PSG allows the detection of subclinical forms of RBD, such as REM sleep without atonia, which can be observed in the absence of behavioral manifestations. In the ICSD-2, PSG features are essential to the RBD diagnosis.[1] The first essential criterion is the presence of REM sleep without atonia, that is, the EMG finding of excessive amounts of either sustained or intermittent elevation of submental EMG activity or excessive phasic submental or limb EMG twitching. The second criterion is the presence of either sleep-related injurious or disruptive behaviors by history, or abnormal REM sleep behaviors documented during PSG recording. Time-synchronized video recording is essential for helping to establish the diagnosis of RBD during PSG. The last two criteria are the absence of epileptiform activity during REM sleep and the absence of other sleep disorders or medical or neurologic disorders that could better explain the sleep disturbance.

One limitation of these new criteria is the absence of a validated and universally accepted method for scoring REM sleep in RBD. Assessing REM sleep without atonia by using standard criteria is impossible—muscle atonia is an essential defining criterion for REM sleep.[188] Lapierre and Montplaisir[183] developed a scoring method for REM sleep based on the EEG and electro-oculography only (Table 35–3). In this method, the occurrence of the first REM is used to determine the onset of the REM sleep period. The termination of the REM sleep period is identified either by the occurrence of specific EEG features of a different sleep stage (K complexes, sleep spindles, EEG signs of arousals), or by the absence of REMs for 3 consecutive minutes. Then, tonic and phasic components of REM sleep are scored separately. Each epoch is scored as tonic or atonic depending on whether tonic chin EMG activity is present for more or less than 50% of the epoch duration. Phasic EMG density is also scored from the submental EMG recording, and is expressed as the percentage of mini-epochs (2 or 3 seconds depending on epoch duration of 20 or 30 seconds) containing phasic EMG events.

TABLE 35–3 Polysomnographic Scoring Criteria for RBD	
REM sleep onset	Occurrence of the first REM
REM sleep termination	Occurrence of a specific EEG feature of another sleep stage (K complex, sleep spindle, EEG sign of arousal) *or* Absence of REMs for 3 consecutive minutes
Muscle atonia	Each 20-sec epoch is scored as tonic or atonic depending on whether chin EMG activity is present for more or less than 50% of the epoch duration. Presence of EMG activity is defined by chin EMG amplitude at least twice that of the background or greater than 10 μV.
Phasic EMG activity	Percentage of 2-sec mini-epochs containing chin EMG events. EMG events are defined by any burst of EMG activity lasting 0.1–5 sec, with amplitude exceeding 4 times the amplitude of background EMG activity.
REM density	Percentage of 2-sec mini-epochs of REM sleep containing at least one REM

EEG, electroencephalogram; EMG, electromyographic; RBM, REM sleep behavior disorder; REM, rapid eye movement.
Modified from Lapierre O, Montplaisir J. Polysomnographic features of REM sleep behavior disorder: development of a scoring method. Neurology 1992;42:1371.

Associated Factors and Pathophysiology: Idiopathic and Secondary RBD

RBD may be associated with a great variety of medical conditions or with the use of various psychotropic medications. Therefore, RBD has been divided into primary and secondary forms.[1] Primary or idiopathic RBD is diagnosed when none of the conditions listed for secondary RBD is present.

Secondary RBD has been classified into acute and chronic subtypes depending on the time course of clinical manifestations.[1] Acute RBD is usually associated with intoxication or withdrawal from psychotropic substances. Caffeine abuse, tricyclics antidepressants, biperidin, and monoamine oxidase inhibitors have been reported to be associated with RBD. Withdrawal from alcohol or from medications such as meprobamate, pentazocine, barbiturates, and nitrazepam can also trigger episodes of acute RBD (for review, see Mahowald and Schenck[179]).

Chronic secondary RBD may occur during long-term use of several medications: cholinesterase inhibitors,[189,190] monoamine oxidase inhibitors,[191,192] tricyclic antidepressants,[193–195] or newer serotoninergic agents such as fluoxetine, paroxetine, citalopram, sertraline, and venlafaxine.[196] Secondary RBD can occur in association with narcolepsy[181,197–199] and other neurologic disorders, such as olivopontocerebellar degeneration, ischemic cerebrovascular disease, multiple sclerosis, Guillain-Barré syndrome, Shy-Drager syndrome, and Arnold-Chiari malformation.[179]

Finally, RBD is strongly associated with neurodegenerative diseases, especially the synucleinopathy subtype,[200] which includes Parkinson's disease (PD),[201,202] dementia with Lewy bodies (DLB),[203–207] and multiple system atrophy (MSA).[208–214] In fact, based on clinical diagnostic criteria, 15–34% of patients with PD have been estimated to have symptoms of RBD.[201,215] In a sleep laboratory study, one-third of patients with PD (11/33) had RBD based on PSG criteria.[202] RBD is also very common in patients with DLB.[205,206] Several studies have shown a very high association between RBD and MSA.[209,210] In a sleep laboratory study of 19 patients with MSA, RBD was detected in 100%.[216] RBD has been shown to coexist with Alzheimer's disease[217] and with progressive supranuclear palsy,[218] two tauopathies.

As more patients with so-called idiopathic RBD are studied over time, it is becoming increasingly clear that more than 50% will eventually develop neurodegenerative disorders, especially PD. For example, Schenck and coworkers[203] found that a parkinsonian syndrome developed in 38% of 29 patients initially diagnosed with idiopathic RBD after 5 years of follow-up. Seven years later, 65% of patients from the same cohort had developed a parkinsonian syndrome.[219] Since RBD patients are at risk of

developing PD, studies have looked at a variety of potential early markers of PD in patients with idiopathic RBD who were free of parkinsonism.

Multiple dysfunctions have been described in the last 5 years for idiopathic RBD patients (Fig. 35–3), such as olfactory deficits, color identification deficits, and decreased motor speed[220]; EEG slowing[185]; mild dysautonomia[186,221,222]; and subtle neuropsychological dysfunctions.[185,223,224] These abnormalities are similar to those found in early stages of PD.[225] Finally, fluorodeoxyglucose–positron emission tomography brain imaging of cognitively normal patients with dream-enacting behaviors revealed lower metabolic activity in several brain regions known to be affected in DLB.[226]

Animal studies using various methodologic approaches (electrophysiology, lesions, and neuropharmacology) have shown that REM sleep muscle atonia results from the interaction of several neuronal systems located in the brain stem. Bilateral tegmentopontine lesions in animals

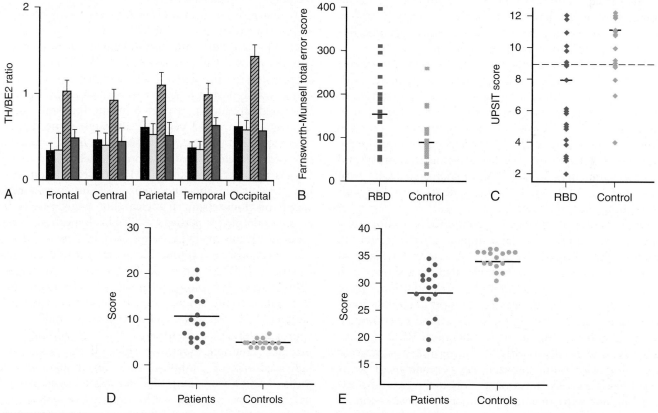

FIGURE 35–3 Electroencephalographic changes and sensory and neuropsychological deficits associated with REM sleep behavior disorder (RBD). **(A)** Electroencephalographic slowing during wakefulness is indicated by a generalized increase in the theta/beta2 ratio in male RBD patients (*hatched bars*) relative to male controls (*black bars*), female controls (*light blue bars*), and female RBD patients (*dark blue bars*). **(B)** Visual discrimination deficits are apparent as higher error scores on the Farnsworth-Munsell 100-Hue Test for RBD patients. **(C)** Olfactory discrimination deficits are apparent as lower average scores on the University of Pennsylvania Brief Smell Identification Test. **(D and E)** Neuropsychological deficits are shown by higher error scores on the Corsi Supraspan Learning Test **(D)** and lower scores on the Rey-Osterrieth Complex Figure Design **(E)**. *(**A** reproduced with permission from Fantini ML, Gagnon JF, Petit D, et al. Slowing of electroencephalogram in rapid eye movement sleep behavior disorder. Ann Neurol 2003;53:774. **B** and **C** reproduced with permission from Postuma RB, Lang AE, Massicotte-Marquez J, Montplaisir J. Potential early markers of Parkinson disease in idiopathic REM sleep behavior disorder. Neurology 2006;66:845. **D** and **E** reproduced with permission from Ferini-Strambi L, Di Gioia MR, Castronovo V, et al. Neuropsychological assessment in idiopathic REM sleep behavior disorder [RBD]: does the idiopathic form of RBD really exist? Neurology 2004;62:41.)*

can produce both a loss of muscle atonia and the presence of motor behaviors during REM sleep,[227–232] a model for human RBD. To produce RBD in animals, two different systems must be involved: the atonia system and the locomotor system. Lesions to the atonia system will produce only REM sleep without atonia, a phenomenon frequently encountered in neurodegenerative diseases and thought to be a form of incomplete RBD. To produce RBD in animals, the lesions should also involve the system that normally suppresses the brain stem motor generators during REM sleep. Therefore, RBD may result from a dysfunction in these two systems: either a loss of REM sleep atonia, excessive locomotor drive, or both.[233]

Neuropathologic analysis and imaging studies of patients with RBD, whether associated with a neurodegenerative disorder or not, have also started to provide answers. Only 10 cases of RBD with autopsy that included examination of the brain stem have been published so far.[51,205,234–238] Histopathologic anomalies (i.e., Lewy bodies, neuronal loss, depigmentation or gliosis) were reported in the locus ceruleus–subceruleus complex and the substantia nigra for all patients. Anomalies have been found less severely or less consistently in the dorsal raphe, dorsal vagus, gigantocellular reticular, and pedunculopontine nuclei.

Magnetic resonance imaging revealed ischemic lesions in pontomesencephalic regions in three patients with RBD.[239] Other studies have also suggested that tumor, ischemic infarct, or surgery in the pontine region may trigger RBD.[240–242] However, neuroimaging is negative in most patients with RBD.[181] Similarly, proton magnetic resonance spectroscopy revealed no anomalies on several metabolic measures in the brain stems of patients with idiopathic RBD,[243] nor between patients with PD with and without RBD.[244]

Single-photon emission computed tomography showed a reduction in striatal dopamine transporters in patients with idiopathic RBD.[245] A reduced density of striatal dopaminergic terminals has also been shown with positron emission tomography.[246] In addition, there appeared to be a continuum of reduction in striatal dopamine transporters on single-photon emission computed tomography from patients with subclinical RBD to clinical RBD, and finally to PD.[247] Moreover, a significant correlation was found between the percentage of REM sleep muscle atonia and striatal dopaminergic transmission, but not with thalamic cholinergic transmission.[248] It remains unclear, however, whether the dysfunction of the nigrostriatal dopaminergic system is the primary cause of RBD or an epiphenomenon.

In conclusion, a dysfunction of one or several neural pathways originating in the brain stem (nigrostriatal dopaminergic neurons, noradrenergic/cholinergic neurons of the locus ceruleus–subceruleus complex, serotonergic neurons of the raphe nucleus, or cholinergic neurons of the pedunculopontine nucleus) is likely responsible for the pathogenesis of RBD.

Prevalence

The overall prevalence of RBD remains largely unknown. A large telephone survey assessing violent behaviors during sleep in the general population (15–100 years of age) suggested a prevalence of about 0.5%.[249] Another study of 1034 individuals (70+ years of age) in the Hong Kong area found a prevalence of PSG-confirmed RBD of 0.4%.[250] There is a male predominance (87%) with primarily men over the age of 50 being affected.[174] Milder forms of RBD with less aggressive behaviors that do not lead to clinical consultation have been postulated for women.[174]

Treatment

To our knowledge, there are no randomized, double-blind, placebo-controlled studies of any treatment for RBD. There are numerous reports of case series of RBD treated with a variety of medications, but these have important methodologic limitations and few have included PSG assessments.

Clonazepam, a sedating benzodiazepine, is considered the treatment of choice for RBD. Two large case series have reported substantial improvement in a majority of patients treated with clonazepam.[180,181] In most cases, a suppression of problematic sleep behaviors and nightmares was reported during the first week of treatment. Sustained efficacy was reported during long-term administration of up to 17 years,[179] although some degree of tolerance did occur. Polysomnographic recordings revealed that clonazepam suppresses behavioral manifestations and decreases phasic EMG activity without restoring REM sleep muscle atonia.[183] The mechanism of action of clonazepam is unclear but likely results from its serotonergic properties.[179,183] This hypothesis is based on observations made in animals where selective destruction of brain stem serotonergic neurons produced a disinhibition of REM sleep phasic activity and triggered hallucinatory behaviors, whereas the administration of serotonin inhibited motor activity in several experimental designs.[251,252] However, clonazepam is ineffective in approximately 10% of patients.[180,181] In addition, some patients experience serious side effects, such as an increased risk of confusion and falls in elderly individuals[253] and a worsening of sleep-related respiratory disturbances in patients with obstructive sleep apnea syndrome.[254] Therefore, alternative treatments must be considered.

A 6-week open-label trial of 3 mg of melatonin given 30 minutes before bedtime demonstrated a dramatic clinical improvement in five of six RBD patients.[255] A PSG recording showed a significant restoration of REM sleep muscle atonia without any significant reduction of phasic motor activity. This initial observation was confirmed in a study of 15 idiopathic RBD patients treated with melatonin 3–9 mg.[256] These authors noted a nearly threefold suppression of REM sleep tonic activity after melatonin therapy. More recently, Boeve and coworkers[257] looked at the efficacy of melatonin in 14 patients with RBD associated with neurologic conditions. RBD was controlled in six patients, significantly improved in four, and initially improved but subsequently returned in two. No improvement occurred in one patient and increased RBD frequency/severity occurred in one patient. The effective melatonin doses ranged from 3 to 12 mg. However, the findings from these studies suggest that melatonin may be less potent than clonazepam. In summary, melatonin can be considered as an alternative therapy in both idiopathic or secondary RBD, but long-term, controlled trials are needed to ascertain the efficacy of melatonin in this condition. The mechanism of action of melatonin in RBD is still unknown; it appears that melatonin restores REM sleep muscle atonia, whereas clonazepam exerts its therapeutic effect by suppressing phasic motor activity.

Another drug family was shown to produce therapeutic benefit in RBD. Indeed, some studies of acetylcholinesterase inhibitors (donepezil and rivastigmine) demonstrated increased sleep quality and reduced motor events in patients with idiopathic RBD[258] and in patients with RBD associated with DLB.[259–261] However, neither of these studies used PSG recordings to confirm treatment efficacy. Other studies of patients with RBD associated with DLB did not find any change in the frequency or the severity of RBD symptoms with donepezil.[257,261]

Other medications have been used to treat RBD. Based on the strong association between RBD and PD, dopaminergic agents have been considered as a treatment of RBD. Pramipexole, a dopamine D_2 receptor agonist with a high affinity for D_3 receptors, was shown to reduce the intensity and the frequency of clinical motor events reported by patients and to decrease the number of simple motor manifestations seen on PSG video recordings.[262] The REM sleep phasic EMG activity was not changed, and there was a paradoxical increase in REM sleep tonic EMG activity. This effect of pramipexole was not found in RBD associated with PD.[263] Another study reported an increase in both REM sleep phasic and tonic EMG activity after treatment with levodopa in patients with PD.[264]

Finally, since injury to the patient or to the bed partner is the most common reason that brings patients to consultation, the treatment program should start with a discussion on risk of accidents, indication of sleeping in different beds and safety measures such as removal of dangerous objects in the room, protection of the windows, and placement of cushions around the bed or the mattress on the floor. These recommendations are important even in treated patients since cases of injuries were reported in patients successfully treated for RBD.

OTHER PARASOMNIAS

Sleep Enuresis

Clinical Presentation

Sleep enuresis is characterized by recurrent involuntary voiding during sleep at least twice a week among individuals who are at least 5 years of age.[1] If the child has never been constantly dry during sleep, it is considered primary. Sleep enuresis is secondary when the child (or adult) had been previously dry for at least 6 consecutive months and started wetting at least twice a week for at least 3 months.

A common belief among parents is that sleep enuresis is the result of sleeping too deeply. However, changes in sleep depth and sleep architecture have not been consistently demonstrated.[265] For most enuretic children, voiding occurs in the first half of the night and is not associated to a specific sleep stage.[265] Conversely, a PSG study has demonstrated that enuretic boys are more difficult to arouse from sleep than are age-matched controls.[266]

Associated Factors and Pathophysiology

A three-system model has been proposed to explain enuresis, which has wide clinical appeal.[267] It identifies three processes that alone or in combination can engender nocturnal enuresis: (1) lack of arginine vasopressin release during sleep (which would normally decrease urine production); (2) overactivity of the bladder (uninhibited bladder contractions) or low functional bladder capacity; and (3) inability of the child to wake up in response to sensations of a full bladder.[268] Tachycardia and short EEG arousals are often present prior to enuretic events.[265]

Some evidence indicates that bed-wetting may reflect delayed development of the central nervous system. It has been shown that premature and/or low-birth-weight children were bed-wetting more often than normal-birth-weight children.[269–272] Moreover, several studies or clinical observations have suggested an association between bed-wetting and developmental delays in motricity,[273–275] language,[275–280] physical growth,[276] and skeletal maturation.[281,282]

Enuresis is not linked with anxiety in preschoolers[67] but is in older children.[283–285] However, anxiety is more likely a consequence than a cause of enuresis, brought about by perplexity or a sense of immaturity, humiliation, social embarrassment, or fear of detection. Hereditary factors have been recognized; it is inherited via an autosomal dominant mode of transmission (for a review, see von Gontard et al.[286]).

Prevalence

Prevalence is 77% when both parents were enuretic as children and 44% when one parent was enuretic.[287] Adult enuresis occurs in about 3% of elderly women

(65 years and older) and in 1% of elderly men living at home.[288] In 5-year-old children, population-based studies[67,278,289] found a prevalence between 20% and 33%. A male predominance in prevalence is well established.[65,67,278,289]

Treatment

Treatments for enuresis differ depending on the suspected cause of enuresis. When bed-wetting is caused by lack of arginine vasopressin release during sleep, an enuresis alarm (a device that alerts and sensitize the child to respond quickly to a full bladder by waking up) or pharmacologic intervention using desmopressin, a synthetic analog of vasopressin, is indicated. The anticholinergic agent oxybutynin is preferred in cases in which the cause is bladder overactivity. Oxybutynin is a smooth muscle relaxant with specific effects on the bladder. Combining treatments is also possible when mixed causes are present (for review, see Butler[290]).

Sleep-Related Bruxism

Clinical Presentation

Sleep related bruxism is the grinding or clenching of one's teeth during sleep, usually in association with sleep arousals.[1] This activity results in tooth wear, headaches, jaw dysfunction, and pain. Orofacial morphology is not likely a causal factor since it has been shown not to differentiate sleep bruxers from controls.[291]

The definitive diagnosis rests on the presence of rhythmic masticatory muscle activity and grinding sounds during all-night PSG recording, although abnormal tooth wear is very indicative of sleep bruxism. Bruxism episodes most frequently occur in stages 1 and 2 but can occur in all stages.[292,293] Surprisingly, bruxers have a normal sleep architecture and high sleep efficiency (>90%).[292]

Associated Factors and Pathophysiology

Various hypotheses have been put forward to explain sleep bruxism. The first one was changes in dental occlusion, but no strong evidence-based data support this hypothesis.[294] Anxiety has been reported as an associated factor in children,[65] adolescents, and adults.[295–298] Smoking also exacerbates bruxism.[299] Finally, a deficiency of the dopaminergic system has been implicated, but that remains to be confirmed since most randomized trials with dopaminergic medications have only marginally reduced sleep bruxism episodes.[300,301]

A clear sequence of cortical to cardiac activation preceding jaw motor activity in bruxism patients[302] suggests that sleep bruxism is secondary to microarousals. In fact, both microarousals and rhythmic masticatory muscle activity/sleep bruxism episodes were shown to increase concomitantly just before each REM sleep period.[303] It has been suggested that the sudden apparition of sleep bruxism is under the influence of brief and transient

activity of the brain stem arousal–reticular ascending system contributing to the increase of activity in autonomic-cardiac and motor modulatory networks (Fig. 35–4).[304]

Finally, as it is the case for many parasomnias, there is a strong genetic influence on bruxism.[305] Children of sleep bruxers are more likely to be affected than those of individuals who never had the problem or who suffer from daytime bruxism only.[306–308] Twin studies in bruxism have suggested that hereditary factors are important to both the genesis and pattern of bruxism.[309,310]

Prevalence

Sleep bruxism is very common in early childhood. A recent longitudinal, population-based study found that the prevalence increases from 2.5 years to reach 33% at 6 years of age.[67] Another longitudinal study reported a progressive decrease toward adolescence, attaining 9% at age 13.[65] An age-related decline in prevalence has also been described throughout adulthood in a population-based study.[311] Overall prevalence in adults has been estimated to be around 8%.[312] No gender difference has been found for either children[65] or adults.[311] The presence of sleep bruxism in childhood is highly predictive of bruxism in adulthood.[305]

Treatment

A meta-analysis study evaluated randomized controlled studies of seven pharmacologic treatments and three oral devices.[313] The mandibular advancement device and clonidine are the most promising experimental treatments, although both are associated with adverse effects (discomfort for the device; REM suppression and morning hypotension for clonidine). Clonazepam appears to be an acceptable short-term alternative. Occlusal appliances (soft mouth guard, occlusal stabilization splint, splint with vibration) can protect orofacial structures.

Sleep-Related Rhythmic Movement Disorder

Clinical Presentation

Sleep-related rhythmic movement disorder is characterized by the repetitive, stereotyped, and rhythmic activity of large muscle groups that occurs predominantly during drowsiness (sleep onset) or sleep.[1] It is largely a parasomnia of infancy and early childhood. The most frequent rhythmic movements are body rocking, head rolling, and head banging, although it can involve any body part. Body rocking may be difficult to distinguish from head banging because the former sometimes includes banging of the head into a solid object. The frequency of movements is more typically around 1 Hz but can range from 0.5 to 2.0 Hz.[314] Episodes of rhythmic movement can last from a few seconds to more than an hour.[314] In most sufferers, they will occur nightly or almost every night.[315] The

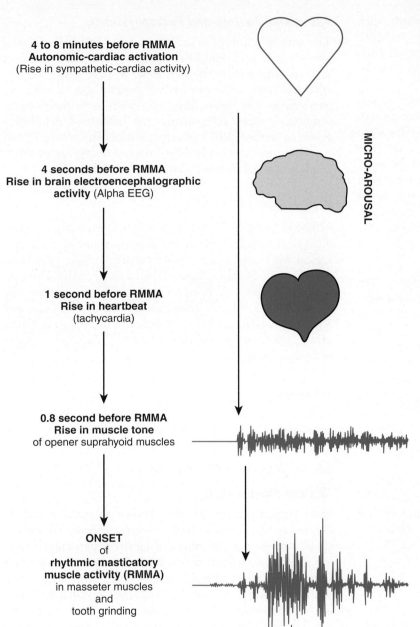

4 to 8 minutes before RMMA
Autonomic-cardiac activation
(Rise in sympathetic-cardiac activity)

4 seconds before RMMA
Rise in brain electroencephalographic
activity (Alpha EEG)

1 second before RMMA
Rise in heartbeat
(tachycardia)

0.8 second before RMMA
Rise in muscle tone
of opener suprahyoid muscles

ONSET
of
rhythmic masticatory
muscle activity (RMMA)
in masseter muscles
and
tooth grinding

MICRO-AROUSAL

FIGURE 35–4 Sequence of physiologic events preceding rhythmic masticatory muscle activity (RMMA) associated with sleep bruxism. *(Reproduced with permission from Lavigne GJ, Huynh N, Kato T, et al. Genesis of sleep bruxism: motor and autonomic-cardiac interactions. Arch Oral Biol 2007;52:381.)*

majority of episodes (around 80%), at least for head banging, occur at sleep onset.[315] When appearing at sleep onset, rhythmic movements are considered to be a self-soothing or tension-releasing behavior linked with pleasurable sensations that have hypnotic properties. However, more violent movements, usually in cases of mental retardation, have been reported to cause head or eye injuries.[316–318]

Polysomnographic recordings show that rhythmic movement disorder can arise from REM sleep, NREM sleep, or sleep onset with persisting activity in light sleep. Longer movements are usually observed at sleep onset and during stage 1 sleep, whereas shorter movements are seen in stages 2, 3, and 4 NREM sleep and in

REM sleep.[314] Rhythmic movements are not preceded by EEG changes, as are nocturnal seizures,[165] and do not provoke arousals or interrupt SWS even in older children.[315,319]

Associated Factors and Pathophysiology

There are no reports of rhythmic movement disorder in association with other parasomnias or sleep problems except for RLS, which is associated with body rocking.[320] Cases of adult rhythmic movement disorder are not usually associated with severe psychiatric disorders as previously believed. However, some studies have reported daytime complaints such as attentional difficulties, sleepiness, morning headaches, fatigue, and poor concentration—and even more serious problems such as anxiety, depression, hyperactivity, and irritability.[314,321,322] Whether the daytime symptoms result from poor sleep caused by the rhythmic movements remains to be determined.

The etiology of rhythmic movement disorder is still unknown. The involvement of the central motor pattern generator in the genesis of motor phenomena during sleep has been suggested.[323] This network is involved in the control of early locomotor function[324] and is thought to be under the inhibitory control of the cortex. Immaturity of the inhibitory cortical system in early infancy might account for rhythmic movements occurring during sleep, coinciding with the acquisition of motor milestones.

Prevalence

This parasomnia is quite common in infancy but decreases rapidly in prevalence with increasing age. Incidences of 66% at 9 months, 26% at 2 years, and 6% at 5 years had been reported using a sample of children,[325] but an epidemiologic study reported lower incidences of about 6% at 2.5 years, 3% at 4 and 5 years, and 2% at 6 years.[67] Body rocking was found to be present in 3% of children ages 11–13 years.[65] In rare cases, rhythmic movement disorder persists into adulthood. No gender difference has been demonstrated.

Treatment

There are no systematic pharmacologic studies or behavioral trials for rhythmic movement disorder; it generally has a benign course and is not usually associated with a severe clinical picture. Benzodiazepines, especially clonazepam, or tricyclic antidepressants can be effective.[326–328]

Somniloquy

Clinical Presentation

Somniloquy, also known as sleeptalking, is defined as talking during sleep "with varying degrees of comprehensibility."[1] Somniloquy is such a prevalent phenomenon that it is considered to be a normal sleep behavior, especially in childhood.

Somniloquy can arise from all sleep stages.[329] Since there are few systematic PSG studies, no clear profiles have been identified. However, EMG-induced artifact is common and may begin several seconds prior to, and continue several seconds following, verbalizations.[330] Temporary suspension of eye movements and occurrence of sustained alpha EEG trains during REM sleep somniloquy episodes have also been noted,[330] as has suppression of theta and alpha activity prior to utterances.[331] Episodes frequently occur in parallel with sleep mentation, but concordance between verbal utterances and ongoing dreamed speech may vary from isomorphic to completely absent.[332]

Associated Factors and Pathophysiology

The pathophysiology is unknown. In addition, since somniloquy is so prevalent, it is virtually impossible to isolate predisposing factors. Nonetheless, a clear genetic influence has been demonstrated.[333] Somniloquy is also the parasomnia that most often co-occurs with other parasomnias. It often accompanies the behavioral manifestations of either RBD or somnambulism. Stereotyped vocalizations can also be heard during nocturnal seizures. In most cases, however, somniloquy is idiopathic.

Prevalence

Although considered the most frequent parasomnia, somniloquy is usually without consequences and thus rarely a reason for consultation. Its prevalence among preschoolers (84%)[67] is much higher than among older children and adolescents. A prevalence of 30% was found for children ages 11–13 years using mainly retrospective reports,[65] while in adults, an estimate of 24% was found using a telephone sampling method.[249] There is no apparent gender difference.

Treatment

There is no known treatment for somniloquy. It is usually considered too benign to treat.

Sleep-Related Groaning

Clinical Presentation

Sleep-related groaning, also known as catathrenia, is defined as "a chronic, usually nightly, disorder characterized by expiratory groaning during sleep, particularly during the second half of the night."[1] Groaning or moaning sounds typically begin 2–6 hours after sleep onset. The sounds produced are usually loud, but the pitch and timbre vary among individuals: groaning, loud humming, roaring, and high-pitched sounds have all been observed. By contrast, within individuals the type of sound is usually fairly constant. Catathrenia is not associated with abnormal motor activity and is qualitatively different from somniloquy. Degree of concordance with sleep mentation is unknown. The affected individual is usually unaware of the problem and, apart from occasional complaints of daytime sleepiness, typically has no other sleep complaints. However, production of the sounds may disturb the bed partner. The identification of this disorder is relatively new, with a total of only 29 cases reported in the literature.[334–340]

Catathrenia occurs during either REM or NREM sleep, but episodes arise predominantly from REM sleep; only one patient presented groaning exclusively in NREM sleep.[338] Polysomnographic tracings reveal bradypneic events, often occurring in clusters, with deep inspirations followed by long expirations and

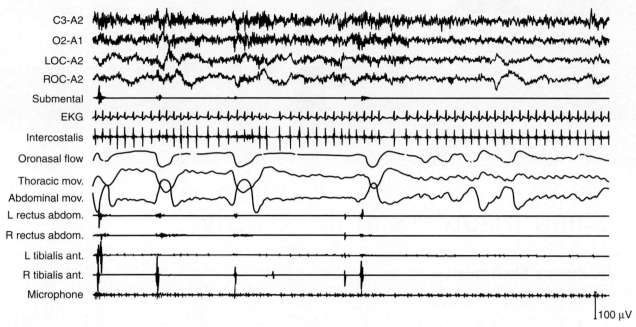

FIGURE 35–5 PSG recording of a nocturnal groaning episode. A deep inspiration is followed by a short expiration and long, relatively flat period of reduced breathing during which the vocal groan is heard. *(Reproduced with permission from Oldani A, Manconi M, Zucconi M, et al. 'Nocturnal groaning': just a sound or parasomnia? J Sleep Res 2005;14:305.)*

monotonous vocalization (Fig. 35–5). There is a high night-to-night consistency of the groaning episodes.[335] Although catathrenia is associated with bradypneic events, only one[339] of the reported cases had significant obstructive apnea-hypopnea, and oxygen saturation remained above 90% across the night; body position does not seem to have any influence.[338] Whereas the loud sounds of snoring or obstructive sleep apneas occur during the inspiratory phase, the vocalizations of catathrenia occur during expiration. Unlike sleep apnea, sleep architecture for nocturnal groaners is usually preserved. However, a few patients will show either reduced total sleep time combined with reduced sleep efficiency, or a reduction of either slow-wave or REM sleep.[338]

Associated Factors and Pathophysiology

No particular anomaly was found on neurologic and physical (including otorhinolaryngologic) examination, on routine laboratory testing, or in the medical history.[335,336,338] There appear to be no associated conditions or obvious predisposing factors.[338] As is the case for many parasomnias, catathrenia is, at least in part, genetically determined. In about 15% of cases, there is at least one family relative also affected, sometimes in a way consistent with an autosomal dominant pattern of inheritance.[338] A possible cause could be a functional REM

sleep–related narrowing of the upper airways during expiration. This would produce the groaning sound.

Prevalence

Nocturnal groaning represents less than 1% of the population consulting at a sleep disorder center.[338] However, since this parasomnia is without major consequences, there are probably a large number of affected individuals who do not seek medical help. It appears to be three times more prevalent in men than in women, although too few cases have been reported so far to be able to determine the gender ratio accurately. Onset is habitually during adolescence or early adulthood, and the parasomnia persists for several years.[338] The precise time course of the condition is unknown due to lack of follow-up on this recently identified condition.

Treatment

A few bedtime treatments have been tried with no sustained therapeutic effect: clonazepam, gabapentin, pramipexole, carbamazepine, trazodone, paroxetine, and dosulepine.[335,338] Treatment with nasal continuous positive airway pressure produced inconsistent effects.[335,340]

⊙ REFERENCES

A full list of references are available at www.expertconsult. com

CHAPTER 36

Sleep Disorders in the Elderly

Sudhansu Chokroverty

INTRODUCTION

To understand the sleep disorders of the elderly, it is important to know what changes in sleep structure and sleep cycle are normal in disease-free aged individuals. It is also important to understand the neurology of aging and, in particular, changes in central nervous system (CNS) physiology and morphology in normal healthy older individuals.

In 1900, 4% of the American population was older than age 65; according to the best current estimate, that figure will be 13% in the year 2000, and 21% by 2050.[1] It is life expectancy that has been increasing rather than the human life span, which is determined biologically and genetically and remains fixed.[2] We do not know what determines aging and the changes associated with aging (see Behnke et al.[3] and Comfort[4] for a review of this topic). Older individuals are at risk for sleep disturbances owing to a variety of factors, including social and psychosocial problems; increasing prevalence of concurrent medical, psychiatric, and neurologic illnesses; increasing use of medications (often sedative-hypnotics) and alcohol; and alterations in circadian rhythms.

NEUROLOGY OF AGING

Clinical Aspects of Central Nervous System Changes

Before discussing the neurology of aging, it is important to define what is meant by *aging*. No standard definition is available, but for this discussion I arbitrarily define age 65 as the start of old age. A normal elderly person is one who is free of obvious diseases of the central and peripheral neurologic systems as well as of general systemic diseases (e.g., cardiovascular, respiratory, renal, metabolic, hematologic, skeletal, and muscular diseases). Accepting this definition, a variety of changes in mental functions and the general nervous system of healthy elderly individuals have been noted. At the outset, I must point out certain difficulties in studying the neurology of aging. It is difficult to get a large number of elderly subjects who meet the criteria by being free of neurologic and other systemic disorders. Even if a number of such subjects can be recruited, without many years' subsequent longitudinal study, it often remains problematic to decide whether certain abnormal findings are related to a subclinical affliction of the nervous system that is expressed in overt manifestations later in life.[5] A large number of elderly individuals have general medical and neurologic disorders, particularly dementia of the Alzheimer's type. In addition, there could be subclinical cerebral infarction, as noted in large series of autopsy examinations[6] in which half the individuals with cerebral infarction remained asymptomatic. The following discussion of the neurologic changes of normal aging was written with these limitations in mind.

On mental function examination, the most striking changes in old age are in learning new information and in central processing of information.[5] In the Wechsler Adult Intelligence Scale,[7] the performance scale declines much more rapidly than the verbal tests.[5,8] This has been confirmed in several cross-sectional and longitudinal studies comparing young and old individuals.[7–11] The past and the immediate memory remain relatively intact until approximately the middle 70s, but recent memory is impaired. There is often forgetfulness and difficulty remembering names and remembering several objects at one time, which suggests impairment of central processing time. Speed of learning is retarded, as is speed of processing new information.[5] The reaction time to simple and complex stimuli is often delayed, and there is impairment of motor speed.[12–16] The cognitive impairment of the normal elderly is often termed *benign forgetfulness of senescence*[17] or *age-associated memory impairment.*[18]

In a classic paper in 1931, Critchley[19] first directed attention to certain changes in the nervous system of normal healthy elderly individuals. Since then, several studies have appeared in the literature documenting the presence of abnormal neurologic signs in a small number of such people,[20,21] but these signs may represent asymptomatic subclinical disease[5] (e.g., cerebrovascular disease or cervical spondylosis), and without longitudinal studies it is impossible to exclude these definitely. Despite this limitation, there is a general consensus about the presence of certain findings in normal elderly individuals. There are changes in both the somatic nervous system and autonomic nervous system (ANS).[5,22,23] In the somatic system, an important finding is impairment of gait and stance.[5,24,25] It is difficult to stand on one leg with the eyes closed.[20,21,25] The so-called senile gait is characterized by stooped posture with flexed attitude, accompanied by short steps, reduced arm swings, shortening of the stride, and impaired speed and balance.[2,5,24] The gait resembles that of patients in the early stage of Parkinson's disease, which may be due to the loss of dopaminergic neurons and striatal dopamine receptors.[5,24] Grip strength declines with age.[21] The ankle reflex may be diminished, which may be related to the loss of large-diameter nerve fibers.[5] In the sensory examination, the striking abnormality is impairment of the vibration sense in the lower extremities.[21] Rowe and Troen[26] suggested that old age represents a hyperadrenergic state. If this is the case, sympathetic overactivity may explain some of the changes noted in the cardiovascular reflex, galvanic skin response, erection, maturation, and pupillary response of elders. Overactivity of the sympathetic nervous system may also interfere with cognitive function.

Physiologic Changes in Old Age

Electroencephalographic Changes

Awake Electroencephalography. The question remains whether electroencephalography (EEG) changes in old age are maturational changes or are related to pathologic alterations of the CNS. Many elderly individuals are afflicted with a variety of dementing illnesses, cerebrovascular disease, or systemic medical disorders that may cause metabolic encephalopathy.[27] Thus it is important to select healthy elderly individuals who are free from any of these diseases for EEG study. Such a selection was made in the study of healthy septuagenarians by Katz and Horowitz.[28] The subjects were screened by careful neurologic, psychiatric, and neuropsychological examination and found to represent normative EEG data. The EEG was normal, with an average alpha frequency of 9.8 Hz, and was therefore similar to that of young and middle-aged adults. This study can be contrasted with the report by Torres and colleagues,[29] in which they found that 52% of a group of normal volunteers with a mean age of 69 years had mild to moderate EEG abnormalities.

Obrist[30] summarized the EEG changes in old age as follows: slowing of the alpha rhythm and an increase of fast activities, diffuse slow activity, and focal slow waves. In an important longitudinal study by Obrist and colleagues,[31] alpha frequency fell from 9.4 Hz at age 79 to 8 Hz intermixed with 6- to 7-Hz theta waves at age 89. Spectral analysis by Matejcek[32] and Nakano and coworkers[33] supported the progressive slowing of the alpha rhythm with aging. Duffy and associates[34] found no significant change in the frequency of the posterior EEG rhythm in a study of 63 men between 30 and 80 years of age. Oken and Kaye[35] analyzed conventional EEG and computerized EEG frequency in 22 extremely healthy subjects between 84 and 98 years old. The posterior peak frequency was higher than 8 Hz in those younger than 84, but between 7 and 8 Hz in 5 of 22 subjects older than 84 years. Alpha slowing appears to be related to the decline in mental function, which may be an early stage of progressive dementia of old age.[36] Alpha blocking and photic driving response to intermittent photic stimulation are also diminished in old age.[37] These findings may be related to the structural CNS alterations in elderly individuals (see *Pathologic Central Nervous System Changes of Normal Aging* later).

An increase of fast activity was noted by Busse and Obrist[38] in elderly volunteer community subjects, especially women. In an EEG spectral analysis, Brenner et al.[39] also found more beta activity in elderly women than men. Kugler[40] also reported an increase of fast activity with increasing age. The significance of this is uncertain, but Kugler[40] stated that the presence of fast activity in old age correlates with preserved mental functioning.

Intermittent focal slow waves in the temporal regions (particularly in the middle and anterior temporal regions and greater on the left side) are noted in 17–59% of healthy elderly individuals (Fig. 36–1).[29,30,35,41–43] This temporal slow activity may be accompanied by sharp transients, which may be related to cerebral vascular disease causing asymptomatic small infarction of the temporal lobe,[36] ventricular enlargement with cerebral atrophy,[44] or white matter hyperintensities on magnetic resonance imaging (MRI).[35] Klass and Brenner[45] listed some of the characteristics of what they called *benign temporal delta transients of the elderly* as follows: slow waves occur in patients older than 60 years and are maximally noted in the left temporal, particularly anterior temporal, region; the voltage is usually less than 70 µV, and these waves do not disrupt background activity; these delta transients are attenuated by mental alerting and eye opening and are increased by drowsiness and hyperventilation; the transients generally occur as single waves or in pairs but not in rhythmic trains; and the transient waves are present for up to 1% of recording time. The elderly may also have an increased amount of theta activity.[41,46]

There is no clear relationship between intellectual deterioration and EEG slowing.[30,35] Whether the EEG changes are correlated with cerebral blood flow (CBF) study remains controversial. There is no correlation, however, between areas that show the maximum blood flow reduction and those that show prominent EEG slowing, or between the blood flow changes and the

alpha frequency changes in normal elderly subjects.[47,48] The other suggestion is that the alpha slowing is related to the loss of choline acetyltransferase, the enzyme for synthesis of acetylcholine.[5]

Sleep EEG Changes, Including Changes in Sleep Architecture and Organization. In addition to awake EEG changes, there are changes during sleep in the elderly.[49,50] It is interesting to note that Liberson[51] in 1945 described paroxysmal bursts of sleeplike EEG lasting 1–10 seconds in the eyes-resting state in elderly subjects, and the incidence of these bursts increased with the age of the subject. Liberson[51] termed these episodes *microsleeps*. Transient bursts of anteriorly dominant rhythmic delta waves are often noted in elderly subjects in the early stage of sleep. Gibbs and Gibbs[52] used the term *anterior bradyrhythmia* for this finding. Katz and Horowitz[53] obtained sleep-onset frontal intermittent

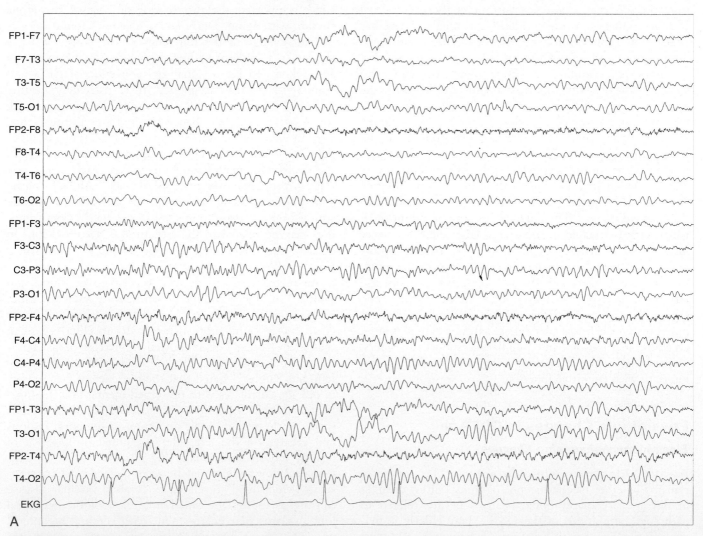

FIGURE 36–1 (A) Electroencephalogram shows transient burst of delta activity in the left temporal, and occasionally also in the right temporal, region in a 94-year-old woman with a history of syncope.

(*Continued*)

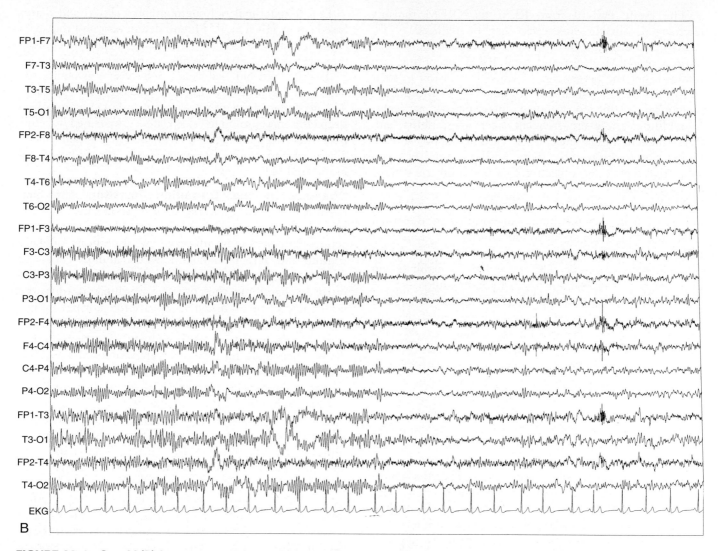

FIGURE 36–1—Cont'd (B) Same subject data as in **A** viewed at a 30-second epoch. *(From Chokroverty S, Bhatt M, Goldhammer T: Electroencephalography for the sleep specialists. In Chokroverty S, Thomas RJ, Bhatt M (eds), Atlas of Sleep Medicine. Philadelphia: Elsevier, 2005:29.)*

rhythmic delta activity in normal elderly subjects, which should be differentiated from that associated with a variety of neurologic disorders. These are highly stimulus-sensitive and disappear in deeper stages of sleep. In demented elders, however, one can see diffuse slow waves in the delta and theta frequencies.

Normal elders show normal sleep patterns with certain modifications. The delta waves during slow-wave sleep (SWS) are reduced in amplitude and incidence.[22,54,55] The amplitude of delta waves decreases, and therefore, in the usual Rechtschaffen and Kales[56] scoring technique, non–rapid eye movement (NREM) stages 3 and 4 decrease. Feinberg and colleagues[57] discussed this point and suggested that quantification of the amount of time spent in a specified frequency be used for scoring SWS in elderly individuals, rather than using an amplitude criterion. Mann and Roschke[58] in a later study using EEG frequency and cross-correlation analysis in a group of 59 healthy young and middle-aged men confirmed

a significant decline of the delta/theta bands during NREM sleep but an increase of EEG power in beta frequency during rapid eye movement (REM) sleep with increasing age. This reduction of amplitude of delta waves could be related to the following factors: (1) reduction of neuronal synchronization in the neocortex,[22,57] (2) alterations in the skull,[22,57] (3) changes in the subarachnoid spaces,[22,57] (4) reduction of specific subpopulation(s) of neurons,[59] (5) a steady decline of synaptic density resulting in a decline of intracerebral connectivity,[60,61] and (6) changes of receptor functions and neurochemical alterations affecting synaptic communication and connectivity.[62]

Sleep spindles may show a variety of changes in old age,[63–65] including decreased frequency, amount, and amplitude. The frequency may decrease from 16 to 14 Hz, and then from 14 to 12 Hz. The spindles are often poorly formed and poorly developed. Sleep spindle changes thus resemble those noted with alpha frequency in old age.

The cyclic pattern from REM to NREM remains unchanged, but the first cycle may be reduced.[22,66–68] REM density (i.e., number of eye movement bursts per minute of REM sleep) and total REM sleep time are reduced, but the percentage of REM in relation to total sleep time (TST) remains unaltered.[22,51,69,70] Sleep fragmentation is due to frequent interruptions at night. In addition, there are frequent sleep stage shifts and, thus, frequent awakenings.[22,51] Regarding nocturnal TST (lights out to lights on), there is discrepancy between subjective report and objective data based on the technician's schedule.[22]

Nighttime sleep of elders usually is reported to be decreased (e.g., 5.5–6.5 hours, in contrast to the usual 7.5-hour TST average of young adults).[71,72] This may not be an accurate observation, because elders often take daytime naps; 24-hour TST of elders probably is no different from the 24-hour TST of young adults.

Increased fragmentation of sleep and increased numbers of transient arousals accompanied by increased daytime sleepiness have been described in the studies by Carskadon and coworkers.[73–75] Kales et al.[76] and Feinberg et al.[55] demonstrated the following changes in sleep with advancing age: state changes; frequent stage shifts; reduction of SWS (NREM stages 3 and 4) and the EEG amplitude of delta waves; and increased NREM stage 1 owing to frequent arousals, decreased total nocturnal sleep, and reduction of total REM sleep time but normal REM percentage in relation to the TST.

Williams and colleagues[77] recruited 120 healthy seniors through advertisements, without mentioning sleep. They tried to carefully screen out sleep disorders by excluding those who had sleep complaints. These authors found that the seniors' sleep quality was poorer than that of young individuals. In particular, there was a decrease of stages 3 and 4 sleep and an increase in nighttime wakefulness.[77,78] Prinz and Vitiello[79] considered these findings as a benchmark level of sleep change associated with aging per se. In another study involving the Veterans Administration Survey, Cashman and colleagues[80] found that nighttime hypoxemia, which correlated with sleep apnea, was worse in several medical disorders (i.e., diabetes, cardiovascular disease, history of alcoholism, and vascular headaches). Thus, the data suggest that the disease states may interact with sleep disorders.

Between the ages of 60 and 90 years, there are differences in the sleep architecture of men and women.[50,65] Between 60 and 70 years, men have more frequent arousals and more decrements in stages 3 and 4 sleep. Between 60 and 80 years, women spend 9% of TST in the slow-wave stage, whereas men spend only 2%. The percentages of REM and total REM sleep are not different for men and women between 60 and 90 years. In a meta-analysis of normative sleep data across the human life span, Ohayon et al.[81] also reported a reduction of SWS beginning in middle age, with complete absence after the age of 90 years.

In a longitudinal polysomnographic (PSG) and diary-based study, Hoch et al.[82] found deterioration of measures of sleep quality, continuity, and depth but not other sleep measures over a 3-year follow-up period in a group of 27 healthy "old old" subjects (75–87 years) as contrasted with a group of 23 "young old" subjects (61–74 years). The decline in sleep measures was manifested by impaired sleep efficiency, prolonged sleep latency, increased wakefulness after sleep onset, and decreased SWS percentage. These changes were accompanied by increased napping in the "old old" group.

Changes in the Circadian Rhythm. Circadian rhythm changes[50,83] in the elderly result from fundamental changes in social activity, including family interaction. Interaction is governed by alterations of daily routine and activities, health needs, and psychosocial factors (e.g., loneliness, divorce).[22] There may also be intrinsic changes in the circadian rhythm related to the pathologic changes noted in apparently normal individuals. Animal studies lend support to this conclusion.[84–88] In long-term care facilities, circadian rhythm disturbances may be related to alterations of *Zeitgebers* (external time cues), such as bedtime, medication time, mealtime, and special institutional regulations on lights out and lights on.[17] Wessler and colleagues[89] made an intensive study of 69- to 94-year-old institutionalized patients under strict environmentally controlled conditions and found a remarkable regularity in circadian synchronization. In a study involving 69- to 86-year-old subjects, however, Scheving et al.[90] did not find support for the other group's conclusion. In all of these studies involving institutionalized patients, the effect of chronic illnesses must be considered in explanations of circadian rhythm disturbances. Thus, these changes may not be related to "normal" old age.

A study of evolution of sleep shows that the strong monophasic circadian rhythm of youth gives way to a polyphasic ultradian rhythm in old age. Frequent awakenings at night, with reduction of wakefulness, are accompanied by increased daytime naps. These physiologic changes may be related to the structural alterations noted in the suprachiasmatic nucleus (SCN) and brain stem hypnogenic neurons in experimental studies in several species of animals.[91–94]

There is also phase advance in the elderly—that is, there is a tendency to go to sleep early and awaken early. These changes may be related to age-related changes in the core body temperature rhythm.[95,96] In elderly individuals, the amplitude of the temperature rhythm is attenuated and phase advanced.[96]

Autonomic Nervous System Changes with Age

There are striking functional and structural changes noted in the elderly in the ANS.[22,23,97–100] Changes are found in autonomic nerves and ganglia; ANS-controlled cardiovascular, respiratory, and gastrointestinal functions; sympathetic nerve activity; thermoregulation; and nocturnal penile tumescence in men. The age-related structural alterations in the human superior cervical ganglia may explain deterioration of neuronal functional capacity and affect neuronal plasticity and regenerative characteristics.[99]

Sympathetic Nerve Activity. The most consistent abnormalities in old age are increased muscle sympathetic nerve activity and elevated plasma concentration of the sympathetic neurotransmitter norepinephrine.[97,101,102] Age-related changes are noted in circulating catecholamine levels and microneurographic recordings from sympathetic nerves of skeletal muscles. In contrast, the reactivity of the sympathetic and parasympathetic activities is reduced with aging.[97]

Thermoregulation. Thermoregulation is impaired in old age.[23] In response to passive heating, the sweating response of elders is impaired.[104] They are susceptible to hypothermia (both postoperatively and in response to low ambient temperature in the environment)[105,106] and hyperthermia.[107] There is a paucity of studies that show ANS changes during sleep in elders.

Cardiovascular Changes. Blood pressure (BP) and pulse rate fall at sleep onset, rise on awakening, and fluctuate during the night.[108] The increased incidence of stroke in elders during sleep may be related to these factors.[22] Orthostatic hypotension is common in elders and may be due to impaired baroreflex responsiveness and neuroeffector function.[23] Aging is associated with decreased cardiovagal baroreflex sensitivity (i.e., blunted reflex changes in the R–R interval in response to a change in BP).[98] These alterations may cause increased levels of BP variability and increased risk of sudden cardiac death.[98] However, baroreflex control of sympathetic outflow is not impaired with age. Baroreflex functional changes with aging may cause an impaired ability to buffer BP changes.

Respiration. Age-related changes in the respiratory system and pulmonary function include a reduction of vital capacity, chest wall compliance, diffusion capacity, elastic recoil, and arterial oxygen tension; mismatch of the ventilation-perfusion ratio; decreased respiratory muscle strength; and respiratory center sensitivity.[22,109–111] There is a higher incidence of periodic breathing, including Cheyne-Stokes breathing and snoring, in elders at night.[108,112–114] Patients with chronic obstructive pulmonary disease, who are often elderly, are at special risk for periodic breathing during sleep (both at night and during the day) because of increasing oxygen desaturation, hypercapnia, and apnea during sleep.[115,116]

Nocturnal Penile Tumescence. Penile erection occurs during REM sleep. This REM-related penile tumescence shows a linear decrease from youth to old age (from 88% at 20–26 years old to 64–74% at 60–90 years old).[117,118]

Gastrointestinal Function. Selective degenerative changes may occur in the aging enteric nervous system, which regulates gastrointestinal functions.[100] These age-associated changes in intestinal innervation may contribute to the gastrointestinal disturbances that increase in incidence in the elderly (e.g., dysphagia, gastroesophageal reflex, constipation).

Endocrine Changes with Age

Plasma Cortisol. Cortisol secretion has a circadian rhythmicity that remains intact in the elderly. There is an age-dependent increase of mean nocturnal cortisol levels and an advancement of the morning rise.[119] However, normal diurnal rhythm of salivary cortisol is maintained in older adults.[120] Magri et al.[121] observed a significant increase in nocturnal cortisol levels in 23 healthy elderly and 23 demented elderly individuals as compared with levels in 10 healthy young subjects. MRI of the brain correlated these higher nocturnal cortisol levels, with a reduction of hippocampal volume in these elderly subjects. Poor sleep in the elderly may be related to an activation of the hypothalamic-pituitary-adrenal (HPA) axis associated with hypersecretion of cortisol and increased inflammatory cytokines (e.g., interleukin-6), which stimulate the HPA axis.

Growth Hormone. Sleep-related growth hormone release is diminished in old age,[122,123] but the response of the growth hormone secretion to insulin hypoglycemia is normal.[124] There is a parallel decrease of SWS and growth hormone in the elderly.[125]

Prolactin Secretion. Prolactin secretion in old age shows a normal pattern of episodic secretion with a sharp rise just after sleep onset and a sharp fall during morning awakening.[22,126,127] Although older subjects wake up several times during the night and have daytime naps, these episodes are not correlated with the prolactin secretion pattern.[22]

Gonadotropins (Follicle-Stimulating Hormone and Luteinizing Hormone). No good studies correlate sleep changes in the elderly with gonadotropin secretion.[22]

Plasma Insulin and Glucose. Insulin secretion shows a clear circadian variation in healthy young adults, but there is no adequate study of aged individuals.[22]

Thyroid-Stimulating Hormone. Plasma thyroid-stimulating hormone shows a circadian periodicity in adults: peak levels occur just before sleep onset at night.[108,128,129] In subjects older than 50 years, there are progressive changes in thyroid function causing a modest decrease in serum triiodothyronine concentration and minimal changes in thyroid-stimulating hormone and thyroxine concentrations.[130]

Melatonin Secretion. Serum melatonin concentration shows an age-related decrease in old age.[131] Impaired melatonin secretion has been reported to be associated with sleep complaints in the elderly.[132,133]

Changes in Cerebral Blood Flow and Cerebral Metabolism

Despite some inconsistent early findings,[5] there is a direct relationship between normal aging, CBF, and cerebral metabolism. The xenon-133 inhalation method related a clear-cut decline in the regional blood flow exclusively to advancing age, without the compounding factors of associated diseases.[134–136] This decline with advancing age was noted more in the gray than in the white matter CBF values.[137] Maximal declines were seen in the prefrontal and parietal regions and minimal declines in the frontal and frontotemporal regions.[5] This decline in old age seems to be related to a progressive decrease in the cerebral metabolic rate,[138,139] and possibly also to the morphologic changes in the neurons in the brains of elderly individuals.[137] It should be noted, however, that the decrease of CBF during SWS and the increase during REM sleep are similar in normal subjects of all ages.[137] In elderly sleep apnea patients, however, this decrease during SWS becomes excessive, placing elderly individuals at increasing risk for sudden death and development of stroke during sleep when combined with hypoxemia related to apnea.[137]

Pathologic Central Nervous System Changes of Normal Aging

Aging represents biologic maturation, which may be accompanied by a variety of pathologic changes in the CNS. The neuropathologic changes of old age can be summarized as follows[5,140]: shrinkage of the brain; alterations in the outline and loss of neurons in various locations; lipofuscin accumulation; collection of corpora amylacea; intraparenchymal vascular changes; loss of dendritic arbor and dendritic spines; and presence of senile plaques and amyloid deposits, neurofibrillary tangles and granulovacuolar degeneration, and Hirano bodies. The presence of senile plaques and amyloid deposits, neurofibrillary tangles and granulovacuolar degeneration, and Hirano bodies is correlated with dementia, but the other neuropathologic changes are considered nonspecific changes of aging.

From the standpoint of sleep disorders medicine, the cell loss in the locus ceruleus, pontine and midbrain reticular formation, selective hypothalamic regions, and SCN, as well as accumulation of neurofibrillary tangles and abnormal pigment in the hypothalamus, are important morphologic correlates for widespread sleep disturbances in the elderly. Animal experiments on the SCN show the relationship between destruction of these nuclei and

alteration of circadian rhythmicity of adrenal cortical secretion, body temperature, activity-rest cycle, and sleep cycle loss.[22]

SLEEP COMPLAINTS IN OLD AGE

In an epidemiologic study, Ford and Kamerow[141] interviewed 7954 subjects and observed that 40% of patients with insomnia and 46.5% of those with hypersomnia had a psychiatric disorder, compared with 16% of those with no sleep complaints. Complaints of persistent insomnia are important late in life. There is a high incidence of depression with insomnia in the elderly. Among the 1801 elderly respondents ages 65 and older, the prevalence of insomnia was 12% and the incidence of insomnia was 7.3%.[141] For hypersomnia, the figures for prevalence and incidence were 1.6% and 1.8%, respectively. There was a strong association between persistent insomnia (longer than 1 month) and the risk of major depression. Clayton and coworkers[142] noted that, in late-life spousal bereavement, there is also a persistent and debilitating complaint of insomnia.

Brabbins et al.[143] noted an overall prevalence of 35% for insomnia complaints (more in women) after an interview of 1070 noninstitutionalized elderly individuals. In contrast, after interviewing 59 institutionalized and 874 community-dwelling residents, Henderson et al.[144] found a prevalence of approximately 12% in the institutionalized and approximately 16% among the community-dwelling elderly at 70 years or older. Insomnia complaints are more prevalent among women; whites; and those with depression, pain, and poor health. In another study from Germany, Hohagen et al.[145] investigated the prevalence of insomnia in 330 patients older than 65 years attending the offices of five general practitioners. Using the *Diagnostic and Statistical Manual of Mental Disorders* (3rd revision) diagnostic criteria, they found severe insomnia in 23%, moderate insomnia in 17%, and mild insomnia in another 17% of the patients. There was a significant association between insomnia, depression, and dementia.

Foley et al.[146] conducted an important epidemiologic study limited to interviews in more than 9000 elderly subjects ages 65 years and older from three communities in the United States in the National Institute on Aging's multicentered study entitled "Established Populations for Epidemiologic Studies of the Elderly." These authors observed at least one of the following complaints in over half the subjects: trouble falling asleep, multiple awakenings, early morning awakening, daytime naps, and tiredness. These complaints are more common in women than in men and are often associated with respiratory symptoms, depression, nonprescription and prescription medications, poor self-esteem, and physical disabilities. The authors observed 33% of men and 19% of women with snoring and 13% of men and 4% of women with observed apneas. In this cross-sectional study, the authors did not find a clear relationship of loud snoring, observed apneas, or daytime sleepiness to hypertension or cardiovascular disease in the elders. In a later epidemiologic study of 6800 persons over 3 years, Foley et al.[147] reported that 28% of older adults had complaints of chronic insomnia but, in the absence of risk factors (e.g., depression, medical disorders, circadian rhythm disorders, medications), only 7% had insomnia. In a 2003 National Sleep Foundation Sleep in America poll, sleep complaints common in older adults are found to be secondary to comorbidities rather than aging per se.[148]

Excessive daytime somnolence (EDS) is often associated with fragmentation of nocturnal sleep, which may have been due to sleep-disordered breathing and periodic leg movements in sleep (PLMS).[149–151] Other factors are changes in the circadian rhythms of temperature, alertness and sleepiness, and social time cues. Frequent daytime sleepiness in older adults is associated with an impairment of physical functioning and decreased exercise frequency.[152] Based on the National Sleep Foundation 2003 Sleep in America poll, Foley et al.[148] reported frequent napping associated with EDS, depression, pain, and nocturia in older adults.

Many other factors can disrupt sleep: nocturia, leg cramps, pain, coughing or difficulty breathing, temperature sensitivity, and dreams.[149–151] There is an increased prevalence of nocturia in the elderly causing sleep disturbance.[153–155] Sleep disturbances, particularly complaints of insomnia, may contribute to increasing risk of falls and fractures in the elderly.[151,156–158] There is controversy whether the increasing risk of falls in the elderly is related to the sleep disturbance per se or greater use of hypnotics by the elderly.[156] In a multicenter community-dwelling questionnaire-based study involving over 8000 white women ages 69 and older (mean = 77 years), self-reported long sleep (at least 10 hours per 24 hours) and daily napping were associated with greater risk of falls and fractures.[157]

Vitiello and Prinz[159] found that CNS degenerative disorders (e.g., dementia of the Alzheimer's type) may cause polyphasic sleep-wake patterns, which constitute a significant problem among old nursing home residents. In demented elderly subjects, nocturnal agitation, night wandering, shouting, and incontinence contribute to a variety of sleep disturbances.[123] There are many factors in the pathogenesis of nocturnal agitation, including loss of social *Zeitgebers* and circadian timekeeping, sleep apnea, REM-related parasomnias, low ambient light, and cold sensitivity.[160]

An important behavioral disturbance during sleep late in life is snoring.[151] According to Koskenvuo and associates,[161,162] habitual snoring was found in 9% of men and 3.6% of women ages 40–69 years in their study done in Finland. Hypertension, ischemic heart disease, and stroke are risk factors for snoring. In an epidemiologic

survey, Lugaresi and colleagues[163] found that approximately 60% of men and 40% of women between the ages of 41 and 64 years were habitual snorers. Enright et al.[164] recruited 5201 adults ages 65 and older who were participants in a cardiovascular health study that enrolled a random sample of Medicare subjects in four U.S. communities. In this study, there was no positive correlation between aging and self-reported snoring. Loud snoring, however, was independently associated with body mass index, diabetes mellitus, and arthritis in older women, and with alcohol use in elderly men.

What is the relationship between sleep duration and mortality in elders? In 1989, Ancoli-Israel[165] re-examined the 1979 data of Kripke and coworkers[166] and concluded that 86% of deaths associated with short (<7 hours) or long (>8 hours) sleep occurred among those older than 60 years. Thus, it could be concluded by extrapolation from these data that older individuals who sleep less than 5 hours or more than 9 hours may be at greater risk for death.

The high frequency of sleep complaints in aged individuals may be related to the physiologic sleep changes of normal aging as well as to concomitant medical, psychiatric, neurologic, and other disorders that are prevalent in this group.[52,150,151] Subjective sleep complaints are common in older subjects, as many reports attest.[166–171] The subjective complaints were corroborated by objective laboratory data. In contrast to the increasing incidence of subjective complaints from women, however, elderly men had more sleep disturbances than elderly women by objective reports.[172]

CLINICAL ASSESSMENT OF SLEEP DISORDERS

Clinical assessment consists of a sleep, medical, drug, and psychiatric history. A general approach for making a clinical assessment is described in Chapter 19; only the points relevant to elders are emphasized in this section.

Sleep History

Kales and coworkers[173] developed excellent guidelines for taking an adequate sleep history, summarized as follows:

1. The specific sleep problem should first be defined from the history. It is important with elders to understand the significance of daytime fatigue, which may result either from insomnia at night or from EDS. The latter condition can be an indirect effect of repeated arousals at night owing to sleep-related respiratory disorders, with or without PLMS. The other important factor to note is that the sleep of elders becomes polyphasic, associated with frequent daytime naps and less sleep at night. Therefore, every daytime nap is not necessarily indicative of EDS.

2. The onset and the clinical course of the condition should be assessed from the history. The course of

the illness in some sleep disorders (e.g., night terrors, nightmares, sleepwalking) is different.[174] Nightmares have a chronic course, whereas night terrors may be of recent onset. It should be noted that the relatively sudden onset of sleepwalking or night terrors in an elderly person is indicative of an organic CNS disorder, and appropriate investigation should be directed toward that diagnosis.[174]

3. Inquiries should be made into a family history of a sleep disorder. Certain sleep disorders (e.g., narcolepsy, hypersomnia, sleep apnea, sleepwalking, night terrors, restless legs syndrome) may have a family history.[173–180]

4. Various sleep disorders should be distinguished from one another, and any previous diagnosis should be reassessed.

5. It is important to obtain a complete 24-hour sleep-wakefulness pattern. This is important in elderly individuals, because in old age the sleep cycle becomes polycyclic, rather than monophasic as in young adults. In elders, because of the tendency to take frequent naps, the sleep-wake schedule becomes irregular and may cause circadian rhythm disorders.

6. It might be important to keep a sleep diary or sleep log, and it is very important to question the bed partner or other caregivers about sleep disturbances of elders. Keeping a sleep diary may help assess the 24-hour sleep-wake cycle pattern.

7. The bed partner or caregivers should be questioned carefully, as they may have clues to the diagnosis of sleep apnea syndrome (SAS). For example, excessively loud snoring, temporary cessation of breathing, or restless movements in the bed are important pointers to the diagnosis of SAS[175] or PLMS.

8. It is essential to evaluate the impact of the sleep disorder and to determine the presence of other sleep disorders. The history may suggest a diagnosis of sleepwalking, night terrors, or REM sleep behavior disorder (RBD). A careful sleep history may also suggest nocturnal epilepsy, which is sometimes mistaken for a sleep disorder.

Medical History

It is vital that a complete medical history be obtained from the patient.[173,181] Elderly individuals often have a variety of medical disorders, including congestive cardiac failure, hypertension, ischemic heart disease, chronic bronchopulmonary disorders, gastrointestinal disorders, arthritis and musculoskeletal pain syndromes, cancer, chronic renal disorders, endocrinopathies, and a variety of neurologic disorders. All of these conditions may disrupt sleep by virtue of the uncomfortable symptoms or because of the medications prescribed for them. Therefore, patients often complain of insomnia, but sometimes also of hypersomnia.

Drug History

It is important to obtain a drug history[173] because many medications can cause insomnia, including[147] CNS stimulants; bronchodilators; β blockers; antihypertensives; benzodiazepines, particularly the short-acting ones; steroids; and theophylline. Withdrawal from short- and intermediate-acting benzodiazepines and nonbenzodiazepine hypnotics causes rebound insomnia. Many CNS depressants, such as hypnotics, sedatives, and antidepressants, may cause EDS. Finally, drinking coffee or cola at night may cause difficulty initiating sleep. Alcohol consumption may cause difficulty maintaining sleep.

Psychiatric History

Psychophysiologic and psychiatric problems are the most common causes of insomnia in elders.[147] Elderly insomniacs can have a variety of psychological and psychiatric problems, such as anxiety, depression, organic psychosis, and obsessive-compulsive neurosis. A patient with depression complains of early morning awakenings, whereas a patient with obsessive-compulsive neurosis has difficulty initiating sleep. Some drugs (e.g., thioridazine) may increase nightmares.[144] Marital and sexual problems may give rise to interpersonal problems that cause sleep disturbances, particularly insomnia.[181]

SLEEP DISORDERS IN OLD AGE

It is well known that the prevalence and intensity of sleep disturbances increase with age.[150,151,181–184] Factors that affect the prevalence of sleep disturbances in the elderly are (1) physiologic (e.g., age-related changes in sleep patterns); (2) medical; (3) psychiatric; (4) pharmacologic (e.g., use, misuse, and abuse of drugs); and (5) social (changing rest-activity schedules, and, therefore, sleep-wake patterns).[150,151,181–186]

The prevalence of sleep-related breathing disorders, PLMS, and snoring are all greater among elders. The prevalence of sleep apnea increases with age and is greater in men than in women, and in menopausal women than in premenopausal women.[165] There is controversy over the exact prevalence of sleep apnea in the older population. The prevalence rates for sleep apnea—defined as repetitive episodes of upper airway obstruction—in elders in various studies have been estimated to range from 5.6% to 70%.[165,187–195] The prevalence is greater in the elderly than in younger adults, and in men than in women.[196,197] There is a lack of consistency in study methods, so it is very difficult to generalize from these studies. In the Sleep Heart Health study involving a large cohort of about 6400 subjects (ages 40–98 years, with a mean of 63.5), Young et al.[195] reported an increased prevalence of SAS by 10-year age groups: 32% of those ages 60–69 years had an apnea-hypopnea index (AHI) of 5–14 and 19% had an AHI of ≥15; 33% of those ages 70–79 years had an AHI of 5–14 and 21% had an AHI of $\geq$15; and 36% of those ages 80–98 years had an AHI 5–14 and 20% had an AHI $\geq$15. Thus there was a small increase of the AHI index by 10-year age groups. In an earlier study, Hoch et al.[189] also found increased AHI and prevalence of SAS from 60 to 90 years. It should be noted, however, that the prevalence of SAS in the population ages 30–60 years has currently been estimated to be 2% in women and 4% in men.[198] Because of the high prevalence of SAS in elders, questions have been raised as to the significance of sleep-disordered breathing in the elderly. Prinz et al.[199] stated that, because apneic episodes in the elderly may not have the same clinical symptoms as noted in younger people, it is more difficult to determine if further investigations are needed. Fleury[200] suggested that SAS in the elderly not be considered different from SAS in middle-aged men, however, assuming that an appropriate diagnostic apnea index (AI) or respiratory disturbance index (RDI) was taken into consideration. Ancoli-Israel and Coy[194] agreed that, if SAS is severe enough to cause symptoms in the elderly, treatment should be similar to that in a younger patient.

The controversy as to whether SAS in the elderly represents a specific entity or the same disease in younger subjects continues.[151,201–203] Further research is needed to resolve this issue. Launois et al.[202] contended that untreated SAS in the elderly appears to have lesser impact on mortality than in middle-aged adults; however, symptomatic elderly SAS patients tolerate continuous positive airway pressure (CPAP) as well as the younger patients. Based on a retrospective study in Poland, Bielicki et al.[203] concluded that SAS is more frequent in elderly than in younger patients but is more severe, requiring higher CPAP titration pressure, in younger patients. In an important longitudinal follow-up study of elderly patients with SAS for 18 years, Ancoli-Israel et al.[204] observed that the AHI did not continue to increase if the patient's body mass index remained stable. Some of the risk factors predisposing the elderly to SAS are as follows[205,206]: age, gender, obesity, smoking, family history, race, upper airway anatomic configuration, use of sedative-hypnotics, and alcohol consumption.

Reasons for the variation in the prevalence of sleep apnea could be the sampling of different populations without using a random sampling method, small sample size, or the use of different criteria to define sleep apnea. An important problem has been the scoring criteria for apnea and hypopnea and the definition of AI, AHI, or RDI. In the current American Academy of Sleep Medicine guidelines for scoring,[207] these questions have been addressed and standardized (see Chapter 18). Another problem has been the clinical significance of an AI or RDI of 5. Some authors have suggested that an AI of 20 or more is related to increased risk of death.[208] In a survey among 427 randomly selected community-dwelling people, 65–95 years of age, in San Diego, California, Ancoli-Israel and coworkers[187] reported that 81% of the

subjects had an AHI of $\geq$5 with a prevalence rate of 62% for an AHI $\geq$10, 44% for an AHI of $\geq$20, and 24% for an AHI of $\geq$40. Night-to-night variability in sleep apnea has been the other confounding problem in the elderly.[187,209–212]

The question of the relationship between sleep apnea or sleep-disordered breathing and increased morbidity or mortality remains controversial. Several studies have found a positive relationship.[208,213,214] In a nearly 10-year follow-up of a randomly selected, population-based probability sample of 426 men and women (65–95 years old), however, Ancoli-Israel et al.[215] found that those with severe sleep-disordered breathing (RDI of 30 or more) had a significantly shorter survival but that the RDI was not an independent predictor of death. Similar results were reported from a sleep disorders clinic patient population study by Lavie et al.[216] Ancoli-Israel et al.[215] stated that other confounding variables such as age, hypertension, and cardiovascular or pulmonary disease might be responsible for the increased morbidity and mortality. Chronologic or biological age (determined by biological markers of physiologic aging) may be the single most important factor for increased morbidity and mortality in sleep-disordered breathing (i.e., sleep apnea may be an age-dependent condition). To address this controversy, well-designed controlled clinical studies are needed.

Diagnosis of Sleep Disorders in Old Age

Recognition of a variety of sleep disorders in elders is important for treatment of sleep disturbances and the associated medical or psychiatric conditions. Some examples of sleep disorders that have been recognized in the aged population[172,199,217] are insomnia; sleep-related respiratory dysfunction with periods of apneas and hypopneas; PLMS; sleep disturbances secondary to a variety of medical or psychiatric illnesses (particularly depression in the elderly); sleep disturbances associated with dementia (particularly of the Alzheimer's type); and sleep disturbances related to the abuse of alcohol and sedative-hypnotic drugs, narcolepsy, restless legs syndrome, parasomnias, and circadian rhythm sleep disorders (Table 36–1).

Insomnia and EDS are the two most common symptoms noted in normal aged individuals.[199] There is a high incidence of insomnia in the elderly, particularly elderly women[149,181] (see Chapter 26 for further details about insomnia).

Sleep Apnea Syndrome

For the diagnosis of SAS, questioning the bed partner is very important. A history of loud snoring with periods of cessation of breathing at night accompanied by EDS and daytime fatigue suggests SAS.[218] The diagnosis is strongly suspected if the patient is also obese and hypertensive. For a definitive diagnosis, and to quantify the severity, an all-night PSG study is essential. The usual

TABLE 36-1 Common Sleep Problems in Old Age

Primary Sleep Disorders

- Insomnia
- Sleep-related breathing disorders
- Restless legs syndrome/periodic limb movements in sleep
- REM sleep behavior disorder
- Advanced sleep phase state

Other Sleep Disorders

- Comorbid psychiatric illnesses
- Comorbid general medical disorders
- Comorbid neurodegenerative and other neurologic disorders
- Medication related
- Abuse of alcohol and use of sedative-hypnotic drugs

type is upper airway obstructive sleep apnea, but often it is mixed with central apnea, giving rise to mixed apnea (see Chapter 24). It is important to diagnose the condition because of possible adverse consequences,[218] such as congestive cardiac failure, cardiac arrhythmias, hypertension, neuropsychological impairment,[194,219] increased risk of traffic accidents,[220,221] and increased mortality related to cardiovascular events.[222–225] In a 6-year follow-up prospective longitudinal study in a population-based cohort of 394 noninstitutionalized elderly subjects (ages 70–100 years, median 77 years; 57% men), Munoz et al.[223] found that severe obstructive sleep apnea-hypopnea (AHI index of ≥30) at baseline had an increased risk of ischemic stroke in the elderly population independent of known confounding factors (e.g., age, sex, smoking, alcohol consumption, body mass index, blood pressure, serum cholesterol levels, presence or absence of diabetes mellitus and atrial fibrillation). Lugaresi and colleagues[163] reported a high prevalence of snoring in elderly individuals, and this can be the forerunner of full-blown SAS.

Periodic Limb Movements in Sleep

PLMS is reported more often in older normal subjects than in younger ones.[190,226–228] According to Coleman and associates,[228] the occurrence of PLMS may be related to disturbance of circadian sleep-wake rhythm in the elderly. In the study by Kripke and coworkers,[227] 20–30% of subjects 65 years and older had PLMS, whereas Ancoli-Israel and colleagues[226] reported an incidence of 37% of PLMS in 24 older subjects. PLMS is often associated with SAS independently of respiratory-related PLMS.

Sleep Disturbances and Medical Illnesses

A variety of medical disorders may be associated with insomnia—congestive cardiac failure; ischemic heart disease; arthritis and musculoskeletal pain syndrome; chronic respiratory disorder associated with bronchospasm; and dyspnea, which is often worse at night (see Chapter 26). Diabetics with autonomic neuropathy may

have SAS.[229] Foley et al.[148] reported more sleep complaints in those with comorbid cardiopulmonary diseases and depression compared with those without associated medical disorders. Wilcox et al.[230] reported difficulty falling asleep in 31% of patients with osteoarthritis and 66% of those with chronic pain, whereas 81% of patients with arthritis and 85% with chronic pain complained of sleep maintenance difficulty. There is an increasing prevalence of sleep maintenance problems in patients with diabetes mellitus.[231] For information on medical disorders that cause sleep-disordered breathing, EDS, and other sleep disturbances, see Chapter 33. Treatment should be directed at the primary condition to alleviate secondary sleep disturbances.

Sleep Disturbances and Comorbid Psychiatric Illness

An important psychiatric illness that causes sleep disturbances in the elderly is depression,[144,149,217,232–236] which should be carefully evaluated through a thorough psychiatric history. The condition is treatable, and misdiagnosis and prescription of hypnotics for insomnia would lead to a vicious cycle of worsening sleep complaints. An important sleep complaint in these patients is early morning awakening, resembling advanced sleep phase syndrome.[232–234] Untreated insomnia is also a strong predictor of depression.[237] Treating insomnia may also improve comorbid depression.[238,239] Anxiety disorders also cause sleep disturbances,[236] and various psychotic disorders may cause both hypersomnolence and insomnia[236] (see Chapter 32).

Sleep Disturbances and Comorbid Neurodegenerative and Other Neurologic Disorders

Alzheimer's disease and related dementias in the elderly may cause sleep disturbances, including nocturnal confusional episodes (sundowning syndrome), which may require antipsychotic medication (see Chapter 29). For information on other neurologic disorders causing sleep disturbances in the elderly, see Chapter 29.

Sleep Disturbances Associated with Drugs and Alcohol

A careful drug and alcohol history is important, as elderly individuals often take a variety of medications, including sedative-hypnotics for associated medical conditions, and over-the-counter drugs to promote sleep.[144,150,151,172,181,217] Sleeping medications produce secondary drug-related insomnia. Alcohol worsens sleep disturbances and may exacerbate existing SAS. Some examples of medications[150] that may cause insomnia include β blockers (probably by interfering with nocturnal melatonin secretion), bronchodilators, corticosteroids, decongestants (e.g., pseudophedrine), and CNS stimulants (e.g., caffeine, theophylline), as well as drugs to treat gastroesophageal reflux (e.g., cimetidine), cardiovascular disorders (e.g., methyldopa, furosemide), neurologic diseases (e.g., phenytoin, modafinil, ritalin, amphetamines, dopaminergic drugs), and depression (e.g., bupropion, fluoxetine, venlafaxine, sertraline, paroxetine). Some antidepressants may cause sedation (e.g., nortriptyline, desipramine, amitriptyline, trazodone). Sedating medications should preferably be administered at bedtime and stimulating medications should be ingested during daytime hours.

Narcolepsy

Narcolepsy is a disease of earlier onset than old age, and the diagnosis will probably have been made much earlier, but it is a lifelong condition. The diagnosis rests on a history of sudden sleep attacks lasting a short time and associated with auxiliary symptoms such as cataplexy, hypnagogic hallucinations, and sleep paralysis. A history of narcoleptic sleep attacks and cataplexy may be sufficient for diagnosis, but an all-night PSG study, followed by the Multiple Sleep Latency Test (MSLT), which will show reduced sleep-onset latency and sleep-onset REM in two out of five recordings, is needed for confirmation.

Restless Legs Syndrome

Restless legs syndrome (see Chapter 28) is primarily a lifelong condition, although it may be secondary to diabetic or uremic peripheral neuropathy. In addition to the characteristic restless movements during the daytime, nighttime sleep is severely disturbed. The prevalence increases with age, and the symptoms may occur initially in old age.

Parasomnias

The important parasomnias in the elderly are RBD, sleepwalking, and night terrors. The latter two conditions usually present in childhood or adolescence, but if they have a relatively sudden onset in an elderly person, an acute neurologic condition should be suspected and excluded by appropriate laboratory investigations.[185,240] RBD can be suspected from the history given by the bed partner and by simultaneous video-PSG evaluation at night. (See Chapter 35 for a general discussion of parasomnias.) RBD is frequently a preclinical manifestation of a neurodegenerative disorder, particularly synucleinopathies (e.g., Parkinson's disease, diffuse Lewy body dementia, and multiple system atrophy) in the elderly.[241]

Disorders of Circadian Function

Morgan and associates[242] reported that occasional sleep complaints are noted by 40% of older individuals, and according to Garma and colleagues,[243] older individuals complain of frequent and prolonged awakenings during the night. It has been speculated by Czeisler and coworkers[244] that these disorders may be due to changes in the human circadian pacemaker with advancing age. Work with light by Czeisler and colleagues[245,246] showed that, with appropriately timed exposure to bright light, one can change the temperature cycle—that is, circadian phase—and may be able to correct the circadian sleep disorder. Further research is needed in this area.

In 1962, McGhie and Russell[168] reported that 15% of older individuals complained of early morning awakenings, and in 1988 Mant and Eyland[247] reported that 33% of elderly individuals woke up early in the morning several times a week. Sleep parameters thus show an advanced phase, which is also noted with other circadian rhythms such as activity rhythm, body temperature rhythm, and timing of REM sleep and the cortisol rhythm.[244] An advance in the circadian phase due to a reduction of the endogenous period of the circadian pacemaker with advancing age is suggested by animal experiments.[84,248] Human data for such studies are lacking, but a cross-sectional study by Weitzman's group[249] documented that the free-running period of the temperature rhythm was significantly shorter in six subjects ages 53–60 years than in six healthy young adults. A study by Czeisler and colleagues[245] suggested a strong relationship between period reduction and phase advance in the circadian rhythms of older people.

The pathophysiologic mechanism of these changes remains speculative. In 1972,[92,250] a cluster of neurons was discovered in the anterior tip of the hypothalamus on either side of the third ventricle, the SCN. This is the circadian pacemaker. With advancing age, the volume of SCN cells shrinks—that is, the number of neurons decreases,[251–253] which may result in functional impairment. Other factors may contribute to circadian dysrhythmia in the elderly[151,254,255]: gradual decrement of nocturnal endogenous melatonin secretion with age; and inadequate time spent in daylight, thus weakening exogenous cues (*Zeitgebers*) to entrain the circadian rhythm, causing sleep fragmentation and circadian dysrhythmia.

LABORATORY ASSESSMENT

The diagnostic evaluation should begin with a thorough history of sleep disturbances, which may be EDS, difficulty initiating or maintaining sleep, and intrusions of unusual behavior during sleep. Physical examination may direct attention to systemic disease. Based on the history and findings of the physical examination, a decision should be made regarding referrals to specialized sleep centers for PSG and MSLT studies. Tests should be performed when clinical interview and examination cannot resolve the problems.

Most of the sleep disturbances of elders can be diagnosed by a careful history and physical examination.

For some conditions, however, laboratory assessment is important. In SAS, it is important to have an all-night PSG study to quantify and determine the severity of sleep-related respiratory disturbances. Sleep apnea is a treatable condition, so it is important to make this diagnosis correctly. In addition, MSLT and PSG studies are important for a narcolepsy diagnosis, although in elderly people this diagnosis may have been made many years earlier. All-night video recordings are necessary to diagnose some conditions, such as RBD, that require the examiner to differentiate from among a number of sleep disorders with similar symptoms. Appropriate tests should be performed if other medical or neurologic disorders are suspected.

TREATMENT

The objective of treatment is to reduce the risk of mortality and morbidity and improve quality of life.[256] The first step is accurate assessment and diagnosis.

Indications for Treatment of Obstructive Sleep Apnea

Indications for treatment of obstructive sleep apnea are reviewed briefly in this section; the reader is referred to Chapters 24 and 25 for details. Obstructive sleep apnea is a major cause of hypersomnia in elders, and it is often a reversible condition if appropriately diagnosed and treated. For moderate to severe obstructive sleep apnea, treatment is recommended. Polysomnography and MSLT studies should be able to decide the severity of the apnea when findings are considered with the RDI, the degree of oxygen saturation, and abnormally short sleep latency. Before instituting any specific treatment, certain general measures are recommended, including weight loss; smoking cessation; avoidance of alcohol, sedatives, and hypnotics; avoidance of the supine sleep position; and management of nasopharyngeal disorders. The majority of patients respond to CPAP treatment. Weaver and Chasens[257] reviewed findings from clinical trials including CPAP therapy for older individuals. These studies clearly showed the benefit of CPAP therapy in an older population, with improvement of cognition, memory, executive function, sleep quality, and cardiovascular function. CPAP treatment is well tolerated by older adults, and patterns of adherence are similar to those noted in younger adults. In general, older patients require lower CPAP titration pressure than younger patients and this may be related to the physiologic differences in respiratory structure and function.

If all measures including CPAP fail, surgical procedures such as uvulopalatopharyngoplasty (UPP) may be appropriate, particularly if the site of obstruction is in the pharyngeal region. The success rate of UPP is variable. Tracheostomy, which is modified to keep the trachea closed during the day and open at night, has been an option in most severe cases. The primary criteria for recommending tracheostomy[173] include severe daytime symptoms that interfere with function, severe hypertension or dangerous cardiac arrhythmias, and an AI of 20 or greater or a decrease in oxygen saturation of more than 10% below average baseline values. Tracheostomy is now rarely used and reserved for morbidly ill patients who cannot tolerate CPAP. In selected patients with a moderate degree of sleep apnea, oral appliances[258] have been tried with moderate success.

Indications for Treatment of Insomnia

Multiple factors are responsible for insomnia in elders, and, therefore, evaluation and treatment of insomnia should be multidisciplinary.[174,181] Elimination or avoidance of factors that are causing insomnia is the first step in treatment. The next important general measure is paying attention to sleep hygiene. See Chapter 26 for more information on the treatment of insomnia.

Insomnia is a very common complaint in the elderly and may be the result of a variety of medical or psychiatric conditions. Insomnia may also result from PLMS, or occasionally from sleep apnea. An important cause is pharmacologic agents (i.e., drugs and alcohol), so a careful history and physical examination are important before any treatment is instituted.

PLMS is an important condition in elders, but its incidence and natural history are unknown. Even the relationship between PLMS and insomnia is not clear. Therefore, any pharmacologic treatment for PLMS is subject to controversy, and the long-term effect of drug treatment on patients is unknown. For selected cases in which PLMS clearly disrupts sleep, therapy may be indicated (see Chapter 28).

Circadian rhythm disorder, another important cause of insomnia, results from changes in the daily routine or sleep pattern, shift work, or trans-meridian travel. Therefore, environmental control and adequate counseling should be the first line of treatment.

When a medical or psychiatric disorder causes insomnia, appropriate treatment should be directed toward the primary condition. In the case of depression, appropriate treatment with tricyclic antidepressants, often those with sedative effect (e.g., amitriptyline, doxepin, trazodone), or with selective serotonin reuptake inhibitors could be used to advantage.

Medical conditions such as cardiac failure, hyperthyroidism, respiratory disorders, arthritis and other painful conditions, and esophageal reflux syndrome should be treated appropriately. It should be remembered, however, that medications themselves may cause sleep disturbance.

For transient or temporary disturbances of sleep, short-term intermittent use of hypnotics and sedatives may be useful. Long-term use of hypnotics is not recommended (see Chapter 26). The National Institutes of

Health State-of-the-Science Conference on Insomnia[259] concluded that there is no systematic evidence for the effectiveness of a variety of medications used to treat insomnia in the past and even now in the elderly (e.g., antihistamines, antidepressants, antipsychotics, anticonvulsants). The conference panel also warned about the risks of using these medications in the elderly. For chronic insomnia, nonpharmacologic treatment (see later and Chapter 26) is the mainstay of therapy.

Currently the drugs of choice for treating insomnia in the elderly are the newer nonbenzodiazepine receptor agonists[150,151,260,261] (see Chapter 26). Before the advent of these agents, intermediate- and short-acting benzodiazepines were used to treat insomnia in the elderly[262,263] (see Chapter 26). The benzodiazepine group of drugs may have to be used even now in some patients if they fail to respond to the newer nonbenzodiazepine agonists or the recently approved ramelteon, a melatonin agonist.[264] However, benzodiazepine hypnotics must be used conservatively and with caution in the elderly because of their adverse side effect profile, including next-day hangover effects with a risk of falls and fractures.[265] The specific type of insomnia (e.g., sleep-onset or sleep-maintenance insomnia) should be assessed first before determining the appropriate type of sleeping medication. The best agent for sleep-onset insomnia should be a short-acting, rapidly absorbing medication (e.g., zolpidem or zaleplon), whereas for sleep-maintenance insomnia an intermediate-acting hypnotic (e.g., zolpidem extended release, eszopiclone) is best.[266,267] Zaleplon is an ultra-short-acting hypnotic that may be used at bedtime and again in the middle of the night if needed, but the patient must remain in bed for at least 4 hours to avoid residual next-morning sedation.

There is a relative lack of data regarding use of nonbenzodiazepine receptor agonists in the elderly. In an earlier report, Reynolds et al.[268] reviewed 1082 patients in 23 randomized, double-blind trials in elderly patients with chronic insomnia and found scientific support for the short-term (up to 3 weeks) efficacy of zolpidem and triazolam in the elderly, as well as temazepam, flurazepam, and quazepam. Triazolam, an ultra-short-acting benzodiazepine hypnotic, has since been restricted by the U.S. Food and Drug Administration and suspended in the United Kingdom because of serious behavioral disturbances. Dolder et al.[260] recently reviewed five drugs: zolpidem, zaleplon, eszopiclone, ramelteon, and zopiclone. Based on limited data, all these drugs are modestly effective and well tolerated for treatment of insomnia in older subjects.[224,225,230,231] Comparative head-to-head trials of these drugs, however, are lacking.

Melatonin, an indoleamine secreted by the pineal gland at night, has received considerable attention as a hypnotic based mostly on anecdotal rather than scientific evidence. Garfinkel et al.[269] found melatonin to be superior to placebo in improving sleep efficiency in the elderly in a double-blind, placebo-controlled study. However, later studies did not find melatonin to be an effective hypnotic.[259] In a subgroup of elderly insomniacs with a melatonin deficiency, Haimov et al.[270] found melatonin replacement therapy to be beneficial in the initiation and maintenance of sleep in these patients.

Special Pharmacologic Considerations

Vestal and Dawson[271] directed attention to the important factor of alterations of drug metabolism, with attendant changes in pharmacokinetics, in the elderly. It is important to start with a dose smaller than younger subjects require and then gradually to increase the dose, depending on the response. It is also extremely important to obtain a drug history, to prevent drug-drug interactions and exacerbation of sleep disturbances by hypnotics or other agents.

Situational and Lifestyle Considerations

Lifestyle factors are different for elders.[217] Retirement, with disturbance of the sleep-wake schedule (e.g., napping in the daytime and consequent inability to sleep at the scheduled night time); so-called empty nest syndrome that develops when children leave home; and bereavement over the death of a spouse or close friend may lead to loneliness and depression with attendant sleep disturbances. Other causes of sleep disturbances in the elderly include institutionalization, prolonged bed rest, poor sleep hygiene, unsatisfactory bed environment, poor dietary habits, and caffeine and alcohol consumption.

Treatment of Sleep Cycle Changes Related to Age

Treatment of sleep cycle changes related to age consists of educating the patient about sleep disruptions in old age, discouraging multiple naps, and urging participation in special interests and other activities and hobbies.[151,185]

For treatment of circadian rhythm disorder in the elderly, bright-light therapy is the treatment of choice[151] as light is the strongest cue for circadian sleep-wake cycle entrainment. In community-dwelling elderly patients and nursing home residents, evening exposure to light is found to delay circadian rhythms, correcting the advanced sleep phase state seen in the elderly.[272] Such patients are advised to avoid bright light in the morning and spend more time outdoors during late afternoon and early evening. Such light exposure outdoors or exposure to artificial light by a bright-light box (5000–10,000 lux) not only may help correct the advanced circadian state in the elderly but also may improve sleep maintenance insomnia in some subjects.[272–274]

Treatment of Situational Stress

Patients should be given supportive psychotherapy and behavior modification treatment, as well as clear explanations, to reduce stress and sleeplessness.[185]

Treatment of Nocturnal Confusional Episodes

Nocturnal confusional episodes are characterized by disorientation, agitation, and wandering at night, and often result from acute or chronic organic neurologic dysfunction (see Chapter 29).[185,275] Relatively sudden onset of night terrors or sleepwalking indicates an organic brain disorder, and an appropriate investigation should be made. Nocturnal confusional episodes can be precipitated by other associated medical illnesses. The treatment should be directed toward the precipitating or causal factors for these confusional episodes. Often episodes are precipitated when the patient is transferred from home to an institution. As much as possible, the home environment of such patients should be preserved. The darkness of night often precipitates episodes, so a night light is helpful. A careful drug history should be obtained, and medications that are not absolutely necessary should be gradually reduced and eliminated. The use of hypnotics may further aggravate the condition. The treatment of choice is high-potency antipsychotics, such as haloperidol and thiothixene, in small doses[217,275] or the newer antipsychotics (e.g., risperdone, olanzapine).

Treatment of Medication-Induced Sleep-Wakefulness Disturbances

Some medications cause insomnia, whereas others cause EDS. Elderly individuals often take a variety of medications because of the increased prevalence of other illnesses. Furthermore, because of their altered metabolism, they are susceptible to the side effects of various medications. The patient should avoid alcohol, caffeine, and cigarettes, and should gradually eliminate drugs that are not essential.

Special Environmental Considerations in Treatment

Treatment should be designed and tailored to different environmental situations (e.g., nursing home, hospital, home), as different types of sleep disturbances have been noted in different environments.[49]

Exercise Program

Exercise, particularly 5–6 hours before sleep, is thought to have a beneficial effect on sleep quality. However, there is a dearth of well-controlled studies.[276] King et al.[277] found that older adults with moderate sleep complaints can improve self-rated sleep quality by initiating a regular, moderate-intensity, endurance exercise program. Sugaya and coworkers[278] reported an improvement of deep sleep and nocturia in 18 (60%) of 30 men (average age 71 years) after walking rapidly for 30 minutes or longer in the evening for 8 weeks. Preliminary study findings by Gary and Lee[279] suggested that a progressive walking program may improve TST and quality of life in older women with diastolic heart failure.

Nonpharmacologic Treatment

Time-limited and sleep-focused nonpharmacologic interventions have been found to improve sleep in many chronic insomniacs[280–282] (see Chapter 26). The nonpharmacologic intervention consists of cognitive behavioral therapy, including stimulus control therapy, sleep restriction therapy, relaxation techniques, and sleep hygiene education. There are some limited studies combining nonpharmacologic interventions with pharmacotherapy to improve the quality of sleep,[282] but none in elderly insomniacs.

⊗ REFERENCES

A full list of references are available at www.expertconsult.com

CHAPTER 37

Sleep Disorders of Childhood

Richard Ferber

INTRODUCTION

The same sleep disorders that occur in adults also occur in children: sleep apnea, narcolepsy, the parasomnias, sleep schedule or circadian rhythm disorders, and the insomnias.[1] All of these disorders have presentations, and most have etiologies, that are peculiar to children, a fact that must be taken into account to assure proper evaluation and treatment. For example, narcolepsy in children may present initially as a form of hypersomnolence with a single prolonged but otherwise normal-appearing sleep period, and only later evolve into the adult pattern of disrupted nighttime sleep and daytime sleepiness with short, refreshing naps and cataplexy (R. Ferber, unpublished data, 1997).[2–5] Sleep apnea in children is rarely caused by a floppy upper airway; instead, the most common cause is adenotonsillar hypertrophy, and the pattern of obstruction often more resembles an upper airway resistance syndrome with partial obstruction and relatively mild desaturations than it does the typical pattern of clear-cut apneas, marked desaturations, and severe sleep disruption as is seen in adults.[6,7] Bed-wetting during the first 5 years of life reflects normal function and maturation, not the "disorder" of enuresis. Confusional arousals are much more frequent in children than sleepwalking or sleep terrors,[8,9] and in young children the causes of the parasomnias and the insomnias may overlap considerably.[10]

The sleep disorders whose childhood presentations are most different from their adult counterparts are the insomnias, particularly the forms of sleeplessness seen in young children, especially if one includes the relevant schedule-related disorders.[10–14] Thus, this chapter focuses primarily on the presentations, causes, and treatments of the young child with difficulty falling or remaining asleep.

Sleep states develop in fetal life, first rapid eye movement (REM) then non-REM (NREM). Thus, newborns enter the world already able to achieve both main states of sleep. At birth, however, NREM sleep is not fully developed and is not yet divisible into substages.[15–20] Although the circadian pacemaker is functional at birth, its full expression is not seen for some months because of state instability (especially REM) and the interference from other physiologic systems (such as the need to eat frequently), and because ultradian rhythms are still quite immature.[18,21–24] As a result, periods of sleeping and waking are spread, initially almost randomly, across the 24-hour day.

After birth, changes continue to occur rapidly, both in the electrophysiologic appearance of sleep and in its circadian control. The tracé alternant electroencephalographic pattern of NREM sleep in the newborn (2- to 6-second bursts of high-amplitude slow waves separated by 4–8 seconds of low-voltage mixed activity) disappears within a few weeks and is replaced by a more continuous pattern.[15,18,20] Division of NREM sleep into substages is clear by 6 months if not before. Sleep spindles appear by age 4–6 weeks and are prominent by 2 months.[17] Vertex waves suggestive of K complexes are usually seen by approximately 4 months, and are clearly defined by 6 months.[16]

The circadian clock is functional at birth but does not become well linked to the sleep rhythm it controls until 6–12 weeks.[24,25] By 3 months there is consolidation of the major sleep period into the night, and there is beginning organization of daytime sleep into a pattern of regularly recurring naps throughout the day.[18-23] By 5–6 months, nighttime sleep usually improves further because of the decrease in the need for nighttime feedings. By now there are usually two main naps in the midmorning and midafternoon, and a small nap in the evening. By the second half of the first year of life, the evening nap is dropped and sleep should be well organized, with good nighttime sleep and two regular daytime naps. Shortly after the first birthday, these naps generally coalesce into a single nap after lunch. Naps are usually given up altogether between the third and fifth birthdays, although the exact time may vary considerably, depending somewhat on imposed schedule.

Most children do not start sleeping through the night before the age of 3 months, and it is not reasonable to try to get such young infants to do so. However, full-term infants who are developing and growing normally should be able to sleep through the night, or at least very nearly so, by age 5–6 months.[26,27] If bedtime difficulties or nighttime awakenings continue to be significant problems after this time, the reasons for these problems can now usually be identified and most often easily corrected, generally by behavioral means and schedule adjustment.[10,11,13,14,28-32]

PROBLEM VERSUS DISORDER, AND PROBLEM VERSUS NO PROBLEM

Youngsters are very adaptable in terms of their ability to vary their sleep patterns, change habits associated with sleep, sleep at different times, and divide their sleep into different numbers of segments. These variations are especially common during the early years of life, when sleep is normally still polyphasic (i.e., divided into daytime and nighttime segments).[1] Certain patterns may present significant problems for family members, although technically these patterns represent variations of normal function, not true dysfunctions of physiologic disorders. The bulk of the complaints of sleeplessness in young children seen in practice fall into this category.

For a problem of sleeplessness to truly represent a disorder, some combination of the following must be present: the child should have difficulty falling asleep even at the correct circadian phase and regardless of environmental setting, there should be increased numbers or lengths of wakings (i.e., not just reflecting normal sleep cycling), total sleep time should be below the sleep requirements of the child, or daytime functioning should be affected.

This symptom of insufficient sleep may be difficult to assess in young children. A 1-year-old child who sleeps only 7 hours a night but naps 5 hours during the day could be viewed as getting a normal amount of sleep but distributed in a manner that is difficult for the family to accommodate. This child could also be viewed as having a disorder preventing him or her from getting sufficient

sleep at night, resulting in excessive sleepiness during the day. The former interpretation is usually the correct one, since such poor distribution of sleep usually is not secondary to a physiologic disorder and also is usually easily corrected. It is also difficult to evaluate the consequences of insufficient sleep in a child because, in young children, mild sleepiness often appears as irritability and attentional difficulty instead of as overt sleepiness (yawning or dozing).[4] If symptoms are chronic, their existence is often inferred only retroactively when behavior improves after adjustment of the sleep pattern.

Unlike adults, children generally do not deal with their sleep problems by themselves. Instead, these problems lead to interactions between the children and their parents (or other caregivers), and it is often the specifics of these interactions that determine whether parents perceive the sleep pattern as a problem.[10,11,29,30,33,34] If parents must wake up at night to help their child return to sleep, the parents may consider this a problem (even if the child sleeps in the parents' room). Also, what is considered to be a problem for one family may not be for the next. Often what determines the perception of a problem's existence is the ability of the parent who gets up at night to go back to sleep quickly after intervening. Even just briefly covering a child after a single nighttime waking may represent a major problem to a parent who cannot then go back to sleep.

Nighttime wakings are not a problem per se. In fact, they occur as part of the normal pattern of sleep cycling from the day a child is born. However, they can develop into problems when parents, misinterpreting these awakenings as abnormal, establish patterns of intervention that end up disrupting what was actually a normal sleep pattern.

Children are different and so are parents. Both have variable needs and temperaments.[35,36] A routine that works well for one family or child may not work at all for another. Although parents may manage their two children the same way at bedtime and at nighttime awakenings, one child may go to sleep quickly and sleep throughout the night (i.e., return to sleep after normal nighttime awakenings without waking the parents) and the other may protest loudly at bedtime and be up three times a night, unable (or unwilling) to go back to sleep without the parents doing something. "Treatment" of the first child is unnecessary (whatever the parents are doing at night is working fine for that child), but changes in management are required for the second. The decision for parents to change their approach should be dictated both by their own desires and by their child's actual sleep pattern.

General Considerations

A major advance in the treatment of insomnia in adults came with the realization that many factors are involved in causing the problem, many diagnoses are possible, and specific treatments can be designed to fit the specific causes of patients' complaints.[37,38] No longer is it appropriate to treat insomnia as a single diagnosis with a single treatment (as was the case with barbiturate prescriptions for adults a half-century ago). By assuming that all sleepless youngsters have the same diagnosis and need the same treatment, a practitioner is sure to treat many children inappropriately and unsuccessfully.

When dealing with an insomniac adult, one must take the history directly from the patient; for children, the history is usually obtained from the parent or caregiver. In the adult, it is the degree of unhappiness of the patient with his or her own sleep pattern that determines the severity of the complaint; in the child, it is the impact on the family that determines it. An insomniac adult may be frustrated by an inability to sleep despite a desire to do so. A sleepless child may not want to sleep at the time or under the conditions the parents have established.

In most cases, a very careful history from the family provides enough information to diagnose the causes of a child's sleep problems and to decide on therapy.[12,14,39,40] The history itself should not be rushed, and it should be extensive and wide ranging, as multiple factors often contribute to a child's sleep difficulties. A physical examination should not be neglected, but it only rarely provides the answers.

It is helpful to obtain the history in a circadian format, finding out what happens and at what time around the clock.[12,39–41] Of course, there must be emphasis on the times of sleep (bedtime, actual time of falling asleep, naptimes) and awakenings, and the exact circumstances under which all sleep transitions take place (after nighttime awakenings as well as at bedtime). Night to night, and weekday versus weekend, schedules should be clarified. Parents often forget to mention short periods of sleep (e.g., in the car or stroller) that may have much impact on the rest of the sleep pattern. The timing and pattern of daytime events are also important: day care, other structured activities, peer interactions, and television viewing. A careful description of the sleeping environment or environments may be crucial, including the organization of the house, the bedroom locations, the proximity of the child's bedroom to the parents', whether there is a night light (and how bright it is), if the child's bedroom door is open or closed, if there is a transitional object, if other children share the room, if the child sleeps with the parents, and if the parents are on the same floor of the house at bedtime and during the night. External stimulation, such as a parent coming home just as a youngster is about to go to sleep or a parent getting up and showering very early in the morning, may also be relevant.

A complete social history should be obtained.[12,39,40] The makeup of the family should be known, marital discord should be probed, alcohol or drug abuse identified, and any other factors that could lead to stress in the home should be investigated.

SPECIFIC DISORDERS

Sleep-Onset Association Disorder

When sleep-onset association disorder is the only problem, the child's ability to fall asleep at the desired time and to sleep the desired number of hours often is not affected.[10,30] The child has come to associate falling asleep with some behavioral pattern that is partially outside his or her control.[10,11,14,28–32,34,42–52] To avoid problems, it is generally necessary for the parents to reestablish this routine both at bedtime and at times of (even normal) nighttime awakening.

The child may fall asleep quickly when the circumstances are to his or her liking (e.g., being rocked in the living room). However, when the parents try to get the child to go to sleep in the location and under the conditions they desire, the process of sleep transition will be extended. Even if bedtime is not believed to be a problem (the parents may be up, in the living room, watching television anyway), the nighttime will be when the child needs help returning to sleep.

A pattern of specific associations with sleep transitions is common at all ages, but most older children and adults are able to take on the responsibility for generating these patterns by themselves (e.g., sleeping on their side, with a heavy blanket, with music playing, and a dim light). Whether by necessity or choice, parents of young children often become entangled in these associations. Such parent-assisted patterns may truly be necessary in the first few months to help a very young infant smoothly negotiate the transition from wakefulness to sleep at bedtimes and after spontaneous interruptions of sleep, and to help a colicky youngster who appears to be in discomfort.[53,54] By the age of 3–4 months, most youngsters have passed the age of colic and, in any case, have matured sufficiently to be able to handle these transitions by themselves.

Bedtime routines that continue through the process of falling asleep may become habitual and have to be repeated during the night. Rocking and back patting or rubbing are perhaps the most common routines for infants. Youngsters may require a bottle or cup of water, juice, or milk. They may be handed a pacifier, walked about, or driven in the car. They may fall asleep quickly and transfer easily to the crib, or they may fall asleep slowly and be difficult to move from arms to mattress until they reach the deepest stage of sleep. Once asleep, children generally do well for several hours (the initial epochs of deep NREM sleep). Although awakenings may begin earlier, they typically start 3–4 hours after the child first falls asleep (at, or shortly after, the time the parents go to bed themselves). This middle third of the night is when sleep is lightest, as youngsters change back and forth among stages of light NREM sleep, REM sleep, and brief periods of waking. If they wake sufficiently to sense that the patterns associated with sleep transitions are no longer present, they arouse more completely and signal the parents of their dissatisfaction by crying or calling. Often a child falls asleep in a parent's arms in the living room with the lights and television on, only to awaken during the night alone, in a crib, in a dark, quiet room. It is not surprising that a youngster in such a situation may have difficulty returning to sleep.

The key diagnostic feature comes from the description of the nighttime awakenings.[10,12,29,30,39,40,44] The youngster goes back to sleep promptly when the parents respond by quickly reinstituting conditions that have become associated with sleep transitions. If simply rocking a child at this point causes him or her to go back to sleep quickly, most other causes of sleeplessness, including pain and schedule disorders, can be ruled out. There certainly can be no problem with the child's inherent ability to sleep if he or she returns to sleep with such minimal intervention. When association are at fault, a youngster may seem angry at the parents if they do not do what he or she wants, but the child does not appear frightened.

Parents of children with sleep-onset association disorder are usually aware of one to three awakenings per night. Often the last several hours of the night are quiet again, reflecting the tendency of young children to return to deep sleep toward morning.

Once sleep-onset associations have been identified as the cause of a child's problem (i.e., interfering with return to sleep after normal nighttime awakenings), and if the parents want to take steps to improve matters, an appropriate pattern of intervention can be designed. Typically, this involves giving the youngster a chance to learn to make the transition from wake to sleep under the conditions that will be present at the time of spontaneous nighttime awakenings.[1,10,29,30,34,50,55–60] If the child will wake at night in the crib alone, in a relatively dark and quiet room, then that is the way the youngster should learn to go to sleep at bedtime. If there is any question about when the child is ready to fall asleep, the time chosen should be somewhat on the late side, to be sure. The youngster simply needs to be put down awake after an appropriate bedtime ritual and given increasing amounts of time to fall asleep, interrupted by brief parental visits for reassurance. The same patterns should be used at times of nighttime awakenings, increasing the waiting times as needed on successive nights.

Although some clinicians begin the training at naptime,[55] it seems reasonable to start at bedtime, when the drive to sleep is greater. Also, although some recommend starting before 2 months of age,[55] it seems appropriate to wait until it is clear that the youngster has the neurologic capacity to manage these transitions smoothly. Because most children show an ability to sleep through the night by the age of 5 or 6 months, this age seems to be a reasonable time to start. Starting the training process from the beginning (i.e., always putting a youngster down awake) in an effort to avoid problems later on makes little sense, as it is unclear why trying to teach a neonate to negotiate the transitions to sleep alone is of any particular value. Parental closeness is more important for neonates than is learning how to sleep alone, and new patterns can be learned later on without much difficulty. The learning process generally takes only 1–3 nights.

Another approach to this problem is that of scheduled awakenings.[61–64] The child is awakened during the night before the expected time of natural awakening. The assumption is that the child will be quite sleepy at that point and able to go back to sleep quickly, with little parental intervention, and by so doing will learn new habits that will allow him or her to sleep through subsequent times of usual awakenings.

In some situations it is best to have the parents sleep in the child's room for 1–2 weeks, so as to be present at times of awakening, but not to reinstitute rocking or other learned associations. This is particularly useful for a child with separation (or other) anxiety. In this case, the reassurance of having a parent in the room is enough to let the child return to sleep. This differs from the situation of a youngster for whom the habitual nighttime interventions, not parental reassurance, is desired. In fact, such a child often finds it more frustrating to have a parent nearby, if the parent refuses to rock or pat him or her.

Nocturnal Eating Disorder

A youngster with nocturnal eating disorder is fed at times of nighttime awakening (and usually also at bedtime).[1,10,26,33,42,49,50,65–67] To some degree, this is analogous to the problem just discussed, sleep-onset associations, if the youngster falls asleep at the breast or while taking a bottle. The difference is that, when there are excessive feedings, the child has more awakenings at night than when the problem is just one of sleep-onset associations.

To make this diagnosis, one must be sure that the number of nighttime awakenings is more than is required for nutritional purposes. Although many children continue to be fed at night beyond age 5 or 6 months, this generally reflects habit, not need. Continued nighttime feeding after 6 months does not define the existence of a problem; this depends on the frequency of awakenings and the number and amount of feedings. Even if the parents are not complaining, an 8-month-old child who is fed six times a night has his or her sleep disrupted to a degree that is unlikely to be in the child's best interests.

Beside the factor of associations, the feedings themselves have a major impact. The amount of milk or juice taken during the night is frequently extraordinary, up to a quart (4 full bottles) or more. It is easy to understand how such intake can disrupt sleep. With intake of food, there is stimulation of digestive processes, increased body temperature and other disruptions of circadian cycling, and increased urine output—all factors that may lead to increased awakenings. In addition, a youngster who *learns* to expect feeding during the night *learns* to get hungry at those times.[1,10,11,27,28,44,50,68] The associated gastric contractions and central signals can also stimulate arousal. The effect on the circadian system should not be underestimated. A youngster who continues to feed multiple times during the night remains on a pattern typical of early infancy, when sleeping, waking, and feeding are all distributed across the 24-hour day.[28,44]

If the family decides to decrease or eliminate the nighttime feedings, there are different ways it can be accomplished,[10,50,68] and these should be discussed with the family so that they can choose the one they feel best suits them. Perhaps the easiest is simply to progressively lengthen the interval between feedings (e.g., by 30 minutes each night), and eliminating the nighttime feedings over approximately 1 week. At the same time, decreasing the amount of milk or juice given per bottle may also help. Some families prefer to water down the formula or juice progressively; once only water is given, the nutritional aspects of nighttime feedings are eliminated, and then the water may be stopped completely the next day.

It is not always necessary to eliminate the bedtime feeding. If bedtime feeding is kept, the youngster should be fed and put into the crib. He or she should not be allowed back to the breast or given another bottle after that (even if he or she wakes at the time of transfer), to prevent the related association problem from developing or persisting. Occasionally, a parent wants to decrease nighttime feedings from several to one. This can be attempted by spacing out the minimum time between feedings and then stopping at a preselected interval (such as 5 hours). This is often, but not always, successful.

Limit-Setting Sleep Disorder

Limit-setting sleep disorder is usually seen in youngsters ages 3–6 years. Problems often start the day a child learns how to climb out of a crib or is moved to a bed for other reasons. With the loss of the controls previously provided by the bars of the crib, the locus of nocturnal control is shifted from the parents to the youngster. The child is now expected to control his or her own urges, including the desire to put off bedtime, make endless requests, and leave the bed and bedroom. The same problems may occur even if the youngster sleeps in the parents' bed. If parents are unable to enforce control by setting appropriate limits, the youngster becomes increasingly anxious,[69–72] limits are further tested, tension increases, and the night becomes more difficult.

A typical scenario is that of a child stalling at bedtime with multiple requests for an extra story, another glass of water, to watch more television, or to make additional trips to the bathroom. The more the parents give in to these requests, the more the child continues to make them. If the parents are not nearby, the child may get out of bed and find them.

Many factors have to be considered in these situations. A parent may not understand the importance of setting limits or that it is actually part of appropriate nurturing and not punishment. This point must be made clear. The tension that exists in the home when parents are distraught at the child's continued demands is certainly not in the youngster's best interest. A little boy who climbs into his parents' bed and kicks his father until his father goes to another room to sleep is made to feel inappropriately powerful and may be frightened by that power rather than happy at getting what he wanted. Parents differ considerably in their understanding of the importance of limits and even how to set them properly.

Setting limits in the context of guilt is especially difficult, for example, for a youngster who has, or has had, significant medical problems (prematurity, chronic illness, deafness). Also, it may be impossible as well as inappropriate to set certain limits in a home where there is ongoing psychosocial stress such as from marital discord, depression, alcoholism, or financial difficulties. A child who is not being appropriately nurtured during the day may use the struggles at night as a way of ensuring interaction with the parents, even though the tone of the interaction is negative.

Finally, to make the diagnosis of a limit-setting disorder, one assumes that the youngster is ready to fall asleep at the designated bedtime. If circadian factors are taken into consideration, what at first appears to be a limit-setting disorder may turn out be to a schedule disorder instead.[41,73–75] A careful history is usually sufficient to make this distinction.

Management must take into account why this disorder exists. If the need is clearly to replace limits that have been lost (or were never present), then considerable time must be spent working with the family. First is the process of education, helping the parents to understand that setting limits is important to a youngster's development. Then a concrete plan for setting limits that the family can follow must be devised.[50,72,76,77] Often this can be done quite easily, such as by replacing the controls previously provided by the bars of the crib with ones created by gates at the doorway. Parents can respond in a progressive manner, coming back to the gates for brief reassurance at increasing intervals. A youngster who can knock gates over or climb over even a double gate may have to be kept in the room with the door held closed temporarily,[10,13] although it is never reasonable lock a child in his or her bedroom for the night. The closed door serves as a passive limit setter, to avoid major confrontation between parents and child while enforcing the parents' rules. This should be done with the parent by the door and starting with very short closure time (approximately 30 seconds). The objective is not to frighten the youngster, only to help him or her learn the newly set rules.

Older children (at least age 3 years) may be motivated with a star chart or some other reward system.[10,30,50]

If the child is motivated and is willing to follow through with such a program, that should be tried; a positive reinforcement system is always better than a negative one.

Often, to the parents' surprise, once limits are firmly set, anxiety decreases markedly[11,70] and the youngster becomes much happier in the evening as nighttime tensions disappear. In fact, such children frequently remind their parents to close the gate before they leave, to be sure the parents remain in control.

In situations involving guilt or psychosocial difficulties, there must be careful evaluation and discussion before proceeding.[11,12,28,40,72] Parents who feel guilty may need to have more gradual limit-setting measures outlined for them, and families with psychosocial difficulties may require very individualized care. In this last setting, a child may actually need more access to the parents at night (as well as during the day), and it may be best to hold off on a strict limit-setting program until the psychosocial issues themselves can be better addressed. Counseling is often indicated.[11,12,72]

Food Allergy Insomnia

Kahn and associates[78–80] have described a condition of food allergy insomnia in which young children with documented allergy to cow's milk protein have severely disrupted sleep. Typically, they have delayed sleep initiation, frequent and prolonged nighttime awakenings, and markedly reduced total sleep time. Typical allergic symptoms such as rash or wheezing may be minimal or absent. There generally is spontaneous resolution by age 2–4 years.

Radioallergosorbent testing in these children shows elevated immunoglobulin E (IgE) against β-lactoglobulin. Eosinophil count, IgE titer, and skin reactivity may be normal, especially before the first birthday. There may be some cross-reactivity with soy-based products.

Switching to a hypoallergenic hydrolyzed formula is followed by resolution of symptoms within days to weeks. A challenge with even small amounts of cow's milk protein causes a return of symptoms until the apparent allergy is outgrown.

This disorder has not frequently been described in the United States, perhaps because of the tendency of U.S. pediatricians to switch formulas empirically when things are not going well. Sensitivity of children's sleep to other dietary agents has also been described.[81]

Circadian Rhythm Sleep Disorders

Delayed or Advanced Sleep Phase

Circadian rhythm disorders have been well described in adults (see Chapter 34).[25,82] The syndromes are conceptually the same in young children, except that it is the parents' dissatisfaction with the schedule that generates the complaint. Strictly speaking, these are situations in which a youngster gets (or is capable of getting) a normal amount of sleep at night but it does not occur during the desired hours; neither the start nor the end of the spontaneous sleep period is at the desired time.[25,41,73,75,82]

A child with an advanced sleep phase may fall asleep by 7:00 PM but awaken at 4:00 or 5:00 AM. The complaint is one of early morning awakening. The parents of a youngster with a delayed sleep phase may complain that it takes him or her several hours to fall asleep (perhaps not until 10:00 PM or later) but that the time of spontaneous morning awakening is later than the desired or appropriate hour (perhaps anywhere from 7:00 to 10:00 AM).

A careful history of a child with an advanced sleep phase usually shows advance of other aspects of the daytime schedule, such as meals and naptimes.[10,73,74] The child who awakens at 5:00 AM may be fed shortly after that and nap as early as 7:00 AM. Both the early feeding and early nap may contribute to persistence of this syndrome.[10,74] The bedtime behavior of a child with a delayed sleep phase may resemble that of a youngster with limit-setting difficulties, but with one major difference: the child with the phase delay is unable to fall asleep at the desired hour, even if the parents set very firm limits. Instead of calling and coming out of bed (as most youngsters would do), some try to "be good" and lie in bed each night for hours, waiting for sleepiness (and sleep) to arrive. During that time, they are generally not allowed to read, listen to the radio, or watch television. They must lie in the dark room, and they have nothing to do but think. Thinking in a dark room may lead to fantasy, and fantasy may lead to scary thoughts. Some of these youngsters end up scaring themselves, and nighttime fears may be the presenting complaint. However, such children will not experience bedtime fears on nights they go to bed late enough.

The youngster with a delayed sleep phase must be distinguished from one with a limit-setting disorder or true nighttime fears. Typically, the time of sleep onset is fairly independent of the bedtime. A youngster who falls asleep at 10:00 PM usually does so regardless of what hour he or she is put to bed; only the sleep latency changes (shortest after the latest bedtimes). On nights the family arrives home after the child's usual hour of sleep onset, the child likely has fallen asleep in the car. Description of weekend and vacation schedules are often critical in recognizing this syndrome.

Often children with phase delays are allowed (or want) to sleep late in the morning. If they are attending school or day care, they may be wakened (with difficulty); late morning sleep is then limited to weekends (but late sleep just on the weekends is still enough to prevent the schedule from normalizing). Children old enough to watch television on their own in the morning may give up the late weekend sleep for cartoons; however, lying in a dark room in front of the television for several hours does little to reset the circadian clock either. Children doing this probably doze by the television; they certainly are not fully awake, and do not get the morning light exposure they need to control their internal clock setting. The child getting up to watch television like this does so before the true end of the sleep phase, which can be identified by the time he or she wakes spontaneously when television watching is not available, or the time the youngster climbs out from under the blanket on the sofa, leaves the television, asks for breakfast, and appears (finally) to be wide awake.

In young children, a delayed sleep phase can usually be corrected easily by controlling the time of morning awakening.[10,41,73-75] It is best to start with a late bedtime, at the time the youngster actually has been falling asleep, to remove the stresses that have been present during the presleep hours and to help the child become accustomed to falling asleep quickly. If he or she is awakened for school or day care 5 days a week, this schedule should be enforced on weekends as well. If he or she usually sleeps late every day, the time of awakening can be easily advanced by 15–30 minutes a day. Once awakening is better controlled, bedtime can be slowly advanced in a similar manner. It is best to ensure that the youngster is up, fed, and moving about in the morning, exposed to as much light as possible. Television as the first morning activity should not be permitted. Formal use of light boxes[83] or around-the-clock progressive phase delay[84] is not usually necessary at this age.

For a child with an advanced sleep phase, ensuring plenty of light in the evening, progressively delaying bedtime, and progressively delaying early morning meal and naptimes should lead to prompt resolution. Avoiding early morning light exposure is also important.

Regular but Inappropriate Schedule

Inappropriately Timed Meal or Nap. It is well known that a regular nap in the late afternoon may delay the onset of sleep in the evening. What is less well known is that a very early meal or naptime may reinforce early morning awakening.[10,73,74] Youngsters who nap very early, perhaps at 6:00 or 7:00 PM, may awaken at 5:00 AM only to return to sleep after 1–2 hours. The youngster acts as if the last sleep cycle was broken off from the night and moved 1–2 hours later. An early feeding, such as at 5:00 AM (given because the youngster is awake anyway), may only reinforce continued early awakening, because the child learns to expect a feedings and feel hunger at that hour, and such sensations can trigger arousal. In these cases, nap and feeding times may need adjustment. The morning nap may be delayed to an appropriate time, such as 10:00 AM, it may be moved into the afternoon as a single nap (if the child is at least 1 year of age), or it may be eliminated altogether (if the child is old enough). Similarly, the first feeding in the morning may be delayed gradually to an appropriate breakfast time (perhaps 6:00 or 7:00 AM). Such interventions allow for later sleep in the morning.

Time in Bed Exceeding the Sleep Requirement. The syndrome of spending too much time in bed is similar to one sometimes seen in elderly individuals, but again, it is not the child's own decision to do so but that of the parents. It is not at all uncommon for parents to incorrectly estimate the amount of sleep their youngster needs.[85] Their estimate is often based on desire or incorrect data. Thus, parents may decide that their 18-month-old child should get 11 hours of sleep at night, and they keep him in the crib from 7:00 PM to 6:00 AM. In fact, this child may need only 11 hours of sleep per 24 hours—that is, night sleep plus naps. If he or she gets 2 hours a day in a regular afternoon nap, he or she is left with only 9 hours to sleep at night. These hours could run from 7:00 PM to 4:00 AM, perhaps, or from 9:00 PM to 6:00 AM, or even from 7:00 PM to 1:00 AM and then (after a 2-hour middle-of-the-night waking) from 3:00 AM to 6:00 AM. In all of these cases the parents leave an unhappy, wakeful child in the crib for 2 unnecessary hours: in the first case after waking early in the morning; in the second case after an inappropriately early bedtime; and in the third case as part of an extended nighttime waking. Older children may be forced to spend too much time in bed as well, but at least sometimes they are allowed to read or play (if they can do so quietly).

The solution to all of these problems is the same: the time in bed should be limited to the sleep requirement.[10,73,74,85,86] In the situations just described, bedtime and awakening should be 9 hours apart, whichever 9 hours the parents find most workable. Daytime naps should continue but be limited to a length appropriate for age.

Sometimes the total sleep time is inappropriately divided between night and day, with a night that is too short and naps that are too long. A 15-month-old may be taking a 3- or 4-hour nap (or two 2-hour naps), leaving time for only 7–8 hours to sleep at night. In this case, part of the treatment involves shortening the naps and moving that sleep back to the night.

Medical and Psychiatric Sleep Disorders

Sleep Disorders Associated with Mental Disorders

In young children, the most common "psychiatric" disorder affecting sleep is anxiety. Fears and worries of various kinds are common in early childhood and are generally a normal part of development. In some children, however, these anxieties become excessive and long lasting.[59,69,87-89]

It is common for children to pass through a period of separation anxiety toward the end of the first year. In addition, as they go through other developmental hurdles such as toilet training, the start of school, and acceptance of a new sibling, transient regression is common with a return of anxiety. Other problems may reflect more general psychosocial or even medical issues in the home.

An anxious child is usually unwilling to separate from parents at night. If this is the only problem, the child is able to fall asleep without difficulty as long as the parents are close by, either in the child's room or the child in theirs (a fact that effectively rules out many of the other potential causes of sleeplessness).

Children who are truly frightened appear so, and most often the parents are able to recognize this and describe it in a convincing manner. Anxious youngsters may become quite panicky as bedtime approaches. They usually do not enjoy the bedtime routines because they are fearful of the separation that will follow, and they become progressively more upset. Some children are sufficiently frightened that they are willing to accept punishment simply to be allowed to be near the parents.

The main challenge in making diagnostic and treatment decisions is to identify the severity (and source, if possible) of the anxiety. If it is very mild, firm reassurance and understanding is often all that is necessary. If the anxiety is generated by a lack of appropriate and consistent limit setting, instituting proper setting limits may be beneficial. However, a child who is truly frightened at night will not be helped by increased limits. In fact, increased limits (and separation from parents) may only increase fears. Whatever is necessary to make such a child feel safe and comfortable at night should be provided. This may require a parent to sleep in the child's room temporarily, or permission for the child to sleep in the parents' room (in a sleeping bag on their floor, or in their bed). If the parent is in the child's room, the child continues to associate his or her room and bed with sleep, making eventual return to sleeping in his or her own room alone that much easier.

A child who is sufficiently verbal can discuss his or her concerns with the examiner, along with options for treatment. Sometimes the youngster only needs the reassurance of having a parent on the same floor of the house when he or she goes to sleep, or the promise that a parent will check on him or her and not go to sleep while he or she is still awake.

If the anxiety is relatively mild, it often can be dealt with by providing negotiated supports and, perhaps, rewards, gradually renegotiating the behaviors required to earn rewards as certain goals are met. Each time the child is successful at one level, he or she may feel more confident and able to attempt the next. When the fears are marked and long standing, however, such methods generally are not enough. Parental presence in the bedroom may be required to alleviate the fears initially, and professional counseling may be required to alleviate them on a longer term basis.

Sleep Disorders Associated with Neurologic Disorders

The list of neurologic disorders associated with sleep problems is large, including neonatal insults, abnormalities in the development of the nervous system, genetic and other syndromic disorders, and epilepsy and associated drug therapy.[90–94] Children with central nervous system dysfunction are subject to the same type of sleep disorders as are other youngsters, perhaps more so because of parents' guilt feelings, which affect the pattern of nighttime intervention.[95] When the disorders are severe and psychomotor retardation marked, normal interaction with family members may not be possible, sleep may become inappropriately distributed across the day, and nighttime sleep may be severely disrupted.[96] Much more careful control of the timing and regularity of sleep may be an important consideration.

Certain children have severe sleep disorders that do not fit into other categories. These sleep abnormalities appear to be directly due to dysfunction of the central systems that control sleep. This may be seen in some youngsters with pervasive developmental delay (autism) and in those with severe malformations, dysfunctions, or central injury. In these cases, total (day plus night) sleep sometimes is severely limited (R. Ferber, unpublished data, 1997).[91–93,97–99] Although the electrophysiologic aspects of sleep in an autistic child are generally normal, this is not necessarily the case when more clear-cut structural abnormalities are present.

Behavioral intervention and schedule adjustment may not be sufficient to treat these children. Such children may be very demanding of parents' time and difficult to manage at home, even if they were sleeping a normal amount. Therefore, efforts at normalizing their sleep may have to include pharmacologic trials. Unfortunately, there are few formal studies of drug interventions for sleep in such children, and it is difficult to generalize from these studies in any case because many of the youngsters needing treatment differ significantly from each other in terms of their underlying structural and physiologic abnormalities, various comorbid factor, and the specifics of the medications they may already be taking. The common sleeping pills used for adults (zolpidem, zaleplon, eszopiclone) often do not seem to help these youngsters. Medications often tried include antihistamines, melatonin, chloral hydrate, benzodiazepines, antihypertensives such as clonidine, antidepressants such as trazodone, and the atypical antipsychotics.[100–107] However, even if there is a good response to a particular drug, one should not assume a lifetime need; repeated attempts at documenting ongoing need and efficacy are important, and one should always be sure the lowest dose needed is the one used.

Sleep Disorders Associated with Other Medical Disorders

Almost any medical problem may be associated with a sleep disorder because of direct effects on the sleep system, associated fever, pain, medication, or parental concern.[108] These are obvious in short-term situations and usually do not demand intervention.

Certain medical problems may be more chronic and problematic. Asthma, with nighttime wheezing (and associated fear), may be disruptive and require medication and possibly counseling.[108,109] The stimulant medications such as theophylline used to treat asthma may be directly responsible for sleep disruption, and switching to inhaled preparations may be helpful. Migraines may directly cause sleep loss at night, or indirectly disrupt sleep at night after extra daytime sleep occurs following headaches during the day.[110]

Gastroesophageal reflux, chronic middle ear disease, or atopic dermatitis may be associated with poor sleep.[50,111–113] Often there are nighttime awakening associated with these conditions, when the child seems to be in discomfort. Parental interventions are slow to aid return to sleep after such awakenings. Treating the underlying condition, medically or surgically, is usually necessary.

Colic is the most common medical cause of sleep difficulties in an infant's early months. Typical symptoms include irritability and inconsolable crying, especially in the late afternoon and evening.[53,54,114–117] Colic usually resolves by 3 months of age, and because nighttime sleep is not expected to consolidate before then, it is actually the consequences of patterns developed during the colicky period that are most relevant. These youngsters often are held, walked, rocked, placed in a swing, or patted in an effort to calm them and help them fall asleep. The patterns may persist after the colic has disappeared, creating a routine that the child associates with sleep. If the child cannot fall asleep without this attention, the habits need to be modified.

Finally, every medication must be considered a potential sleep disrupter in a given child. Probably even certain additives in liquid preparations affect youngsters in undesirable ways. In addition, the underlying medical problem that requires a child to take medication routinely, as well as associated psychosocial effects, must be considered. For example, a young leukemia patient on chemotherapy has many reasons for sleeping poorly: the effects of the illness itself, the medication, concerns about the illness, family concerns about the illness, and altered patterns of parent-child interaction. Separating these variables and designing appropriate therapy are the greatest challenges to the sleep clinician.

REFERENCES

A full list of references are available at www.expertconsult.com

Evolution of Sleep from Birth through Adolescence, and Sleep-Disordered Breathing in Children

Timothy F. Hoban

INTRODUCTION

The maturational changes that occur in sleep between infancy and adolescence exhibit complex interrelationships with the other physical and developmental changes that occur during this time. For example, the night-time sleep of young infants is necessarily interrupted by the frequent feedings required at this age. Conversely, the tendency toward delayed sleep phase exhibited by many adolescents can make morning waking difficult for teenagers whose classes begin at an early hour. The first part of this chapter examines the evolution of sleep from birth through adolescence, with particular focus upon how sleep changes with age and developmental level, and how these influences may affect vulnerability to the common sleep problems of childhood. The second part of the chapter reviews sleep-related breathing disorders in children, including obstructive sleep apnea, hypoventilation, upper airway resistance syndrome, and snoring. Epidemiology, clinical features, and diagnostic testing are reviewed with particular emphasis upon how these differ for children compared to adults. Treatment options and outcomes are likewise examined.

THE EVOLUTION OF SLEEP FROM BIRTH THROUGH ADOLESCENCE

Infant Sleep

For premature infants, sleep and wakefulness do not always represent distinct or easily recognizable states. Behavioral assessment of these states becomes possible after 28 weeks of gestation, when infants begin to demonstrate episodes of spontaneous alerting and when gentle stimulation during apparent sleep results in several minutes of increased alertness and activity.[1] Longer periods of alertness become apparent by 32 weeks, and are accompanied by crying or are otherwise easily recognized by 36 weeks.

Electroencephalography (EEG) in premature infants does not clearly distinguish between wakefulness and sleep prior to 36 weeks of gestation.[2] Between 36 and 38 weeks of gestation, periods of quiet behavioral sleep come to be accompanied by *tracé alternant*, a distinctive EEG background in which bursts of high-amplitude slow waves lasting several seconds alternate with 3- to 15-second periods of lower amplitude faster frequencies. This activity represents the major EEG marker of *quiet sleep*, the infant equivalent of non–rapid eye movement (NREM) sleep. Quiet sleep is additionally characterized by regular respiration, regular heart rate, and a paucity of body movements.

The EEG activity of *active sleep*, the precursor of rapid eye movement (REM) sleep, resembles that of wakefulness in many respects. Both states are characterized by a continuous, low- to medium-voltage background with less regular respiration and increased variability of heart rate. The presence of REMs and low electromyographic tone during active sleep usually allows the polysomnographer to distinguish this state from wakefulness, but concurrent video or behavioral assessment is sometimes required for complete certainty. This is particularly true for infants of less than 37 weeks of gestation, whose inhibition of muscle tone during active sleep may be variable or incomplete.[3]

Healthy infants who are born at term usually sleep in excess of 16 hours daily in the form of short sleep periods lasting 2–4 hours distributed throughout the daytime and nighttime hours. The fragmented nature of sleep in the newborn infant is thought to be related to both the biologic necessity for frequent feedings at this age and the fact that circadian regulatory mechanisms may not yet be sufficiently strong or well entrained to have substantial impact.[4] Although there is initially little day-to-day consistency in the timing and duration of sleep periods for most newborns, subtle changes in the length and organization of sleep periods begin within weeks after birth.[5] Over a span of several months, recurring environmental and social cues foster gradual lengthening and consolidation of nighttime sleep in a process known as *settling*. The majority of healthy infants achieve prolonged nighttime sleep periods—interrupted only briefly for feedings—by 3 months of age, but 10% fail to achieve uninterrupted nighttime sleep during the first year of life.[6]

As the first year of life progresses, daytime sleep diminishes and consolidates into several daily naps. Total duration of daily sleep declines to an average of 14.2 hours at 6 months of age and 13.9 hours at 1 year.[7] As napping and nighttime sleep achieve greater regularity, many families establish regular bedtime and naptime routines that provide cues and structure that supplement underlying circadian mechanisms in promoting the transition to sleep. Nighttime feedings gradually diminish and disappear during the first year for most infants. Although nocturnal feedings are no longer a biological necessity for most healthy infants after 5–6 months of age, they may persist after that age as a learned habit for some.[8] Between 6 and 12 months of age, the normal developmental milestones of teething and separation anxiety have the potential to disrupt previously well-established sleep routines.[9]

Electroencephalographic and polysomnographic (PSG) studies of infant sleep reveal profound differences in the character and organization of sleep compared to those of older children and adults. Within the first month of life, the tracé alternant pattern of quiet sleep evolves into more clearly recognizable NREM patterns, including the high-amplitude delta activity of slow-wave sleep.[10] Sleep spindles are first seen by about 4 weeks of age and are well developed by 6–8 weeks.[8,11] K complexes become evident by 6 months of age and demonstrate mature forms by 2 years.[12]

REM sleep also evolves considerably during the first year of life. Newborns spend 50% of total sleep time in REM sleep, declining to 40% at 3–5 months and 30% at 6–23 months.[13,14] The question of whether the high proportion of REM sleep serves a vital function in the newborn remains unanswered; however, it has been postulated that the REM sleep may play an important role in brain maturation during early development.[15,16] Newborns typically enter sleep via an initial REM period, but by 3 months enter sleep through NREM stages.[8] The recurring ultradian cycling of REM and NREM states is shorter for infants (50–60 minutes) than for adults (90–100 minutes), and lengthens gradually through childhood and adolescence.[13]

Sleep in Toddlers and Preschoolers

Sleep during the toddler and preschool years is characterized by further evolution of sleep duration and architecture. Total daily sleep duration declines from an average of 13.2 hours at age 2 to 11.8 hours at age 4.[7] Daytime napping diminishes to a single daytime nap during the second year of life, and most children stop regular daytime naps after about age 3.

Sleep for toddlers and preschoolers is also strongly influenced by a variety of developmental and environmental influences. Intrinsic aspects of a child's temperament, particularly the ability to self-settle, may substantially affect the ease with which a child is able to fall asleep independently at bedtime or following nighttime waking.[17] Sleep may be transiently disturbed during the minor illnesses common at these ages or more persistently disrupted if well-established sleep routines and sleep schedule are suddenly changed. Co-sleeping—sleeping with a parent or sibling—is especially common in this age group and may be associated with increased risk of night waking or bedtime struggles.[18]

Polysomnographic changes during these years are somewhat more modest and gradual than those seen during infancy. REM sleep declines to 20% of total daytime sleep by age 5, approximating the proportion exhibited by older children and adults.[14] Despite a decline in total sleep time, the duration of NREM sleep increases by about 1 hour daily between infancy and age 3, with gradual reductions thereafter. Polysomnograms of toddlers and preschoolers often exhibit lengthy and highly consolidated periods of slow-wave sleep during the early portions of the night.

Sleep cycles in toddlers and preschoolers remain somewhat shorter than those of older children and adults, but overall sleep architecture rapidly assumes a mature pattern in which slow-wave sleep is predominantly distributed during the first third of the night and REM sleep is more prominent in the last third. The temporal distribution of these sleep states is additionally reflected by the parasomnias commonly exhibited by toddlers and preschoolers. Sleep terrors, confusional arousals, and other NREM arousal parasomnias tend to occur during the first hours of sleep, whereas nightmares—which arise from REM sleep—more often transpire during the latter hours of the child's habitual sleep period.

Sleep in Preadolescent Children

Overall sleep duration continues to decline for school-age, preadolescent children, diminishing from a mean of 11.4 hours at 5 years of age to 9.3 hours by age 12.[7] Napping is uncommon in children of this age, and the presence of habitual napping is often an indication of insufficient nighttime sleep or other sleep disorders. Declining sleep duration results in later bedtimes for most children as they grow older, but morning waking times may be concurrently impacted by the child's school schedule as well.[19]

Other social and environmental factors also frequently impact the sleep of school-age children. For some, evening activities such as homework, television viewing, or athletic pursuits may be stimulating enough to cause delayed bedtime or delayed sleep onset even if the regular bedtime can be maintained. Consumption of caffeinated beverages and use of sleep-influencing medications (e.g., antidepressants, stimulants prescribed for attention-deficit/hyperactivity disorder) may also disrupt sleep onset or continuity.

There are few data regarding the evolution of PSG findings for healthy normals in this age group. It is thought that the relative proportion of REM sleep remains fairly constant at 18.5–20% of total sleep time.[14] Although total NREM sleep also remains relatively constant, slow-wave sleep declines from 24% of total sleep time for 6- and 7-year-olds to 21% for 10- and 11-year-olds, while stage 2 sleep increases from 47% to 52%.[20] By ages 10 and 11, the average sleep cycle length of 87 minutes is close to that exhibited by mature sleepers.

Multiple Sleep Latency Test (MSLT) data for healthy school-age children reveal mean sleep latencies that are substantially higher than those for adolescents and adults, suggesting that preadolescents may be intrinsically less sleepy than teenagers and adults.[21-23] It has been postulated that this may represent one of the reasons why children with sleep disorders do not always "act sleepy" and are more likely to exhibit daytime symptoms of inattention, hyperactivity, or behavioral disturbances rather than frank somnolence.

Adolescent Sleep

Total sleep time declines further during adolescence, from a mean of 9.0 hours at the age of 13 years to 8.1 hours by age 16 in one large cohort.[7] Despite only gradual reduction in sleep duration during the adolescent years, mean sleep latency on the MSLT for healthy normals rapidly declines during early adolescence and remains at a reduced level during later adolescence, suggesting that sleepiness and sleep need may actually increase by midpuberty.[22,24] Reductions in mean sleep latency on the MSLT are more closely linked with Tanner stage of sexual development than age, and detailed MSLT norms for children have been reported.[21,22]

Polysomnographic changes during adolescence are relatively modest. REM sleep remains fairly constant at about 20% of total sleep time.[24,25] Slow-wave sleep diminishes by 35% during adolescence, balanced by proportionate increases in stage 2 sleep.[22,24] Sleep cycling and overall sleep architecture otherwise approximate that of young adults.

Although a detailed review of sleep disorders affecting adolescents is provided elsewhere in this volume, several developmental and environmental influences that often impact adolescent sleep patterns deserve brief discussion. Foremost among these is the well-recognized tendency toward delayed sleep phase that characterizes the sleep of many adolescents and young adults.[26] While many individuals successfully adapt their sleep times to meet the needs of their school schedule despite this tendency, others adapt less well and may experience difficulty falling asleep at their desired bedtime or waking up at the time necessary in the morning. It is also common for adolescents to have longer sleep periods on non-school days, typically accompanied by delay of both bedtime and waking times compared to the school day schedule.[22,24] This irregularity of sleep schedule may contribute to sleep problems for some adolescents, particularly when the sleep schedule on non-school days reinforces an underlying phase delay that is already problematic.

Adolescents usually have much greater autonomy in determining their sleep schedules than younger children, whose bedtimes are more closely regulated by parents and caregivers. This often results in irregular sleep habits, habitually insufficient sleep, or otherwise suboptimal sleep hygiene. Evening activities including television watching, Internet use, and computer game playing may be associated with decreased time in bed and higher levels of daytime tiredness.[27] Consumption of caffeinated beverages—on average three times higher for adolescents than for preadolescents—may also disrupt sleep for some teenagers.[28] As is the case for younger children, prescription medications may disturb nighttime sleep or daytime alertness for adolescents. In addition, alcohol and drugs of abuse represent under-recognized but common causes of tiredness and sleep problems in this population.[29]

SLEEP-DISORDERED BREATHING IN CHILDREN (see also Chapter 24)

It is not at all uncommon to find children who suffer from... enlargements of the lymphoid (tonsillar) tissues of the nasopharynx and fauces, described by their parents and teachers as backwards and stupid. ... The fact, however, that children, the victims of nasal and pharyngeal obstructions, often suffer from headaches, especially when engaged in study, and frequently evince marked inability to fix their attention on their lessons or work for any length of time, has in recent years led many to suspect that these symptoms [are] in part a reflection of some evident hampering of the cerebral functions.[30]

History and Classification of Sleep-Disordered Breathing in Children

Astute observations regarding the clinical manifestations of sleep-disordered breathing (SDB) in children date from the late 19th century, including that of William Hill in 1889.[30] Sir William Osler eloquently reported: "At night, the child's sleep is greatly disturbed; the respirations are loud and snorting, and there are sometimes prolonged pauses, followed by deep noisy inspirations."[31] It is thought that Charles Dickens may have provided a description of daytime somnolence secondary to SDB in the *Posthumous Papers of the Pickwick Club*, wherein the character Joe is described as an obese, red-faced, and perpetually sleepy child.[32]

Modern descriptions of childhood SDB date from 1965, with initial reports of reversible cor pulmonale in children with upper airway obstruction due to adenotonsillar enlargement.[33,34] *Obstructive sleep apnea* (OSA) affecting eight children between 5 and 14 years of age was described by Guilleminault and colleagues in 1976.[35] Subjects in this series had relatively severe SDB—exhibiting 78–824 apneic episodes per night during PSG—with referable daytime symptoms including headache, behavioral disturbances, poor school performance, hypertension, and excessive somnolence. This and subsequent reports initially characterized childhood OSA as consisting of episodic partial or complete airway obstruction resulting in hypoxemia, hypercapnia, or arousal from sleep in a fashion that resembles the "classic" OSA of adults (Figs. 38–1 and 38–2).

Over time, it was discovered that children with SDB often exhibit nonapneic respiratory disturbances, and it is now thought that prolonged partial airway obstruction (Fig. 38–3), as opposed to discrete events such as apneas and hypopneas, may be the predominant form of respiratory disturbance for many children.[36,37] *Obstructive hypoventilation* is characterized by prolonged partial obstruction resulting in diminished pulmonary ventilation causing hypoxemia and/or hypercapnia.[38] *Upper airway*

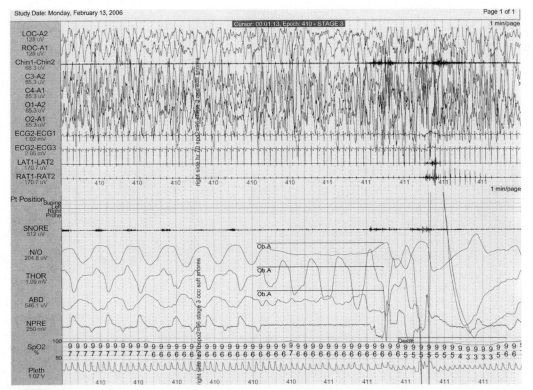

FIGURE 38–1 Obstructive apnea (60-second PSG epoch). The event is characterized by cessation of nasal/oral (N/O) and nasal pressure (NPRE) airflow with preserved thoracic and abdominal respiratory effort (THOR and ABD). Obstruction lasts the length of 4 respiratory cycles and is followed by brief arousal from sleep.

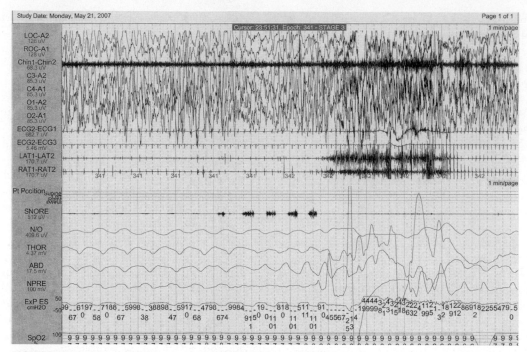

FIGURE 38–2 Obstructive hypopnea (60-second PSG epoch). The event is characterized by diminished nasal pressure airflow (NPRE) and crescendo snoring leading to arousal. Excessively negative esophageal pressure fluctuations (ExPES) increase during the hypopnea and resolve following arousal.

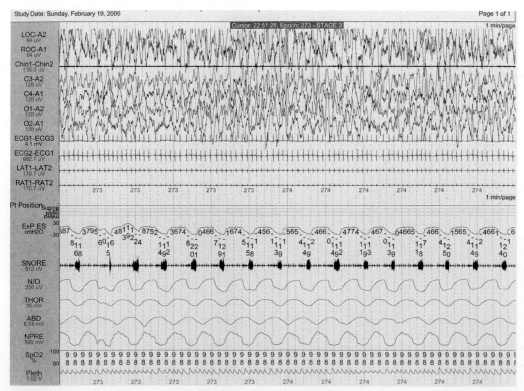

FIGURE 38–3 Prolonged partial airway obstruction (60-second epoch). Continuous snoring and excessively negative esophageal pressure fluctuations (measured peak-to-trough on ExPES) indicate prolonged partial airway obstruction. Note normal oxygen saturation (SpO2) and lack of obvious changes on nasal/oral and nasal pressure airflow tracings (N/O and NPRE).

resistance syndrome (UARS) represents a form of prolonged partial airway obstruction in which increased work of breathing disrupts the quality or continuity of sleep even in the absence of gas exchange abnormalities.[39] It is not unusual for children with SDB to exhibit variable or complex disturbances of respiration during PSG that may include features of both chronic partial obstruction and "classic" OSA.

SDB without upper airway obstruction is substantially less common than obstructive SDB in children. *Nonobstructive hypoventilation* during sleep usually occurs in the context of diminished respiratory drive, weakness of the respiratory muscles, intrinsic lung disease, or a combination of these factors. Ventilation or gas exchange during sleep becomes insufficient to meet the body's needs, resulting in hypercapnia and/or hypoxemia. Predisposing conditions include disorders of the brain stem and cranial nerves (e.g., Chiari's malformation type I), cervical spinal cord injuries, neuromuscular disorders (e.g., Duchenne's muscular dystrophy), and restrictive lung disease (e.g., severe scoliosis).

Congenital central hypoventilation syndrome (CCHS) is a distinct variety of nonobstructive hypoventilation that is usually present—but not always recognized—at birth. Affected children exhibit impaired ventilatory responses to hypercapnia and occasionally to hypoxemia.[40] As a result, ventilation during wakefulness may be normal or only modestly impaired, whereas ventilation during sleep is characterized by hypoventilation of a degree that may be life threatening if the condition is not promptly identified and treated. Mutations of the *PHOX2B* gene have been identified in the majority of cases studied, and CCHS may be associated with Hirschsprung's disease, neural crest tumors, and disturbances of cardiac autonomic regulation.[41,42] CCHS is thought to be a heterogeneous disorder, and late-onset forms with hypothalamic dysfunction have been described.[43]

Central sleep apnea affecting children is identified most frequently in the context of *primary sleep apnea of infancy*, formerly called apnea of prematurity. This condition is characterized by prolonged central, mixed, or obstructive apneas associated with significant hypoxemia or bradycardia, or associated with a need for stimulation or resuscitation by caregivers in order for normal respiration to resume.[44] Respiratory disturbances in affected children are variable in duration. Central apneas usually last in excess of 20 seconds, whereas obstructive and mixed events are sometimes shorter. Primary sleep apnea in small or premature infants is thought to result primarily from dysmaturity of respiratory control mechanisms, and usually improves with maturation. Apnea in infants may also occur as an associated manifestation of gastroesophageal reflux, infection, metabolic disturbance, upper airway obstruction, or other serious illness.

Central sleep apnea is otherwise uncommon in children and has received little formal study. Brief central apneas may be observed during REM sleep or following arousals in otherwise healthy children, but seldom are accompanied by significant oxygen desaturation. Central apneas may also be encountered in the context of *periodic breathing*—recurring cycles of regular respiration interrupted by pauses lasting several seconds (Fig. 38–4). This well-stereotyped respiratory pattern is frequently observed in young infants, in whom it is usually benign, and is occasionally seen in older children during sleep/wake transitions.

Primary snoring in children is defined as snoring that does not disrupt sleep, cause gas exchange abnormalities, or result in pathologic daytime symptoms.[45] Although this condition by definition should not be associated with any secondary symptoms, subtle deficits in mood, behavior, and cognitive function have been reported in children with primary snoring compared to non-snoring controls.[46,47] It is not precisely known how often or how quickly primary snoring may progress to more serious varieties of SDB. In one small series of children with PSG-documented primary snoring, 10% were found to have developed OSA when reassessed 1–3 years later.[48]

Epidemiology of Childhood SDB

Prevalence rates for SDB in children remain uncertain because of the lack of universally accepted diagnostic criteria for these conditions and because large population-based studies using PSG have not been undertaken. It is estimated that between 5% and 12% of children snore habitually, with some reports suggesting increased risk for children exposed to tobacco smoke.[49-53] The prevalence of OSA in children has been traditionally estimated to be 1–3%.[54,55] Substantially higher prevalence was identified among a population-based sample of 126 children selected as control subjects for a study assessing risk factors in childhood SDB. In this cohort, 10.3% of subjects fulfilled a commonly used adult criterion for OSA: an apnea-hypopnea index (AHI) exceeding 5 respiratory events per hour of sleep.[56]

Data are not available regarding the prevalence of UARS, central sleep apnea, and hypoventilation in children. CCHS is a rare disorder conservatively estimated to affect at least 300 children worldwide.[40] The prevalence of primary sleep apnea of infancy varies with size and gestational age. Symptomatic apnea affects 84% of newborns weighing less than 1000 g, 25% of newborns weighing less than 2500 g, and less than 0.5% of term infants.[44]

Clinical Features of Childhood SDB

The clinical manifestations of SDB in children differ from those exhibited by adults, as summarized in Table 38–1. Children with obstructive SDB tend to be noisy breathers during sleep, but severity may range from heroic snoring or stridor to only minimally loud respiration.

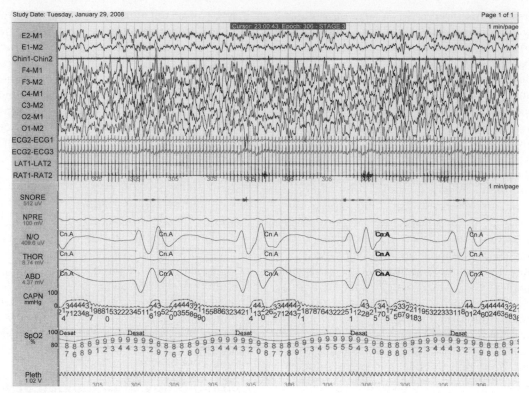

FIGURE 38–4 Periodic respiration (60-second epoch). Repetitive, stereotyped central apneas separated by several breaths (nasal/oral [N/O] and capnography [CAPN]) are accompanied by desaturation (SpO2) without arousal.

TABLE 38–1 Sleep-Disordered Breathing in Children Compared to Adults

	Children	Adults
Physical Characteristics		
Gender	Younger children: sexes equally affected Adolescents: males > females	Primarily males
Peak age	2–8 yr	Middle age and older
Body weight	Usually normal, occasionally obese	Most often obese
Upper airway	Adenotonsillar enlargement frequent Redundant soft tissue occasional	Adenotonsillar enlargement occasional Redundant soft tissue frequent
Symptoms During Sleep		
Snoring	Frequent, often continuous	Frequent, often interrupted by pauses
Witnessed apnea	Occasional	Frequent
Polysomnographic Characteristics		
Obstruction	Prolonged partial obstruction > intermittent	Cyclical intermittent obstruction
Sleep architecture	Normal > fragmented	Frequent arousals with sleep fragmentation
Secondary Symptoms		
Daytime sleepiness	Most often absent or intermittent	Frequent
Neurobehavioral	Inattention, hyperkinesis, disturbed behavior	Cognitive slowing
Cardiovascular	Hypertension, cor pulmonale	Hypertension, cor pulmonale, stroke

Snoring for many children is nearly continuous, but for others may be intermittent or vary with body position. Snoring often worsens during upper respiratory infections or with exacerbations of allergic rhinitis and sometimes improves during treatment with decongestants or nasal steroids. Snoring in children with obstructive SDB is often accompanied by prominent mouth breathing and unusual sleeping positions such as neck hyperextension or excessive propping upon pillows, which represent compensatory mechanisms that may improve airway patency.

Witnessed apneas are only occasionally reported for children with obstructive SDB. This observation is consistent with the premise that prolonged partial airway obstruction during sleep is more common in children than the recurring episodes of brief obstruction followed by arousal that characterize typical adult OSA. When witnessed apnea is present in a child with obstructive SDB, parents may report paradoxical chest wall motion during events or the presence of snorting or gasping noises as respiration resumes.

Children with obstructive SDB demonstrate greater degrees of restlessness, enuresis, and perspiration during sleep than healthy controls.[57] Several reports additionally suggest that obstructive SDB may be associated with increased risk for parasomnias.[58,59]

In contrast to the prominent snoring and restlessness exhibited during the sleep of children with obstructive SDB, children with nonobstructive SDB tend to be quiet sleepers who seldom exhibit obvious respiratory symptoms during sleep. The lack of easily recognizable nighttime symptoms may lead to delays in diagnosis and treatment, particularly if sleepiness or other daytime symptoms are misattributed to other causes.

Children with obstructive SDB often complain of sore throat, dry mouth, headache, or grogginess upon morning waking, although these symptoms are often transient and self-limited. Daytime mouth breathing is frequently seen in children with obstructive SDB, particularly when adenotonsillar hypertrophy is present.[57] Daytime somnolence is usually not prominent unless a child's underlying SDB is severe.[60] When excessive somnolence is present, it is often subtle or intermittent, and may only be evident during sedentary activities such as riding in an automobile.

Neurobehavioral deficits represent the most common and most variable daytime symptoms of childhood SDB. Early reports of childhood OSA, documenting relatively severe cases, identified a high prevalence of school problems, behavioral disturbances, and hyperactivity among affected children.[35,61,62] More recent reports have suggested that even less severe varieties of childhood SDB may be associated with the same problems. Children with mild or moderate SDB have been reported to have higher rates of parentally reported behavior problems, lower scores on tests of sustained attention, and lower scores on neuropsychometric assessments of executive function.[63,64] Subtle neurocognitive deficits have also been reported in children with primary snoring.[46,47,65]

There is also limited evidence that SDB is overrepresented in children with attention-deficit/hyperactivity disorder (ADHD) and learning problems. Snoring was reported to be three times as frequent among children with ADHD compared to non-ADHD controls drawn from general pediatric and child psychiatry clinics, with higher snoring scores being associated with greater levels of inattention and hyperactivity.[66] Among 297 first-grade children performing poorly in school, 54 (18%) were

found to have evidence of nocturnal hypoxemia or hypercapnia during limited, home-based sleep studies.[67]

Physical Features Associated with Childhood SDB

The physical examination is sometimes completely normal in children with SDB, but predisposing anatomic features are frequently identified in affected children. Adenotonsillar enlargement, which is most common between 2 and 8 years of age, is associated with several physical findings.[68] In addition to visible tonsillar hypertrophy, "adenoid facies"—visible mouth breathing, pinched nose, and elongated facial appearance—is often observed. A narrow and high-arched hard palate, maxillary or mandibular hypoplasia, and macroglossia represent occasional findings in otherwise healthy children with SDB.

Obesity may accompany SDB for some children, but this association is less robust for children than for the adult population. Obese adolescents represent a particularly high-risk population. In a group of 22 obese adolescents without sleep complaints, 10 (46%) were reported to have abnormal PSGs.[69] Daytime sleepiness and AHI for this group both correlated with degree of obesity.

Some children with SDB—particularly infants and young children with severe airway obstruction—may present with decreased growth, low body weight, or failure to thrive. Treatment of these children has been reported to result in improved growth parameters and insulin-like growth factor-I levels.[70–72]

A variety of medical, genetic, and craniofacial conditions are associated with increased risk of SDB during childhood (Table 38–2). Detailed epidemiologic data are not available for most of these conditions; however, it is estimated that at least 30% of children with Down syndrome may exhibit SDB.[73,74]

Secondary Complications of Childhood SDB

The long-term effects of childhood SDB are not well understood apart from limited data regarding cardiovascular effects. Reversible cor pulmonale and congestive heart failure have been reported in children with severe SDB.[75,76] In addition, evidence of heart strain was reported in 3.3% of 92 children referred for adenotonsillectomy.[77] The frequency with which hypertension affects children with SDB remains unknown, but obesity and respiratory disturbance index were found to be independently associated with increased blood pressure in a large cohort of 6- to 11-year-old children.[78]

The public health impact of childhood SDB has also received little scrutiny. The extent to which affected children's neurobehavioral symptoms limit their long-term academic achievement and adult socioeconomic status has not been studied, although the effect is suspected to

TABLE 38–2 Conditions Associated with Sleep-Disordered Breathing in Children

Craniofacial Syndromes Associated with Maxillary or Mandibular Hypoplasia

- Apert's syndrome
- Crouzon's disease
- Goldenhar's syndrome (hemifacial microsomia)
- Hallermann-Streiff syndrome
- Robin sequence (Pierre Robin syndrome)
- Treacher-Collins syndrome

Other Syndromes with Prominent Craniofacial Involvement

- Achondroplasia
- Klippel-Feil syndrome
- Saethre-Chotzen syndrome
- Velocardiofacial syndrome (Shprintzen's syndrome)

Conditions Associated with Macroglossia

- Beckwith-Wiedemann syndrome
- Down syndrome
- Hypothyroidism
- Mucopolysaccharide storage disorders (Hunter's, Hurler's, and Scheie's syndromes)

Conditions Causing Congenital Upper Airway Abnormalities

- Cleft palate
- Choanal atresia
- Fetal warfarin syndrome
- Pfeiffer syndrome

Systemic Neurologic Disorders

- Structural lesions of the brain stem and medulla (e.g., Chiari's malformation)
- Cranial neuropathies (e.g., Fazio-Londe disease)
- Neuromuscular disorders (e.g., myasthenia gravis, Duchenne's muscular dystrophy, myotonic dystrophy)

Miscellaneous Conditions

- Prader-Willi syndrome

TABLE 38–3 Clinical Assessment of the Child with Suspected Sleep-Disordered Breathing

Sleep History

- Snoring: volume, frequency, character, changes over time
- Mouth breathing
- Unusual sleeping positions (e.g., neck hyperextension, propping on pillows)
- Restlessness, limb movements
- Excessive perspiration
- Night waking: frequency, duration, and patterns
- Enuresis
- Symptoms upon waking: grogginess, headache, sore throat, dry mouth
- Sleep schedule
- Family history of sleep-disordered breathing or other sleep disorders

Daytime Symptoms

- Mouth breathing
- Headache
- Behavior: irritability, distractibility, hyperkinesis, temperamental behavior
- School: attention, academic performance, decline in grades
- Sleepiness, especially in sedentary situations (e.g., automobile rides)

Medical History

- Ear-Nose-Throat: adenotonsillar disease, allergic rhinitis, congenital anatomic abnormalities
- Endocrine: obesity, growth, thyroid disease
- Cardiovascular: hypertension, congenital heart disease
- Pulmonary: asthma, other intrinsic lung disease
- Neurologic: disorders affecting brain stem and cranial nerves or causing muscle weakness
- Development: developmental delay, infant failure to thrive
- Other: craniofacial disorders, genetic syndromes (e.g., Prader-Willi syndrome, Down syndrome)

Physical Examination

- Vital signs: Weight, height, body mass index, blood pressure, percentile ranks
- Oropharynx: tonsillar size, airway patency, palate, dentition, occlusion, tongue
- Nasopharynx: polyps, septal deviation, airflow, "pinched-nose" appearance
- Craniofacial: micrognathia, maxillary hypoplasia, occlusion, cleft palate or other craniofacial syndrome
- Neck: thyroid, masses, circumference
- Thorax: cardiac auscultation, lung auscultation, evidence of scoliosis
- Neurologic: cranial nerve palsies, evidence of muscular weakness or neuropathy
- Behavior: attention, hyperkinesis, evidence of irritability or sleepiness
- Other: mouth breathing, noisy respiration, "adenoid facies"

be substantial for at least some children with SDB. Perhaps the most dramatic evidence illustrating the public health impact of childhood SDB is current data reporting substantially higher health care utilization for children with OSA compared to controls, including higher rates for hospitalization, medication use, and emergency department visits.[79] Treatment of children with OSA with adenotonsillectomy resulted in a reduction of total annual health care costs by one-third, compared to no change for controls and untreated OSA children.[80]

Clinical and Laboratory Assessment of Children with SDB

The assessment of a child with suspected SDB should begin with a detailed history and physical examination as outlined in Table 38–3. The sleep history should

thoroughly screen for the symptoms of SDB already discussed, but also include limited assessment for other sleep disorders whose clinical manifestations may mimic those of SDB. The medical history and physical examination should focus on screening for other conditions that might cause or predispose to SDB.

The history and physical examination are sometimes supplemented by other assessment tools that are less expensive and more easily administered than PSG. A variety of standardized questionnaires have been developed with the goal of predicting whether sleepiness or SDB is likely to be present based on the presence and severity of specific symptoms. Questionnaires such as the Epworth Sleepiness Scale and Stanford Sleepiness Scale are of limited usefulness in the assessment of children with suspected SDB due to limited validation data for this age group and because the symptom that these measures assess—sleepiness—is often not obvious in affected children.[81,82] Several questionnaires have been developed specifically for use in children, and limited validation data have been obtained regarding use of the Pediatric Sleep Questionnaire and OSA-18 as screening tools for childhood SDB in clinical and research populations.[83,84]

Although audiotapes recording a child's snoring have been recommended as a "$5 sleep study," this technique did not reliably distinguish primary snoring from SDB (AHI ≥5) in a blinded study assessing 29 snoring children.[85] Although home videotapes of a child's sleep are an easy and usually inexpensive supplement to the clinical history during evaluation of a child with suspected SDB, the reliability of this technique has not been rigorously assessed.

Overnight oximetry is generally not indicated in the assessment of children with suspected SDB. Although the technique is unobtrusive, inexpensive, and well tolerated by most children, it reliably detects SDB only when arterial oxygen desaturation is prominent and does not identify those children whose SDB is characterized primarily by hypercapnia or obstruction without desaturation. Among 210 children with PSG-documented OSA (AHI ≥1), 120 (57%) had normal or inconclusive nocturnal oximetry, confirming that normal oximetry cannot be used to rule out SDB in children.[86]

Other non-PSG diagnostic tests are used on a selective basis for children with suspected SDB, primarily in children with predisposing conditions and children presenting with severe symptoms. Anatomic obstruction of the upper airway is often demonstrable on radiographic or endoscopic assessment.[87,88] Children suspected to have severe SDB or cardiorespiratory complications sometimes require chest radiographs, an electrocardiogram (ECG), an echocardiogram, and formal pulmonary function testing for complete assessment. Children with prominent learning or behavior problems usually benefit from referral for more formal assessment and intervention, even when these symptoms are secondary to SDB.

Polysomnography in Childhood SDB

Laboratory-based PSG represents the most sensitive and reliable tool presently available for the detection and classification of SDB in children. It is also a test that can be easily customized based on the clinical presentation of each patient. For example, end-tidal carbon dioxide (ET_{CO_2}) is often monitored during PSG for patients with neuromuscular disorders and other conditions associated with high risk of hypoventilation, and esophageal pressure monitoring (P_{es}) is often performed for children believed to be at risk for UARS and other SDBs characterized by prolonged partial airway obstruction.

Polysomnography also has several limitations when used in children. The test itself is lengthy, expensive, and potentially stressful for both children and their parents. Laboratories having experience in performing and interpreting PSG for children are limited in number and sometimes have lengthy waiting lists. Finally, routine PSG is not always sensitive for the detection of prolonged partial airway obstruction (e.g., UARS), but tools such as P_{es} make the study more invasive and are not available in all sleep laboratories.

Polysomnography should be performed when a child's symptoms, medical history, and physical examination suggest a substantial risk for clinically significant SDB. Isolated snoring—especially when it is only soft and occasional—is seldom a sufficient indication for PSG unless other risk factors are also present. Practice guidelines that address indications for PSG in children have been issued by the American Academy of Pediatrics and the American Thoracic Society.[89,90] Although it is common for otolaryngologists to perform adenotonsillectomy for suspected SDB without preoperative PSG, the safety and cost-effectiveness of this practice have been vigorously debated.[91-93] In addition, this practice can potentially result in children with noisy respiration but no clinically significant SDB having unnecessary surgery. Until better validated practice guidelines address these issues, the author's practice is to apply the same standards presently used for adults: to obtain a baseline PSG for patients with clinically suspected SDB before decisions are made with respect to treatment.

Polysomnography in children is performed in a manner comparable to adult studies, utilizing frontal, central, and occipital EEG channels, an electro-oculogram, and an ECG, as well as a chin and limb electromyogram. Respiratory monitoring at minimum includes oral and nasal airflow, chest and abdominal movement, and arterial oxygen saturation. Most laboratories use nasal pressure transducers—thought to be sensitive to flow limitation and subtle decrements in flow—to assess nasal airflow, but since many children breathe through their mouths, thermistor or thermocouple sensors to monitor oral or oral-nasal airflow remain necessary as well.

Many sleep laboratories have the capability to supplement standard recording techniques with additional modes of respiratory monitoring when clinically indicated. ET_{CO_2} monitoring by nasal cannula provides added sensitivity for hypoventilation, which is sometimes characterized by more prominent hypercapnia than hypoxemia. Likewise, P_{es} may be added to improve sensitivity of the study for partial airway obstruction and increased work of breathing. P_{es} is minimally invasive, requiring insertion of a thin catheter through the nasopharynx into the esophagus, but the technique has negligible impact upon children's sleep and is the most sensitive method presently available for the measurement of increased upper airway resistance.[94,95] Several less invasive techniques for assessment of partial airway obstruction are being investigated for use in children, including pulse transit time, respiratory inductance plethysmography, peripheral arterial tonometry, respiratory cycle–related EEG changes, and intercostal electromyographic monitoring, but none of these techniques is yet available for routine clinical use.[96–100]

Scoring of sleep stages, movements, and arousals during pediatric PSG is performed in the same manner used for adult studies. Thirty-second epochs are reviewed and scored manually using standard criteria revised by the American Academy of Sleep Medicine.[101] Scoring of respiratory events for children using these new criteria differs slightly from that for adults. Whereas scoring of apneas, hypopneas, and respiratory effort–related arousals requires a minimum event duration of 10 seconds in adult studies, scoring of these events for pediatric studies requires only that the event last at least the duration of two missed breaths. This rule permits scoring of brief events in children whose baseline respiratory rate during sleep exceeds 12 breaths/min.

Standards for interpreting the results of pediatric PSG are less well established than those for adults. Normative PSG data for 50 healthy, asymptomatic children between 1 and 18 years of age were reported in 1992, and are summarized in Table 38–4.[102] Although these data have helped define the statistical limits of normality in healthy children, the point at which abnormal PSG parameters become associated with pathologic symptoms and outcomes has not been precisely determined. An AHI exceeding 5 events/hr is generally considered to be abnormal for adults, but the fact that children frequently demonstrate concerning SDB-related symptoms with AHIs below 5 has long suggested that a lower threshold is more appropriate for children.[103,104] Further

outcomes-based research is required to better define the precise points at which abnormal respiratory parameters on PSG become associated with clinically significant SDB.

The criteria in the second edition of the International Classification of Sleep Disorders (ICSD-2) for the diagnosis of pediatric OSA require a minimum of 1 respiratory event per hour of sleep in conjunction with other clinical and PSG findings as outlined in Table 38–5.[44] These revised criteria now permit many children who previously would have been classified as having nocturnal hypoventilation or UARS to be classified as having OSA, provided that an AHI of at least 1 is documented during PSG.

The ICSD-2 did not establish separate pediatric criteria for hypoventilation, which for children had been traditionally defined as ET_{CO_2} >45 mm Hg for more than 60% of total sleep time, ET_{CO_2} >50 mm Hg for more than 10% of total sleep time, or peak ET_{CO_2} ≥55 mm Hg during PSG.[102,105] The scoring rules revised by the American Academy of Sleep Medicine in 2007 now define sleep-related hypoventilation as consisting of ET_{CO_2} or transcutaneous CO_2 levels exceeding 50 mm Hg for greater than 25% of total sleep time[101] (Fig. 38–5).

Diagnostic criteria for UARS in children were not addressed in the ICSD-2, although proposed criteria have been published elsewhere.[104]

TABLE 38–4 Polysomnographic (PSG) Parameters in 50 Healthy Children Ages 1–18 Years

PSG Parameter	Mean ± SD
Apnea index (events/hour)	0.1 ± 0.5
Minimum Sa_{O_2} (%)	96 ± 2
Desaturations ≥4% (per hour of total sleep time)	0.3 ± 0.7
Maximum ET_{CO_2} (mm Hg)	46 ± 4
Duration of hypoventilation (ET_{CO_2} > 45 mm Hg) (percentage of total sleep time)	6.9 ± 19.1

ET_{CO_2}, end-tidal carbon dioxide; Sa_{O_2}, arterial oxygen saturation.
Adapted from Marcus CL, Omlin KJ, Basinki DJ, et al. Normal polysomnographic values for children and adolescents. Am Rev Respir Dis 1992;146(5 Pt 1):1235.

TABLE 38–5 ICSD-2 Criteria for Pediatric Obstructive Sleep Apnea

1. Parent or caregiver report of snoring or other obstructive symptoms during sleep.
2. Parent or caregiver report of at least one associated symptom:
   a. Paradoxical chest wall motion during inspiration
   b. Movement arousals
   c. Excessive perspiration
   d. Unusual sleeping positions (e.g., neck hyperextension)
   e. Daytime symptoms: hyperactivity, aggressive behavior, or sleepiness
   f. Impaired growth
   g. Headache upon waking
   h. Secondary enuresis
3. PSG documents at least one scoreable respiratory event per hour of sleep (events lasting at least 2 respiratory cycles in duration).
4. PSG demonstrates either *a* or *b*:
   a. At least one of the following findings:
      i. Frequent arousals associated with increased respiratory effort
      ii. Desaturation with apneic events
      iii. Hypercapnia in sleep
      iv. Excessively negative esophageal pressure fluctuations
   b. Periods of abnormal gas exchange during sleep (hypoxemia, hypercapnea, or both) with snoring, paradoxical chest wall motion, and at least one of the following:
      i. Frequent arousals during sleep
      ii. Excessively negative esophageal pressures swings
5. The disorder is not better explained by other sleep disorders, by medical or neurologic conditions, or by medication or substance use.

ICSD-2, International Classification of Sleep Disorders, second edition; PSG, polysomnography.
Adapted from Diagnostic Classification Steering Committee; M Sateia (Chairperson). The International Classification of Sleep Disorders: Diagnostic and Coding Manual, 2nd ed. Westchester, IL: American Academy of Sleep Medicine, 2005.

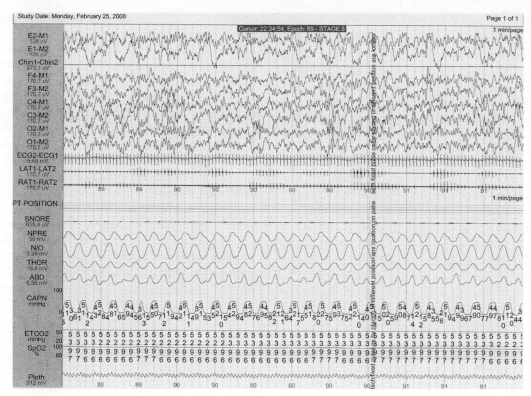

FIGURE 38–5 Sleep-related hypoventilation (60-second epoch). Capnography (CAPN) and average end-tidal CO_2 (ETCO2) demonstrate persistent elevations above 50 mm Hg in the absence of desaturation and scoreable respiratory events.

Treatment of SDB in Children

Adenotonsillectomy

Adenotonsillectomy is the most commonly administered treatment for obstructive SDB in children.[106] Although this procedure is thought to be effective in alleviating upper airway obstruction for many symptomatic children, it is not precisely known how often adenotonsillectomy "cures" SDB. This uncertainty is the result of widely variable intake and outcome measures within existing research as well as a lack of large, randomized, controlled studies assessing long-term clinical outcome.

Early case series assessing response of childhood OSA to adenotonsillectomy reported surgical cure rates exceeding 70%; however, these studies were limited by substantial variability in patient selection and in the PSG criteria used to define OSA.[107,108] More recent case series have reported more modest operative success rates. Among one group of 110 children with OSA (AHI >1; mean AHI, 22.3), complete postoperative normalization of the AHI was observed in only 27 subjects (25%).[109] In another large cohort of successively seen children with OSA (AHI >1), 94 of 199 subjects (47%) demonstrated abnormal PSGs postoperatively.[110] These and other data suggest that children with high Mallampati scores, obesity, or atypical anatomy of the upper airway may be at elevated risk for residual SDB following adenotonsillectomy.

In addition to improvements in obstructive symptoms and PSG parameters, adenotonsillectomy for children with SDB may also be associated with visible improvements in behavior, school performance, and quality-of-life measures.[111–113]

The potential clinical benefits of adenotonsillectomy in children with OSA should be considered with due attention to the possible complications of the procedure. Postoperative hemorrhage may occur in up to 8% of pediatric patients.[114] Reports documenting the frequency of postoperative respiratory complications range from 0% to 27% of children, with greatest risk for children who are young (especially < age 2), exhibit high baseline AHIs, or have associated craniofacial or medical problems.[115–117] Children who fall into this high-risk group often require close or prolonged cardiorespiratory monitoring in the immediate postoperative period.

Follow-up for children treated via adenotonsillectomy should commence with a postoperative clinic visit. Repeat PSG is usually indicated for children who have residual symptoms postoperatively or whose preoperative SDB was severe. Delayed recurrence of SDB following childhood adenotonsillectomy has also been reported, with recurrence in 20 of 40 children reassessed 1 year postoperatively in one report and in 3 of 13 patients reassessed during adolescence in another small series.[118,119]

Nasal Continuous Positive Airway Pressure

Nasal continuous positive airway pressure (CPAP) represents the most common nonsurgical treatment for childhood SDB. Although children with adenotonsillar hypertrophy are most often treated via adenotonsillectomy, CPAP represents the most common treatment for children with nonobstructive varieties of SDB and for children with obstructive disease who are not appropriate surgical candidates or whose obstruction persists following adenotonsillectomy. CPAP has not been formally approved by the U.S. Food and Drug Administration for use in children weighing <30 kg, but is nonetheless generally considered to be a first-line treatment for pediatric SDB, with reports of successful use in hundreds of children.[54] CPAP in children may be customized using a variety of interfaces, including nasal pillows and nasal or oral-nasal masks.

Effective use of CPAP for the treatment of obstructive SDB has been reported in children of all ages (Table 38–6), although long-term compliance and outcome data have not been well documented for the pediatric age group. Side effects are generally mild, most often consisting of skin irritation, mask leak, or pressure sores, which are easily remedied by improving mask fit. Nasal dryness or congestion often improves with addition of a heated humidifier. Central apnea may occasionally complicate treatment with CPAP, particularly at higher pressure settings. Serious side effects are uncommon, but isolated cases of pneumothorax have been reported in children with concomitant neuromuscular

disorders.[120,121] Midface hypoplasia has been also been reported as a rare long-term complication of therapy.[122]

A child's compliance with use of CPAP is influenced by several important factors. Infants and disabled children who are physically unable to remove the CPAP mask will usually tolerate nighttime CPAP once acclimated. Children and adolescents who are old enough to understand and accept the need for CPAP are also likely to achieve consistent long-term use. Compliance is most problematic for toddlers, preschoolers, and older disabled children who are facile enough to remove their mask independently. Sustained parental effort or age-appropriate desensitization programs with experienced providers are sometimes required to achieve consistent use.[123]

Data regarding use of CPAP for treatment of nonobstructive SDB are extremely limited, addressing a small number of patients. Standard or bilevel CPAP may be effective in the treatment of hypoventilation, with most reports focusing on children with CCHS.[124–126]

Alternative Surgical Treatments for Childhood SDB

Other surgical treatments besides adenotonsillectomy are only occasionally performed in children. *Septoplasty* and *turbinectomy* can sometimes alleviate nonadenoidal nasal obstruction. *Uvulopalatopharyngoplasty* (UPPP) is sometimes performed for children with low-lying soft palates or redundant lateral pharyngeal tissue. Despite reports of clinical improvement in several small series of children treated with UPPP, efficacy as determined by PSG

TABLE 38–6   Major Pediatric Reports Assessing CPAP in the Treatment of Sleep-Disordered Breathing

Study	Population	Successful Use	Effective Pressures
Marcus et al.[140]	94 patients Age: infants–19 yr OSA: PSG-documented, not otherwise defined	Successful: 86% Unsuccessful: 1% Noncompliant: 13%	Median 8 cm H_2O (range 4–20 cm H_2O)
Guilleminault et al.[141]	74 patients Age: infants 2–12 mo SDB: AHI >5 or abnormal P_{es}	Successful: 97% Unsuccessful: 3%	Not reported
Waters et al.[142]	80 patients Age: 12 days–15 yr (mean 5.7 ± 0.5 yr) SDB: AHI generally >10	Successful: 86% Unsuccessful: 14%	Mean 7.9 ± 3.2 cm H_2O (range 4–16 cm H_2O)
McNamara and Sullivan[143]	24 patients Age: infants 1–51 wk OSA: obstructive and mixed apnea index >5	Successful: 75% Unsuccessful: 25%	Range 4–6 cm H_2O
Downey et al.[144]	18 patients Age: children <2 yr SDB: Average AHI 12.8 ± 20	Successful: 78% Unsuccessful: 22%	Mean 7.6 cm H_2O (range 6–11 cm H_2O)
Massa et al.[123]	66 patients Age: infants–19 yr SDB: Obstructive apnea index ≥5 or desaturation index (10 sec <90%) ≥ 4	Successful: 67% Unsuccessful: 33%	Mean 8.5 ± 3.2 cm H_2O (range 4–16 cm H_2O)
O'Donnell et al.[145]	79 patients Age: 6 mo–18 yr OSA: AHI >1	Successful: 82% Unsuccessful: 18%	Mean 6.8 ± 1.9 cm H_2O
Uong et al.[146]	27 patients Age: 7–19 yr OSA: AHI ≥5 or abnormal SaO_2/$ETcO_2$	Adherent: 70% Nonadherent: 30%	Mean 8.8 ± 2.1 cm H_2O

AHI, apnea-hypopnea index; CPAP, continuous positive airway pressure; $ETcO_2$, end-tidal carbon dioxide; OSA, obstructive sleep apnea; P_{es}, esophageal pressure; PSG, polysomnography; SaO_2, arterial oxygen saturation; SDB, sleep-disordered breathing.

measures is not well established for the procedure.[127,128] Soft tissue procedures such as *lingual tonsillectomy* and lingual reduction surgery have not been formally studied in children. *Radiofrequency ablation* procedures involving the tongue base and soft palate are rarely undertaken in children, and potential complications include abscess, neuralgia, and mucosal sloughing.[129]

For children having significant micrognathia, maxillary hypoplasia, or other craniofacial deformity, several skeletal procedures have the potential to alleviate upper airway obstruction. Mandibular reconstruction techniques used in children include *distraction osteogenesis* and, for older children, *mandibular advancement* via sagittal osteotomy.[130] For children with maxillary hypoplasia, *Le Fort advancement procedures* can correct cosmetic deformity and sometimes alleviate nasal obstruction. These procedures should only be considered in the context of significant skeletal deformity, since effectiveness for the purpose of treating childhood SDB has not been rigorously assessed.

Tracheostomy for treatment of childhood SDB is performed only when the condition is severe and refractory to conventional therapy. The procedure is highly effective in alleviating upper airway obstruction but carries significant trade-offs in the form of ongoing stoma care, increased risk of infection or bacterial colonization involving the lower respiratory tract, and adverse impact upon overall quality of life.[131,132] Because of these trade-offs, aggressive use of CPAP and skeletal or soft tissue surgery has been advocated to reduce reliance upon tracheostomy.[133]

Alternative Medical Treatments for Childhood SDB

Supplemental oxygen has a limited role in the treatment of childhood SDB and is used most often for children who have failed first-line therapies or who have underlying pulmonary disease. A randomized, double-blind study assessing the response of children with OSA to oxygen at 1 L/min reported modest improvements in oxygen saturation but no change in the frequency or severity of apnea.[134] In addition, 2 of 23 patients became significantly hypercapnic with treatment, consistent with the postulation that some children may be reliant upon hypoxic respiratory drive during sleep to maintain adequate ventilation.[54] For this reason, and also because many varieties of SDB disrupt sleep and produce secondary symptoms even in the absence of hypoxemia, this therapy should be used cautiously and with due recognition of its limitations and side effects.

Respiratory stimulants are used frequently in the treatment of apnea of infancy but are seldom used and largely unstudied outside of this context. Methylxanthine agents—most frequently theophylline and caffeine—produce short-term improvement of infant apnea and reduce the need for mechanical ventilation, but their impact upon long-term outcome is unknown.[135] *Oral appliances* are seldom used for treatment of childhood SDB due to concerns that this therapy could result in orthodontic problems. *Positional therapy*—affixing a small ball to the back of patients' pajamas or nightclothes to prevent them from comfortably assuming a supine position—is sometimes recommended for children with OSA when obstructive symptoms are problematic only in that position. Although this technique has been reported to improve the AHI for adults with OSA, no pediatric trials have been undertaken.[136]

Some reports suggest that use of *nasal steroids* may be associated with improvements in the AHI for some children with SDB. Trials of budesonide in children with OSA reported improvement of mean AHI from 5.2 to 3.2 following 4 weeks of treatment in one uncontrolled series and reduction of AHI from 8.4 to 1.2 following 6 weeks of treatment in another.[137,138] In a randomized, placebo-controlled trial, 6 weeks of treatment using fluticasone propionate was associated with reduction of the obstructive AHI from 10.7 to 5.8 for children with OSA versus an increase in the placebo group. Because the post-treatment AHIs in these reports might still be considered abnormal as determined by current pediatric criteria for the diagnosis of OSA (AHI ≥ 1), and because no long-term studies have been performed, nasal steroids cannot yet be recommended as a primary treatment for children with SDB. *Systemic steroids* have been found to be ineffective in treating OSA in children with adenotonsillar hypertrophy.[139]

⊘ REFERENCES

A full list of references are available at www.expertconsult.com

CHAPTER 39

Women's Sleep

Helen S. Driver and Eileen P. Sloan

INTRODUCTION

Reproductive and hormonal status influences sleep and sleep-related problems in women.[1–4] There is a growing recognition of gender differences in symptom reporting, for example, in sleep-related breathing disorders.[5–7] During a woman's reproductive life, complex changes occur with varying levels of two hormones in particular—estrogen and progesterone. As reviewed in this chapter, changes in hormone concentration or sensitivity to these hormones underlie many of the symptoms experienced by women. Ideally, fluctuations in hormone levels and their influence on the body and brain are delicately balanced so as not to disrupt sleep. However, there are periods when sleep is adversely affected, such as sleep disturbance caused by pain at menstruation, physical changes particularly in the last trimester of pregnancy, or menopausal hot flashes. In addition, gynecologic conditions and a higher incidence of some medical disorders in women (such as obesity and depression) are associated with increased risk of certain sleep disorders. Possible gender differences in such factors as need for sleep, perception, and symptom reporting should also be considered. In this chapter, we outline normal changes in sleep across a woman's adult life, gynecologic conditions associated with sleep disorders, and sleep disorders that may manifest at certain times.

THE MENSTRUAL CYCLE AND THE EFFECTS ON SLEEP

Hormonal and Sleep-Related Changes Across the Menstrual Cycle

Cyclical changes in four reproductive hormones—luteinizing hormone (LH), follicle stimulating hormone (FSH), estrogen, and progesterone—and in body temperature occur in a normal, ovulatory menstrual cycle. The cycle lasts 28 days on average (Fig. 39–1) but may range from 25 to 35 days. When menstruation starts (day 1), levels of all four key reproductive hormones are low. As FSH and estrogen rise, ovarian follicles develop and mature. This follicular phase precedes ovulation and may vary in length. LH peaks about 16 hours prior to ovulation, and the appearance of LH in urine is a reliable marker of ovulation. At ovulation, an oocyte is released from the follicle. The corpus luteum then evolves from the ruptured follicle and secretes progesterone and estrogen during the luteal phase. If ovulation occurs, body temperature, measured at the same time every morning, increases by about 0.4° C; this effect is mediated by progesterone.[4,8,9] In the absence of pregnancy, about 7 days after ovulation, the corpus luteum degenerates and hormone production begins to decline. The luteal phase lasts 14–16 days. Most negative menstrual symptoms are experienced as hormone concentrations decline toward the end of the luteal phase and during the first days of menstruation.

Subjective Reports of Sleep Across the Menstrual Cycle

Normally, subjective sleep quality is reduced both premenstrually and at menstruation.[10–12] Retrospective surveys have found that 16–32% of women report increased fatigue, difficulty in concentrating, or lethargy in the premenstrual period.[1–4] A telephone survey of 514 women for the National Sleep Foundation (NSF) in

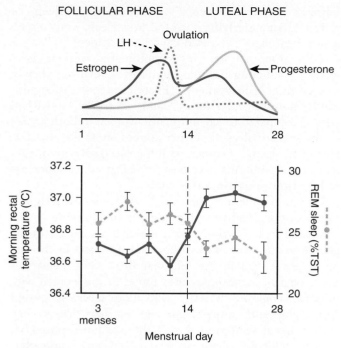

FOLLICULAR PHASE   LUTEAL PHASE

FIGURE 39–1 Menstrual cycle changes across a 28-day ovulatory cycle. The day menstruation begins is generally considered the first day of the menstrual cycle, and ovulation occurs around day 14. **(Top)** The profile for luteinizing hormone (LH), which peaks before ovulation (*dotted line*), and the ovarian hormones estrogen and progesterone. **(Bottom)** Morning core body temperature (*solid line, axis on the left*) and REM sleep as a percentage of total sleep time (TST; *dashed line, axis on the right*).(Modified from Driver et al.[8] and Driver and Baker.[4])

1998 found that approximately 70% of women report that their sleep is adversely affected on average 2½ days every month by menstrual symptoms such as cramps, bloating, tender breasts, and headaches.[13]

Increased sleep disturbance around menstruation have been confirmed in some, but not all, prospective studies.[10–12] In a study of 32 women who kept daily diaries across two menstrual cycles, although there was no change in sleep duration in the late luteal compared to the midfollicular phase, sleep disturbances increased, with poorer sleep quality. In the premenstrual period, sleep onset was delayed and there was an increased number of awakenings.[11] In contrast, Laessle et al.[12] found no change in sleep quality or sleep duration in 30 young women with normal menstrual cycles. Our study, in which ovulatory cycles were confirmed in 26 young women without significant menstrual-associated complaints, sleep quality was reduced 3–6 days premenstrually and during the first 4 days of menstruation.[10] These studies, and other reviews,[1–4] highlight the challenges inherent in studying menstrual cycle effects, including variability in cycle length, the presence of ovulation, individual and cycle-to-cycle differences, changes with age, and the frequency of data sampling. Given the cyclical, though modest, reduction in sleep quality around the time of menstruation in women without sleep complaints, investigation of insomnia in naturally cycling women should consider the temporal relationship of sleep complaints and the phase of the menstrual cycle.

Polysomnographic Studies Across the Menstrual Cycle

Early laboratory studies were based on small sample sizes, usually in young women (<30 years of age), with heterogeneous groups including those with affective symptoms or those taking oral contraceptives (OCs), often without verification that ovulation had occurred.[1,3,5] Two studies addressed these issues[8,14] by conducting more frequent recordings, at 3 nights per week[14] and every other night,[8] in nonsymptomatic good sleepers with verified ovulatory cycles. These polysomnographic (PSG) studies included spectral analysis of the sleep electroencephalogram (EEG) and core body temperature measurements. Both studies revealed an increase in sleep spindle frequency[8,14] in the mid- to late luteal phase compared with the follicular phase. This effect on sleep spindles was reflected in a menstrual-associated variation in stage 2 sleep (higher in the luteal phase), and may represent an interaction between endogenous progesterone metabolites and γ-aminobutyric acid (GABA) type A membrane receptors.[8] A lack of an effect on slow-wave sleep (SWS)[8,14,15] or EEG slow-wave spectral activity[8] suggests that sleep homeostatic mechanisms are not altered by menstrual phase. With the higher nocturnal temperature of the luteal phase, rapid eye movement (REM) sleep is slightly reduced,[8,9,15] with the effect evident over the first 4 cycles if not the whole night.[16] No significant menstrual phase effect on sleep latency or sleep efficiency based on PSG has been reported. The few controlled PSG studies in young women with no menstrual-associated complaints show that sleep across the menstrual cycle is remarkably stable, aside from variation in sleep spindles and subjectively disturbed sleep in the premenstrual and menstrual periods.[1–4,8–10,14]

Oral Contraceptives and Their Effect on Sleep

OCs are used by approximately 100 million women worldwide,[17,18] yet few studies have examined their effects on sleep. Studies are complicated by different levels of synthetic estrogen and progestin within the various OCs, which are available as monophasic and triphasic pills.[17,18] OCs contain synthetic estrogen and/or progestin that prevent ovulation by suppressing endogenous reproductive hormones. While the progestin is responsible for the contraceptive effects, the estrogen component is included for cycle control, and ethinyl estradiol is a potent suppressor of pituitary gonadotropins. Side effects are reported by about half of the women who start taking OCs. Among the most commonly reported are weight gain, painful periods, swollen legs, and heavy menstrual bleeding; a change in sleep is not a commonly reported side effect.[17,18]

Women taking monophasic combination OCs, which provide the same dosage of hormones through the entire 21-day active cycle followed by 7 days of inactive placebo, had persistently raised body temperatures when taking either the active OC or the placebo.[9] This increase in temperature with OCs has also been reported in a study of circadian rhythms during 24 hours of sleep deprivation with 8 women in the follicular phase, 9 in the luteal phase, and 8 who were taking OCs (pseudo-luteal phase) in an environment free of time cues using a modified constant routine procedure.[19] There was also an increase in melatonin levels in the OC group when compared to the women studied in the follicular phase.[19] Women taking OCs had significantly more stage 2 sleep in the active phase of the OC compared to the placebo, and more stage 2 compared to the naturally cycling women in both menstrual cycle phases.[9] OC users also had less SWS than naturally cycling women in the luteal phase.[9] A reduction in SWS with OC use was reported based on an archival analysis that compared women diagnosed with major depressive disorder and healthy controls, although menstrual phase or type of contraceptive was not controlled.[20] Reduced REM latency has also been reported in healthy women taking OCs,[20] but OC use does not affect sleep efficiency[9,20] or subjective sleep quality.[9]

On balance, because OC effects on sleep appear modest, for women with premenstrual and menstrual symptoms as described in the next sections, attenuation of pain and mood symptoms by OCs may improve sleep.

Premenstrual-Related Effects on Sleep: Premenstrual Syndrome and Premenstrual Dysphoric Disorder

Starting from puberty and lasting until menopause, women are at twice the lifetime risk of developing major depression as are men.[21,22] Approximately 60% of women experience mild premenstrual symptoms, referred to as premenstrual syndrome (PMS), but for 3–8% of women the cyclical pattern of symptoms is severe enough to be diagnosed as premenstrual dysphoric disorder (PMDD).[23] Common symptoms that occur in the last week of the luteal phase and lessen after the onset of menstruation include irritability/anger, anxiety/tension, depression and mood swings, change in appetite, bloating, weight gain, fatigue, and problems with sleep.[21] Complicating the comparison of studies of sleep in premenstrual mood disturbance is the fact that definitions and severity of symptoms vary considerably.[23–25] Sleep disturbances include problems falling or staying asleep, hypersomnia, unpleasant dreams, awakenings during the night, failure to wake at the expected time, and tiredness in the morning. Women with PMS perceive their sleep to be poor, with more unpleasant dreams.[26] These women report tossing and turning, frequent awakenings, and taking a long time to fall back asleep after an awakening during the night.

Perhaps as a consequence of the disturbed sleep, or reflecting an underlying need for more sleep, women with severe PMS have increased daytime sleepiness.[26–30]

Laboratory studies in symptomatic women have yielded conflicting findings, and only a small number of women have been studied.[25] There are reports of significantly more stage 2 sleep[15,28] and less SWS[15] and REM sleep[28] compared to asymptomatic women in both phases of the menstrual cycle. Other studies show no objective change in sleep.[29] Women with increased severity of premenstrual symptoms have been found to have an increase in luteal-phase daytime sleepiness.[11]

In a study by Lamarche et al.,[30] 10 women with significant emotional/behavioral premenstrual symptoms when compared with 9 women with minimal symptoms (mean age 26 years) were more sleepy and less alert in the late luteal phase than in the follicular phase. No menstrual-phase change in sleepiness was found in the women with minimal symptoms. Women with more severe symptoms were significantly more sleepy and less alert than women with minimal symptoms during the late luteal phase but not the follicular phase of the cycle. Using a midafternoon 40-minute nap intervention, there were no group differences in sleep-onset latency, with both groups falling asleep within an average of 7 minutes. The short sleep-onset latency found for both groups of women suggests a high sleep need during the late luteal phase regardless of symptom severity, but also suggests a measure of chronic sleep restriction as may be expected in this age group.

Changes in nocturnal temperature rhythms and melatonin secretion suggest that women with PMDD have underlying circadian rhythm abnormalities that could impact sleep.[22] As reviewed by Baker et al.,[25] in the symptomatic (luteal) phase, women with PMDD tend to have higher nocturnal temperatures and decreased melatonin secretion than normal controls; compared to their follicular phase, women with PMDD have delayed and decreased melatonin secretion. Therapeutic mood benefit has been found from 1 night of partial sleep deprivation (4 hours of sleep, either 9:00 PM to 1:00 AM or 3:00 AM to 7:00 AM), with further improvements reported after a subsequent recovery night of sleep (11:00 PM to 7:00 AM).[31] Initial findings indicate that appropriately timed light therapy may be a treatment strategy for PMDD, reducing depression, irritability, and physical premenstrual symptoms compared to a placebo condition. Thirty minutes of light therapy in the evening for 2 weeks during the luteal phase resulted in a significant improvement in premenstrual symptoms in women with PMS compared to baseline levels.[32] Larger trials with light therapy in this population are needed.

Painful Menstrual Conditions: Dysmenorrhea and Endometriosis

As many as 50% of women suffer from dysmenorrhea and experience extremely painful cramps during menstruation;

the pain is very severe in approximately 10–25% of women.[25,33] Similarly, women with endometriosis—who have misplaced uterine (endometrial) tissue in the abdominal and pelvic area—suffer extreme menstrual pain. Not surprisingly, these women report poorer sleep quality and higher anxiety during menstruation compared to symptom-free women.

Baker et al.[34] found that dysmenorrheic women had more disturbed sleep and subjective sleepiness than controls. Their sleep efficiency was reduced when experiencing menstrual pain, with increased wakefulness, movement, and stage 1 sleep compared with pain-free phases of their cycle. Women with dysmenorrhea (like those with PMS/PMDD) had decreased REM sleep and increased core temperature during the luteal and menstrual phases compared to normal controls. Although progesterone concentrations in the luteal phase were similar to those in asymptomatic women, dysmenorrheic women had elevated morning estrogen levels in the follicular and luteal phase and higher prolactin levels in the luteal phase.[23,34] Prostaglandins have been implicated as the mediators of the pain of primary dysmenorrhea, with the most common pharmacologic treatment for dysmenorrhea being nonsteroidal anti-inflammatory drugs.[35]

Polycystic Ovarian Syndrome

Women with polycystic ovary syndrome (PCOS), a condition of irregular or anovulatory menstrual cycles, increased androgen production, and metabolic consequences related to insulin resistance and weight gain,[36,37] are more likely to develop obstructive sleep apnea (OSA).[36–39] OSA is described in more detail in the next section on sleep-disordered breathing (SDB).

Four percent to 10% of women of reproductive age may suffer from PCOS.[36–38] About half of these women are overweight[40] with metabolic-related disorders and visceral obesity. Approximately 15% of obese normal women have OSA,[41] but in obese women with PCOS the incidence of OSA is markedly increased at 41–58%,[36] although body mass index (BMI) itself does not correlate with their OSA severity.[37–39] In obese women with PCOS, fat distribution follows a male pattern, with increased waist-to-hip ratio.[39] A relationship of OSA severity with waist-to-hip ratio, elevated serum testosterone,[38] and higher fasting insulin levels[39] indicates the contribution of androgenization and insulin resistance to the higher prevalence of OSA in women with PCOS.[36]

Sleep-Disordered Breathing in Women

The range of SDB includes snoring, the upper airway resistance syndrome (UARS), OSA, and the obesity-hypoventilation syndrome as well as central sleep apnea and periodic breathing (Cheyne-Stokes respiration). Women with SDB may report snoring less frequently than men[42] but report more fatigue[43] and nonspecific complaints.[44,45] One study found that women were also more likely than men to be treated for depression and have hypothyroidism at the time of diagnosis.[6] As reviewed by Banno and Kryger,[5] women with a diagnosis of OSA had higher obesity and comorbid psychiatric conditions, and received more antidepressants, hypnotics, and anxiolytics before OSA diagnosis, compared to men with OSA matched for age, BMI, and apnea-hypopnea index.[7]

The prevalence of central sleep apnea in women and OSA in premenopausal women is quite low, with women showing about half the prevalence of OSA as men, although this discrepancy declines in postmenopausal women.[46–48] More recent large cohort studies in the general population, coupled with changes in technology (e.g., more accurate airflow measurement via nasal cannula pressure transducers than with thermocouples), the increase in obesity with higher prevalence in women than men,[40] and the referral bias in favor of men,[6] indicate that OSA is more common in women than previously recognized.

There is evidence that upper airway resistance (UAR) during sleep is higher in men[49] and the male airway is more collapsible than in women. Premenopausally, women are protected from developing sleep apnea. Indeed, there is a menstrual phase effect on UAR, with UAR being lower during the luteal phase than in the follicular phase,[50] possibly related to progesterone effects. A number of other factors may contribute to the gender differences in SDB, such as differences in anatomy, upper airway collapsibility, the arousal response to increased inspiratory resistance, and ventilatory control.[49,50] The clinical effect of lower airway resistance and less collapsibility in women is apparent in PSG differences: women with OSA have more hypopneas than frank apneas with a shorter duration of apneas than in men,[51] and lower apnea severity in the luteal versus follicular phase.[52] Women with OSA tend to have a clustering of respiratory events during REM sleep,[53,54] the frequency of which is related to BMI in both men and women.[54] The magnitude of the increase in blood pressure after apnea termination compared with immediately prior to apnea termination was higher during the luteal phase than during the follicular phase, despite lower OSA severity in the luteal phase.[52] The augmented luteal phase pressor response to apneas may effectively be enhancing the arousal response due to a combination of centrally mediated and peripheral sympathetic responses.[52] The arousal response in UARS to airflow limitation results in daytime sleepiness due to fragmented sleep.[44] Excessive sleepiness is a key presenting complaint for OSA. However, in women with recently diagnosed OSA, insomnia was more likely to be a presenting complaint than it was in men.[6,55]

Clinically there is the potential that in some women polysomnographically significant SDB may manifest in the follicular phase, and could be missed by a diagnostic study in the luteal phase. Menstrual-related variability in the severity of sleep apnea may require a corresponding adjustment in management, such as varying the pressure requirement of continuous positive airway pressure (CPAP) therapy.

Fibromyalgia and Functional Somatic Syndromes

Fibromyalgia has been associated with a high prevalence of inspiratory flow limitation.[56] Conceivably, cortical arousability in response to increased UAR may be reflected as increased EEG frequency and sleep fragmentation, causing more somatic symptoms than those more commonly associated with OSA (excessive daytime sleepiness and snoring).

Fibromyalgia is more common in women than in men, as are the other chronically widespread and regional painful, multisymptom syndromes: irritable bowel syndrome, chronic pelvic pain, low back pain, temporomandibular joint disorder, and tension-type headache.[57] These conditions are sometimes referred to as functional somatic syndromes when pain hypersensitivity and stress-immune dysregulation are evident with emotional arousal and physiologic activation but no clear pathologic indicators.[57] Complaints of pain and insomnia are more prevalent in women than in men, though little is known about the physiologic and behavioral mechanisms involved.[58] With fibromyalgia, painful regions and tender points have been associated with poorer sleep and increased alpha EEG.[57,58] In chronic pain conditions, objective PSG measures show lighter and less consolidated sleep, possibly with more arousals, but no specific marker aside from a characteristic alpha EEG (7.5- to 11-Hz) intrusion into non-REM delta sleep (alpha-delta sleep) that was first described in 1975 by Moldofsky and colleagues.[59]

Sleep Disorders Associated with the Menstrual Cycle

Three forms of "menstrual-associated" sleep disorders—premenstrual insomnia, premenstrual hypersomnia, and menopausal insomnia—were listed under the category of Proposed Sleep Disorders in the revised International Classification of Sleep Disorders (ICSD) published in 1997.[60] In the second edition of the ICSD from 2005,[61] the only two disorders carried over are menstrual-related hypersomnia and menopausal insomnia. There is very limited research on premenstrual sleep disorders and its inclusion is based on isolated case reports.

Difficulty falling asleep or staying asleep, usually in the week before menstruation (premenstrual insomnia), should be distinguished from PMS and PMDD. Insomnia as the only premenstrual symptom is not considered sufficient to receive a diagnosis of PMS. Premenstrual hypersomnia occurring periodically around menses, preceding

and into the early follicular phase, has been successfully treated with hormonal treatment (conjugated estrogen or oral contraceptives).[62] In another case of periodic hypersomnia, prolactin was elevated but did not respond to hormone replacement therapy and was symptomatically treated with methylphenidate.[63]

SLEEP DURING PREGNANCY

Sleep disruption during pregnancy is a common and multifaceted problem.[64,65] Contributing factors include hormonal changes, fetal movement, bladder distention, gastrointestinal discomfort, vomiting, and temperature fluctuations. There are significant changes in sleep architecture, and primary sleep disorders such as OSA and restless legs syndrome may be more common. Most women accommodate to the changes in sleep, but for a proportion of them the disruption will prove problematic and may result in medical and psychiatric complications.

Subjective Changes in Sleep

A large percentage (66–94%) of women note alterations in their sleep during pregnancy.[66,67] During the first trimester, subjective sleep quality decreases and the number of nocturnal awakenings increases. Daytime sleepiness is more problematic. During the second trimester, women report that sleep normalizes, although 19% of women continue to experience difficulties at this stage.[66] By the third trimester, women experience worsening insomnia, increased daytime sleeping, and decreased alertness. Reasons cited for the increased sleep disturbances were mainly urinary frequency, backache, fetal movement, abdominal discomfort, leg cramps, and heartburn. A survey of sleep disruption across pregnancy found that 97% of women identified themselves as having disrupted sleep, while a third felt they had a "sleep disorder."[68] The latter group may be biologically or psychologically more vulnerable to the detrimental effects of disrupted sleep. Factors such as a prior history of a psychiatric disorder, lack of a social support network, poor coping skills, and difficulty adjusting to the impending role of motherhood are likely important in this regard.

The 1998 NSF survey found that 79% of women reported that their sleep was, or had been, disturbed during pregnancy.[13] Women who were currently pregnant or had been pregnant recently were more likely to report frequent insomnia (64%) when compared to premenopausal or menopausal women. Of the women reporting sleep disturbance during pregnancy, 70% reported that it interfered with daily functioning on at least a few days per month. It is unclear for what proportion it represented a *serious* problem. There are limitations to this survey, such as the fact that not all women were pregnant at the time of reporting and were hence providing retrospective accounts of their sleep during pregnancy, but it does shed light on the extent of subjective sleep disruption during pregnancy. The NSF 2007 "Sleep in America" telephone poll of 1,003 women included 150 pregnant (second trimester, $n = 47$; third trimester, $n = 91$) and 151 postpartum women.[69] More pregnant women (84%) experienced insomnia symptoms at least a few nights a week, compared to 67% of the overall group. In response to whether they were getting a good night's sleep at least a few nights a week, 82% of pregnant women felt they were doing so before their current pregnancy, compared to 60% who felt this to be the case during their ongoing pregnancy. More women in their second trimester (72%) said they got a good night's sleep at least a few nights a week than those in their third trimester (54%). Reasons for sleep disturbance were to go to the bathroom (92% in the third trimester and 75% in the second trimester), and pain in their back, neck, or joints (66% and 47% of third- and second-trimester women, respectively). Two other reasons for disturbed sleep in the third trimester are leg cramps (54%) and heartburn (51%).

Objective Changes in Sleep

Pregnancy has a significant impact on sleep architecture and on the quantity and quality of sleep. Several excellent reviews[3,70–72] show that the findings are not fully consistent and that more research into the changes in sleep architecture that accompany pregnancy is necessary. However, there is consensus that there is a "lightening" of sleep as pregnancy progresses, with a decrease in sleep efficiency, decreased total sleep time, increased wakefulness after sleep onset, and decreased REM sleep. Most studies show a decrease in SWS, especially in the third trimester.[73,74] One study reports an *increase* in SWS from early to late pregnancy.[75] This last finding may relate to the fact that only primiparous women were included, while the other studies included both primiparous and multiparous subjects. The sleep of these two groups of women appears to differ; exactly in what way remains to be determined. According to one study, multiparous women have lower sleep efficiency at all time points across pregnancy.[74] Immediately postpartum, primiparous women have lower sleep efficiency, but at 3 months postpartum their sleep had improved but did not revert to its prepregnancy baseline. This finding would suggest that pregnancy and childrearing has a prolonged impact on sleep architecture. Another study, following women's sleep using actigraphy during pregnancy and at 1 and 6 weeks postpartum, reported that primiparous women have lower sleep efficiency in general during pregnancy and postpartum, when they also had fewer sleep episodes than their multiparous counterparts.[76] Again, the discrepancy in findings could be secondary to varying assessment techniques (PSG, actigraphy) and relatively small sample sizes.

Primary Sleep Disorders Associated with Pregnancy

The risk for OSA increases substantially with obesity[40,77] but the prevalence with the weight gain during pregnancy is unclear. Changes in respiratory physiology during pregnancy, such as decreased functional residual capacity,[78] changes in the airway mucosa,[79] and hyperventilation with increased sensitivity to CO_2,[80] may predispose to obstructive or central apneic events. Some investigators have found no decrease in nocturnal arterial oxygen saturation during pregnancy.[81,82] Others, however, report significantly more nocturnal desaturation in pregnant women compared with controls.[83,84] Hypertension in the mother at the time of birth and lower Apgar scores in the infant are significantly more common in women who reported snoring during pregnancy as compared to nonsnorers.[85] A number of case series, using small numbers and relying on clinical examination rather than PSG, indicate that OSA may be associated with intrauterine growth retardation, especially if other complications such as maternal obesity and diabetes mellitus are present.[86] The control of partial upper airway obstruction and snoring using nasal CPAP in women with preeclampsia, has been shown to decrease blood pressure significantly.[87] Edwards and Sullivan[88] have reviewed the risks and treatment options of SDB during pregnancy and with preeclampsia.

Restless legs syndrome (RLS) and periodic limb movements in sleep (PLMS) increase during pregnancy.[71,89] Women cite restless legs as a common cause of sleep disruption during pregnancy.[65] Complaints of leg cramps during waking should raise the possibility of PLMS, especially if the woman is experiencing daytime sleepiness or fatigue.

Risks Associated with Sleep Disruption During Pregnancy

The role of sleep disturbance in the development of psychiatric illness is a grave concern. Patients with persistent insomnia are at significant risk for developing depression.[90] This holds true even when there is a medical cause, such as sleep apnea, for the insomnia. Women with sleep disruption during pregnancy and in the weeks postpartum may be at higher risk for postpartum mood disorders, especially where there is a previous history of mental illness. Sleep disruption often heralds the onset of a manic or hypomanic episode among patients in the general population who suffer from bipolar illness.[91] The risk of new-onset mania or recurrence of a preexisting illness during the postpartum period is significant. Women with a history of bipolar affective disorder (BAD) have a twofold increase in risk for symptom exacerbation during the immediate postpartum period. Furthermore, women with no prior history of BAD have a sevenfold increase in risk for a psychiatric admission in the puerperum when compared with non-postpartum and nonpregnant women.[92] Even fathers with BAD are at increased risk of relapse in the postpartum period.[93] This suggests that the sleep disruption associated with caring for a neonate may play an important role in the development or recurrence of postpartum psychiatric illness. The challenge for the clinician is to identify those women for whom sleep loss, an inevitable part of childbearing, will have serious consequences.

Patients with insomnia often resort to the use of alcohol and over-the-counter remedies. The NSF report[13] found that 7% of pregnant women used over-the counter medications and 7% used alcohol at some point in the pregnancy to help them sleep, while 4% used prescription medications for this purpose. The use of such sleep aids during pregnancy could have significant consequences for the developing fetus.

Research is being carried out on the impact of pregnancy-related and inflammatory markers. A study by Okun et al.[94] on 19 women during mid- and late-trimester pregnancy examined subjective sleep reports and levels of interleukin-6 (IL-6) and tumor necrosis factor-α. Complaints of shorter sleep duration and poor sleep efficiency at both stages of pregnancy were associated with higher levels of stimulated IL-6, while in late pregnancy sleep complaints were also associated with higher levels of circulating IL-6. The implications of these findings for maternal well-being and fetal development remain to be determined.

Management of Pregnancy-Related Sleep Disruption

Significant sleep disruption during pregnancy is likely underreported by women. Hence, it is imperative that the primary caregiver inquire about it and determine to what extent it warrants further assessment and intervention. Potential medical causes should be considered (e.g., medications, thyroid problems, psychiatric illness) and treated where appropriate. Primary sleep disorders such as OSA and RLS/PLMS should be ruled out.

Significant respiratory disturbance can be treated with CPAP, which has been shown to be safe during pregnancy.[86,87] Milder respiratory disturbances may respond to conservative measures such as positional therapy.

There is a relationship between low serum ferritin levels and RLS/PLMS. Iron supplementation should be instituted where this is the case. Conservative measures such as reducing caffeine intake or wearing supportive stockings should be implemented. The use of any form of medication during pregnancy must be approached with caution, and the patient must be made fully aware of the risks and benefits. Pregnant women are rarely included in drug trials, and the safety of many medications during pregnancy has not been determined. The safety of certain medications used to treat RLS/PLMS (e.g., pramipexole, gabapentin, ropinirole) is unknown. The benzodiazepine clonazepam carries concern about possible teratogenicity

when used in the first trimester. However, judicious use in the second and third trimesters may be warranted. Some patients with RLS/PLMS respond well to opioids such as codeine and oxycodone, and there is no evidence of teratogenicity, although there is a risk of a withdrawal syndrome or respiratory depression in the neonate.

During the postpartum period, the sleep of women with a history of a mood disorder must be protected since a recurrence at this time can have disastrous consequences for both mother and infant. Prolongation of the hospital stay to enable the new mother to recover from the impact of labor and birth may be beneficial. The patient's partner and other family members should be encouraged to play an active role in nocturnal feeding.

Where no primary cause for the sleep disruption can be determined, nonpharmacologic treatments should be the primary intervention. Attention to sleep hygiene factors, such as a regular sleep-wake schedule, avoiding caffeinated beverages, reducing the amount of fluids consumed in the evening, and ensuring the temperature in the bedroom is comfortable, should be highlighted. There are no data concerning the efficacy of cognitive and behavioral techniques, such as cognitive behavioral therapy or stimulus control therapy, for insomnia during pregnancy. However, given that they are efficacious for insomnia in general, we would expect that they would be beneficial when applied during pregnancy.

The majority of women are likely to resist the use of sleeping medications, but where insomnia is having a severe effect, the use of a sleep aid may be warranted. The antihistamine dimenhydrinate and the nonbenzodiazepine hypnotic zolpidem (not available in Canada) have not shown fetal effects in animal studies. Zolpidem has the advantage of being less anticholinergic. The use of the other nonbenzodiazepine hypnotics, zopiclone and zaleplon, should be limited during pregnancy until more data are available. However, a study of pregnancy outcome in 40 women exposed to zopiclone during the first trimester did not find an increase in the rate of major malformations when compared with a nonexposed group.[95]

The antidepressant trazodone may be beneficial for reducing sleep-onset latency and improving sleep quality in depressed patients.[96] The American Academy of Pediatrics (AAP) stated that data are too limited to provide a recommendation on the use of this and other sedating antidepressants, such as mirtazapine and nefazadone (not available in Canada), during pregnancy.[97] No difference in pregnancy outcome (including rate of major malformations and gestational age at birth) has been found between patients taking nefazadone and trazadone during the first trimester when compared with women taking other nonteratogenic antidepressants or other nonteratogenic drugs (e.g., sumatriptin, dextromethorphan), matched for age, smoking, and alcohol use.[98] Both antidepressant groups, however, had a trend toward a higher rate of spontaneous abortion, although the difference was not statistically significant.

The tricyclic antidepressant amitriptyline has considerable sedating properties, does not appear to have teratogenic effects, and is considered safe for use in pregnancy.[97]

Benzodiazepines are frequently used to treat insomnia in the general population. The AAP[97] recommends that their use be limited during pregnancy since they can induce sedation, withdrawal signs (including restlessness, hypertonia, irritability, seizures, and abdominal distention), and floppy baby syndrome (muscular hypotonia, low Apgar scores, neurologic depression) in the neonate, effects that can last for up to 3 months. Hence, when benzodiazepines are used, they should be slowly tapered over a number of weeks prior to delivery. Use during the first trimester should be avoided if possible because of concerns about congenital malformations such as cleft palate.[99] However, no congenital defects have been associated with lorazepam or alprazolam.[97] Use of the former is preferred since it lacks active metabolites and is less likely to be associated with a withdrawal syndrome in the neonate.

MENOPAUSE AND THE CLIMACTERIC

Changes in menstrual cycle frequency and menstrual flow reflect the changing hormone milieu in the perimenopausal period. Menstrual cycle length decreases from 28 days for women in their 20s to 26 days for women in their 40s.[100] Between the ages of 45 and 55 years, production of estrogen and progesterone decreases, FSH levels increase, and menstrual cycles become irregular.[100] This transition occurs over a few years (mean 3.8 years) prior to the last menstrual period. There is no definitive way to distinguish transient amenorrhea from menopausal amenorrhea, and generally menopause is only confirmed when menstrual periods have stopped for a year (average age 51 years).[101] The term *climacteric* is used to refer to the transition period (usually 7–10 years) preceding the last menses when ovarian function decreases, and afterward, when women experience hormonally induced physical and or psychological changes.[100]

Sleep Disturbance and Climacteric Symptoms

Women of any age are more likely than men to report dissatisfaction with their sleep and to experience daytime consequences. Insomnia is more prevalent in women than men,[102] and this gender disparity increases with age—the female:male ratio of insomnia symptoms after 45 years of age is 1.7:1.[103] Menopause is often cited as the underlying cause for the gender disparity in middle-aged individuals. Complaints of sleep disruption are higher in perimenopausal than in premenopausal women.[103,104] Sleep disturbances include waking at night (the most common problem), waking early, and difficulty falling asleep.[104] Trouble sleeping has been associated with more depressive symptoms, mood swings, higher levels of stress, tension and anxiety, hot flashes, and palpitations, particularly during perimenopause.[100,104–107] Other menopausal symptoms that can be disruptive to sleep either directly or indirectly include weight gain, vaginal dryness and irritation, and urinary problems. Nocturia in postmenopausal women is reportedly improved with estrogen therapy.[108] However, as in men, the prevalence of nocturia increases with age (9% in women <39 years old to 51% of women ≥80 years old),[108] and OSA can increase nocturnal diuresis through increased atrial natriuretic peptide production. Thus, aside from menopausal symptoms disturbing sleep, underlying chronic physical conditions or sleep disorders should also be considered.

The terms *hot flush*, *hot flash*, and *vasomotor symptoms* are used to describe the same phenomenon. Nocturnal hot flashes (also called night sweats) that can soak bedclothes, followed by chills as the body cools down, lead to sleep disruption.[107,109] Up to 85% of women experience hot flashes,[100,107,109] with variation depending on ethnicity and culture.[107,109] In a large (n = 14,906) multisite, multiethnic study in the United States of women's health across the nation (SWAN), the population group with the lowest incidence of night sweats were Japanese women at 9% and the highest was African women at 32%.[110] A further analysis from the SWAN study found that 38% of all women reported subjective difficulty sleeping; the incidence was lowest in Japanese women (28%) and highest in Caucasian women (40%), and difficulty sleeping was associated with hot flashes.[109] In the SWAN study, an odds ratio for sleep problems in women with vasomotor symptoms was 2.0 compared to asymptomatic women.[109] Furthermore, in a smaller study (n = 63) based on healthy women who had undergone hysterectomy, those with subjectively impaired sleep had more hot flashes and palpitations as well as mood-related symptoms (anxiety, depression, mood instability, memory problems).[111] Perimenopausal women (n = 15) who reported increased awakenings and dissatisfaction with sleep quality compared to age matched premenopausal controls (n = 13) showed an increased number and duration of arousals and more movement activity on wrist actigraphy.[105]

Interestingly, PSG studies do not consistently show worse sleep quality peri- and postmenopausally than premenopausally,[106,114,115] or an association with climacteric vasomotor, somatic, or mood symptoms.[111,113,114] Although no significant differences in sleep were apparent, for 39 symptomatic versus 32 nonsymptomatic women there was a trend toward lower sleep efficiency.[112] Young et al.[113] compared objective sleep data from a single night in 589 women of known menopausal status but, despite postmenopausal women reporting more dissatisfaction with their sleep than premenopausal women, PSG sleep efficiency was not lower in peri- and postmenopausal women. Indeed, the proportion of SWS was higher in postmenopause than premenopause. A study by Freedman and Roehrs[114] also found that 12 symptomatic women, versus 8 asymptomatic postmenopausal women and 11 premenopausal women, did not have more sleep disturbance. Clearly there is a disconnect between objective and subjective sleep that merits further investigation.

Potential factors contributing to the disparity between subjective dissatisfaction with sleep and objective measures include (1) the severity of climacteric symptoms and the presence of hot flashes during the sleep recording, (2) effects on sleep microstructure—arousals, alpha EEG intrusion,[58] and cyclic alternating pattern (CAPS)[115]—rather than macrostructure, and (3) sympathetic activation. The association of hot flashes with subjectively poorer sleep suggests they should be monitored during PSG studies. One study that used skin conductance to monitor hot flashes in women with nightly complaints of sweating found a reduction in hot flashes associated polysomnographically with a reduced CAPS rate and improved sleep efficiency after 4 weeks of conjugated estrogens (0.625 mg).[115] Similarly, when monitoring hot flashes in breast cancer survivors with insomnia ($n = 24$), more sleep disruption and wake time around the time of hot flashes was observed; sleep efficiency was lower on nights with than on nights without hot flashes.[116] However, Freedman and Roehrs[114] did not find any association of sleep disturbance around the time of hot flashes measured by skin conductance.

Hormone and Estrogen Replacement Therapy: A Role for Improving Sleep?

Vasomotor symptoms are reduced with estrogen alone (estrogen replacement therapy [ERT])[115,117,118] or in combination with progesterone therapy (hormone replacement therapy [HRT]),[119–122] but in laboratory studies they have not been found consistently to improve sleep. Findings from three studies highlight these inconsistencies. Polo-Kantola et al.[117] reported subjective sleep improvement with transdermal estrogen preparations compared with placebo ($n = 70$), associated with reduced hot flashes and sweating, but estrogen was no better than placebo in terms of sleep on PSG. Antonijevic et al.,[123] in contrast, found reduced wakefulness and increased REM sleep with an estradiol patch ($n = 11$). In a third study, an HRT with estrogen (Premarin 0.625 mg) and two different progesterone preparations—either micronized progesterone (Prometrium 200 mg) ($n = 10$), which gives rise to sedative metabolites, or medroxyprogesterone (Provera 5 mg) ($n = 11$)—showed improved sleep efficiency with micronized progesterone.[122] Despite the sleep improvement, daytime vigilance was unchanged with the micronized progesterone, whereas it improved with medroxyprogesterone. Clearly more detailed studies of the effects of HRT are needed before firm conclusions can be drawn regarding their effects on sleep.

For those women whose menopausal symptoms and sleep may be alleviated on hormone therapy, safety concerns with HRT from the Women's Health Initiative (WHI)[118] posed a dilemma. The large ($n = 16,608$),

randomized, placebo-controlled WHI trial on the effect of conjugated equine estrogens (0.625 mg) combined with medroxyprogesterone acetate (2.5 mg), revealed increased risks for stroke, venous thromboembolism, coronary heart disease, and breast cancer.[118] These risks have been subsequently confirmed in other clinical trials that used a variety of estrogen and progestin products.[124] Given the fear of adverse events, over 50% of women stop therapy after 1 year.[125] However, in the WHI trial, women with severe menopausal symptoms were excluded, yet symptom relief is the reason most women initiate HRT. The choice of whether to use hormone therapy or not is a balance between current quality of life and potential risk.[126]

Subsequent analysis of health-related quality of life in nonsymptomatic women from the WHI trial[127] showed there was only a small and not clinically meaningful reduction in sleep disturbance in the first year that was not evident after 3 years. Indeed, women with flushing from the Heart and Estrogen/Progestin Replacement Study—another large ($n = 2,763$) randomized, placebo-controlled trial of the same hormone concentrations as the WHI trial—had improved mental health and depressive symptoms.[128] Thus the effects of HRT on quality of life appear to depend on the presence of menopausal symptoms with negative effects in women without flushing and improvements in women with flushing.[128] For women who experience significant disruptive menopausal symptoms, the smallest effective dose of estrogen may serve a useful short-term role in symptom management.[124,126,129] Family history and potential risk of disease should be taken into account when considering HRT for relief from disturbed sleep.[124,129]

Alternatives to Hormone Replacement Therapy for Sleep Disruption

Given the safety concerns related to hormone therapy, many women seek alternative therapies to relieve sleep disturbances. Hot flashes occur more frequently in warmer than cooler environments[107]; reducing ambient temperature (to 16–19° C) may provide relief from hot flashes and sleep disruption.[121,126]

A telephone survey ($n = 866$) on the use of eight alternative therapies to manage menopause symptoms found that 76% of women had used at least one type of alternative therapy.[130] Women who experienced trouble sleeping were more likely to use alternative therapies such as dietary soy and stress management. Soy isoflavones are estrogen-like substances that have been investigated as an alternative therapy to relieve menopausal symptoms but have not been found consistently to have an appreciable effect.[131]

With a decrease in HRT prescriptions since July 2002, there has been an increase in prescriptions of serotonergic antidepressants.[132] Some antidepressants that block the release of serotonin and norephinephrine (e.g., fluoxetine, paroxetine, venlefaxine) have been reported to alleviate climacteric symptoms.[132,133] Norepinephrine and serotonin have a central role in the pathophysiology of hot flashes[126]; clonidine, an α_2-adrenergic agonist, has also been found to alleviate climacteric symptoms and accordingly related sleep problems. Though not well studied, black cohosh (a root extract from a North American perennial plant) may relieve hot flash symptoms, and gabapentin (a GABA analog) has been found to have a favorable effect compared to placebo.[133] Hypnotic drugs such as zolpidem (10 mg) in women with menopause-related insomnia ($n = 141$) reduced wake after sleep onset and improved subjective sleep quality.[134]

Sleep-Disordered Breathing in the Menopause

Menopause increases the risk of SDB by three to four times, even after adjusting for known risk factors such as age and BMI, compared to premenopausal women.[47,135] Increased age, hormone-related changes, and weight gain—including a change in fat distribution[100] with more visceral adiposity—are all contributing factors for increased OSA. Older, overweight women with high blood pressure, insomnia, disturbed sleep, or "fatigue" should be considered at high risk for having OSA.

Progesterone is a respiratory stimulant and, in women receiving HRT, the prevalence of OSA and SDB was found to be lower than women not taking HRT.[47] This finding needs to be confirmed in larger clinical trials. The prevalence of moderate to severe OSA in women in the Sleep Heart Health Study ($n = 2,994$, age ≥ 50 years) among women using hormone replacement (either ERT or HRT) was half the prevalence in nonusers.[136] The reduction in SDB (estimated odds ratio, 0.55) for hormone users corresponded to the predicted effect of reducing BMI by $6.8 \, kg/m^2$.[136] Before recommending menopausal hormone replacement to treat apnea in women, however, many other factors need to be considered. The focus should instead be on using standard therapy such as weight loss, CPAP, an oral appliance, or positional therapy (side sleep) for milder OSA.

Other Factors Influencing Sleep During Menopause

The secretion of other endogenous hormones, such as thyrotropin, decreases with age: 25% of postmenopausal women show clinical or subclinical thyroid disease, which often causes symptoms similar to those of the climacteric.[126] The cause of sleep problems around menopause is not always evident. Factors aside from menopause—such as systemic diseases, medications, depressed mood, stress, behavioral or cognitive factors, pain, and aging-associated increases in RLS and PLMS—may explain, or contribute to, decreases in sleep quality.

CONCLUSION

The changing hormone profile across the reproductive life of a woman, from puberty through the reproductive period to the postmenopausal years, has a significant influence on sleep. Abrupt changes in, or withdrawal of, female hormones may lead to sleep disruption. During pregnancy, however, multiple factors contribute to sleep disruption, and these will vary according to the stage of pregnancy. Certain sleep disorders such as OSA and RLS are influenced by stage of menstrual cycle or life cycle. This chapter has highlighted the impact of the reproductive and menstrual cycles on sleep. It is imperative that sleep clinicians take these factors into account when working with women. Women should be encouraged to track whether there is a cyclical change in their symptoms in association with hormone changes or if the symptom changes are due to age-related changes in hormonal profile.

⊗ REFERENCES

A full list of references are available at www.expertconsult.com

CHAPTER 40

Sleep-Related Violence: Forensic Medicine Issues

Mark W. Mahowald and **Carlos H. Schenck**

In all of us, even in good men, there is a lawless, wild-beast nature which peers out in sleep. — Plato
(*The Republic*)

Acts done by a person asleep cannot be criminal, there being no consciousness.[1]

INTRODUCTION

Increasingly, practitioners are asked to render legal opinions regarding legal issues pertaining to violent or injurious behaviors arising from the sleep period. Automatic behaviors (automatisms) resulting in acts that may result in illegal behaviors have been described in many different conditions. Those automatisms arising from wakefulness are reasonably well understood. Recent advances in sleep medicine have made it apparent that some complex behaviors, occasionally resulting in forensic science implications, are exquisitely state dependent, meaning that they occur exclusively, or predominately, during the sleep period.

Case Example

A 24-year-old single white male who had enjoyed a stellar college academic and athletic record, with no history of psychiatric disease or drug or substance abuse, had no history of any sleep disorder, and absolutely no prior history of interpersonal violence. In December 1993 he was living in Japan and working as a teacher. He was very sleep deprived prior to returning to the United States, and estimates that he had received no more than 15 hours of sleep during the preceding 4 days. He went to a friend's house upon his return, where he drank 1.5 beers and took one hit of marijuana. He was noticed to be acting "peculiar" while riding with his friends. When they stopped, he got out of the car and saw a policeman approaching. He told his friends it was "OK," as he knew the officer (not true).

He walked over toward the officer and then sat down in the police car. The officer then drove him to where his friends were waiting. Each got out and met behind the car. He viciously attacked the officer, fracturing his jaw and knocking him unconscious. Another officer arrived. The subject was finally subdued by a number of people. According to his friends, his behavior was extremely inappropriate, irrational, and completely out of character for him.

He had no recollection of any of the event from riding in the car until he "came to" in a hospital. He does remember "dream-like" images. He stated: "I remember thinking I was in hell." He remembers being held down by a number of arms, but could not identify bodies or faces. He believes he thought he was in hell because of the burning sensation on his face. In retrospect, he thinks this may have been fragmentary imagery of being held down by the policemen, and having been sprayed in the face with Mace. Extensive psychiatric and chemical dependency evaluations performed after the incident were unrevealing.

He was charged with a felony. If convicted, it would destroy his developing business in Japan. Based upon reports from his friends and the police, and upon his fragmentary memories, he never denied having committed the violent act. He wished to have his behavior declared a "noninsane automatism"—which would have very different legal implications.

NEUROPHYSIOLOGY OF SLEEP-RELATED VIOLENCE

The State-Dependent Nature of Violence

The concept that sleep is simply the passive absence of wakefulness is no longer tenable. Not only is sleep an active rather than passive process, it is now clear that sleep comprises two completely different states: non–rapid eye movement (NREM) sleep and rapid eye movement (REM) sleep. Therefore, our lives are spent in three entirely different states of being: wakefulness, REM sleep, and NREM sleep. Studies have indicated that bizarre behavioral syndromes can occur as a result of the incomplete declaration or rapid oscillation of these states.[2,3] Although the automatic behaviors of some "mixed states" are relatively benign (i.e., shoplifting in narcolepsy),[4] others may be associated with violent behaviors.

The fact that violent or injurious behaviors may arise in the absence of conscious wakefulness and without conscious awareness raises the crucial question of how such complex behavior can occur. Examination of extensive animal experimental studies provides preliminary answers. The widely held concept that the brain stem and other more "primitive" neural structures primarily participate in elemental/vegetative rather than behavioral activities is inaccurate. There are overwhelming data documenting that extremely complex emotional and motor behaviors can originate from these more primitive structures—without involvement of "higher" neural structures such as the cortex.[5–11]

SLEEP-RELATED DISORDERS ASSOCIATED WITH VIOLENCE

Violent sleep-related behaviors have been reviewed in the context of automatized behavior in general. There are well-documented cases of (1) somnambulistic homicide, attempted homicide, and suicide; (2) murders and other crimes with sleep drunkenness (confusional arousals); and (3) sleep terrors/sleepwalking with potential violence/injury. A wide variety of disorders may result in sleep-related violence.[12,13] Conditions associated with sleep period–related violence are listed in Table 40–1. These conveniently fall into two major categories: neurologic and psychiatric.

Neurologic Conditions Associated with Violent Behaviors

Extrapolating from animal data to the human condition, it has been shown that structural lesions at multiple levels of the nervous system may result in wakeful violence.[14–17]

TABLE 40–1 Conditions Associated with Sleep-Related Violent Behavior

Neurologic Sleep Disorders

- Disorders of arousal (confusional arousals [sleep drunkenness], sleepwalking, sleep terrors)*
- REM sleep behavior disorder*
- Nocturnal seizures*
- Automatic behavior
  - Narcolepsy and idiopathic central nervous system hypersomnia
  - Sleep apnea
  - Sleep deprivation (including jet lag)

Psychiatric Sleep Disorders

- Psychogenic dissociative states (may arise exclusively from sleep)
  - Fugues
  - Multiple personality disorder
  - Psychogenic amnesia
- Malingering
- Munchausen syndrome by proxy

*Obstructive sleep apnea may mimic or trigger these parasomnias.

The animal studies provide insights into violent behaviors in the disorders of arousal, REM sleep behavior disorder (RBD), and sleep-related seizures.

Disorders of Arousal (Confusional Arousals, Sleepwalking, Sleep Terrors)

The disorders of arousal comprise a spectrum ranging from confusional arousals (sleep drunkenness) to sleepwalking to sleep terrors.[18] Although there is usually amnesia for the event, vivid dream-like mentation may be experienced and reported.[19] Contrary to popular opinion, these disorders may actually begin in adulthood, and are most often *not* associated with psychopathology.[19] The commonly held belief that sleepwalking and sleep terrors are always benign is erroneous: the accompanying behaviors may be violent, resulting in considerable injury to the individual or others, or damage to the environment.

Febrile illness, prior sleep deprivation, and emotional stress may serve to trigger disorders of arousal in susceptible individuals.[20–22] Sleep deprivation is well known to result in confusion, disorientation, and hallucinatory phenomena.[23] Medications such as sedative-hypnotics, neuroleptics, minor tranquilizers, stimulants, and antihistamines, often in combination with each other or with alcohol, may also play a role.[18]

Confusional arousals (also termed *sleep drunkenness*) occur during the transition between sleep and wakefulness and represent a disturbance of cognition and attention despite the motor behavior of wakefulness, resulting in complex behavior without conscious awareness.[24–26] These may be potentiated by prior sleep deprivation or the ingestion of sedative-hypnotics before sleep onset.[27] These episodes of "automatic behavior" occur in the setting of chronic sleep deprivation or other conditions associated with state admixture (shoplifting has been reported during a period of automatic behavior in a narcoleptic).[4,28,29]

Numerous associations exist between obstructive sleep apnea (OSA) and confusional arousals. Patients suffering from OSA may experience frequent arousals that may serve to trigger arousal-induced precipitous motor activity.[30] Therefore, the observed clinical behavior—a confusional arousal—is actually the result of another underlying primary sleep disorder, OSA. Guilleminault and Silvestri have made the following observations[30]:

> It is well known that adult patients with OSA syndrome present nocturnal wandering during sleep. These patients frequently demonstrate yelling and screaming during sleep, as well as confusion, disorientation, and sleepwalking...The nocturnal hypoxia and the repetitive sleep disruptions secondary to the OSA syndrome readily explain these symptoms.

This is another example of why overnight polysomnographic (PSG) studies with extensive physiologic monitoring are mandatory in the evaluation of problematic motor parasomnias. Disorders of arousal may also be precipitated by adequate or incomplete treatment of sleep apnea with nasal continuous positive airway pressure.[31,32]

To remind us that apparently criminal acts without conscious awareness occurring during sleep drunkenness (formerly termed *somnolentia*) are not a recently described condition, dramatic cases were described in a classic book on sleep well over a century ago. The author's conclusion regarding sleep drunkenness was: "It is a natural phenomenon, to which all are liable."[33] Treatment of the disorders of arousal includes both pharmacologic (benzodiazepines and tricyclic antidepressants) and behavioral (hypnosis) approaches.[34]

The behavioral similarities between documented sleepwalking and sleep terrors violence in humans and "sham rage," as seen in the "hypothalamic savage" syndrome, are striking.[35] Although it has been assumed that the "sham rage" animal preparations are "awake," there is some suggestion that similar preparations are behaviorally awake and yet (partially) physiologically asleep, with apparent "hallucinatory" behavior possibly representing REM sleep dreaming occurring during wakefulness, dissociated from other REM state markers.[36]

The neural bases of aggression and rage in the cat have been reviewed, indicating that there is clearly an anatomic basis for some forms of violent behavior.[37] The prosencephalic system may serve to control and elaborate, rather than initiate, behaviors originating from deeper structures.[10] In humans, during confusional arousals (sleep drunkenness), which can result in confusion or aggression, there is clear electroencephalographic (EEG) evidence of rapid oscillations between wakefulness and sleep.[26,38] It may be that such behaviors occurring in states other than wakefulness are the expression of motor/affective activity generated by lower structures—unmonitored and unmodified by the cortex. Keeping in mind that not only is sleep a very active process, but the generators or effectors of many components of both REM and NREM sleep reside in the brain stem and other "lower" centers, it is not surprising that, during sleep, prominent motoric and affective behaviors do occur.

Some very dramatic cases have been tried using the confusional arousal defense. In one, the "Parks" case in Canada, the defendant drove 23 km, killed his mother-in-law, and attempted to kill his father-in-law. Somnambulism was the legal defense, and he was acquitted.[39] In another, the "Butler, PA" case, a confusional arousal attributed to underlying OSA was offered as a criminal defense for a man who fatally shot his wife during his usual sleeping hours. He was found guilty.[40] In a recently highly publicized case, a man stabbed his wife to death. He was found guilty and sentenced to life in prison.[41]

Inappropriate sexual behaviors during the sleep state, presumably the results of an admixture of wakefulness and sleep, have been well described.[42–51] Conversely, recurrent sexually oriented hypnagogic hallucinations experienced by patients with narcolepsy may be so vivid and convincing to the victim that they may serve as false accusations.[52]

Sleep talking has also been addressed by the legal system; it is interesting to ponder whether utterances made during sleep are admissible in court.[53]

Specific incidents of violence associated with disorders of arousal include[13]

1. Somnambulistic homicide and attempted homicide
2. Murders and other crimes during sleep drunkenness, including sleep apnea and narcolepsy
3. Suicide or suicide attempts[54,55]
4. Violence/injury during sleep terrors or sleepwalking; these episodes may be drug-induced

Violent sleep behaviors may result in post-traumatic stress disorder in the spouse or bed partner.[56]

Other, very important factors beyond the scope of this chapter include (1) the known effect of genetics on violence, and (2) the well-demonstrated effects of environmental and social factors upon the structure and function of the nervous system.[57] (In one study of 31 individuals awaiting trial or sentencing for murder, none was neurologically or psychiatrically normal.[15]) The plasticity of the nervous system is greater than previously thought.[58,59] These factors are undoubtedly operant in both wakeful and sleep-related violence.

REM Sleep Behavior Disorder

RBD represents an experiment of nature, predicted in 1965 by animal experiments[60] and more recently identified in humans.[61] Normally, during REM sleep, there is active paralysis of all somatic muscles (sparing the diaphragm and eye movement muscles). In RBD, there is the absence of REM sleep atonia, which permits the "acting out" of dreams, often with dramatic and violent or injurious behaviors. The oneiric (dream) behavior demonstrated by cats with bilateral peri–locus ceruleus lesions and by humans with spontaneously occurring RBD clearly arises from and continues to occur *during* REM sleep. These oneiric behaviors displayed by patients with RBD are often misdiagnosed as manifestations of a seizure or psychiatric disorder. RBD is usually idiopathic, but may be associated with underlying neurologic disorders.[62] The overwhelming male predominance (90%) of RBD raises interesting questions about the relationship of sexual hormones to aggression and violence.[63,64] The violent and injurious nature of RBD behaviors has been extensively reviewed elsewhere.[62] Treatment with clonazepam is highly effective.[62]

As with the disorders of arousal, underlying sleep apnea may simulate RBD, again underscoring the necessity for thorough formal PSG evaluation of all bothersome complex behaviors arising during the sleep period.[65]

Nocturnal Seizures

The association between seizures and violence has long been debated. It is plain that, on occasion, seizures may result in violent, murderous, or injurious behaviors.[2,66] Of particular note is the frantic and elaborate nocturnal motor activity that may result from seizures originating in the orbital, mesial, or prefrontal region.[67] "Episodic nocturnal wanderings," a condition clinically indistinguishable from other forms of sleep-related motor activity such as complex sleepwalking, but that is responsive to anticonvulsant therapy, has also been described.[68–70] Aggression and violence may be seen pre-ictally, ictally, and postictally. The postictal violence is often induced or perpetuated by the good intentions of bystanders trying to "calm" the patient following a seizure.[71] As with disorders of arousal, OSA may masquerade as nocturnal seizures.[72–74]

Psychiatric Conditions

Psychogenic Dissociative States

Waking dissociative states may result in violence.[75] It is now apparent that dissociative disorders may arise exclusively or predominately from the sleep period.[2,76] Virtually all patients with nocturnal dissociative disorders evaluated at our center were victims of repeated physical and/or sexual abuse beginning in childhood.[77]

Malingering

Although uncommon, malingering must also be considered in cases of apparent sleep-related violence. Our center has recently seen a young adult male who developed progressively violent behaviors, apparently arising from sleep, directed exclusively at his wife. This behavior included beating her and chasing her with a hammer. Following extensive neurologic, psychiatric, and PSG evaluation, it was determined that this behavior represented malingering.

Munchausen Syndrome by Proxy

In this syndrome, a child is reported to have apparently medically serious symptoms that, in fact, are induced by an adult—usually a caregiver, often a parent. The use of surreptitious video monitoring in sleep disorder centers during sleep (with the parent present) has documented the true etiology for reported sleep apnea and other unusual nocturnal spells.[78–80]

MEDICOLEGAL EVALUATION

Clinical and Laboratory Evaluation of Waking and Sleep Violence

The history of complex, violent, or potentially injurious motor behavior arising from the sleep period should suggest the possibility of one of the previously mentioned conditions. Our experience with over 200 adult cases of sleep-related injury/violence has repeatedly indicated that clinical differentiation, without PSG study, among RBD, disorders of arousal, sleep apnea, and sleep-related psychogenic dissociative states and other psychiatric conditions may be impossible.[13] It is likely that violence arising from the sleep period is more frequent than previously assumed.

The legal implications of automatic behavior have been discussed and debated in both the medical and legal literature.[1,81–83] As with nonsleep automatisms, the identification of a specific underlying organic or psychiatric sleep violence condition does not establish causality for any given deed.

These conditions are diagnosable, and most are treatable. Clinical evaluation should include a complete review of sleep/wake complaints from both the victim and bed partner (if available). This should be followed by a thorough general physical, neurologic, and psychiatric examination. The diagnosis may only be suspected clinically. Extensive polygraphic study employing a full EEG montage, electromyographic monitoring of all four extremities, and continuous audiovisual recording is mandatory for correct diagnosis in atypical cases; and clinical and laboratory evaluations are best performed by experienced clinicians.[13]

Establishing the diagnosis of nocturnal seizures may be extremely difficult, as the motor activity associated with the spell often obscures the EEG pattern. Further, there may be no scalp-EEG manifestation of the seizure activity. Numerous well-documented cases of scalp electrode EEG–negative but depth electrode EEG–positive electrical seizure activity or video-documented clinical seizure activity have been reported.[84–86] Another possible explanation for "scalp electrode EEG–negative" seizures is that some seizures manifest electrically with only generalized low-voltage fast activity, not followed by postictal slowing.[87] Such activity arising from EEG-recorded sleep may be misinterpreted as an "arousal," rather than as electrical seizure activity. Seizure activity arising in the limbic system may spread to other more "primitive" structures, with resultant clinical behaviors, without EEG involvement of the neocortex.[9] The treatment of nocturnal seizures is similar to that of diurnal seizures. The previously mentioned difficulties in evaluating nocturnal seizures (obscuring of the record by movement artifact, absence of surface EEG abnormality or electrical seizure activity, lack of postictal slowing, misinterpretation of electrical seizure activity as an "arousal") emphasize the necessity of extensive, in-person laboratory monitoring. (Scantily channeled "ambulatory" EEG monitoring has led to the misdiagnosis of functional psychiatric disease in a number of our patients subsequently demonstrated to have bona fide nocturnal seizures). If the history or physical examination suggests underlying neurologic disease, further studies such as magnetic resonance imaging or computed tomography scanning of the brain, multimodal (visual, auditory, and somatosensory) evoked potentials, and/or formal neuropsychometric evaluation are indicated.

While it is often possible to state that a given violent act may conceivably have arisen from the sleep period or from a mixed state of wakefulness and sleep, it is usually impossible to prove that a given incident did, in fact, represent a sleep-related phenomenon. To assist in the determination of the putative role of an underlying sleep disorder in a specific violent act, we have proposed guidelines, modified from Bonkalo (sleepwalking),[21] Walker (epilepsy),[88] and Glasgow (automatism in general)[89] and formulated from our clinical experience[2]:

1. There should be reason (by history or formal sleep laboratory evaluation) to suspect a bona fide sleep disorder. Similar episodes, with benign or morbid outcome, should have occurred previously.
2. The duration of the action is usually brief (minutes).
3. The behavior is usually abrupt, immediate, impulsive, and senseless—without apparent motivation. Although ostensibly purposeful, it is inappropriate to the total situation, out of (waking) character for the individual, and without evidence of premeditation.
4. The victim is someone who merely happened to be present, and who may have been the stimulus for the arousal.
5. Immediately following return of consciousness, there is perplexity or horror, without attempt to escape,

conceal or cover up the action. There is evidence of lack of awareness on the part of the individual during the event.
6. There is usually some degree of amnesia for the event; however, this amnesia need not be complete.
7. In the case of sleep terrors, sleepwalking, or sleep drunkenness, the act may (a) occur upon awakening (rarely, immediately upon falling asleep or, usually, at least 1 hour after sleep onset); (b) occur upon attempts to awaken the subject; or (c) have been potentiated by sedative-hypnotic administration or prior sleep deprivation.

The proposition that sleep disorders may be a legitimate defense in cases of violence arising from the sleep period has been met with much skepticism.[90] For credibility, evaluations of such complex cases are best performed in experienced sleep disorders centers with interpretation by a veteran clinical polysomnographer. Due to the complex nature of many of these disorders, a multidisciplinary approach is highly recommended.

One fortunate, and unexplained, fact is that nocturnal sleep-related violence is seldom a recurrent phenomenon.[90] Very rarely, recurrence is reported, and possibly should be termed a "noninsane automatism." Thorough evaluation and effective treatment are mandatory before the patient can be regarded as no longer a menace to society.[91] In other cases, clear precipitating events can be identified, and must be avoided to be exonerated from legal culpability. This concept has led to the proposal of two new forensic categories: (1) "parasomnia with continuing danger as a noninsane automatism" and (2) "(intermittent) state-dependent continuing danger."[91]

Legal and Forensic Medicine Evaluation

With the identification of ever-increasing causes, manifestations, and consequences of sleep-related violence comes an opportunity for neurologists and sleep medicine specialists to educate the general public and practicing clinicians as to the occurrence and nature of such behaviors, and as to their successful treatment. More importantly, the onus is on the sleep medicine professional to educate and assist the legal profession in cases of sleep-related violence that result in forensic medicine issues. This often presents difficult ethical problems, as most "expert witnesses" are retained by either the defense or the prosecution, leading to the tendency for expert witnesses to become advocates or partisans for either one side or the other. Historically, this has been fertile ground for the appearance of "junk science" in the courtroom[92]—from Bendectin to triazolam to breast implants. Junk science leads to junk justice, and altered standards of care.[93] Recently, much attention has been paid to the existence and prevalence of junk science in the courtroom, with recommendations to minimize its occurrence. Prior to accepting any given case, the sleep professional should familiarize him/herself with this most important issue. A good starting point is the highly informative book, *Galileo's Revenge: Junk Science in the Courtroom*.[92] There is some hope that the judicial system is paying more attention to the process of authentic science and may move to accept only valid scientific evidence.[94,95] To address the problem of junk science in the courtroom, many professional societies are calling for, and some have developed guidelines for, expert witness qualifications and testimony. Similarly, the American Sleep Disorders Association and the American Academy of Neurology have adopted their own guidelines, which include[96,97]:

A. Expert witness qualifications
  1. Must have a current, valid, unrestricted license.
  2. Must be a Diplomat of the American Board of Sleep Medicine.
  3. Must be familiar with the clinical practice of sleep medicine and should have been actively involved in clinical practice at the time of the event.
B. Guidelines for expert testimony:
  1. The practitioner must be impartial: the ultimate test for accuracy and impartiality is a willingness to prepare testimony that could be presented unchanged for use by either the plaintiff or the defendant.
  2. Fees should relate to time and effort, not be contingent upon the outcome of the claim. Fees should not exceed 20% of the practitioner's annual income.
  3. The practitioner should be willing to submit such testimony for peer review.
  4. To establish consistency, the practitioner should make records from his or her previous expert witness testimony available to the attorneys and expert witnesses of both parties.
  5. The practitioner must not become a partisan or advocate in the legal proceeding.

Familiarizing oneself with these guidelines may be helpful in a given case, as the expert witnesses for each side should be held to the same standards.[98]

The current legal system unfortunately must consider a parasomnia case strictly in terms of choosing between "insane" or "noninsane" automatism. Such a choice results in two very different consequences for the accused: either commitment to a mental hospital for an indefinite period of time if "insane," or acquittal without any mandated medical consultation or follow-up, or without any stipulated deterrent concerning a recurrence of the behavior with criminal charges that was induced by a recurrence of the high-risk behavior. One reasonable approach in dealing with these automatisms from a legal standpoint would be to add a category of acquittal that allowed for innocence based on lack of guilt consequent to set diagnoses—specific illnesses that could be categorized by a group of subspecialty clinicians in consultation with the legal profession.[99] Another suggestion has been a two-stage trial, which would first establish who committed the act, and then deal separately with the issue of culpability. The first part would be held before a jury; the second would be held in front of a judge with medical advisors present.[100]

Forensic Sleep Medicine Experts as Impartial Friends of the Court (Amicus Curae)

One infrequently used tactic to improve scientific testimony is to use a court-appointed "impartial expert."[92] When approached to testify, volunteering to serve as a court-appointed expert, rather than one appointed by either the prosecution or defense, may encourage this practice. Other proposed measures include the development of a specific section in scientific journals dedicated to expert witness testimony extracted from public documents with request for opinions and consensus statements from appropriate specialists, or the development of a library of circulating expert testimony that could be used to discredit irresponsible "professional witnesses."[92] Good science is determined not by the credentials of the expert witness, but rather by scientific consensus.[93]

SUMMARY AND DIRECTIONS FOR THE FUTURE

It is abundantly clear that violence may occur during any one of the three states of being. That which occurs during REM or NREM sleep may have occurred without conscious awareness and may be due to one of a number of completely different disorders. Violent behaviors during sleep may result in events that have forensic science implications. The apparent suicide (e.g., leaping to death from a second-story window), assault, or murder (e.g., molestation, strangulation, stabbing, shooting) may be the unintentional, nonculpable but catastrophic result of disorders of arousal, sleep-related seizures, RBD, or psychogenic dissociative states. The majority of these conditions are diagnosable and, more importantly, are treatable. The social and legal implications are obvious.

The fields of neurology and sleep medicine must pursue further productive study and discourse, and request adequate funding to objectively study the following important questions: What is the true prevalence of these disorders? How are they best and most accurately diagnosed? How can the usually present prodromes be taken seriously? Why the male predominance in many? How can they best be treated or, better yet, prevented? Are "social stressors" truly more prevalent in this population? What is the best way to deal with forensic science issues? What to do with the offender? What is the likelihood of recurrence? Is such behavior a sane or an insane automatism?[101] How to protect the potential victim?

More research, both basic science and clinical, is urgently needed to further identify and elaborate upon the components of both waking and sleep-related violence, with particular emphasis upon neurobiologic, neuroplastic, genetic, and socioenvironmental factors.[15,16,102] The study of violence and aggression will be greatly enhanced by close cooperation among clinicians, basic science researchers, and social scientists.

REFERENCES

A full list of references are available at www.expertconsult.com

Index

Note: Page numbers followed by *f* refer to figures; those followed by *t* refer to tables.